LeMone & Burke's
Adult Nursing

Visit the *Adult Nursing* Companion Website at www.pearsoned.co.uk/lemone
to find valuable **student** learning material including:

- Interactive Case Studies
- Multiple Choice Questions
- Weblinks
- Searchable Glossary
- Flashcards

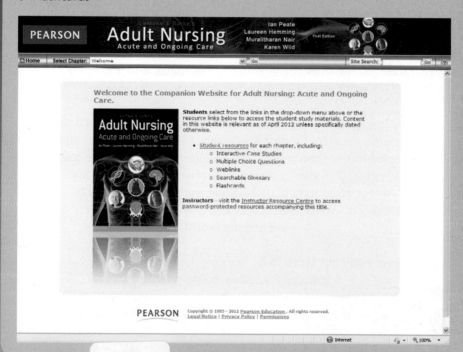

LeMone & Burke's

Adult Nursing
Acute and Ongoing Care

Ian Peate
EN(G), RGN, DipN (Lond), RNT, BEd (Hons), MA (Lond), LLM

Professor of Nursing
Editor in Chief, *British Journal of Nursing*

Muralitharan Nair
SRN, RMN, DipN (Lond), RNT, Cert Ed, Cert in Counselling, BSc (Hons), MSC (Surrey), FHEA

Senior Lecturer, School of Nursing, Midwifery and Social Work
University of Hertfordshire

Laureen Hemming
RGN, DipN (Lond), RCNT, BA, PGCEA, RNT, BPhil Complementary Health Studies, HEA Fellow

Senior Lecturer and Programme Tutor, School of Nursing, Midwifery and Social Work
University of Hertfordshire

Karen Wild
RGN, HV, RNT, MA

Senior Lecturer and Widening Participation Lead, School of Nursing, Midwifery and Social Work
University of Salford

Priscilla LeMone
RN, DSN, FAAN

Associate Professor Emeritus, Sinclair School of Nursing
University of Missouri–Columbia
Columbia, Missouri

Karen Burke
RN, MS

Education Consultant, Oregon State Board of Nursing
Portland, Oregon

PEARSON

Harlow, England • London • New York • Boston • San Francisco • Toronto • Sydney
Auckland • Singapore • Hong Kong • Tokyo • Seoul • Taipei • New Delhi
Cape Town • São Paulo • Mexico City • Madrid • Amsterdam • Munich • Paris • Milan

Pearson Education Limited

Edinburgh Gate
Harlow
Essex CM20 2JE
England

and Associated Companies throughout the world

Visit us on the World Wide Web at:
www.pearson.com/uk

First published 2012

© Pearson Education Limited 2012

ISBN: 978-0-273-71999-1

British Library Cataloguing-in-Publication Data
A catalogue record for this book is available from the British Library

Library of Congress Cataloging-in-Publication Data
LeMone & Burke's adult nursing: acute and ongoing care / Ian Peate . . . [et al.].
    p. ; cm.
  LeMone and Burke's adult nursing
  Adult nursing
  Adapted from: Medical-surgical nursing: critical thinking in client care / [edited by] Priscilla LeMone, Karen Burke. 4th ed. c2008.
  Includes bibliographical references and index.
  ISBN 978-0-273-71999-1
  I. Peate, Ian. II. Medical-surgical nursing: critical thinking in client care. III. Title: LeMone and Burke's adult nursing. IV. Title: Adult nursing.
  [DNLM: 1. Nursing Process–Great Britain. 2. Acute Disease–nursing–Great Britain. 3. Adult–Great Britain.
4. Chronic Disease--nursing–Great Britain. 5. Nursing Care–Great Britain. WY 150]
  610.730941--dc23

                                                                    2012001444

10 9 8 7 6 5 4 3 2 1
16 15 14 13 12

Typeset in 9.75/12pt Minion by 35
Printed and bound by Grafos SA, Barcelona, Spain

Brief contents

Supporting resources

Visit **www.pearsoned.co.uk/lemone** to find valuable online resources

Companion Website for students
- Interactive Case Studies
- Multiple Choice Questions
- Weblinks
- Searchable Glossary
- Flashcards

For instructors
- PowerPoint slides of the key diagrams from the text

Also: The Companion Website provides the following features:

- Search tool to help locate specific items of content
- E-mail results and profile tools to send results of quizzes to instructors
- Online help and support to assist with website usage and troubleshooting

For more information please contact your local Pearson Education sales representative or visit **www.pearsoned.co.uk/lemone**

Contents in detail

List of figures

Preface

Nursing is changing: career pathways for nurses are opening up into domains hitherto forbidden, the way care is being delivered is being transformed; there is an ageing population and, as such, your knowledge and skills will be in great demand to meet healthcare needs well into the future. This book has been written to help you build those skills. The book also contains the help you need to ensure that you meet the competencies demanded by the Nursing and Midwifery Council (NMC) to enable you to register as a nurse. On registration as a nurse, you will have the privilege to care for the public. As well as this, you must also work within the confines of the Code of Professional Practice (NMC 2008).

In order to register with the NMC to practise as a nurse, students have to follow and complete an education programme that meets the NMC's standards set out for pre-registration nursing education. The standards lay out what must be achieved when the student is at the point of registration. It takes at least three years to become a nurse in the UK.

Nurse education is based in universities, and is delivered in direct partnership with NHS Trusts and other organisations such as the private and independent and voluntary sectors that provide practice learning opportunities for nursing students.

Fifty per cent of the education programme is spent in practice, with the aim of ensuring that students can learn how to provide direct nursing care. The other half of the programme is spent learning about the knowledge and technical abilities required to underpin and support practice.

Some nursing students currently complete their education with at least a Diploma in Higher Education – the equivalent of two-thirds of a degree. This is changing.

Nursing in the 21st century

The challenges facing nurses and nursing in the 21st century are much more complex than they have hitherto been, and the way healthcare is delivered is changing. The depth of knowledge and level of skill people will expect nurses to have will have to change to meet these challenges.

In the future, nurses will have to practise differently. Adult and children's nurses will have to have the knowledge and skills needed to meet the needs of people with mental health problems, and mental health and learning disability nurses will need to be able to demonstrate that they are better able to care for people with complex physical needs.

To meet these challenges and to seize new opportunities, nurse education programmes will have to demonstrate that nurses, when they graduate in their field of practice, are in possession of the high-level skills essential to care safely and effectively for people in their particular field, as well as possessing the knowledge and range of skills required to deliver essential care to others in alternative settings.

Nursing students will continue to learn in hospitals and residential care settings and increasingly in the wider community where care ranging from fundamental to highly complex is being delivered more often.

Nursing education in the 21st century

For a student to complete their programmes of study successfully, they will have to demonstrate knowledge and competence in practice at degree level, justifying their actions based on sound evidence.

Learning to be a nurse of the future requires that you have the specialised skills to care for specific groups of people, as well as having the knowledge and skills essential in providing the fundamental aspects of care to all patient groups. The NMC have decided that, in future, nurse education programmes will have a blend of generic learning and learning which is specific to the student's chosen specialism (field), with the proportion of field-specific learning growing as the programme progresses.

Both generic and field-specific aspects of the programme will be combined, providing the opportunity to develop shared learning between fields. Opportunities will also be made available for shared learning with members of other healthcare professions. This approach provides students with a chance to meet the required generic and field competencies in a wide range of settings, in all places where nurses provide care.

To meet the new competencies set by the NMC and, in effect, to register as a nurse, a student must demonstrate competence in specific skills (NMC 2010a). These specific skills are included in the essential skills clusters (ESCs) and they have to be met at various points in the programme.

The new programmes

New programmes will still be at least three years' long, with half the time spent learning how to give direct care in practice settings. There will be two progression points as opposed to the current one. Progression points will usually separate the programme into three equal parts; each part will have specific criteria that must be met prior to the student progressing from one part of the programme to the next.

Competencies that have to be achieved for progression point 1 are associated with achieving the criteria related to the fundamental aspects of care and safety, as well as demonstrating professional behaviours expected of a nursing student (NMC 2010b). Learning outcomes for progression point 2 will enable the student to demonstrate an ability to work in a more independent and confident way.

Minimum academic level

The NMC made a decision in October 2008 that the minimum academic level for pre-registration nursing education would be degree. There will only be degree-level pre-registration nursing programmes offered in the UK from September 2013.

The NMC's decision was based on a number of factors, including the need to prepare nurses to have critical thinking skills in the increasingly diverse and complex arena of healthcare delivery. Raising the minimum level of nursing education to degree level will bring the UK in line with other countries as well with other healthcare professions. This might help to encourage more interprofessional learning across pre-registration programmes.

Nursing students are expected to build on knowledge of basic sciences, social sciences and the fundamentals of nursing to synthesise and critically analyse new skills necessary to ensure clinical competence. Our text provides you with the knowledge and skills you need to care for adult patients to promote health, facilitate recovery from illness and injury, and provide support when coping with disability or loss.

Throughout the text, we make every effort to communicate that both nurses and adult patients may be male or female; and that patients require holistic, individualised care regardless of their age or racial, cultural or socio-economic background.

Our goal: helping you achieve clinical competence by building on your skills

Our focus in writing this book is to offer you the knowledge that provides a base for clinical judgement and that can be applied to provide safe, individualised and competent clinical nursing care. Our easily understood, straightforward style will help you integrate concepts in pathophysiology, pharmacology and interdisciplinary healthcare interventions into prioritised nursing care. We have developed multiple learning strategies to help you succeed, including boxes, tables, special features and illustrations, as well as synthesis and critical thinking exercises, so you can build your skills for class and for clinical practice.

We believe that students learn best within a nursing model of care with consistent organisation and understandable text.

This textbook:

- maintains a strong focus on nursing care as the essential element in learning and doing nursing, regardless of the age of the patient or the setting for care;

- provides a proper balance of physiology, pathophysiology, pharmacology and interdisciplinary care on which to base safe, competent and individualised nursing care;

- emphasises the nurse's role as an essential member of the interdisciplinary healthcare team;

- uses functional health patterns and the nursing process as the structure for providing nursing care in today's world by prioritising nursing diagnoses and interventions specific to altered responses to illness;

- fosters critical thinking and decision-making skills as the basis for nursing excellence in clinical practice;

- continues to believe that the person receiving care has not only a personal experience with health and illness, but is also an active participant in maintaining and/or regaining health.

Organisation

The book is organised into 17 chapters. Each part opens with an introduction setting the scene. A comprehensive review of anatomy and physiology is provided related to the chapter content, drawing upon the student's prerequisite knowledge and reinforcing basic principles of anatomy and physiology as applied to physical assessment.

Each chapter provides case studies related to the chapter with the intention of contextualising and reinforcing learning. The chapters follow a consistent format and include the following components:

- *Pathophysiology.* The discussion of each major illness or condition begins with incidence and prevalence with an overview of pathophysiology, followed by manifestations and complications. The use of pathophysiology illustrated art brings physiological processes to life.

- *Interdisciplinary care.* This considers treatment of the illness or condition by the healthcare team. The section includes information about specific tests necessary for diagnosis, medications, surgery and treatments, fluid management, dietary management and complementary and alternative therapies.

- *Nursing care.* Because illness prevention is critical in healthcare today, this section provides health promotion information. Nursing care is discussed within a context of priority nursing diagnoses and interventions, with rationales provided for intervention. Boxes that present information essential to care are community care, in practice, practice alerts, fast facts and consider this.

A comment on terminology

There have been a number of moves on the part of government and regulatory bodies to enhance direct community involvement in all types of public services, and several terms are used to ensure this happens when working with people.

A number of terms are used in the health service and in this book to describe the people we care for. Terms you may see in this book will include patient, individual or person. Some people choose specific terms such as survivor, as in some mental health settings, to describe their relationship with services. Each term has a different emphasis, with overlap; some people identify with one more than another, or use some terms only in particular situations. The terms used can be very powerful in defining relationships and, as such, much thought needs to be given to them.

It is important that in making a selection of terms of address and pronouns the nurse considers the delicate nuances of the options available so that the status of the person is not compromised. When addressing the person individually, best practice would dictate that you ask that person for their preferred title.

References

Nursing and Midwifery Council (2008) *The Code: Standards of Conduct, Performance and Ethics for Nurses and Midwives*. London, NMC.

Nursing and Midwifery Council (2010a) *Standards for Pre-registration Nursing Education*. London, NMC. Available at: http://standards.nmc-uk.org/PublishedDocuments/Standards%20for%20pre-registration%20nursing%20education%2016082010.pdf (accessed September 2011).

Nursing and Midwifery Council (2010b) *Guidance on Professional Conduct for Nursing and Midwifery Students*. London, NMC.

About the authors

Ian Peate is a highly dedicated and driven educator with 20 years cumulative experience in a variety of education and healthcare settings in the UK. He is enthusiastic and determined, with a passion for inclusive education for all. Ian began his nursing career in 1981 at Central Middlesex Hospital, becoming an enrolled nurse working in an intensive care unit. He later undertook three years' student nurse training at Central Middlesex and Northwick Park Hospitals, becoming a staff nurse then a charge nurse. He has worked in nurse education since 1989. His key areas of interest are nursing practice and theory, men's health, sexual health and HIV/AIDS. He is dedicated to pursuing and developing the art and science of nursing care. Ian is Professor of Nursing and Editor in Chief, *British Journal of Nursing*.

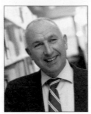

Muralitharan Nair commenced his nursing career in 1971 at Edgware General Hospital becoming a staff nurse. In 1975, he commenced his mental health nurse training at Springfield Hospital and worked as a staff nurse for approximately one year. He has worked at St Mary's Hospital Paddington and Northwick Park Hospital, returning to Edgware General Hospital to take up the post of senior staff nurse and then charge nurse. He has worked in nurse education since 1989. His key interests include physiology, diabetes, surgical nursing and nurse education. Muralitharan has published in journals, written a chapter on elimination and co-edited textbooks.

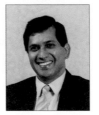

Laureen Hemming is currently a senior lecturer in Oncology Nursing and Palliative Care at the University of Hertfordshire. Her nursing career commenced in the 1960s at Addenbrooke's Hospital, Cambridge, and she has held various posts in medical and surgical nursing, elderly care and orthopaedic nursing before settling in St Albans and focusing on end-of-life care. Laureen's interests in complementary therapies led to further study at Exeter University. She has published in various journals and contributed to a number of texts and has presented at national and international conferences on various aspects

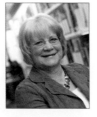

of cancer, palliative care and nurse education, the most recent being a poster on preparing staff working with people with dementia to help their patients and families cope with imminent death for the European Association of Palliative Care Conference held in Lisbon.

Karen Wild is a senior lecturer in the School of Nursing and Midwifery at the University of Salford. She is a member of the directorate of Adult Nursing and Knowledge Acquisition in that school. As a registered nurse and health visitor, she became involved in supporting health education at a number of levels: as an invited teacher to teenagers with special needs; as a staff trainer in sexual health; as a founder member of community-based well woman's health sessions; and as a family health visitor supporting health needs across the adult lifespan. She is interested in a variety of subjects that support nursing, including human relations. These skills and the knowledge to support them have extended into her role with students on pre- and post-qualifying programmes of nursing. Her current position as widening participation champion within the school supports the notion of fair opportunity of access to nursing and midwifery courses to those who have high levels of potential and ability.

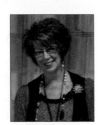

Mary Braine is currently a lecturer in adult nursing at the University of Salford. Mary began her nursing career at University College Hospital, London. She has held various posts in orthopaedic and gastroenterology before moving into the specialist field of neuroscience nursing. She has over 20 years of experience in neuroscience, and has been published in various journals and presented nationally and internationally on topics related to neuroscience nursing practice. Mary is an executive board member of the British Association of Neuroscience Nurses and the national lead for Neuroscience Nursing Benchmarking group. Her interests include various aspects of neuroscience care, in particular acquired brain injury, culminating in her doctorate thesis on families' experiences following acquired brain injury; and within nurse education she has focused on personal development planning and reflection.

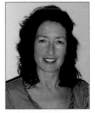

Marvelle Brown has been in the NHS and nurse education for over 30 years. In 1991, she developed the first professionally and academically recognised haematology course in England. She went on to further develop this into both a diploma and degree. She was a member of one of the 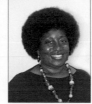 working groups, which led to the development of the NICE Guidance in Haemato-Oncology. She was chair of the RN Haematology/BMT Forum and is currently chair of the Acute Nurses Forum for Sickle Cell and Thalassaemia. Marvelle was a non-executive director for a North West London Hospital Trust and is currently a non-executive director for Milton Keynes PCT. Marvelle has written a number of articles and chapters on haematology. She is an invited speaker nationally and internationally on a wide number of issues in haematology nursing and is currently completing her PhD.

Melanie Stephens is an adult nursing lecturer at Salford University who teaches on the pre-registration diploma and degree and post-registration nurse programmes. Melanie also leads the tissue viability modules within the school. Her nursing career has spanned many 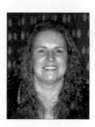 specialities such as medical endocrinology, gynaecology, oncology, burns and plastic surgery, intensive care and tissue viability. Melanie has worked as a lecturer for the last nine years and during this time has developed simulated wounds for use in her teaching, based on real patients nursed in the clinical area. This has led to work with the discovery channel and a programme about her work with special effects and make-up artist Davy Jones. Melanie has an interest in many aspects of nursing, but in particular tissue viability, internationalisation of the curricula and blended learning.

Peter Vickers Following a career in teaching, Peter commenced his nursing career in 1980 at the York District Hospital, followed shortly afterwards by studying and working at the Hospital for Sick Children, Great Ormond Street, London. He later obtained his first degree in Biosciences and 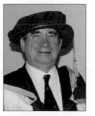 Health Studies and then obtained a doctorate in his specialty, immunology nursing – for which he has a passion – concentrating on the long-term development of children with SCID in the UK and Germany. He has worked in nurse education for several years, and has recently completed a research study into adult palliative care. The author of books on children's responses to early hospitalisation, and research

methodology/proposals, he has also written chapters for several nursing bioscience and pathophysiology books, as well as presented papers at many national and international conferences. His key areas of interest are all aspects of immunology and immunology nursing, infectious diseases, genetics and research. Although officially retired, he continues to work part-time at the University of Hertfordshire, as well as continuing with his writing and presenting at conferences.

Priscilla LeMone spent most of her career as a nurse educator, teaching medical-surgical nursing and pathophysiology at all levels from diploma to doctoral students. She has a diploma in nursing from Deaconess College of Nursing 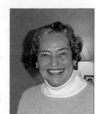 (St Louis, Missouri), baccalaureate and master's degrees from Southeast Missouri State University, and a doctorate in nursing from the University of Alabama–Birmingham. She is retired as an Associate Professor Emeritus, Sinclair School of Nursing, University of Missouri–Columbia, but continues to keep up to date in nursing as an author of nursing textbooks. Dr LeMone had numerous awards for scholarship and teaching during her more than 30 years as a nurse educator. She is most honoured for receiving the Kemper Fellowship for Teaching Excellence from the University of Missouri–Columbia, the Unique Contribution Award from the North American Nursing Diagnosis Association, and for being selected as a Fellow in the American Academy of Nursing.

Karen Burke has practised nursing in direct care and as a nurse educator and administrator. She is currently the Education Consultant for the Oregon State Board of Nursing. In this role, she serves as a consultant to new and existing nursing 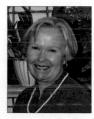 education programmes in the state. Ms Burke entered nursing with a diploma from Emanuel Hospital School of Nursing in Portland, Oregon, later completing baccalaureate studies at Oregon Health & Science University (OHSU), and a master's degree at the University of Portland. She retired as the Director of Health Occupations at Clatsop Community College in Astoria, Oregon. Ms Burke currently is a member of the steering committee for the Oregon Consortium for Nursing Education, and is actively involved in the Education Committee of the Oregon Nursing Leadership Council. Ms Burke strongly values the nursing profession and the importance of providing a strong education in the art and science of nursing for all students preparing to enter the profession.

Guided tour

Learning outcomes

- Describe, identify and relate the anatomy, physiology and functions of the eye and the ear.
- Explain change processes related to vision and hearing.
- Identify specific topics for consideration during a health history.
- Describe normal variations in assessment findings for the older adult and discuss some of the diagnostic tests.
- Identify abnormal findings indicating impairment of the eye and the ear.
- Describe surgical and other invasive procedures.

Clinical competencies

- Assess vision, hearing and functional health of persons with eye and ear disorders.
- Conduct and document a health history.
- Monitor the results of diagnostic tests reporting abnormal findings.
- Conduct and document physical assessment.
- Implement individualised nursing interventions.

Learning outcomes and **Clinical competencies** outline the topics which will be covered in the chapter for you to track your learning and assess your clinical skills.

CASE STUDIES

Below are three case studies that you may wish to consider before, during or after you have read this chapter. There are no right or wrong answers to these care studies, but you should think about the physical, psychological and social implications. For example, can you identify the major anatomical structures of the lower respiratory tract? You may also want to think about what nursing observations you are familiar with to assess people with respiratory problems.

Case Study 1 – Jim

Jim Hunter, aged 58, was an emergency admission to the medical admissions unit (MAU) with a diagnosis of right lower lobe **pneumonia**. Jim is a cigarette smoker, with a history of acute chest infections (acute **bronchitis**)

Case Study 2 – Gemma

Gemma Watson is a 24-year-old single woman who works as an office cleaner. She is admitted to the medical ward with an acute **asthma** attack.

Case Study 3 – Alan

Alan Hoyle is 74. Living in the North West of Britain, all of his working life was spent in the textile industry and, like many of his peers, he smoked cigarettes from starting employment at the age of 15. Alan has a diagnosis of **chronic obstructive pulmonary disease** (COPD) and has been prescribed a variety of inhalers over the years by his GP. On most occasions he abandons them; in fact, at home he has a drawer full of part and unused medication. Alan is isolated because of his condition and relies on the support of his close neighbours for shopping. His daughter visits a

Case studies about different patients are introduced at the start of every chapter and revisited throughout the discussion to illustrate practical nursing care in real-world settings. They can be used for your own personal reflection or for group discussion.

FAST FACTS

Sudden cardiac death

- 74 000 people in the UK die this way every year
- 74% of SCD happens outside of hospitals
- A bystander giving CPR can triple the chance of survival

Source: Gregory and Quinn 2010.

- 84% of patients in hospital who have a cardiac arrest show signs of deterioration before the arrest.

Fast facts pinpoint key statistics and research and can form the basis for personal reflection or group discussion.

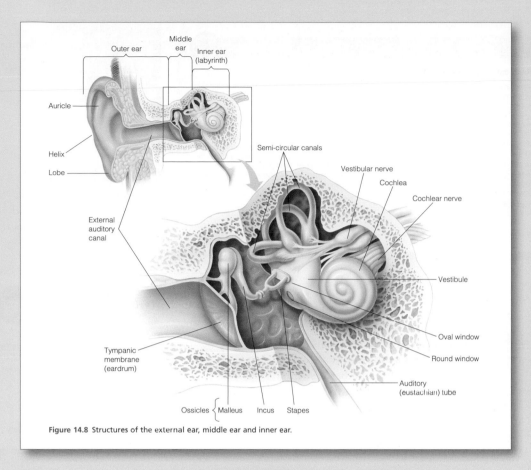

Figure 14.8 Structures of the external ear, middle ear and inner ear.

Photos and illustrations bring theory to life, and demonstrate key concepts clearly.

Signs and symptoms of conjunctivitis

Signs and symptoms of conjunctivitis include:

- redness and itching;
- feelings of scratching or burning;
- photophobia may occur;
- tearing and discharge – this may be watery, purulent (pus) or mucoid (mucus), depending on the cause;
- associated signs and symptoms such as sore throat, fever, malaise and swollen lymph nodes near the ears.

Signs and symptoms are listed in clear and straightforward bullet points throughout.

PRACTICE ALERT

- The person in AHF will feel cold and clammy; this is a classical sign.
- Their breathing will be laboured and short of breath, they will have a rapid pulse and a low blood pressure, and they may not be passing urine (oliguria).
- If the skin is pressed, it will blanch and take time to regain its colour, denoting poor peripheral circulation.
- They may also appear 'blue' (cyanotic) because the blood is not being oxygenated sufficiently due to the sluggish circulation.

Practice alerts emphasise pertinent areas of nursing practice where particular care must be taken including, for example, risk assessment, drug administration and infection control.

Consider this . . .

Why might it be better to investigate tuberculosis in a clinic environment as opposed to hospital admission?

Consider this boxes of key points and ideas for you to consider are highlighted in yellow throughout each chapter. They present triggers for reflection, debate and discussion.

IN PRACTICE

Care following post-cardiac catheterisation

- Following cardiac catheterisation, these observations are recorded after the procedure:
  - blood pressure;
  - heart rate and rhythm;
  - respiration rate and pulse oximetry;
  - checking the wound site for seepage of blood;
  - checking the patient's colour, warmth and sensation in the extremities.
- Complications may develop up to several hours after the procedure; therefore, bedrest is recommended for three hours after the procedure if the femoral artery was used and for two hours if the radial artery was the insertion site.
- The person is advised to report if they experience shortness of breath, chest pain or discomfort and bleeding that may occur at the insertion site.

- The person needs to drink plenty of fluids to flush the dye out of their body and only have a light diet to avoid nausea and vomiting.
- If the person having the cardiac catheterisation was on anticoagulant therapy, this may be recommened.
- They are advised to avoid strenuous activity for 24 hours, which may dislodge the clot which has formed over the insertion site, and to have showers rather than hot baths, which would raise their blood pressure and increase peripheral dilatation of the capillaries, which may leave them feeling faint.

Source: Bowden 2009.

In practice boxes give examples of procedures and diagnostic tests with pertinent tips and hints relating to practice.

Community-based care features provide information, recommendations and advice about caring for individuals in a community or home-based setting, including teaching patients self-care practices, and communication skills with patients and with wider multidisciplinary team members.

COMMUNITY-BASED CARE

People with conjunctivitis are usually cared for in the community, reinforcing the need for effective teaching for home care. Emphasise ways to prevent transmission of infection. If unable to administer eye medications, involve the family in teaching. Include:

- Safety and medical asepsis when cleansing the eye
- Instillation of prescribed eyedrops and ointments
- Comfort measures such as reducing lighting intensity and wearing sunglasses

CHAPTER HIGHLIGHTS

- Hormones regulate growth, development and metabolism. Homeostasis is dependent on a balanced level of each type of hormone. Not only do hormones affect organ function, they interact and, when excesses or deficits occur, signs and symptoms are manifested.
- Thyroid disorders are the most common endocrine disorders. Occurring mainly among women, these diseases change body image and impose upsets to energy levels creating fatigue and exhaustion.
- Diabetes mellitus (DM) is a chronic and progressive illness affecting people of all age groups. There are 1.8 million people in the UK with diagnosed diabetes, and this figure is increasing every year. The estimated cost to the NHS is £5 million per day for treatment. With an ageing population, the number of males and

females with diagnosed diabetes is projected to rise by 37% for males and 24% for females by 2023.
- Type 2 DM has a hereditary link and is characterised by obesity and sedentary lifestyles. Unlike type 1 DM, in which the onset is often sudden, the development of symptoms that bring persons to their healthcare providers for evaluation is slow.
- Tighter, more intensive blood glucose control is increasingly the focus of care for hospitalised persons with hyperglycaemia.
- Treatment for persons with DM includes insulin, non-insulin hypoglycaemics and blood glucose monitoring devices. Nurses must be familiar with these products and help persons become proficient in their use.

Chapter highlights summarise the main ideas discussed in each chapter. Ideal for quick reference and revision.

TEST YOURSELF

1. What component of the brain protects it from harmful substances?
   a. the circulation of cerebrospinal fluid
   b. the large oxygen demand
   c. the structure of neurones
   d. the blood–brain barrier

2. What pathophysiology results from damage to the lower motor neurones?
   a. loss of cognitive ability
   b. inability to communicate verbally
   c. loss of reflexes
   d. decreasing levels of consciousness

3. Which of the following statements about cerebrospinal fluid (CSF) is true?

4. Your body responses to stress are caused by which division of the autonomic nervous system?
   a. sympathetic
   b. parasympathetic
   c. cholinergic
   d. adrenergic

5. Which position best describes decorticate posturing?
   a. neck extended, arms extended and pronated, feet plantar flexed
   b. arms close to sides, elbows and wrists flexed, legs extended
   c. in prone position with arms and knees sharply flexed
   d. in supine position, spine extended, legs extended

6. Which of the following pathophysiological events

Test yourself questions appear at the end of each chapter to assess your learning and help with revision.

Further resources

British Obesity Surgery Person Association (BOSPA)
www.bospa.org
BOSPA has information on many types of weight-loss surgery. We think that you will find this website useful as it provides information on different types of surgery for obese people, information on support groups and patients' experiences after the surgery.

National Institute for Health and Clinical Excellence (NICE)
http://guidance.nice.org.uk/CG43/Guidance/Section
This link provides you with information on obesity from NICE. We think it is useful website for all nursing students and qualified nurses. As you are aware, obesity in the UK is alarmingly high and even in children this is a big problem. The government is committed to reducing obesity in children and adults as it has an impact on health and public resources.

NICE
http://guidance.nice.org.uk/CSGCC
This link provides information on NICE guidance on improving

BUPA
http://www.bupa.co.uk/health-information/directory/s/stomach-cancer
This is a BUPA website. It has useful information about stomach cancer. We think that you will find this link very useful as it gives an overview of the causes, signs and symptoms, treatment and some preventative measures for stomach cancer. They also give a link to other websites which deal with cancer and references for journal articles which deal with cancer.

Cancer Research UK
http://cancerhelp.cancerresearchuk.org/type/bowel-cancer/
We think that this website gives some insight into colorectal cancer. The information on this website should give you some insight into colorectal cancer. They also provide some useful journal links on colorectal cancer. This site may be useful for your studies.

Department of Health (DoH)
http://www.dh.gov.uk/en/Publichealth/Obesity/index.htm
This is a Department of Health website on obesity. Here you will find the latest Health Survey for England (HSE). It is alarming to find that

Further resources provide guidance towards additional print and electronic materials to promote further study and research.

Glossary

accommodation the process by which the eyes focus

acquired immunity immunity acquired by coming into contact with infectious micro-organisms

acute coronary syndrome (ACS) an umbrella term for a group of conditions that result in coronary artery disease

acute illness describes an illness with a sudden/rapid onset which is severe in nature

acute respiratory distress syndrome (ARDS) severe difficulty in getting adequate oxygenation despite significant effort to breathe

acute wound a wound that is new or relatively new in injury and occurs suddenly

afterload the force required by the ventricles when they

atelectasis the failure of part of the lung to expand

atherosclerosis a progressive disease characterised by atheroma (plaque) formation, which affects the intimal and medial layers of large and mid-sized arteries

aura a symptom experienced before a migraine or seizure e.g. flashing lights

autoimmunity an abnormal immune response to the body's own cells, which act as self-antigens

autosome a non-sex chromosome

azotaemia an elevation of blood urea nitrogen

bacterial vaginosis a common cause of vaginal discharge

benign prostatic hyperplasia (BPH) an overgrowth of cells in the prostate gland

A **Glossary** of key terms and definitions, highlighted in the text, is included at the end of the book for quick reference.

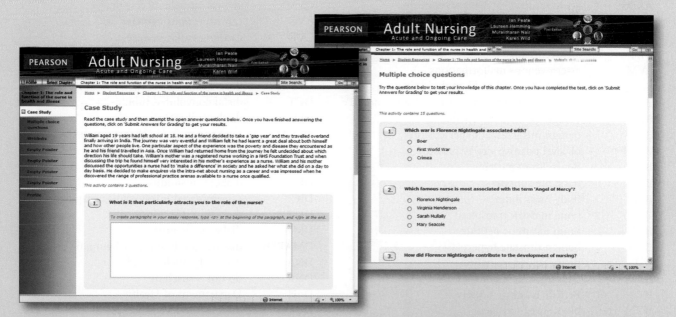

Electronic resources are available online at **www.pearsoned.co.uk/lemone** including Interactive Case Studies, Multiple Choice Questions and Flashcards to measure learning and understanding as you progress through the book.

List of acronyms

ABGs	arterial blood gases
ABPI	ankle brachial pressure index
ABR	auditory brainstem response
ACE	angiotensin-converting enzyme
ACh	acetylcholine
ACS	acute coronary syndrome
ACTH	adrenocortitropic hormone
AD	Alzheimer's disease
ADCH	adrenocorticotropic hormone
ADH	antidiuretic hormone
AEDs	antiepileptic drugs
AEP	auditory evoked potential
AER	auditory evoked response
AFP	alpha-fetoprotein
AHA	alpha-hydroxy acid
AHF	acute heart failure
AIHA	autoimmune haemolytic anaemia
AKI	acute kidney injury
ALL	acute lymphoblastic leukaemia
ALs	activities of living
AML	acute myeloid leukaemia
ANS	autonomic nervous system
APC	antigen-presenting cells
APTT	activated partial thromboplastin time
ARDS	acute respiratory distress syndrome
ARF	acute renal failure
ATN	acute tubular necrosis
AV	atrioventicular
AVM	arteriovenous malformations
BALT	bronchial-associated lymphoid tissue
BASHH	British Association for Sexual Health and HIV
BEN	benign ethnic neutropenia
BIH	benign intracranial hypertension
BiPAP	bi-level positive airway pressure
BJPs	Bence Jones proteins
BLS	basic life support
BMI	body mass index
BMT	bone marrow transplant
BNP	brain naturetic peptide
BPH	benign prostate hyperplasia
BSE	breast self-examination
BTM	beta thalassaemia major
BTS	British Thoracic Society
BUN	blood urea nitrogen
CABG	coronary artery bypass graft
CAD	coronary artery disease
CAD	continuous analgesia delivery

CAPD	continuous ambulatory peritoneal dialysis
CBE	clinical breast examination
CBF	cerebral blood flow
CH	cluster headache
CHD	coronary heart disease
CHF	chronic heart failure
CIN	cervical intraepithelial neoplasia
CIS	carcinoma in situ
CKD	chronic kidney disease
CLL	chronic lymphoblastic leukaemia
CML	chronic myeloid leukaemia
CMV	cytomegalovirus
CNS	clinical nurse specialist
CO	cardiac output
COPD	chronic obstructive pulmonary disease
CPAP	continuous positive airway pressure
CPP	cerebral perfusion pressure
CPR	cardiopulmonary resuscitation
CRF	chronic renal failure
CRH	corticotropin-releasing hormone
CRP	C reactive protein
CSF	cerebrospinal fluid
CT	computed tomography
CTA	CT angiography
CVAD	central vascular access device
CVC	central venous catheter
CVD	cardiovascular disease
CVID	common variable immunodeficiency
CVP	central venous pressure
DBS	deep-brain stimulation
DCT	distal convoluted tubule
DES	diethylstilbesterol
DEXA	dual energy x-ray absortiometry
DFA	direct fluorescent antibody
DHT	dihydrotestosterone
DI	diabetes insipidus
DIC	disseminated intravascular coagulation
DKA	diabetic ketoacidosis
DM	diabetes mellitus
DMARDs	disease modifying antirheumatic drugs
DNA	deoxyribonucleic acid
DNR	do not resuscitate
DoH	Department of Health
DOT	directly observed therapy
DRE	digital rectal examination
DSS	Durie–Salmon staging system
DTR	deep tendon reflexes

DUB	dysfunctional uterine bleeding	HLA	human leukocyte antigen
DVT	deep vein thrombosis	HPA	Health Protection Agency
ECF	extracellular fluid	HPLC	high-performance liquid chromatography
ECG	electrocardiogram	HPV	human papillomavirus
EBCT	electron beam computed tomography	HR	heart rate
ED	erectile dysfunction	HRT	hormone replacement therapy
EDH	extradural haematoma	HSE	Health Survey for England
EEG	electroencephalogram	HSV	herpes simplex virus
ELISA	enzyme-linked immunosorbent assay	HU	hydroxyurea
EMG	electromyogram	IBD	inflammatory bowel disease
EPUAP	European Pressure Ulcer Advisory Panel	IBS	irritable bowel syndrome
ERV	expiratory reserve volume	ICF	intracellular fluid
ESR	erythrocite sedimentation rate	ICH	intracerebral haematoma
ESRD	end-stage renal disease	ICP	intracranial pressure
ESWL	extracorporeal shock wave lithotripsy	ICP	integrated care pathway
Fab	fragment antigen-binding	ICU	intensive care unit
FBC	full blood count	IDA	iron deficiency anaemia
Fc	fragment crystallisable	IF	intrinsic factor
FCC	fibrocystic changes	Ig	immunoglobulin
FDPs	fibrin degradation products	IICP	increased intracranial pressure
FES	fat embolism syndrome	IM	intramuscular
FEV1	forced expiratory volume in 1 second	INR	International Normalised Ratio
FFP	fresh frozen plasma	IPSS	International Prognostic Scoring System
FIGO	International Federation of Gynecology and Obstetrics	IRV	inspiratory reserve volume
		ISS	International Staging System
fMRI	functional MRI	ITP	idiopathic thrombocytopenic purpura
FRC	functional residual capacity	IUD	intrauterine device
FSH	follicle-stimulating hormone	IV	intravenous
FTA-ABS	fluorescent treponemal antibody absorption	LABA	long-acting beta2 agonist
FVC	forced vital capacity	LAVH	laparascopy-assisted vaginal hysterectomy
FVD	fluid volume deficit	LCP	Liverpool Care Pathway
FVE	fluid volume excess	LCR	ligase chain reaction
GABA	gamma aminobutyric acid	LDH	serum lactic acid dehydrogenase
GALT	gut-associated lymphoid tissues	LDL	low-density lipoprotein
GCS	Glasgow Coma Scale	LEEP	loop electrosurgical excision procedure
GDC	Guglielmi detachable coil	LEETZ	loop electrosurgical excision of transformation zone
GFR	glomerular filtration rate		
GH	growth hormone	LH	luteinising hormone
GHRH	growth hormone-releasing hormone	LHRH	luteinising hormone-releasing hormone
GnRH	gonadotrophin-releasing hormone	LOC	loss of consciousness
GSF	Gold Standards Framework	LP	lumbar puncture
GTN	glyceryltrinitrate	LRP	laparascopic radical prostatectomy
GUM	genitourinary medicine	LSMDT	local hospital skin cancer multidisciplinary team
HAART	highly active antiretroviral therapy	LTRA	leukotriene receptor antagonists
HADS	Hospital Anxiety and Depression Scale	LVEF	left ventricular ejection fraction
HAV	hepatitis A virus	MALT	mucosal-associated lymphoid tissue
HBV	hepatitis B virus	MAO	monoamine oxidase
HCA	healthcare assistant	MAP	mean arterial pressure
HCl	hydrochloric acid	MAU	medical admissions unit
HCV	hepatitis C virus	MDS	myelodysplastic syndrome
HDL	high-density lipoprotein	MCH	mean cell haemoglobin
HDV	hepatitis B-associated delta virus	MCHC	mean cell haemoglobin concentration
HEV	hepatitis E virus	MCV	mean cell volume
HHS	hyperosmolar hyperglycaemic state	MGUS	monoclonal gammopathy of undetermined significance
HIT	heparin-induced thrombocytopenia		
HL	Hodgkin's lymphoma	MI	myocardial infarction

MM	multiple myeloma		PIs	protease inhibitors
MMSE	mini-mental status examination		PICC	peripherally inserted central catheter
MPS	myocardial perfusion scintigraphy		PID	pelvic inflammatory disease
MRA	magnetic resonance angiography		PIN	prostate intraepithelial neoplasia
MRI	magnetic resonance imaging		PMDD	premenstrual dysphoric disorder
MS	multiple sclerosis		PMS	premenstrual syndrome
MUST	Malnutrition Universal Screening Tool		PNES	psychogenic non-epileptic seizures
MV	minute volume		PNS	peripheral nervous system
NAATs	nucleic acid amplification tests		POS	polycystic ovary syndrome
NCSP	National Chlamydia Screening Programme		PPC	Preferred Priorities of Care
NE	norepinephrine		PPCI	primary PCI
NES	non-epileptic seizures		PPI	proton-pump inhibitor
NG	nasogastric		PRL	prolactin
NHL	non-Hodgkin's lymphoma		PSA	prostate specific antigen
NHS	National Health Service		PTH	parathyroid hormone
NHSCSP	NHS Cervical Screening Programme		PTK	phototherapeutic keratectomy
NICE	National Institute for Health and Clinical Excellence		PUD	peptic ulcer disease
			PUSH	Pressure Ulcer Scale for Healing
NIPPV	non-invasive positive pressure ventilation		PV	polycythaemiavera
NIV	non-invasive ventilation		PVR	pulmonary vascular resistance
NJ	nasojejunal		RA	rheumatoid arthritis
NK	natural killer		RAS	reticular activating system
NMC	Nursing and Midwifery Council		RBCs	red blood cells
NNRTIs	non-nucleoside reverse transcriptase inhibitors		RDW	red cell distribution width
NPSA	National Patient Safety Agency		RES	reticuloendothelial system
NPTR	nocturnal penile tumescence and rigidity		RLS	restless leg syndrome
NPUAP	National Pressure Ulcer Advisory Panel		RLS	Reporting and Learning System
NRS	numerical rating scale		ROM	range-of-motion
NRTIs	nucleoside reverse transcriptase inhibitors		RPR	rapid plasmin reagin
NSAID	non-steroidal anti-inflammatory drugs		RSV	respiratory syncytial virus
NSCLC	non-small cell lung cancer		RV	reserve volume
NSF	National Service Framework		SAARDs	slow-acting antirheumatic drugs
NSTEMI	non-ST elevated MI		SAH	subarachnoid haemorrhage
NYHA	New York Heart Association		SCA	sickle cell anaemia
OA	osteoarthritis		SCC	spinal cord compression
OAFs	osteoclast activating factors		SCC	squamous cell carcinoma
ONS	Office for National Statistics		SCD	sickle cell disease
OPCAB	off-pump coronary artery bypass		SCD	sudden cardiac death
ORIF	open reduction and internal fixation		SCLC	small-cell lung cancer
PA	pernicious anaemia		SCT	spinal cord tumour
PBC	polychlorinated biphenyl		SCT	stem cell transplantation
PBI	penetrating brain injury		SDH	subdural haematoma
PCA	patient-controlled analgesia		SER	somatosensory evoked response
PCI	percutaneous coronary intervention		SERMs	selective oestrogen receptor modulators
PCLI	plasma cell labelling index		SHOT	Severe Hazards of Transfusion
PCP	pneumocystis carinii pneumonia		SIADH	syndrome of inappropriate ADH secretion
PCR	polymerase chain reaction		sIgA	secretory immunoglobulin A
PCS	post-concussion syndrome		SIRS	systemic inflammatory response syndrome
PCT	primary care trust		SLE	systemic lupus erythematosus
PCT	proximal convoluted tubule		SPECT	single photon emission computed tomography
PCV	packed cell volume		SSRIs	selective serotonin reuptake inhibitors
PD	Parkinson's disease		STEMI	ST elevated MI
PEG	percutaneous endoscopic gastrostomy		STI	sexually transmitted infection
PEJ	percutaneous endoscopic jejunostomy		SV	stroke volume
PET	positron emission tomography		SVR	systemic vascular resistance
PFT	pulmonary function tests		TAA	tumour-associated antigen

TBI	traumatic brain injury		TURP	transurethral resection of prostate
TBI	total body irradiation		TV	total volume
TBSA	total body surface area		UC	ulcerative colitis
TCA	trichloroacetic acid		URTI	upper respiratory tract infection
TCC	transitional cell carcinoma		UTI	urinary tract infection
TEDS	thromboembolic deterrent stockings		VAD	vascular access device
TENS	transcutaneous electrical nerve stimulation		VAS	visual analogue scale
TH	thyroid hormone		VC	vital capacity
TIA	transient ischaemic attack		VCAM	vascular cell adhesion moelcule
TIBC	total iron binding capacity		VCD	vacuum constriction device
TLC	total lung capacity		VD	venereal disease
TLS	tumour lysis syndrome		VDRL	venereal disease research laboratory
TPN	total parenteral nutrition		VEP	visual evoked responses
TNM	Tumour, Node, Metastases		VLDL	very low-density lipoproteins
TRAM	transverse rectus abdominis myocutaneous		VNS	vagus nerve stimulation
TRANCE	TNF-related activation-induced cytokine		VOC	vaso-occlusive crisis
TRUS	transrectal ultrasound		vWD	von Willbrand disease
TSH	thyroid-stimulating hormone		vWF	von Willebrand factor
TTH	tension-type headache		WBCs	white blood cells
TTP	thrombotic thrombocytopenic purpura		WHO	World Health Organization
TUIP	transurethral incision of the prostate		YAG	yttrium aluminium garnet
TUNA	transurethral needle ablation			

Acknowledgements

The editors would like to thank the contributors for their input, insight, skills and knowledge. We would also like to thank our families, colleagues and students for their support and tolerance whilst we undertook this challenging and worthwhile task.

Publisher's acknowledgements

We would like to thank the review panel who helped us with the development of this book:

David Barrett, University of Hull
Dolores Bahn, University of Hull
Juliet Bostwick, Oxford Brookes University
Kathy Curtis, University of Surrey
Hora Ejtehadi, Birmingham City University
Maureen Gale, Anglia Ruskin University
Di Halliwell, University of Bournemouth
Lynne Henshaw, University of Middlesex
Fiona Heskins, Anglia Ruskin University
Peter Hirskyj, Cardiff University
Julia Hubbard, University of East Anglia
Jim Jolly, University of Leeds
Maria Kisiel, Birmingham City University
Roger McFadden, Birmingham City University
Barbara MacFarlane, University of Dundee
Julia Mingay, King's College, London
Owena Simpson, University of Glamorgan
Annetta Smith, University of Stirling
Swaleh Toofany, University of West London

We are grateful to the following for permission to reproduce copyright material:

Figures
Figure 2.5 from The McGill Pain Questionnaire: Major properties and scoring methods, *Pain*, Vol. 1, No. 3, pp. 277–299 (Melzack, R. 1975), with the kind permission of Dr Melzack; Figure 14.8 from Todd Buck © Todd Buck Illustration, Inc.

Tables
Table 15.3 adapted *from International Journal of Gynaecology and Obstetrics*, Vol. 7, No 2, Benedet, J.L., Bender, H., Jones, H. Ngan, H.Y. and Percorelli, S., FIGO Staging Classifications and Clinical Practice Guidelines in the Management of Gynecologic Cancers. FIGO Committee on Gynecologic Oncology, pp. 209–62, 2000, with permission from Elsevier

Text
Box 1.3 and extract on page 648 from *The code: Standards of conduct, performance and ethics for nurses and midwives*, Nursing and Midwifery Council (2008), The Nursing and Midwifery Council. Available at www.nmc-uk.org/Publications/Standards/; Box 1.10 from *Ambitions for Health: A strategic framework for maximising the potential of social marketing and health-related behaviour, Department of Health* (2008) pp. 27–28, Crown Copyright; Extract on page 169 adapted from www.nice.org.uk/nicemedia/pdf/CG029quickrefguide.pdf, © NICE 2005, National Institute for Health and Clinical Excellence (2005) Adapted from *CG 29 Pressure ulcers: the prevention and treatment of pressure ulcers*. London: NICE. Available from www.nice.org.uk/guidance/CG29 Reproduced with permission.; Extract on page 314 adapted from Reducing the incidence of coronary heart disease, *British Journal of Nursing*, Vol. 19, No.14, pp. 865–70 (Chummum, H. 2009); Extract on page 325 adapted from Reducing the incidence of coronary heart disease, *British Journal of Nursing*, Vol. 19, No. 14, pp. 865–70 (Chummum, H. 2009); Extract on page 412 adapted from *Fundamental Aspects of Nursing Adults with Respiratory Problems*, Quay Books (Scullion, J. 2007).

Photographs
Norman Collinge 12; Steve Horton 412; Bernard Seddon 419; Stuart M. Levitz, M.D. 148.

In some instances we have been unable to trace the owners of copyright material, and we would appreciate any information that would enable us to do so.

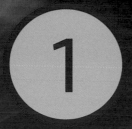

1

The role and function of the adult nurse in health and illness

Learning outcomes

- Be able to describe the core proficiencies of the nurse in **health** and **illness** management and to apply the attitudes and skills necessary for **critical thinking** when using the **nursing process** in person care.

- Be able to explain the importance of the Nursing and Midwifery Council (NMC) 'The Code' of conduct and standards as guidelines for clinical nursing practice (NMC 2008).

- Explain the activities and characteristics of the nurse as caregiver, educator, advocate, leader and manager, and researcher.

- Explain factors affecting functional health status and discuss the nurse's role in health promotion, and describe the primary, secondary and tertiary levels of illness prevention.

- Describe characteristics of health, **disease** and illness, and describe illness behaviours and needs of the person with **acute illness** and **chronic illness**.

- Compare and contrast the physical status, risks for alterations in health, assessment guidelines and healthy behaviours of the adult through the lifespan.

Clinical competencies

- Demonstrate critical thinking when using the nursing process to provide knowledgeable, safe client care.

- Provide clinical care within a framework that integrates, as appropriate, the medical–surgical nursing roles of caregiver, educator, advocate, leader/manager and researcher.

- Include knowledge of developmental levels and of activities to promote, restore and maintain health when planning and implementing care for adults and their families.

- Apply the theory to practice settings.

CASE STUDY

Below is a case study that you may wish to consider before, during or after you have read the chapter. There are no right or wrong answers, but you should think about the physical, psychological and social implications. For example, can you identify the psychological impact that admission for surgery has on the individual? You may also want to think about what nursing observations you are familiar with to assess people in the pre- and post-operative stages of care.

Case Study 1 – Wendy

Ms Wendy Xin is admitted to hospital for surgery to explore a possible malignancy. What emerges is the experiences that Wendy has as she embarks upon her journey as a patient during the pre-, peri- and post-operative stages of care.

INTRODUCTION

Adult nurses are at the forefront of a wealth of different types of care in a variety of healthcare settings. People and the associated health issues that they present with are diverse. The role of the adult nurse is both demanding and rewarding and carries with it a high degree of responsibility.

Aspects of the role include health promotion, health and illness care of adults based on knowledge derived from the arts and sciences, and shaped by knowledge (the science) of nursing. It focuses on the adult's response to actual or potential alterations in health. The wide range of ages and the variety of healthcare needs specific to individual people make the field of adult nursing an ever-changing and challenging area of nursing practice.

Adults requiring healthcare services may access and use the system through a variety of providers and settings, including hospital-based outpatients care, community-based offices and clinics and home care. In the healthcare system of the 21st century, hospitals are primarily acute care providers with services focused on high-technological care for severely ill or injured people or for people having major surgery. Even those people rarely remain in the hospital for long. They are moved as rapidly as possible to less acute care settings within the hospital and then to community-based and home care. Healthcare has become a managed care, community-based system. Although many nurses are still employed in hospitals, they are increasingly providing nursing care outside of the acute care, in-hospital setting. Those settings include clinics, schools, prisons, day care centres, offices and homes, and also the facility for instantaneous responses to problems via NHS Direct.

Regardless of the type of healthcare service or setting, nurses in the field of adult care must use knowledge and skills to be competent and safe when providing person support. Nursing care is structured by the activities planned and carried out through critical thinking within the nursing process, is based on ethics and standards established by nursing organisations, and is focused on returning the person to their best state of functional health.

Claire, a third year student nurse said: *'If you can make a difference to one person (adult) as a nurse then you have achieved something special.'*

The first part of this chapter provides a broad overview of the context of nursing in acute and ongoing care. An overview of the nurse as a caregiver, and critical and ethical thinker is presented. The next part of the chapter explores aspects of health and illness. Prevention of illness and disease are highlighted, and adult development is explored with an overview of the types of health breakdown that are characteristic of the developing adult. To finish the chapter, there is a section that considers the role of the nurse when caring for patients undergoing surgery. Here you will see aspects of care in both the pre- and post-operative period.

Consider this . . .

● 'This area requires the care of adults, from 18-year-olds to older people, in a variety of settings for individuals with wide ranging levels of dependency. The ethos of adult nursing is person centred and acknowledges the differing needs, values and beliefs of people from ethnically diverse communities.

● Nurses engage in and develop therapeutic relationships that involve individuals and their carers in ongoing decision-making that informs nursing care. Adult nurses have skills to meet the physical, psychological, spiritual and social needs of individuals, supporting them through care pathways and working with other health and social care professionals to maximise opportunities for recovery, rehabilitation, adaptation to ongoing disease and disability, health education and health promotion.

● New ways of working provide enhanced opportunities for adult nurses to provide safe and effective care that meets the defined needs of this group in partnership with them. Their ability to be self-directed throughout their professional careers to support lifelong learning, in turn, contributes to continuous quality improvement in care delivery.'

Source: NMC 2004, *Standards of Proficiency for Pre-registration Nursing Education*, 23–24.

In this textbook, the human response to health and illness is structured within the framework of functional health patterns, and nursing care is presented within the context of nursing case studies and intervention. To assist your understanding and development, case studies are presented at the start of each chapter. You will notice that the cases guide you into thinking about what you already know in relation to the illnesses presented and the nursing care required. Opportunities for you to stop and consider broader issues of the subjects presented are given. These are in the form of Practice Alerts, which provide quick summaries of aspects of care, and Consider This boxes like the one above to give you the opportunity to think and reflect. Fast Facts aim to give you some up-to-date food for thought to support the more detailed information within each chapter. The pedagogical features within the book aim to support the idea of lifelong learning, and to stimulate the reader into further investigation.

The nurse in acute and ongoing nursing practice

Contemporary healthcare is a vast and complex system. It reflects changes in society, changes in the populations requiring nursing care and a philosophical shift toward health promotion and illness prevention. The roles of the adult nurse have broadened and expanded in response to these changes. Adult nurses are not only caregivers but also educators, advocates, leaders and managers, and researchers. The nurse assumes these various roles to promote and maintain health, to prevent illness and to facilitate coping with disability or death for the adult patient (a person requiring healthcare services) in any setting.

TYPES OF HEALTHCARE IN THE UNITED KINGDOM

The National Health Service (NHS) Plan (DoH 2000) set out to improve the performance of healthcare and to invest in both the facilities for health and in the staff who support health in the UK. The main overarching principle of healthcare which is predominantly free at the point of delivery still remains. We will now look at primary and secondary care and who receives healthcare in the UK.

Primary care

Primary care is often thought of as the first point of contact for people seeking healthcare, and primary care offers a wide variety of services. You may be familiar with the examples below as these typically include:

- NHS walk-in centres, providing quick and accessible (often on the high street) care and advice. They are often nurse-led

services and provide treatment, advice and referral for minor injuries and illness.
- General Practitioner (GP) practices, that cover a wealth of services to promote, educate, treat and support healthcare. Examples include screening services, e.g. cervical screening; smoking cessation; diagnosis and treatment of health problems; referral for specialist medical assessment, e.g. consultants in hospitals. A variety of healthcare staff support GP services including practice nurses, district nurses, health visitors, school health advisors, physiotherapists and midwives.
- Opticians, dentists and pharmacists provide support to persons in the primary care setting and can be part of the NHS provision or offer independent services which are fee based.
- NHS Direct offers a 24-hour confidential service over the telephone, providing information and advice on a wide range of health topics. The service also has an on-line link.

Secondary care

Secondary care (or acute care) takes place in the hospital setting. This can be NHS Trust provision or within the independent sector (for example private hospitals). Here, there is provision for both emergency and elective care. Elective care is the care which is planned in negotiation with the person – a typical example of this might be elective surgery for a hip joint replacement.

Who receives acute and ongoing nursing care?

Nurses support and care for a number of different people. Recipients of care and support are often referred to as consumers and service users (defining care as a commodity). The terms person and client can be used to define a person who is within the system of healthcare. *Patient* arises from the Latin 'to suffer' or 'to bear'. Because of this, the use of 'patient' has been criticised as being a submissive term implying acceptance of the decisions of health professionals and a lack of negotiation with consumers of healthcare. As such, the term *client* is often adopted to express the notion of consumers of health who are self-directed and responsible for their own health. Within this text you will see the terms 'person' and 'individual' used to describe consumers of care.

> ### Consider this . . .
>
> The report, *Nursing in Society: Starting the debate*, was commissioned by the Chief Nursing Officer for England and was undertaken in the spring and early summer of 2008 to support and inform the nursing contribution to Lord Darzi's NHS Next Stage Review. The driving force behind the report was the sense that nursing had lost its way; that there was unacceptable variation in the quality of care that nurses delivered. While the standard of nursing is generally high, when it falls short it has a marked impact on how individuals

experience the whole of their contact with the health service. The report defines what patients and nurses want, in terms of good-quality care in all healthcare settings, and identifies a series of proposals to improve the quality of care in the NHS in England.

Source: Maben 2008.

Within this textbook, there will be opportunities for you to think about the nurse's role in providing and managing good-quality contemporary nursing care in an acute and ongoing setting and about health and ill health in general, and to be aware of the professional status of the nurse.

THE NURSE AS CAREGIVER

Nurses have always been identified as caregivers. However, the activities carried out within the caregiver role changed tremendously in the 20th century to inform and subsequently influence the development of contemporary nursing. From 1900 to the 1950s, from Nightingale to the introduction of the NHS, the nurse was almost always female and was regarded primarily as the person who gave personal care and carried out the physician's orders. This dependent role has changed completely, due in part to the increased education of nurses, research in and the development of nursing knowledge, and the recognition that nurses are autonomous and informed professionals.

Consider this . . .

Florence Nightingale (1820–1910) was a pioneer in bringing respectability to nursing. The public image viewed nurses as *guardian angels* and *angels of mercy*. Middle class women were encouraged into this moral, compassionate, self-sacrificing role. Nightingale defined nursing in relation to the environment in which recovery took place and set great store by the cleanliness, quietness and airiness of the care setting.

Later theorists considered nursing in relation to health as well as ill health and began to define nursing in these terms. In 1966 Virginia Henderson wrote:

the unique function of the nurse is to assist the individual, sick or well, in the performance of those activities contributing to health or its recovery (or to peaceful death) that he would perform unaided if he had the necessary strength, will, or knowledge, and to do this in such a way as to help him gain independence as rapidly as possible (Henderson 1966, 3).

In the Consider This box, you will note that Henderson (1966) implies that nursing is more than a matter of carrying out the doctor's orders. Instead, nursing involves a special relationship with the person (and often the family). According to Henderson, the nurse intervenes with knowledge and skills

to meet those needs that individuals and family would not normally be able to provide.

The caregiver role for the nurse today is both independent and collaborative. Nurses independently make assessments and plan and implement care based on nursing knowledge and skills. Nurses also collaborate with other members of the healthcare team to implement and evaluate care.

As a caregiver, the nurse is a practitioner of nursing both as a science and as an art. Using critical thinking in the nursing process as the framework for care, the nurse provides interventions to meet not only the physical needs but also the psychosocial, cultural, spiritual and environmental needs of individuals and families. As such, nurses have to understand the complex nature of what it is to be human, in order to respect and value the beliefs and diverse needs of individuals.

PRACTICE ALERT

Samira is a 42-year-old woman admitted to a busy surgical ward for cholecystectomy (removal of the gall bladder). She asks for a facility to pray in private.

Nursing care should be provided within a multicultural setting that respects diversity. Nurses should consider the care needs of people with similar and differing values, beliefs and cultures in order to provide meaningful and beneficial healthcare (Leininger and McFarland 2002).

Whatever social customs characterise the ethnic group being cared for (be it dietary and religious practices, dress, social interactions or health rituals etc.), nurses should value and facilitate these (Peate 2006).

Healthcare systems support individuals who are culturally diverse. This diversity can include differences in country of origin, health beliefs, sexual orientation, race, socioeconomic level and age. Nurses need to deliver care which is culturally sensitive. However, there can be barriers to this such as the view that one's own cultural values and beliefs are the preferred ones. The healthcare system itself is a culture, primarily managed by white middle class people, and this in itself can be interpreted as a barrier to culturally sensitive care.

The nursing process

Consider this . . .

The nursing process is the series of critical thinking activities nurses use as they provide care. These activities define a nursing model of care, differentiating nursing from other healthcare professions, and can be used in any setting. The purpose of care may be to promote and maintain health, restore health or manage disability or death. Regardless of the purpose of care, the planned process of nursing allows for the inclusion of specific, individualised and holistic caring activities.

Application of the Nursing Process to a variety of health and ill health nursing situations is a feature of the subsequent chapters of this book

The nursing process is referred to as a systematic approach to the delivery of person-centred nursing care. This process involves the collection and analysis of an individual's information in order to identify actual or potential health problems, to develop a plan of nursing care and intervention and to constantly review this process in the light of current evidence-based nursing practice. This is achieved through a systematic application of the five phases of the nursing process (see Box 1.1 and Figure 1.1). Information from each phase inputs to the next phase, for example, the evaluation phase will discover findings to feed back into the assessment phase, and so the cycle of the process continues.

The recurring nature of the nursing process encourages the revisiting of the phases. There is a real focus on the person at the heart of this process. Returning to the distinct phases of the nursing process encourages the nurse to be responsive to the person's needs and changing health status.

COLLECTING DATA AS PART OF THE NURSING PROCESS

Data collection is the process of gathering the relevant information in relation to the person's state of ongoing health. Data should reflect both current and past information, and rely on

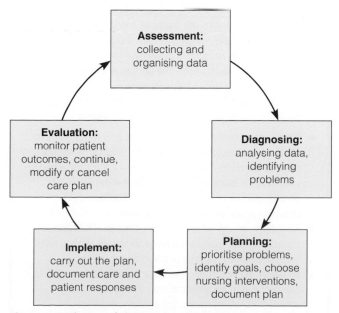

Figure 1.1 Phases of the nursing process.

Box 1.1

The phases of the nursing process

- *Assessing* involves the collection and organising of information. Assessment is usually listed as the first step of the nursing process, but in actuality it is a critical element in each of the steps. Data collected are validated with the individual by reviewing nursing and/or interdisciplinary team records and by conducting physical examinations. The individual's view of health and illness and their ability to self-care are considered. To make accurate and holistic assessments, nurses must have and use a wide variety of knowledge and skills. The ability to assess the physical status of the individual is essential, as is the ability to use effective communication techniques.

- *Diagnosing* is the analysis and interpretation of the data collected. In this phase, the nurse identifies the individual's health problems, making comparisons against the expected norms. In this way, the nurse determines the person's strengths, risks, problems and nursing diagnosis. The nurse formulates diagnostic statements.

- *Planning* determines how to promote individual strengths and prevent, reduce or resolve problems and how to intervene and implement nursing care. Goals are set in an individualised nursing care plan, and desired outcomes are identified. Care is organised in a way that prioritises goals and interventions and these, in turn, are communicated to other healthcare workers in the form of a collaborative care plan. The nursing interventions planned must be specific and individualised. If, for example, the nurse identifies that a person is at risk of dehydration, it is not enough for the nurse to simply encourage the person to drink increased amounts of fluid. The nurse and the person together must identify those liquids preferred, the times that will be best for drinking them and the amount of fluid required; this information must be documented on the written care plan. Only then does care truly become a part of the plan of care.

- *Implementing*. Planned interventions take place to help the individual meet the desired negotiated and identified goals and outcomes. In this phase, the care plan is updated by documenting the care given. Collaboration is maintained with the individual and interdisciplinary team. For example, the nurse would not be able to encourage fluids if the person was feeling sick or vomiting.

- *Evaluating* measures the degree to which goals and outcomes have been achieved. This helps the nurse determine which interventions have had a positive or negative effect. Again, collaboration with the person is paramount, and care plans can be continued, modified or even cancelled.

Source: adapted from Kozier *et al.* 2008.

Table 1.1 Types of data: objective and subjective

Objective data	Subjective data
Weight	Pain
Height	Anxiety
Temperature	Emotion
Urinalysis	Tiredness
Blood analysis	Depression
Heart rate	Anticipation

the participation of both the nurse and the individual. Recording of data is an integral part of the process, and can inform the development of a framework for care such as a nursing model.

The data collected can be broadly divided into two types: objective or subjective (Table 1.1). Objective data are those which you observe and measure, for example height and weight measurement. Subjective data are those which the person feels and perceives, for example the symptoms that an individual has. The usual primary source of data is the person; however, secondary sources can include family members, past and current medical and nursing records and other members of the healthcare team.

Data are used to support the nurse in decision-making in each phase of the nursing process. Nurses make independent and individual responses to individual needs, resulting in the development of individualised care plans. Skills inherent within the nursing process are problem-solving, the therapeutic relationship with individuals, interdisciplinary working and critical thinking.

Critical thinking and evidence-based care in adult nursing

Critical thinking is self-directed thinking that is focused on what to believe or do in a specific situation. It involves attitudes, skills and knowledge and happens when the nurse uses scientific knowledge combined with the stages of the nursing process to consider a care situation. Judgements and decisions develop through this framework.

> Emma, a third year student nurse said: *'To practise within the framework of evidence-based care, you need to have the best information available.'*

Consider this . . .

Critical thinking is essential to skilled nursing and is therefore essential to nursing. Skilled nursing develops in an atmosphere that is rich in debate, questioning and evidence-based care. Critical thinking becomes an integral component of the nurse's attitudes and skills within the practice setting.

ATTITUDES AND THOUGHT PROCESSES NECESSARY FOR CRITICAL THINKING

Thinking critically involves more than just cognitive (knowledge) skills. It is strongly influenced by your attitudes and thought processes. To think critically, you must focus your attention on your attitudes and how they affect your thinking. The skills necessary for critical thinking are outlined in Box 1.2.

Have a look at the following attributes that can support you as a nurse to:

- *Be able to think independently.* This enables you to make clinical decisions based on sound thinking and judgement.
- *Be willing to listen to and be fair in your evaluation of others' ideas and beliefs.* Listening carefully to other ideas and thoughts, and making a decision based on what you learn instead of how you feel.
- *Have empathy.* For example, if you put yourself in the place of the person with severe pain, you are better able to understand why he or she is so upset when medication to alleviate pain is late.

Box 1.2

Skills for critical thinking

The major critical thinking skills are divergent thinking, reasoning, clarifying and reflection.

- *Divergent thinking* is having the ability to weigh up the importance of information. This skill involves weighing up the relevance of data from which you draw conclusions, for example, information which is abnormal is usually considered relevant; normal data can be helpful but may not change the care you provide.
- *Reasoning* is having the ability to discriminate between facts and guesses. By using known facts, problems are solved and decisions are made in a systematic, logical way. For example, when you take a pulse you must know the facts of normal pulse rate for a person of this age, types of medications the person is taking that may alter the pulse rate and the emotional and physical state of the person. Based on these facts, you are able to decide if the pulse rate is normal or abnormal.
- *Clarifying* involves noting similarities and differences to sift out unnecessary information to help focus on the present situation. For example, when caring for a person with chronic pain, you must know the definition of chronic pain and the similarities and differences between acute pain and chronic pain.
- *Reflection* occurs when you take time to think about something, comparing different situations with similar solutions. It cannot take place in an emergency situation. As you reflect on your experiences in nursing, many of those experiences may in turn become alternatives when caring for a different person.

- *Be fair minded and consider all viewpoints.* Consider the viewpoints of others that may be different from yours before reaching a conclusion.
- *Learn from others.* You are not afraid to say, 'I don't know the answer to that question, but I will find out and let you know.'
- *Be disciplined.* Don't stop at easy answers, but continue to consider alternatives.
- *Be creative and self-confident.* Consider different ways of providing care and constantly look for better, more cost-effective methods. Confidence in one's decisions is gained through critical thinking.
- *Reflect and take time to think about situations.* As you reflect on your experiences in nursing, many of those experiences may in turn become alternatives in different care scenarios.

In essence, the ability to apply critical thinking is expected of all nurses. Using critical thinking to provide care that is structured by the nursing process allows the nurse to provide safe, effective, holistic and individualised care.

Helen, a staff nurse on a surgical ward shared her view by stating: *'Don't just do things because that is the way things are done – make your own decisions based on the best nursing evidence available.'*

The science (knowledge base) of nursing is translated into the art of nursing through caring. Caring is the means by which the nurse is connected with and concerned for the individual. Thus, the nurse as caregiver is knowledgeable, skilled, empathic and caring.

Applying ethics to nursing practice

Nursing practice is structured by codes of ethics (shown in Box 1.3) and standards that guide nursing practice and protect the public. Individual nursing practice can be held to these standards in a court of law. The guidelines are especially important because nurses encounter legal and ethical problems almost daily. The large number of ethical issues facing nurses in clinical practice makes the standards for nurses and midwives critical to moral and ethical decision-making. These standards also help to define the roles of nurses.

A standard is a statement or criterion that can be used by a profession and by the general public to measure quality of practice. Established standards of nursing practice make each individual nurse accountable for practice. This means that each nurse providing care has the responsibility or obligation to account for his or her own behaviours within that role. Professional nursing organisations develop and implement standards of practice to help clarify the nurse's responsibilities to society. In the UK, the Nursing and Midwifery Council (NMC) (2008) identify standards of conduct, performance and ethics for nurses and midwives.

Box 1.3

The code: Standards of conduct, performance and ethics for nurses and midwives (NMC 2008) (The code)

'The code' states that:

The people in your care must be able to trust you with their health and wellbeing. To justify that trust, you must:

- Make the care of people your first concern, treating them as individuals and respecting their dignity:
  - treat people as individuals
  - respect people's confidentiality
  - collaborate with those in your care
  - ensure you gain consent
  - maintain clear professional boundaries.
- Work with others to protect and promote the health and wellbeing of those in your care, their families and carers, and the wider community:
  - share information with your colleagues
  - work effectively as part of a team
  - delegate effectively
  - manage risk.
- Provide a high standard of practice and care at all times:
  - use the best available evidence
  - keep your skills and knowledge up to date
  - keep clear and accurate records.
- Be open and honest, act with integrity and uphold the reputation of your profession:
  - act with integrity
  - deal with problems
  - be impartial
  - uphold the reputation of your profession.

As a professional, you are personally accountable for actions and omissions in your practice and must always be able to justify your decisions.

You must always act lawfully, whether those laws relate to your professional practice or personal life.

Source: adapted from The code: Standards of conduct, performance and ethics for nurses and midwives (NMC 2008).

An established code of ethics is one criterion that defines a profession. Ethics are principles of conduct, and ethical behaviour is concerned with moral duty, values, obligations and the distinction between right and wrong. Codes of ethics for nurses provide a frame of reference.

Ethics is relevant to all areas of nursing practice, and even the wider aspects of research, management and education fall under this umbrella. Active involvement in ethical decision-making is an integral part of being a nurse, because the primary aims of caring are to do good and to minimise harm. These two fundamental considerations when engaging in caring are significant overarching ethical principles, and are linked together with justice and the belief in avoiding harm to those in our care (see Box 1.4).

Box 1.4

Ethical principles

There are four principles which are the essential core of ethics.

- Autonomy (the respect for rights of individuals and for their self-determination; holding self-determination and self-governance over one's actions).
- Beneficence (doing good, providing benefits & measuring benefits against risks & costs; the prevention of harm and the promotion of good).
- Non-maleficence (to do no intentional harm).
- Justice (derived from the general rule of human conduct to treat others fairly/distributing benefits, risks & costs fairly).

Source: Beauchamp and Childress 2001, Glass and Cluxton 2004.

Of course, many high-profile discussions about ethics will focus on the big debates about life and death (for example, Assisted Dying for the Terminally Ill Act 2005). However, in everyday encounters, ethical issues are constantly played out in a subconscious way. Moral decision-making can be as fundamental as whether or not to tell your friend that 'no, she really doesn't suit that colour'! When applied to the care setting, this subconscious decision-making can be influenced by our opinions and personal values, a sense of what is right or wrong, our understanding of our obligations and duties as a nurse and the subsequent consequences of our actions. **Nursing ethics** is about asking ourselves whether something that can be done, should be done, or should not be done. Some answers can be considered more socially or morally acceptable than others, depending on the context in which they exist.

Consider this . . .

Everyday sayings that involve ethical thinking:

'I demand to be treated with respect.'

'You shouldn't behave like that.'

'You've got no right to say that to me.'

'Well, at least there was no harm done.'

'You can't say fairer than that.'

'He is a really good person.'

'We will treat her first because her needs are greater.'

Source: adapted from Chaloner 2007.

Ethical discussion will often focus around the balance between rights and obligations in healthcare. In essence, this means that if we acknowledge the right to a healthy life, we should also acknowledge the obligation to support that right. Nurses are in a position to promote, maintain and support healthy living, and to provide appropriate care when a person's

health breaks down. This is also echoed in the Health Act of 2009 which endorses the principle of supporting the population in the UK in its right to healthcare. Here the NHS Constitution values, for example, the right for persons to be treated with a professional standard of care, by appropriately qualified and experienced staff.

Theories might include:

- *Deontology*. Universal moral rules that everyone should follow – the idea that rights must be defined regardless of the consequences of actions.
- *Consequentialism* (often referred to as utilitarianism). Actions produce the greatest good for the greatest number of people. In this theory, rights should not be granted without examination of the possible results (or consequences).

Consider this . . .

100 people are on a sinking ship, but the lifeboats will only carry half that number. How do you decide who will get the safety of the lifeboat?

- Deontologists would apply the rule that everybody has the right to a place on a lifeboat (one option might be to draw short and long straws to decide).
- Consequentialists would consider the individual merits of each person and debate the best outcome (or consequence) of choosing who would get a place (for example, a scientist on the brink of developing a life-saving vaccine).

The same types of theories can be applied to decisions in healthcare.

Legal and ethical dilemmas in nursing

A dilemma is a choice between two unpleasant, ethically troubling alternatives. Nurses who provide acute and ongoing nursing care face dilemmas almost daily – so many, in fact, that a complete discussion of them is impossible here. However, many commonly experienced dilemmas involve confidentiality, a person's rights, and issues of dying and death. The nurse must use ethical and legal guidelines to make decisions about moral actions when providing care in these and in many other situations.

Nurses respect the right to confidentiality of information found in the person's record or noted during assessment. Rights of the person as an individual, however, can result in dilemmas for the nurse in the clinical setting. For example, the right to privacy and confidentiality creates a dilemma when it conflicts with the nurse's right to information that may affect personal safety.

The right to refuse treatment (including surgery, medication, medical therapy and nourishment) is another individual right that raises nursing dilemmas. The situation, the alternatives and the potential harm from refusal must be carefully explained.

The issues surrounding dying and death have become increasingly pressing as advances in technology extend the lives of people with chronic debilitating illness and major trauma. These changes have altered concepts of living and dying, resulting in ethical conflicts regarding quality of life and death with dignity versus technologic methods of preserving life in any form. Even if the person is competent and requests that no heroic measures be used to maintain life, many questions arise related to nursing care. What constitutes a heroic measure? Should nursing interventions to provide comfort include administering medication at a level known to stop breathing? Should a feeding tube be placed in the person who is terminally ill? These and other questions are being debated not only within the healthcare system but also in the British and European courts.

THE NURSE AS ADVOCATE

The person entering the healthcare system may be unprepared to make independent decisions. However, today's healthcare consumer is better educated about options for care, and may have very definite opinions. The nurse as an advocate actively promotes the person's rights to autonomy and free choice (see Box 1.5). Speaking for the person, the nurse mediates between the person and others, and/or protects the person's right to self-determination.

> Nathan, a Charge Nurse, notices that patients will often willingly agree with what the doctor says, and then ask for support and clarity from the nurses. *'Nurses are viewed more as equals and are less threatening than those who are seen as powerful. Often patients will turn to the more junior student nurse for support and clarification of their position.'*

The nurse must practise advocacy based on the belief that individuals have the right to choose treatment options, based on information about the results of accepting or rejecting the treatment, without coercion. The nurse must also accept and respect the decision of the individual, even though it may differ from the decision the nurse would make. According to MIND, the National Association for Mental Health, *'An advocate is someone who can both listen to you and speak for you in times of need.'* (inyo@mind.org.uk)

THE NURSE AS LEADER AND MANAGER

All nurses are leaders and managers. They practise leadership and they manage time, people, resources and the environment in which they provide care. Nurses carry out these roles by directing, delegating and coordinating nursing activities. Nurses must be knowledgeable about how and when to delegate, as well as the legal requirements of delegation. Nurses also evaluate the quality of care provided.

Models of care delivery

Nurses are leaders and managers of care within a variety of models of care delivery. Examples are primary nursing, team nursing, case management and **integrated care pathways**. Terms commonly used in the management of clinical care processes are shown in Box 1.6.

PRIMARY NURSING

Primary nursing allows the nurse to provide individualised direct care to a small number of people during their entire in-patient stay. This model was developed to reduce the fragmentation of care experienced by individuals and to facilitate family-centred continuity of care. In primary nursing, the nurse provides care, communicates with individuals, families and other healthcare providers and carries out discharge planning.

TEAM NURSING

Team nursing is practised by teams of variously educated healthcare workers. For example, a team may consist of a registered nurse, a student nurse and two healthcare assistants. The registered nurse is the team leader. The team leader is responsible for delegating care and has overall responsibility for individual care delivered by team members. All team members work together, each performing the activities for which he or she is best prepared.

Box 1.5

Goals of the nurse as advocate

The goals of the nurse as advocate are to:

- Assess the need for advocacy.
- Communicate with other healthcare team members.
- Provide individual and family teaching.
- Assist and support individual decision-making.
- Serve as a change agent in the healthcare system.
- Participate in health policy formulation.

Box 1.6

Common terms used for the management of clinical care processes

Common terms used for the management of clinical care processes include:

- Anticipated recovery path – clinical pathway.
- Care map – clinical protocol.
- Care pathway – critical paths.
- Case management plan – expected recovery path.
- Clinical guidelines – integrated care pathway.

CASE MANAGEMENT

Case management focuses on management of a caseload (group) of people and the members of the healthcare team caring for them. The purpose of case management is to maximise positive outcomes and contain costs. The nurse who is case manager is usually a clinical specialist, and the caseload consists of individuals with similar healthcare needs. As case manager, the nurse makes appropriate referrals to other healthcare providers and manages the quality of care provided, including accuracy, timeliness and cost. The case manager is also in contact with people after discharge, ensuring continuity of care and health maintenance.

Delegation

Delegation is carried out when the nurse allocates appropriate and effective work activities to other members of the healthcare team. When the nurse delegates nursing care activities to another person, that person is authorised to act in the place of the nurse, although the nurse retains the accountability for the activities performed.

> Danny, a Band 5 Staff Nurse, said: *'As a newly qualified staff nurse, I found delegation to be one of the most difficult challenges, however, I soon realised that my priorities were to manage and to carry out the activities that others were not legally able to do. I now know that I can legitimately delegate in those situations.'*

IN PRACTICE

Enhancing delegation skills

- Be aware of the level of competence of each member of the healthcare team, the complexity of the work to be allocated and the amount of time available to supervise the work.
- Understand the level of nursing judgement and evaluation required for the work.
- Consider the potential harm and difficulty of performing the work.
- Be aware of the job descriptions for each member of the care team.
- Assign the right job to the right person.
- Give clear directions. Ask questions to ensure that instructions have been understood.
- Give the team member the authority to complete the work.
- Monitor the outcomes of the care provided and give constructive evaluation if necessary.

INTEGRATED CARE PATHWAYS

Integrated care pathways (also called clinical pathways, critical pathways or treatment protocols) are designed to provide a coordinated approach to care within a multidisciplinary health service. Such pathways are generally developed for specific diagnoses – usually common, high-risk and high-cost type problems – with the collaboration of members of the healthcare team. The goals of critical pathways are listed in Box 1.7.

Typically, care pathways will include protocols for the care and treatment of a variety of health problems including:

- Cardiovascular problems, e.g. rehabilitation following a coronary episode.
- Stroke rehabilitation.
- Surgical pathways, e.g. total abdominal hysterectomy.
- Orthopaedic problems, e.g. joint replacement.

This care management tool describes how resources will be used to achieve predetermined outcomes. It also establishes the sequence of multidisciplinary interventions, including education, discharge planning, consultations, medication administration, diagnostics, therapeutics and treatments.

Box 1.7

The goals of critical pathways

The goals of critical pathways are to:

- Achieve realistic, expected person and family outcomes.
- Promote professional and collaborative practice and care.
- Ensure continuity of care.
- Guarantee appropriate use of resources.
- Reduce costs and length of stay.
- Provide the framework for continuous improvement.

Nurses and quality assurance

You will recall earlier in the chapter the NMC Code which states that you must *'Work with others to protect and promote the health and wellbeing of those in your care, their families and carers, and the wider community'* (NMC 2008). As a leader and manager, the nurse is responsible for the quality of person care through a process called **quality assurance**. This process consists of the quality control activities that evaluate, monitor or regulate the standard of services provided to the consumer. Three components of care are evaluated: *structure*, to assess the impact of the environment in which care takes place; *process*, to consider how care is given; and *outcome*, to question the changes in the person's health status as a result of nursing interventions.

As such, quality assurance methods evaluate person care. They commonly evaluate actual care against an established set of standards of care. Nurses and other healthcare providers make this evaluation by reviewing documentation, by conducting patient surveys and nurse interviews and/or by direct observation of nurse or patient performance. The data are then used to identify differences between actual practice and established standards and to develop a plan of action to resolve any differences found.

The operating framework for the NHS for 2010/11 sets out the priorities for the NHS for the year ahead to enable them to begin their planning (see Box 1.8).

Box 1.8

The NHS in England: The operating framework for 2009/10

The national priorities in the operating framework remain the same, providing important stability. The five priorities are:

- improving cleanliness and reducing healthcare-associated infections;
- improving access through achievement of the 18-week referral to treatment pledge and improving access (including at evenings and weekends) to GP services;
- keeping adults and children well, improving their health and reducing health inequalities;
- improving patient experience, staff satisfaction and engagement;
- preparing to respond in a state of emergency such as an outbreak of pandemic flu, learning from our experience of swine flu.

During 2010/11, the NHS has pledged to continue its work to reduce local variation and eliminate poor performance.

Source: DoH 2010.

THE NURSE AS RESEARCHER

Nurses have always identified problems in person care. Although they have developed interventions to meet specific needs, the activities often have not been conducted within a scientific framework or communicated to other nurses through nursing literature. To develop the science of nursing, nursing knowledge is established through clinical research and then published, so that the findings can be used by all nurses to provide evidence-based person care.

To be relevant, nursing research must have a goal to improve the care that nurses provide to persons. This means that all nurses must consider the researcher role to be integral to nursing practice. Safe and effective nursing care is based on the best evidence available.

PRACTICE ALERT

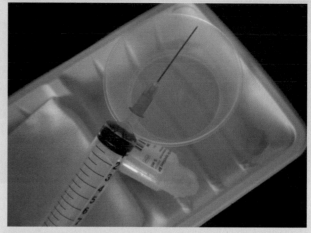

Figure 1.2 Unsheathed hypodermic needle.

The evidence base has demonstrated that most needle-stick injuries in the healthcare setting can be prevented (RCN 2005b, Casey and Elliott 2007, NPSA 2007, Pratt et al. 2007). As a result, nursing practice has responded to minimise the risks of needle-stick injury as follows:

Precautions to reduce the risk of sharps injuries include:

- Never re-sheath or re-cap needles.
- Immediate and safe disposal of sharps into appropriate containers.
- Correct use of sharps containers: do not overfill, and replace containers as required.
- Convenient access to sharps containers.
- Regular collections of used sharps containers.
- Use of pre-filled syringes where possible.
- Use of needle-free systems where possible.
- Use of cannulae with integral sharps protection.
- Avoidance of suturing where possible.
- Appropriate anchoring and management of vascular access devices (VADs).
- Ongoing education for staff involved in handling and disposal of sharps.
- Mandatory reporting of all sharps and needle-stick injuries.

Source: Gabriel 2008.

THE NURSE AS EDUCATOR

The nurse's role as educator (see Figure 1.3) is becoming increasingly important for several reasons. Healthcare providers and consumers and the government are placing greater emphasis on health promotion and illness prevention; hospital stays are becoming shorter; and the number of people with chronic

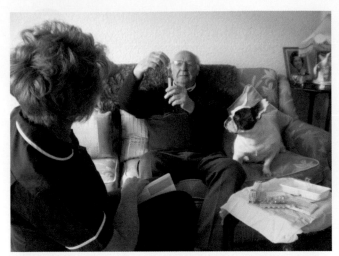

Figure 1.3 The nurse's role as educator is an essential component of care.

illnesses in our society is increasing. Early discharge of patients from the hospital setting to home care means that family carers must learn how to perform complex skills. All of these factors make the educator role essential to maintaining the health and wellbeing of individuals. A major component of the health educator role today is discharge planning. Discharge planning, which begins on admission to a healthcare setting, is a systematic method of preparing the person and family for exit from the healthcare agency and for maintaining continuity of care after the patient leaves the care setting. Discharge planning also involves making referrals, identifying community and personal resources and arranging for necessary equipment and supplies for home care.

The framework for the role of educator is the teaching–learning process, something that nurses often do intuitively. Within this framework, the nurse assesses learning needs, plans and implements teaching methods to meet those needs and evaluates the effectiveness of the teaching. To be an effective educator, the nurse must have effective interpersonal skills and be familiar with adult learning principles.

Jane, a Junior Sister, Neurology, said: *'I love it when student nurses ask me to tell them about this and that! It challenges me to think and it really opens me up to new learning.'*

Health and illness

The human responses that nurses must consider when planning and implementing care result from changes in the structure and/or function of all body systems, as well as the interrelated effects of those changes on the psychosocial, cultural, spiritual, economic and personal life of the individual.

A useful starting point to understand the complexities of health and illness is to begin to define what health is. You could start by considering a definition of your own health. You might consider freedom from disease or the ability to work and socialise as being aspects of your health. Others might include eating a healthy diet and exercising within their definition. How we define health will depend on a complex relationship between our physical makeup, genetics, culture and education and, to some extent, the powerful influences around us from, for example, the media and our social group.

The World Health Organization (WHO) defines health as *'a state of complete physical, mental, and social well-being, and not merely the absence of disease or infirmity'* (WHO 1974, 1). However, this definition does not take into account the various levels of health a person may experience, or that a person may be clinically described as ill yet still think of themselves as well. These additional factors, which greatly influence nursing care, include the health–illness continuum and high-level wellness.

THE HEALTH–ILLNESS CONTINUUM AND HIGH-LEVEL WELLNESS

The **health–illness continuum** (Figure 1.4) represents health as a dynamic process, with high-level wellness at one extreme of the continuum and death at the opposite extreme. Individuals place themselves at different locations on the continuum at specific points in time.

Dunn (1959) expanded the concept of a continuum of health and illness in his description of high-level wellness. Dunn conceptualised wellness as an active process influenced by the environment. He differentiated good health from wellness:

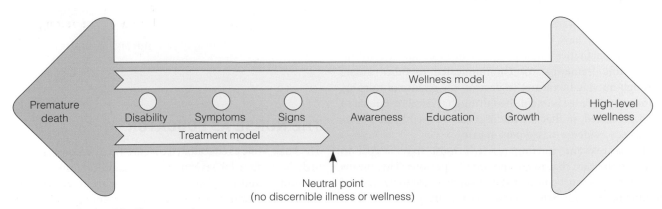

Premature death — Disability — Symptoms — Signs — Awareness — Education — Growth — High-level wellness

Wellness model

Treatment model

Neutral point
(no discernible illness or wellness)

Figure 1.4 The health–illness continuum.

Good health can exist as a relatively passive state of freedom from illness in which the individual is at peace with his environment . . . Wellness is an integrated method of functioning, which is oriented toward maximizing the potential of which the individual is capable, within the environment where he is functioning. (Dunn 1959, 4)

A variety of factors influence wellness, including self-concept, environment, culture and spiritual values. Providing care based on a framework of wellness facilitates active involvement by both the nurse and the individual in promoting, maintaining or restoring health. It also supports the philosophy of **holistic healthcare**, in which all aspects of a person (physical, psychosocial, cultural, spiritual and intellectual) are considered as essential components of individualised care.

FACTORS AFFECTING HEALTH

Many different factors affect a person's health or level of wellness. These factors often interact to promote health or to become risk factors for alterations in health. Factors that can contribute to health are numerous – here are just a few:

- age;
- gender;
- education;
- religion;
- culture;
- social circumstances can contribute;
- lifestyles are partly determined by income;
- social inequalities can affect choices.

Other influences:

- media;
- peers;
- own experience;
- knowledgeable others;
- significant happenings in our (or others') health career.

> **Consider this . . .**
> You might want to stop at this point and think about what other factors influence your health and wellbeing.

You might have considered how each person's genetic makeup influences health status throughout life. Genetic makeup affects personality, temperament, body structure, intellectual potential and susceptibility to the development of hereditary alterations in health. Examples of chronic illnesses that are associated with genetic makeup include sickle cell disease, haemophilia, diabetes mellitus and cancer.

Although cognitive abilities (our ability to understand, reason and perceive information) are determined prior to adulthood, the level of cognitive development affects whether people view themselves as healthy or ill; cognitive levels may also affect health practices. Injuries to and illnesses affecting the brain may alter cognitive abilities. Educational level affects the ability to understand and follow guidelines for health. For example, if an individual is functionally illiterate (can't read or write), written information about healthy behaviours and health resources can be of little use.

Certain diseases occur at a higher rate of incidence in some races and ethnic groups than in others. For example, in the UK, cancer of the prostate is more prevalent in older men and those from the Afro–Caribbean communities.

Age, gender and developmental level are factors in health and illness. Cardiovascular disorders are uncommon in young adults, but the incidence increases after the age of 40. Myocardial infarctions are more common in men than women until women are past the menopause. Some diseases occur only in one gender or the other (e.g., prostate cancer in men and cervical cancer in women). The older adult often has increased incidence of chronic illness and increased potential for serious illness or death from infectious illnesses such as influenza and pneumonia.

The components of a person's lifestyle that affect health status include patterns of eating, use of chemical substances (alcohol, nicotine, caffeine, legal and illegal drugs), exercise and rest patterns and coping methods. Examples of altered responses are the relationship of obesity to hypertension, cigarette smoking to chronic obstructive pulmonary disease, a sedentary lifestyle to heart disease and a high-stress career to alcoholism. The environment has a major influence on health. Occupational exposure to toxic substances (such as asbestos and coal dust) increases the risk of pulmonary disorders. Air, water and food pollution increase the risk of respiratory disorders, infectious diseases and cancer. Environmental temperature variations can result in hypothermia or hyperthermia, especially in the older adult.

Socioeconomic background

Both lifestyle and environmental influences are affected by one's income level. The culture of poverty, which crosses all racial and ethnic boundaries, negatively influences health status. Living at or below the poverty level often results in crowded, unsanitary living conditions or homelessness. Housing often is overcrowded, lacks adequate heating or cooling. Crowded living problems increase the risk of transferring communicable diseases. Other problems include lack of infant and child care, lack of medical care for injuries or illness, inadequate nutrition, use of addictive substances and violence.

Health behaviour

Health behaviour is mediated by the circumstances and environments in which individuals live their lives, in their community, work, school or other settings. Lifestyle choices do not happen in isolation from other factors which may limit either the availability of healthy options in the first place, or the skills of

FAST FACTS

Geographic area and health status

Among the population of working age within the UK in 2005:

● In Wokingham, Windsor and Maidenhead one half of the population were in higher managerial and professional occupations whereas in Blaenau Gwent half of the population were in routine and manual occupations.

Source: Hall 2009.

This is further illustrated by the gap between the best and the worst areas for life expectancy:

● *Life expectancy – females*

Living in Kensington & Chelsea = 87.2 years
Living in Liverpool = 78.3 years

● *Life expectancy – males*

Living in Kensington & Chelsea = 83.1 years
Living in Manchester = 73 years

Source: DoH 2007.

individuals to make and carry out those healthy choices. It has been suggested that 50% of mortality from the 10 leading causes of death results from individual behaviour. Behaviour such as smoking, alcohol consumption, poor diet and risky sexual behaviour has been identified as highly significant.

Individual beliefs about health and illness are a significant factor in the way persons behave in relation to their health status. Beliefs imply that there are certain assumptions that we trust to be true or accept as truth. A belief can be thought of as a 'convinced opinion'. You might like to consider if you believe in the power of paracetamol. Placebo effects (the positive response to medication simply because the recipient believes it will work) can arise not only from a conscious belief in a drug, but also from subconscious associations between recovery and the past experience of being treated. Such subconscious thoughts can control our bodily processes without us being aware, such as immune responses and the release of hormones to make us feel better.

Attitudes to health

Why is it useful as nurses to consider attitudes, behaviour and beliefs in health? Attitudes can be central to health promotion because they determine how people behave in relation to their health. Attitudes directly influence how we make choices about health. As nurses engaging in health promotion activities, it is important to understand why some people opt for more healthy behaviour than others, i.e. those who actively seek screening activities against those who decline screening opportunities.

Smoking-related behaviour and attitudes surveyed by the Office for National Statistics (ONS) released results from the *Opinions Survey Report No. 40: Smoking-related Behaviour and*

Attitudes 2008/09 (Lader, 1999). The survey, carried out on behalf of the Department of Health and the NHS Information Centre for health and social care, monitors changes in the general attitude towards smoking and towards smoking in public places as well as smoking behaviour and habits, giving up and stopping smoking. Key findings from the report show that 67% of smokers said they would like to give up, which was significantly lower than 2007 (74%). It also demonstrated that the proportion of those polled who supported the smoking ban in restaurants was 93%, compared with 75% who agreed with the ban in pubs. This suggests that the attitude of drinkers is proportionately different from the attitudes of those enjoying a restaurant environment when it comes to smoking in public.

So, our beliefs about health can influence the way we react to healthcare and the way we adopt lifestyle behaviours. For example, a strong belief in the risk of certain behaviours might in turn alter our actions in relation to them. In a survey conducted by the Food Standards Agency in February 2007, 88% of people in the UK said that they believe that parents should be strict with children and make them eat healthily. In the same study, 89% of people claim that healthy eating is important to them (FSA 2007).

HEALTH PROMOTION AND MAINTENANCE

For many years, the emphasis in nursing was on care of the acutely ill in the hospital setting. With changes in society and in healthcare, this emphasis is shifting toward preventive, community-based care. The importance of teaching health-promoting behaviours is an essential component of health and ill-health nursing. In 2008, Lord Darzi's review of the NHS highlighted the need for a shift in emphasis from a curative approach in healthcare to a model that views health promotion as a key priority (DoH 2008). In promoting this aim Lord Darzi outlined the requirement for primary care trusts (PCTs) to commission and provide comprehensive health promotion services that are aligned to the specific needs of their local populations (DoH 2008).

Healthy living

Promoting healthy lifestyles for people in England and Wales is an important governmental responsibility. The DoH runs initiatives to help people quit smoking, eat better and exercise more, as well as health screening projects and training and skills programmes. The DoH is committed to tackling obesity, sexually transmitted infections, alcohol and substance misuse and smoking.

The DoH 5 A DAY logo and portion indicator is an example of an important part of this programme, and has been developed in consultation with industry, local and national health, education and consumer organisations, and through several stages of consumer research. Use of the logo and portion indicator have to comply with strict criteria which take into account portion size, as well as fat, sugar and salt levels.

The government's success in these campaigns may be reflected in the prevalence of obesity in England. It is the highest in the European Union (EU) and, in conjunction with this, the UK is seeing increased levels of diabetes. However, premature mortality rates from the two biggest killers, circulatory diseases and cancer, are reducing faster in England than the average for the EU (DoH 2007).

The Change4life campaign, published in 2008, focuses on promoting healthy behaviours in a 'Swap it – don't stop it' message aimed at overweight adults. The idea behind the message is not to give up the things you enjoy, but to consider a healthier option. There is a direct link between health promotion and preventive healthcare, where adults are supported because of their associated risk factors for ill health. The next section will discuss this in more detail.

Disease and illness

Disease and *illness* are terms that are often used interchangeably, but in fact they have different meanings. In general, nursing is concerned with illness, whereas medicine is concerned with disease.

DISEASE

Disease (literally meaning 'without ease') is a medical term describing alterations in structure and function of the body or mind. Diseases may have mechanical, biologic or normative causes, and some common causes are listed in Box 1.9. Mechanical

Box 1.9

Causes of disease

The following are generally accepted as common causes of disease:

- genetic defects;
- developmental defects resulting from exposure to viruses, chemicals or drugs that affect the developing foetus;
- biologic agents or toxins (including viruses, bacteria, fungi, etc.);
- physical agents such as temperature extremes, radiation and electricity;
- chemical agents such as alcohol, drugs, strong acids or bases, and heavy metals;
- generalised response of tissues to injury or irritation;
- alterations in the production of antibodies, resulting in allergies or hypersensitivities;
- faulty metabolic processes (e.g., a production of hormones or enzymes above or below normal);
- continued stress.

Table 1.2 Disease classifications and definitions

Classification	Definition
Acute	A disease that has a rapid onset, lasts a relatively short time and is self-limiting
Chronic	A disease that has one or more of these characteristics: (1) is permanent, (2) leaves permanent disability, (3) causes non-reversible patho-physiology, (4) requires special training of the person for rehabilitation, (5) requires a long period of care
Communicable	A disease that can spread from one person to another
Congenital	A disease or disorder that exists at or before birth
Degenerative	A disease that results from deterioration or impairment of organs or tissues
Functional	A disease that affects function or performance but does not have signs and symptoms of organic illness
Malignant	A disease that tends to become worse and cause death
Psychosomatic	A psychological disease that is manifested by physiological symptoms
Idiopathic	A disease that has an unknown cause
Iatrogenic	A disease that is caused by medical intervention

causes of disease result in damage to the structure of the body and are the result of trauma or extremes of temperature. Biologic causes of disease affect body function and are the result of genetic defects, the effects of ageing, infestation and infection, alterations in the immune system and alterations in normal organ secretions. The cause of many diseases is still unknown.

Diseases may be classified as acute or chronic, communicable, congenital, degenerative, functional, malignant, psychosomatic, idiopathic or iatrogenic (see Table 1.2). In all types of disease, alterations in structure or function cause signs and symptoms that prompt a person to seek treatment. Although both subjective symptoms and objective signs commonly appear with disease, objective signs often predominate. Examples of objective signs include bleeding, vomiting, diarrhoea, limitation of movement, swelling, visual disturbances and changes in elimination. However, pain (a subjective symptom) is often the primary reason that prompts a person to seek healthcare.

ILLNESS

Illness is the response a person has to a disease. This response is highly individualised, because the person responds not only to his or her own perceptions of the disease but also to the perceptions of others. Illness integrates patho-physiological alterations; psychological effects of those alterations; effects on roles, relationships and values; and cultural and spiritual beliefs. A person may have a disease and not categorise himself or

IN PRACTICE

A sequence of illness behaviours

1. *Experiencing symptoms.* In the first stage of an acute illness, a person experiences one or more signs and symptoms that serve as cues for an awareness that a change in normal health is occurring. The most significant manifestation is pain. Examples of other symptoms that signal an illness are bleeding, swelling, fever or difficulty with breathing. If the signs and symptoms are mild or are familiar (such as symptoms of the common cold or influenza), the person usually uses over-the-counter medications or a traditional remedy for self-treatment. If the symptoms are relieved, no further action is taken; however, if the symptoms are severe or become worse, the person moves to the next stage.

2. *Assuming the sick role.* In the second stage, the person assumes the sick role. This role assumption signals acceptance of the symptoms as proof that an illness is present. The person usually validates this belief with others and seeks support for the need to have professional treatment or to stay at home from school or work. Self-preoccupation is characteristic of this stage, and the person focuses on alterations in function resulting from the illness. If the illness is resolved, the person validates a return to health with others and resumes normal activities; however, if signs and symptoms remain or increase in severity and others agree that no improvement has occurred, the person moves to the next stage by seeking medical care.

3. *Seeking medical care.* In our society, a doctor or other healthcare provider most often provides validation of illness. People who believe they are ill (and who are encouraged by others to contact a healthcare provider) seek medical contact for diagnosis, prognosis and treatment of the illness. If the medical diagnosis is of an illness, the person moves to the next stage. If the medical diagnosis does not support illness, the individual may return to normal functioning or may seek validation from a different healthcare provider.

4. *Assuming a dependent role.* The stage of assuming a dependent role begins when a person accepts the diagnosis and planned treatment of the illness. As the severity of the illness increases, so does the dependent role. It is during this stage that the person may enter the hospital for treatment and care. The responses of the person to care depend on many different variables: the severity of the illness, the degree of anxiety or fear about the outcome, the loss of roles, the support systems available, individualised reactions to stress and previous experiences with illness care.

5. *Achieving recovery and rehabilitation.* The final stage of an acute illness is recovery and rehabilitation. Institutional healthcare focuses on the acute care needs of the ill person, with recovery beginning in the hospital and completed at home. This focus makes person education and continuity of care a major goal for nursing. It has also contributed to the shift in settings for nursing care, with increasing numbers of nurses providing care in community settings and the home. The person now gives up the dependent role and resumes normal roles and responsibilities. As a result of education during treatment and care, the person may be at a higher level of wellness after recovery is complete. There is no set timetable for recovery from an illness. The degree of severity of the illness and the method of treatment both affect the length of time required, as does the person's compliance with treatment plans and motivation to return to normal health.

Source: based on Suchman 1972.

herself as ill, or may validate feelings of illness through the comments of others ('You don't look as though you feel well today').

Acute illness

An **acute illness** occurs rapidly, lasts for a relatively short time and is self-limiting. The problem responds to self-treatment or to medical–surgical intervention. People with uncomplicated acute illnesses usually recover and return to normal functioning.

Illness behaviours are the ways people cope with the alterations in health and function caused by a disease. Illness behaviours are highly individualised and are influenced by age, gender, family values, economic status, culture, educational level and mental status. The study of illness behaviour has shaped our understanding of how persons might react when they are ill. The study summarised in the In Practice box is dated but is still a valuable source of evidence to inform nurses of how persons behave in contemporary society.

Chronic illness

Chronic illness is a term that encompasses many different lifelong pathological and psychological alterations in health. Current trends affecting an increased incidence of chronic illnesses include diseases of ageing, diseases of lifestyle and behaviour and environmental factors. Chronic illness can be characterised by impaired function in more than one body system; responses to this impaired function may occur in sensory perception, self-care abilities, mobility, cognition and social skills. The demands on the individual and family as a result of these responses are often lifelong.

The intensity of a chronic illness and its related signs and symptoms range from mild to severe, and the illness is usually characterised by periods of remission and exacerbation. During periods of remission, the person does not experience symptoms, even though the disease is still clinically present. During periods of exacerbation, the symptoms reappear.

These periods of change in symptoms do not appear in all chronic diseases.

Each person with a chronic illness has a unique set of responses and needs. The response of the person to the illness is influenced by the following factors:

- the point in the life-cycle at which the onset of the illness occurs;
- the type and degree of limitations imposed by the illness;
- the visibility of impairment or disfigurement;
- the pathophysiology causing the illness;
- the relationship between the impairment and functioning in social roles;
- pain and fear.

These factors are highly complex. They are interrelated within each person, resulting in individualised illness behaviours and needs. Because there are so many different chronic diseases and because the experience of each person with the illness is a composite of individualised responses, it is difficult to generalise about needs.

In the Fast Facts box, Miller (2000) uses the term 'comply' to describe how people with chronic illness should adhere to medical advice (e.g. correctly taking medication, or following instructions for a healthy diet). Literature to investigate why individuals may or may not comply will often use a combination of the terms adherence, compliance and **concordance** to describe this behaviour.

Concordance has been defined as 'a new approach to the prescribing and taking of medicines' (Medicines Partnership 2003). An agreement is reached after negotiation between the individual and healthcare professional. This implies acknowledgement of the person's rights, beliefs and wishes when determining whether, how and when medicines are to be taken.

CARING FOR THE PSYCHOLOGICAL NEEDS OF ILL PEOPLE

Disease and illness can result in a high level of vulnerability and dependency in our persons, and nurses in the adult field of acute and ongoing care are ideally placed to support the psychological needs of those in their care. Many theorists identify two main elements of care: one is the need for practical and technical activities, and the other is focused on the way in which those activities are carried out by individual nurses.

In the case below, there is little consideration of the individual's need for information, or evidence of a kind approach, someone to listen and to provide basic reassurance in the initial time of arriving at the ward. It was not until the named nursed became involved that Wendy began to experience some degree of psychological support.

Psychological needs of adults who are experiencing healthcare can be influenced by a variety of factors. For example, in the case study below, Wendy has limited understanding of the formal healthcare setting, and she has no experience of major illness. We cannot assume that her social and emotional support is effective, despite the presence of her husband. In this scenario, the culture and priorities of staff in the care setting can negatively influence the way Wendy perceives care provision.

Case Study – Wendy

Return to Wendy at the beginning of the chapter. Wendy, aged 53, is scheduled for surgical investigations of possible malignancy (cancer). She is normally well, works in a supermarket and is an active woman with two grown up sons both away at university. Her husband is with her as she arrives to the surgical unit for admission. This is her first experience of hospital admission since she had her second son 19 years ago.

A healthcare assistant (HCA) hurriedly shows her to her bed and leaves her there. The ward is alive with activity but nobody acknowledges Wendy and she is unsure of what to do; her husband patiently waits outside of the ward.

Some two hours later another HCA asks Wendy what she ordered for her lunch and despite Wendy trying to explain that she has just arrived that day, nobody listens. Wendy wanders out to look for her husband and eventually, some four hours after her arrival, a staff nurse comes to find her. Wendy is met with an awkward encounter as the staff nurse implies that the bed that was allocated was nearly given over to someone else and that Wendy should have arrived on time!

It is not until Wendy's named nurse sits down and introduces himself by name and role, and discusses fully what Wendy might expect that she begins to relax a little.

FAST FACTS

Chronic illness

Almost all people with a chronic illness will need to:

- live as normally as possible, despite the symptoms and treatment that make the person with a chronic illness feel alienated, lonely and different from others without the illness;
- learn to adapt activities of daily living and self-care activities;
- grieve the loss of physical function and structure, income, status, roles and dignity;
- comply with a medical treatment plan;
- maintain a positive self-concept and a sense of hope;
- maintain a feeling of being in control;
- confront the inevitability of death.

Source: Miller 2000.

Individuals will differ in the amount and level of care needed, and their reactions may range from stress and distress to poor or prolonged recovery from illness. Adult nurses can offer their unique knowledge and skill coupled with good communication and a genuine empathic approach to support the emotional needs of individuals.

Tracey, Junior Sister, Women's Health Unit, said: *'From the first step onto the ward, patients should be made to feel welcome and encouraged to explore how they feel.'*

HEALTH PROMOTION AND ILLNESS PREVENTION

Consider this . . .

Prevention is better (and cheaper) than cure!

Securing Good Health for the Whole Population (written by Sir Derek Wanless and published by HM Treasury in February 2004) set out a challenge to move towards a 'fully engaged scenario' in which most people were taking active steps to improve their own health. The document made it clear that increases in NHS funding would be cancelled out by increasing numbers of people with chronic diseases and largely preventable ill health unless we can reach this position. The potential cost of inaction was said in the review to run to a staggering £187 billion.

Cutting costs in healthcare provision can be interpreted as a classic reason for preventative medicine (Tones and Tilford 2001).

Health promotion and illness prevention has at its core the focus of improving people's health and quality of life. Health promotion is concerned with promoting health at all levels, from the individual to society and indeed worldwide (as evidenced by the onset of global 'swine flu' in 2009). The Ottawa Charter (1989) presented a practical approach to health promotion by identifying five key strategies (WHO 1986):

- reorienting health services;
- developing personal skills;
- building a healthy public policy;
- strengthening community action;
- creating supportive environments for health.

Health promotion and illness prevention have become an important aspect of public health policy. Key areas of prevention, derived from evidence of epidemiology, have focused the UK government in their plans to reduce morbidity (the incidence of illness) and mortality (the incidence of death from illness). An example of this is the *Saving Lives: Our Healthier Nation* campaign (DoH 1999), which suggests that a reduction in smoking and the adoption of a diet rich in fruit, vegetables and cereals would reduce the number of deaths from cancer by 10% in people under the age of 75.

Saving Lives: Our Healthier Nation (DoH 1999) was the government's action plan for tackling poor health by improving the health of everyone, the economically worst off in particular. 'Our Healthier Nation' looked at a new approach to saving lives and at the aims and advances in public health. It also discussed individuals and health and tackling the wider causes of ill health within communities. 'Saving Lives' dealt with the specific issues of cancer, coronary heart disease and stroke, accidents and mental health. These are deemed to be the major causes of morbidity and mortality and the most responsive to prevention. It also looked at wider issues such as sexual health, tackling drug and alcohol problems, communicable disease, genetics and improving ethnic minorities' health. The Marmot Review (Marmot *et al.* 2010) is a review of health inequalities in England that demonstrates the link between the hierarchy of social class and the prevalence of disease.

As nurses, we promote health by teaching the activities that maintain wellness, by providing information about the characteristics and consequences of diseases when risk factors have been identified and by supplying specific information about decreasing risk factors.

The term 'prevention' implies an action to stop something, or act in a way that creates a barrier or an obstacle to events (in this case illness). Three levels of prevention are identified to classify interventions that promote health (see Table 1.3):

1. *Primary prevention* to reduce the onset of ill health.
2. *Secondary prevention* – early intervention to minimise illness.
3. *Tertiary prevention* to limit disability in established illness.

Behaviour and lifestyle have a profound effect on health and wellbeing. Having an understanding of this can help health promoters focus resources in the most efficient way (i.e. in terms of people and finance and the right kinds of tools). Health promotion activities that can harness elements of group behaviour can have value in the identification, prevention and management of illness. One way of doing this is health needs assessment.

HEALTH NEEDS ASSESSMENT

Health needs assessment is a systematic method of assessing the health issues faced by a particular population to provide evidence about a population on which to plan services and address health inequalities. Following assessment, priorities are agreed and resources allocated with the goal of improving health and reducing inequalities. Person involvement and partnership working across the voluntary, independent, health and social care sectors are key to this approach. Have a look at Box 1.10 for an example of effective insight into the health behaviour of men in the North West of England.

A wide range of lifestyle choices are marketed to people (this is referred to as 'social marketing'), but health itself has not been marketed. Previous attempts to sell a healthy lifestyle have been criticised by focus groups as being preachy, boring and too much like hard work. Promoting health on the principles that commercial markets use – making it something

Table 1.3 The preventive model of health

Level of prevention	Function of health promotion	Examples in nursing practice
Primary prevention	*Health education*: concerned with health behaviour to prevent future health problems. *Aims*: to promote the adoption of healthy behaviours. *Policy focus*: around legislation and fiscal measures, e.g. the law around compulsory seatbelts, health and safety legislation.	Promoting healthy lifestyles around diet, smoking, exercise, risky sexual behaviours and accident prevention. Other examples: immunisation, genetic screening and promoting infection control. Empowering people to make healthy choices.
Secondary prevention Aims to prevent the development of existing disease and enable the person to return to his or her former state of health as soon as possible.	*Health education*: concerned with illness behaviour, for example identifying those at risk from health breakdown. *Aims*: to support people in the uptake of screening services, adopt self-care activities and concord with any treatments offered. *Policy focus*: availability of and access to health services.	Supporting the provision of screening to identify the onset of disease, e.g. cervical cytology, screening for hypertension, measuring body mass index (BMI). Educating individuals in relation to their health status, the disease process and treatment options. Supporting concordance with treatments.
Tertiary prevention Aims to stop the disease process, prevent deterioration and return the affected individual to a useful place in society within the constraints of any disability.	*Health education*: concerned with sick role behaviour and adjustment to accept the effects of disease on the individual. *Aims*: to support individuals to adjust and concord with treatments and care, to resume lifestyle within the limitations of illness or disability and to provide terminal care when needed. *Policy focus*: the provision of and access to relevant health and social care.	Providing specific nursing care, this can include educating significant others in the provision of that care, e.g. family members. Supporting rehabilitation of people. Provision of effective end-of-life nursing care. Pain management.

Box 1.10

Health Promotion

Humour drives home health behaviour change.

Knowsley's PITSTOP initiative helps men to get their health checked out.

Knowsley PCT and Knowsley Council employed insight effectively when raising awareness of health among local men aged 50–65 by encouraging and supporting positive behavioural change.

THE APPROACH

- First, desk research revealed some key insights: men don't like talking about their health, they are reluctant to go to a doctor and late diagnosis can be a factor in early death. The team then held focus groups, which revealed that any health campaign for this group must be hard-hitting, humorous and non-judgemental, and that NHS and local authority branding needed to be very subtle.
- A programme of health checks called PITSTOP was set up in 'non-health' venues (including pubs, social clubs, community centres and workplaces) and publicised with a motoring-inspired publicity campaign. Spoof road signs carried the message 'Endangered species – it's never too late to get healthier' and 'Don't ignore the warning signs – get a free health check', and there was further ambient publicity in the form of beer mats, washroom posters, stickers, pens, stress toys and car air fresheners.

OUTCOMES AND LEARNING

- Over 3000 local men had health checks, with 85% of them reporting lifestyle changes some weeks later.
- Awareness of men's health campaigns was shown to have increased overall. Major long-term social marketing-driven programmes in adult stop smoking services, cardiovascular disease prevention services and a range of other public health and corporate business areas are now under way as a result of the success of PITSTOP.

Source: DoH 2008.

Table **1.4** Theories of adult development

	Theorist	Age	Task
Psychosocial development	Erikson	18–25	• Identity versus role confusion. • Establishing an intimate relationship with another person. • Committing oneself to work and to relationships.
		25–65	• Generativity versus stagnation. • Accepting one's own life as creative and productive. • Having concern for others.
		65–death	• Integrity versus despair. • Accepting worth of one's own life. • Accepting inevitability of death.
Spiritual development	Fowler	After 18	• Having a high degree of self-consciousness. • Constructing one's own spiritual system.
		After 30	• Being aware of truth from a variety of viewpoints.
	Westerhoff	Young adult	• Searching faith. • Acquiring a cognitive and an affective faith through questioning one's own faith.
		Middle–older adult	• Owned faith. • Putting faith into action and standing up for beliefs.
Moral development	Kohlberg	Adult	• Post-conventional level. • Social contract/legalistic orientation. • Defining morality in terms of personal principles. • Adhering to laws that protect the welfare and rights of others. • Universal ethical principles. • Internalising universal moral principles. • Respecting others; believing that relationships are based on mutual trust.
Developmental tasks	Havighurst	18–35	• Selecting and learning to live with a mate. • Starting a family and rearing children. • Managing a home. • Starting an occupation. • Taking on civic responsibility. • Finding a congenial social group.
		35–60	• Achieving civic and social responsibility. • Establishing and maintaining an economic standard of living. • Assisting teenage children in becoming responsible and happy adults. • Developing leisure-time activities. • Relating to one's spouse as a person. • Accepting and adjusting to the physiologic changes of middle age. • Adjusting to ageing parents.
		60 and over	• Meeting civic and social obligations. • Establishing an affiliation with one's own age group. • Establishing satisfactory physical living arrangements. • Adjusting to decreasing physical strength, health, retirement, reduced income, death of spouse.

Sources: Erickson 1963, Fowler 1981, Havighurst 1972, Kohlberg 1979, Westerhoff 1976.

people aspire to and making healthy choices enjoyable and convenient – will, it is felt, create a stronger demand for health.

An example of this is the government's response to the rise in obesity in the UK. The '*Change 4 Life–Eat well, Move more, Live longer*' campaign aims to inspire a societal movement in which individuals, groups and health organisations can play a part.

Meeting the health needs of adults

The adult years commonly are divided into three stages: the young adult (ages 18–40), the middle adult (ages 40–65) and the older adult (over age 65). Although developmental markers are not as clearly delineated in the adult as in the infant or child, specific changes do occur with ageing in intellectual, psychosocial and spiritual development, as well as in physical structures and functions.

The developmental theories specific to the adult, with related stages and tasks, are listed in Table 1.4. Applying a variety of developmental theories is important to the holistic care of the adult client as nurses perform assessments, implement care and provide teaching.

THE YOUNG ADULT

From ages 18–25, the healthy young adult is at the peak of physical development. All body systems are functioning at maximum efficiency, and the main risks to health are those listed in Box 1.11. Then, during the 30s, some normal physiological changes begin to occur (see Table 1.5).

Assessment guidelines

The following guidelines are useful in assessing the achievement of significant developmental tasks in the young adult. Does the young adult:

- feel independent from parents?
- have a realistic self-concept?
- like oneself and the direction in which life is going?
- interact well with family?
- cope with the stresses of constant change and growth?
- have well-established bonds with significant others, such as marriage partners or close friends?
- have a meaningful social life?
- have a career or occupation?
- demonstrate emotional, social and economic responsibility for own life?
- have a set of values that guide behaviour?
- have a healthy lifestyle?

Physical assessment of the young adult includes height and weight, blood pressure and vision. During the health history, the nurse should ask specific questions about substance use,

Box 1.11

Risks for alterations in health in young adults age 18–25 years

The young adult is at risk for alterations in health from accidents, sexually transmitted infections, substance abuse and physical or psychosocial stressors. These risk factors may be interrelated and include injuries, sexually transmitted infections, substance abuse, physical and psychological stressors outlined below.

INJURIES

Unintentional injuries are the leading cause of injury and death in people between ages 15 and 24. Most injuries and fatalities occur as the result of motor vehicle crashes; but injuries and death also result from assaults, drowning, fire, guns, occupational accidents and exposure to environmental hazards. Accidental injury or death is often associated with the use of alcohol or other chemical substances, or with psychological stress.

SEXUALLY TRANSMITTED INFECTIONS

Sexually transmitted infections include genital herpes, chlamydia, gonorrhoea, syphilis and HIV/AIDS. The young adult who is sexually active with a variety of partners and who does not use condoms is at greatest risk for development of these diseases. Nursing care of clients with sexually transmitted infections is discussed in Chapter 17.

SUBSTANCE ABUSE

Substance abuse is a major cause for concern in the young adult population. Although alcohol abuse occurs at all ages, it is greater in the 20s than during any other decade of the lifespan. Heavy drinking (exceeding a daily intake of eight units for men and six for women) was most common in the 16–24 and 25–44 age groups (ONS 2010b). Alcohol contributes to motor vehicle crashes and physical violence, and it is damaging to the developing foetus in pregnant women. It can also cause liver disease and nutritional deficits. Other substances that are commonly abused include nicotine, marijuana, amphetamines, cocaine and crack. Smoking increases the risk of respiratory and cardiovascular diseases. Cocaine and crack can cause death from cardiovascular effects (increased heart rate and ventricular arrhythmias), and can lead to addiction and health problems in the baby born to an addicted mother.

PHYSICAL AND PSYCHOSOCIAL STRESSORS

Physical stressors that increase the risk of illness include environmental pollutants and work-related risks (e.g., electrical hazards, mechanical injuries or exposure to toxins or infectious agents). Other physical stressors include exposure to the sun, ingestion of chemical substances (e.g., caffeine, alcohol, nicotine) and pregnancy.

sexual activity and concerns, exercise, eating habits, menstrual history and patterns, coping mechanisms, any familial chronic illnesses and family changes.

Table 1.5 Physical status and changes in the young adult years

Assessment	Status during the 20s	Status during the 30s
Skin	Smooth, even temperature	Wrinkles begin to appear
Hair	Slightly oily, shiny Balding may begin	Greying may begin Balding may begin
Vision	Snellen 20/20	Some loss of visual acuity and accommodation
Musculoskeletal	Strong, coordinated	Some loss of strength and muscle mass
Cardiovascular	Maximum cardiac output 60–90 beats/min Mean BP: 120/80	Slight decline in cardiac output 60–90 beats/min Mean BP: 120/80
Respiratory	Rate: 12–20 Full vital capacity	Rate: 12–20 Decline in vital capacity

THE MIDDLE ADULT

The middle adult, ages 40–65, has physical status and function similar to that of the young adult. However, many changes take place between ages 40 and 65. Table 1.6 lists the physical changes that normally occur in the middle years, and the main risks to health are those shown in Box 1.12.

NHS health checks for the middle adult

NHS health checks are being made available across the country for all 40–74-year-olds. These will check an individual's risk of heart disease, stroke, diabetes and kidney disease, and will offer support in reducing or managing that risk, with the necessary lifestyle advice and effective interventions (such as NHS Stop Smoking Services or weight management programmes) or through medication. This is a world-leading programme to prevent heart disease, stroke, diabetes and chronic kidney disease. The programme will save thousands of lives by preventing stroke and heart attacks, and at least 4000 people will not develop diabetes as a result. It is expected that some one million checks will have been performed by the end of 2011, with complete roll-out planned by 2012/13. Around three million persons will be checked every year (DoH 2009a, 26).

Assessment guidelines

The following guidelines are useful in assessing the achievement of significant developmental tasks in the middle adult. Does the middle adult:

Table 1.6 Physical changes in the middle adult years

Assessment	Changes
Skin	• Decreased moisture and subcutaneous fat result in wrinkles. • Fat is deposited in the abdominal and hip areas.
Hair	• Loss of melanin in hair shaft causes greying. • Hairline recedes in males.
Sensory	• Visual acuity for near vision decreases (presbyopia) during the 40s. • Auditory acuity for high-frequency sounds decreases (presbycusis); more common in men. • Sense of taste diminishes.
Musculoskeletal	• Skeletal muscle mass decreases by about age 60. • Thinning of inter-vertebral discs results in loss of height (about 2.5 cm [1 inch]). • Postmenopausal women may have loss of calcium and develop osteoporosis.
Cardiovascular	• Blood vessels lose elasticity. • Systolic blood pressure may increase.
Respiratory	• Loss of vital capacity (about 1 L from age 20–60) occurs.
Gastrointestinal	• Large intestine gradually loses muscle tone; constipation may result. • Gastric secretions are decreased.
Genitourinary	• Hormonal changes occur: menopause, women (↓oestrogen); andropause, men (↓testosterone).
Endocrine	• Gradual decrease in glucose tolerance occurs.

Box 1.12

Risks for alterations in health in the middle adult

The middle adult is at risk for alterations in health from obesity, cardiovascular disease, cancer, substance abuse and physical and psychosocial stressors. These factors may be interrelated.

OBESITY

The middle adult often has a problem maintaining a healthy weight. Weight gain in middle adulthood is usually the result of continuing to consume the same number of calories while decreasing physical activity and experiencing a decrease in basal metabolic rate. Obesity affects all of the major organ systems of the body, increasing the risk of atherosclerosis, hypertension, elevated cholesterol and triglyceride levels and diabetes. Obesity is also associated with heart disease, osteoarthritis and gallbladder disease.

CARDIOVASCULAR DISEASE

The major risk factors, especially for coronary artery disease, include age, male gender, physical inactivity, cigarette smoking, hypertension, elevated blood cholesterol levels and diabetes. Other contributing factors include obesity, stress and lack of exercise. The middle adult is at risk for peripheral vascular, cerebrovascular and cardiovascular disease.

CANCER

The Office for National Statistics (ONS) reports that 'Rates of cancer rose more quickly with age in females than in males up to the 50–54 age group. In the 40–44 age group, the rate in females was more than double that for males' (ONS 2010a).

Cancers of the breast, colon, lung and reproductive system are common in the middle years. The middle adult is at risk for cancer as a result of increased length of exposure to environmental carcinogens, as well as alcohol and nicotine use.

SUBSTANCE ABUSE

Although the middle adult may abuse a variety of substances, the most commonly abused are alcohol, nicotine and prescription drugs. Excess alcohol use in the middle adult contributes to an increased risk of liver cancer, cirrhosis, pancreatitis, hyperlipidaemia and anaemia. Alcoholism also increases the risk of accidental injury or death and disrupts careers and relationships. Cigarette smoking increases the risk of cancer of the larynx, lung, mouth, pharynx, bladder, pancreas, oesophagus and kidney; of chronic obstructive pulmonary disorders; and of cardiovascular disorders.

PHYSICAL AND PSYCHOSOCIAL STRESSORS

The middle adult years are ones of change and transition, frequently resulting in stress. Both men and women must adapt to changes in physical appearance and function and accept their own mortality. Children may leave home or choose to remain at home longer than they are welcome. Parents are ageing, with illness probable and death inevitable. The middle adult thus becomes caught between the need to care for both children and ageing parents. Both men and women may make career changes, and approaching retirement becomes a reality. Divorce in the middle years is a major emotional, social and financial stressor.

- accept the ageing body?
- feel comfortable with and respect him- or herself?
- enjoy some new freedom to be independent?
- accept changes in family roles?
- enjoy success and satisfaction from work and/or family roles?
- interact well and share companionable activities with a partner?
- expand or renew previous interests?
- pursue charitable and altruistic activities?
- consider plans for retirement?
- have a meaningful philosophy of life?
- follow preventive healthcare practices?

Physical assessment of the middle adult includes all body systems, including blood pressure, vision and hearing. Monitoring for risks and onset of cancer symptoms is essential. During the health history, the nurse should ask specific questions about food intake and exercise habits, substance abuse, sexual concerns, changes in the reproductive system, coping mechanisms and family history of chronic illnesses.

FAST FACTS

Body mass index

In the Health Survey for England (DoH 2003) overweight and obesity is measured in terms of body mass index or BMI. BMI is a widely accepted measure of weight for height and is defined as:

$$weight\ (kg)/(height\ (m))^2$$

Height and weight data used to calculate BMI are collected in each year of the Health Survey. Adult informants can be classified into the following BMI groups:

BMI (kg/m^2)	Description
18.5 or less	Underweight
Over 18.5–25	Normal
Over 25–30	Overweight
Over 30	Overweight

However, BMI does not distinguish between mass due to body fat and mass due to muscular physique. It also does not take account of the distribution of fat.

THE OLDER ADULT (OVER 65)

Consider this . . .

Life expectancy at birth in the UK has reached its highest level on record for both males and females. A newborn baby boy could expect to live 77.4 years and a newborn baby girl 81.6 years if mortality rates remain the same as they were in 2006–08.

As far back as 1875, in Britain, the Friendly Societies Act enacted the definition of old age as 'any age after 50', yet pension schemes mostly used age 60 or 65 years for eligibility. The increase in numbers of older adults has important implications for nursing. People needing healthcare in all settings will be older, requiring nursing interventions and teaching specifically designed to meet needs that differ from those of young and middle adults. Although care of the older adult is a nursing specialty area, it is also an integral component of acute and ongoing care in adult nursing. Life expectancy from birth continues to improve across England for both men and women, but there is still a wide variation across the country. Table 1.7 lists the physical changes that normally occur in the older years and some of the risks to health associated with older adults are shown in Box 1.13.

The National Service Framework for Older People

The National Service Framework (NSF) for Older People (DoH 2001) sets national standards and service models of care across health and social services for all older people, whether they live at home, in residential care or are being looked after in hospital. It was developed to deliver improved lives for older people and greater value for money. Work to redesign services and systems incorporates five key areas:

- early intervention for old age problems;
- streaming to specialist care in crisis situations;
- early transfer to the community for rehabilitation in intermediate care;
- multidisciplinary assessment prior to care home placement;
- partnership working across health and social care.

Box 1.13

Risks for alterations in health in the older adult

The older adult is at risk for alterations in health from a variety of causes. Most older adults have one chronic health problem, while many have multiple illnesses. The most frequently occurring problems in the older adult are hypertension, arthritis, heart diseases, cancer, respiratory disease and diabetes. The leading causes of death are heart disease, cancer and stroke. Like the middle adult, the older adult is at risk for alterations in health from obesity and a sedentary lifestyle. Other risk factors specific to this age group include accidental injuries, pharmacologic effects and physical and psychosocial stress.

INJURIES
Injuries in the older adult cause many different problems: illness, financial burdens, hospitalisation, self-care deficits, loss of independence and even death. The risk of injury is increased by normal physiologic changes that accompany ageing, pathophysiological alterations in health, environmental hazards and lack of support systems. The three major causes of injury in the older adult are falls, fires and motor vehicle crashes. Of these, falls with resultant hip fractures are the most significant in terms of long-term disability and death.

PHARMACOLOGIC EFFECTS
A number of risk factors predispose the older adult to experiencing drug toxicity. Age-related changes in tissue and organ structure and function alter the absorption of both oral and parenteral medications. Low nutritional levels and decreased liver function may alter drug metabolism. The ageing kidney may not excrete drugs at the normal clearance rate. Self-administration of both prescribed and over-the-counter medications presents risks for error resulting from confusion, forgetfulness or misreading the directions. The older adult may take several drugs at once, and it is difficult to know how drugs interact with each other.

PHYSICAL AND PSYCHOSOCIAL STRESSORS
The older adult is exposed to the same environmental hazards as the young and middle adult, but the accumulation of years of exposure may now appear. For example, exposure to the sun in earlier years may be manifested by skin cancer, and the long-term effects of exposure to noise pollution can result in impaired hearing. The older adult (especially the older male) is at increased risk for respiratory disorders as a result of years of smoking, or from such pollutants as coal or asbestos dust. Living problems and economic constraints may prevent the older adult from having necessary heating and cooling, contributing to thermal-related illnesses and even death. Elder abuse and neglect further increase the risk of injury or illness.

Psychosocial stressors for the older adult include the illness or death of a spouse, decreased or limited income, retirement and isolation from friends and family because of lack of transportation or distance, return to the home of a child or relocation to a long-term healthcare facility. A further stressor may be role loss or reversal – for example, when the wife becomes the caretaker of her chronically ill husband.

Table 1.7 Physical changes in the older adult years

Assessment	Changes
Skin	• Decreased sebaceous gland activity results in dry, wrinkled skin. • Melanocytes cluster, causing 'age spots' or 'liver spots'.
Hair and nails	• Scalp, axillary and pubic hair thins; nose and ear hair thickens. • Women may develop facial hair. • Nails grow more slowly; may become thick and brittle.
Sensory	• Visual field narrows and depth perception is distorted. • Pupils are smaller, reducing night vision. • Lenses yellow and become opaque, resulting in distortion of green, blue and violet tones and increased sensitivity to glare. • Production of tears decreases. • Sense of smell decreases. • Age-related hearing loss progresses, involving middle- and low-frequency sounds. • Threshold for pain and touch increases. • Alterations in proprioception (sense of physical position) may occur.
Musculoskeletal	• Loss of overall mass, strength and movement of muscles occurs; tremors may occur. • Loss of bone structure and deterioration of cartilage in joints results in increased risk of fractures and in limitation of range of motion.
Cardiovascular	• Systolic blood pressure rises. • Cardiac output decreases. • Peripheral resistance increases, and capillary walls thicken.
Respiratory	• Continued loss of vital capacity occurs as the lungs become less elastic and more rigid. • Anteroposterior chest diameter increases; kyphosis. • Although blood carbon dioxide levels remain relatively constant, blood oxygen levels decrease by 10–15%.
Gastrointestinal	• Production of saliva decreases, and decreased number of taste buds decrease accurate receptors for salt and sweet. • Gag reflex is decreased, and stomach motility and emptying are reduced. • Both large and small intestines have some atrophy, with decreased peristalsis. • The liver decreases in weight and storage capacity; gallstones increase; pancreatic enzymes decrease.

Genitourinary	• Kidneys lose mass, and the glomerular filtration rate is reduced (by nearly 50% from young adulthood to old age).
	• Bladder capacity decreases, and the micturition reflex is delayed.
	• Urinary retention is more common.
	• Women may have stress incontinence; men may have an enlarged prostate gland.
	• Reproductive changes in men occur:
	  – testosterone decreases.
	  – sperm count decreases.
	  – testes become smaller.
	  – length of time to achieve an erection increases; erection is less full.
	• Reproductive changes in women occur:
	  – oestrogen levels decrease.
	  – breast tissue decreases.
	  – vagina, uterus, ovaries and urethra atrophy.
	  – vaginal lubrication decreases.
	  – vaginal secretions become alkaline.

Endocrine	• Pituitary gland loses weight and vascularity. • Thyroid gland becomes more fibrous, and plasma T_3 decreases. • Pancreas releases insulin more slowly; increased blood glucose levels are common. • Adrenal glands produce less cortisol.

The NSF leads with plans to:

- tackle age discrimination to make it a thing of the past, and ensure older people are treated with respect and dignity;
- ensure older people are supported by newly integrated services with a well-coordinated, coherent and cohesive approach to assessing individuals' needs and circumstances and for commission and providing services for them;
- specifically address those problems which are particularly significant for older people – stroke, falls and mental health problems associated with older age;
- promote the health and wellbeing of older people through coordinated actions of the NHS and councils.

Assessment guidelines

The following guidelines are useful in assessing the achievement of significant developmental tasks in the older adult. Does the older adult:

- adjust to the physiologic changes related to ageing?
- manage retirement years in a satisfying manner?
- have satisfactory living arrangements and income to meet changing needs?
- participate in social and leisure activities?
- have a social network of friends and support persons?
- view life as worthwhile?
- have high self-esteem?
- have the abilities to care for self or to secure appropriate help?
- gain support from a value system or spiritual philosophy?
- adapt lifestyle to diminishing energy and ability?
- accept and adjust to the death of significant others?

Physical assessment of the older adult includes a careful examination of all body systems. During the health history, the nurse should ask specific questions about usual dietary patterns; elimination; exercise and rest; use of alcohol, nicotine, over-the-counter medications and prescription drugs; sexual concerns; financial concerns; and support systems.

The family

DEFINITIONS AND FUNCTIONS OF THE FAMILY

The definitions of a family are changing as society changes. A family is composed of two or more people who are emotionally involved with each other and live in close geographical proximity. In a global society, it may not be possible for family members to live in close proximity, but they do remain emotionally involved.

Although every family is unique, all families have certain structural and functional features in common. Family structure (family roles and relationships) and family function (interactions among family members and with the community) provide the following:

- *Interdependence.* The behaviours and level of development of individual family members constantly influence and are influenced by the behaviours and level of development of all other members of the family.
- *Maintaining boundaries.* The family creates boundaries that guide its members, providing a distinct and unique family culture. This culture, in turn, provides values.
- *Adapting to change.* The family changes as new members are added, current members leave and the development of each member progresses.
- *Performing family tasks.* Essential tasks maintain the stability and continuity of the family. These tasks include physical maintenance of the home and the people in the home, the production and socialisation of family members and the maintenance of the psychological wellbeing of members.

FAMILY DEVELOPMENTAL STAGES AND TASKS

The family, like the individual, has developmental stages and tasks. Each stage brings change, requiring adaptation; each new stage also brings family-related risk factors for alterations in health. The nurse must consider the needs of the person both at a specific developmental stage and within a family with specific developmental tasks. Family developmental stages and developmental tasks are described next; related risk factors and health problems for each stage are listed in Table 1.8.

Family with adolescents and young adults

The developmental tasks of the family with adolescents and young adults focus on transition. While providing a supportive home base and maintaining open communications, parents must balance freedom with responsibility and release adult children as they seek independence.

Family with middle adults

The family with middle adults (in which the parents are middle-aged and children are no longer at home) has the developmental tasks of maintaining ties with older and younger generations and planning for retirement. If the family consists of just the middle-aged couple, they have the developmental task of re-establishing the relationship and (if necessary) acquiring the role of grandparents.

Family with older adults

The older adult family has the developmental tasks of adjusting to retirement, adjusting to ageing and coping with the loss

Table 1.8 Family-related risk factors for alterations in health

Stage	Risk factors	Health problems
Couple or family with infants and preschoolers	• Lack of knowledge about family planning, contraception, sexual and marital roles. • Inadequate prenatal care. • Altered nutrition: inadequate nutrition, overweight, underweight. • Smoking, alcohol/drug abuse. • First pregnancy before age 16 or after age 35. • Low socioeconomic status. • Lack of knowledge about child health and safety. • Rubella, syphilis, gonorrhoea, AIDS.	• Premature pregnancy. • Low-birth-weight infant. • Birth defects. • Injury to infant or child. • Accidents.
Family with school-age children	• Unsafe home environment. • Working parents with inappropriate or inadequate resources for child care. • Low socioeconomic status. • Child abuse or neglect. • Multiple, closely spaced children. • Repeated infections, accidents and hospitalisations. • Unrecognised and unattended health problems. • Poor or inappropriate nutrition. • Toxic substances in the home.	• Behaviour problems. • Speech and vision problems. • Learning disabilities. • Communicable diseases. • Physical abuse. • Cancer. • Developmental delay. • Obesity, underweight.
Family with adolescents and young adults	• Family values of aggressiveness and competition. • Lifestyle and behaviour leading to chronic illness (substance abuse, inadequate diet). • Lack of problem-solving skills. • Conflicts between parent and children.	• Violent death and injury. • Alcohol/drug abuse. • Unwanted pregnancy. • Suicide. • Sexually transmitted infections. • Domestic abuse.
Family with middle adults	• High-cholesterol diet. • Overweight. • Hypertension. • Smoking, alcohol abuse. • Physical inactivity. • Personality patterns related to stress. • Exposure to environment: sunlight, radiation, asbestos, water or air pollution. • Depression.	• Cardiovascular disease (coronary artery disease and cerebral vascular disease). • Cancer. • Accidents. • Suicide. • Mental illness.
Family with older adults	• Age. • Depression. • Drug interactions. • Chronic illness. • Death of spouse. • Reduced income. • Poor nutrition. • Lack of exercise. • Past environment and lifestyle.	• Impaired vision and hearing. • Hypertension. • Acute illness. • Chronic illness. • Infectious diseases (influenza, pneumonia). • Injuries from burns and falls. • Depression. • Alcohol abuse.

of a spouse. If a spouse dies, further tasks include adjusting to living alone or closing the family home.

THE FAMILY OF THE PERSON WITH A CHRONIC ILLNESS

The person with a chronic illness may be hospitalised for diagnosis and treatment of acute exacerbations, but care is primarily provided at home. Chronic illness in a family member is a major stressor that may cause changes in family structure and function, as well as changes in performing family developmental tasks.

Many different factors affect family responses to chronic illness; family responses in turn affect the person's response to and perception of the illness. Factors influencing response to chronic illness include personal, social and economic resources; the nature and course of the disease; and demands of the illness as perceived by family members.

Support for the family is essential. The following information should be considered when performing any family assessment and developing a plan of care:

- cohesiveness and communication patterns within the family;
- family interactions that support self-care;
- number of friends and relatives available;
- family values and beliefs about health and illness;
- cultural and spiritual beliefs;
- developmental level of the person and family.

It is important to remember that standardised teaching plans may not be effective. Rather, individuals with chronic illnesses and their families should be given the freedom to choose appropriate literature, self-help or support groups and interactions with others who have the same illness.

The person undergoing surgical intervention

Case Study 1 – Wendy

You will recall Wendy Xin from earlier in the chapter (the case study). She is normally well, works in a supermarket and is an active woman with two grown up sons both away at university. This is her first experience of hospital admission since she had her second son 19 years ago. Wendy had previously attended a pre-operative assessment clinic where the nurse was able to assess her general health and to highlight any risk factors that might impact upon Wendy's recovery from surgery.

Surgery is an invasive procedure performed to diagnose or treat illness, injury or deformity. Throughout the process, the nurse assumes an active role in caring for the individual before, during and after surgery; this is referred to collectively as the peri-operative period. Interdisciplinary care and nursing care together prevent complications and promote optimal recovery. Interdisciplinary care refers to healthcare services provided by professionals in addition to physicians and surgeons, including nurses, pharmacists, social workers, technologists, dieticians, chaplains, physiotherapists and occupational therapists.

Peri-operative nursing is a specialised area of practice. It incorporates the three phases of the surgical experience: pre-operative, intra-operative and post-operative. The pre-operative phase begins when the decision for surgery is made and ends when the person is transferred to the operating room. The intra-operative phase begins with the person's entry into the operating room and ends with admittance to the recovery room. The post-operative phase begins with the person's admittance to the recovery room and ends with the individual's complete recovery from the surgical intervention.

SETTINGS FOR SURGERY

Surgical patients may be in-patients or out-patients. The complexity of the surgery and recovery and the expected recovery of the individual following the surgery are the major differences. Sometimes out-patients (i.e., people intending to be discharged home immediately following surgery) are admitted to the hospital. Cataract removal with or without lens implants, hernia repairs, tubal ligations, vasectomies, dilation and curettage (D&C), haemorrhoidectomies and biopsies are commonly performed in day-surgeries.

Table 1.9 shows how surgical procedures can be classified and, according to the table, Wendy's surgery would be termed 'diagnostic', intended to determine the cause of her medical problem. (To find out more about nursing the person with cancer, please refer to Chapter 2.)

INFORMED CONSENT

Consent is the principle that a person must give their permission before they receive any type of medical treatment. Consent is required from a patient regardless of the type of treatment being undertaken, from a blood test to an organ donation. Prior to receiving surgical care, Wendy must give her informed consent. The principle of consent is based on the following:

For consent to be valid, it must be:

- *Voluntary.* The decision to consent or not consent to treatment must be made alone, and must not be due to pressure by medical staff, friends or family.
- *Informed.* The person must be given full information about what the treatment involves, including the benefits and risks, whether there are reasonable alternative treatments, and what will happen if treatment does not go ahead.

Table 1.9 Classification of surgical procedures

	Classification	Function	Examples
Purpose	Diagnostic	Determine or confirm a diagnosis.	Breast biopsy, bronchoscopy.
	Ablative	Remove diseased tissue, organ, or extremity.	Appendectomy, amputation.
	Constructive	Build tissue/organs that are absent (congenital anomalies).	Repair of cleft palate.
	Reconstructive	Rebuild tissue/organ that has been damaged.	Skin graft after a burn, total joint replacement.
	Palliative	Alleviate symptoms of a disease (not curative).	Bowel resection in client with terminal cancer.
	Transplant	Replace organs/tissue to restore function.	Heart, lung, liver, kidney transplant.
Risk factor	Minor	Minimal physical assault with minimal risk.	Removal of skin lesions, dilation and curettage (D&C), cataract extraction.
	Major	Extensive physical assault and/or serious risk.	Transplant, total joint replacement, cholecystectomy, colostomy, nephrectomy.
Urgency	Elective	Suggested, though no foreseen ill effects if postponed.	Cosmetic surgery, cataract surgery, removal of bunions.
	Urgent	Necessary to be performed within one to two days.	Heart bypass surgery, amputation resulting from gangrene, fractured hip.
	Emergency	Performed immediately.	Obstetric emergencies, bowel obstruction, ruptured aneurysm, life-threatening trauma.

● *Capacity.* The person must be capable of giving consent, which means that they understand the information given to them, and they can use it to make an informed decision.

RISK FACTORS FOR SURGERY

Risks are associated with all surgical interventions; these may be complex and involve high levels of blood loss and prolonged time under anaesthetic, increasing the risk for complication following surgery. The degree of risk can be categorised into two areas; health problems that increase surgical risk, and general factors that contribute to that risk. Table 1.10 highlights these.

PRACTICE ALERT

Remind people with diabetes that the stress of surgery increases rather than decreases blood sugar.

Table 1.10 Factors and risks associated with surgery

Factor	Associated risk
Age	Older adults have age-related changes that affect physiologic, cognitive and psychosocial responses to the stress of surgery; decreased tolerance of general anaesthesia and post-operative medications; and delayed wound healing.
Nutritional status	The obese person is at increased risk for delayed wound healing, chest infections, wound separation (dehiscence) and infection. Obese and underweight people are more at risk of pressure ulcer development (see Chapter 5).
Dehydration/electrolyte imbalance	Depending on the degree of dehydration and/or type of electrolyte imbalance, cardiac dysrhythmia or heart failure may occur. Liver and renal failure may also result (see Chapter 3).
Cardiovascular problems	Presence of cardiovascular disease increases the risk of haemorrhage and shock, hypotension, thrombophlebitis, pulmonary embolism, stroke (especially in the older person), and fluid volume overload (see Chapter 9).
Respiratory problems	Respiratory complications such as bronchitis, atelectasis and pneumonia are some of the most common and serious post-operative complications. Respiratory depression from general anaesthesia and acid–base imbalance may also occur. People with pulmonary problems are more at risk for developing these complications (see Chapter 11).

Table 1.10 (continued)

Factor	Associated risk
Diabetes mellitus	Diabetes causes an increased risk for fluctuating blood glucose levels, which can lead to life-threatening hypoglycaemia or ketoacidosis. Diabetes also increases the risk for cardiovascular disease, delayed wound healing and wound infection (see Chapter 6).
Renal and liver dysfunction	The person with renal or liver dysfunction may poorly tolerate general anaesthesia, have fluid/electrolyte and acid–base imbalances, decreased metabolism and excretion of drugs, increased risk for haemorrhage and delayed wound healing (see Chapters 7 and 8).
Alcoholism	The person may be malnourished and experience delirium tremens (acute withdrawal symptoms). More general anaesthesia may be required. Haemorrhage and delayed wound healing can result from liver damage and poor nutritional status.
Smoking	Cigarette smokers are at increased risk of respiratory complications such as pneumonia, atelectasis and bronchitis because of increased mucous secretions and a decreased ability to expel them.
Medications	Anaesthesia interaction with some medications can cause respiratory difficulties, hypotension and circulatory collapse. Other medications can produce side-effects that may increase surgical risk.
Neurological problems	Uncontrolled problems such as epilepsy may result in seizures during surgery or recovery (see Chapter 13).

Case Study 1 – Wendy
NURSING CARE PLAN The person undergoing surgery

Pre-operative nursing care

Pre-operative care is the assessment and preparation of a person for surgery. The individual's response to planned surgery varies greatly. Discharge planning should be considered as early as possible and will incorporate specific care pathways that map the expected recovery following specific surgical procedures.

When planning and implementing nursing care, consider individual psychological and physical differences, the type of surgery and the circumstances surrounding the need for surgery. A thorough nursing assessment is needed to determine the most appropriate care for each person undergoing surgery. Sources of information to support the initial assessment of the individual can include medical and nursing records, the individual's relatives and other members of the interdisciplinary team.

In Wendy's case, she has been assessed for the following physical, psychological and social needs:

+ **Current health**. Wendy is physically fit. 'I like to exercise and keep reasonably fit, so I aim to walk the dog at least once a day. Luckily my dog is young and doesn't mind if I power walk.' The nurse checks for Wendy's ability to communicate after surgery (this might include noting any prosthesis, for example a hearing aid). Allergies are discussed, particularly in relation to latex allergy, penicillin and food allergies. Wendy's mental state is assessed to look for signs of dementia, mental illness, excessive anxiety and depression.

Tools such as the Hospital Anxiety and Depression Scale (HADS) can help to measure psychological distress in people.

+ **Physical assessment**. Measurements of blood pressure, respiratory rate and temperature are made to determine baseline information that can be compared post-operatively to evaluate Wendy's condition.

+ **Medications.** A list of Wendy's current medication is made. The nurse should be alerted to people taking anticonvulsants that affect conscious levels, anticoagulants that may affect bleeding.

PRACTICE ALERT

Assess information about use of over-the-counter medications including herbal supplements. These drugs can interact with medications administered in the peri-operative period.

+ **Smoking and alcohol intake.** Wendy is a non-smoker. She enjoys a 'social drink' with friends and estimates her intake at 6–8 units of alcohol per week.

+ **Psychological status.** Surgery is a significant and stressful event. Regardless of the nature of the surgery (whether major or minor), the individual and family will be anxious. Some individuals and their families seek care from a spiritual

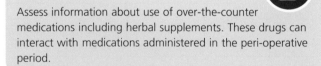

Case Study 1 – Wendy	NURSING CARE PLAN The person undergoing surgery

provider during this time. The degree of anxiety they will feel is not necessarily proportional to the magnitude of the surgical procedure. For example, In Wendy's case, being scheduled to have investigations to rule out cancer, which is considered minor surgery, may be more anxiety provoking than undergoing major surgery. Therapeutic communication can help Wendy and her family identify fears and concerns. The nurse can then plan nursing interventions and supportive care to reduce her anxiety level and assist her to cope successfully with the stressors encountered during the peri-operative period.

Investigations can typically include a range of the following:

+ *full blood count (FBC)* to assess the oxygen-carrying capacity of red blood cells. White blood cells can indicate infection;

+ *blood grouping and cross matching* in case of need for transfusion;

+ *serum electrolytes* to evaluate fluid status;

+ *fasting blood glucose* – high levels may be an indication of undiagnosed diabetes;

+ *blood urea, nitrogen and creatinine* to determine renal function;

+ *liver function tests*;

+ *serum albumin and protein* to determine nutritional status;

+ *urinalysis* can highlight a number of abnormalities, for example glucose and infection;

+ *chest x-ray* can highlight enlarged heart and respiratory problems;

+ *electrocardiogram (ECG)*, a diagnostic tool to show evidence of cardiac problems.

Pre-operative teaching

Teaching the individual is an essential nursing responsibility in the pre-operative period. Education and emotional support have a positive effect on the individual's physical and psychological wellbeing, both before and after surgery. There is a wealth of evidence that supports the benefits of this in surgical care, where people experience reduced anxiety and post-operative complications, and quicker discharge and return to normal activities. These positive outcomes may be attributed in part to the sense of control the individual gains through the nurse's teaching.

Wendy is given information about what and when things will take place, for example, the estimated time of her surgery, what she can expect following surgery in terms of pain relief, and how soon she is likely to eat and drink following surgery.

Those people undergoing major surgery should be supported in their recovery by teaching them how best to move and deep breathe, how to hold themselves to cough and how to help

prevent the onset of post-operative complications, for example leg exercises to minimise the risk of deep vein thrombosis (DVT).

Pre-operative fasting

General anaesthesia carries the risk of Wendy inhaling gastric contents. With this in mind, she will be kept 'nil by mouth' long enough for the stomach to empty.

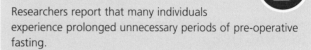

PRACTICE ALERT

Researchers report that many individuals experience prolonged unnecessary periods of pre-operative fasting.

The Royal College of Nursing recommend that individuals can have clear water or fluids for up to three hours before surgery and light solid foods up to six hours. Wendy prefers not to eat but would like to keep her mouth moist before surgery.

Anti-embolic stockings (graduated elastic compression stockings)

Sometimes referred to as thromboembolic deterrent stockings (TEDS), they are used to help prevent the onset of DVT. They compress the veins of the legs and help to facilitate the return of blood to the heart, helping to reduce swelling and oedema. National Institute for Health and Clinical Excellence guidelines (NICE 2010) state that thigh-length antiembolic stockings should be fitted from admission to hospital and until the individual has returned to their usual level of activity. Regular checking of the feet and skin will alert the nurse to any redness or skin breakdown.

Pre-operative checklist

A pre-operative surgical checklist serves as an outline for finalising preparation of the individual for surgery. Complete the checklist before Wendy is transported to surgery as follows:

+ Assist with bathing, grooming and changing into operating room gown.

+ Ensure that the individual takes nil by mouth three hours for fluids prior to surgery, six hours for light food.

+ Remove nail polish, lipstick and make-up to facilitate circulatory assessment during and after surgery.

+ Ensure that identification and allergy bands are correct, legible and secure.

+ Remove hair pins and jewellery; a wedding ring may be worn if it is removed from the finger, covered with gauze, replaced and then taped to the finger.

Case Study 1 – Wendy   **NURSING CARE PLAN** **The person undergoing surgery**

+ Complete skin or bowel preparation as required.

+ Remove dentures, prosthesis and contact lenses, and store them in a safe place.

+ Leave a hearing aid in place if the client cannot hear without it, and notify the theatre nurse.

+ Verify that the informed consent has been signed prior to administering pre-operative medications.

+ Verify that all ordered diagnostic test reports are in the chart.

+ Have the individual empty the bladder immediately before the pre-operative medication is administered (unless an indwelling catheter is in place).

+ Administer pre-operative medication as prescribed.

+ Ensure the safety of the individual once the medication has been given by placing them on bed rest and by placing the call button within reach.

+ Obtain and record vital signs.

+ Provide ongoing supportive care to the individual and their family.

IN PRACTICE

Pre-operative teaching – leg, ankle and foot exercises

Leg exercises are taught to the person who is at risk for developing thrombophlebitis (inflammation of a vein, which is associated with the formation of blood clots). Risk factors for developing thrombophlebitis include decreased mobility pre-operatively and/or post-operatively; a history of difficulties with peripheral circulation; and cardiovascular, pelvic or lower extremity surgery.

The purpose of leg exercises is to promote venous blood return from the extremities. As the leg muscles contract and relax, blood is pumped back to the heart, promoting cardiac output and reducing venous stasis. These exercises also maintain muscle tone and range of motion, which facilitate early ambulation.

Teach the individual to perform the following exercises while lying in bed:

1. *Muscle pumping exercise*: contract and relax calf and thigh muscles at least 10 times consecutively.

2. *Leg exercises*:
   a. bend the knee and raise it toward the chest (see Figure 1.5a);
   b. straighten out leg and hold for a few seconds before lowering the leg back to the bed;
   c. repeat exercise five times consecutively prior to alternating to the other foot.

3. *Ankle and foot exercises*:
   a. rotate both ankles by making complete circles, first to the right and then to the left (see Figure 1.5b);
   b. repeat five times and then relax;
   c. with feet together, point toes toward the head and then to the foot of the bed (see Figure 1.5b);
   d. repeat this pumping action 10 times, and then relax.

Encourage the individual to perform leg, ankle and foot exercises every one to two hours while awake, depending on their needs and how mobile they are.

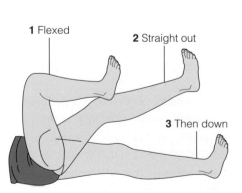

(a) Leg exercises.

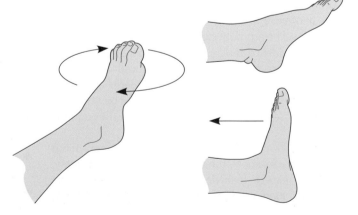

(b) Ankle and foot exercises.

Figure 1.5 Leg and ankle exercises.

Case Study 1 – Wendy   **NURSING CARE PLAN The person undergoing surgery**

✦ Document all pre-operative care in the nursing notes.

✦ Verify with the surgical team the individual's identity, and verify that all information is documented appropriately.

✦ Help the surgical team transfer the individual from the bed to the trolley.

✦ Prepare the individual's bed and surrounding area for post-operative care, including making the surgical bed and ensuring that the anticipated supplies and equipment are within reach.

Intra-operative nursing care

The intra-operative phase of surgery begins when the client enters the operating room and ends when the individual is transferred to the recovery area. Nursing care in this phase focuses on keeping the individual and the environment safe and providing physiological monitoring and psychological support. Theatre nurses, according to specific role definitions, support and care for the individual during this critical period.

Post-operative nursing care

Immediate post-operative care

Immediate post-operative care begins when the individual has been transferred from the operating room to the recovery room. Here, the recovery nurse is part of the surgical team and monitors the individual's vital signs and surgical site to determine the response to the surgical procedure and to detect significant changes. Assessing mental status and level of consciousness is another ongoing nursing responsibility, and the individual may require repeated orientation to time, place and person. Emotional support is also essential, because the individual is in a vulnerable and dependent position. Assessing and evaluating hydration status by monitoring intake and output is crucial to detecting cardiovascular or renal complications. In addition, the recovery nurse assesses the individual's pain level. Careful administration of analgesics provides comfort without compounding the potential side-effects from the anaesthesia (see Chapter 2).

Post-operative recovery is focused on the prevention and detection of potential complications arising from surgery and anaesthesia (see Table 1.11).

During the post-operative period, Wendy will be closely monitored every 15 minutes during the first hour and, if stable, every 30 minutes for the next two hours, and then every hour during the subsequent four hours. Assessments are then carried out every four hours, subject to change according to Wendy's condition.

Table 1.11 Common post-operative complications

Problem	Cause
Cardiovascular complications:	
Shock	Shock is a life-threatening post-operative complication. It results from an insufficient blood flow to vital organs, an inability to use oxygen and nutrients or the inability to rid tissues of waste material. Hypovolaemic shock, the most common type in the post-operative individual, results from a decrease in circulating fluid volume. Decreased fluid volume develops with blood or plasma loss or, less commonly, from severe prolonged vomiting or diarrhoea (see Chapter 3).
Haemorrhage	Haemorrhage is an excessive loss of blood. A concealed haemorrhage occurs internally from a blood vessel that is no longer sutured or cauterised or from a drainage tube that has eroded a blood vessel. An obvious haemorrhage occurs externally from a dislodged or ill-formed clot at the wound. Haemorrhage may also result from abnormalities in the blood's ability to clot; these abnormalities may result from a pathologic condition, or they may be a side-effect of medications.
	Haemorrhage from a venous source oozes out quickly and is dark red, whereas an arterial haemorrhage is characterised by bright red spurts of blood pulsating with each heartbeat. Whether the haemorrhage is from a venous or an arterial source, hypovolaemic shock will occur if sufficient blood is lost from the circulation.
DVT	DVT is the formation of a thrombus (blood clot) in association with inflammation in deep veins. This complication most often occurs in the lower limbs. It may result from the combination of several factors, including trauma during surgery, pressure applied under the knees and sluggish blood flow during and after surgery.
Pulmonary embolism	Pulmonary embolism is a dislodged blood clot or other substance that lodges in a pulmonary artery. For the post-operative person with DVT, the threat that a portion of the thrombus may dislodge from the vein wall and travel to the lung, heart or brain is a constant concern. Early detection of this potentially life-threatening complication depends on the nurse's astute, continuing assessment of the post-operative client.
	Common assessment findings of the individual experiencing a pulmonary embolism include mild to moderate dyspnoea, chest pain, diaphoresis, anxiety, restlessness, rapid respirations and pulse, dysrhythmias, cough and cyanosis. Sudden death can occur if a major pulmonary artery becomes completely blocked.

Case Study 1 – Wendy	NURSING CARE PLAN The person undergoing surgery

Table 1.11 (continued)

Problem	Cause
Respiratory complications:	
Pneumonia	Pneumonia is an inflammation of lung tissue. Inflammation is caused either by a microbial infection or by a foreign substance in the lung, which leads to an infection. Numerous factors may be involved in the development of pneumonia, including aspiration infection, retained pulmonary secretions, failure to cough deeply and impaired cough reflex and decreased mobility (see Chapter 11).
Atelectasis	Atelectasis is an incomplete expansion or collapse of lung tissue resulting in inadequate ventilation and retention of pulmonary secretions. Common assessment findings include dyspnoea, diminished breath sounds over the affected area, anxiety, restlessness, crackles and cyanosis. Promoting lung expansion and systemic oxygenation of tissues is a goal in the care here.
Wound healing	From the time the surgical incision is made until the wound is completely healed, all wounds progress through four stages of healing. However, healing time varies according to many factors, such as age, nutritional status, general health and the type and location of the wound (see Chapter 5).
Complications of elimination	Common post-operative complications associated with elimination include urinary retention and altered bowel elimination. The inability to urinate with urinary retention may occur post-operatively as a result of the lying down position, effects of anaesthesia and narcotics, inactivity, altered fluid balance, nervous tension or surgical manipulation in the pelvic area. Bowel elimination frequently is altered after abdominal or pelvic surgery and sometimes after other surgeries. Return to normal gastrointestinal function may be delayed by general anaesthesia, narcotic analgesia, decreased mobility or altered fluid and food intake during the peri-operative period.
Acute post-operative pain	Pain is expected after surgery. It is neither realistic nor practical to eliminate post-operative pain completely. Nevertheless, the individual should receive substantial relief from and control of this discomfort. Controlling post-operative pain not only promotes comfort but also facilitates coughing, turning, deep-breathing exercises, earlier ambulation and decreased length of hospitalisation, resulting in fewer post-operative complications. It is usually worse 12–36 hours following surgery, decreasing after the 2nd and 3rd day post-operation (see Chapter 2).

Hydration and nutrition

It is common for individuals to be hydrated by intravenous infusion. In Wendy's case, she is able to take small sips of water initially to combat her dry, sticky mouth. Hydration is important to maintain cardiovascular and renal function and to moisten mucous membranes and secretions.

Providing there is no feeling of nausea, Wendy can be offered small amounts of food. Normally this would take place after assessing the presence of peristalsis. Handling of the intestines during surgery and inactivity combined with pre-operative fasting can all inhibit peristalsis.

COMMUNITY-BASED CARE

Because the post-operative phase does not end until the individual has recovered completely from the surgical intervention, the nurse plays a vital role as the person nears discharge. As Wendy prepares to recuperate at home, the nurse will provide information and support to help her successfully self-care. All aspects of teaching should be accompanied by written guidelines, directions and information. This is particularly helpful when a large amount of unfamiliar, detailed information is presented. Teach Wendy:

- How to perform wound care. Teaching is more effective if the nurse first demonstrates and explains the procedure to Wendy. To evaluate the effectiveness of the teaching, ask Wendy to demonstrate the procedure in return.

- The signs and symptoms of a wound infection. She should be able to determine what is normal and what should be reported to her doctor.

- The method and the frequency of taking her temperature.

- The limitations or restrictions that may be imposed on such activities as lifting, driving, bathing, sexual activity and other physical activities.

- The control of pain. If analgesics are prescribed, instruct Wendy in the dosage, frequency, purpose, common side-effects and other side-effects. Reinforce the use of relaxation or other pain control techniques that she has found useful in controlling post-operative pain.

CHAPTER HIGHLIGHTS

In this chapter, you are introduced to Wendy Xin, who is admitted to hospital for surgery to explore a possible malignancy (for detailed information about cancer see Chapter 2). What emerges is the experiences that Wendy has as she embarks upon her journey as a patient during the pre-, intra- and post-operative stages of care. As such, you will be encouraged to review the aspects of the nurse's role in health and ill health in relation to the following:

- Adult nursing is diverse in terms of where, how and to whom it is delivered.
- The nursing process consists of five phases: assessing, diagnosing, planning, implementing and evaluating.
- Critical thinking uses scientific knowledge combined with the nursing process to consider a care situation.
- Ethics should be applied to nursing care within the framework of the four ethical principles and 'The Code' (NMC 2008).

- The nurse acts as a leader and manager of care and how care is delivered.
- Quality assurance is a tool to measure effectiveness of care delivery.
- The nurse is a researcher and evidence-based care underpins care management and delivery.
- The health and illness continuum is explored.
- Factors that influence health are considered and you are invited to consider your own health in the light of this.
- Health beliefs and behaviour are defined and examples shared.
- Health promotion activities are highlighted.
- Health and illness through the lifespan are explored in detail and the physical changes that occur in adulthood are identified.
- Pre-, intra- and post-operative care is explored in the case study of Wendy Xin who is admitted for surgery.

TEST YOURSELF

1. Which of the following is a true representation of the term *primary care*?
   a. healthcare which is free at the point of delivery
   b. the first point of contact for people seeking healthcare
   c. care in the hospital setting
   d. general practitioner practices

2. The nursing process:
   a. is the series of critical thinking activities nurses use to provide care
   b. is a process to sort out the best procedures for moving and handling
   c. delivers planned care only
   d. implements multidisciplinary activities

3. The phases of the nursing process are:
   a. implementing, planning, evaluating, diagnosing and assessing
   b. assessing, planning, evaluating, diagnosing and implementing
   c. assessing, diagnosing, planning, implementing and evaluating
   d. assessing, evaluating, planning, diagnosing and implementing

4. Evaluating care involves:
   a. collaborating with the patient in relation to the care given
   b. identifying risks that the patient might have
   c. formulating diagnostic statements
   d. measuring the degree to which goals and outcomes have been achieved

5. An example of objective data is:
   a. pain
   b. temperature
   c. depression
   d. tiredness

6. An example of subjective data is:
   a. heart rate
   b. urinalysis
   c. weight
   d. anxiety

7. Which of the following is an example of beneficence?
   a. promotion of good and the prevention of harm
   b. to do no intentional harm
   c. to respect the rights of people
   d. to treat people fairly

8. To which theory in ethics does the term *utilitarianism* belong?
   a. deontology
   b. non-maleficence
   c. consequentialism
   d. moral debate

9. Obtaining a pre-operative blood pressure measurement serves the following purpose:
   a. fulfils a legal requirement
   b. informs anaesthetist so proper level of anaesthesia can be given

c. prevents atelectasis
d. provides a baseline to compare post-operative blood pressure levels

10. Deep vein thrombosis is:
   a. the formation of a blood clot in the vein
   b. formation of a blood clot in the pulmonary artery
   c. a condition that only affects women
   d. the pulse sensation felt in the blood vessels

Further resources

Healthtalkonline
www.healthtalkonline.org
Listen to persons talking about their experiences of taking medication for a variety of problems by visiting this website.

Immunisations
www.immunisation.nhs.uk
Access a list of immunisation schedules, use these resources to update your knowledge about vaccinations and immunisations.

Department of Health (DoH)
www.dh.gov.uk
Access the full range of policy, guidance and publications from the Department of Health website.

Nursing and Midwifery Council (NMC)
www.nmc.org.uk
Access this site to get the latest update and guidance from our professional body.

Bibliography

Beauchamp T L and Childress J F (2001) *Principles of Biomedical Ethics*. Oxford, Oxford University Press.

Benner P and Wrubel J (1989) *The Primacy of Caring: Stress and coping in clinical nursing practice*. Redwood City, CA, Addison-Wesley Nursing.

Bindless L (2000) Identifying ethical issues in nursing research. *Journal of Community Nursing*, 14(4), 27–30.

Casey A L and Elliott T S (2007) The usability and acceptability of a needleless connector system. *British Journal of Nursing*, 16(5), 267–271.

Chaloner C (2007) An introduction to ethics in nursing. *Nursing Standard*, 21(32), 42–46.

Currie L and Harvey G (1998) Care pathways development and implementation. *Nursing Standard*, 12(30), 35–38.

Dahlgren G and Whitehead M (1991) *Policies and Strategies to Promote Social Equity in Health*. Stockholm, Institute of Futures Studies.

Davies M and MacDowell W (2006) *Health Promotion Theory*. Maidenhead, Open University Press.

DoH (1999) *Saving Lives: Our healthier nation*. London, Department of Health.

DoH (2000) *The NHS Plan – A Plan for investment. A Plan for Reform*. London: Department of Health.

DoH (2001) *The National Service Framework for Older People*. London, Department of Health.

DoH (2003) *Health Survey for England 2002*. London, Department of Health.

DoH (2004) *Choosing Health: Making healthier choices easier*. London, Department of Health.

DoH (2007) *Executive Summary. What the health profile of England 2007 shows – the general picture*. London, Department of Health.

DoH (2008) *Ambitions for Health. A strategic framework for maximising the potential of social marketing and health-related behaviour*. London, Department of Health.

DoH (2009a) *NHS 2010–2015: From good to great. Preventative, people-centred, productive*. London, Department of Health.

DoH (2009b) *The NHS Constitution: A consultation on new person rights*. London, Department of Health.

DoH (2010) *The NHS in England: The operating framework for 2009/10*. London, Department of Health.

Downie R S, Tannahill C and Tannahill A (1996) *Health Promotion: Models & values*. Oxford, Oxford Medical Publications.

Dunn H (1959) High-level wellness for man and society. *American Journal of Public Health*, **49**, 786–972.

Edwards S D (1996) *Nursing Ethics. A principle-based approach*. London, Macmillan.

Ellis J and Hartley C (2004) *Managing and Coordinating Nursing Care* (4th edn). Philadelphia, PA, Lippincott.

Erickson E (1963) *Childhood and Society* (2nd edn). New York, Norton.

FSA (2007) *Consumer Attitudes to Food Survey*. London, Food Standards Agency.

Fowler J W (1981) *Stages of Faith: The psychology of human development and the quest for meaning*. New York, Harper and Row.

Gabriel J (2008) Infusion therapy part two: prevention and management of complications. *Nursing Standard,* 22(32), 41–48.

Glass E and Cluxton D (2004) Truth-telling. Ethical issues in clinical practice. *Journal of Hospice and Palliative Nursing*, 6(4), 232–242.

Hall C (2009) *A Picture of the United Kingdom using the National Statistics Socio-economic*

Classification. London, Office for National Statistics.

Havighurst R J (1972) *Human Development and Education* (3rd edn). New York, Longman.

Henderson V (1966) *The Nature of Nursing: A definition and its implications for practice, research and education*. New York, Macmillan.

Kohlberg L (1979) *The Meaning and Measurement of Moral Development*. New York, Clark University.

Kozier B, Erb G, Berman A, *et al*. (2008) *Fundamentals of Nursing: Concepts, process and practice*. Harlow, Pearson Education.

Lader D (1999) *Opinions Survey Report No. 40. Smoking-related behaviour and attitudes 2008/09*. London, Office for National Statistics.

Leininger M and McFarland M (2002) *Transcultural Nursing* (3rd edn). New York, McGraw Hill.

Loewy E H (1996) *Textbook of Healthcare Ethics*. New York, Plenum Press.

Maben J (2008) *Nursing in Society: Starting the debate. What is high quality nursing care and how can we best ensure its delivery?* London, National Nursing Research Unit, Florence Nightingale School of Nursing and Midwifery.

Marmot M, Atkinson T, Bell J, *et al*. (2010) *Fair Society, Healthy Lives; The Marmot Review*. London, Department of Health.

Medicines Partnership (2003) *Project Evaluation Toolkit*. London, Medicines Partnership.

Miller C (2003) Safe medication practices: Nursing assessment of medications in older adults. *Geriatric Nursing*, **24**(5), 314–315, 317.

Miller J (2000) *Coping with Chronic Illness: Overcoming powerlessness* (3rd edn). Philadelphia, PA, F A Davis.

Mitchell M (2010) A person-centred approach to day surgery nursing. *Nursing Standard*. **24**(44), 40–46.

NICE (2010) *Reducing the Risk of Venous Thromboembolism (Deep Vein Thrombosis and Pulmonary Embolism) in Patients Admitted to Hospital*. CG92, London, National Institute for Health and Clinical Excellence.

NMC (2004) *Standards of Proficiency for Pre-registration Nursing Education*. London, Nursing and Midwifery Council.

NMC (2008) *'The Code'*. London, Nursing and Midwifery Council.

NPSA (2007) *Promoting Safer Use of Injectable Medicines*. London, National Patient Safety Agency.

Ogden J (2001) Health psychology. In Naidoo J and Wills J (eds), *Health Studies. An Introduction*, Basingstoke, Palgrave Macmillan, 147–184.

ONS (2010a) *Cancer Statistics Registrations*. Office for National Statistics. Crown Copyright.

ONS (2010b) *Professionals Drink More Than Manual Workers*. News Release. Office for National Statistics. Crown Copyright.

Peate I (2006) *Becoming a Nurse in the 21st Century*. Chichester, Wiley.

Pender N, Parsons M and Murdaugh C (2006) *Health Promotion in Nursing Practice* (5th edn). Upper Saddle River, NJ, Prentice Hall.

Pratt R J, Pellowe C M, Wilson J A *et al*. (2007) epic2: national evidence-based guidelines for preventing healthcare-associated infections in NHS hospitals in England, *Journal of Hospital Infection*, **65**(Suppl 1), S1–S64.

Priest H (2010) Effective psychological care for physically ill persons in hospital. *Nursing Standard*, **24**(44), 48–56.

Pritchard M J (2011) Using the Hospital Anxiety and Depression Scale in surgical patients, *Nursing Standard*, **25**(34), 35–41.

RCN (2005a) *Perioperative Fasting in Adults and Children. An RCN Guideline for the multidisciplinary team*. London, Royal College of Nursing.

RCN (2005b) *Standards for Infusion Therapy*. London, Royal College of Nursing.

Roebuck J (1979) When does old age begin?: the evolution of the English definition. *Journal of Social History*, **12**(3), 416–428.

Suchman E (1972) Stages of illness and medical care. In Jaco E (ed.), *Persons, Physicians and Illness*. New York, Free Press.

Tones K and Tilford S (2001) *Health Promotion: Effectiveness, efficiency and equity* (3rd edn). Cheltenham, Nelson Thornes Ltd.

Wanlass D (2004) *Securing Good Health for the Whole Population*. HMSO. Crown Copyright.

Westerhoff J (1976) *Will Our Children Have Faith?* New York, Seabury Press.

WHO (1974) *Constitution of the World Health Organization: Chronicle of the World Health Organization*. Geneva, World Health Organization.

WHO (1986) *Ottawa Charter for Health Promotion*. Geneva, World Health Organization.

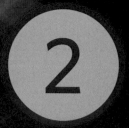

Caring for people with cancer

Learning outcomes

- In defining cancer, explain the theories of carcinogenesis, the risk factors and the causative agents and promoting factors.

- Examine the physical, psychological and social effects of cancer on individuals and society and how this impacts on them throughout their cancer experience.

- Describe the role of palliative care as disease progresses.

- Examine the range of responses to **loss**, considering implications these have for the person and those supporting them.

Clinical competencies

- Undertake a holistic assessment of the person with cancer, identifying their physical and psychosocial needs.

- Incorporate evidence-based research into the planning of nursing care for the person with cancer throughout the disease trajectory.

- Evaluate the management of symptoms that arise from both the disease process and as a result of treatment of the cancer, recognising the need for a palliative approach at the appropriate time.

- Provide sensitive, individualised care for those experiencing loss, **grief** and death.

CASE STUDIES

Below are three case studies that you may wish to consider before, during or after you have read the chapter. There are no right or wrong answers to these case studies, but you should think about the physical, psychological and social implications.

Case Study 1 – Susan

Mrs Susan Stone, a 30-year-old beauty consultant, has always had sunshine holidays with the family from being a young child and even now likes to maintain a year-round tan using tanning beds to top up her colour. She notices that a mole on her shoulder has changed colour and shape recently and when it was knocked recently, it bled. She is hoping to get married in a month's time on a Caribbean island and is worried that this might be something serious. Susan represents someone at the start of their cancer journey.

Case Study 2 – Brian

Mr Brian Smith is a 55-year-old publican. He has cancer of the colon which was treated surgically, and did not have a colostomy fashioned. He has now had two cycles of **chemotherapy**. He has telephoned the nurse in the chemotherapy suite as he does not feel very well and does not want to attend for treatment. He is not eating or sleeping and feels very tired. He has developed mouth ulcers which are very painful and is feeling very dispirited.

Case Study 3 – Molly

Mrs Molly McKenzie, aged 75 years and widowed, had a mastectomy performed for breast cancer 20 years previously. She has been well since her treatment and enjoys seeing her grandchildren and helping with childcare. She presents at the doctors with severe **pain** in her back and tingling sensation down her left leg, and is looking very thin. When questioned about her weight loss, she has not been dieting and the weight has changed rapidly over the last three months. She represents someone who requires palliative care.

INTRODUCTION

Although the incidence and mortality rates of cancer have continued to decline since the 1990s, it remains one of the most feared diseases. The fear engendered by the suggestion of a cancer diagnosis often evokes feelings of hopelessness and helplessness. Cancer results when normal cells mutate into abnormal cells, and it can affect any body tissue; it is a disruptive and life-threatening process that affects the whole person and that person's family, friends and acquaintances. Nursing interventions are based on the understanding that cancer is a chronic disease with acute episodes, and that the person is often treated as an out-patient and is usually treated with a combination of therapies. Equally important, the nurse recognises that caring for the person with cancer involves health education, early detection and treatment, together with supportive care, long-term follow-up and possibly end-of-life care.

Oncology is the study of cancer. The term is derived from the Greek word *oncoma* ('bulk'). Oncologists specialise in caring for people with cancer; they may be medical doctors, surgeons, radiologists, immunologists or researchers. The oncology nurse (or clinical nurse specialist – CNS) is an important and significant member of the oncology team, who has received specialised training in cancer care and treatment and in assisting the person with the psychosocial problems. Specialist palliative care nurses are skilled in the management of symptoms that develop as the illness progresses when cure is not the main intent. Many of these nurses are known as Macmillan nurses in the UK because their posts and education have been supported by the Macmillan Cancer Relief charity. Collaboration among health-care professionals (e.g., surgeons, oncologists, nurses, social workers) ensures the most effective care and treatment for the person with cancer.

This chapter focuses on the patho-physiology of cancer; identifies current diagnostic and treatment modalities; and discusses nursing care appropriate for people with cancer throughout their journey. Most people with cancer experience a range of symptoms, including pain, which is explored. The chapter concludes by addressing the needs of the dying person and the support they and those closest to them require. Cancers that affect specific body systems (e.g., leukaemia, lung cancer) are dealt with in more detail in other chapters of the book.

Incidence and mortality

In 2008, 410 500 new cases of cancer were registered (ONS 2010) and there were 156 723 deaths attributed to cancer in the UK (Cancer Research UK 2010a). Cancer Research UK (2010b) claim that 1:4 or 27% of deaths occurring in 2006 were from cancer, with lung cancer accounting for the largest number of deaths, followed by colorectal and breast cancer. Mortality rates for different cancers vary. The UK, in the 1980s and 1990s, had cancer survival rates that were the poorest in Western Europe, with people waiting a long time for diagnosis and treatment. In response, the government launched its Cancer Plan in 2000 and since then outcomes have improved, so much so that cancer mortality in those younger than 75 years of age fell by 17% during the period of 1996–2005, representing 60 000 lives saved (DoH 2007). Whilst survival rates are increasing, so too are the number of people presenting with cancer and this number will increase by a third by 2020. Despite the improvements, the UK still has not closed the gap with the best European countries.

Since the introduction of the NHS Cancer Plan in 2000, the DoH (2007) claims that the UK now has better prevention because:

- The number of people smoking has fallen.

- More cancers are detected through screening, especially breast cancers.

- People are diagnosed and treated sooner with approximately 99% of those people with cancer receiving their first treatment within a month of diagnosis.

FAST FACTS

Cancer in the UK

- 30 cancer networks coordinate services and all aspects of care.

- Someone is diagnosed with cancer every two minutes in the UK.

- Breast cancer is the most common cancer in the UK with around 125 new cases diagnosed each day.

- There are four cancers – breast, lung, colorectal and prostate – that make up over half of all newly diagnosed cases.

- Cancer survival is lower for people living in deprived areas of England and Wales.

- Highest male survival rate is seen for those with testicular cancer.

- Highest female survival is seen for women with melanoma.

Source: www.cancerresearch.co.uk.

- People are receiving better treatment since guidelines have been issued by the National Institute for Health and Clinical Excellence (NICE) ensuring greater conformity between those providing care.

However, survival rates in those cancers that are difficult to detect – like lung cancer – remain the same.

Risk factors

Risk factors make an individual or a population vulnerable to a specific disease and can be divided into those that are controllable and those that are not. Knowledge and assessment of risk factors are especially important in counselling the person and their families about measures to prevent cancer. However, cancer is multifactorial, that is, it develops from a combination of events, and it is difficult to categorically state which factors contribute most to cancer development. Trends can be identified, but explanations for these trends are more difficult to ascertain. According to statistics (Cancer Research UK 2010c) we know that:

- Men are at greater risk of developing cancer than women, except for breast cancer.

- Generally, men and women from Asian, Chinese and mixed ethnic groups are significantly less likely to get cancer than the white population.

- Asian and black women under the age of 65 years who develop breast cancer have a lower survival rate than the white population.

- Black men and women are less likely to get lung, breast or colorectal cancers.

- Black men and women are more at risk of developing cancer of the stomach.

> **Consider this . . .**
> Why might people from different populations be at risk of developing certain cancers?
>   Why might men be at more risk than women?

There is evidence supporting the following risk factors.

HEREDITY

It is estimated that 5–10% of cancers may have a hereditary component. The familial pattern of some breast and colon cancers has been documented; and there is some evidence supporting the theory in lung, ovarian and prostate cancers. Although further research is needed to identify cancers that are due to heredity, familial predisposition should be counted among risk factors so that people at risk can reduce behaviours that promote cancer. For example, a person with a family history of lung cancer should be counselled to avoid smoking, areas where smoking is allowed and working in an occupation that may expose them to carcinogens. All cancers are a genetic disease because it results from mutations of the genes in the cells, but they are not all inherited diseases.

AGE

Cancer is a disease associated with ageing; three quarters of cases are aged over 60 years and only 1% of cancers are seen in children and teenagers (Cancer Research UK 2010d). It is believed that if people changed their lifestyle habits, e.g. stopped smoking, reduced alcohol intake, avoided sun exposure and reduced weight, then half of all cancers would be avoided. Another problem is that free radicals (molecules resulting from the body's metabolic and oxidative processes) tend to accumulate in the cells over time, causing damage and mutation. Hormonal changes that occur with ageing can be associated with cancer. Post-menopausal women receiving exogenous oestrogen, as in hormone replacement therapy (HRT), have an increased risk for breast and uterine cancers. Older men are at risk of prostate cancer, possibly due to breakdown of testosterone into carcinogenic (cancer-making) forms.

POVERTY

The poor are at higher risk for cancer than the population in general. This is attributed in part to delays in seeking treatment and poor compliance with health advice. They have more difficulty in getting time away from work for medical consultations, and time away from work usually results in a loss of wages that they cannot afford. Other factors that may be involved such as diet and stress, which usually come under the category of controllable risks, are frequently uncontrollable in this population (Cancer Research UK 2010e).

DIET

Diet has been implicated in most cancers. A diet that is predominantly high in fat and meat and low in vegetables can increase the risk of bowel cancer, and obesity is associated with breast cancer. Excessive body fat has been linked to an increase of hormone-dependent cancers. Diets that include a high salt component are thought to lead to stomach cancer; certain vegetables, such as brassicas (broccoli and cabbage), have a protective function, and a diet that contains a large proportion of fruit and vegetables does seem to prevent cancers of the stomach, bowel and oesophagus.

OCCUPATION

Occupational risk might be considered to be either controllable or uncontrollable. For many people, education and ability limit their choice of occupation. During times of high unemployment, changing occupation poses a risk so this may not be a viable option. Government standards are designed to protect workers from hazardous substances, but many believe that these standards are not strict enough and that inspections are not frequent enough to prevent violations.

Specific risks vary according to the occupation. Outdoor workers such as farmers and construction workers are exposed to solar radiation; healthcare workers such as x-ray technicians and biomedical researchers are exposed to ionising radiation and carcinogenic substances; and exposure to asbestos is a problem for people who work in old buildings with asbestos insulation in the walls.

INFECTION

A range of bacterial infections and viruses increase the risk of cancer:

- Human papillomavirus (HPV) causes 80% of cervical cancers.
- Hepatitis B and C results in 81% hepatocellular (liver) carcinomas.
- Epstein Barr virus results in Hodgkin's lymphoma (60%) or Burkitt's lymphoma (90%).
- HIV infections can result in Kaposi sarcomas and lymphomas.

Bacteria and viruses can alter the genetic makeup of the cells; exposure usually has to be over a period of time, and other factors play a role such as an impaired immunological response. Papillomaviruses cause plantar, common and flat warts, which are benign and usually regress spontaneously; however, they also cause genital warts and laryngeal papillomas, which are associated with malignant melanoma and cervical, penile and laryngeal cancers.

TOBACCO USE

Lung cancer is considered highly preventable because of its relationship to smoking. The carcinogenic substances in tobacco are weak; therefore, stopping smoking can reverse the damage it causes. Many other substances in tobacco which are not in themselves carcinogenic promote cancer changes so that the larger the dose and longer the use, the higher the risk for developing cancer. Research has shown a significantly lower lung cancer death risk for former smokers compared to current smokers. Smokers who stop before middle age lessen the risk of lung cancer by 90%.

Tobacco is also related to other forms of cancer. Smokers face an increased risk for oropharyngeal, oesophageal, laryngeal, gastric, pancreatic and bladder cancers. Pipe and cigar smokers are susceptible to oropharyngeal and laryngeal cancers. Oral and oesophageal cancers are more common among those who chew tobacco or use snuff.

Research has documented the harmful effects of second-hand tobacco smoke. Tobacco-specific nitrosamines were recovered in the urine of children living with smokers. It is now accepted that non-smokers exposed to tobacco smoke over long periods of time, whether in the workplace or the home, have an increased risk for lung or bladder cancers.

ALCOHOL USE

Alcohol promotes cancer by enhancing the contact between carcinogens such as those in tobacco and the stem cells that line the oral cavity, larynx and oesophagus. People who both smoke and drink a considerable amount of alcohol daily have an increased risk for oral, oesophageal and laryngeal cancers.

SUN EXPOSURE

As the protective ozone layer thins, more of the sun's damaging ultraviolet radiation reaches the earth. The rate of skin cancers has increased; evidence suggests that 90% of malignant melanomas are a result of overexposure to solar radiation. Sun-related skin cancers are now considered to be a problem for all people, regardless of skin colour, but people of Northern European extraction with very fair skin, blue or green eyes, and light-colour hair are most vulnerable. It is the second most common cancer to occur in 15–30-year-olds; however, 90% of the non-melanoma skin cancers are curable. Elderly people with decreased pigment in their skin are also more at risk.

Case Study 1 – Susan

Susan in Case Study 1 has had holidays abroad most of her life; she likes the tanned look and has maintained or supplemented her tan with frequent use of sunbeds. She has not used high factor sun lotions to protect her skin on sunny days in the UK; only using them when on holiday; she does remembering burning her shoulders on a couple of occasions when working in her garden in hot weather. Knowing that her lifestyle may be a contributing factor does not help Susan to cope with the news that a mole changing shape, colour and size could be bad news and signify that she has skin cancer.

Skin cancer is common, with 76 500 new cases presenting each year in the UK; this accounts for 20% of all new cancers being reported. There are three main skin cancers – basal cell carcinoma, squamous cell carcinoma (which tend to occur more in older people) and malignant melanomas (which tend to occur more in younger people aged between 19 and 39 years of age). Skin cancers are not usually life-threatening; however, the majority of those who do die have malignant melanomas.

If the primary healthcare professionals consider Susan to have cancer, then the 'two week wait' rule applies and an urgent referral is made for her to see a specialist. The 'two week wait' rule is a target that the current UK government has decided on as part of its strategy to improve cancer care. It means that people who are seen by their GP should not wait longer than two weeks before seeing a specialist consultant.

Photographs will be taken of the mole, and its dimensions will be drawn on graph paper so that changes to size and shape can be monitored. If the GP does not think the changes to the mole are cancerous, they will monitor the person over eight weeks to see whether any further changes are noted.

IN PRACTICE

Skin cancer

National Institute for Health and Clinical Excellence (NICE 2006) have issued a seven-point scale clinicians can use to assess whether a mole is potentially cancerous.

There are three major changes and if all three are present the score is 6 (two points for each change):

● change in size;

● change in colour;

● change in shape.

There are four minor features which score one point each:

● measures 7 mm or more across in any direction;

● inflammation;

● oozing or bleeding;

● change in sensation – itching or pain, for example.

If the score is 3 or more, then the person needs to be referred to a specialist dermatologist. However, if only one item scores in a worrying manner, then referral is indicted.

Susan will be referred to the local hospital skin cancer multidisciplinary team, who will assess Susan and determine her care because she scores 5 points. Susan is very anxious and it is important not to give false reassurances. Providing Susan with factual information about who she is being referred to, what will happen when she sees the specialist, what kind of tests will be undertaken, etc. will help lessen some of her anxieties (NICE 2006).

Pathophysiology

Cancer is an eclectic term that is used for a number of diseases which have a similar way of developing. Cancer develops from one ancestral cell so it is called monoclonal. The changes that occur in a 'normal' cell to a 'malignant' (cancer) one occur over time and involve many stages or mutations, and several factors are implicated. This may take years and is the reason why cancer is principally a disease of older people. Before a discussion of the various theories of the causes of cancer, it is useful to review how normal cells divide and adapt to changing conditions.

NORMAL CELL GROWTH

Mature normal cells are uniform in size and have nuclei that are characteristic of the tissue to which the cells belong. Within the nucleus of normal cells, chromosomes containing deoxyribonucleic acid (DNA) molecules carry the genetic information that controls the synthesis of polypeptides (proteins). Genes are subunits of chromosomes and consist of portions of DNA that specify the production of particular sets of proteins. Thus, genes control the development of specific traits. The genetic code in the DNA of every gene is translated into protein structures that determine the type, maturity and function of a cell. Any change or disruption in a gene can result in an inaccurate 'blueprint' that can produce an aberrant cell, which may then become cancerous. Normal cells replicate in a controlled manner, and only when conditions such as space and nutrients are available. There is a balance between mature and maturing cells; if all cells changed at the same time we would be like snakes shedding a skin.

The cell cycle

The cell cycle (Figure 2.1) consists of four phases. In the G_1 phase, the cell enlarges and prepares for replication by building proteins which helps prepare the DNA for change. During the synthesis (S) phase, DNA is copied and the chromosomes in the cell are duplicated. During the next phase, (G_2), the cell prepares itself for mitosis (splitting in two). Finally, with all preparations complete, the cell begins mitosis (M). This phase culminates in the division of the parent cell into two exact copies called daughter cells, each having identical genetic material. The cells then immediately enter G_1 where they begin the cell cycle again, or divert into a resting phase called G_0. Cells that line the mouth change rapidly, bone cells less frequently. The cell cycle is controlled by cyclins (chemical messengers), which combine with and activate enzymes called cyclin-dependent kinases.

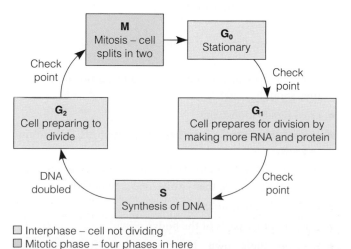

☐ Interphase – cell not dividing
☐ Mitotic phase – four phases in here

Figure 2.1 The cell cycle.

Some cyclins cause a 'braking' action and prevent the cycle from proceeding. Checkpoints in the cell cycle ensure that it proceeds in the correct order; if there are any abnormalities, apoptosis (or cell death) occurs through the action of certain enzymes. A malfunction of any of these regulators of cell growth and division can result in the rapid proliferation of immature cells. In some cases, these cells become cancerous. Knowledge of the cell cycle is used in the development of chemotherapeutic drugs, which are designed to disrupt the cancer cells during different stages of their cycle and kill them.

Differentiation

Cells in the body originated from 'stem' cells differentiate as the embryo grows; that is, they take on different shapes so that they can fulfil specific roles, some becoming skin cells and others becoming nerve cells. It is possible to determine where a cell has originated from microscopically because it has its own specific characteristics. When cells become cancerous, they alter so that they are not a copy of the parent cell. When a sample of tissue is taken, as in a biopsy, it is possible to see how much of the tissue has changed and how much of the tissue no longer represents the original.

If more than 75% of the tissue has changed, it is said to be poorly differentiated or undifferentiated; that is, most of it has altered and become cancerous. If only 50% of the tissue has changed, it is said to be moderately differentiated and if less than 25% has changed it is minimally differentiated. The significance of this is that it determines how progressive the disease is and it impacts on a person's cancer diagnosis. The less the tissue has changed, the more likely it is to respond to cancer treatment.

Aetiology of cancer

Intensive research efforts during the past decades have led to an increased understanding of how cancer develops. Cancer research has brought new options for treatment and improved overall survival rates. Factors that cause cancer are both external (chemicals, radiation and viruses) and internal (hormones, immune conditions and inherited genetic mutations). Causal factors may act together or in sequence to initiate or promote carcinogenesis (the development of cancer). Ten or more years often pass between exposures to substances or mutations of cells and detectable cancer.

THEORIES OF CARCINOGENESIS

There are various theories for how cancer develops, and all have certain credence. One theory is that a specific substance, a carcinogen, affects a cell's DNA causing it to mutate. Another theory is that specific genes, called oncogenes, trigger the development of cancer. Several oncogenes have been identified; for example, *BRCA-1* and *BRCA-2* which are associated with breast cancer. It is thought a decrease in the body's immune response may allow the development of oncogenes; this can occur during times of stress or in response to certain carcinogens.

Another explanation is that tumour suppressor genes that normally suppress oncogenes can become inactive. An example is p53, a suppressor gene that causes apoptosis during the cell cycle if there is a problem detected during that process. Half of human cancers exhibit mutations of p53; unfortunately, it is not absent in all cancers, so measuring for this cannot be used in diagnosis.

Central to these theories are two important concepts about the aetiology of cancer. First, damaged DNA, whether inherited or from external sources, sets up the necessary initial step for cancer to occur. Second, impairment of the human immune system, from whatever cause, lessens its ability to destroy abnormal cells.

CARCINOGENS

A number of substances have a clear link with the development of certain cancers and they can be categorised in two groups:

- genotoxic carcinogens directly altering DNA and causing mutations; and
- promoter substances causing other adverse biological effects, such as hormonal imbalances, altered immunity or chronic tissue damage, which then go onto cause cancer.

Promoter substances do not cause cancer in the absence of previous cell damage (initiation) and often require high-level and long-term contact with the altered cells.

Other factors, such as genetic predisposition, impairment of the immune response and repeated exposure to the carcinogen, are necessary for a cancer to develop. Known carcinogens are:

- viruses because they weaken the immune system;
- drugs such as chemotherapy drugs which can affect normal cells as well as cancer cells;
- hormones such as those found in contraceptive pills which can cause breast cancer;
- chemical agents such as those found in soot or arsenic which is used in pesticides;
- physical agents such as sunshine or solar radiation.

> ### Consider this . . .
> - Why is it that some people who smoke escape from getting cancer?
> - We all come into contact with carcinogenic substances, yet we do not all develop cancer; Why?

TYPES OF NEOPLASMS (NEW GROWTHS)

The term *neoplasm* is often used interchangeably with *tumour*, from the Latin word meaning 'swelling.' Neoplasms can be either benign or malignant. Benign neoplasms are localised growths that form a solid mass with well-defined borders, and are encapsulated with connective tissue. They respond to the body's normal control which means they often stop growing when they reach the boundaries of another tissue (a process called *contact inhibition*). They are easily removed and tend not to recur. Although harmless, benign neoplasms can be destructive if they crowd surrounding tissue and obstruct the function of organs. For example, a benign meningioma (from the meninges of the brain and spinal cord) can cause increased intracranial pressure (ICP), which progressively impairs the person's cerebral function. Unless the meningioma can be successfully removed, the rising ICP will eventually lead to coma and death.

Malignant neoplasms grow aggressively and do not respond to the body's controls. They are not cohesive (do not stick together, break apart easily) and present with an irregular shape (normal cells have a defined shape and purpose). Instead of slowly crowding other tissues aside, malignant neoplasms invade surrounding tissues, causing bleeding, inflammation and necrosis (tissue death) as they grow. This invasive quality of malignant neoplasms is reflected in the word origin of *cancer*, from the Greek *karkinos*, meaning 'crab'. Malignant neoplasms are either primary, that is they have originated in that tissue, or secondary, where the tumour started in one tissue and is now spread elsewhere. A person who has a primary breast cancer can develop a secondary neoplasm in the bone. Besides growing into adjacent tissue, malignant cells can travel through the blood and lymph and seed themselves in other parts of the body. A secondary tumour is usually identified by the cells that have not totally mutated, that is they still bear a semblance to the original parent cell and these cells do not resemble the tissue in which they are found. Highly differentiated cancer cells try to mimic the specialised function of the parent tissue, but undifferentiated cancers, consisting of immature cells, have almost no resemblance to the parent tissue and so perform no useful function. To make matters worse, undifferentiated cancers rob the body of its energy and nutrition as they grow. To summarise, malignant cancer cells:

- lose the regulation of mitosis, they divide and grow rapidly;
- lose their specialist characteristics and do not perform as they should;
- cross tissue boundaries;
- are not subject to signals that cause apoptosis, so continue to grow;
- do not revert back to their normal function once the stimulus that made them cancerous is removed;
- develop different nuclei;
- travel to other parts of the body;
- develop their own blood supply, which is called angiogenesis.

TUMOUR INVASION AND METASTASIS

The ability of cancer cells to invade adjacent tissues and travel to distant organs is considered their most ominous characteristic. For metastasis to occur, the cancerous cells must avoid detection by the immune system. A damaged immune system is a major factor in the establishment of metastatic lesions. Cells may escape detection in different ways:

- Aggressive cancer cells may form a large mass (greater than 1 cm) so quickly that the immune system is unable to overcome the tumour before it takes a hold.
- The tumour cells are not recognised as foreign by the immune system because they do not have a special antigen called tumour-associated antigen (TAA). TAA marks tumour cells for destruction by the lymphocytes. Some oncogenic viruses depress the expression of TAA.
- The person's immune response is weakened or altered and unable to deal with malignant cells.

Between 50 and 60% of all cancers have already metastasised by the time the primary tumour is identified, which supports the need for public health raising awareness of the benefits of screening. The time it takes for metastasis to occur is variable and often difficult to predict. The aggressiveness and location of the tumour, and the state of the person's immune system, can determine whether and how rapidly metastasis takes place.

Physiological and psychological effects of cancer

Cancer may vary with the type and location but it impacts on several levels. The following effects are usually observed.

DISRUPTION OF PHYSIOLOGICAL FUNCTION

Tumours can disrupt function by causing an obstruction (as in cancer of the colon which can lead to bowel obstruction) or pressing on adjacent organs and tissue. This pressure may cause anoxia (lack of oxygen) to the area causing it to die (necrosis).

INFECTION

Some tumours are less efficient in creating capillaries (angiogenesis); as a consequence, the centre of the tumour becomes necrotic and infected. When a tumour grows near the surface of the body, it may erode through to the surface, thus breaking down the natural defences of the skin, providing a site for the entry of micro-organisms as seen in fungating breast tumours.

HAEMORRHAGE

Tumours can grow into blood vessels causing bleeding as in gastric tumours. The loss of blood can result in anaemia. Haemorrhage can be serious enough to cause life-threatening hypovolaemic shock, this occurs more with head and neck cancers, where an artery is breached and the blood loss is so severe it causes shock and death.

ANOREXIA – CACHEXIA SYNDROME

Cachexia is often associated with anorexia (loss of appetite) and asthenia (weakness) and fatigue; and, although these conditions can interplay and aggravate each other, they are separate entities. In cancer, the tumour requires amino acids (proteins) for growth and development and obtains these through the breakdown of skeletal muscle. In cachexia, the resting metabolic rate is raised; cytokines (chemical messengers) block the transformation of glycogen in the liver to glucose by blocking the action of insulin. Without energy supplied from the usual source (glucose), the cells break down proteins to meet their energy requirements. The raised serum blood sugar levels trigger the hypothalamus to secrete a neuropeptide, leptin, which depresses the appetite and induces anorexia. The muscle wastage resulting from cachexia increases the person's sense of asthenia and fatigue. People may have already lost a considerable amount of weight before seeing their GP. Loss of 1/5th of body weight is indicative of a poor prognosis; people do not respond well to either chemotherapy or **radiotherapy** and surgery may not be possible because their disease is too advanced as is seen in Case Study 3.

Molly has lost a great deal of weight over a short period of time and is cachectic; this would indicate a poor prognosis. If she has a poor prognosis, there is little point in instigating strict dietary regimens that makes her and her family overly distressed. Allowing her to eat what she feels like eating and presenting food in small manageable portions is less distressing both for her and for those caring for her. The diet can be supplemented by special high-protein feeds rich in omega 3 oils. Unfortunately, some ready-made brands cause unpleasant side-effects, like a fishy aftertaste and fishy burps. Parenteral (intravenous) or enteral (nasogastric) feeding does not improve symptoms or prolong life and may actually cause discomfort. As weakness and difficulty in swallowing progress, the gag reflex is decreased and people are at increased risk for aspiration if oral foods or fluids are given.

PAIN

Cancer has the potential to generate more pain than other conditions; 75% of cancer patients experience pain. Pain is the symptom most associated with describing oneself as ill, and it is the most common reason for seeking healthcare. The International Association for the Study of Pain defines pain as an unpleasant sensory and emotional experience associated with actual or potential tissue damage (damage that occurs

IN PRACTICE

Cachexia

When caring for a person with cachexia:

- Assess current eating patterns, including usual likes and dislikes, and identify factors that impair food intake.
- Weigh the patient to establish their current weight. They may find this acutely distressing, but it does provide a baseline and enables the nurse to estimate the percentage of body weight lost.
- Provide the person with an honest explanation for the loss of weight and plan care that meets with their own agendas.
- Provide advice on nutritional supplements like Ensure Plus.
- Provide space and time for the person with cachexia and their carers to talk through their concerns.

Families may spend a great deal of time in food preparation that is not eaten; this can become frustrating, and can result in arguments and recriminations at a time when spending quality time together is more important.

when pain is ignored, as in a repetitive strain injury; e.g., we may adopt a poor posture when using a computer and ignore the pain until inflammation sets in) or described in terms of such damage. Although there are many definitions and descriptors of pain, the one most relevant is that pain is:

> whatever the person experiencing it says it is, and existing whenever the person says it does (McCaffery 1979, 11).

This definition acknowledges the person as the only one who can accurately define and describe his or her own pain. It also supports the values and beliefs about pain necessary for holistic nursing care, including the following:

- Only the person affected can experience pain; that is, pain has a personal meaning.
- If the person says he or she has pain, they have pain. All pain is real.
- Pain has physical, emotional, cognitive, sociocultural and spiritual dimensions.
- Pain affects the whole body, usually negatively.
- Pain may serve as both a response to and a warning of actual or potential trauma.

Types of cancer pain

Cancer pain can be divided into three main types:

- acute, because it starts suddenly;
- chronic, because it persists over a long period of time;
- episodic or **breakthrough pain**.

Most people with cancer cite acute pain as the primary symptom that led to the diagnosis and therefore tend to associate pain with the introduction to their disease. If these people experience pain after their treatment has ended, they often perceive it as introducing another cancer or as a recurrence of the original cancer and can be frightened by this, the anxiety increasing the pain experience.

Chronic pain may be related to treatment or may indicate progression of the disease. Identifying the pain as treatment-related rather than tumour-related is extremely important because it has a definite effect on the person's psychological outlook. For the person whose pain is due to the advancement of the disease, psychological factors play an even more important role.

Hopelessness and fear of impending death intensify physiological pain and contribute to overall suffering (which goes well beyond just physical pain).

Episodic or breakthrough pain is a different pain to the one brought on by the cancer. It can start suddenly and be brought on by a sudden movement or coughing fit, and it requires different treatment to acute or **chronic pain**. This is why it is important to establish the type of pain a person is experiencing.

Causes of cancer pain

The primary cause of pain experienced by people with cancer is the tumour which presses on nerves and other tissues. The tumour itself also produces chemicals called cytokines and these activate and sensitise **nociceptors** (small nerve endings throughout the body).

Side-effects or toxic effects of cancer treatments (e.g., surgery, radiotherapy and chemotherapy) may also cause pain. These are usually the result of traumatised tissue; one example of this is the oropharyngeal ulcerations that occur with some types of chemotherapy. However, these treatments may also be used to manage pain, such as radiotherapy to decrease pain caused by bone metastasis. Pain management is discussed later in the section on palliative care.

PHYSICAL STRESS

When the immune system discovers a neoplasm, it tries to destroy it using the resources of the body. The body mounts an all-out assault on the foreign invader, calling on many resources:

- chemical mediators;
- hormones and enzymes;
- blood cells;
- antibodies;
- proteins;
- inflammatory and immune responses.

These protective responses mobilise fluid, electrolytes and nutritional systems which requires energy. If the neoplasm is small enough (i.e., microscopic), the immune system can destroy it, and a tumour will never develop. A neoplasm of 1 cm is large enough to overwhelm most immune systems; however, the body will continue to try to fight it until it reaches the stage of exhaustion and is no longer capable. Thus, many people with cancer present with fatigue, weight loss, anaemia, dehydration and altered blood chemistries (e.g., decreases in electrolytes).

PSYCHOLOGICAL STRESS

People confronted with the diagnosis of cancer exhibit a variety of psychological and emotional responses. Some people see cancer as a death sentence and experience overwhelming grief, often giving up. Others may feel guilt, considering the cancer a punishment for past behaviours, such as smoking or unhealthy eating habits, or for delaying diagnosis or treatment. The person may experience anger, especially if the person believes that he or she had been practising a healthy lifestyle or has been to the doctor several times with symptoms that have not been heeded; beneath that anger may reside feelings of powerlessness.

Fear is common: fear of the outcome of the illness, fear of the effects of treatment, fear of pain, fear of death. Some people feel isolated because of the stigma of cancer and old beliefs that it is contagious. Concerns about body image and sexual dysfunction may be present but often are unexpressed, especially if the cancer is of the breast or sexual organs or causes visible body changes. Some people feel abandoned or punished by God, cancer challenges their belief systems and values.

INTERDISCIPLINARY CARE FOR THE PERSON WITH CANCER

Making a cancer diagnosis

Making a diagnosis consists of naming the tumour (classification), describing its aggressiveness (**grading**) and spread within or beyond the tissue of origin (staging). This is achieved through diagnostic testing.

CLASSIFICATION

Tumours are classified and named by the tissue or cell of origin, often incorporating the Latin stem identifying the tissue. For example, a smooth muscle cancer is a leiomyosarcoma. A cancer coming from epithelial tissue is called a carcinoma. A tumour from supportive connective tissues is called a sarcoma; for example, a cancer of fibrous connective tissue is called a fibrosarcoma. Other names for tumours incorporate the name of the discoverer of that particular cancer, such as Burkitt's lymphoma or Hodgkin's disease. Haematopoietic malignancies (also known as 'liquid tumours') are usually named by the type of immature blood cell that predominates. An example is myelocytic leukaemia, named for the immature form of the granulocyte that is predominant in this malignancy.

GRADING

Grading depends on cell differentiation, see p. 43. Cells that are the most differentiated, that is, most like the parent tissue and where less than 25% have changed, are described as grade 1 tumour. They are associated with a better prognosis. Grade 4 is reserved for the least poorly differentiated and most aggressively malignant cells, where more than 75% of the tissue has changed and become cancerous.

STAGING

Staging is used to classify solid tumours and refers to the relative size of the tumour and extent of the disease spread. The Tumour, Node, Metastases (TNM) classification system first devised in the 1950s has been adopted by all countries and is an internationally recognised staging system for most cancers:

- T stands for the relative tumour size, depth of invasion and surface spread.
- N indicates the presence and extent of lymph node involvement.
- M denotes the presence or absence of distant metastases.

Table 2.1 shows the basic outline of the TNM system.

Table 2.1 TNM staging classification system

	Stage	Manifestations
Tumour	T_0 T_1, T_2, T_3, T_4	• No evidence of primary tumour. • Ascending degrees of tumour size and involvement.
Nodes	N_0 N_{1a}, N_{2a} N_{1b}, N_{2b}, N_{3b}	• No abnormal regional nodes. • Regional nodes – no metastasis (1 = one node; 2 = two nodes involved). • Regional lymph nodes – metastasis suspected.
Metastasis	M_0 M_1, M_2, M_3	• No evidence of distant metastasis. • Ascending degrees of metastatic involvement of the host including distant nodes.

DIAGNOSTIC TESTING

Cytological examination

For the malignant tissues to be identified by name, grade and stage, they must first be subjected to histological and cytological examination by light or electron microscope. Specimens are collected by three basic methods:

- scraping cells from an epithelial surface, for example collecting a smear from the cervix;

- taking a blood or fluid sample, for example to assess white blood cells for evaluation of haematopoietic cancers, pleural fluid and cerebrospinal fluid for cancer cells;

- needle aspiration of solid tumours where a needle is placed in a tumour site and a small amount of tissue is drawn up into a syringe to determine breast, lung or prostate cancers.

Cytological examination is also carried out on specimens from biopsied tissues or tumours and on collected body secretions, such as sputum or urine.

After collection, specimens are spread on a glass slide, fixed chemically and stained if necessary. The morphological features of the cells are examined, with special attention to the nucleus and cytoplasm.

Tumour markers (proteins that are elevated in cancer)

Tumour markers are chemicals that can be detected in the blood and are used for early diagnosis, for tracking responses to therapy and for devising immunological treatments. They are useful to identify tumours when a biopsy cannot be performed as in some brain tumours; to screen for certain cancers as in the measurement of PSA levels (prostate specific antigen – the prostate normally secretes this protein, but if it

Table 2.2 Different imaging procedures used to detect cancer

Procedure	Key points
X- ray imaging	• Least expensive and invasive of these procedures. • They do not distinguish between calcifications, benign cystic growths and malignancies. • When screening for lung cancer, only 80% of the lung is visible and tumours have to be at least 1 cm in size to be detected.
Computed tomography (CT)	• Produces pictures of cross-sections of the anatomy. • Reveals subtle differences in tissue density and is more accurate in identifying tumours. • Shows up lymph node involvement.
Magnetic resonance imaging (MRI)	• Pulsed radio waves directed at the person produce signals which computers interpret to give detailed pictures of the tumour. • Positron emission tomography (PET) and single photon emission computed tomography (SPECT) also create visible images from electrical images. • Can be a claustrophobic experience for the person as they are encased in a tube. • When imaging is in progress, the machine is noisy, which can be frightening.
Ultrasonography	• Relatively safe and non-invasive. • Measures sound waves which bounce off the body. • Outlines normal structure as well as tumours. • Can be used to guide needle biopsies. • Useful in detecting tumours in young women with breast cancer as the breast tissue is denser and tumours are not detected on x-ray imaging as well.
Nuclear imaging	• Following ingestion or injection of radioactive isotopes, a scintillation scanner picks up areas of greatest uptake of the isotopes. • This is an invasive but safe procedure. • The isotopes do not damage normal cells. • The person has to lie still during the scan which may be difficult for some. • Nothing should be eaten for at least four hours beforehand.
Angiography	• Expensive and invasive procedure. • Used before surgery to identify precise site of the tumour. • Radio-opaque dye is injected into a major blood vessel near the tumour. • As the dye flows through an organ's blood vessels, its progress is traced through a series of x-ray films or fluoroscopy. • The person is prepared as for surgery. • When dye is inserted, a hot flushing sensation may be felt. • Observations are recorded following the procedure to ensure there is no bleeding before the person can be discharged home.

is present in large amounts, 4–10 nanograms per millilitre – it could indicate cancer of the prostate).

Oncological imaging

Because physical assessment usually cannot detect cancer until the tumour has reached a size that poses a major risk for metastasis, radiological examination is extremely important in early diagnosis. This diagnostic process may involve routine x-ray imaging (usually for screening only), CT, MRI, ultrasonography, nuclear imaging, angiography and positron emission tomography. Table 2.2 explains the key points for each procedure.

People attending for investigations are usually anxious about the forthcoming results. They may not verbalise their fears and they do not wish to be patronised. A clear explanation about the procedures enables them to feel empowered and in control, but it is cruel to give false hope and reassurance, and rude not to acknowledge that they are concerned and worried.

Direct visualisation

Some cancers are diagnosed from procedures that enable the healthcare professional to examine the growth more closely and obtain biopsies from suspicious tissue growths:

- *Sigmoidoscopy.* Viewing the sigmoid colon with a fibre-optic flexible sigmoidoscope.
- *Cystoscopy.* Viewing the urethra and bladder.
- *Endoscopy.* Viewing the upper gastrointestinal tract.
- *Bronchoscopy.* Inspecting the tracheobronchial tree.

Flexible fibre-optic scopes, such as bronchoscopes and sigmoidoscopes, allow deeper penetration than do traditional scopes. These procedures all require some preparation (see Table 2.3), can cause moderate to considerable discomfort and may require sedation or even anaesthesia, as in the case of bronchoscopy. Some procedures, such as sigmoidoscopy and cystoscopy, may be performed in an out-patient clinic, making them more accessible screening procedures.

PSYCHOLOGICAL SUPPORT DURING DIAGNOSIS

Preparing for and awaiting the results of diagnostic tests can create extreme anxiety. It has been compared to the experience of a prisoner awaiting trial and sentencing: After they know what the 'sentence' is, then they can prepare for the future. In addition to coping with the possibility of a life-threatening disease, or at least a life-altering one, people often also face the prospect of uncomfortable, even painful, diagnostic procedures. They have important decisions to make that depend on the outcome of those tests.

Many unspoken questions may exist, including the following:

- Do I have cancer?
- If so, what kind, and how serious?
- Has it spread?
- Will I survive?
- What kind of treatment is needed?
- How will this affect my lifestyle?
- How will this affect family members and friends?

Denial serves some people well, but others display signs of anxiety and stress as they attempt to cope.

Case Studies 1 and 3

Case studies 1 and 3 may well need psychological support as Susan and Molly may either have ignored or been in denial about their signs and symptoms for some time before seeking help. Molly may feel her initial weight loss is of a benefit to her, particularly if she has tried to lose weight in the past. It may take some time before she acknowledges that there is something wrong.

Similarly, Susan may feel that moles are 'normal' and that there is little to worry about, especially if the mole has only recently changed shape. When people delay seeking help, they may feel guilty and foolish and may avoid discussing this. When talking to the person who suspects cancer, it is important to establish what they know or already suspect, rather than launch into lengthy explanations that they may not need or be able to hear. A useful strategy is to use the format set out in the Cambridge Calgary guide (see Figure 2.2) (Silverman *et al.* 2005).

Table 2.3 Preparation for investigative procedures

Procedure	Preparation
Sigmoidoscopy and cystoscopy	• Bowel preparation is essential so that the views are not obscured by faeces. • The person should not eat on the day of the procedure to ensure the bowel remains clear.
Bronchoscopy and endoscopy	• The person may require preparing as for a surgical procedure because they may require anaesthesia.
Frozen section biopsies	• These are usually performed under general anaesthesia and the person remains on the operating table until the results are confirmed.

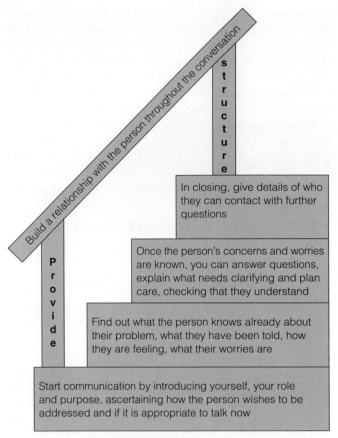

Figure 2.2 Steps to building a relationship through communication.

Reflecting questions back and seeking views helps the nurse to find out how much the person knows or suspects already. It is not necessary to always have an answer, because someone else who does know can be brought into the conversation,

but it is always important to acknowledge that the question has been heard.

It is essential that people understand the preparation required for their tests and comply with instructions given to ensure that the results are the best they possibly can be. Visits to clinics and departments undertaking the investigations provide people with an opportunity to verbalise their concerns.

The nurse should engage in active listening and avoid giving false reassurance. Some people may not wish to discuss their concerns with you and this should be respected. Some may appear angry and upset; the best approach here is to recognise that their anger may well be justified, be non-judgemental, calm and listen to them as this may well help defuse the situation.

Cancer treatment

The goals of cancer treatment are aimed at cure, control of the disease process or palliation of symptoms. These goals may overlap. Cancer may be treated through surgery, chemotherapy, radiotherapy, **biotherapy**, bone marrow and stem cell transplants. Treatment options are discussed at multidisciplinary team meetings and are dependent on tumour staging, grading and classification as discussed above. The goals of treatment are:

- eliminating the tumour or malignant cells;
- preventing metastasis developing;
- reducing cellular growth and the tumour burden;
- promoting functional abilities and providing pain relief to those whose disease has not responded to treatment.

IN PRACTICE

Caring for the person with altered body image

Loss of a body part (e.g., amputation, prostatectomy or mastectomy) or creation of unnatural openings on the body for elimination (e.g., colostomy or ileostomy) have a major effect on the person's self-image. They may fear rejection from those they love and, to pre-empt this, may reject any caring advances made towards them. They may verbalise negative feelings about their body, refuse to look at the affected site and depersonalise the body change or lost part (e.g., by calling the colostomy 'that thing'). Nurses need to:

- Discuss what the change means for that person. Small, seemingly trivial losses may have a huge impact on some people; similarly, major loss may not be perceived as important as might be imagined. Therefore, an individualised approach is needed.

- Observe and evaluate the person's interaction with significant others. People who are important to them may unintentionally reinforce negative feelings about body image; on the other hand, the person may perceive rejection where none exists.
- Allow denial as it may be the person's preferred manner of coping, but do not participate in the denial.
- Teach the person how to care for the afflicted body area, providing support and validation of their efforts.
- Teach strategies for minimising physical changes, such as providing dressings to enhance appearance and minimise change in the body part.

SURGERY

Surgical resection is used for diagnosis and staging of more than 90% of all cancers and for primary treatment of more than 60% of cancers. It is also used for reconstruction (as in breast cancer), and prophylactically (to prevent cancers growing). As a primary treatment for cancer, the aim is to remove the entire tumour, a clear margin of unaffected surrounding tissue and lymph nodes (if suspicious). This sometimes necessitates mutilation of the body and the creation of new structures to assume function of the lost structures as in the removal of the distal sigmoid colon and rectum which requires a new means of bowel elimination, so the remaining healthy segment of the bowel is brought out through a created opening (stoma) in the abdominal wall, resulting in a permanent colostomy.

Surgery can also destroy sensitive nerve plexuses, resulting in alteration or loss of normal functioning; for example, prostate surgery may result in incontinence and impotence. Surgical removal of involved regional lymph nodes can also lead to long-term lymphoedema (swelling in the affected area) that greatly impacts cancer survivors' quality of life, for instance, lymphoedema of the arm following surgery for breast cancer.

If the tumour is inoperable or there are widespread metastases, surgery may be only palliative to allow the involved organs to function as long as possible, to relieve pain and provide comfort or to bypass an obstruction. Surgery may also be performed to reduce the bulk of the tumour to enhance the ability to control the remaining disease through other modalities, like chemotherapy and radiotherapy. Surgery is often used in conjunction with these other treatments to effect a cure.

In cases when extensive removal of tissue is contraindicated (e.g., in surgical removal of a brain tumour), radiotherapy may be used prior to surgery to shrink the tumour before it is removed. Laser technology is being explored for use in different types of cancer surgery because it minimises blood loss, reduces deformity, increases the accuracy of tissue resection and enhances healing. Lasers are currently being used to the prostate in order to preserve urinary continence and sexual functioning.

Nursing responsibilities focus on preparing the person physically and psychologically for the specific surgery, as well as teaching them what to expect post-operatively. Before surgery, the nurse should give the person the opportunity to ask questions and to discuss concerns and fears. In some cases, the person may want to discuss alternative treatment options. In this case, the nurse should avoid trying to persuade the person to accept any one option; rather, the nurse should contact the oncologist and the surgeon and set up a conference before surgery to review all options again.

CHEMOTHERAPY

During the First World War, chemicals like mustard gas were used as a weapon against the troops in the trenches. During the Second World War, some allied troops were accidently poisoned by the gas and found to have a low white blood cell count as a result. It was hypothesised that mustard gas might be useful to treat diseases like cancers of the blood, where the cells divide and multiply quickly. Mustard gas was given intravenously to people with advanced lymphomas (a cancer resulting in the overproduction of white blood cells – see Chapter 10) and it was found to improve their condition for a short time. Since then, more drugs have been developed and found to disrupt the cell cycle at various points during its replication (which is why it is important to understand how cells divide normally). These drugs are also called cytotoxic because they kill cells. Chemotherapy agents are either:

- *phase-specific*, working at specific points of the cell cycle, like the S and M phase (see p. 43); or

- *non-phase-specific*, working throughout the entire cell cycle (see Figure 2.3).

Chemotherapy agents are often used in combination to increase the potential cell kill. This is because tumours consist of cells replicating at different rates so a combination of drugs affecting the cell at different points in the cell cycle have a greater potential of effectiveness. Combinations of drugs are also used when a cancer exhibits drug resistance which develops when cells mutate rapidly; an example is CHOP (cyclophosphamide, doxorubicin, vincristine and prednisone) used to treat lymphomas.

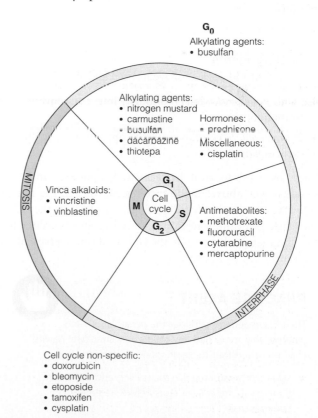

Figure 2.3 Chemotherapeutic drugs useful in each phase of the cell cycle.

Researchers have examined the possibility of basing chemo-therapy administration on the body's circadian rhythms (day to night patterns). Some drugs work better if they follow the normal cyclic fluctuations of body hormones during the night, whereas others are more effective when given during daytime hours. There are fewer side-effects with this pattern of delivery.

The cell-kill hypothesis explains why several courses of chemotherapy are necessary. A 1 cm tumour contains about 10^9 (10 billion) cells, most of which are viable (working). During each cell cycle, the chemotherapy kills a fixed percent-age of cells, always leaving some behind. With each reduction, the tumour burden of cells decreases until the number of viable, clonogenic cells (i.e., those that are able to clone daughter cells) becomes small enough to allow the body's immune system to finish the job. For this reason, oncologists usually give the maximum amount of chemotherapy that can be tolerated by the person.

Classes of chemotherapy drugs

Chemotherapeutic agents can be classified either by the effects of the agent on the cell or by the pharmacological properties of the agent. They are usually grouped as:

- alkylating agents;
- antimetabolites;
- anti-tumour antibiotics;
- mitotic inhibitors;
- hormone and hormone antagonists.

Alkylating agents
These are the oldest class of agents used and are either:

- *mono-functional*, which means they target one part of DNA formation; or
- *bifunctional*, where there are two opportunities in the cell cycle of working.

They are used to treat leukaemias, lymphomas and solid cancers. Cyclophosphamide requires enzymes in the liver to activate it. They are called alkylating agents because they affect the DNA so it cannot replicate and cell apoptosis occurs. It is thought that this happens in the $G_1 - S$ transition phase of the replicating cell (see p. 43).

PRACTICE ALERT

The nurse needs to consider the person's age and whether they have had any children or anticipate having children, given that these drugs result in infertility.

- Does the person require counselling and advice on banking sperm cells or eggs before treatment commences?
- Do they wish to see a geneticist?

Alkylating agents affect stem cells and lead to infertility; other side-effects are nephrotoxicity (renal failure) and haem-orrhagic cystitis (inflammation of the bladder that causes bleeding).

Antimetabolites
These are phase specific, working best in the S phase (see p. 43). They interfere with the making of DNA causing the cells to die. Side-effects occur when high levels of the drug are administered and it mostly affects rapidly dividing cells, such as those in the gastrointestinal tract, the hair, skin and white blood cells.

Examples of antimetabolites are: folic acid analogues (methotrexate) – used to treat breast cancer, osteogenic sarcomas and choriocarcinoma; pyrimidine analogues (5-fluorouracil) – used to treat colorectal and pancreatic cancers; cytosine arabinoside (ARA-C) – used to treat acute myeloid leukaemia; gemcitabine – used for pancreatic cancer; and purine analogues (6-mercaptopurine) – used for lympho-mas and leukaemias.

Anti-tumour antibiotics
These are originally derived from natural sources that are generally too toxic to be used as antibacterial agents. They are not phase specific and act in several ways:

- disrupt DNA replication and RNA transcription;
- create free radicals, generating breaks in DNA;
- interfere with DNA repair;
- bind to cells and kill them, probably by damaging the cell membrane.

They also damage the cardiac muscle which limits the amount and duration of treatment. Examples of these antibiotics include actinomycin D, doxorubicin, bleomycin, mitomycin-C and mithramycin.

Mitotic inhibitors
Mitotic inhibitors are drugs that act to prevent cell division during the M phase and include the plant alkaloids and taxoids.

Plant alkaloids are extracted from plant sources:

- vinca alkaloids (for example, vincristine and vinblastine);
- etoposide.

The vinca alkaloids are phase specific, acting during mitosis, binding to a specific protein in tumour cells that promotes chromosome migration during mitosis. The side-effects are:

- depression of deep tendon reflexes;
- paresthesias (pain and altered sensation);
- motor weakness;
- cranial nerve disruptions;
- paralytic ileus (where the ileus goes into spasm leading to projectile vomiting).

Etoposide acts in all phases of the cell cycle, causing breaks in DNA. Although etoposide may cause bone marrow suppression and nausea and vomiting, the most common toxic effect is hypotension when the intravenous administration is too rapid.

The taxoids act during the G_2 phase to inhibit cell division. Paclitaxel is used for the treatment of Kaposi's sarcoma and metastatic breast and ovarian cancer. Taxotere is used for breast cancer. The side-effects of these drugs include alopecia (hair loss), bone marrow depression and severe hypersensitivity reactions [e.g., hypotension (low blood pressure), dyspnoea (breathlessness), and urticaria (an itchy rash on the skin)].

Hormones and hormone antagonists

The main hormones used in cancer therapy are the corticosteroids (e.g., prednisone), which are phase specific (G_1). These have side-effects which can impair healing, and they may also lead to:

- hyperglycaemia (high blood sugar levels);
- hypertension (high blood pressure);
- osteoporosis (thinning of the bone);
- hirsutism (growing hair).

Hormone antagonists work with hormone-binding tumours of the breast, prostate and endometrium. They block the hormone's receptor site on the tumour and prevent it from receiving normal hormonal growth stimulation. These drugs do not cure, but cause regression of the tumour in about 40% of breast and endometrial tumours and 80% of prostate tumours. Tamoxifen blocks oestrogen receptors in breast tumours. Anti-androgen (flutamide) and luteinising hormone-releasing hormone block testosterone synthesis in prostate cancers. They may result in alterations of sexual characteristics – women may grow facial hair, men may develop breasts.

Effects of chemotherapeutic drugs

The side-effects of chemotherapy vary with the drug used and the length of treatment. As most of these drugs act on fast-growing cells, the side-effects impact on normally rapidly dividing cells. Tissues usually affected by cytotoxic drugs include the following:

- Mucous membranes of the mouth, tongue, oesophagus, stomach, intestine and rectum. This may result in anorexia, loss of taste, aversion to food, painful ulcerations in any portion of the gastrointestinal tract, called mucositis or stomatitis, and nausea, vomiting and diarrhoea.
- Hair cells, resulting in alopecia.
- Bone marrow depression affecting most blood cells (for example, granulocytes, lymphocytes thrombocytes and erythrocytes). This results in an impaired ability to respond to infection, a diminished ability to clot blood and severe anaemia.

- Organs, such as heart, lungs, bladder and kidneys. This kind of damage is related to specific agents, such as cardiac toxicity with doxorubicin or pneumonitis with bleomycin.
- Reproductive organs, resulting in impaired reproductive ability or altered foetal development.
- Nerve damage, resulting in neuropathies and loss of sensation in the soles of the feet and palms of the hands.

Mucositis

The most common adverse effect of chemotherapy (and radiotherapy) is mucositis. The mouth, throat and oesophagus are lined with mucous membrane and these cells divide rapidly so are most susceptible to many chemotherapeutic drugs. Small ulcers occur on the tongue and mucous membranes in the mouth and throat, which become infected with fungal infections such as thrush that appear as a white, yellow or tan coating on the tongue. Gums can become red, swollen and bleed.

IN PRACTICE

Mouth care

- Advise the person to use a soft toothbrush when cleaning their teeth and to clean their teeth after every intake of food or at least three times a day and at bedtime.
- Non-alcoholic mouthwashes are useful to keep the mouth clean and moistened.
- Sucking chunks of pineapple also helps to keep the mouth clean and fresh and prevents fungal infections.
- People are usually advised to see a dentist before treatment commences and have dental caries filled or teeth extracted to reduce risk of infection.

Hair loss

Hair loss (or alopecia), when it occurs, can be very distressing for the person having chemotherapy, as they lose all their body hair. Some people claim it is the most distressing feature of having cancer. Not all chemotherapy treatments result in hair loss and it can be minimised by scalp cooling. The person who wishes to opt for scalp cooling has to wear a cold cap for 30–40 minutes before treatment starts and maintain the cooling whilst they have treatment. However, the caps can feel heavy as they have to fit snugly and can be uncomfortable. They are not effective in all chemotherapy treatments, and people may still lose their hair.

Having hair cut short before the treatment starts can result in the hair loss seeming less dramatic. Men tend to shave their heads. Alternatively, the person may wish to invest in a wig before treatment starts; acrylic wigs are free to some who registered with the NHS, and the Cancer Research website gives a list of suppliers. Hats and scarves are another solution, as hair does grow back after treatment stops; it may, however, change in colour and texture.

Preparation and administration of chemotherapy agents

Special training is generally required to administer chemotherapy. Pharmacists usually prepare chemotherapeutic drugs for parenteral administration under specific safety guidelines established by the government or local policy guidelines. Because of the potential carcinogenic effects, it is usually recommended that the healthcare professional wear gloves, a mask and apron while preparing and administering the drug and disposing of equipment. The nurse must use care when handling excretory products of persons undergoing chemotherapy. Oral medications pose a lesser risk of exposure, but a risk nonetheless, primarily through excretion in the urine.

COMMUNITY-BASED CARE

People receiving chemotherapy usually receive their drugs as out-patients. Chemotherapy agents remain in the body for up to seven days and are excreted in urine and faeces. Good hygiene practices, i.e. hand washing following toileting, is all that is usually required. There is no danger to the rest of the family.

If a person is incontinent, soiled pads need double bagging before disposal in appropriate waste containers. Nurses will have to provide appropriate bags for clinical waste.

Chemotherapeutic drugs such as cyclophosphamide and chlorambucil can be given orally. Other drugs, such as hormones or hormone-blocking agents, may be given intramuscularly. However, many drugs require intravenous infusion or direct injection into intraperitoneal or intrapleural body space. Intravenous preparations can be given through large peripheral veins, but the risk of extravasation (drugs leaving the vein and going into the surrounding tissue because of damage to the vein) or irritation to the vein may preclude this method for long-term therapy. Most people have a central vascular access device (CVAD) fitted, especially if their treatment requires several cycles over weeks or months. Different types of CVADs are available:

- Catheters that are inserted non-surgically by threading them through a large peripheral vein. Called peripherally inserted central catheters (PICCs), they have multiple lumens that facilitate blood drawing. The placement is usually monitored by fluoroscopy.
- Catheters tunnelled under the skin on the chest into a major vein, such as the subclavian vein. Hickman or Groshong catheters may be used.

- Surgically implanted ports, which are placed under the skin with a connected catheter inserted into a major vein. These are accessed by means of a special needle with a 90-degree angle inserted through the skin directly into the rubber dome of the port, which has a hard plastic back to prevent tissue damage.

The main problems associated with CVADs and peripheral lines are:

- risk of infection;
- catheter obstruction;
- extravasation (become dislodged).

Nurses therefore must teach patients and family members to observe for redness, swelling, pain, or seepage at the insertion site. During each encounter with the person, the nurse inspects the site; observes for infection, infiltration, and catheter occlusion; and provides site care when necessary.

PRACTICE ALERT

Neutropenia is an oncological emergency that can occur with chemotherapy treatment, which depresses the bone marrow and the white blood cells leaving the person at risk to infection which can prove fatal if not treated properly (see Chapter 10). The nurse should ensure that the person has a thermometer and can keep a record of their temperature as a raised temperature is an indication either that infection is present or that the person may have developed neutropenia. The nurse advises the person to seek medical attention immediately if their temperature is raised.

Management of people receiving chemotherapy

Nurses help identify and manage side-effects of the drugs and provide psychosocial support. Careful assessment and monitoring of the person's signs and symptoms, including appropriate laboratory tests, alert the nurse to the onset of toxicity. Indicators of organ toxicities, such as nephrotoxicity, neurotoxicity or cardiac toxicity, must be reported immediately to the physician.

Case Study 2 – Brian

Case Study 2 is an example of a person experiencing problems during his cycle of chemotherapy. Brian has been trying to manage his pub whilst having chemotherapy. He has his treatment in the morning and then works in the afternoon and evening in the pub, but the late nights are beginning to take their toll. He did not realise just how debilitating having chemotherapy could be. Fatigue is a major problem for him.

It is only by taking time to talk to Brian that the nurse realises the financial problems he is experiencing, and the impact they are having for him whilst he is undergoing treatment. The nurse must first identify the physical causes that are affecting him, but also recognise the importance of the other factors that are affecting his ability to cope with the treatment.

Brian should be advised:

✚ to increase fluid intake to flush out the drugs;

✚ to get extra rest, which can assist therapy;

✚ to limit exposure to those who have minor infections like coughs and colds (maybe working in an environment like the pub puts him at risk);

✚ to identify major complications of his particular drug protocol;

✚ to contact his doctor if he spikes a temperature or feels unwell.

Brian should try to:

✚ plan activities around his treatments;

✚ delegate tasks to others;

✚ make time for more relaxing activities like a short walk;

✚ discuss his problems with a Macmillan nurse.

In addition to dealing with the side-effects of chemotherapy, the nurse refers Brian to the Macmillan team who are able to offer advice and secure some financial support that enables him to employ someone to take over the duties in the pub whilst he continues with the chemotherapy.

RADIOTHERAPY

Radiotherapy may be used to kill the tumour, to shrink it, to decrease pain or to relieve obstruction. Lymph nodes and adjacent tissues are also irradiated if metastases are suspected. The goal is to achieve maximum tumour control with a minimum of damage to normal tissue. It consists of delivering ionising radiations of gamma and x-rays in one of two ways:

● *Teletherapy*, or external radiation, involving delivery of radiation from a source at some distance from the person. A relatively uniform dosage is delivered to the tumour over a period of days, the total dose being divided up into fractions (called fractionation).

● *Brachytherapy*, where the radioactive material is placed directly into or adjacent to the tumour, delivering a high dose to the tumour and a lower dose to the normal tissues, thus sparing adjacent tissue from damage. Brachytherapy may be referred to as internal, interstitial or intracavity radiation.

For many common neoplasms, a combination of these two therapies is used.

Implanted or ingested radiation can be dangerous for those living with, taking care of or treating the person and certain measures need to be taken:

● Maintain distance from and limit time spent near the source of radiation.

● Provide protection with lead gloves and aprons.

● If you work routinely near radiation, wear a monitoring device to measure exposure.

● Keep the person with implanted radioisotopes in a private room with private hygiene facilities.

● Dispose of body fluids with unsealed implanted radioisotopes with special care and in specially marked containers.

● Handle bed linen and clothing with care and according to agency protocol.

● Use long-handled forceps to place any dislodged implants into a lead container.

● Consult with the radiotherapy department if any problems occur when caring for the person with radioactive implants.

Some tumours, such as neuroblastomas, lymphomas and chronic leukaemias, are very sensitive to radiotherapy; others, such as adencarcinomas and fibrosarcomas, are not responsive. Those that are moderately sensitive are:

● lung cancers;

● oesophageal cancers;

● squamous cell carcinoma;

● prostate cancer;

● testicular cancer;

● cervical cancer.

Side-effects of radiotherapy

Whilst external radiotherapy is aimed at penetrating through the body to the tumour, the skin and normal tissue that the radiation passes through may also be damaged. The skin can blanch (look white), become red (erythematosus), slough (desquamation, which can be either wet or dry) or haemorrhage, and it may burn. Ulcerations of mucous membranes may cause severe pain; oral secretions can decrease, causing xerostomia (dry mouth) which can then become infected. Gastrointestinal effects include nausea and vomiting, diarrhoea or bleeding. Lungs may develop interstitial exudate, a condition called radiation pneumonia. Occasionally, external radiation therapy may cause fistulas or necrosis of adjacent tissues. Implanted radioactive materials can lead to similar problems.

Nursing care of the person receiving radiotherapy

The nurse will need to provide psychological support for the person having external radiotherapy because the machines can be noisy and claustrophobic and the person has to remain still for the treatment duration, which may prove stressful. The site that is going to be treated is usually marked on the skin with a semi-permeable marker. This should not be washed off, otherwise all the measurements for positioning of the radio-therapy beam will have to be recalculated.

The nurse should also advise the person:

- not to wash the treated area with soap or apply creams, talcum powder or other topical preparations as this may lead to skin damage;
- avoid rubbing, scratching, shaving or exposing the area to sunlight;
- not to apply hot or cold packs to the area;
- to wear loose cotton clothing;
- check the skin condition daily and report any changes to a member of the team.

BIOTHERAPY

Biotherapy uses the knowledge gained about cell biology and immunology to control cancers. It is used for both haemato-logical malignancies and solid tumours. Most tumour cells have an altered structure because they carry a TAA which is recognised by the immune cells; a person with a competent immune system destroys or inhibits tumour growth. Monoclonal antibodies are developed in a genetic laboratory where they are cloned from inoculating an animal with a tumour antigen and collecting the antibodies that this action produces.

The antibodies are then given to the person with that cancer to assist in the destruction of the tumour. A number of cytokines (normal growth-regulating molecules) with anti-tumour activity, such as alpha interferon (IFN-a), bacillus Calmette-Guérin (BCG, which has been used for many years as an inoculation against tuberculosis) and interleukin-2 (IL-2), have been made and have been beneficial in treating cancer. Natural killer (NK) cells have a cytotoxic effect on some types of cancer. These cells are like large granular lymphocytes, but have a cell surface different from that of T lymphocytes or macrophages that occur naturally in the body's immune system and provide a strong resistance to metastases.

Since the early 1990s, the combination of cytokines, particularly IFN-a and IL-2, with chemotherapy has been used in metastatic melanoma patients. The rationale for biochemo-therapy is based on the independent anti-tumour activity of both IFN-a and IL-2 against melanoma. IL-2 can cause acute alterations in renal, cardiac, liver, gastrointestinal and mental functioning. IFN-a causes mental slowing, confusion and lethargy and, when used in combination with 5-fluorouracil or IL-2, severe flu-like symptoms – chills and fever of 103–106°F (39.4–41.1°C), nausea, vomiting, diarrhoea, anorexia, severe fatigue and stomatitis.

BONE MARROW AND PERIPHERAL BLOOD STEM CELL TRANSPLANTATIONS

Bone marrow transplantation (BMT) is an accepted treatment to stimulate a non-functioning marrow or to replace marrow. BMT is given as an intravenous infusion of bone marrow cells from a donor to the person. Most commonly used in leukae-mias, this therapy is being expanded to include treatment of other cancers including melanoma and testicular cancer.

COMPLEMENTARY THERAPIES

Although advances in cancer treatment have increased five-year survival rates, the uncertainty of cure of cancer and reoccurrence often compels some people to look for com-plementary or alternative therapies rather than undergo what they perceive to be aggressive treatment with awful side-effects. It is estimated that approximately 30–50% of people with cancer may have had the experience of using some kind of complementary therapy. Complementary therapies that are commonly used are:

- Herbal remedies such as echinacea and Essiac preparations for which there is little research-based evidence to support their efficacy. There is evidence that aromatherapy massage helps to reduce anxiety, thus enabling the person with cancer to sleep better and wake feeling more refreshed than fatigued.
- Dietary regimens, like the carrot juice diet, eating only organically produced food and the use of such nutritional supplements as vitamins or shark cartilage, which may help the immune system but can prove expensive and beyond the reach of some sections of the population.
- Mind–body modalities like meditation and visualisation which help reduce stress levels and so indirectly help the person with cancer cope.
- Energy therapies like non-contact therapeutic touch, Reiki, where universal energy is directed at the person, or spiritual healing, which involves laying on of hands; again reducing stress and anxiety and thus helping indirectly to manage the symptoms brought on either by the illness or its treatment.

It is important for nurses to provide truthful, non-judgmental responses to the questions or inquiries about complementary therapies from people with cancer. Nurses should encourage people to report the use of any complementary therapies to their oncologist to prevent potential interactions of the com-plementary therapies with their medical treatment.

Oncological emergencies

There are a number of oncological emergency situations that can occur as a result of cancer treatment:

- *Pericardial effusions and neoplastic cardiac tamponade* where an accumulation of excess fluid builds up in the pericardial sac around the heart, compressing it, restricting movement and resulting in cardiac tamponade. Signs include hypotension, tachycardia, tachypnoea, dyspnoea, cyanosis, increased central venous pressure, anxiety, restlessness and impaired consciousness.

- *Superior vena cava syndrome* where tumours (e.g. lung) cause an obstruction resulting in backup of the blood flowing into the superior vena cava leading to increased venous pressure, venous stasis and engorgement of veins that are drained by the superior vena cava. The person has respiratory distress, is breathless and cyanosed (looks blue).
- *Spinal cord compression* where metastases destroy the vertebral column. Back pain is the initial symptom in 95% of cases. This may progress to leg pain, numbness, paresthesias and coldness. Later, bowel and bladder dysfunction occur

and, finally, neurological dysfunction progressing from weakness to paralysis. Treatment often consists of radiotherapy and steroids, but early detection is essential.

- *Hypercalcemia* results from the activity of osteoclasts in the bone which releases calcium into the bloodstream. People often present with non-specific symptoms of fatigue, anorexia, nausea, polyuria and constipation. Neurological symptoms include muscle weakness, lethargy, apathy and diminished reflexes. Without treatment, hypercalcemia progresses to alterations in mental status, psychotic behaviour, cardiac arrhythmias, seizures, coma and death.

NURSING CARE FOR THE PERSON WITH CANCER

Nursing care for the person with cancer focuses on health promotion, rehabilitation and survivorship, palliative care and end-of-life and bereavement care.

Health promotion

Early detection and treatment are considered the most important factors influencing the prognosis of those who have cancer. Nurses can be instrumental in encouraging members of the public to access screening programmes and participate in activities such as self-examination of breast or testicles which will help detect tumours early. There are seven warning signs to note which can be summarised with the acronym CAUTION:

- **C**hange of bowel habits.
- **A** sore that does not heal.
- **U**nusual bleeding or discharge.
- **T**hickening or a lump growing in the breast or testicle or in the axilla.
- **I**ndigestion or difficulty in swallowing.
- **O**bvious changes in size, shape or colour of moles or warts or mouth ulcers.
- **N**agging cough or hoarseness of the throat.

DIETARY ADVICE

Nurses can also help by promoting healthy eating. A diet that reduces the risk of cancer consists of:

- low-fat, high-fibre;
- ample amounts of antioxidant foods, such as those containing beta carotene (a vitamin A precursor), vitamins E and C and omega-3 oils;
- foods without carcinogenic additives, dyes or chemicals used in processing.

COMMUNITY-BASED CARE

Screening programmes are usually undertaken in the community.

The NHS offers screening for certain cancers:

- *Breast cancer.* Currently women aged between 50 and 70 years are invited every three years to have an x-ray taken of their breast (mammography). This is being extended to women aged between 47 and 73 years from 2012. It is a painless and relatively quick procedure to detect tumours.
- *Bowel cancer.* All men and women aged over 60 years are sent faecal occult blood testing kits in the post. Five consecutive specimens are collected and smeared on a card which is then returned to a laboratory for testing. If the tests are found to be positive, the person is then invited to out-patients for a colonoscopy.
- *Cervical cancer.* Women aged between 25 and 65 years of age are invited every three years to their local GP centres so that a smear test can be taken.

Source: www.cancerscreening.nhs.uk, accessed August 2011.

Rehabilitation and survivorship

Rehabilitation and survival from cancer not only involves regaining strength, recovering from surgery or chemotherapy and learning to live with an altered body part or appliance, but also entails recovering from associated psychological and emotional turmoil. It is evident that as treatments become more successful there are growing numbers of people who have had or are living with cancer that can be classified as cancer survivors and who experience similar issues and require support. They may need help to return to work, obtain financial support, cope with negative reactions from acquaintances and come to terms with their own feelings and emotions. Having had cancer, people may see the experience as a 'wake up' call and alter their lifestyle accordingly; alternatively, they may need professional help in coming to terms with their experience.

Palliative care

Palliative care has been defined by the WHO as:

> an approach that improves the quality of life of patients and their families facing problems associated with life-threatening illness, through the prevention and relief of suffering by means of early identification and impeccable assessment and treatment of pain and other problems, physical, psychological and spiritual (Sepulveda *et al.* 2002).

Therefore, palliative care:

- affirms life, and regards dying as a normal process;
- provides relief from pain and other symptoms;
- enhances quality of life;
- provides psychological and spiritual support;
- supports the family up to the person's death and;
- provides bereavement support.

Palliative care provision varies across the world with some countries using palliative care services at the end of life; however, in the UK specialist palliative care may start at any point of the cancer journey and the team provides advice on symptomatology that is difficult to manage. Palliative care is not only available for cancer patients but for all people where medicine cannot cure but mainly relieves symptoms and enables a better quality of life.

In the UK, palliative care teams operate in hospitals, hospices and the community. They are usually multiprofessional and, since palliative care has been a medical speciality for over a decade, they are usually headed up by a palliative care consultant. Initially, nurses were supported by the Macmillan Cancer Relief charity and many are known as 'Macmillan nurses'. Now the charity may help set up a post for a 'Macmillan Specialist' – medical, nursing or other – but they expect the local health trusts to pick up the funding and continue to employ the person. Many nurses are not funded in this manner and are known as clinical nurse specialists (CNSs). To obtain a post as a Macmillan nurse or a CNS requires further education and most hold a degree in either palliative care or oncology nursing. Macmillan Cancer Relief offers ongoing education as do several other charities such as Marie Curie and Help the Hospices in the form of on-line education and conferences and study days. Most palliative care teams include social workers and family therapists, a member of the clergy, physiotherapists and complementary therapists.

However, as Koffman *et al.* (2008) point out, those who most require palliative care services are less likely to gain services. There is evidence demonstrating that those who are living in poverty, suffering from dementia or learning disabilities and from ethnic minority groups are more likely to die in hospital than in a hospice and less likely to receive specialist palliative care services.

HOSPICE CARE

The hospice movement in the UK owes its resurgence to Cicely Saunders, who set up St Christopher's Hospice in Sydenham, London; however, hospices have been in existence since medieval times and have a long history of providing care for those who need it. In those days, hospice care was based on charity and linked to religious houses or establishments. Many of the hospices in the UK are set up as independent charities, the services largely funded by public donations and bequests with some support from government where local primary care trusts have contracted with the hospices for palliative care services. Hospices have evolved and the services include day care and hospice at home services, where home care teams cooperate with community care to enable the person deemed to be in the palliative stage of their disease to remain at home rather than be hospitalised for their care.

Palliative care mainly consists of symptom management; the key focus is usually pain management, but other symptoms such as breathlessness are equally distressing. People can receive palliative care for months or years as it is possible to stabilise disease without curing disease, reinforcing the notion that cancer is now regarded as a chronic illness. Molly, who represents Case Study 3, is an example of palliative care where the disease trajectory may not be very long.

Case Study 3 – Molly

Molly, aged 75 years, presents at the surgery complaining of pain and having lost more than a fifth of her body weight in less than three months. Her prognosis is poor. Whilst some investigations may be performed, such as bone scans and blood screening, she will be referred by her doctor to the specialist palliative care team for pain management and psychological support. The Macmillan nurses or CNS will discuss with Molly her options for pain management, having first assessed her thoroughly. The nurses will also discuss with Molly what her preferences are regarding her care, whether home is her favoured option. Advance care plans can be drawn up at this point to ensure that the healthcare team have a record of Molly's preferences.

Pain may be her key concern, which the specialist palliative care team will aim to treat, and this may require a short time in a hospice while this is stabilised. Once her pain is under control with appropriate medication, Molly can be discharged home and she will be supported by district/community nurses and hospice at home teams which could also include Marie Curie twilight nurses covering evening care.

PAIN MANAGEMENT

In advanced stages of cancer, pain can be difficult to manage for a variety of reasons. Many people fear dying in pain. Cicely Saunders, who founded the modern hospice movement in the UK, believed in the concept of total pain; in other words, pain had physical, psychological, social and spiritual components. Focusing on one aspect at the expense of the others would result in pain that is poorly managed. It is estimated that 20–50% of people with early-stage cancer and up to 95% of patients with advanced cancer experience pain that requires analgesia.

Physical aspects of pain

Pain is perceived through the sensory neurons (nerves) and responded to through the motor neurons. Nerve receptors that sense pain are called nociceptors and consist of two different types of nerve fibres: one of these is myelinated, called A-delta fibres, and are covered with a myelin sheath that conducts impulse quickly; and one is unmyelinated, called C fibres, and has no sheath and conduction is slower. The pain from deep body structures (such as muscles and viscera) is primarily transmitted by C fibres, producing diffuse burning or aching sensations. C fibres are associated with chronic pain as from cancer. Both A-delta and C fibres are involved in most injuries. For example, if a person bangs their elbow, A-delta fibres transmit this pain stimulus within 0.1 second. The person feels this pain as a sharp, localised, smarting sensation. One or more seconds after the blow, the person experiences a duller, aching, diffuse sensation of pain impulses carried by the C fibres. Pain arising from these fibres is called nociceptive pain (Figure 2.4), which can be either somatic (from the skin and muscle) or visceral (from the internal organs). There are fewer receptors in the viscera which is why it is much harder to be exact about the pain location. When nerves themselves are damaged, for example when they become trapped following spinal damage, the pain is described as neuropathic.

The gate theory of pain transmission

It is believed that pain messages travel via A-delta and C fibres into the dorsal horn of the spinal cord, an area referred to as the substantia gelatinosa; it is in this area that the 'gating' takes place. Here, chemical substances produced by the body help relay the pain message up to the brain; however, the messages can be either intensified or attenuated by these chemicals, e.g. substance P exaggerates the pain message, whereas endorphins (the body's own painkillers) lessen the pain. The gate accommodates only one message at a time and is opened wider by substance P or closed by the endorphins. In the brain, neurones carry the pain messages to the sensory and motor

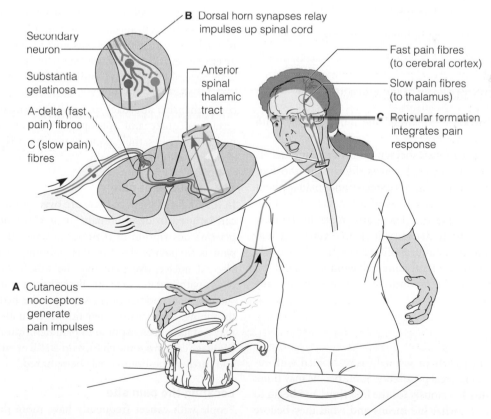

Figure 2.4 Transmission of nociceptive pain.

cortex of the brain, so we know where the pain is and can act to move away from the stimulus causing pain, which is why when we prick a finger on a rose bush, we withdraw quickly. A message from the brain has been transmitted via the nerves to the muscles to make us move. It is believed that our understanding of where the pain is coming from, which we develop from previous pain experiences, also affects the gating mechanism and alters our perception of the pain.

Psychological pain

Fear and anxiety cause tension and stress which can result in pain or aggravate the perception of physical pain. Psychological pain is real and left untreated results in depression. The distinction drawn between physical and psychological pain is arbitrary; stress affects hormone levels and produces a physiological reaction in the body which results in pain.

Social pain

It is important to consider family and cultural influences in order to effectively assess and treat people in pain because they affect the way in which a person tolerates pain, interprets the meaning of pain and reacts verbally and non-verbally to the pain. Cultural standards also teach an individual how much pain to tolerate, what types of pain to report, to whom to report the pain and what kind of treatment to seek. Behaviours vary greatly within a culture and from generation to generation so assumptions should not be drawn – nothing replaces good individual assessment. Being ill may result in:

- loss of earnings, resulting in financial worries;
- a change of role within the family;
- feeling isolated;
- not being able to address usual responsibilities;

all of which contribute to stress and intensify the pain experience.

The nurse also has a set of sociocultural values and beliefs about pain. If these values and beliefs differ from those of the person in their care, the assessment and management of pain may be based on the values of the nurse rather than on the needs of that person. The nurse must be familiar with ethnic and cultural diversity in pain expression and management and respect cultural differences. It is particularly important to remember that pain behaviours are not an objective indicator of the amount of pain present for any individual person.

Spiritual pain

A cancer diagnosis, rightly or wrongly, is associated with recognition that death is a real possibility. Some people may think about their own death seriously for the first time, and begin to review their past life, what life means and what they believe in. Some people have a religious faith, and the experience of cancer may challenge their beliefs or, conversely, give them hope and courage. Some people may have no religious beliefs and question the purpose of life, their lives and their contribution to society. In this review they may feel that they have 'unfinished' business, e.g. broken relationships they wish to mend, which can lead to feelings of spiritual distress and aggravate the intensity of pain.

Factors affecting responses to pain

The individualised response to pain is shaped by many factors, including age, sociocultural influences, emotional status, past experiences with pain and knowledge gained from those experiences, the source and meaning of the pain. Pain tolerance is the amount of pain a person can endure before outwardly responding to it. The ability to tolerate pain may be decreased by repeated episodes of pain, fatigue, anger, anxiety and sleep deprivation. Medications, alcohol, hypnosis, warmth, distraction and spiritual practices may increase pain tolerance. The sensation of pain may be blocked by intense concentration (during sports activities, for example; distraction is a learnt coping mechanism) or may be increased by anxiety or fear. Pain is often increased when it occurs in conjunction with other illnesses or physical discomforts such as nausea or vomiting. The presence or absence of support people or caregivers that genuinely care about pain may alter emotional status and the perception of pain.

Assessing pain

As seen in the section on the physiological and psychological effects of cancer, p. 46, cancer causes different types of pain. It may be acute, chronic and episodic; it may be nociceptive in origin or neuropathic. Given that pain is a complex symptom with several causes and individualised levels of tolerance and because its intensity is influenced by many factors, a comprehensive approach to pain assessment is essential to ensure adequate and appropriate interventions. The way a person describes their pain experience may well give clues about the nature of the pain.

The language of pain

In the English language there are over 77 different words that can be used to describe pain, so it is useful to listen to the person's description of their pain. Acute somatic nociceptive pain is frequently described as stabbing, sharp, whilst acute visceral nociceptive pain may be described as a dull ache. Neuropathic pain may be described as burning, tingling, shooting pain and bone pain is described as being gnawing, deep, throbbing. Some people may not have a pain vocabulary, they may not have been exposed to pain descriptor words, so whilst language can give some clues, pain is still open to interpretation and further questioning may be required.

Locating the pain site

People with cancer frequently have more than one pain experience at a time, so it is important to assess the site of their pain. Many pain assessment tools have a picture of a body, so the pain site can be marked. Acute somatic nociceptive pain is usually fairly easy to pinpoint; however, acute visceral nociceptive pain is more difficult to place because the viscera contains fewer nociceptors. Pain may be referred; that is, felt elsewhere. Pain under the diaphragm may be experienced as pain in the shoulders; pain in the appendix is felt over the umbilicus because the nerves sensing the pain belong to a particular dermatome (area that is served by a given nerve) and, whilst it receives the message, in the spinal cord it is sensed as coming from elsewhere.

Pain intensity

There is no accurate measure of pain intensity; the person with pain has to be believed. Numerical rating scales (NRS) do give some indication of efficacy of treatment. Sometimes called a visual analogue scale (VAS), NRS ask the person with pain to rate their pain on a scale of 1 to 10, where 1 is no pain and 10 is the worst pain imaginable. Unfortunately, NRS are not foolproof and people with pain can pick a midpoint for a variety of reasons; they may want to appear stoic and brave or they may perceive that they may need higher figures if their condition deteriorates. So whilst it is useful, on its own, it has limited value as an assessment tool. VAS may be a vertical or horizontal line or a series of faces going from happy to sad. The person with pain picks a face whose expression depicts how they are feeling, which is useful for people who have limited understanding of language, or they pick a spot on the line where one end is no pain and the other is the worst pain imaginable.

Pain behaviours

Pain behaviours may be learnt and are therefore culturally determined, and can be influenced by a person's coping mechanisms. Some people in pain may withdraw, curl up or lie still; whilst others may find comfort in moving, pacing the floor. Their behaviour may not match what they record on the NRS. People with dementia also get cancer; unfortunately 67% of this pain is neither recognised nor treated. Their behaviour may be the only ways of knowing that they are in pain; they may shout, become aggressive or self-harm by banging their heads.

Past coping strategies

People experiencing cancer pain or any other type of pain may well have strategies that they use which offer them relief and may well rely on these so that they avoid taking too much medication. Therefore, it is useful to know what helps them to be more comfortable. With their past experience of pain, people also develop beliefs about pain and pain medication. Some beliefs may need to be challenged to ensure that good pain control is achieved.

Pain assessment tools

There are a variety of pain assessment tools; good ones incorporate each of the above: especially a body map, key descriptor

words, NRS. Most owe their development to the pioneering work of McGill and are called McGill pain questionnaires (see Figure 2.5).

If pain is not assessed properly and not recorded in a person's medical records, there is no way to determine the efficacy of treatment given and the person remains with uncontrolled pain and may die in pain.

Treating pain

The most common drugs used to treat pain are:

- *non-opioid analgesics*, for example acetaminophen (paracetamol) – used to treat mild to moderate pain and particularly useful in musculoskeletal pain and reducing fever;
- *non-steroidal anti-inflammatory drugs* (NSAIDs), for example aspirin and ibuprofen – act on peripheral nerve endings, minimising pain by interfering with prostaglandin synthesis (chemicals that enhance pain);
- *opioids*, for example morphine – a strong opioid used to treat severe pain, morphine is still the drug of choice despite the advent of newer preparations because it is cheaper and as effective as the synthetic opioids;
- *synthetic opioids*, for example codeine, tramadol and fentanyl.

In the 1990s the WHO estimated that four million people with cancer experienced pain that was not treated properly. In 1996, it published the analgesic ladder (Figure 2.6) as a guide for clinicians treating cancer pain, which still remains a mainstay of good practice.

For people who have not used opioid analgesics, the advice is to start low with a non-opioid analgesic. Adjuvant drugs (that is, drugs not primarily used as analgesics but which help the analgesics to be more effective) can be added. If this is not sufficient to control a person's pain, then the clinician needs to move up the ladder, using stronger preparations to ensure adequate pain relief. Table 2.4 summarises the main adjuvant drugs used in pain management. The WHO also added two more key principles to optimal pain management:

- Where possible, analgesics should be given orally.
- Pain medication should be given regularly.

Administering pain relief

Most people prefer to take their medication orally and most analgesics are dispensed in pill form; however, they do cause gastric irritation so need to be taken with food. For people who cannot swallow there are alternative methods of drug delivery:

- Transdermal patches, for example fentanyl, which are long lasting (usually 72 hours), painless and easy to apply. Additional short-acting medication is often needed for breakthrough pain. It is important to start with a low dose and titrate (which means to increase or decrease the dose in

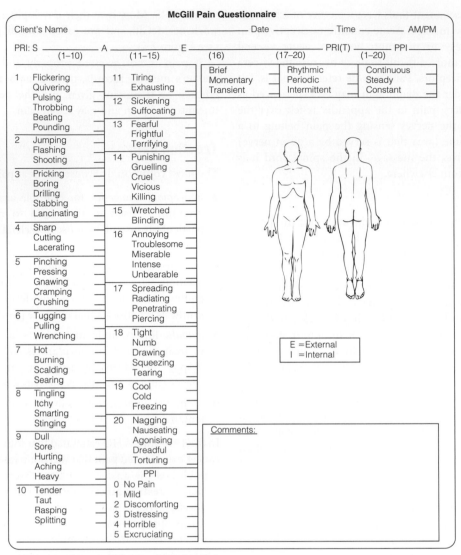

Figure 2.5 The McGill Pain Questionnaire.

small increments) to the effective level. It is lipid soluble and may be stored in fat cells longer than expected. When a person has a fever or inflammation of the skin, expect increased rate of absorption. Exercise and use of electric blankets or heating pads also may accelerate absorption.

- Rectally, for example suppositories.
- Subcutaneously, through a syringe driver. Syringe drivers are set up to administer the drugs over 24 hours; a small pump depresses the plunger of a syringe slowly releasing the drug so that the levels of the drugs remain consistent in the bloodstream. The advantage of syringe drivers are that other medication (such as drugs that dry up secretions when someone is dying) can be added. There are a variety of different syringe drivers available in the UK, all calibrated differently, so it is important to check with a qualified healthcare professional who will have had special training in the use of syringe drivers and be guided by them in the management of pain using these devices.

Timing of pain relief

For optimum pain relief in cancer, drugs need to be given regularly and not on an 'as needed' (or PRN which is short for the Latin term 'pro re nata') basis. Unlike pain from acute trauma, where tissues heal, cancer pain does not magically

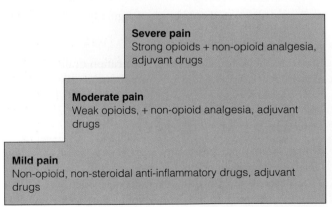

Figure 2.6 Analgesic ladder.

Table 2.4 Adjuvant drugs used in pain management and their mode of action

Drugs that assist with pain management	Mode of action
Antidepressants – tricyclics and related drug groups	Retains serotonin (a chemical that enhances pain messages) in the CNS, thus inhibiting pain sensation. They also promote normal sleeping patterns, further alleviating the suffering. They are useful with neuropathic pain.
Anticonvulsants, e.g. gabapentin, carbamazepine	Anti-spasmodics that are useful in neuropathic pain including shingles (herpes zoster) and migraines.
Local anaesthetics, e.g. benzocaine and xylocaine	Block the initiation and transmission of nerve pulses locally.
Bisphosphonates and radiopharmaceuticals, e.g. pamidronate and zoledronic acid	Stabilise the bone and slow down the growth of bone tumours (osseous metastases).

disappear. The tumour itself as it grows produces cytokines (chemical messengers) that can intensify pain (among other things). To achieve good pain control, the person needs to maintain a fairly constant level of analgesia in the bloodstream, so that there are no peaks and troughs. Many of the opioids now in use come in controlled release tablets, which means the person need only take medication twice a day; however, it is important to keep to the same time each day and for fentanyl patches, it is important that these get changed at exactly the same time every 72 hours. Failure to adhere to this principle will result in the person with cancer developing chronic pain syndromes and pain that is then difficult to control.

Side-effects of analgesic treatment

All analgesic preparations have the capacity to cause constipation. Pain receptors are present in the colon and when analgesia binds with these receptors its action is to slow and weaken the peristaltic action, which means faeces remains in the bowel longer and become drier. If not treated prophylactically (to prevent the condition occurring) the person with pain may have a bigger problem than the original pain. It is good practice to administer a laxative with the analgesia.

Strong opioids like morphine can cause nausea, but this side-effect lessens after a few days. If it persists, then the doctor will prescribe a synthetic opioid. People can develop resistance to certain drugs and changing drugs can be effective.

Myths in pain management

The public and healthcare professionals are wary of the use of strong opioids, believing that long-term use will result in addiction; however, there is no evidence to support this belief. There is ample evidence that pain that is poorly managed results in chronic pain syndromes that are extremely difficult to treat. People with cancer pain may need increasing doses of strong opioid analgesia because the tumour burden continues to grow and they may not be drinking enough fluid to flush out the inactive metabolites (waste products) of morphine.

Other myths are that:

● Older people do not feel as much pain as younger people.
● People with dementia do not feel pain; 55% of people with dementia do not have their pain recognised.

Non-pharmacological management of pain

Whilst pharmacological management is the predominant way to manage pain, relief can be achieved through other methods. The list below is not exhaustive but offers a few examples of complementary or alternative approaches to managing pain.

● *Acupuncture* is an ancient Chinese system involving the stimulation of certain specific points on the body to enhance the flow of vital energy (chi) along pathways called meridians. Acupuncture points can be stimulated by the insertion and withdrawal of needles, the application of heat, massage or a combination of these methods. Only care providers with special training can use this method.
● *Relaxation* involves learning activities that deeply relax the body and mind, lessening the effects of stress from pain, increasing pain tolerance and increasing the effectiveness of other pain relief measures. By teaching relaxation techniques, the nurse acknowledges the person's pain and provides reassurance that they will receive help in managing the pain. Examples of relaxation activities include:
  a. *diaphragmatic breathing* which can relax muscles, improve oxygen levels and provide a feeling of release from tension;
  b. *progressive muscle relaxation* which may be used alone or in conjunction with deep breathing to help manage pain;
  c. *guided imagery*, also called creative visualisation, where the imaginative power of the mind creates a scene or sensory experience that relaxes the muscles and moves the attention of the mind away from the pain experience;
  d. *meditation* whereby the person empties the mind of all sensory data and concentrates on a single object, word or idea producing a deeply relaxed state in which oxygen consumption decreases, muscles relax and endorphins are produced – its deepest level, the meditative state may resemble a trance.

- *Distraction* involves the redirection of the person's attention away from the pain and onto something more pleasant. Examples of distracting activities are listening to music, or doing some form of rhythmic activity to music.

- *Laughing* for 20 minutes or more is known to produce an increase in endorphins that may continue pain relief even after the person stops laughing, so participating in an activity that promotes laughter, such as reading a joke book or viewing a comedy, has been found to be highly effective in pain relief.

End-of-life care

A distinction has been made between palliative care and end-of-life care, with end-of-life care representing the final few days (maybe weeks) of life. Despite a well-established tradition of palliative and hospice care, the reality is that many people (58%) die in acute hospitals rather than in their own homes, the latter tending to be their usual preference. In an effort to change this dynamic, the UK government published its End of Life Care Strategy (DoH 2008) which charges all those working in healthcare to improve services. The strategy aims to provide high-quality end-of-life care by:

- accurately identifying those people who are reaching the end of life and initiating discussions to ascertain their preferences for care at this time;

- planning and delivering care according to the person's needs and preferences and reviewing and adapting accordingly as time progresses and needs change;

- coordinating care amongst all agencies involved to provide a seamless and rapid response to the person's needs;

- caring for the bereaved after the person has died.

DETERMINING CARE

There are three tools that help determine care:

- The Liverpool Care Pathway (LCP).
- The Gold Standards Framework (GSF).
- Preferred Priorities of Care (PPC), which has been included in the documentation of the LCP and GSF.

The Liverpool Care Pathway (LCP)

The LCP is so named because it was developed by nurses and doctors working in Liverpool who wanted to help professionals working in acute care recognise when people were dying. The LCP provides a framework which prompts 'end-of-life' discussions with people and their families, the key points being:

- Where they wish to die; can the person be transferred to their place of preference?

- Are there any special observances needed, for example religious rituals such as the last sacrament being given?

- Are there any special funeral arrangements? For example is the body to be washed?

- What care is currently being given? Does the person need all the medication they are being given or could some of the drugs be stopped?

The Gold Standards Framework (GSF)

The GSF is very similar to the LCP in that it aims to reduce hospitalisation for people who are dying and offers GPs guidelines for their decision-making. There are six key areas for consideration:

- communication between families and professionals;

- coordination of care, referring to specialist palliative care services;

- control of symptoms;

- continuity of care including the provision of 'out of hours' services and points of contact;

- carer support – often hospitalisation occurs because of carer fatigue;

- care in the dying phase, which may include helping the person who is dying to terminate their relationships and supporting the family to be present at the death.

DECISIONS ABOUT END-OF-LIFE CARE

In the UK, the Mental Capacity Act was passed to clarify the legal position when people are making decisions about their care and treatment. The key principles are:

- A person is assumed to have capacity unless it is established that they do not.

- A person is not treated as unable to make a decision unless all practical steps have been taken to help them come to a decision.

- A person is not treated as unable to make a decision on the basis of them having made an unwise decision.

- Decisions made by someone else must be in the person's best interest not anyone else's.

- Decisions made by others have to be 'least restrictive' of the person's rights and freedom.

People can make decisions in advance so that if they do lose the capacity to make decisions, their wishes are already known. These are referred to as Advance Care Plans which are legal documents and may include living wills, healthcare surrogates and durable power of attorney. Advance Care Plans are reviewed frequently to ensure that the person has not changed their mind and the person making the plans ensures that their views are known by their carers, both lay and professional.

WHEN THE PERSON IS DYING

As the person approaches the end of life, they do not require as much in the way of fluids and nutrition but they do need oral hygiene, the mouth being kept moist. There will be changes in their levels of consciousness because the organs of the body are working less efficiently, their breathing becomes shallow, oxygen saturation in the blood declines and the person becomes hypoxic, which affects the brain function. The kidneys shut down as a result of the falling blood pressure. This results in a build of toxins in the body which may cause terminal delirium where the person may be confused, restless or agitated. Moaning, groaning and grimacing often accompany the agitation and may be misinterpreted as pain, which is distressing for the family. Level of consciousness often decreases to the point where the person cannot be aroused.

IN PRACTICE

End-of-life care

- Dame Cicely Saunders believed that the way people died stayed in the memory of those who knew them forever and impacted on their grief response and their abilities to come to terms with their loss.

- When it is deemed a person is dying, a tool such as LCP or GSF may guide discussions and decisions. Paramount to good care is the management of symptoms.

- It is usual to set up a syringe driver pump, in which morphine is added for pain relief, a drug like midazolam, a sedative, and glycopyrronium or hyoscine, drugs that dry up secretions if the person's respirations sound 'bubbly', cyclizine or haloperidol, drugs that prevent nausea, may also be included. The aim of the medication is to make the person comfortable.

- Nursing care involves maintaining the person's hygiene needs, providing fluids as they are required, turning the person from side to side or altering their position in bed so that they do not become stiff and uncomfortable.

- The families are usually encouraged to stay with the person whether they are in hospital or at home. This vigil can be very tiring and people need to be encouraged to take breaks.

AT THE TIME OF DEATH

It is usually the doctor who certifies that a person has died, although where death is expected at home, specialist palliative care nurses who have received specialist training may also verify death. Death notifications have to be taken to the Registry Office by the next of kin where the death is formerly registered and a certificate is issued. People may need several copies of these to close bank accounts, obtain insurance policies, etc. The nurse usually performs 'last offices', a term used for preparing the body after the death. Some people, usually because of religious beliefs, do not require nurses to do this as it is disrespectful to the person. Last offices usually involves washing the person, removing jewellery, if that is in accord

with the family's wishes, putting on clean clothes or a shroud and wrapping the person in a sheet ready for the person's removal to the hospital mortuary or to the funeral directors.

It is the final act of caring for a person and, as such, is a very important part of nursing care, performed with reverence and respect. Sharing grief with the family after the death of a loved one helps both the nurse and family to cope with their feelings. Taking time to grieve after the death provides a release that can help prevent 'blunting' of feelings, a problem often experienced by nurses who care for people who are terminally ill. Some families appreciate support from the nurse's presence when they express grief, but grief reactions are individual and the nurse needs to be aware that their presence might be intrusive.

Bereavement care

People with cancer may have had to adjust to various losses along the disease trajectory; loss of control of their lives, loss of independence, loss of hair, loss of body parts, loss of their role in the family are a few examples. People adapt and assimilate these losses in different ways according to the significance they place on that which is lost. Machin (2009) argues that people have three main reactions in grief situations; some people are resilient, they cope well with grief, largely because they have good support systems, can access that support readily and have a balanced view on life; some people exhibit control in situations of grief, they have no wish to break down and cry publicly and try and maintain composure until in a place they feel safe to release their emotions; finally, there are those who are overwhelmed by their emotions, they cannot regain control easily and remain focused on their grief and loss.

The significance is that those who are resilient do not require professional help in adjusting to their loss. However, those in the other two groups may well benefit from professional help. Some people grieve before the loss occurs, this is called **anticipatory grieving**, and they may feel their grief will be less as a result, but it is often not the case.

FACTORS AFFECTING RESPONSES TO LOSS

Grieving is painful and lonely. One's social support system is important because of its potentially positive influence on the successful resolution of grief. Some losses may lead to social isolation, placing people at risk for dysfunctional grief reactions. People may not be able to grieve because they feel:

- Others do not share the loss.
- People do not recognise the loss, for example a person with dementia has died.
- Their relationship with the person who has died was difficult, for example an abuser has died.
- The person should not have died.

Most people have good social support networks and recover from their experience of loss, although it may take time. It was once believed that people recover from their loss and move on, but the reality is that the person who has died is never forgotten, the grief remains but the displays of grief lessen and the person adjusts to life without the person who has died.

CASE STUDY SUMMARIES

Many people's lives are touched by cancer; they may suffer from cancer themselves or cancer may affect someone close to them. The same is true for nursing staff. Regardless of whether they are working in hospitals or in the community and in whatever specialty, nurses will find themselves caring at some stage in their career for adults with cancer. They have a central role to play in caring for people who have cancer and their families and loved ones.

The case studies at the beginning of the chapter have provided you with examples of how cancer can impact on a number of different people in a number of different ways. Each person in each case must be treated holistically. Susan in *Case Study 1* was at the beginning of her cancer journey whereas Molly in *Case Study 3* was progressing to the end of her life. The skills required by the nurse must encompass caring, kindness and compassion, paying attention to a range of factors including the important issue of spirituality. Brian in *Case Study 2* will require a different approach to his care and treatment; he must be given options and his decisions, whatever they may be, must be respected.

CHAPTER HIGHLIGHTS

- The term cancer is an eclectic term and is often used for a number of diseases which have a similar way of developing. Cancer develops from one ancestral cell and is called monoclonal. The changes occurring in a 'normal' cell to a 'malignant' (cancer) one happen over time; this involves a number of stages or mutations and several factors are implicated. The process can take years, which is why cancer is principally a disease of older people.

- There are a number of risk factors that predispose people to developing cancer. Knowledge and assessment of risk factors are important, particularly in counselling the person and their families about measures to prevent cancer. As cancer is multifactorial, developing from a combination of events, it is difficult to state categorically which factors contribute most to cancer development.

- The physiology of cancer may vary with the type and location, but it impacts on several levels. The following effects are usually observed:
  - *Disruption of physiological function* can occur when tumours cause an obstruction. This may lead to anoxia to the area causing it to die.
  - *Infection.* Some tumours are less efficient in creating capillaries; as a consequence, the centre of the tumour becomes necrotic and infected.
  - *Haemorrhage.* Tumours can grow into blood vessels causing bleeding and loss of blood which can result in anaemia and hypovolaemic shock.
  - *Anorexia–cachexia syndrome* is frequently associated with anorexia and asthenia and fatigue; although these conditions can interplay and aggravate each other, they are separate entities.

  - *Pain.* Cancer has the ability to cause more pain than other conditions, and three quarters of cancer patients experience pain. Pain is the symptom most associated with describing oneself as ill, and it is the most common reason for seeking healthcare.

- Cancers are classified according to degree of differentiation, spread and tissue affected. Tumours are classified and named by the tissue or cell of origin, usually incorporating the Latin stem identifying the tissue. A smooth muscle cancer, for example, is a leiomyosarcoma. A cancer coming from epithelial tissue is called a carcinoma; a tumour from supportive connective tissues is called a sarcoma.

- For malignant tissues to be identified by name, grade and stage, they must first be subjected to histological and cytological examination by light or electron microscope. Specimens are collected by three basic methods: scraping cells from an epithelial surface; taking a blood or fluid sample; and needle aspiration of solid tumours where a small amount of tissue is drawn up into a syringe to determine cancer type. Cytological examination is carried out on specimens from biopsied tissues or tumours and on collected body secretions.

- Treatments for cancer vary and treatment decisions must take into account a variety of factors including patient choice, for example with respect to surgery, chemotherapy, radiotherapy and biotherapy.

- Each person must be treated as an individual; the effects of cancer on the person vary and a holistic perspective is essential. Pain and pain management will depend on a number of factors and the nurse must always undertake a holistic assessment, plan care accordingly and carry out interventions using an evidence-based approach. The nurse must also evaluate care interventions and adjust care needs if needed.

● A distinction has been made between palliative care and end-of-life care, with end-of-life care representing the final few days (maybe weeks) of life. The nurse provides end-of-life care that will incorporate care of the dying, providing psychological and spiritual support to the family up to the person's death and offering bereavement support.

TEST YOURSELF

1. In which phase of the cell cycle does the DNA form two sets of chromosomes?

   a. G_1
   b. G_2
   c. S
   d. M

2. Oncogenes are genes that:

   a. block cell growth
   b. regulate cell growth
   c. promote cell growth
   d. have a complex signalling process

3. You are asked to explain chemotherapy, which of the following is most accurate?

   a. chemotherapy uses drugs that kill cancer cells but do not affect normal cells
   b. chemotherapy uses a single drug to kill the cancer cells
   c. chemotherapy has fewer side-effects than radiotherapy
   d. chemotherapy are drugs that affect all the cells in the body when they are replicating

4. People having radiotherapy care for their skin in the following way:

   a. wash it daily with soap and water
   b. keep it dry and avoid rubbing it
   c. apply talcum powder daily
   d. apply aromatherapy massage oils

5. Which of the following cancers is not currently routinely screened for in the UK?

   a. breast cancer
   b. prostatic cancer
   c. bowel cancer
   d. cervical cancer

6. The preferred route for opioid administration in a person with cancer pain is:

   a. oral
   b. transdermal
   c. syringe driver
   d. intramuscular injection

7. The most common side-effect of taking opioid analgesics regularly is:

   a. respiratory depression
   b. itchy skin
   c. constipation
   d. hallucinations

8. Which of the following statements demonstrates a misconception about pain management?

   a. anxiety can cause pain and pain causes anxiety
   b. pain medication should only be given when a person is in pain
   c. if people are laughing and joking they cannot be in pain
   d. if the person is lying still and is not restless, they are not in pain

9. Palliative care can be described as:

   a. care that hastens the dying process
   b. care that occurs for all cancer patients
   c. care that focuses on symptom management
   d. care that is only given in hospices

10. People recover from a loss when

   a. the loss is not talked about openly
   b. only when they grieve publicly
   c. when they have been able to view the body
   d. when they have support from their family and friends

Further resources

Macmillan Cancer
http://www.macmillan.org.uk
The Macmillan Cancer support website provides useful explanations about all cancers, how they develop, and the treatments used, and it is useful for anyone interested in learning more about cancer. It has an education programme which is free, but you do have to register.

Cancer Research UK
http://www.cancerresearchuk.org
The Cancer Research website has information for professionals and is a useful resource for the latest statistics and current research news. It enables you to keep up to date with all that is developing.

National Council for Palliative Care (NCPC)
http://www.ncpc.org.uk
The NCPC website has publications and education packages for professionals, although there is a small charge for some of its services. It also provides details of its latest campaigns as it is key in lobbying the government on behalf of vulnerable people.

Patient.co.uk
http://www.patient.co.uk
This website produces useful information for people interested in health topics; it has direct links to charitable organisations such as Help the Hospices which also produces educational material for healthcare professionals.

National End of Life Care Programme
http://www.endoflifecareforadults.nhs.uk
This website provides on-line education about end-of-life care that has been developed by clinicians who have specialised in the field of palliative medicine. The units take between 30 and 45 minutes to complete and certificates are available on successful completion.

Liverpool Care Pathway
http://www.nursingtimes.net/online-nurse-training-courses/Liverpool-Care-Pathway-for-End-of-Life-Care?T=130 8912569&JTID=152709107&OGID=459&network=GAW
This website offers a training package on the Liverpool Care Pathway that can be completed on-line (there is a small charge). As there are now 12 versions of this tool, it is imperative that the latest version is accessed.

Bibliography

Alkner S, Bendahl P, Fernö M, Nordenskjöld B and Rydén L (2009) Tamoxifen reduces the risk of contralateral breast cancer in premenopausal women: results from randomised controlled trials. *European Journal of Cancer*, **45**, 2496–2502.

Blows W T (2005) Pain and analgesia. In *The Biological Basis of Nursing: Cancer*, Chapter 10. London, Routledge, Taylor Francis 255–284.

Cancer Research UK (2009) *Cancer Incidence Projections to 2024*. Available at: http://info.cancerresearchuk.org/cancerstats/projections/?a=5441 (accessed September 2011).

Cancer Research UK (2010a) *Cancer mortality – UK statistics*. London, available at: http://info.cancerresearchuk.org/cancerstats/mortality/ (accessed September 2011).

Cancer Research UK (2010b) *Common cancers – UK mortality statistics*. London, available at: http://info.cancerresearchuk.org/cancerstats/mortality/cancerdeaths/ (accessed September 2011).

Cancer Research UK (2010c) *Cancer Inequalities and Ethnicity*. London, available at: http://info.cancerresearchuk.org/cancerstats/inequalities/ (accessed September 2011).

Cancer Research UK (2010d) *Cancer Mortality by Age – UK statistics*. London, available at: http://info.cancerresearchuk.org/cancerstats/mortality/age/ (accessed September 2010).

Cancer Research UK (2010e) *Deprivation Underlies Thousands of Cases of Cancer Every Year*, press release. Available at: http://info.cancerresearchuk.org/news/archive/pressrelease/2010-06-14-deprivation-cancer-cases (accessed September 2011).

Cassidy J, Blisset D, Spence R A J and Payne M (2006) *Oxford Handbook of Oncology* (2nd edn). Oxford, Oxford University Press.

Davies A (2007) *Cancer Related Breakthrough Pain*. Oxford, Oxford University Press.

Davies N J (2009) Cancer survivorship: living with or beyond cancer. *Cancer Nursing Practice*, **8**(7), 29–34.

Davis M (2005) Introduction. In Davis M, Glare P and Hardy J (eds) (2005) *Opioids in Cancer Pain*. Oxford, Oxford University Press, 1–10.

Dein S (2006) *Culture and Cancer Care: Anthropological insights in oncology*. Maiden-head, Open University Press.

Dewey A and Dean T (2009) Nurses' management of patients with advanced cancer and weight loss: Part 2. *International Journal of Palliative Nursing*, **14**(3), 132–138.

DoH (2007) *Cancer Reform Strategy*. London, Department of Health.

DoH (2008) *End of Life Care Strategy: Promoting high quality care for all adults at the end of life*. London, Department of Health.

Dunlop R J and Campbell C W (2000) Cytokines and advanced cancer. *Journal of Pain & Symptom Management*, **20**(3), 214–232.

Ellershaw J E and Ward C (2003) Care of the dying patient: the last hours or days of life. *BMJ*, January 4th, **32**(6), 30–34.

Ellershaw J E and Murphy D (2005) The Liverpool Care Pathway influencing the UK national agenda on care of the dying. *International Journal of Palliative Nursing*, **11**(3), 132–134.

Gage H, Storey L, McDowell C, *et al.* (2009) Integrated care: utilisation of complementary and alternative medicine within a conventional cancer treatment centre. *Complementary Therapies in Medicine*, **17**, 84–91.

Harrold K (2010) Effective management of adverse effects while on oral chemotherapy: implications for nursing practice. *European Journal of Cancer Care*, **19**, 12–20.

Hemming L J and Maher D (2005a) Understanding cachexia and excessive weight loss in cancer. *British Journal of Community Care*, **10**(10), 492–495.

Hemming L J and Maher D (2005b) Cancer pain in palliative care: why is management so difficult? *British Journal of Community Nursing*, **10**(8), 362–367.

Keeney S, McKenna H, Fleming P and Mclifatrick S (2009) Attitudes, knowledge and behaviours with regard to skin cancer: a literature review. *European Journal of Oncology Nursing*, **13**, 29–35.

Klein J and Griffiths P (2004) Acupressure for nausea and vomiting in cancer patients receiving chemotherapy. *British Journal of Community Nursing*, **9**(9), 383–387.

Koffman J, Harding R, Higginson I (2008) Palliative care: the magnitude of the problem. In Mitchell G (ed.), (2008) *Palliative Care: A patient centered approach*. Abingdon, Radcliffe Publishing, 7–34.

Kyle G (2007) Constipation and palliative care – where are we now? *International Journal of Palliative Nursing*, **13**(1), 6–16.

Li S and Arber A (2006) The construction of troubled and credible patients: a study of emotion talk in palliative care settings. *Qualitative Health Research*, **16**(1), 27–46.

Machin L (2009) *Working with Loss and Grief*. London, Sage.

Mann E M and Carr E C J (2009) *Pain: Creative Approaches to Effective Management* (2nd edn). Basingstoke, Palgrave Macmillan.

McCaffery M (1979) *Nursing Management of the Patient with Pain*. Philadelphia, PA, Lippincott.

Metcalfe A, Werrett J, Burgess L and Clifford C (2007) Psychosocial impact of the lack of information given at referral about familial risk for cancer. *Psycho-oncology*, **16**, 458–465.

NICE (2006) *Guidance on Cancer Services: Improving outcomes for people with skin tumours including melanoma: the manual*. London, National Collaborating Centre for Cancer.

ONS (2010) *Cancer Statistics Registration*, series MB1 No 39, London, Office for National Statistics, available at: http://www.ons.gov.uk/ons/rel/vsob1/cancer-statistics-registrations--england--series-mb1-/no--39--2008/index.html (accessed September 2011).

Poole K and Froggatt K (2002) Loss of weight and loss of appetite in advanced cancer: a problem for the patient, the carer or health professional? *Palliative Medicine*, **16**(6), 499–506.

Randall J and Ream E (2005) Hair loss with chemotherapy: at a loss over its management? *European Journal of Cancer Care*, **14**, 223–231.

Reid J, McKenna H, Fitzsimmons D and McCance T (2009) The experience of cancer cachexia: a qualitative study of advanced cancer patients and their family members. *International Journal of Nursing Studies*, **46**, 606–616.

Sepulveda C, Marln A, Yoshida T and Ullrich A (2002) Palliative Care: the World Health Organization's global perspective. *Journal of Pain and Symptom Management*, **24**(2), 91–96.

Silverman J, Kurtz S M and Draper J (2005) *Skills for Communicating with Patients*. Abingdon, Radcliffe Publishing.

Stone P C and Minton O (2008) Cancer related fatigue. *European Journal of Cancer*, **44**, 1097–1104.

Tadman M and Roberts D (2007) *Oxford Handbook of Cancer Nursing*. Oxford, Oxford University Press.

Watson M, Lucas C and Hoy A (2006) *Adult Palliative Care Guidance* (2nd edn). South West London, Surrey, West Sussex & Hampshire, Mount Vernon & Sussex Cancer Networks & Northern Ireland Palliative Medicine Group.

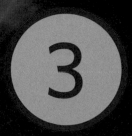

3

Caring for people with altered fluid, electrolyte, acid–base balance and shock

Learning outcomes

- Describe the functions and regulatory mechanisms that maintain water and electrolyte balance in the body.

- Compare and contrast the causes, effects and care of the person with fluid and electrolyte imbalance.

- Explain the pathophysiology of electrolyte imbalance.

- Discuss the risk factors, aetiologies and pathophysiologies of hypovolaemic, cardiogenic, obstructive and distributive shocks.

- Use the nursing process as a framework for providing individualised care to persons experiencing fluid and electrolyte imbalance and shock.

Clinical competencies

- Assess and monitor fluid and electrolyte for assigned persons.

- Determine priority nursing diagnoses, based on assessment data, to select and implement individualised nursing interventions.

- Provide person and family teaching about diet and medications used to restore, promote and maintain fluid and **electrolytes**.

- Integrate interdisciplinary care into care of persons with altered fluid and electrolyte.

CASE STUDIES

Below are three case studies that you may wish to consider before, during or after you have read the chapter. There are no right or wrong answers to these case studies, but you should think about the physical, psychological and social implications. Also consider what questions you would ask the person so that you can help alleviate their anxieties.

Case Study 1 – Martha

Mrs Martha Spearman, a 67-year-old female, with a three-day history of abdominal pain, abdominal bloating and **nausea** and **vomiting**, came to the Accident and Emergency department. Mrs Spearman is not tolerating any liquid or solids. She moved from South Africa to join her grandson and his family only two months ago. Mrs Spearman speaks very little English. All information was obtained through her grandson. Her grandson stated that his grandmother was treated for inflamed pancreas in South Africa. This condition occurred after her gallbladder was removed. Although Mrs Spearman is happy to be with her grandson, she feels lonely and misses her life in South Africa. She says that she does not like the food and climate over here. She is a very active lady but feels that she is unable to do things she used to do.

Case Study 2 – Suresh

Mr Suresh Joshi, a 48-year-old man, went to see his GP complaining of severe back pain, nausea and vomiting. Mr Joshi described his pain as 'a horse kicking me on my back. I feel sick and vomit a lot. I cannot eat or drink any water because of the pain'. His wife, who accompanied him to the doctor, stated that her husband did not sleep in the night and she found him crying in bed. He has taken all kinds of home remedies but nothing helps. Mr Joshi was doubled up with pain in the surgery and his GP found it difficult to communicate or examine him.

Case Study 3 – May Sew

Mr Tan May Sew is a 70-year-old Chinese gentleman who collapsed on the road while walking with his wife. A passerby stopped to help and called for an ambulance to take Mr Tan to the local hospital. In the Accident and Emergency department, Mr Tan was examined by the student nurse who found that Mr Tan was breathless and finding it difficult to breathe and that his bladder was distended and he was in lots of pain. The student nurse also observed that both his legs were swollen and that he had very little sensation to touch. In agony Mr Tan cried out, 'I want to pass water.' The student nurse also noticed some blood in his underpants.

INTRODUCTION

Fluid and electrolytes are essential for body function and to maintain homeostasis. Fluid and electrolytes are not stationary in the body. There is constant movement of fluid and electrolytes between the **intracellular** and **extracellular compartments**. The movement of fluid and electrolytes ensures that the cells are constantly supplied with electrolytes such as sodium, chloride, potassium, magnesium, phosphates, bicarbonate and calcium for cellular function. Nurses are in the forefront to deliver high-quality care for persons and therefore they should recognise subtle changes of fluid and electrolytes that may cause harm to the person. Changes in the movement of fluid and electrolytes between compartments occur as a result of disease. This chapter will consider fluid and electrolyte balance and some diseases resulting from fluid and electrolyte imbalance.

Body fluid compartments

The fluid in the body forms approximately 60% of the body weight in an adult male, 50% in an adult female and 70% in an infant. The percentage of fluid distribution varies with age and gender. Women have less body fluid compared to men as women have more body fat and men have more muscle mass. Fat cells contain less water compared to muscle cells.

The two principal body fluid compartments are intracellular and extracellular. The intracellular compartment is the space inside a cell and the fluid inside the cell is called intracellular fluid (ICF). The extracellular compartment is found outside the cell and the fluid outside the cell is called extracellular fluid (ECF). However, the extracellular compartment is further divided into the **interstitial** compartment and the intravascular compartment (see Figure 3.1). Two thirds of body fluid is found inside the cell and one third of the fluid outside the cell. Eighty per cent

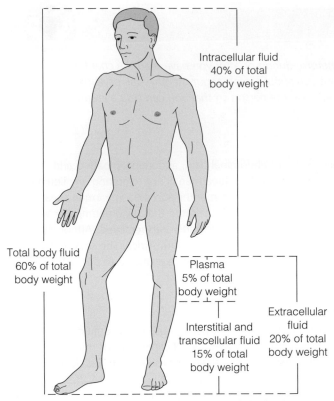

Figure 3.1 The major fluid compartments of the body.

of the ECF is found in the interstitial compartment and 20% in the intravascular compartment as **plasma** (see Figure 3.2).

COMPOSITION OF BODY FLUID

The body fluid is composed of water and dissolved substances such as electrolytes (sodium, potassium and chloride), gases (oxygen and carbon dioxide), nutrients, enzymes and hormones. Water is essential for the body as it:

- acts as a lubricant;
- transports nutrients, gases such as oxygen, hormones and enzymes to the cells and waste products of **metabolism**, for example, carbon dioxide, urea and uric acid from the cells for excretion;
- helps in the regulation of body temperature;
- provides an optimum medium for the cells to function;
- provides a medium for chemical reactions;
- breaks down food particles in the digestive system.

BODY FLUID BALANCE

The term fluid balance indicates that the body's required amount of water is present and distributed proportionally among the compartments. Generally, water intake equals water loss and

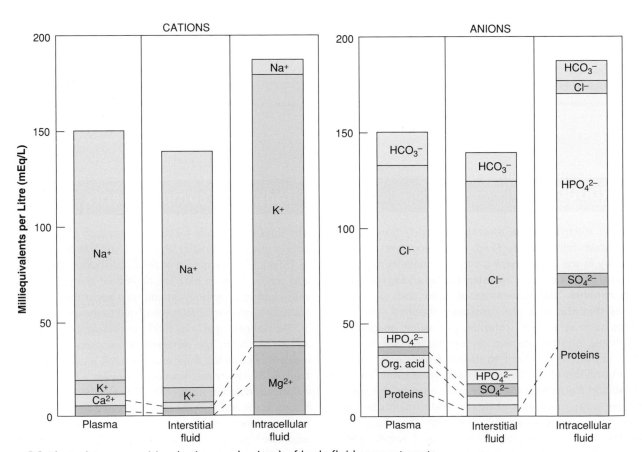

Figure 3.2 Electrolyte composition (cations and anions) of body fluid compartments.

Table 3.1 Fluid intake and output

	Intake		Output
Drinking	1500–2000 ml	Urine	1500–2000 ml
Water from food	700–1000 ml	Faeces	100 ml
Cellular metabolism	300–400 ml	Expiration	600–800 ml
		Skin	300–600 ml
Total balance	2500–3400 ml		2500–3400 ml

the body fluid remains constant. However, fluid intake varies with individuals; but the body regulates fluid volume to maintain homeostasis. Most of the water essential for body function is obtained from drinking water, some from the food consumed and some from cellular metabolism. The kidneys play a vital role in fluid balance as water is excreted in the urine. Some water is lost in respiration, through the skin and in faeces. See Table 3.1 for fluid intake and output.

OSMOSIS

Osmosis is a process by which water moves from an area of high volume to an area of low volume through a selective permeable membrane. The selective permeable membrane will allow water molecules to move across but is not permeable to solutes such as sodium, potassium and other substances. Water accounts for the **osmotic pressure** in tissues and cells of the body. Water movement between the intracellular and the extracellular compartments occurs through osmosis (see Figure 3.3).

ELECTROLYTES

Electrolytes are chemical compounds that dissociate in water to form charged particles called ions. They include potassium (K), sodium (Na), chloride (Cl), magnesium (Mg) and phosphate (HPO_4). The composition of electrolytes differs between the intracellular and the extracellular compartments (see Figure 3.2).

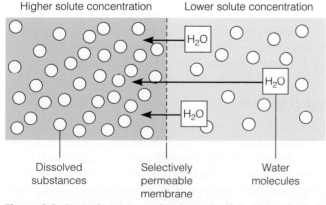

Figure 3.3 Osmosis. Water molecules move through a selectively permeable membrane from an area of low solute concentration to an area of high solute concentration.

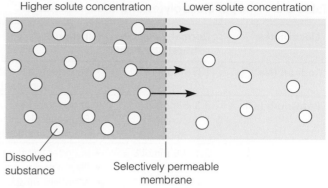

Figure 3.4 Diffusion. Solute molecules move through a selectively permeable membrane from an area of high solute concentration to an area of low solute concentration.

Functions of the electrolytes

Electrolytes have numerous functions in the body. They:

● regulate fluid balance;
● regulate acid–base balance;
● are essential in neuromuscular excitability;
● are essential for neuronal function;
● are essential for enzyme reaction.

See Table 3.2 for a summary of the principal electrolytes and their functions.

DIFFUSION

Diffusion describes the movement of particles from regions of higher concentration to regions of lower concentration. Solutes such as sodium, potassium, urea and uric acid move from an area of high concentration to an area of low concentration (see Figure 3.4). Diffusion is further subdivided into simple and facilitated diffusion. Liquid soluble molecules and gases move by a process of simple diffusion through a concentration gradient while larger molecules such as glucose and amino acids are transported across cell membrane by facilitated diffusion.

When there is severe loss of fluid and electrolytes all the organs of the body are affected. The heart is unable to pump enough blood to the organs, which can cause many organs to stop working. Now let us consider the different types of shock.

Acid–base balance

Homeostasis and optimal cellular function require maintenance of the hydrogen ion (H^+) concentration of body fluids within a relatively narrow range. Hydrogen ions determine the relative acidity of body fluids. Acids release hydrogen ions in solution; bases (or alkalis) accept hydrogen ions in solution. The hydrogen ion concentration of a solution is measured as its pH. The relationship between hydrogen ion concentration

Table 3.2 Principal electrolytes and their functions

Electrolytes	Normal values in extracellular fluid	Function	Main distribution
Sodium (Na^+)	135–145 mmol/L	• Important cation in generation of action potentials. • Plays an important role in fluid and electrolyte balance.	Main cation of the extracellular fluid.
Potassium (K^+)	3.5–5 mmol/L	• Important cation in establishing resting membrane potential. • Regulates pH balance. • Maintains intracellular fluid volume.	Main cation of the intracellular fluid.
Calcium (Ca^{2+})	2.1–2.6 mmol/L	• Important clotting factor. • Plays a part in neurotransmitter release in neurons. • Maintains muscle tone and excitability of nervous and muscle tissue.	Mainly found in the extracellular fluid.
Magnesium (Mg^{2+})	0.5–1.0 mmol/L	• Helps to maintain normal nerve and muscle function, maintain regular heart rate, regulate blood glucose and blood pressure. • Essential for protein synthesis.	Mainly distributed in the intracellular fluid.
Chloride (Cl^-)	98–117 mmol/L	• Maintains a balance of **anions** in different fluid compartments.	Main anion of the extracellular fluid.
Hydrocarbons (HCO_3^-)	24–31 mmol/L	• Main buffer of hydrogen ions in plasma. • Maintains a balance between **cations** and anions of intracellular and extracellular fluids.	Mainly distributed in the extracellular fluid.
Phosphate – organic (HPO_4^{2-})	0.8–1.1 mmol/L	• Essential for the digestion of proteins, carbohydrates and fats and absorption of calcium. • Essential for bone formation.	Mainly found in the intracellular fluid.
Sulphate (SO_4^{2-})	0.5 mmol/L	• Involved in **detoxification** of phenols, alcohols and **amines**.	Mainly found in the intracellular fluid.

and pH is inverse; that is, as hydrogen ion concentration increases, the pH falls and the solution becomes more acidic. As hydrogen ion concentration falls, the pH rises and the solution becomes more alkaline or basic. The pH of body fluids is slightly alkaline, with the normal pH ranging from 7.35–7.45 (a pH of 7 is neutral).

REGULATION OF ACID–BASE BALANCE

A number of mechanisms work together to maintain the pH of the body within this normal range. Metabolic processes in the body continuously produce acids, which fall into two categories: volatile acids and non-volatile acids. Volatile acids can be eliminated from the body as a gas. Carbonic acid (H_2CO_3) is the only volatile acid produced in the body. It dissociates (separates) into carbon dioxide (CO_2) and water (H_2O); the carbon dioxide is then eliminated from the body through the lungs. All other acids produced in the body are non-volatile acids that must be metabolised or excreted from the body in fluid. Lactic acid, hydrochloric acid, phosphoric acid and sulphuric acid are examples of non-volatile acids. Most acids and bases in the body are weak; that is, they neither release nor accept a significant amount of hydrogen ions.

Buffer systems

Buffers are substances that prevent major changes in pH by removing or releasing hydrogen ions. When excess acid is present in body fluid, buffers bind with hydrogen ions to minimise the change in pH. If body fluids become too basic or alkaline, buffers release hydrogen ions, restoring the pH. Although buffers act within a fraction of a second, their capacity to maintain pH is limited. The major buffer systems of the body are the bicarbonate–carbonic acid buffer system, phosphate buffer system and protein buffers.

Respiratory systems

The respiratory system (and the respiratory centre of the brain) regulates carbonic acid in the body by eliminating or retaining carbon dioxide. Carbon dioxide is a potential acid; when combined with water, it forms carbonic acid, a volatile acid. Acute increases in either carbon dioxide or hydrogen ions in the blood stimulate the respiratory centre in the brain. As a result, both the rate and depth of respiration increase.

Renal system

The renal system is responsible for the long-term regulation of acid–base balance in the body. Excess non-volatile acids produced during metabolism normally are eliminated by the kidneys. The kidneys also regulate bicarbonate levels in ECF by regenerating bicarbonate ions as well as reabsorbing them in the renal tubules. Although the kidneys respond more slowly to changes in pH (over hours to days), they can generate bicarbonate and selectively excrete or retain hydrogen ions as needed.

Acidosis and alkalosis

Disorders of acid–base balance are primarily respiratory or metabolic in origin. Respiratory acidosis is caused by a buildup of carbon dioxide in the body. It is caused by primary disorders of the respiratory tract or other conditions affecting the respiratory centre. Respiratory alkalosis, on the other hand, results from an anxiety attack whereby the person hyperventilates resulting in the excess removal of carbon dioxide from the body.

Metabolic acidosis is as a result of low pH and low levels of bicarbonate ions. Metabolic alkalosis, by contrast, occurs when there is an excess of bicarbonate ions. The pH then rises above 7.45. The management of these conditions depends on identifying and treating the underlying cause.

Shock

TYPES OF SHOCK

Any condition that leads to a reduction in cardiac output can lead to circulatory shock; consequently the effects of shock are not limited to one organ system and can be considered to be a general systemic reaction. For multisystem effects of shock see Figure 3.5. However, shock is typically classified by its causative factors and includes the following.

Hypovolaemic shock

Hypovolaemic shock is the most common type of shock and occurs as a result of fluid loss, including blood loss, plasma loss and/or loss of interstitial fluid. Blood can be lost from a bleeding organ or wound; however, the circulating volume can also be reduced as a result of plasma loss, e.g. from extensive burns or damaged tissues, or excessive loss of fluids from either renal impairment or inadequate fluid intake, e.g. **dehydration**. This loss of fluid leads to a reduction in circulatory fluid in the blood vessels leading to insufficient quantities of blood returning to the heart. This poor venous return results in a decrease in cardiac output and subsequent decrease in blood pressure leading to a decrease in tissue perfusion resulting in impaired cellular metabolism and shock. Figure 3.6 outlines the physiological events leading to hypovolaemic shock.

Physiologically, hypovolaemic shock is divided into three stages:

1. *Compensated shock* is when baroreceptor reflexes result in increase in myocardial contractility, tachycardia and vasoconstriction. They maintain cardiac output and blood pressure and lead to the release of antidiuretic hormone (ADH), aldosterone and renin.
2. *Progressive or uncompensated shock* occurs with myocardial depression, failure of vasomotor reflexes and failure of the microcirculation, with increase in capillary permeability,

sludging and thrombosis, resulting in cellular dysfunction and lactic acidosis.
3. *Irreversible shock* means failure of vital organs with inability to recover.

Cardiogenic and obstructive shock

Cardiogenic shock occurs when the heart 'fails' as a pump, resulting in abnormal cardiac functioning. Obstructive shock happens when a mechanical or physical obstruction impedes the flow of blood, e.g. a pulmonary embolism or tension pneumothorax.

Distributive shock

The next three types of shock (septic, neurogenic and anaphylactic) are collectively known as distributive shock in which (irrespective of the causative factors) widespread vasodilatation and decreased peripheral vascular resistance are a common feature. This type of shock differs from hypovolaemic shock in that the circulating blood volume remains normal.

Septic shock

Septic shock is a life-threatening condition that occurs when a person's blood pressure drops to a dangerously low level (severe hypotension). The fall in blood pressure is a reaction to a serious bacterial infection that develops in the blood, causing an inflammatory response from the body that is known as sepsis. If sepsis is not treated, it will lead to septic shock.

Neurogenic shock

Neurogenic shock is a type of shock caused by the sudden loss of the autonomic nervous system signals to the smooth muscle in vessel walls. This results in loss of background sympathetic stimulation, which is responsible for maintenance of tone of blood vessels. As a result of loss of vascular tone, the vessels suddenly relax resulting in a sudden decrease in peripheral vascular resistance and decreased blood pressure.

Anaphylactic shock

This form of shock (also known as anaphylaxis) occurs following a widespread allergic or hypersensitivity reaction to the presence of an allergen or antigen that can lead to severe circulatory collapse within seconds.

Anaphylactic shock does not occur with the first exposure to an allergen. With the first exposure to a foreign substance (the antigen), the body produces specific immunoglobulin E (IgE) antibodies against this antigen. The person is thus sensitised to that specific antigen. With subsequent exposure, the antigen reacts with the already formed IgE antibodies, disrupting cellular integrity. In addition, large amounts of histamine and other vasoactive amines are released and distributed through the circulatory system. These substances cause increased capillary permeability and massive vasodilation, resulting in profound hypotension and eventual vascular collapse.

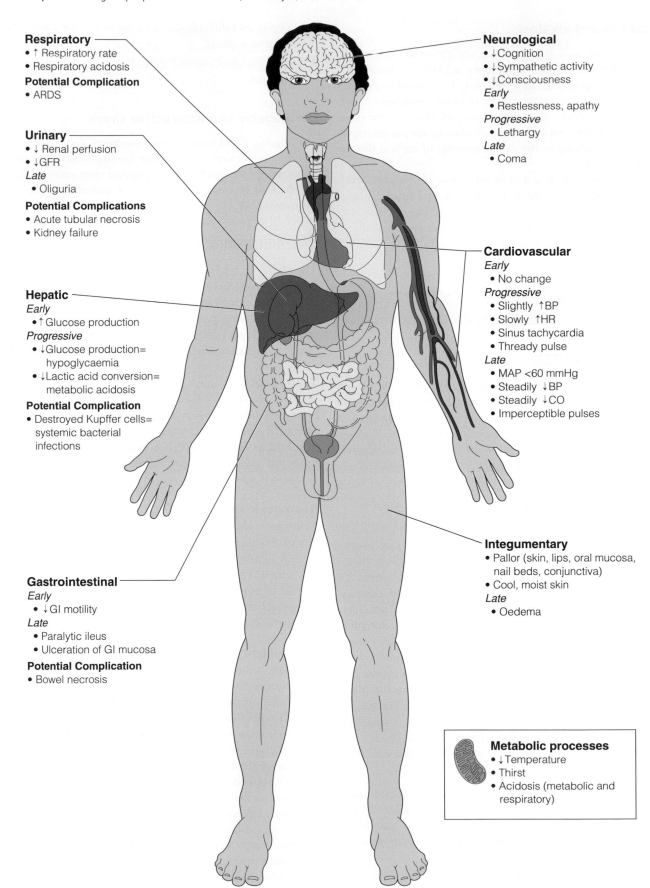

Respiratory
- ↑ Respiratory rate
- Respiratory acidosis

Potential Complication
- ARDS

Urinary
- ↓ Renal perfusion
- ↓GFR

Late
- Oliguria

Potential Complications
- Acute tubular necrosis
- Kidney failure

Hepatic
Early
- ↑Glucose production

Progressive
- ↓Glucose production=
  hypoglycaemia
- ↓Lactic acid conversion=
  metabolic acidosis

Potential Complication
- Destroyed Kupffer cells=
  systemic bacterial
  infections

Gastrointestinal
Early
- ↓GI motility

Late
- Paralytic ileus
- Ulceration of GI mucosa

Potential Complication
- Bowel necrosis

Neurological
- ↓Cognition
- ↓Sympathetic activity
- ↓Consciousness

Early
- Restlessness, apathy

Progressive
- Lethargy

Late
- Coma

Cardiovascular
Early
- No change

Progressive
- Slightly ↑BP
- Slowly ↑HR
- Sinus tachycardia
- Thready pulse

Late
- MAP <60 mmHg
- Steadily ↓BP
- Steadily ↓CO
- Imperceptible pulses

Integumentary
- Pallor (skin, lips, oral mucosa,
  nail beds, conjunctiva)
- Cool, moist skin

Late
- Oedema

Metabolic processes
- ↓Temperature
- Thirst
- Acidosis (metabolic and
  respiratory)

Figure 3.5 Multisystem effects of shock.

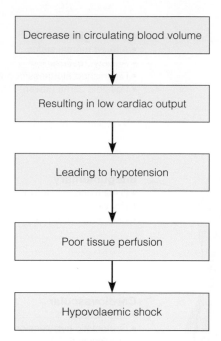

Figure 3.6 Hypovolaemic shock.

Anaphylactic shock begins and progresses rapidly. Symptoms may begin within 20 minutes of contact with an antigen. Unless appropriate intervention is provided, death can occur within a matter of minutes. Because anaphylaxis is rapid and potentially lethal, persons with known allergies should carry some form of warning (such as a Medic-Alert bracelet) informing others of their susceptibility. Nurses should be extremely careful to assess and document all allergies or previous drug reactions in the nursing care plan.

Cellular homeostasis and haemodynamics

To maintain cellular metabolism, cells of all body organs and tissues require a regular and consistent supply of oxygen and the removal of metabolic wastes. This homeostatic regulation is maintained primarily by the cardiovascular system and depends on four physiologic components:

- a cardiac output sufficient to meet bodily requirements;
- an uncompromised vascular system, in which the vessels have a diameter sufficient to allow unimpeded blood flow and have good tone (the ability to constrict or dilate to maintain normal pressure);
- a volume of blood sufficient to fill the circulatory system and a blood pressure adequate to maintain blood flow;
- tissues that are able to extract and use the oxygen delivered through the capillaries.

In a healthy person, these components function as a system to maintain tissue perfusion. During shock, however, one or more of these components is disrupted. An understanding of basic haemodynamics is necessary to understand the pathophysiology of shock:

- Stroke volume (SV) is the amount of blood pumped into the aorta with each contraction of the left ventricle.
- Cardiac output (CO) is the amount of blood pumped per minute into the aorta by the left ventricle. CO is determined by multiplying the stroke volume (SV) by the heart rate (HR): $CO = SV \times HR$.
- Mean arterial pressure (MAP) is the product of cardiac output and systemic vascular resistance (SVR): $MAP = CO \times SVR$. When CO, SVR or total blood volume rises, MAP and tissue perfusion increase. Conversely, when CO, SVR or total blood volume falls, MAP and tissue perfusion decrease.
- The sympathetic nervous system maintains the smooth muscle surrounding the arteries and arterioles in a state of partial contraction called *sympathetic tone*. Increased sympathetic stimulation increases vasoconstriction and SVR; decreased sympathetic stimulation allows vasodilatation, which decreases SVR.

Now let us consider some of the common problems associated with fluid and electrolyte balance.

DISORDERS OF FLUID BALANCE

The person with fluid volume deficit (FVD)

FVD is a decrease in intravascular, interstitial and/or intracellular fluid in the body. Fluid volume deficits may be due to excessive fluid losses, insufficient fluid intake or failure of regulatory mechanisms and fluid shifts within the body. FVD is a relatively common problem that may exist alone or in combination with other electrolyte or acid–base imbalances. The term *dehydration* refers to loss of water alone, even though it is often used interchangeably with fluid volume deficit. For the effects of FVD on systems, see Figure 3.7.

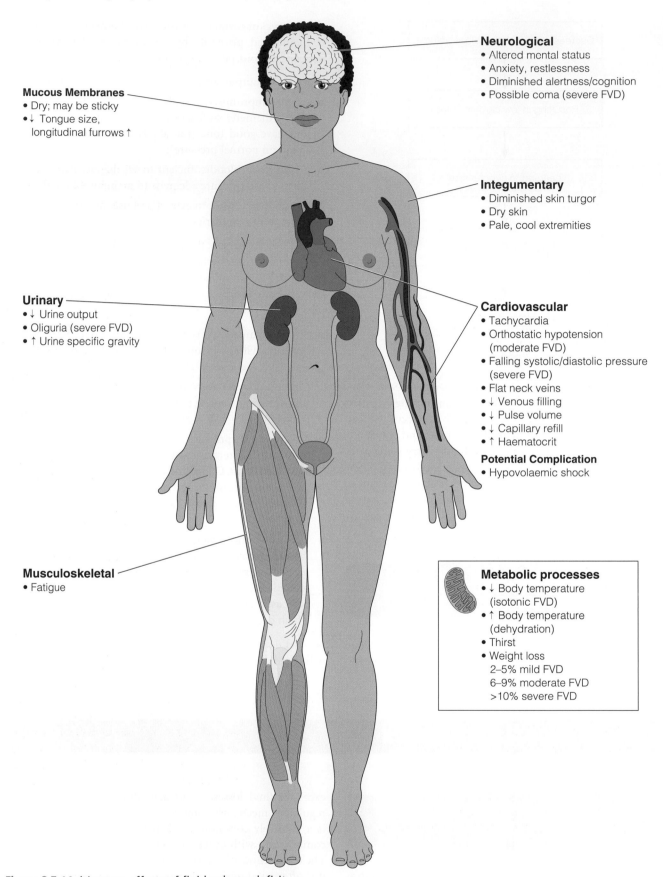

Neurological
- Altered mental status
- Anxiety, restlessness
- Diminished alertness/cognition
- Possible coma (severe FVD)

Mucous Membranes
- Dry; may be sticky
- ↓ Tongue size, longitudinal furrows ↑

Integumentary
- Diminished skin turgor
- Dry skin
- Pale, cool extremities

Urinary
- ↓ Urine output
- Oliguria (severe FVD)
- ↑ Urine specific gravity

Cardiovascular
- Tachycardia
- Orthostatic hypotension (moderate FVD)
- Falling systolic/diastolic pressure (severe FVD)
- Flat neck veins
- ↓ Venous filling
- ↓ Pulse volume
- ↓ Capillary refill
- ↑ Haematocrit

Potential Complication
- Hypovolaemic shock

Musculoskeletal
- Fatigue

Metabolic processes
- ↓ Body temperature (isotonic FVD)
- ↑ Body temperature (dehydration)
- Thirst
- Weight loss
  2–5% mild FVD
  6–9% moderate FVD
  >10% severe FVD

Figure 3.7 Multisystem effects of fluid volume deficit.

FAST FACTS

FVD

- Water loss of as little as 1–2% impairs cognition and physical performance.
- Loss of 7% of body water can lead to circulatory collapse.
- Dehydration is one of the ten most common hospital admitting diagnoses for older adults.

PATHOPHYSIOLOGY OF FVD

The most common cause of FVD is excessive loss of gastro-intestinal fluids from vomiting, diarrhoea, gastrointestinal suctioning, intestinal fistulas and intestinal drainage. Other causes of fluid losses include:

- excessive renal losses of water and sodium from diuretic therapy, renal disorders or endocrine disorders;
- water and sodium losses during sweating from excessive exercise or increased environmental temperature;
- haemorrhage;
- chronic abuse of laxatives and/or enemas.

Inadequate fluid intake may result from lack of access to fluids, inability to request or to swallow fluids, oral trauma or altered thirst mechanisms. The elderly are at particular risk for FVD. Fluid volume deficit can develop slowly or rapidly, depending on the type of fluid loss. Electrolytes are often lost along with fluid, resulting in an **isotonic** FVD. When both water and electrolytes are lost, the serum sodium level remains normal, although levels of other electrolytes such as potassium may fall. Fluid is drawn into the vascular compartment from the interstitial spaces as the body attempts to maintain tissue perfusion. This eventually depletes fluid in the intracellular compartment as well.

Third spacing

Third spacing is a shift of fluid from the vascular space into an area where it is not available for normal fluid exchange. The trapped fluid represents a volume loss and is unavailable for normal physiologic processes. Fluid may be sequestered in the abdomen or bowel or in such other actual or potential body spaces as the pleural or peritoneal space. Fluid may also become trapped within soft tissues following trauma or burns.

Assessing the extent of FVD resulting from third spacing is difficult. It may not be reflected by changes in weight or intake-and-output records, and it may not become apparent until after organ malfunction occurs.

SIGNS AND SYMPTOMS OF FVD

Signs and symptoms of FVD include:

- hypovolaemia;
- weight loss;
- loss of skin turgor (elasticity);
- hypotension;
- tachycardia;
- pale appearance;
- low urine output.

Tongue turgor is not generally affected by age; therefore, assessing the size, dryness and longitudinal furrows of the tongue may be a more accurate indicator of FVD.

INTERDISCIPLINARY CARE FOR FVD

Oral rehydration

Oral rehydration is the safest and most effective treatment for fluid volume deficit in alert persons who are able to take oral fluids. Adults require a minimum of 1500 mL of fluid per day or approximately 30 mL per kg of body weight (ideal body weight is used to calculate fluid requirements for obese persons) for maintenance. Fluids are replaced gradually, particularly in older adults (to prevent rapid rehydration of the cells). In general, fluid deficits are replaced at a rate of approximately 30–50% of the deficit per 24 hours.

For mild fluid deficits in which the loss of electrolytes has been minimal (e.g., moderate exercise in warm weather), water alone may be used for fluid replacement. When the fluid deficit is more severe and when electrolytes have also been lost (for example, FVD due to vomiting and/or diarrhoea, strenuous exercise for longer than an hour or two), a carbohydrate/electrolyte solution such as a sports drink or a rehydrating solution is more appropriate. These solutions provide sodium, potassium, chloride and calories to help meet metabolic needs.

Intravenous therapy

When the fluid deficit is severe or the person is unable to ingest fluids, the intravenous route is used to administer replacement fluids. Isotonic electrolyte solutions (0.9% NaCl or Ringer's solution) are used to expand plasma volume in hypotensive persons or to replace abnormal losses, which are usually isotonic in nature. Normal saline (0.9% NaCl) tends to remain in the vascular compartment, increasing blood volume. When administered rapidly, however, this solution can precipitate acid–base imbalances, so balanced electrolyte solutions such as lactated Ringer's solution are preferred to expand plasma volume.

Case Study 2 – Suresh

Now, look at Suresh in Case Study 2. He is unable to eat or drink as a result of severe pain. What you also need to bear in mind is that Mr Joshi may vomit as a result of his pain.

Therefore, he is going to lose fluid and electrolytes, which could result in dehydration and other health risks such as urinary tract infection and hypotension. Think about the types of fluid required and how these will be administered to Mr Joshi.

NURSING CARE FOR FVD

Nurses are responsible for identifying persons at risk for FVD, initiating and carrying out measures to prevent and treat FVD and monitoring the effects of therapy. The aim in FVD is to identify the cause of FVD and replace the fluid loss.

Health promotion

Health promotion activities focus on teaching persons to prevent FVD. Discuss the importance of maintaining adequate fluid intake, particularly when exercising and during hot weather. Advise persons to use commercial sports drinks to replace both water and electrolytes when exercising during warm weather. Advise persons to maintain fluid intake when ill, particularly during periods of fever or when diarrhoea is a problem.

Discuss the increased risk for FVD with older adults and provide information about prevention. Advise the elderly (and their caregivers) that thirst decreases with ageing and urge them to maintain a regular fluid intake of about 1500 mL per day, regardless of perception of thirst.

Carefully monitor persons at risk for abnormal fluid losses through routes such as vomiting, diarrhoea, nasogastric suction, increased urine output, fever or wounds. Monitor fluid intake in persons with decreased level of consciousness, disorientation, nausea and anorexia, and physical limitations.

> ### Consider this . . .
> If a large volume of fluid, say one litre, is trapped in the third space, such as the peritoneal or pleural cavities, does it mean that the person is overhydrated or dehydrated? Think about fluid movement between compartments.

The person with fluid volume excess (FVE)

FVE results when both water and sodium are retained in the body. It may be caused by fluid overload (excess water and sodium intake) or by impairment of the mechanisms that maintain homeostasis. The excess fluid can lead to excess intravascular fluid (hypervolaemia) and excess interstitial fluid (**oedema**).

PATHOPHYSIOLOGY OF FVE

Fluid volume excess usually results from conditions that cause retention of both sodium and water. These conditions include heart failure, cirrhosis of the liver, renal failure, adrenal gland

IN PRACTICE

FVD will arise when the person's fluid intake is less than fluid loss. The effects are more acute in the elderly than in a younger adult. The elderly may suffer from conditions such as arthritis or other illnesses that may prevent them from drinking adequate amounts of fluid. Nurses need to be aware that sometimes symptoms of FVD may not be detected until it is quite severe. Thus nurses need to use a wide range of skills to detect significant change before it becomes a problem for the person. These include:

- utilising their knowledge in how the fluid is distributed in the body and recognising some of the symptoms of dehydration;
- obtaining a comprehensive nursing history from the person or their relatives;
- having the knowledge in the different types of fluid used to treat FVD so that they can evaluate the effectiveness of the fluid treatment;
- being able to plan, implement and evaluate nursing care as the condition of the person changes;
- Communicating effectively during handover and reporting any changes with the person so that prompt action can be taken.

disorders, corticosteroid administration and stress conditions causing the release of ADH and aldosterone. Other causes include an excessive intake of sodium-containing foods, drugs that cause sodium retention, and the administration of excess amounts of sodium-containing intravenous fluids (such as 0.9% NaCl or Ringer's solution). This iatrogenic (induced by the effects of treatment) cause of FVE primarily affects persons with impaired regulatory mechanisms.

Stress responses activated before, during and immediately after surgery commonly lead to increased ADH and aldosterone levels, leading to sodium and water retention. In the immediate post-operative period, however, this additional fluid tends to be sequestered in interstitial tissues and unavailable to support cardiovascular and renal function (see 'Third spacing' section on page 79). This sequestered fluid is reabsorbed into the circulation within about 48–72 hours after surgery. Although it is then normally eliminated through a process of diuresis, persons with heart or kidney failure are at risk for developing fluid overload. Conditions such as heart failure and chronic renal failure could result in fluid overload as these organs are not able to get rid of excess fluid from the body which could lead to multisystem failure.

PRACTICE ALERT

Critically ill persons are at higher risk for fluid and electrolyte imbalance. Careful monitoring of the critically ill person is vital.

Signs and symptoms of FVE

Excess extracellular fluid leads to hypervolaemia and circulatory overload. Excess fluid in the interstitial space causes peripheral or generalised oedema. The following symptoms of FVE relate to both the excess fluid and its effects on circulation. Circulatory overload causes symptoms such as:

- distended neck and peripheral veins;
- increased central venous pressure (>11–12 cm of water);
- cough, dyspnoea (laboured or difficult breathing), orthopnoea (difficulty breathing when supine);
- moist crackles (rales) in the lungs – pulmonary oedema (excess fluid in pulmonary interstitial spaces and alveoli) if severe;
- increased urine output (polyuria);
- ascites (excess fluid in the peritoneal cavity);
- peripheral oedema;
- possible cerebral oedema (excess fluid in brain tissues) which can lead to altered mental status and anxiety.

INTERDISCIPLINARY CARE FOR FVE

Medication

Diuretics are commonly used to treat FVE. Diuretics are medicines that remove water from the body by increasing the amount of urine the kidneys produce. They are often known as 'water tablets' because they remove excess water. Medications such as bendroflumethiazide, furosemide and amiloride are some of the diuretics that may be used to treat FVE.

Fluid and dietary management

Fluid intake may be restricted in persons who have FVE. The amount of fluid allowed per day is prescribed by the primary care provider. All fluid intakes must be calculated, including meals, and the information used to administer medications orally or intravenously.

A mild sodium restriction can be achieved by instructing the person and primary food preparer in the household to reduce the amount of salt in recipes by half, avoid using the salt cellar during meals and avoid foods that contain high levels of sodium (either naturally or because of processing). In moderate and severely sodium-restricted diets, salt is avoided altogether, as are all foods containing significant amounts of sodium.

NURSING CARE FOR FVE

Health promotion

Health promotion related to FVE focuses on teaching preventive measures to persons who are at risk (for example, persons who have heart or kidney failure). Discuss the relationship between sodium intake and water retention. Provide guidelines for a low-sodium diet, and teach persons to carefully read food labels to identify 'hidden' sodium, particularly in processed foods. Instruct persons at risk to weigh themselves on a regular basis, using the same scales, and to notify their primary care provider if they gain more than 5 lb in a week or less.

Nursing care focuses on preventing FVE in persons at risk and on managing problems resulting from its effects. Carefully monitor persons receiving intravenous fluids for signs of hypervolaemia. Reduce the flow rate and promptly report symptoms of fluid overload to the doctor.

Nursing diagnoses and interventions

Nursing care for the person with FVE includes collaborative interventions such as administering diuretics and maintaining a fluid restriction, as well as monitoring the status and effects of the FVE. This is particularly critical in older persons because of the age-related decline in cardiac and renal compensatory responses.

Risk for excess fluid volume

✦ Assess vital signs, heart sounds, central venous pressure and volume of peripheral arteries. *Hypervolaemia can cause hypertension, bounding peripheral pulses, a third heart sound (S3) due to the volume of blood flow through the heart and high central venous pressure (CVP) readings.*

✦ Assess for the presence and extent of oedema, particularly in the lower extremities, the back, sacral and periorbital areas. *Oedema in lower extremities can lead to complications such as poor circulation to the legs and development of pressure sores.*

> ### PRACTICE ALERT
>
> Assess urine output hourly and maintain accurate intake and output records. Note urine output of less than 30 mL per hour or a positive fluid balance on 24-hour total intake and output calculations. Heart failure and inadequate renal perfusion may result in decreased urine output and fluid retention.

✦ Obtain daily weights at the same time of day, using approximately the same clothing and a balanced scale. *Daily weights are one of the most important gauges of fluid balance. Acute weight gain or loss represents fluid gain or loss. Weight gain of 2 kg is equivalent to 2 L of fluid gain.*

✦ Administer oral fluids cautiously, adhering to any prescribed fluid restriction. Discuss the restriction with the person and their relatives, including the total volume allowed, the rationale and the importance of reporting all fluid taken. *All sources of fluid intake, including ice cubes, are recorded to avoid excess fluid intake.*

+ Provide oral hygiene at least every two hours. *Oral hygiene contributes to a person's comfort and keeps mucous membranes intact; it also helps relieve thirst if fluids are restricted.*

+ Teach the person and significant others about the sodium-restricted diet, and emphasise the importance of checking before bringing foods to the person. *Excess sodium promotes water retention; a sodium-restricted diet is ordered to reduce water gain.*

+ Administer prescribed diuretics as ordered, monitoring the person's response to therapy. *Loop or high-ceiling diuretics such as furosemide can lead to rapid fluid loss and signs of hypovolaemia and electrolyte imbalance.*

+ Promptly report significant changes in serum electrolytes or osmolality or abnormal results of tests done to determine contributing factors to the FVE. *Gradual correction of serum electrolytes and osmolality is expected; however, aggressive diuretic therapy can lead to over-correction.*

Risk for impaired skin integrity

Tissue oedema decreases oxygen and nutrient delivery to the skin and subcutaneous tissues, increasing the risk of injury.

+ Frequently assess skin, particularly in pressure areas and over bony prominences. *Skin breakdown can progress rapidly when circulation is impaired.*

+ Reposition the person at least every two hours. Provide skin care with each position change. *Frequent position changes minimise tissue pressure and promote blood flow to tissues.*

+ Provide a pressure relieving mattress or alternating pressure mattress and other devices to reduce pressure on tissues. *These devices, which distribute pressure away from bony prominences, reduce the risk of skin breakdown.*

Risk for impaired gas exchange

With FVE, gas exchange may be impaired by oedema of pulmonary interstitial tissues. Acute pulmonary oedema is a serious and potentially life-threatening complication of pulmonary congestion. As a nurse, you should:

+ Listen to the lungs for presence or worsening of crackles and wheezes; listen to the heart for extra heart sounds. *Crackles and wheezes indicate pulmonary congestion and oedema.*

+ Place the person in a semi-upright sitting position if dyspnoea or orthopnoea is present. *This position helps lung expansion by decreasing the pressure of abdominal contents on the diaphragm.*

+ Monitor oxygen saturation levels, using pulse oximetry and arterial blood gases (ABGs) for evidence of impaired gas exchange. Administer prescribed oxygen as indicated. *Oedema of interstitial lung tissues can interfere with gas exchange and delivery of oxygen to body tissues. Supplemental oxygen promotes gas exchange across the alveolar–capillary membrane, improving tissue oxygenation.*

Case Study 3 – May Sew
NURSING CARE PLAN FVE

Tan May Sew has been admitted to the Accident and Emergency department (A/E) after collapsing while walking with his wife. Now, let us consider the nursing care of Mr Tan.

Assessment

In A&E the doctor notices that Mr Tan has pulmonary oedema and that he is in early stages of heart failure. Mr Tan has only passed approximately 250 mL of urine and this low output has been constant for the past eight days. This diagnosis is confirmed by a 12 lead ECG rhythm of the heart.

During the nursing assessment, the student nurse notes the following:

+ BP 160/100 mmHg; P 102 beats per minute, with obvious neck vein distension; R 28 breaths per minute, with crackles and wheezes and T 36° Celsius.

+ Periorbital and sacral oedema present, skin cool, pale and shiny.

+ Alert oriented; responds appropriately to questions.

+ Person states he is thirsty, slightly nauseated and extremely tired.

Mr Tan is immediately prescribed oxygen to improve gas exchange, diuretics to get rid of excess fluid from the body and antihypertensives to lower his blood pressure.

Diagnosis

Persons with heart failure will need a full clinical assessment of cardiac functions such as cardiac output and a fluid and nutritional assessment. Investigations such as full blood count, blood urea and nitrogen levels and electrolyte levels are done to assess renal function and the effects of any medications that may be administered. Other tests that may be done for heart failure include:

+ exercise testing (to see how the heart performs under stress);

+ electrocardiograph (ECG);

+ chest x-ray;

+ echocardiograph (an ultrasound scan of the heart muscles and valves);

+ MRI (imaging technique);

+ coronary angiography (a dye is injected into the bloodstream so arteries can be seen on an x-ray).

Case Study 3 – May Sew

Medications

The following medications are used to treat heart failure.

+ *angiotensin converting enzyme inhibitors* which relax the muscles of the blood vessels and reduce the workload of the heart, helping to lower blood pressure;
+ *diuretics* to get rid of excess body fluid;
+ *cardiac glycosides* (such as digoxin) to strengthen and slow the heartbeat;
+ *cholesterol lowering medication* (lipid lowering drugs);
+ *beta blockers* which can be used to protect the heart muscle – they slow the heartbeat, improve the blood flow and help the heart pump effectively.

Nursing care

In FVE the aim is to remove excess fluid from the person and at the same time ensure that the person does not develop any complications such as hypotension as a result of the treatment. For detailed nursing care of heart failure see Chapter 9. Specific care for Mr Tan includes:

+ Weigh him daily to ensure that he is losing weight as a result of his treatment.
+ Take and record his vital signs every two to four hours. Changes in his vital signs should be reported immediately.
+ Measure intake and output every two hours and maintain a fluid balance chart.
+ Turn every two hours and inspect and provide skin care as needed.
+ Document all care provided for Mr Tan.
+ Use your verbal and non-verbal communication skills to assess the progress of the person.

Remember that rapid removal of fluid from the body can lead to complications such as dehydration, hypotension or urinary tract infection. Remember what you have learned about FVD. You need to monitor Mr Tan regularly and ensure that he is responding to the treatment well without complications.

Evaluation

At the end of the shift, the student nurse evaluates the effectiveness of the plan of care and continues all diagnoses and interventions. Mr Tan has gained no weight and his urinary output is 170 mL. His vital signs are unchanged, but his crackles and wheezes have decreased slightly. His skin and mucous membranes are intact. Mr Tan has sat in the bedside chair without dyspnoea or fatigue.

> **Consider this . . .**
> ● What is the pathophysiological basis for Mr Tan's increased respiratory rate, blood pressure and pulse?
> ● Explain how elevating the head of the bed 30 degrees facilitates respirations.
> ● Suppose Mr Tan says, 'I would really like to have all my fluids at once instead of spreading them out.' How would you reply, and why?
> ● Outline a plan for teaching Mr Tan about compliance to his prescribed medications.

DISORDERS OF ELECTROLYTE BALANCE

Where there is an imbalance, the aim is to restore the normal electrolyte levels in the person as soon as possible; otherwise it could prove to be a serious health risk for the person.

The person with sodium imbalance (hypernatraemia)

Sodium is the most plentiful electrolyte in the ECF, with normal serum sodium levels ranging from 135–145 mmol/L. Sodium is the primary regulator of the volume, osmolality and distribution of ECF. It also is important to maintain neuromuscular activity. Because of the close interrelationship between sodium and water balance, disorders of fluid volume and sodium balance often occur together. Sodium imbalances affect the osmolality of ECF and water distribution between the fluid compartments. When sodium levels are low (hyponatraemia), water is drawn into the cells of the body, causing them to swell. In contrast, high levels of sodium in ECF (hypernatraemia) draw water out of body cells, causing them to shrink.

PATHOPHYSIOLOGY OF HYPONATRAEMIA

Excess sodium loss can occur through the kidneys, gastrointestinal tract or skin. Diuretic medications, kidney diseases or adrenal insufficiency with impaired aldosterone and cortisol production can lead to excessive sodium excretion in urine. Vomiting, diarrhoea, excessive sweating, exercise and gastrointestinal aspirations are common causes of excess sodium loss through the gastrointestinal tract. Sodium may also be lost when gastrointestinal tubes are irrigated with water instead of saline, or when repeated tap water enemas are administered. Excessive sweating or loss of skin surface (as with an extensive burn) can also cause excessive sodium loss.

Some of the possible causes of hyponatraemia are:

- systemic diseases such as heart failure, renal failure or cirrhosis of the liver;
- syndrome of inappropriate secretion of antidiuretic hormone (SIADH), in which water excretion is impaired;
- excessive administration of **hypotonic** intravenous fluids.

Hyponatraemia causes a drop in serum osmolality. Water shifts from ECF into the intracellular space, causing cells to swell and reducing the osmolality of ICF. Many of the manifestations of hyponatraemia can be attributed to cellular oedema and hypo-osmolality.

SIGNS AND SYMPTOMS OF HYPONATRAEMIA

The manifestations of hyponatraemia depend on the rapidity of onset, the severity and the cause of the imbalance. If the condition develops slowly, manifestations are usually not experienced until the serum sodium levels reach 125 mmol/L. Symptoms include:

- nausea and vomiting;
- abdominal cramp;
- anorexia;
- diarrhoea.

As sodium levels continue to decrease, the brain and nervous system are affected by cellular oedema. Neurological manifestations progress rapidly when the serum sodium level falls below 120 mmol/L. The person may present with headache, depression, personality changes, irritability, lethargy, hyperreflexia, muscle twitching and tremors. If serum sodium falls to very low levels, convulsions and coma are likely to occur.

INTERDISCIPLINARY CARE FOR HYPONATRAEMIA

Medication

When both sodium and water have been lost (hyponatraemia with hypovolaemia), sodium-containing fluids are given to replace both water and sodium. These fluids may be given by mouth, nasogastric tube or intravenously. Isotonic Ringer's solution or isotonic saline (0.9% NaCl) solution may be administered. Cautious administration of intravenous 3% or 5% NaCl solution may be necessary in persons who have very low plasma sodium levels (110–115 mmol/L). Loop diuretics are administered to persons who have hyponatraemia with normal or excess ECF volume. Loop diuretics promote an isotonic diuresis and fluid volume loss without hyponatraemia. Thiazide diuretics are avoided because they cause a relatively greater sodium loss in relation to water loss.

Fluid and dietary management

If hyponatraemia is mild, increasing the intake of foods high in sodium such as ham and meat loaf may restore normal sodium balance. Fluids are often restricted to help reduce ECF volume and correct hyponatraemia.

NURSING CARE FOR HYPONATRAEMIA

Nursing care of the person with hyponatraemia focuses on identifying persons at risk and managing problems resulting from the systemic effects of the disorder.

Health promotion

People at risk for mild hyponatraemia include those who participate in activities that increase fluid loss through excessive perspiration (diaphoresis) and then replace those losses by drinking large amounts of water. This includes athletes, people who do heavy labour in high environmental temperatures and elderly living in non-air-conditioned settings during hot weather. Teach the following to persons who are at risk:

- ✚ symptoms of mild hyponatraemia, including nausea, abdominal cramps and muscle weakness;
- ✚ the importance of drinking liquids containing sodium and other electrolytes at frequent intervals when perspiring heavily, when environmental temperatures are high and/or if watery diarrhoea persists for several days.

Nursing diagnoses and interventions

Risk for imbalanced fluid volume

Because of its role in maintaining fluid balance, sodium imbalances are often accompanied by water imbalances. In addition, treatment of hyponatraemia can affect the person's fluid balance.

- ✚ Monitor intake and output, weigh daily and calculate 24-hour fluid balance. *Fluid excess or deficit may occur with hyponatraemia.*

PRACTICE ALERT

Carefully monitor persons receiving sodium-containing intravenous solutions for signs of increased blood pressure and CVP, tachypnoea, tachycardia, shortness of breath or crackles. **Hypertonic** saline solutions can lead to hypervolaemia, particularly in persons with cardiovascular or renal disease.

- ✚ Use an intravenous flow control device to administer hypertonic saline (3% and 5% NaCl) solutions; carefully monitor flow rate and response. *Hypertonic solutions can increase the risk of pulmonary and cerebral oedema due to water retention. Careful monitoring is vital to prevent these complications and possible permanent damage.*

✚ If fluids are restricted, explain the reason for the restriction, the amount of fluid allowed and how to calculate fluid intake.

Risk for ineffective cerebral tissue perfusion

The person with severe hyponatraemia experiences fluid shifts that cause an increase in ICF volume. This can cause brain cells to swell, increasing pressure within the cranial vault.

✚ Monitor serum electrolytes and serum osmolality. Report abnormal results to the nurse in charge. *As serum sodium levels fall, the manifestations and neurologic effects of hyponatraemia become increasingly severe.*

✚ Assess for neurological changes, such as lethargy, altered level of consciousness, confusion and convulsions. Monitor mental status and orientation. Compare baseline data with continuing assessments. *Serum sodium levels of 115–120 mmol/L can cause headache, lethargy and decreased responsiveness; sodium levels less than 110–115 mmol/L may cause seizures and coma.*

✚ Assess muscle strength and tone, and deep tendon reflexes. *Increasing muscle weakness and decreased deep tendon reflexes are manifestations of increasing hyponatraemia.*

For additional nursing interventions that may apply to the person with hyponatraemia, review the discussions of fluid volume deficit and fluid volume excess.

PRACTICE ALERT

Maintain a quiet environment, and institute seizure precautions in persons with severe hyponatraemia. Severe hyponatraemia can lead to seizures. A quiet environment reduces neurologic stimulation. Safety precautions, such as ensuring that side rails are up and having an airway readily available, reduce risk of injury from seizure.

The person with sodium imbalance (hypernatraemia)

Hypernatraemia is a serum sodium level greater than 145 mmol/L. It may develop when sodium is gained in excess of water, or when water is lost in excess of sodium. Either FVD deficit or FVE often accompanies hypernatraemia.

Pathophysiology of hypernatraemia

Two regulatory mechanisms protect the body from hypernatraemia: (1) Excess sodium in ECF stimulates the release of ADH so more water is retained by the kidneys; and (2) the thirst mechanism is stimulated to increase the intake of water. These two factors increase extracellular water, diluting the excess sodium and restoring normal levels. Because of the effectiveness of these mechanisms, hypernatraemia almost never occurs in persons who have an intact thirst mechanism and access to water.

Water deprivation is a cause of hypernatraemia in persons who are unable to respond to thirst due to altered mental status or physical disability. Excess water loss may occur with watery diarrhoea, fever, hyperventilation, excessive perspiration or massive burns. Unless water is adequately replaced, persons with diabetes insipidus may also develop hypernatraemia.

Signs and Symptoms of hypernatraemia

Signs and symptoms of hypernatraemia include:

● Excessive thirst.

● Hyperosmolality of ECF.

● Water is drawn out of cells, leading to cellular dehydration. The most serious effects of cellular dehydration are seen in the brain. As brain cells contract, neurological manifestations develop. The brain itself shrinks, causing mechanical traction on cerebral vessels.

● Altered neurologic function such as lethargy, weakness and irritability can progress to seizures, coma and death in severe hypernatraemia.

INTERDISCIPLINARY CARE FOR HYPERNATRAEMIA

Medication

The principal treatment for hypernatraemia is oral or intravenous water replacement. Hypotonic intravenous fluids such as 0.45% NaCl solution or 5% dextrose in water (which is isotonic when administered, but provides pure water when the glucose is metabolised) may be administered to correct the water deficit. Diuretics may also be given to increase sodium excretion.

NURSING CARE FOR HYPERNATRAEMIA

The primary focus of nursing care related to hypernatraemia is prevention. Measures to prevent hypernatraemia include identifying risk factors, teaching persons and caregivers, monitoring laboratory test results and working with the interdisciplinary team to reduce the potential for hypernatraemia.

Health promotion

Persons at risk for hypernatraemia, as well as their care providers, need teaching to prevent this electrolyte disorder. Instruct caregivers of elderly persons who are unable to perceive thirst or unable to respond to thirst to offer fluids at regular intervals.

If the person is unable to maintain adequate fluid intake, contact the primary care provider about an alternative route for fluid intake (for example, a feeding tube). Teach care providers the importance of providing adequate water for persons receiving tube feedings (many of which are hypertonic).

Nursing diagnoses and interventions

Risk for injury

Mental status and brain function may be affected by hypernatraemia itself or by rapid correction of the condition that leads to cerebral oedema. In either case, closely monitor the person and take precautions to reduce risk of injury.

✚ Monitor and maintain fluid replacement to within the prescribed limits. Monitor serum sodium levels and osmolality; report rapid changes to the care provider. *Rapid water replacement or rapid changes in serum sodium or osmolality can cause fluid shifts within the brain, increasing the risk of bleeding or cerebral oedema.*

✚ Monitor neurological function, including mental status, level of consciousness and other manifestations such as headache, nausea, vomiting, elevated blood pressure and decreased pulse rate. *Both hypernatraemia and rapid correction of hypernatraemia affect the brain and brain function. Careful monitoring of the person is vital to detect changes in mental status that may indicate cerebral bleeding or oedema.*

✚ Keep persons personal effects and familiar objects at bedside. Orient to time, place and circumstances as needed. Allow significant others to remain with the person as much as possible. *An unfamiliar environment and altered thought processes can further increase the person's risk for injury. Significant others provide a sense of security and reduce the person's anxiety*

COMMUNITY-BASED CARE

When preparing the person who has experienced hypernatraemia for home care, nurses should discuss the following topics with the person and their relatives:

● the importance of responding to thirst and consuming adequate fluids (if the person is dependent on a caregiver, stress the importance to the caregiver of regularly offering fluids);

● if prescribed, guidelines for following a low-sodium diet;

● use and effects (intended and unintended) of any prescribed diuretic or other medication;

● the importance of following a schedule for regular monitoring of serum electrolyte levels and reporting manifestations of imbalance to the care provider.

Consider this . . .

A person after transurethral resection of prostate (TURP) had hypotonic solution for bladder irrigation over 24 hours. Can this person develop hypo- or hypernatraemia? Explain your answer.

The person with potassium imbalance (hypokalaemia)

Hypokalaemia (low serum potassium levels) is a lower-than-normal amount of potassium in the blood. The normal serum (ECF) potassium level is 3.5–5.0 mmol/L. Potassium is needed for cells, especially nerve and muscle cells, to function properly. Potassium, the primary intracellular cation, plays a vital role in cell metabolism, and cardiac and neuromuscular function. For multisystem effects of hypokalaemia, see Figure 3.8.

Pathophysiology of hypokalaemia

Excess potassium may be lost through the kidneys or the gastrointestinal tract. These losses deplete total potassium levels in the body.

● Excess potassium loss through the kidneys is often secondary to drugs such as non-potassium-sparing diuretics, corticosteroids and large doses of some antibiotics. Hyperaldosteronism, a condition in which the adrenal glands secrete excess aldosterone, also causes excess elimination of potassium through the kidneys. Glucosuria and osmotic diuresis (for example, associated with diabetes mellitus) also cause potassium loss through the kidneys.

● Gastrointestinal losses of potassium result from severe vomiting, gastric suction or loss of intestinal fluids through diarrhoea or ileostomy drainage.

Potassium intake may be inadequate in persons who are unable or unwilling to eat for prolonged periods. Hospitalised persons are at risk, especially those on extended parenteral fluid therapy with solutions that do not contain potassium. Persons with anorexia nervosa or alcoholism may develop hypokalaemia due to inadequate intake and loss of potassium through vomiting, diarrhoea, laxative or diuretic use.

Signs and symptoms of hypokalaemia

Hypokalaemia affects the transmission of nerve impulses, interfering with the contraction of smooth, skeletal and cardiac muscle, as well as the regulation and transmission of cardiac impulses.

● Characteristic ECG changes of hypokalaemia include flattened or inverted T waves and a depressed ST segment. The

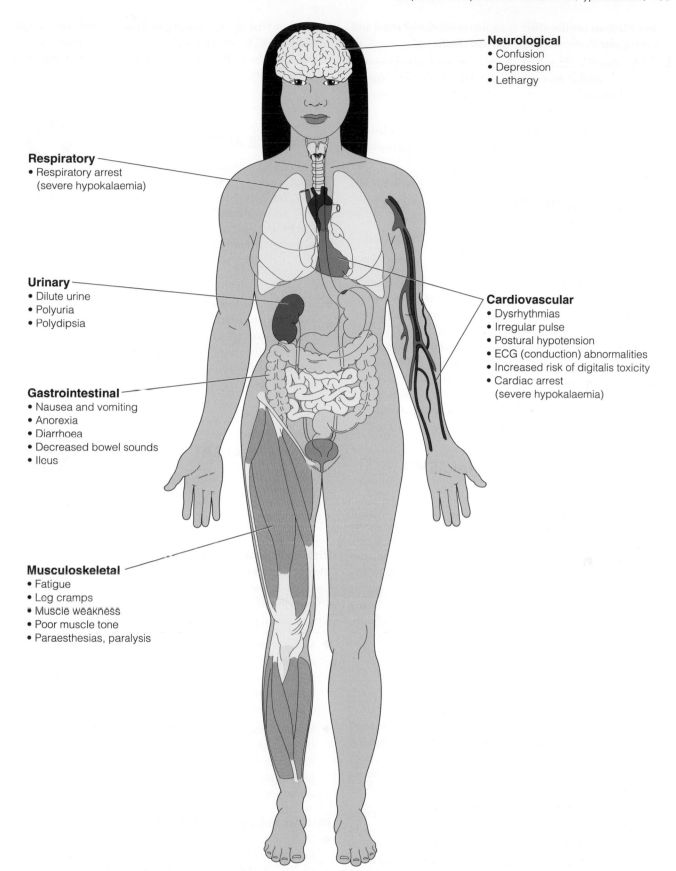

Neurological
- Confusion
- Depression
- Lethargy

Respiratory
- Respiratory arrest
  (severe hypokalaemia)

Urinary
- Dilute urine
- Polyuria
- Polydipsia

Cardiovascular
- Dysrhythmias
- Irregular pulse
- Postural hypotension
- ECG (conduction) abnormalities
- Increased risk of digitalis toxicity
- Cardiac arrest
  (severe hypokalaemia)

Gastrointestinal
- Nausea and vomiting
- Anorexia
- Diarrhoea
- Decreased bowel sounds
- Ileus

Musculoskeletal
- Fatigue
- Leg cramps
- Muscle weakness
- Poor muscle tone
- Paraesthesias, paralysis

Figure 3.8 Multisystem effects of hypokalaemia.

most serious cardiac effect is an increased risk of atrial and ventricular *dysrhythmias* (abnormal rhythms).

● Hypokalaemia affects both the resting membrane potential and intracellular enzymes in skeletal and smooth muscle cells. This causes skeletal muscle weakness and slowed peristalsis of the gastrointestinal tract.

● Carbohydrate metabolism is affected by hypokalaemia. Insulin secretion is suppressed, as is the synthesis of glycogen in skeletal muscle and the liver.

INTERDISCIPLINARY CARE FOR HYPOKALAEMIA

Medication

Oral and/or parenteral potassium supplements are given to prevent and, as needed, treat hypokalaemia. To prevent hypokalaemia in the person taking nothing by mouth, 40 mmol of potassium chloride per day may be added to intravenous fluids. The dose used to treat hypokalaemia includes the daily maintenance requirement, replacement of ongoing losses (e.g., gastric suction) and additional potassium to correct the existing deficit. Several days of therapy may be required. A diet high in potassium-rich foods is recommended for persons at risk for developing hypokalaemia or to supplement drug therapy.

NURSING CARE FOR HYPOKALAEMIA

Health promotion

When providing general health education, discuss using balanced electrolyte solutions to replace abnormal fluid losses. Provide diet teaching and refer persons with anorexia nervosa for counselling. Stress the potassium-losing effects of taking diuretics and using laxatives to enhance weight loss. Discuss the potassium-wasting effects of most diuretics with persons taking these drugs, and encourage a diet rich in high-potassium foods, as well as regular monitoring of serum potassium levels.

Nursing diagnoses and interventions

Risk for decreased cardiac output

Hypokalaemia affects the strength of cardiac contractions and can lead to dysrhythmias that further impair cardiac output. Hypokalaemia also alters the response to cardiac drugs, such as digitalis and the antidysrhythmics. Antidysrhythmic drugs such as quinidine sulphate prevent cardiac arrhythmias.

✚ Monitor serum potassium levels, particularly in persons at risk for hypokalaemia (those with excess losses due to drug therapy, gastrointestinal losses or who are unable to consume a normal diet). *Potassium must be replaced daily, because the body is unable to conserve it. Either lack of intake or abnormal losses of potassium in the urine or gastric fluids can lead to hypokalaemia.*

✚ Monitor vital signs, including orthostatic vitals and peripheral pulses. *As cardiac output falls, the pulse becomes weak and thready. Orthostatic hypotension may be noted with decreased cardiac output.*

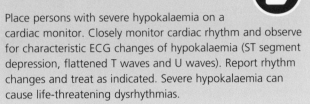

PRACTICE ALERT

Place persons with severe hypokalaemia on a cardiac monitor. Closely monitor cardiac rhythm and observe for characteristic ECG changes of hypokalaemia (ST segment depression, flattened T waves and U waves). Report rhythm changes and treat as indicated. Severe hypokalaemia can cause life-threatening dysrhythmias.

✚ Dilute intravenous potassium and administer using an electronic infusion device. In general, potassium is given no faster than 10–20 mmol/h. Closely monitor intravenous flow rate and response to potassium replacement. *Rapid potassium administration is dangerous and can lead to hyperkalaemia and cardiac arrest.*

PRACTICE ALERT

Never administer undiluted potassium directly into the vein as it can cause severe cardiac problems.

Risk for activity intolerance

Muscle cramping and weakness are common early manifestations of hypokalaemia. The lower extremities are usually affected initially. This muscle weakness can cause the person to fatigue easily, particularly with activity.

✚ Monitor skeletal muscle strength and tone, which are affected by moderate hypokalaemia. *Increasing weakness, paraesthesias or paralysis of muscles or progression of affected muscles to include the upper extremities or trunk can indicate a further drop in serum potassium levels.*

✚ Monitor respiratory rate, depth and effort; heart rate and rhythm; and blood pressure at rest and following activity. Report changes to the care provider. *Tachypnoea, dyspnoea, tachycardia and/or a change in blood pressure may indicate decreasing ability to tolerate activities.*

Risk for imbalanced fluid volume

✚ Maintain accurate intake and output records. *Gastrointestinal fluid losses can lead to significant potassium losses.*

✚ Monitor bowel sounds and abdominal distention. *Hypokalaemia affects smooth muscle function and can lead to slowed peristalsis and paralytic ileus.*

COMMUNITY-BASED CARE

The focus in preparing the person with or at risk for hypokalaemia is prevention. Discharge planning focuses on teaching self-care practices. Include the following topics when preparing the person and family for home care.

- recommended diet, including a list of potassium-rich foods;
- prescribed medications and potassium supplements, their use and desired and unintended effects;
- using salt substitutes (if recommended) to increase potassium intake; avoiding substitutes if taking a potassium supplement or potassium-sparing diuretic;
- manifestations of potassium imbalance (hypokalaemia or hyperkalaemia) to report to healthcare provider;
- recommendations for monitoring serum potassium levels;
- if taking digitalis, manifestations of digitalis toxicity to report to healthcare provider;
- managing gastrointestinal disorders that cause potassium loss (vomiting, diarrhoea, ileostomy drainage) to prevent hypokalaemia.

The person with potassium imbalance (hyperkalaemia)

Hyperkalaemia (high serum potassium levels) is an abnormally high serum potassium (greater than 5 mmol/L). Hyperkalaemia can result from inadequate excretion of potassium, excessively high intake of potassium or a shift of potassium from the intracellular to the extracellular space. Hyperkalaemia affects neuromuscular and cardiac function.

Pathophysiology of hyperkalaemia

The major causes of hyperkalaemia are kidney dysfunction, diseases of the adrenal gland, potassium shifting out of cells into the blood circulation and medications. A shift of potassium ions from the intracellular space can occur in acidosis, with severe tissue trauma, during chemotherapy and due to starvation. In acidosis, excess hydrogen ions enter the cells, displacing potassium and causing it to shift into the extracellular space. The extent of this shift is greater with metabolic acidosis than with respiratory acidosis.

Hyperkalaemia alters the cell membrane potential, affecting the heart, skeletal muscle function and the gastrointestinal tract. The most harmful consequence of hyperkalaemia is its effect on cardiac function. The cardiac conduction system is affected first, with slowing of the heart rate, possible heart blocks and prolonged depolarisation (change in cell membrane voltage between the interior and exterior of a cell). Skeletal muscles become weak, and paralysis may occur with very high serum potassium levels. Hyperkalaemia causes smooth muscle hyperactivity, leading to gastrointestinal disturbances.

Signs and symptoms of hyperkalaemia

Signs and symptoms of hyperkalaemia include:

- nausea and vomiting;
- fatigue;
- muscle weakness or twitching;
- tingling sensations;
- diarrhoea;
- irritability.

INTERDISCIPLINARY CARE FOR HYPERKALAEMIA

Medication

Medications are administered to lower the serum potassium and to stabilise the conduction system of the heart. For moderate to severe hyperkalaemia, calcium gluconate is given intravenously to counter the effects of hyperkalaemia on the cardiac conduction system. While the effect of calcium gluconate lasts only for one hour, it allows time to initiate measures to lower serum potassium levels. Calcium gluconate is used as a cardioprotective drug in hyperkalaemia. Though it does not have an effect on potassium levels in the blood, it reduces the excitability of cardiomyocytes (heart muscle cells) thus lowering the likelihood of developing cardiac arrhythmias. To remove potassium from the body, sodium polystyrene sulfonate (Kayexalate), a resin that binds potassium in the gastrointestinal tract, may be administered orally or rectally. If renal function is normal, diuretics such as furosemide may be prescribed to promote potassium excretion.

NURSING CARE FOR HYPERKALAEMIA

Nursing care focuses related to hyperkalaemia include identifying persons at risk, preventing hyperkalaemia and addressing problems resulting from the systemic effects of hyperkalaemia.

Health promotion

Persons at the greatest risk for developing hyperkalaemia include those taking potassium supplements (prescribed or over-the-counter), using potassium-sparing diuretics or salt substitutes and experiencing renal failure. Athletes participating in competition sports such as body building and using anabolic steroids, muscle-building compounds or 'energy drinks' also may be at risk for hyperkalaemia.

Nurses should encourage all persons to carefully read food and dietary supplement labels. Discuss the importance of taking prescribed potassium supplements as ordered, and not increasing the dose unless prescribed by the care provider. Advise persons taking a potassium supplement or potassium-sparing diuretic to avoid salt substitutes, which usually contain potassium. Discuss the importance of maintaining an adequate fluid intake (unless a fluid restriction has been prescribed) to maintain renal function to eliminate potassium from the body.

Nursing diagnoses and interventions

Risk for decreased cardiac output

Hyperkalaemia affects depolarisation of the atria and ventricles of the heart. Severe hyperkalaemia can cause dysrhythmias with ventricular fibrillation and cardiac arrest. The cardiac effects of hyperkalaemia are more pronounced when the serum potassium level rises rapidly. Low serum sodium and calcium levels, high serum magnesium levels and acidosis contribute to the adverse effects of hyperkalaemia on the heart muscle.

PRACTICE ALERT

Monitor the ECG pattern for development of peaked, narrow T waves, prolongation of the PR interval, depression of the ST segment, widened QRS interval and loss of the P wave. Notify the doctor of changes. Progressive ECG changes from a peaked T wave to loss of the P wave and widening of the QRS complex indicate an increasing risk of dysrhythmias and cardiac arrest.

+ Observe the person closely for the side-effects of intravenous calcium gluconate, such as dysrhythmia, palpitations and confusion, particularly in persons taking digitalis. *Calcium increases the risk of digitalis toxicity.*

Risk for activity intolerance

Both hypokalaemia and hyperkalaemia affect neuromuscular activity and the function of cardiac, smooth and skeletal muscles.

+ Monitor skeletal muscle strength and tone. *Increasing weakness, muscle paralysis or progression of affected muscles to affect the upper extremities or trunk can indicate increasing serum potassium levels.*

+ Monitor respiratory rate and depth. Regularly assess lung sounds. *Muscle weakness due to hyperkalaemia can impair ventilation. In addition, medications such as sodium bicarbonate can cause fluid retention and pulmonary oedema in persons with pre-existing cardiovascular disease.*

+ Assist with self-care activities as needed. *Increasing muscle weakness can lead to fatigue and affect the ability to meet self-care needs.*

Risk for imbalanced fluid volume

Kidney injury is a major cause of hyperkalaemia. Persons with kidney injury are also at risk for fluid retention and other electrolyte imbalances.

+ Closely monitor serum potassium, blood urea nitrogen (BUN) and serum creatinine. Notify the physician if serum potassium level is greater than 5 mmol/L, or if serum creatinine and BUN levels are increasing. *Serum creatinine and BUN are the primary indicators of renal function. Levels of these substances rise rapidly in acute kidney injury, more slowly in chronic kidney disease.*

+ Maintain accurate intake and output records. Report an imbalance of 24-hour totals and/or urine output less than 30 mL/hour. *Oliguria (scanty urine output) or anuria (no urine output) may indicate kidney injury and an increased risk for hyperkalaemia and FVE.*

+ Monitor persons receiving sodium bicarbonate for FVE. *Increased sodium from injection of a hypertonic sodium bicarbonate solution can cause a shift of water into the extracellular space.*

+ Monitor persons receiving cation exchange resins and sorbitol for FVE. *The resin exchanges potassium for sodium or calcium in the bowel. Excessive sodium and water retention may occur.*

Case Study 2 – Suresh
NURSING CARE PLAN Electrolyte imbalance

Suresh is in severe pain and perhaps is experiencing nausea and vomiting. If you recall from what we discussed about the possible causes of electrolyte imbalance, you can picture how and why he may develop electrolyte imbalance.

Assessment

A full assessment should be carried out to establish the possible cause of Suresh's nausea and vomiting and his back pain. Assessments should include person history, physical assessment,

recording vital signs and noting any abnormal changes and evaluating laboratory blood results of the person.

Person history is important to identify persons who are at risk of developing electrolyte imbalance. It may reveal conditions such as renal problems, heart diseases and diabetes mellitus that may lead to fluid and electrolyte imbalances. Certain medications such as diuretics may also affect fluid and electrolyte balances if they are not monitored regularly. A thorough physical assessment of skin condition, neurological status, oral cavity to identify any infection, heart, lungs and the kidneys should be done to plan appropriate care for Suresh.

Changes in the vital signs will indicate the status of the person. For example, if Suresh is pyrexial, this may indicate that he may have an infection as a result of dehydration. Respiration rate may indicate problems with acid–base balance; rapid pulse (tachycardia) may be the result of hypovolaemia, which could also result in low blood pressure (hypotension).

Diagnosis

Laboratory tests of urea and electrolytes will show if there is any abnormal electrolyte values as far as Suresh is concerned. These can then be corrected to re-establish his electrolyte values within the normal range.

Nursing care

+ Monitor intake and output.

+ Monitor signs and symptoms, for example, confusion and decreased cardiac function as a result of electrolyte imbalance.
+ Promote healthy eating to maintain electrolyte balance.
+ Discuss different types of food and their electrolyte values.

Evaluation

The goals are evaluated on a daily basis. Some of the goals, for example electrolyte values, may need to be reviewed more often depending on the severity of the imbalance. Nurses must check with Suresh that he is able to mobilise without any assistance. The nurse should provide verbal and written information regarding electrolyte imbalance, the importance of eating a healthy diet and the importance of maintaining fluid balance. It is also important that nurses document all care given to Suresh in accordance with the Nursing and Midwifery code for Record keeping (NMC 2010).

The person with calcium imbalance (hypocalcaemia)

Calcium is one of the most abundant ions in the body. The normal adult total serum calcium concentration is 8.5–10.0mg/dL.

Pathophysiology of hypocalcaemia

Common causes of hypocalcaemia (low serum calcium levels) are hypoparathyroidism resulting from surgery (parathyroidectomy, thyroidectomy, radical neck dissection) and acute pancreatitis. In the person who has undergone this type of surgery, symptoms of hypocalcaemia usually occur within the first 24–48 hours, but may be delayed.

PRACTICE ALERT

Carefully monitor persons who have undergone neck surgery for manifestations of hypocalcaemia. Check serum calcium levels and report changes to the care provider.

Extracellular calcium acts to stabilise neuromuscular cell membranes. This effect is reduced in hypocalcaemia, increasing neuromuscular irritability. The threshold of excitation of sensory nerve fibres is lowered as well, leading to paraesthesias (altered sensation). The nervous system becomes more excitable and muscle spasms develop. In the heart, this change in cell membranes can lead to dysrhythmias such as ventricular tachycardia and cardiac arrest. Hypocalcaemia decreases the contractility of cardiac muscle fibres, leading to decreased cardiac output.

Signs and symptoms of hypocalcaemia

Signs and symptoms of hypocalcaemia include:

- low blood calcium;
- tetany (tonic muscular spasm);
- painful muscle spasm of hands;
- painful muscle spasm of feet;
- facial muscle spasms;
- facial grimacing;
- lip paraesthesias (tingling, pricking or numbness of the lip);
- tongue paraesthesias;
- finger paraesthesias;
- foot paraesthesias;
- muscle aches.

INTERDISCIPLINARY CARE FOR HYPOCALCAEMIA

Medication

Hypocalcaemia is treated with oral or intravenous calcium. The person with severe hypocalcaemia is treated with intravenous calcium to prevent life-threatening problems such as airway obstruction. The most common intravenous calcium preparations include calcium chloride and calcium gluconate. Although calcium chloride contains more elemental calcium than calcium gluconate, it is also more irritating to the veins and may cause venous sclerosis (hardening of the vein walls) if given into a peripheral vein. Intravenous calcium preparations can cause necrosis and sloughing of tissue if they extravasate (to exude from or pass out) into subcutaneous tissue. Rapid drug administration can lead to bradycardia and possible cardiac arrest due to over-correction of hypocalcaemia with resulting hypercalcaemia.

Oral calcium preparations (calcium carbonate, calcium gluconate, or calcium lactate) are used to treat chronic, asymptomatic hypocalcaemia. Calcium supplements may be combined with vitamin D, or vitamin D may be given alone to increase gastrointestinal absorption of calcium. A diet high in calcium-rich foods may be recommended for persons with chronic hypocalcaemia or with low total body stores of calcium.

NURSING CARE FOR HYPOCALCAEMIA

Health promotion

Because of the large stores of calcium in bones, most healthy adults have a very low risk of developing hypocalcaemia. A deficit of total body calcium is often associated with ageing, however, increasing the risk of osteoporosis, fractures and disability. Women have a higher risk for developing osteoporosis than men due to lower bone density and hormonal influences. Teach women of all ages the importance of maintaining adequate calcium intake through diet and, as needed, calcium supplements. Stress the relationship between weight-bearing exercise and bone density, and encourage women to engage in a regular aerobic and weight-training exercise regime. Discuss hormone replacement therapy and its potential benefits during and after menopause.

Nursing diagnoses and interventions

Risk for injury

The person with hypocalcaemia is at risk for injury from possible laryngospasm, cardiac dysrhythmias or convulsions. In addition, too rapid administration of intravenous calcium or extravasation of the medication into subcutaneous tissues can lead to injury.

+ Frequently monitor airway and respiratory status. Report changes such as respiratory stridor (a high-pitched, harsh inspiratory sound indicative of upper airway obstruction) or increased respiratory rate or effort to the doctor. *These changes may indicate laryngeal spasm due to tetany.*

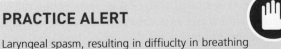

PRACTICE ALERT

Laryngeal spasm, resulting in diffiuclty in breathing in, is a respiratory emergency, requiring immediate intervention to maintain ventilation and gas exchange.

+ Monitor cardiovascular status including heart rate and rhythm, blood pressure and peripheral pulses. *Hypocalcaemia decreases myocardial contractility, causing reduced cardiac output and hypotension. It also can cause bradycardia or ventricular dysrhythmias. Cardiac arrest may occur in severe hypocalcaemia.*

+ Continuously monitor ECG in persons receiving intravenous calcium preparations, especially if the person is also taking digitalis. *Rapid administration of calcium salts can lead to hypercalcaemia and cardiac dysrhythmias.*

+ Provide a quiet environment. *A quiet environment reduces central nervous system (CNS) stimuli and the risk of convulsions in the person with tetany.*

COMMUNITY-BASED CARE

In preparing the person with hypocalcaemia for discharge and home care, consider the circumstances leading to low serum calcium levels. Discuss risk factors for hypocalcaemia specific to the person, and provide information about managing these risk factors to avoid future episodes of hypocalcaemia. Teach about prescribed medications, including calcium supplements. Provide a list of foods high in calcium, as well as sources of vitamin D if recommended. Discuss symptoms to report to the care provider, and stress the importance of follow-up care as scheduled.

The person with calcium imbalance (hypercalcaemia)

Hypercalcaemia is a serum calcium value greater than 10.0 mg/dL. Excess ionised calcium in ECF can have serious widespread effects.

Pathophysiology of hypercalcaemia

Hypercalcaemia usually results from increased resorption of calcium from the bones. The two most common causes of bone resorption are hyperparathyroidism and malignancies. In hyperparathyroidism, excess parathyroid hormone (PTH) is produced. This causes calcium to be released from bones, as well as increased calcium absorption in the intestines and retention of calcium by the kidneys. Hypercalcaemia is a common complication of malignancies. It may develop as a result of bone destruction by the tumour or due to hormone-like substances produced by the tumour itself. Prolonged immobility and lack of weight bearing also cause increased resorption of bone with calcium release into extracellular fluids. Self-limiting hypercalcaemia may also follow successful kidney transplant. Levels of PTH may be altered in chronic renal failure, leading to increased serum calcium levels.

Increased intestinal absorption of calcium can also lead to hypercalcaemia. This may result from excess vitamin D, overuse of calcium-containing antacids or excessive milk ingestion. Renal failure and some drugs such as thiazide diuretics and lithium can interfere with elimination of calcium by the kidneys, causing high serum calcium levels.

The effects of hypercalcaemia largely depend on the degree of serum calcium elevation and the length of time over which it develops. In general, higher serum calcium levels are associated with more serious effects. Calcium has a stabilising effect on the neuromuscular junction; hypercalcaemia decreases neuromuscular excitability, leading to muscle weakness and depressed deep tendon reflexes. Gastrointestinal motility is reduced as well. In the heart, calcium exerts an effect similar to digitalis, strengthening contractions and reducing the heart rate. Hypercalcaemia affects the conduction system of the heart, leading to bradycardia and heart blocks. The ability of the kidneys to concentrate urine is impaired by hypercalcaemia, causing excess sodium and water loss and increased thirst.

Extremely high serum calcium levels affect mental status. This is thought to be due to increased calcium in cerebrospinal fluid. Behavioural effects range from personality changes to confusion, impaired memory and acute psychoses.

Signs and symptoms of hypercalcaemia

Symptoms of hypercalcaemia relate to its effects on neuromuscular activity, the CNS, the cardiovascular system and the kidneys. Decreased neuromuscular excitability causes muscle weakness and fatigue, as well as gastrointestinal manifestations such as anorexia, nausea, vomiting and constipation. Central nervous system effects may include confusion, lethargy, behaviour or personality changes and coma. Cardiovascular effects include dysrhythmias, ECG changes and possible hypertension. Hypercalcaemia causes polyuria and, as a result, increased thirst.

INTERDISCIPLINARY CARE FOR HYPERCALCAEMIA

Medication

Measures to promote calcium elimination by the kidneys and reduce calcium resorption from bone are used to treat hypercalcaemia. In acute hypercalcaemia, intravenous fluids are given (see below) with a loop diuretic such as furosemide to promote elimination of excess calcium. Calcitonin, which promotes the uptake of calcium into bones, may also be used to rapidly lower serum calcium levels.

Glucocorticoids (cortisone), which compete with vitamin D, and a low-calcium diet may be prescribed to decrease gastrointestinal absorption of calcium, inhibit bone resorption and increase urinary calcium excretion. Also, calcitonin may be prescribed to decrease skeletal mobilisation of calcium and phosphorus and to increase renal output of calcium and phosphorus.

Fluid management

Intravenous fluids, usually isotonic saline, are administered to persons with severe hypercalcaemia to restore vascular volume and promote renal excretion of calcium. Isotonic saline is used because sodium excretion is accompanied by calcium excretion. Careful assessment of cardiovascular and renal function is done prior to fluid therapy; the person is carefully monitored for evidence of fluid overload during treatment.

NURSING CARE FOR HYPERCALCAEMIA

Health promotion

Identify and monitor persons at risk for hypercalcaemia. Promote mobility in persons when possible as it helps the uptake of calcium. Assist hospitalised persons to ambulate as soon as possible. In the home setting, discuss the benefits of regular weight-bearing activity with persons, families and caregivers. Encourage a generous fluid intake of up to three to four litres per day. Encourage persons at risk to limit their intake of milk and milk products, as well as calcium-containing antacids and supplements. In addition, persons with prolonged immobility or hypercalcaemia are encouraged to consume fluids that increase the acidity of urine (which inhibits calcium stone formation), such as cranberry or prune juice.

Nursing diagnoses and interventions

Risk for injury

Persons with hypercalcaemia are at risk for injury due to changes in mental status, the effects of hypercalcaemia on muscle strength and loss of calcium from bones.

✚ Administer safety precautions if confusion or other changes in mental status are noted. *Changes in mental status may impair judgement and the person's ability to maintain their own safety.*

PRACTICE ALERT

Monitor cardiac rate and rhythm, treating and/or reporting dysrhythmias as indicated. Prepare for possible cardiac arrest; keep emergency resuscitation equipment readily available. Hypercalcaemia can cause bradycardia, various heart blocks and cardiac arrest. Immediate treatment may be necessary to preserve life.

✚ Observe for manifestations of digitalis toxicity, including vision changes, anorexia and changes in heart rate and rhythm. Monitor serum digitalis levels. *Hypercalcaemia increases the risk of digitalis toxicity.*

✚ Promote fluid intake (oral and/or intravenous) to keep the person well hydrated and maintain dilute urine. Encourage fluids such as prune or cranberry juice to help maintain acidic urine. *Acidic, dilute urine reduces the risk of calcium salts precipitating out to form kidney stones.*

✚ If excess bone resorption has occurred, use caution when turning, positioning, transferring or ambulating. *Bones that have lost excess calcium may fracture with minimal stress or trauma (pathological fractures).*

Risk for excess fluid volume

Large amounts of isotonic intravenous fluid often are administered to help correct acute hypercalcaemia, leading to a risk for hypervolaemia. Persons with pre-existing cardiac or renal disease are at particular risk.

✚ Closely monitor intake and output. *A loop diuretic such as furosemide may be necessary if urinary output does not keep up with fluid administration.*

✚ Frequently assess vital signs, respiratory status, and heart sounds. Report any changes immediately to the person in charge. *Vital signs may indicate if the person is improving, stable or getting worse.*

✚ Administer diuretics as ordered, monitoring response. *Loop diuretics may be ordered to help eliminate excess fluid and calcium.*

COMMUNITY-BASED CARE

Discuss the following topics when preparing the person for discharge:

● Avoid excess intake of calcium-rich foods and antacids.
● Ensure that the person understands why they have to continue taking the prescribed medications.
● Encourage the person to increase dietary fibre and fluid intake to prevent constipation.
● Encourage the person to maintain weight-bearing physical activity to prevent hypercalcaemia.
● Report early manifestations of hypercalcaemia to the care provider.

We have now looked at some of the common problems related to fluid and electrolytes and what the nurse's role is with regard to them. It is difficult to discuss all the electrolytes in our body but you now have some idea relating to three of the major electrolytes of the body. Earlier on we looked at different types of shock and now let us consider the person with shock.

The person with shock

Shock is a clinical syndrome characterised by a systemic imbalance between oxygen supply and demand. This imbalance

IN PRACTICE

The aim of fluid and electrolyte treatment is to ensure that the person's fluid and electrolytes are in balance. The therapy could be given orally if the person is able to take oral fluids or by intravenous route. The management of the person's fluid and electrolyte status depends on the nursing and medical assessment. Identifying the cause of the fluid and electrolyte imbalance is important. For example, if a person is losing fluid and electrolytes as a result of diarrhoea and vomiting, then this problem needs to be treated as well as correcting the imbalance. Nurses should:

● maintain a strict fluid balance chart;
● advise the person to inform them of any changes within themselves such as feeling nauseous and sick so that they can monitor the person closely;
● monitor urine out and inform the person that all urine voided needs to be recorded in the fluid balance chart;
● inform the doctors of any fluid excess over the 24-hour period;
● unless contraindicated encourage two to three litres of fluid intake over the 24-hour period.

results in a state of inadequate blood flow to body organs and tissues, causing life-threatening cellular dysfunction.

Pathophysiology of shock

When one or more cardiovascular components do not function properly, the body's haemodynamic properties are altered. Consequently, tissue perfusion may be inadequate to sustain normal cellular metabolism. The result is the clinical syndrome known as shock. The manifestations of shock result from the body's attempts to maintain vital organs (heart and brain) and to preserve life following a drop in cellular perfusion. However, if the injury or condition triggering shock is severe enough or of long enough duration, then cellular hypoxia (diminished amount of oxygen) and cellular death can occur.

Shock is triggered by a sustained drop in mean arterial pressure. This drop can occur after a decrease in cardiac output, a decrease in the circulating blood volume, or an increase in the size of the vascular bed due to peripheral vasodilatation. If intervention is timely and effective, the physiological events that characterise shock may be stopped; if not, shock may lead to death.

Stages in shock

Stage I: early, reversible and compensatory shock
The initial stage of shock begins when baroreceptors in the aortic arch and the carotid sinus detect a sustained drop in MAP of less than 10 mmHg from normal levels. The circulating blood

volume may decrease (usually to less than 500 mL), but not enough to cause serious effects. The body reacts to the decrease in arterial pressure as it would to any physical stressor. The cerebral integration centre initiates the body's response systems, causing the sympathetic nervous system to increase the heart rate and the force of cardiac contraction, thus increasing cardiac output. Sympathetic stimulation also causes peripheral vasoconstriction, resulting in increased SVR and a rise in arterial pressure. The net result is that the perfusion of cells, tissues and organs is maintained.

Symptoms are almost imperceptible during the early stage of shock. The pulse rate may be slightly elevated. If the injury is minor or of short duration, arterial pressure is usually maintained and no further symptoms occur.

- Stimulation of the sympathetic nervous system results in the release of epinephrine (adrenaline) from the adrenal medulla and the release of norepinephrine (noradrenaline) from the adrenal medulla and the sympathetic fibres.

- The renin–angiotensin response occurs as the blood flow to the kidneys decreases. Renin released from the kidneys converts a plasma protein to angiotensin II, which causes vasoconstriction and stimulates the adrenal cortex to release aldosterone. Aldosterone causes the kidneys to reabsorb water and sodium and to lose potassium. The absorption of water maintains circulating blood volume while increased vasoconstriction increases SVR, maintaining central vascular volume and raising blood pressure.

- The hypothalamus releases adrenocorticotropic hormone, causing the adrenal glands to secrete aldosterone. Aldosterone promotes the reabsorption of water and sodium by the kidneys, preserving blood volume and pressure.

- The posterior pituitary gland releases ADH which increases renal reabsorption of water to increase intravascular volume. The combined effects of hormones released by the hypothalamus and posterior pituitary gland work to conserve central vascular volume.

Working together, these compensatory mechanisms can maintain MAP for only a short period of time. During this period, the perfusion and oxygenation of the heart and brain are adequate. If effective treatment is provided, the process is arrested, and no permanent damage occurs. However, unless the underlying cause of shock is reversed, these compensatory mechanisms soon become harmful, and shock perpetuates shock.

Stage II: intermediate or progressive shock

The progressive stage of shock occurs after a sustained decrease in MAP of 20 mmHg or more below normal levels and a fluid loss of 35–50% (1800–2500 mL of fluid). Although the compensatory mechanisms in the previous state remain activated, they are no longer able to maintain MAP at a level sufficient to ensure perfusion of vital organs.

Throughout this period, the heart rate and vasoconstriction increase; however, perfusion of the skin, skeletal muscles, kidneys and gastrointestinal organs is greatly diminished. Cells

in the heart and brain become hypoxic while other body cells and tissues become ischaemic (term related to conditions affected by lack of blood supply) and anoxic (absence of oxygen). Unless this stage of shock is treated rapidly, the person's chances of survival are poor.

Stage III: refractory or irreversible shock

If shock progresses to the irreversible stage, tissue anoxia becomes so generalised and cellular death so widespread that no treatment can reverse the damage. Even if MAP is temporarily restored, too much cellular damage has occurred to maintain life. Death of cells is followed by death of tissues, which results in death of organs. Death of vital organs contributes to subsequent death of the body. You need to be aware that all the body systems are affected by shock.

Types of shock

Hypovolaemic shock

Hypovolaemic shock occurs when the volume of the circulatory system is too depleted to allow adequate circulation to the tissues of the body. The aim is to correct the hypovolaemia and hypoperfusion of vital organs such as the heart and the kidneys before irreversible damage occurs.

In adults, hypovolaemic shock is classified as:

- Class 1: 10–15% blood loss with no physiological compensation and clinical changes.

- Class 2: 15–30% blood loss resulting in generalised vasoconstriction and reduction in urine output to 20–30 ml/h.

- Class 3: 30–40% blood loss with urine output under 20 ml/h and the person is confused.

- Class 4: 40% blood loss resulting in marked hypotension, tachycardia and tachypnoea (rapid shallow respiration). No urine output and the person is unconscious.

Signs and symptoms
- The person may feel cold, unwell, anxious, faint and short of breath.
- Postural hypotension and tachycardia.
- The person will probably look pale and sweaty.
- Tachypnoea.
- The periphery will be cold from poor perfusion, and capillary refill time will be prolonged.
- Young adults may show little rise in pulse rate and no fall in blood pressure despite significant exsanguination (to become bloodless); it is very easy to underestimate the severity of loss in a young person.
- If untreated could result in confusion or even coma.

Cardiogenic shock

Cardiogenic shock occurs when the heart's pumping ability is compromised to the point that it cannot maintain cardiac output and adequate tissue perfusion. Myocardial infarction is the most common cause of cardiogenic shock. Persons admitted to the hospital for treatment of myocardial infarction or cardiac surgeries are at risk for cardiogenic shock. The severity and progression of shock are related to the amount of myocardial damage.

Signs and symptoms

- Chest pain.
- Nausea and vomiting.
- Dyspnoea.
- Profuse sweating.
- Confusion and disorientation.
- Palpitations.
- Pale, mottled, cold skin with slow capillary refill and poor peripheral pulses.
- Hypotension.
- Tachycardia or bradycardia.
- Peripheral oedema.
- Oliguria (catheterisation is a useful early monitoring intervention).
- Altered mental state.

Obstructive shock

Obstructive shock is caused by an obstruction in the heart or great vessels that either impedes venous return or prevents effective cardiac pumping action. Obstructive shock is a life-threatening condition involving insufficient blood flow to the body tissues. Obstructive shock is caused by obstruction of the blood flow. Causes include cardiac tamponade, pulmonary embolism and narrowing of the aortic artery. The signs and symptoms are the result of decreased cardiac output and blood pressure, with reduced tissue perfusion and cellular metabolism.

Signs and symptoms

- Low blood pressure.
- Tachycardia but weak.
- Cool and clammy skin.
- Rapid breathing.
- Hypothermia.
- Confusion.
- Dry mouth.
- Fatigue.

Septic shock

Septic shock, the leading cause of death for persons in intensive care units, is one part of a progressive syndrome called *systemic inflammatory response syndrome* (SIRS). This condition is most often the result of gram-negative bacterial infections (i.e., *Pseudomonas*, *E. coli*, *Klebsiella*), but may also follow gram-positive infections from *Staphylococcus* and *Streptococcus* bacteria. Gram-negative sepsis has greatly increased since year 2000, with a 60% mortality rate despite treatment. This may be due to inappropriate use of antibiotics, bacteria becoming

resistant to antibiotics and more invasive treatments being carried out. The pathophysiology of septic shock is complex and not completely understood.

Persons at risk for developing infections leading to septic shock include those who are hospitalised, have debilitating chronic illnesses or have poor nutritional status. The risk is heightened after invasive procedures or surgery. Other persons at risk of septic shock include older adults and those who are immunocompromised. Portals of entry for infection that may lead to septic shock are as follows:

- *Urinary system:* catheterisations, suprapubic catheters, cystoscopy.
- *Respiratory system:* suctioning, aspiration, tracheostomy, endotracheal tubes, respiratory therapy, mechanical ventilators.
- *Gastrointestinal system:* peptic ulcers, ruptured appendix, peritonitis.
- *Integumentary system:* surgical wounds, intravenous catheters, intra-arterial catheters, invasive monitoring, decubitus ulcers, burns, trauma.
- *Female reproductive system:* elective surgical abortion, ascending infections from transmission of bacteria during the intrapartal and postpartal periods, tampon use, sexually transmitted infections.

Septic shock has an early phase and a late phase. In early septic shock (sometimes called the *warm phase*), vasodilatation results in weakness and warm, flushed skin, and the septicaemia often causes high fever and chills. In late septic shock (sometimes called the *cold phase*), hypovolaemia and activity of the compensatory mechanisms result in typical shock manifestations, including cold, moist skin, oliguria and changes in mental status. Death may result from respiratory failure, cardiac failure or renal failure. Manifestations of septic shock are listed in the box below.

FAST FACTS

Septic shock

- The death rate for septic shock is high.
- There are an estimated 31 000 cases a year of severe sepsis in England and Wales.
- Between 30 and 50% of people with severe sepsis will die from it.

Source: http://www.nhsdirect.wales.nhs.uk/encyclopaedia/s/article/septicshock (accessed August 2011).

Signs and symptoms

Early (warm) septic shock:

- blood pressure: normal to hypotensive;
- pulse: increased, thready;

- respirations: rapid and deep;
- skin: warm, flushed;
- mental status: alert, oriented, anxious;
- urine output: normal;
- increased body temperature, chills, weakness, nausea, vomiting, diarrhoea.

Late (cold) septic shock:
- blood pressure: hypotensive;
- pulse: tachycardia, arrhythmias;
- respirations: rapid, shallow, dyspnoeic;
- skin: cool, pale, oedematous;
- mental status: lethargic to comatose;
- urine output: oliguria to anuria.

Neurogenic shock

Neurogenic shock is the result of an imbalance between parasympathetic and sympathetic stimulation of vascular smooth muscle. If parasympathetic overstimulation or sympathetic understimulation persists, sustained vasodilatation occurs, and blood pools in the venous and capillary beds.

Neurogenic shock causes dramatic reduction in systemic vascular resistance as the size of the vascular compartment increases. As systemic vascular resistance decreases, pressure in the blood vessels becomes too low to drive nutrients across capillary membranes, and cellular metabolism is impaired.

Signs and symptoms
- Blood pressure: hypotensive.
- Pulse: slow and bounding.
- Respirations: vary.
- Skin: warm, dry.
- Mental status: anxious, restless, lethargic progressing to comatose.
- Urine output: oliguria to anuria.
- Other: lowered body temperature.

Anaphylactic shock

Anaphylactic shock is a life-threatening condition where a severe allergic reaction causes bronchial airways to constrict. Narrowing of the airways can also occur at the same time, with or without the drop in blood pressure. This can cause breathing difficulties and wheezing.

Signs and symptoms
- Blood pressure: hypotensive.
- Pulse: increased, dysrhythmias.
- Respirations: dyspnoea, stridor, wheezes, laryngospasm, bronchospasm, pulmonary oedema.
- Skin: warm, oedematous (lips, eyelids, tongue, hands, feet, genitals).

- Mental status: restless, anxious, lethargic to comatose.
- Urine output: oliguria to anuria.
- Paraesthesias, pruritus, abdominal cramps, vomiting, diarrhoea.

INTERDISCIPLINARY CARE FOR SHOCK

Medication

When fluid replacement alone is not sufficient to reverse shock, vasoactive drugs (drugs causing vasoconstriction or vasodilatation) and inotropic drugs (drugs improving cardiac contractility) may be administered. When used to treat shock, these drugs increase venous return through vasoconstriction of peripheral vessels; they also improve the pumping ability of the heart by facilitating myocardial contractility and by dilating coronary arteries to increase perfusion of the myocardium.

Oxygen therapy

Establishing and maintaining a patent airway and ensuring adequate oxygenation are critical interventions in reversing shock. All persons in shock (even those with adequate respirations) should receive prescribed oxygen therapy (usually by mask or nasal cannula) to maintain the PaO_2 at greater than 80 mmHg during the first four to six hours of care. Nurses need to be aware that all oxygen to be administered is prescribed and that they adhere to the local and national policies in the safe administration of oxygen.

Fluid replacement

The most effective treatment for the person in hypovolaemic shock is the administration of intravenous fluids or blood. Fluids also treat septic and neurogenic shock. However, the person with cardiogenic shock may require either fluid replacement or restriction, depending on pulmonary artery pressure.

Various fluids may be administered alone or in combination as part of fluid replacement therapy in treating shock. Whole blood or blood products increase the oxygen-carrying capacity of the blood and thus increase oxygenation of cells. Fluid replacements, such as crystalloid and colloid solutions, increase circulating blood volume and tissue perfusion. Fluid replacements are administered in massive amounts through two large-bore peripheral lines or through a central line.

Blood and blood products

If hypovolaemic shock is due to haemorrhage, the infusion of blood and blood products may be indicated. The goal of blood administration is to keep the haematocrit (the relative volume of blood occupied by red blood cells) at 30–35% and the haemoglobin level between 12.5 and 14.5 g/100 ml. Available blood and blood products include fresh whole blood, stored whole blood, packed RBCs, platelet concentrate, fresh-frozen plasma and cryoprecipitate. Often, packed RBCs are given to provide haemoglobin concentration and are supplemented with crystalloids to maintain an adequate circulatory volume.

NURSING CARE FOR SHOCK

Nursing care for the person in shock focuses on treating the underlying cause, increasing arterial oxygenation and improving tissue perfusion. Depending on the cause and type of shock, interventions include emergency care measures, oxygen therapy, fluid replacement and medications.

Nursing diagnoses and interventions

Risk for decreased cardiac output

Decreased cardiac output is the primary problem for the person in shock. Although much of the care related to this diagnosis is collaborative, many independent nursing interventions are critical to the care of the person in shock.

✚ Assess and monitor cardiovascular function via the following:

   a. blood pressure;
   b. heart rate and rhythm;
   c. pulse oximetry;
   d. peripheral pulses;
   e. haemodynamic monitoring of arterial pressures, pulmonary artery pressures and CVPs.

   A baseline assessment is necessary to establish the stage of shock. If palpable peripheral pulses and audible (to auscultation) blood pressure are lost, inserting central arterial, venous and pulmonary artery catheters is essential to establish progression of shock accurately and to evaluate the person's response to therapy.

✚ Measure and record intake and output (total output and urinary output) hourly. *A decrease in circulating blood volume with hypotension and the effect of the compensatory mechanisms associated with shock can cause renal failure. Urinary output of < 30 mL/h in an acutely ill adult indicates reduced renal blood flow.*

✚ Monitor bowel sounds, abdominal distention and abdominal pain. *Decreased splanchnic blood flow reduces bowel motility and peristalsis; paralytic ileus may result.*

✚ Monitor for sudden sharp chest pain, dyspnoea, cyanosis, anxiety and restlessness. *Haemoconcentration and increased platelet aggregation may result in pulmonary emboli.*

✚ Maintain bedrest and provide (to the extent possible) a calm, quiet environment. Place in a supine position with the legs elevated to about 20 degrees, trunk flat and head and shoulders elevated higher than the chest (about 10 degrees). *Limiting activity and ensuring rest decreases the workload of the heart. The supine position with legs elevated increases venous return; however, this position should not be used for persons in cardiogenic shock.*

Risk for ineffective tissue perfusion

As shock progresses, diminished tissue perfusion causes ischaemia and hypoxia of major organ systems. As shock worsens, blood flow and oxygenation of the lungs, heart and brain are also impaired. Hypoxia and ischaemia result from decreased tissue perfusion in the kidneys, brain, heart, lungs, gastrointestinal tract and the periphery.

✚ Monitor skin colour, temperature, turgor and moisture. *Decreased tissue perfusion is evidenced by the skin becoming pale, cool and moist; as haemoglobin concentrations decrease, cyanosis occurs.*

✚ Monitor cardiopulmonary function by assessing/monitoring the following:

   a. blood pressure (by auscultation or by haemodynamic monitoring);
   b. rate and depth of respirations;
   c. lung sounds;
   d. pulse oximetry;
   e. peripheral pulses (brachial, radial, dorsalis pedis and posterior tibial); include presence, equality, rate, rhythm and quality (If unable to palpate pulses, use a device such as a Doppler ultrasound flow meter to assess peripheral arterial blood flow.);
   f. jugular vein distention;
   g. CVP measurements.

   Baseline vital signs are necessary to determine trends in subsequent findings. As shock progresses, the blood pressure decreases, and the pulse becomes rapid, weak and thready. As perfusion of the lungs decreases, crackles, wheezes and dyspnoea are commonly assessed. Capillary refill is prolonged, and peripheral pulses are weak or non-palpable. Neck veins that cannot be seen when the person is in the supine position indicate decreased intravascular volume. CVP is an accurate means of determining fluid status in the person in shock; the findings will be low (5–15 cm of water is normal) in hypovolaemic shock because of the decreased blood volume.

✚ Monitor body temperature. *An elevated body temperature increases metabolic demands, depleting reserves of bodily energy. It also increases myocardial oxygen demand and may place the person with previous cardiac problems at even greater risk for hypoperfusion.*

FAST FACTS

Shock

The most common symptoms of shock include:

● a fast, weak pulse;
● low blood pressure;
● feeling faint, weak or nauseous;
● dizziness;
● cold, clammy skin;
● rapid, shallow breathing;
● blue lips.

+ Monitor urinary output per urinary catheter hourly, using an urometer. *Urine output is a reliable indicator of renal perfusion.*
+ Assess mental status and level of consciousness. *The appropriateness of the person's behaviour and responses reflects the* adequacy of cerebral circulation. Restlessness and anxiety are common in shock; in later stages, the person may become lethargic and progress to a comatose state. Altered levels of consciousness are the result of both cerebral hypoxia and the effects of acidosis on brain cells.

Case Study 1 – Martha
NURSING CARE PLAN Septic shock

Martha Spearman was admitted to A&E with abdominal pain and generally feeling unwell. She was examined by the duty doctor in the A & E department. After a physical examination, a provisional diagnosis of septic shock was made. Her grandson was informed that Mrs Spearman will be admitted to the intensive care unit (ICU) for more investigations, treatment and nursing care and that she is unwell.

Assessment

When Mrs Spearman was admitted to the intensive care unit, the nurse recorded her vital signs as T 37.5 °C, P 130 bpm, R 30 rpm, BP 100/48 mmHg and oxygen saturation 96% on air. Her skin is hot, dry and flushed with poor turgor. She is alert and oriented, but is restless and appears anxious. She has only passed 50 ml of urine in the previous four hours. Her grandson states that Martha is nauseated and she suddenly begins vomiting and is incontinent of liquid stool. Laboratory tests indicate leukocytosis, respiratory alkalosis and reduced platelet count. Blood cultures, as well as cultures of Mrs Spearman's sputum and urine, are carried out. She is diagnosed as having septic shock.

Intravenous broad-spectrum antibiotics are prescribed and administered immediately. Despite treatment, Mrs Spearman's condition worsens. Her blood pressure continues to drop, her skin becomes cool and cyanotic and she begins to have periods of disorientation. She begins to cry and asks her grandson, 'Am I going to die?'

Diagnoses

+ *Deficient fluid volume* related to vomiting, diarrhoea, high fever and shift of intravascular volume to interstitial spaces.
+ *Ineffective breathing pattern* related to rapid respirations and progression of septic shock.
+ *Ineffective tissue perfusion* related to progression of septic shock with decreased cardiac output, hypotension and massive vasodilatation.
+ *Anxiety* related to feelings that illness is worsening and is potentially life-threatening, and the transfer to the intensive care unit.

Expected outcomes

+ Maintain adequate circulating blood volume.
+ Regain and maintain blood gas values within normal limits.
+ Regain and maintain stable haemodynamic levels.
+ Verbalise increased ability to cope with stressors.

Planning and implementation

+ Monitor neurological status, including mental status and level of consciousness.
+ Monitor cardiovascular status, including arterial blood pressure; rate, rhythm and quality of pulses; CVP; pulmonary artery pressure; and cardiac output.
+ Monitor colour and condition of skin.
+ Monitor results of ABGs, blood counts, clotting times and platelet counts.
+ Monitor respiratory status, including respiratory rate, rhythm and breath sounds.
+ Monitor body temperature every two hours.
+ Monitor urinary output hourly, reporting any output of < 30 ml/h.
+ Explain procedures and provide comfort measures (oral care, skin care, turning, positioning).

Evaluation

Despite intensive nursing and medical care, Mrs Spearman's condition remains critical but stable. The nursing care and interventions are continued as planned and to be reviewed later that day.

> ### Consider this . . .
>
> Septic shock is a dangerous, life-threatening condition that can affect anyone and is caused by bacterial infections that cannot be controlled by antibiotics alone or even the best supportive medical care. Pneumonia, avian flu, meningitis, hospital super-bug MRSA and AIDS-related infections, for instance, can all induce septic shock. Cancer sufferers are particularly vulnerable to sepsis and septic shock, because their immune systems are badly weakened by chemotherapy. It is estimated that 67% of cancer persons die from infections brought on by a poor immune system. Post-operative and transplant persons, the old and the very young are also very susceptible.

CASE STUDY SUMMARIES

Case Study 1. Mrs Spearman was transferred to ICU because she needs careful monitoring and any changes can be treated promptly. The condition is serious and, if not treated promptly, could lead to complications such as respiratory and heart failure. Mrs Spearman should recover from her illness, but she will need careful monitoring; hence, her admission to ICU.

Her treatment will include oxygen therapy, antibiotics and careful monitoring of her vital signs. Mrs Spearman will also need a lot of psychological care and support from the nurses and her grandson to come to terms with her condition.

Case Study 2. Mr Joshi has lost a lot of electrolytes as a result of nausea and vomiting. This condition could happen to anyone who suffers from severe bouts of vomiting. We lose valuable salts such as sodium and fluid from our body. Mr Joshi's condition needs careful monitoring. His vital signs need to be recorded regularly to ensure that his condition is not getting worse.

His electrolytes need careful monitoring. Fluid intake needs to be maintained with sips of water and gradually increasing free fluids. When calculating Mr Joshi's fluid balance, you need to take into account his insensible losses which are estimated according to standard norms.

Case Study 3. Remember that in FVE the aim is to identify the cause of the problem and treat accordingly. Mr Tan's fluid intake and output needs careful monitoring. In the initial period nurses need to take and record his vital signs hourly to ensure that he is not developing any complications such as breathlessness and any changes to his condition reported immediately so that prompt action can be taken. It is also vital to ensure that Mr Tan is not dehydrated as a result of his treatment for FVE.

On discharge Mr Tan should be advised to monitor his fluid intake and to ensure that he is voiding a sufficient amount of urine each time. Advise the patient to take programmed light exercise and to see his GP or practice nurse if he is unduly worried.

CHAPTER HIGHLIGHTS

- The volume and composition of body fluid is normally maintained by a balance of fluid and electrolyte intake; elimination of water, electrolytes and acids by the kidneys; and hormonal influences. Change in any of these factors can lead to a fluid, electrolyte or acid–base imbalance that adversely impacts health.

- Fluid, electrolyte and acid–base imbalances can affect all body systems, especially the cardiovascular system, the central nervous system and the transmission of nerve impulses. Conversely, primary disorders of the respiratory, renal, cardiovascular, endocrine or other body systems can lead to an imbalance of fluids, electrolytes or acid–base status.

- The most common electrolyte imbalances relate to sodium, potassium and calcium.

- Potassium imbalances are commonly seen in persons with acute or chronic illnesses. Both hypokalaemia and hyperkalaemia affect cardiac conduction and function. Carefully monitor cardiac rhythm and status in persons with very low or very high potassium levels.

- Calcium imbalances primarily affect neuromuscular transmission: hypocalcaemia increases neuromuscular irritability; hypercalcaemia depresses neuromuscular transmission. Magnesium imbalances have a similar effect.

- Careful monitoring of respiratory and cardiovascular status, mental status, neuromuscular function and laboratory values is an important nursing responsibility for all persons with fluid, electrolyte or acid–base imbalances.

- Shock is a clinical condition in which there is an imbalance between oxygen supply and demand. This imbalance results in inadequate blood flow to organs and tissues causing life-threatening cellular dysfunction.

- An early sign of shock is a change in the level of consciousness with restlessness being a common symptom of cerebral hypoxia.

- Hypovolaemic shock is the most common type of shock and is caused by a decrease in the circulating blood volume of 15% or more. Treatment consists of stopping the bleeding, getting oxygen to the cellular level and restoring blood volume. This is accomplished by providing high-flow oxygen to the person, surgical intervention and transfusion of blood products.

- Cardiogenic shock is caused when the pumping ability of the heart is compromised to the point that the heart cannot maintain adequate cardiac output and tissue perfusion.

- Septic shock is a part of a progressive syndrome called systemic inflammatory response syndrome (SIRS), a condition most often caused by gram-negative infections.

- Anaphylactic shock results in vasodilatation, pooling of blood in the periphery and hypovolaemia which leads to altered cellular metabolism. This condition is the result of a fulminating hypersensitivity reaction to a foreign substance.

TEST YOURSELF

1. A person is admitted to the emergency department with hypovolaemia. Which intravenous solution would the nurse anticipate administering?

    a. Ringer's solution
    b. 10% dextrose in water
    c. 3% sodium chloride
    d. 0.45% sodium chloride

2. When assessing a person with fluid volume deficit, the nurse would expect to find:

    a. increased pulse rate and blood pressure.
    b. dyspnoea and respiratory crackles.
    c. headache and muscle cramps.
    d. orthostatic hypotension and flat neck veins.

3. The nurse caring for a person with acute hypernatraemia includes which of the following in the plan of care? (Select all that apply.)

    a. Conduct frequent neurologic checks.
    b. Restrict fluids to 1500 ml per day.
    c. Orient to time, place and person frequently.
    d. Maintain intravenous access.

4. Laboratory results for a person show a serum potassium level of 2.2 mmol/L. Which of the following nursing actions is of highest priority for this person?

    a. Keep the person on bedrest.
    b. Initiate cardiac monitoring.
    c. Start oxygen at 2 L/min.
    d. Initiate seizure precautions.

5. A person who is known to be an alcoholic presents with confusion, hallucinations and a positive Chvostek's sign. Which medication(s) should the nurse anticipate administering?

    a. magnesium sulfate
    b. calcium chloride
    c. insulin and glucose
    d. sodium bicarbonate

6. A person undergoing mechanical ventilation following a severe chest wall injury and flail chest complains of chest tightness, anxiety, and feeling as though she cannot get enough air. She is afraid she is having a heart attack. The nurse should first

    a. administer prescribed analgesic.
    b. contact respiratory therapy to evaluate ventilator settings.
    c. obtain arterial blood gases.
    d. notify the doctor.

7. You are monitoring blood administration to a trauma victim in shock. Which of the following assessments indicate a dangerous transfusion reaction?

    a. red raised areas (wheals) on the skin that itch
    b. an increase in body temperature by 3°C
    c. decreasing blood pressure and dyspnoea
    d. increasing blood pressure and pulse

8. What type of shock causes widespread vasodilatation and decreased peripheral resistance?

    a. cardiogenic shock
    b. septic shock
    c. hypovolaemic shock
    d. obstructive shock

9. Distributive shock is caused by:

    a. blood loss.
    b. widespread vasodilatation.
    c. ineffective cardiac pumping action.
    d. hypersensitivity reaction.

10. Shock is defined as:

    a. a systemic imbalance between oxygen supply and demand.
    b. sufficient cardiac output.
    c. haemorrhage.
    d. abnormal blood pressure.

Further resources

NHS Choices
http://www.nhs.uk/Conditions/Anaphylaxis/Pages/Introduction.aspx
This website is called NHS choices. Here you are able to browse through symptoms, causes, diagnosis, treatments and complications of anaphylactic shock. A good source for quick reference for your assignments.

Mondofacto
www.mondofacto.com/facts/dictionary?electrolyte+imbalance
The mondofacto study skills kits contain many topics including electrolyte imbalance. We think you'll find these most useful when you've got a specific goal to achieve.

Emedicine
http://www.emedicinehealth.com/shock/article_em.htm
This website is called *emedicinehealth*. Another useful site for looking up medical conditions for you to study. This particular link considers SHOCK: Shock Overview, Causes, Shock – Specific Types, Shock Symptoms, Exams and Tests, Shock Treatment, Self-Care at Home, Medical Treatment, Follow-up and Outlook. You will find this useful for when providing health promotion to your patients in practice.

National Institute for Health and Clinical Excellence (NICE)
http://www.nice.org.uk/nicemedia/live/11546/32957/32957.pdf
This website provides you with a link to the National Institute for Health and Clinical Excellence. Understanding NICE guidance – information for the families and carers of people with severe sepsis, and the public.

British Association for Parenteral and Enteral Nutrition
http://www.bapen.org.uk/pdfs/bapen_pubs/giftasup.pdf
This web link is a BPEN medical site. In this link you will find the recommendations from doctors on fluid therapy for surgical patients. The title is, 'British Consensus Guidelines on Intravenous Fluid Therapy for Adult Surgical Patients'. We think that this website is useful for any nursing student who is looking after surgical patients who need fluid and electrolyte therapy.

Asthma and Allergy Information and Research
http://www.users.globalnet.co.uk/~aair/anaphylaxis.htm
This is the Asthma, Allergy Information & Research site. We think you will find this site useful, as it discusses anaphylaxis. It is a common condition which can affect adults and children of all ages. Knowing what to do is important and this site gives information on treatment with regards to anaphylaxis.

Bibliography

Chang E (2006) *Pathophysiology Applied to Nursing*. St Louis, MO, Mosby-Yearbook.

Kozier B, Erb G, Berman A, *et al.* (2008) *Fundamentals of Nursing: Concepts, process and practice*. Harlow, Pearson Education.

LeMone P and Burke K (2008) *Medical-Surgical Nursing: Critical thinking in client care*. (4th edn). Upper Saddle River, NJ, Pearson Education.

Lindsay B (2007) *Understanding Research and Evidence-based Practice*. Exeter, Reflectpress.

Martini, F H and Nath J L (2011) *Fundamentals of Anatomy and Physiology* (9th edn). San Francisco, CA, Pearson Benjamin Cummings.

McCance K L, Huether S E, Brashers V L and Rote N S (2010) *Pathophysiology: The biologic basis for disease in adults and children* (6th edn). St Louis, MO, Mosby.

Metheny N M (2000) *Fluid and Electrolyte Balance: Nursing Considerations* (4th edn). Philadelphia, PA: Lippincott.

Migliozzi M (2009) Shock. In Nair M and Peate I (eds). *Fundamentals of Applied Pathophysiology: An essential guide for nursing students*. Chichester, Wiley-Blackwell, 86–100.

Monahan F D, Neighbors M, Sands J K and Marek J F (2007) *Phipps' Medical and Surgical Nursing – Health and Illness Perspectives* (8th edn). St Louis, MO, Mosby.

Nair M (2009) Fluid and electrolyte balance and associated disorders. In Nair M and Peate I (eds), *Fundamentals of Applied Pathophysiology: An essential guide for nursing students*. Chichester, Wiley-Blackwell, 439–460.

NICE (2004) *Pre-hospital Initiation of Fluid Replacement Therapy in Trauma*. London, National Institute for Health and Clinical Excellence.

NMC (2010) *Guidelines for Record and Record Keeping*. London, Nursing and Midwifery Council.

Porth C M (2009) *Pathophysiology: Concepts of altered health states* (9th edn). Philadelphia, PA, Lippincott.

Resuscitation Council UK (2010) *The Emergency Medical Treatment of Anaphylatic Reactions: Guidelines for healthcare providers*. London, Resuscitation Council (UK).

Wise L C, Mersch J, Racioppi J, Crosier J and Thompson C (2000) Evaluating the reliability and utility of cumulative intake and output, *Journal of Nursing Care Quality* **14**(3), 37–42.

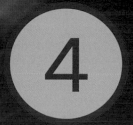

Caring for people with immune problems

Learning outcomes

- Understand the fundamental anatomy, physiology and functions of the **immune system**.
- Demonstrate the differences between innate and **acquired immunity**.
- Provide an understanding of primary and secondary immunity.
- Describe the pathophysiology of wound healing, **inflammation** and infection.
- Identify routes of infection.
- Be aware of the nurse's role in caring for people with altered immunity.

Clinical competencies

- Conduct and document an assessment of skin integrity.
- Monitor the results of diagnostic tests linked to alterations in the immune system and report abnormal findings.
- Assess the psychosocial impact of a diagnosis of HIV.
- Conduct and document a health history of a person with altered immunity.
- Use evidence-based research to provide teaching on skin care.

CASE STUDIES

Below are two case studies that you may wish to consider before, during or after you have read the chapter. There are no right or wrong answers to these case studies, but you should consider the physical, psychological and social implications.

Case Study 1 – Kate

Ms Kate Stable, aged 21, was admitted to a genito-urology ward with the following: pain at the site of her kidneys; she had pain in her joints and was passing small amounts of urine; urinalysis revealed proteinuria. Ms Stable reported she had noticed hair loss over the last six months. Ms Stable's blood pressure was 185/110 mm/Hg. There were colour changes in her fingers and these altered according to external temperature. The nurse observed a 'butterfly' rash on Kate's face. Kate said she was feeling down and depressed. A diagnosis of systemic lupus erythematosus (SLE) was made after a health history and various tests.

Case Study 2 – Thomas

Mr Thomas Worthington, aged 19, a first year physiotherapy student, lives in the halls of residence on the university campus. He has arrived in his local Accident and Emergency department with one of his student friends. He is struggling to breathe, and his face, particularly his mouth, is very swollen. He tells you that he was enjoying a picnic with friends when he was stung on his face by a wasp. Thomas and his friend who accompanied him are very scared and worried.

The treatment of choice for somebody in Thomas's condition is epinephrine (formerly known in the UK as adrenaline – a name change occurred in early 2000), as well as antihistamines and steroids. Epinephrine is given because there are no contraindications (i.e. will not cause the person any harm) and it improves airway patency (reduces any oedema – swelling – in the airway). In addition, it also improves the blood pressure by increasing it. These two positive effects of epinephrine may well be life-saving. Because **anaphylaxis** can lead to huge losses of fluids, large doses of intravenous fluids are given to counteract this symptom.

INTRODUCTION

The immune system is the police force for the body. Practically every cell and space in the body is patrolled for intruders and abnormalities. The immune system works 24 hours a day in thousands of different ways, with most of its work going largely unnoticed. Often we only really notice our immune system when it fails for some reason.

A thorough knowledge of the immune system increases understanding of the local and systemic inflammatory response, resistance to infectious disease and the importance of **immunisation**. This foundation of knowledge can help the nurse to teach people and families to follow recommended treatment regimens, to promote and maintain health and to prevent disease. In addition, the nurse can prescribe appropriate rehabilitative measures, such as increased rest and attention to optimal nutrition.

ANATOMY, PHYSIOLOGY AND FUNCTIONS OF THE IMMUNE SYSTEM

The immune system is an intricate system of cells, enzymes and proteins which protects by making us resistant (immune) to infections caused by different micro-organisms. However, as you have seen from the short case studies above, and as you will find out by reading this chapter, the immune system does more for us than just protect us from infectious diseases. Amongst other functions, it includes:

- the removal and destruction of damaged or dead cells;
- the identification and destruction of malignant cells, thereby preventing their further development into tumours.

The role of the cells of the immune system is to seek out and destroy any damaged cells and foreign tissues and to recognise and preserve host tissues. The main function of the immune system is to protect the body from harm caused by micro-organisms.

The immune system is a very complicated system, so what follows is a very much simplified account.

TYPES OF IMMUNITY

The immune system is activated by infectious micro-organisms, minor injuries, such as small lacerations or bruises, or by major injuries, such as burns and major surgery. There are two types of immunity in humans – the innate and the acquired.

Innate immunity is immunity possessed from birth. Acquired immunity is not present at birth; this is acquired as we go through life. A major role of the innate immune response is to prevent or limit the entrance of micro-organisms into the body, so as to limit tissue damage. This inflammation often destroys any microbes or toxins before the full immune system is activated. However, if the inflammatory process is unable to destroy any of these invading organisms or toxins and repair the damage, then the acquired immune response is activated.

Another name for innate immunity is non-specific immunity – these defences start to work no matter what infectious or non-self material (i.e. material that does not belong in the body, including splinters, dirt, toxins) has entered our bodies. These are non-specific because they are not specifically linked to a particular infectious micro-organism. Acquired immunity is also known as specific immunity because it only responds to known, specific organisms, that we have previously encountered.

BLOOD CELLS OF THE IMMUNE SYSTEM

Blood cells initially develop into one of two different stem cells; all our different blood cells develop from one or other of these stem cells. One branch develops into one of three different types:

- thrombocytes (platelets);
- erythrocytes (red blood cells);
- leucocytes (white blood cells).

However, myeloid cells only develop into particular types of white blood cells:

- **neutrophils;**
- monocytes;
- macrophages;
- basophils;
- eosinophils.

These are the white cells that are involved in innate immunity (see Figure 4.1).

The second type of multipotent stem cells become the lymphoids which further develop into **lymphocytes**. Lymphocytes are the cells involved in acquired immunity. There are two types of lymphocytes – the B-cells and the T-cells.

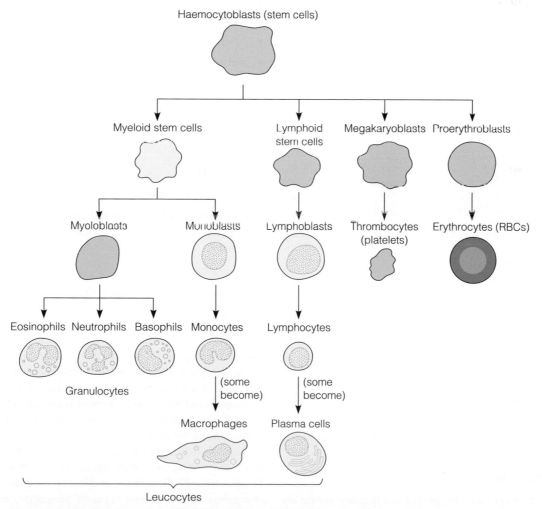

Figure 4.1 The development and differentiation of leucocytes from haemocytoblasts.

Many of our blood cells play diverse and essential roles in the functioning of the immune system. White blood cells (leucocytes) and platelets form a major part of the immune system. The only blood cells that are not considered to be part of the immune system are the red blood cells (erythrocytes); however, they have a vital role to play in our immunity, providing oxygen to cells and tissues. To sum up, the cells of the immune system are the white blood cells and the platelets. The white blood cells can be categorised as:

- *myeloid cells* – neutrophils, monocytes, macrophages, basophils and eosinophils;
- *lymphoid cells* – the lymphocytes.

The activities of white cells can be divided into three main processes:

- **Phagocytosis** – destroying infectious micro-organisms or non-self matter by engulfing and ingesting them.
- *Cytotoxity – cyto* means 'cell' and *toxicity* means 'poisonous' ('lethal to'), so cytotoxicity is the killing of infectious organisms by damaging cell membranes.
- *Inflammation* – white cells are involved in the response of body tissue to infection and injury.

White blood cells play many roles, but we will concentrate on the three roles mentioned above.

THE INNATE IMMUNE SYSTEM

The innate immune system is concerned with preventing any infectious micro-organisms or non-self matter from invading the body. Barrier protection is the body's first line of defence against infection:

- physical barriers;
- mechanical barriers;
- chemical barriers;
- blood cells.

The various parts of the body that make up the innate immune system include:

- skin;
- mucosal membrane;
- tears;
- breast milk;
- sweat;
- saliva;
- stomach acid;
- semen;
- cilia;
- phagocytes and other blood cells.

Physical barriers

The physical barriers that form part of our immune system are the skin and the mucosal membranes; intact skin prevents invasion by external micro-organisms. When skin is damaged or lost (e.g., as a result of injury or surgery) infection may occur. The membranes lining the inner surfaces of the body are protected by a barrier of mucus, which traps micro-organisms and other foreign substances (Rink and Gabriel 2000, Porth 2009, Vickers 2009a).

Mechanical barriers

These includes cilia, coughing, sneezing and tears. Cilia, the tiny hairs found in the nose, for example, are constantly moving to remove dirt, micro-organisms and mucus. Sneezing and coughing force out any micro-organisms or irritants in the respiratory tract. Tears form a mechanical barrier, washing any dirt particles or micro-organisms away from the eyes and also a chemical barrier, containing a bactericidal enzyme – lysozyme.

Chemical barriers

Chemical barriers include:

- tears;
- breast milk;
- sweat;
- saliva;
- acidic secretions – (stomach acid, and semen).

Most of these secretions contain either bactericidal enzymes such as lysozymes, or antibodies (immunoglobulins). Bacteria cannot survive in acidic secretions and are killed if the environment is too acidic.

Blood cells

The blood cells within the innate immune system are the leucocytes (white blood cells) and the thrombocytes (platelets). The white cells that are involved in the innate immune system are:

- neutrophils;
- monocytes and tissue macrophages;
- eosinophils;
- basophils.

The remaining white blood cells are the lymphocytes, the white blood cells which operate within the acquired immune system. This is discussed later on in the chapter. The neutrophils, eosinophils and basophils are known as granulocytes, when seen through a powerful microscope these cells appear to be full of little granules (or grains).

The cells that make up the innate immunity have two major functions – they are either phagocytes or **mediator cells**. Phagocytes are cells that kill and ingest any infectious micro-organisms. There are two types of phagocyte, mononuclear phagocytes and polymorphonucleocytes (see Figure 4.2).

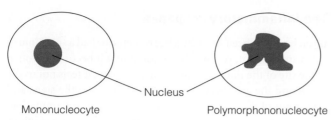

Figure 4.2 Two types of phagocytes.

Phagocytosis

The role of a phagocytic cell is to phagocytose, or consume, any infectious micro-organism or non-self matter that evades our external barriers (see Figure 4.3). Phagocytic cells recognise the bacterium as non-self matter and send out pseudopodia (false arms) which surround the bacterium. Once completely surrounded by the phagocyte, the bacterium comes into contact with the vacuoles inside the phagocytic cell; this then surrounds the bacterium and breaks it, killing the bacterium. Following this, the phagocyte uses (recycles) what it can from the bacterium for its own functions – growth, nutrition – and then ejects the non-usable parts to be excreted from the body. The phagocytes also remove pus and other non-self matter (dirt, splinters).

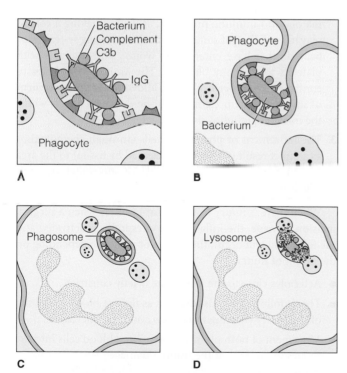

Figure 4.3 The process of phagocytosis. (A) Opsonisation coats the surface of the bacterium with IgG (an antibody) and complement. **(B)** The bacterium is bound to and engulfed by the phagocyte. **(C)** The phagosome is ingested into the cytoplasm of the phagocyte. **(D)** Lysosomes fuse with the phagosome releasing digestive enzymes and destroying the antigen.

Mediator cells

Mediator cells of immunity are monocytes, macrophages and dendritic cells. These recognise non-self matter (molecules/cells) and initiate immune responses.

- Monocytes are the largest of the leucocytes and circulate for one to two days, following which they migrate to various tissues throughout the body.

- Monocytes mature into macrophages after settling into the tissues and are found in loose connective tissue, the lungs, the brain, the spleen, tonsils, lymph nodes and bone marrow.

- Dendritic cells are star-shaped cells originating in both the myeloid and the lymphoid cell lines. Langerhans cells are specialised dendritic cells in the skin.

Monocytes, macrophages and dendritic cells are **antigen**-presenting cells (APCs), activating immune responses in the lymphocytes. They process and present non-self antigens to T-cell lymphocytes, forming part of the acquired immune system. Antigens are proteins triggering off an **antibody** response (antigen stands for antibody generating). Thus a bacterium is an antigen; an immunogen is something that generates an immune response.

Macrophages are also drawn to an inflamed area by chemicals released from damaged tissue, a process known as chemotaxis. Monocytes and macrophages activate the immune response against chronic infections such as tuberculosis, viral infections; dendritic cells activate T-cells against cancer and assist B lymphocytes to produce antibodies (DeMeyer and Buchsel 2005). Following our discussion of the cells that make up the innate immune system, we will now briefly consider the **complement** system.

The complement system

The complement system works with some of the white blood cells helping in the destruction of invading micro-organisms. It consists of more than 30 proteins found in blood plasma and on cell surfaces and works closely with antibodies, hence its name 'complement', because the proteins in the system 'complement' antibodies in the destruction of bacteria (Walport 2001).

There are three pathways which enable complement to carry out their function of fighting infections: classical, alternative and mannan-binding pathways.

Classical pathway

The classical pathway consists of nine factors/proteins (see Figure 4.4), numbered not in sequential order, but in the order in which they were discovered. Of all these complement proteins, C3 can be considered as being the pivotal one, as the other two pathways join the classical pathway at this stage.

The classical pathway is activated by a combination of antigen and antibody – known as antigen–antibody immune complexes. A bacterium is an antigen because it stimulates the production of antibodies by the immune system. A bacterium

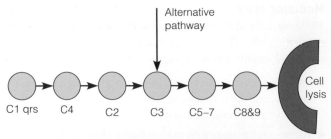

Figure 4.4 The classical pathway of the complement system.

is also an immunogen because it generates an immune response. Not all immunogens are antigens – for example, a virus is an immunogen, but not an antigen – it does not stimulate an antibody response because it stimulates an immune response from another part of the immune system – the T-cell lymphocytes (Murphy *et al.* 2008). The other roles of the complement system, particularly of the **opsonins** and of inflammation (which make their appearance before the membrane attack unit is formed), are of much more importance, because these roles help in the destruction of all species of infectious micro-organisms (Walport 2001).

As well as the complement system being activated by antigen–antibody complexes, where immunoglobulins are bound to bacteria; this pathway can also be activated by other means:

- The presence of apoptic cells – cells that have committed suicide because there are defects within them (for example, they may be old or poorly formed).
- Certain viruses (syncytial respiratory virus).
- Gram-negative bacteria (gram-negative bacteria are bacteria which do not turn purple in the Gram staining process used as a basic step in the identification of bacteria) – one of two major classes of bacteria that can cause very serious disease.
- When C-reactive protein (levels rise when there is inflammation) binds to a bacterium, it is able to opsonise it, as well as activating the complement system.

Alternative pathway
This pathway is activated by a variety of antigens, such as many bacterial, viral and fungal species, and tumour cells. The alternative pathway does not require a specific antibody to commence, and because of this can be effective much faster than if antibody synthesis had to take place, as in the classical pathway. This pathway joins the classical pathway at C3, and it functions because C3 is unstable and can be spontaneously activated on the cell surfaces of pathogenic organisms, such as bacteria (Walport 2001).

Mannan-binding lectin pathway
This pathway is initiated by mannan-binding lectin binding to carbohydrates on the surface of bacteria. The complex formed above indirectly activates the complement components C4 and C2, which then proceed to activate C3, and then continue from there as the classical pathway.

The inflammatory response

If you have ever been stung by a bee or nettle or had a small injury, for example a cut, you will have noted that it becomes swollen at the site of the injury, accompanied by pain, it feels hot to the touch and the area becomes reddish – these are the signs and symptoms of the immune system responding to inflammation. Inflammation is the body's immediate reaction to tissue injury or damage. There may also be nausea, sweating, raised pulse, lowered blood pressure and even loss of consciousness.

Inflammation is usually initiated by injury to our cells. Following this injury or damage, three simultaneous processes occur:

1. Mast cell degranulation. Mast cells are connective tissue cells which contain granules (vacuoles) in their cytoplasm, containing serotonin and histamine which, during the process of degranulation (or the breakup of the cell), are released into the tissues. Together with the other two processes, this provides the full inflammatory signs and symptoms of pain, heat, redness and swelling.

2. The activation of four plasma protein systems. These four systems are:
   a. complement;
   b. clotting;
   c. kinin system;
   d. immunoglobulins (antibodies).

   The complement system activates and assists both the inflammatory and immune processes, as well as having a role to play in the killing of some bacteria. The clotting system traps bacteria that have entered the wound and interacts with platelets to stop any bleeding. The kinin system helps to control vascular permeability – allowing for the movement of immune system elements to the damaged area – whilst the immunoglobulins destroy bacteria.

3. The movement of phagocytic cells (through chemotaxis – as a direct result of chemicals released by tissue) to the area in order to phagocytose bacteria or any other non-self débris in the wound.

When there is injury to tissue, for example when a surgical incision is made, the inflammatory response is activated and the following will occur, the degree of response depending on the extent of injury:

- Arterioles close to the injury site briefly constrict.
- This is followed by vasodilation as flow of blood to the site of the injury (leading to redness and heat) increases.
- Movement of both plasma proteins and blood cells into the tissues in the area of the trauma/damage.
- Swelling occurs.
- Nerve endings in the area become stimulated, causing pain.
- Components of the clotting system, the kinin system and the platelets move into the damaged area blocking any further risk of blood loss or infection by beginning the clotting process.

- The white blood cells (phagocytes and lymphocytes) move into the damaged area and start to kill any infectious micro-organisms. Other elements of the immune system act at the site of the trauma assisting phagocytosis.
- These systems/blood cells/tissue cells will remain in the area until tissue regeneration (repair) takes place, known as resolution.

Inflammation and chronic wounds

Inflammation is a key phase in the process of wound healing. Tissue damage and the activation of the various clotting factors during the vascular phase (when vascular changes take place) stimulate the release of inflammatory mediators, prostaglandins and histamine, and these cause the blood vessels in the area to become more permeable. The walls of the blood vessels stretch and the small pores in them enlarge allowing more fluid and cells to pass into them.

The proliferative stage

During this phase of healing, the damaged area is filled with new connective tissue, and a decrease in the area of damage is achieved by a combination of the physiological processes of granulation, contraction and epithelialisation:

- *Formation of granulation tissue* – provides the scaffolding for the new capillaries that will develop and will help to form connective tissue. 'Angiogenesis' (the growth of new blood vessels) is stimulated by the activity and by tissue hypoxia, resulting from the disruption of blood flow at the time of the injury/trauma.
- *Wound contraction* – following the production of connective tissue, fibroblasts (a type of cells that make extracellular matrix and collagen and which play a major role in the structure of connective tissue, an important factor in wound healing) congregate around the margin of the damaged area, contracting and pulling the edges of the damaged area together.
- *Re-epithelialisation* – the regrowth of epithelial cells across the surface of the damaged area.

The maturation stage

In healthy people, this stage will begin approximately 20 days after injury, lasting for many months or years in complex wounds. Although the scar tissue is initially raised and reddish, as it matures, blood supply decreases, and it becomes paler and smoother.

Factors that might delay healing

Many factors can significantly delay healing (Flanagan 2000), including:

- The person's health, for example stress, malnutrition, infection.
- Chronic diseases, for example conditions such as metabolic disturbances, e.g., hyperglycaemia (high blood sugar) or malabsorption syndromes (inability to absorb nutrients).

- Local factors such as wound infection, physical stress, the use of toxic cleansing agents and presence of foreign bodies prolong healing.
- Socioeconomic and psychological factors can also slow the rate of tissue repair, e.g. poverty, anorexia and bulimia.

Chronic wounds

Chronic wounds are those that fail to heal within an expected timescale. All chronic wounds tend to be characterised by non-resolving inflammation, and this inability to resolve inflammation is the most significant delaying factor in the healing of chronic wounds. Some causes of protracted inflammation (Flanagan *et al.* 2000) are as follows:

- Bacterial infection.
- Sub-clinical bacterial contamination – thought to elicit inflammatory responses within the wound.
- Contamination of wounds with non-self materials, for example dressing components.
- Recurrent physical trauma – leading to the re-initiation of inflammatory activity, for example pressure sores.
- Ischaemia–reperfusion injury – the release of pro-inflammatory **cytokines** (see below), tissue-degrading enzymes and tissue-damaging free radicals from leucocytes trapped in tissues cyclically exposed to periods of blood stasis (ischaemia) and flow.
- Age is probably the most significant factor in abnormal inflammation resulting in a disordered inflammatory response to acute injury.

Pressure ulcers are a type of chronic wound which is widespread and often underestimated in the UK. It has been suggested (NHS Choices 2010a) that as many as 1 in 20 people admitted to hospital with an acute (sudden) illness will develop a pressure ulcer. Pressure ulcers are discussed in Chapter 5.

Cytokines

This section explains what cytokines are and what they do.

- Cytokines are hormone-like polypeptides produced primarily by cells of the immune system.
- Cytokines act as messengers of the immune system, facilitating communication between the cells to adjust or vary the inflammatory reaction or to initiate immune cell proliferation and differentiation.
- Cytokines are an essential component of an adequate immune response. *Interferons* are a class of cytokine with broad antiviral and anticancer effects. A number of different forms of interferon exist, broadly grouped as alpha, beta and gamma interferons, and are synthesised by cells infected with a virus and secreted into extracellular fluid binding to specific **receptors** on uninfected neighbouring cells, protecting them from infection.

We have looked at the many parts of the innate immune system in this section and this has provided a comprehensive overview of the innate immune system and the diversity of systems, molecules and organs that form it. In the next section, we will move on to the acquired immune system, which is acquired throughout our lifetime as opposed to being innate in our bodies from birth.

THE ACQUIRED IMMUNE SYSTEM

The second arm of the immune system – the acquired immune system – is that part of the immune system acquired through-out life, giving extra immunity to pathogenic micro-organisms and non-self matter. In order to acquire this immunity, the body has to come into contact with particular (specific) infectious organisms and other non-self matter (another name for acquired immunity is specific immunity). With acquired immunity, the body achieves specific immunity to a specific threat. A third name for acquired immunity is adaptive immunity, because it adapts to specific immunological threats.

Acquired immunity has the ability to remember when a particular immunological threat (e.g. a pathogenic bacterium or virus) has been met and overcome. The next time the body comes into contact with this specific micro-organism, it remembers how to defeat it and so can mobilise the immune system to counter that threat (immunological memory). The acquired immune system is based upon the lymphocytes, and these are closely allied to the lymphatic system, so we will start this section by describing how this system works.

The lymphatic system

This system consists of a specialised system of lymph vessels (similar to blood vessels) as well as specialised lymph nodes and tissue. A combination of contractions of the smooth muscular walls of the lymph vessels allows drainage of lymph as well as the flexing and relaxing of striated muscle in the body due to the movement of the individual.

The peripheral lymphatic system consists of lymphatic vessels, lymphatic capillaries and encapsulated organs:

- spleen;
- tonsils;
- lymph nodes.

In addition, there are areas of unencapsulated, diffuse lymphoid tissue found in the:

- gastrointestinal tract;
- urinary tract;
- lungs.

The lymph vessels and capillaries form an extensive network throughout the body connecting the organs of the body to the lymphoid organs.

Lymph originates from plasma which moves into the lymphatic vessels from the blood capillaries, and then drains into the lymphoid organs. The lymphatic capillary walls are permeable allowing substances of relatively large sizes, such as plasma proteins, to enter and leave them. Lymph formation and lymph flow takes place at the rate of two to four litres every two hours, with a constant turnover of lymph into and out of the lymph vessels. This ensures effective migration of cells of the immune system into and out of the lymphatic system, and also the filtering of harmful toxins and infectious organisms out of the blood.

Lymphatic capillaries lead to larger lymphatic vessels, and situated throughout the lymphatic system are lymph glands – a little like railway stations on a railway network. There are two types of lymphatic vessels:

- *afferent lymphatic vessels* – carrying lymph into the gland;
- *efferent lymphatic vessels* – draining the lymph from the lymph glands.

Eventually all the lymph enters two large lymph glands within the thoracic cavity (the chest):

- thoracic duct;
- right lymphatic duct.

These two lymph ducts then empty into large veins within the neck, restoring fluid and proteins to the venous circulation (Figure 4.5).

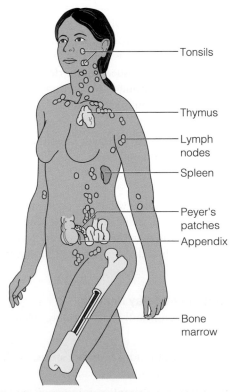

Figure 4.5 The lymphoid system. The central organs of the thymus and bone marrow, and the peripheral organs, including the spleen, tonsils, lymph nodes and Peyer's patches.

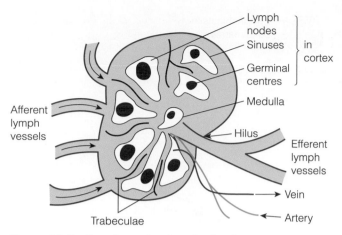

Figure 4.6 Section through a lymph gland.

Lymphoid tissue

Lymphoid tissue consists of:

- lymph nodes;
- lymphoid tissue found in specific organs such as the spleen, bone marrow, lung and liver.

Antigens entering the body enter the lymph system and are trapped in a lymphoid organ or lymph node. The lymph gland comprises a meshwork of reticular cells (these cells are essential for immune function), and the lymph containing antigens from infected tissues, along with antigen-bearing cells, pass through this meshwork, where the antigens are trapped (see Figure 4.6). Within the lymph gland are B-cell and T-cell lymphocytes (specialist white blood cells) as well as macrophages, and these cooperate to destroy the antigens by phagocytosis.

Other lymphoid organs

There are other lymphoid organs which are important parts of the acquired immune system providing immunological cover for parts of the body that are not covered by the lymph nodes.

- The spleen collects antigen from the blood for presentation to phagocytes and lymphocytes, as well as collecting dead red blood cells and disposing of them.
- The gut-associated lymphoid tissues (GALT) are a group of lymphoid tissues including the tonsils, adenoids, appendix, as well as the Peyer's patches in the small intestine.
- Bronchial-associated lymphoid tissue (BALT) and mucosal-associated lymphoid tissue (MALT) are similar to the gut-associated lymphoid tissues and they protect the respiratory tract.

The lymph nodes, spleen and MALT share the same basic design and function, trapping infectious micro-organisms (pathogens) from anywhere in the body where there is an infection and presenting these pathogens to lymphocytes in order to stimulate the immune system, leading to the destruction of these and other pathogens.

Lymphocytes

Lymphocytes are the cornerstone of our acquired immune systems, with two major classes of lymphocytes, which are essential to the functioning of the acquired immune system. These are T-cells and B-cells, each of which is responsible for certain functions:

- T-cell lymphocytes are concerned with cell-mediated immunity (the cells themselves kill the invading micro-organisms).
- B-cell lymphocytes are concerned with humoral immunity (concerned with the antibodies that are soluble in blood and lymph).

In addition to the T-cells and B-cells, there are also lymphocytes called plasma cells, a development of some of the B-cell lymphocytes which occurs following an encounter with an infectious micro-organism (pathogen).

Finally, there are a group of lymphocytes called natural killer (NK) cells. Although these are lymphocytes, they are not really a part of the acquired immune system as they attack any antigens, not just specific ones, so they can be considered to be part of the innate immune system. The development and differentiation of lymphocytes from the lymphoid stem cell can be seen in Figure 4.7.

Cell-mediated immunity (T-cell lymphocytes)

T-cell lymphocytes originate in the bone marrow and leave as immature lymphocytes moving to the thymus, where they are known as thymocytes. Whilst in the thymus, the immature lymphocytes mature, and are called T-cells (T for thymus). T-cell lymphocytes differentiate into various subclasses (see Figure 4.8):

- CD4 (T helper cells);
- CD8 (T suppressor cells);
- T **cytotoxic cells**;
- T **memory cells.**

Within the thymus, the T lymphocytes learn to recognise and differentiate 'self' cells from 'non-self' cells. This distinction is important because when the T lymphocytes have learned to differentiate between our own cells and cells that come from outside of us they can then attack anything that enters our body without damaging our own cells.

Differentiation occurs because all cells possess surface receptors that aid the cells in carrying out their various functions. However, some of the receptors are identification (ID) receptors and are peculiar to each individual, all the cells of an individual carry the same identification receptors. If T lymphocytes meet cells that do not carry our own unique identification receptors on their surfaces, they will attempt to destroy them. This is normally a very good arrangement, except if the occasion should arise that we require an organ or bone marrow transplant; in that eventuality, our T-cells perceive the transplant as 'non-self' and try to destroy it.

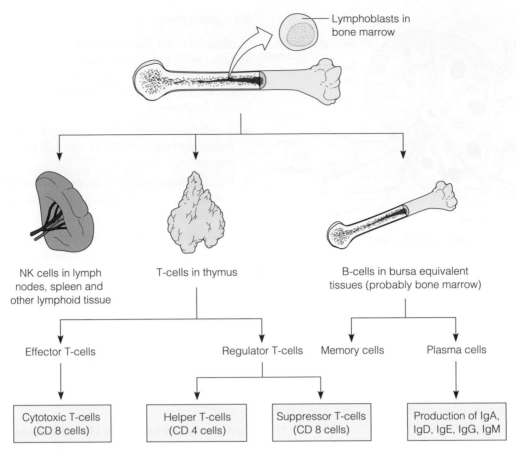

Figure 4.7 The development and differentiation of lymphocytes from the lymphoid stem cell (lymphoblasts).

Inside the thymus, the thymocyte goes through many different stages of development. In addition, the thymus produces several hormones acting on the thymocytes stimulating them to proliferate and generate the ability to recognise the huge numbers of antigens (pathogens) that the host will encounter throughout life (Rote and Huether 2010). However, most of the immature lymphocytes that enter the thymus will die there because they are programmed to die unless they instantly receive signals for them to start to differentiate and fight off pathogens (Klein and Sato, 2000).

As well as maturing in the thymus, the T-cells differentiate there, doing this because different subgroups of T-lymphocytes have to carry out different functions. The type of CD receptor that a T-cell carries determines that cell's function, and the major functions performed by T-cell lymphocytes are:

- cytotoxicity;
- immune system control;
- memory;
- delayed **hypersensitivity**.

Cytotoxicity (cell destruction) (see Figure 4.9)

This function is performed by the T-cytotoxic lymphocyte (Tc). T-cytotoxic lymphocytes possess many CD8 receptors and they mediate the direct killing of target cells by these T-cells themselves – 'cell-mediated immunity' (Rote and Huether 2010). The target cells may be our own cells infected by viruses, or cancerous tumours or even organ grafts from another person, i.e. kidney transplants. The T-cytotoxic cells bind to the target cell and release toxic substances into it, killing the target cell.

Immune system control

The control of the immune system depends upon two types of T-cell lymphocytes - the T-helper (Th) and T-suppressor (Ts) lymphocytes. T-helper cells are coated with many CD4 receptors, and the role of these cells is to stimulate the immune system to proliferate (i.e. to produce more of the correct types of immune cells and other substances associated with the immune system such as complement) in response to antigens in the body. There are two types of T-helper cell.

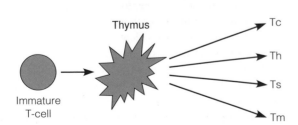

Figure 4.8 Differentiation of T-cell lymphocytes.

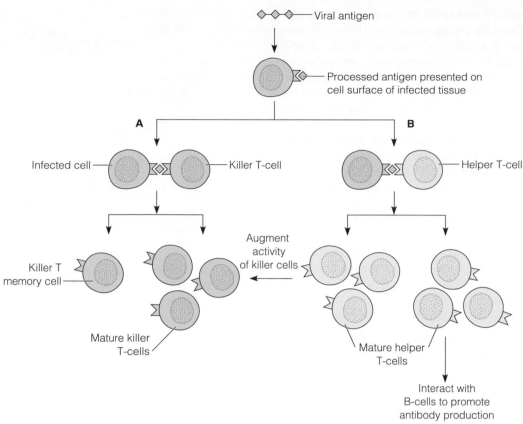

Figure 4.9 Cellular immune response. (A) An infected cell, abnormal cell or phagocyte presents antigen on its surface that binds with a receptor site on a killer T-cell or a helper T-cell. The killer T-cell is activated to proliferate into memory cells or mature cytotoxic cells. **(B)** The helper T-cell is activated to augment the cytotoxic response and stimulate the antibody-mediated immune response.

- Type 1 T-helper cells help to commence cell-mediated activity (directing both macrophages and T-cytotoxic cells to fight invading pathogens).
- Type 2 T-helper cells facilitate humoral (B-cell) immunity causing the production of more plasma B-cells which carry the correct antibodies (immunoglobulins) on their surfaces.

The body stimulates the immune system, but there is a need for checks and balances so that the immune system is neither overactive nor underactive. The T-suppressor lymphocytes (working together with the T-helper lymphocytes) do this.

Memory

What makes the acquired immune system particularly important is its ability to remember receptors on pathogenic micro-organisms with which it has previously come into contact. Because of this, the immune system can immediately stimulate the parts of the immune system which can respond to and attack these same pathogenic micro-organisms if they infect us again. It is the T-memory lymphocytes (Tm) which are responsible for remembering previous antigenic receptors on micro-organisms (Rote and Huether 2010). T-memory cells are long-lived; otherwise we would have to be constantly being

infected to maintain our ability to make a rapid response to a previously encountered antigen. This also is what underpins immunisations.

Delayed hypersensitivity

It is thought that delayed hypersensitivity is due to an imbalance between T-helper type 1 lymphocytes and T-helper type 2 lymphocytes (Kay 2001). Delayed hypersensitivity is the cause of such disorders as contact dermatitis.

B-cell immunity – humoral immunity

The second type of acquired immunity is humoral (or soluble) immunity. B-cell lymphocytes originate and mature in the bone marrow, hence their name of B-cells. Once matured they leave the bone marrow, travelling to the peripheral lymphoid organs, for example the lymph nodes; here they have the opportunity of encountering non-self antigens for which they have specificity (i.e. they have receptors that fit together and match – just like pieces of a jigsaw). The B-cells also have many receptors on their cell surface – they possess greater numbers and more diverse ones than are to be found on the T-cells. Because of this greater diversity, it is thought that more than 10^8 different antigens may be recognised by the receptors on B-cells.

Once the B-cells have met their specific antigen (for example, a bacterial species) they can become activated if they encounter the same antigen at a later date – they have similar memory capabilities as do the T-cell lymphocytes, remembering a previous micro-organism that has infected us and also remembering how to kill it. Those B-cells that do not encounter their matching specific antigen will die within a few weeks (Nairn and Helbert 2007).

In addition, further maturation of the B-cells as well as some differentiation take place at this time, some of the B-cells become memory cells which, like the T memory cells, carry a 'blueprint' of the specific antigenic receptors throughout their lives, whilst others become plasma cells – which produce, carry on their surfaces and secrete the immunoglobulins (or antibodies) when necessary. As the B memory cells divide and reproduce, then that memory is carried in future generations of B memory cells which means that they can quickly produce the correct immunoglobulins to fight previously encountered antigens, such as bacteria (Vickers 2006).

To summarise, mature B-cells are of two types:

● B memory cells memorise a blueprint of the receptors of specific antigens and how to fight them.

● Antibody-secreting plasma cells are produced by the plasma cells and are known as immunoglobulins.

Natural killer lymphocytes

These are the natural killer (NK) cells. They do not bind to an antigen and neither do they proliferate when they come into contact with an antigen – instead they bind to chemicals that occur as a result of chemical changes on the surfaces of cells that have been infected by viruses, such as rotavirus or measles, or cells that have become malignant (Rote and Huether 2010).

Immunoglobulins

Immunoglobulins/antibodies are mediators and assist other components of the immune system in the destruction of pathogens and other non-self matter. The plasma cells carry the immunoglobulins, and are much larger than the immature B-cells. They have a very short life which they spend in lymphoid tissue.

Role of immunoglobulins

The primary function of an antibody is to bind to antigen and inactivate it through one of the processes described below (Roitt 2001) (see Figure 4.10). Within this primary function, the role of immunoglobulins (Rote and Huether 2010) is to protect the host by:

● neutralising bacterial toxins;

● neutralising viruses;

● opsonising bacteria;

● activating components of the inflammatory response.

The immunoglobulins, of which there are five different classes, are soluble molecules and are produced by the plasma

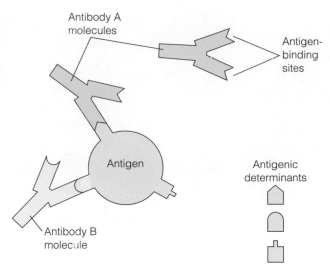

Figure 4.10 Antigen–antibody binding. The unique Fab site on the antibody binds with specific receptor sites on the antigen. As shown, more than one kind of antibody may be produced to an antigen.

cells in response to the immune system coming into contact with an immunogen (an immunogen is anything that generates an immune response). They rarely act in isolation: rather, they join forces with other components of the immune system to help with the destruction of antigens. Immunoglobulins are able to neutralise viruses by binding with receptors on the surface of the viruses, preventing the viruses from binding with the infected host cells prior to entering them.

Immunoglobulin structure

All immunoglobulins have the same basic structure made up of light and heavy molecular chains (Nairn and Helbert 2007). These chains differ in structure, location and amino acid components.

Although the basic immunoglobulin consists of two heavy chains and two light chains, each of the five different classes have slightly different structures. The heavy chains differentiate these five classes, each class being named after its respective heavy chain. These names are:

● immunoglobulin G (IgG) – subdivided into IgG1, IgG2, IgG3 and IgG4;

● immunoglobulin A (IgA) – subdivided into IgA1 and IgA2;

● immunoglobulin M (IgM);

● immunoglobulin D (IgD);

● immunoglobulin E (IgE).

There are two distinct ends to the shape of the basic immunoglobulin unit. One end, containing only heavy chains, is known as the Fc (fragment crystallisable) end, and it is this end that can bind with surface receptors on phagocytes and various other cells of the immune system as well as being able to combine with complement, stimulating complement activity. This occurs due to the B-cell being able to rearrange the genes which code for the variable region of the immunoglobulin

(Vickers 2006). The other end of the immunoglobulin, the Fab (fragment antigen-binding) end, binds with antigens (micro-organisms).

One end can bind onto an antigen, and the other onto a phagocytic cell, with the immunoglobulin holding on to the antigen and forming a 'bridge' between the antigenic organism and the phagocyte, allowing the slow-moving phagocyte enough time to engulf and ingest it. Once held in this way, the antigen cannot get away.

The Fab region includes the variable region – this end of an immunoglobulin can easily change the organisation of its receptors in order to fit the many different and varied antigen receptors – whilst the Fc end is at the end of the constant region of the immunoglobulin. The Fc end cannot change its receptors; it can only bind with the receptors of certain cells of the immune system.

Classification of immunoglobulins

Let us now look at the individual structures and roles of these five classes of immunoglobulins.

Immunoglobulin G (IgG)

Also known as 'gammaglobulin', IgG is an important class of immunoglobulin involved in the secondary immune response to infection. It is the most abundant immunoglobulin found in serum – it constitutes approximately 75% of the total immunoglobulins in serum (blood) (Seymour *et al.* 1995). IgG has the smallest molecular weight and is present in all parts of the body – intravascular (blood) and extravascular (tissues) areas – playing a major role against both blood-borne and tissue infections.

Its small molecular weight means that IgG is the only immunoglobulin that can cross the placental barrier. This is important because, at full-term birth, a baby has only recently begun to produce its own IgG, and is vulnerable to infections. The new-born baby is protected against any infections to which the mother is immune because it receives the maternal IgG. This is known as **passive immunity**. The amount and type of antibodies passed to the baby depends on the mother's immunity. For example, if the mother has had chickenpox, she will have developed immunity against the disease, and some of the chickenpox antibodies will be passed on to her baby. However, if the mother has never had chickenpox, then the baby will not be protected. Maternal IgG in the baby disappears about the age of 9 months (Vickers 2006).

IgG plays several important roles in mediating the immune system:

- IgG activates the complement system.
- IgG enhances phagocytosis.
- IgG assists the T-cytotoxic cells.
- IgG binds to platelets.
- IgG is important in immune responses against encapsulated bacteria.

IgG is often given as therapy to people with immunodeficiencies.

Immunoglobulin M (IgM)

IgM is important in the primary immune response and also the early stages of secondary immune response. It has the largest molecular weight of the five immunoglobulins and is composed of five immunoglobulin units (a pentamer).

IgM is an efficient immunoglobulin for combining bacteria together (a process known as agglutination); it is also capable of activating the classical pathway of the complement system. IgM is restricted almost entirely to the intravascular spaces and is often involved with the immune response to complex blood-borne infectious organisms.

Immunoglobulin A (IgA)

There are two types of IgA – serum and secretory. Secretory IgA is particularly important (Roitt 2001) as this is the major immunoglobulin found in external body secretions:

- saliva;
- breast milk;
- colostrum;
- tears;
- nasal secretions;
- sweat;
- respiratory tract secretions;
- gastrointestinal tract secretions;
- urinary tract secretions.

Secretory IgA (sIgA) is composed of two immunoglobulin molecules and includes a molecule of a secretory component allowing for the easy transfer of secretory IgA across the epithelial cells of the body into the secretions, protecting IgA from attacks by bacterial secretions. IgA has a half-life of seven days and is the last immunoglobulin to develop in children, usually taking about 12 years to reach adult levels.

The main function of sIgA is to prevent bacteria and other antigens from crossing the epithelium into the deeper tissues of the body. SIgA, once combined with bacteria, is able to activate the alternative pathway of the complement system.

Immunoglobulin E (IgE)

IgE makes up less than 1% of total serum immunoglobulin levels, although they rise when someone has an atopic disease (for example, eczema), and it has a half-life of two days. IgE is found on the surfaces of tissue mast cells and circulating basophils. When IgE binds to these target cells (mast cells and basophils) in the presence of antigen, it can trigger off an allergic reaction, activating the mast cells, degranulating them (releasing granules of histamine from cells that carry them). This causes an acute inflammatory response, leading to the signs and symptoms of allergic reactions found in such diseases as hay fever and asthma. IgE is also responsible for sensitising cells on mucosal surfaces, such as the conjunctival, nasal and bronchial mucosa, giving rise to allergic symptoms such as rhinitis and conjunctivitis.

Consider this . . .

What are the differences between **allergy**, sensitivity and intolerance?

- *Allergy*. This is a reaction produced by the body's immune system when it encounters an ordinarily harmless substance.
- *Sensitivity*. This is the exaggeration of a normal side-effect produced by contact with a substance. For example, the caffeine in a cup of coffee may result in extreme symptoms, such as palpitations and trembling, when it would usually only have this effect when taken in much larger doses.
- *Intolerance*. This is where a substance, such as lactose, causes unpleasant symptoms (for example, diarrhoea) for a number of reasons, but this does not involve the immune system. Those people who have an intolerance to particular foods can usually eat a small amount and have no problems. However, those with a food allergy will have a bad reaction even if they come into contact with a very small amount of the food they are allergic to.

Immunoglobulin D (IgD)

Little is known about the functions of IgD. It is chiefly located on B-cell surface membranes as a receptor molecule and is found in very low concentrations in the body. It is thought to be involved in antigen-triggered lymphocyte differentiation, but more research is needed to fully understand the role of IgD (Seymour *et al.* 1995, Roitt 2001, Nairn and Helbert 2007).

FACTORS IMPACTING ON THE IMMUNE SYSTEM

There are a number of factors which can affect our immune system, both innate and acquired; here is a list of just a few of them:

- *Age*. The very young have an immature immune system.
- *Hormones and stress*. An excess of certain hormones, or a lack of them can reduce the effectiveness of the immune system. Stress causes an imbalance in the hormonal system.
- *Drugs and chemicals* including recreational drugs, prescribed drugs and alcohol. These can affect the balance of the immune system. For example, although antibiotics are very useful in helping us to fight bacterial infections, many of them can also kill commensal micro-organisms on and in our bodies, such as those coating the gastrointestinal tract, so leading to diarrhoea and oral fungal infections, such as candida.
- *Malnutrition*. Components of the immune system are protein-based and, as they are dying off or being used up fighting infections, they need to be replenished. People who are malnourished are more at risk of infections, many of which can be fatal.
- *Infections*. Everyone is aware of the effects of **human immunodeficiency virus** (HIV) infection on the immune system but, more mundane infections can also cause a reduction in the functioning effectiveness of the immune system. This is because many components of the immune system are destroyed and used up whilst fighting the micro-organisms causing an infection.

DISORDERS OF THE IMMUNE SYSTEM

The person with a primary immunodeficiency

Primary immunodeficiencies occur as a result of problems with the genes that code for the immune system and are almost all inherited conditions. There are over 170 different types of primary immunodeficiency, of which common variable immunodeficiency (CVID) is the most commom.

Signs and symptoms of CVID

Signs and symptoms of CVID include the following (Toolan 2006):

- recurrent infection of chest/sinuses;
- chronic infection of chest/sinuses;
- incomplete clearing of infections following antimicrobials;
- lung damage – especially bronchiectasis (an abnormal widening of one or more of the airways).

There is a possible association between CVID and asthma/bronchitis.

INTERDISCIPLINARY CARE FOR A PRIMARY IMMUNODEFICIENCY

Diagnosis

Diagnosis is based on an assessment of indicative symptoms and on laboratory tests.

Features frequently present and highly suspicious of immunodeficiency include:

- chronic infection;
- recurrent infection;
- opportunistic infections;
- incomplete clearing of infection;
- incomplete response to infection.

Features frequently present and moderately suspicious of immunodeficiency include:

- skin rash/eczema;
- chronic diarrhoea;
- hepatosplenomegaly (enlarged liver and spleen);
- recurrent abscesses;
- recurrent osteomyelitis (bone infection);
- evidence of **autoimmunity** (production of antibodies against the tissues of your own body).

Laboratory tests for a primary immunodeficiency include the following:

- full blood count and differential (platelet volume, absolute lymphocyte count, neutrophil and eosinophil counts);

- IgG, IgA, IgM numbers;
- antibody counts for certain antigens (for example, anti-tetanus toxoid antibodies);
- lymphocyte subpopulations;
- HIV antibodies to diagnose HIV or to exclude other diagnoses.

Following these diagnostic tests, diagnosis of a primary immunodeficiency such as CVID can be made.

Treatment

Following a diagnosis of CVID, intravenous immunoglobulin therapy may be commenced and prophylactic antibiotics. This treatment is usually life long; currently there is no cure for these primary immunodeficiency disorders.

IN PRACTICE

Administration of IV immunoglobulin

- Good verbal and written information, covering benefits and risks of treatment (for example, transmissible diseases from donors) and adverse reactions, should be given so that a decision can be made as to whether or not to commence treatment. Consent must be obtained.

- Individuals need to be assessed prior to each infusion. It is unwise to infuse IgG if there is an acute infection as an adverse reaction may occur (Misbah and Chapel 1993).

- The immunoglobulin should be made up according to the manufacturer's instructions.

- Asepsis (performing procedures under sterile conditions) should be maintained.

- Blood samples need to be taken before the first infusion and serum saved – this is for testing for hepatitis C. Some centres test for HIV/HBV – consent must be obtained.

- Blood samples also need to be taken every 6–12 weeks for immunoglobulin (IgG, IgA and IgM) levels, for specific

antibodies as indicated and for liver function (LFTs). Serum immunoglobulin levels need to be maintained within the normal/local range (7–14 g/L).

- In addition, blood samples need to be taken for C reactive protein (CRP) and full blood count (FBC).

- During and just after the first infusion, the person should be observed for adverse reactions. Steroids, antihistamines and resuscitation equipment should be available.

- The rate of infusion should be as per the manufacturer's recommendations, especially for the first two infusions (when people with bacteraemia are prone to experience reactions).

- Some people can tolerate faster rates once a treatment regimen based on individual needs has been established.

Source: Toolan 2006.

NURSING CARE FOR A PRIMARY IMMUNODEFICIENCY

Although those with a primary immunodeficiency are being successfully treated with immunoglobulin therapy, the nurse must constantly consider the psychosocial effects that may be experienced by a person of relying on a drug for the rest of their lives. Even if on home therapy, there is still some disruption to

their normal lives, it can prove a challenge to combine a normal life with their disorder and dependence upon a drug product.

Having looked at primary immunodeficiencies, we will now discuss **secondary immunodeficiencies**. Unlike the case with primary immunodeficiencies, you are almost certainly aware of at least one type of secondary immunodeficiency – acquired immunodeficiency syndrome (AIDS), which will be discussed in the next section.

COMMUNITY-BASED CARE

Subcutaneous infusions of immunoglobulins have become popular and many people prefer to infuse at home, although some prefer intravenous self-infusions at home following a period of training (Hansen *et al.* 2002, Henderson 2003, Gardulf *et al.* 2004). Those who are not happy self-infusing at home, or who do not have support at home, will still go to hospital for immunoglobulin infusions.

The person must be carefully assessed prior to being accepted on a training programme that will enable them to undertake treatment at home. People who are antibody deficient should be trained at a recognised training centre. They will be taught all aspects of the infusions including the importance of documentation.

Home therapy saves time missed from work and school, reduces time spent travelling to and from hospital and encourages freedom and autonomy in the family. Home infusions are considerably more cost-effective to the National Health Service and can reduce the stress associated with repeated hospital visits. Subcutaneous therapy is safe and easy to administer and as such is an ideal treatment for home therapy.

Secondary immunodeficiencies

Secondary immunodeficiencies are so-called because, unlike primary immunodeficiencies which are the result of a faulty gene, they are secondary to an external factor, such as drugs or infections. In the following section we will concentrate on **human immunodeficiency virus** (HIV)/AIDS which is a major cause of secondary immunodeficiency, but there are many other causes of secondary immunodeficiences (Vickers 2005).

Globally, one of the major causes of secondary immunodeficiency is protein deficiency due to malnutrition or disorders such as Kwashiorkor disease. Improving calorie and protein intake can correct kwashiorkor, provided that treatment is not commenced too late. Full height and growth potential will never be achieved in children who have had this condition.

In the UK apart from HIV, the major causes of secondary immunodeficiencies are iatrogenic, i.e. caused by medical personnel/treatment, including immunodeficiencies following steroid or cytotoxic drug therapy for various diseases which can damage the components of the immune system (Seymour *et al.* 1995).

Causes of secondary immunodeficiencies

Secondary immunodeficiencies can be caused by a multitude of factors. They are associated with defects in antibodies and T-cells including (Vickers 2005):

- infections, including HIV, hepatitis, measles, mumps, TB, congenital rubella, cytomegalovirus (CMV) and glandular fever;
- medications, including corticosteroids, cytotoxic drugs, immunosuppressive drugs and even antibiotics;
- stress – psychological and physical;
- malnutrition – either by lack of food, the wrong type of food or Kwashiorkor;
- recreational drugs, for example cocaine, heroin and alcohol;
- cancers, for example, Hodgkin's lymphoma, leukaemia;
- disorders of the endocrine system, such as diabetes;
- autoimmune diseases;
- ageing;
- environmental chemicals such as polychlorinated biphenyls (PBCs) and dioxin;
- trauma – particularly burns;
- pregnancy (Weinberg 1987);
- anaesthesia and surgery – stress related;
- kidney disease (Crew *et al.* 2004);
- irradiation – either accidental (job-related) or irradiation therapy to treat malignancies.

Treatment of secondary immunodeficiencies consists of removing or treating the cause (if possible), along with therapy. For example, if an infection is the cause, then the relevant antibiotics or other antimicrobial drugs need to be given. If the cause is drugs or surgery, once the drugs are discontinued, or recovery from surgery is underway, the immune system will usually right itself.

The person with HIV infection

In 1981, five cases of *Pneumocystis carinii (PCP)* (now renamed *Pneumocystis jiroveci*) pneumonia and 26 cases of a rare

FAST FACTS

HIV

- In 2009, the number of people living with HIV in the UK reached an estimated 86 500. A quarter of these people were unaware of their infection.
- New diagnoses among men who have sex with men remained high (2760); four out of five probably acquired their infection in the UK.
- Of the people newly diagnosed in 2009, 1130 probably acquired their infection heterosexually within the UK, accounting for a third of heterosexuals diagnosed.

Source: HPA 2010.

PRACTICE ALERT

HIV can be found in blood and other body fluids, for example, semen and vaginal fluids. It cannot live for long when outside of the body. The virus can enter the body via contact with the bloodstream or by passing through delicate mucous membranes, such as inside the vagina, rectum or urethra.

The main ways people may become infected with HIV are:

● having sexual intercourse with an infected person;

● injecting drugs using a needle or syringe that has been used by someone who is infected;

● as a baby of an infected mother.

There are policies and procedures that have to be adhered to in all settings if spillage of any body fluids occurs. You must ensure that you adhere to these policies and procedures in order to protect yourself and others.

cancer, Kaposi's sarcoma, were diagnosed in young, previously healthy homosexual males in Los Angeles and New York City. In 1983, a common antibody was identified in men with AIDS. The human immunodeficiency virus (HIV) was isolated in 1984. It then became apparent that AIDS was the final, fatal stage of HIV infection.

HIV infection and AIDS

The cause of AIDS is HIV, which is a retrovirus. Retroviruses copy their genetic material into the genetic material of human cells which means that once a cell is infected it stays infected. HIV is transmitted by direct contact with infected blood and body fluids. Significant concentrations of the virus are present in blood, semen, vaginal and cervical secretions and cerebrospinal fluid (CSF) of infected individuals, and it is also found in breast milk and saliva.

Pathophysiology of HIV infection

Viruses are very simple organisms consisting generally of a length of DNA surrounded by a lipoprotein coat – or 'envelope'. When a virus infects a cell, this envelope breaks down, releasing the DNA, which is then transported to the cell nucleus. Here the viral DNA insinuates itself into the cell DNA and, in effect, hijacks the cell DNA in order for it to serve the virus's purpose – that is to make hundreds of copies of the virus. Once all the cell's contents have been used up, the hundreds of viruses break out of the cell. Each of the new viruses then goes on to infect other cells, and so the cycle continues.

Because HIV is a retrovirus, instead of the envelope surrounding viral DNA, it surrounds viral RNA. Before production of the infected cell DNA can be taken over, the viral RNA has to become viral DNA. Fortunately for the HIV, there

is a viral gene, called *pol*, in its RNA, and this gene codes for an enzyme called *reverse transcriptase* which is capable of transcribing viral RNA into viral DNA. In effect, it reverses the normal pathway of protein formation – DNA to RNA to protein. In HIV infection, the pathway is RNA to DNA. Once the viral DNA is present, it integrates with the infected cell's DNA.

This simple fact is the reason why HIV is such a dangerous virus and causes major problems to the immune system. CD4 receptors are present in large numbers on the surface membranes of T-helper cells, and T-helper cells are the cells that help to regulate the immune system and stimulate it to proliferate in response to an infection. As HIV infects T-helper cells and kills them, the immune system cannot respond properly to other infectious organisms. The more the CD4 T-helper cells are destroyed, the more effective the HIV infection becomes, and the sicker the infected person becomes. Eventually there will be too few T-helper cells in the body to be able to fight an infection, such as TB, *Pneumocystis carinii* pneumonia and other opportunistic infections, as well as more common infections.

In addition to T-helper cells, other cells also carry CD4 receptors and they also may be infected – these include antigen-presenting cells, macrophages and monocytes.

In summary, this process of infection from HIV to full-blown AIDS is linked to the spread of HIV from the initial site of infection through to lymphoid tissues throughout the body. The immune response of the infected person initially controls acute infection, but this is only a temporary state, and it does not prevent chronic infection of lymphoid cells (Abbas and Lichtman 2004).

Signs and symptoms of HIV infection

The signs and symptoms of HIV infection may not become apparent for several years after the actual infection. Initially, the infected person may get flu like symptoms (a transient fever that may develop into a lymphadenopathy – abnormally enlarged lymph nodes, also called swollen glands). For several years after infection, the virus may be dormant; although the infected person may not show any symptoms during this time, the virus may be reproducing, and the infected hosts will themselves be infectious to others within two weeks of being infected.

The period from initial infection to seroconversion (this is the time when antibodies to HIV occur) is known as the 'window period' and lasts for about two to four weeks. These antibodies remain detectable for life. During the time when the infected person is showing no signs or symptoms of infection, the HIV integrates into the host cells, but does not replicate. However, they provide a 'reservoir of infection' because, whilst they are not replicating, they cannot be recognised by the immune system and destroyed by it.

When the immune system responds to infection by another infectious organism, HIV replication will then take place because signals are sent to the infected T-cell DNA from T-cell receptors or from cytokines, the number of CD4 T-cells (i.e. T-helper cells) gradually declines until levels of T-helper cells reach a critical threshold. At the same time, because of the decline in T-helper cells – which leads to an overall lessening of the effectiveness of the immune system – the development of opportunistic infections can occur (Male 2004). Eventually the numbers of HIV will have grown so much because of such high levels of replication that the infected host will start to experience the signs and symptoms of AIDS itself.

The signs and symptoms of AIDS are the same as for any immune deficiency:

● chronic and recurring infections;

● candida (thrush);

● rashes;

● loss of weight;

● recurrent abscesses;

● evidence of autoimmunity;

● neoplasms (cancers).

INTERDISCIPLINARY CARE FOR HIV INFECTION

The treatment of HIV infection and AIDS is by means of a four-pronged attack on the disease. These four prongs are:

● medication;

● vaccine;

● immunomodulation;

● palliative therapy.

In addition, measures to prevent infection are an essential component in the care strategy.

Medication

Over the past few years, there have been many advances in medication for the treatment of HIV infection using anti-retroviral drugs. These antiretroviral drugs are now used in combinations and include three major different types:

● *Nucleoside reverse transcriptase inhibitors (NRTIs)* act by competing with the cell nucleosides (DNA) for reverse transcriptase binding. NRTIs interfere with the action of an HIV protein called reverse transcriptase, which the virus needs to make new copies of itself.

● *Non-nucleoside reverse transcriptase inhibitors (NNRTIs)* interfere with reverse transcriptase activity by disrupting the catalytic site of the enzyme. NNRTIs also stop HIV from replicating within cells by inhibiting the reverse transcriptase protein.

● *Protease inhibitors* (PIs) interfere with the cleavage (splitting) of proteins by the viral protease, and cause the production of non-infectious viruses. PIs inhibit protease,

which is another protein involved in the HIV replication process.

For treatment of HIV, three or four drugs may be used in combination. These are collectively known as HAART – highly active antiretroviral therapy – and they have been able to arrest the progress of HIV infection, and even reverse the poor immune functioning (Candy *et al.* 2001). Research is very much ongoing in this area and there can easily be changes to the drug regimen of people with HIV – almost overnight. Therefore, it is important to keep up to date with these changes.

Vaccine

So far the difficulties in developing a vaccine have proven insurmountable. There is no single vaccine produced that can cope with all the variations and mutations of HIV. Most of the present research is geared to finding a vaccine against the glycoprotein gp120, which allows the virus to bind to CD4 receptors on the T-helper cells. Because of the rapid and frequent mutations, and the different subtypes, finding a definitive vaccine has not so far been possible because the vaccine needs to be effective against a range of mutations that may be present at any one time, in addition to new mutations which constantly arise.

There are two major types of HIV – HIV-1 and HIV-2 – and these are distinguished by their genetic differences, global distribution and clinical signs and symptoms. HIV-1 is the cause of the global AIDS epidemic, whereas HIV-2, found in West Africa, has a slower development and a milder course.

Whilst a human has about 40 000 genes in his/her DNA, HIV-1 has only nine genes. Also HIV-1 has a very variable genetic structure, with at least 10 clades (or subtypes). These different subtypes are found in different parts of the world. This has implications when looking for successful drug therapies and vaccines, because what will work in one part of the world may not work in another. The ability of HIV to mutate rapidly means that trying to treat HIV and AIDS brings many problems. This ability to mutate rapidly – and often – enables the virus to evade the immune system, because the initial immune response to any novel infectious organism is slow and weak, but becomes much stronger with subsequent exposures (Vickers 2005).

Immunomodulation

Immunomodulation is an attempt to boost the immune system. It has been found that a combination of both interleukin-2 and antiretroviral drugs can reduce the number of infected T-cells and also reduce the levels of HIV RNA in the body. Immunomodulation is currently under development, but many drug trials are needed to demonstrate that the clinical improvements it brings would outweigh any potential side-effects. Another form of immunomodulation to boost the immune system is the use of glucocorticosteroids (a type of steroid).

Palliative therapy

This includes the use of antibiotic, antiviral and antifungal drugs to deal with infections and to try to prevent them becoming fatal. Other palliative measures include addressing:

- nutritional needs;
- social and psychological care – to improve wellbeing and hence strengthen the immune system;
- stress reduction;
- immunisations;
- maintaining CD4 counts;
- education.

Prevention

Prevention is a crucial component in halting the spread of infection. There are certain definable risks for HIV infection that are based upon the major modes of spread:

- as a sexually transmitted infection (STI);
- through injected drug use;
- as a perinatal infection.

In addition, in places where blood products are not screened, there is potentially a risk to blood/blood product transfusion recipients.

Potential preventative measures include the following:

- Treat HIV infection as an illness, not as a social stigma – people may then be more accepting of people with HIV and this may allow for open dialogue and more discussion of how to prevent it.
- Screening – provide HIV testing in order to identify those persons who are infected, reducing risk to others.
- Provide educational programmes describing how to avoid STIs.
- Promote safer sex activity.
- Provide clean needles for injecting drug users.
- Offer HIV-infected pregnant women antiretroviral therapy in order to reduce the risk of perinatal HIV transmission.

NURSING CARE FOR HIV INFECTION

The nursing care needs for the person with HIV infection change over the course of the disease and include:

- early identification of the infection;
- promoting health-maintenance activities to prolong the asymptomatic period (i.e. avoiding infections);
- prevention of opportunistic infections;
- treatment of disease complications;
- providing emotional and psychosocial support.

We should not think of HIV or indeed any illness as just a collection of symptoms that have to be treated. We have to consider the effect on a person within a holistic framework, and that includes the quality of life experienced by someone with HIV.

HIV infection impacts upon an individual's life in a number of ways. Currently there is no cure for HIV infection. Coping strategies will need to be devised along with the support of:

- family;
- neighbours;
- health professionals;
- politicians, researchers;
- the pharmacological industry;
- society.

HIV is a long-term condition. The person with HIV may have many care needs, including both physical and psychosocial support. Many of these needs fall within the realm of nursing to promote knowledge and understanding, self-care, comfort, and improving or maintaining quality of life. Nursing care needs for the person with HIV infection change over the course of the disease. Preventive healthcare measures, health maintenance activities, education and support of coping mechanisms are important. Counselling the person with a new diagnosis of HIV infection is vital. HIV infection continues to carry a social stigma that may interfere with the person's usual support systems and coping mechanisms. As the disease progresses and the person experiences more physical symptoms, direct care needs become more important while the need for psychosocial support continues. Acute exacerbation of opportunistic infections may necessitate hospitalisation, but typically the person is nursed at home. It may not be just the person who will need support and possibly counselling; the family as well as healthcare professionals may need reassurance and counselling. Support, education and counselling should be in place so that they can be offered to those who may need it.

This discussion of immune system disorders leads us on to a discussion of the very important role the immune system plays in protecting us from infections. When discussing acquired immunity, emphasis was put on its ability to remember previous infectious agents, preventing previously experienced infections from recurring again (the primary and secondary response to infection). We will begin by looking at infectious diseases themselves, before discussing the role of vaccinations and immunisations in helping to protect us.

Hypersensitivity

Another problem that can arise in relation to the immune system is the development of hypersensitivity. Hypersensitivity occurs when an immune response damages the body's own tissues.

Normally, the immune system works well in maintaining its effectiveness and its functions. To do this, it uses a system of checks and balances to maintain homeostasis, although these sometimes fail, and an excessive or an inefficient immune response occurs. This then causes problems, some of them very severe, but all of them debilitating in some way. Inappropriate immune responses can manifest in one of four ways:

1. an exaggerated response against environmental antigens such as grass pollen or pollutants (allergies);

2. a misdirected response against the host's own cells, which can destroy some of the host's own tissues and organs (autoimmunity);

3. an immune response that is directed against non-self antigens, such as blood transfusions and organ transplants, which are actually of benefit to the host (this process comes under the name of alloimmunity);

4. an immune response that is not good enough to protect the host, or is absent (immune deficiency).

Three of these above conditions – allergy, autoimmunity and alloimmunity – come under the heading of hypersensitivity. Hypersensitivity refers to a changed 'immunological reaction to an antigen causing disease or damage to the host' (Rote 2010a).

Pathophysiology of hypersensitivity

Hypersensitivity can be classified into four types, using Gell and Coombs (1968) classification. The first three types involve the humoral system, whilst the fourth type is a function of cellular immunity.

Type I hypersensitivity – immediate hypersensitivity

This type of hypersensitivity is linked to the immunoglobulin known as IgE and is mediated through the degranulation of mast cells and basophils. This produces an allergic response such as allergic rhinitis, asthma, hay fever and atopic eczema (see Figure 4.11).

Atopy is another word, as well as allergy, to describe an IgE-mediated allergic disease. People with atopy have a hereditary predisposition to produce IgE antibodies against common environmental allergies, and may have one or more atopic diseases, such as asthma and eczema (Kay 2001).

With immediate hypersensitivity:

● Reactions occur when an environmental antigen, for example house dust mite faeces, peanuts or grass pollen, interacts with IgE bound to tissue mast cells or basophils.

● The first time this occurs, there are no symptoms and the individual becomes sensitised to the antigen.

● With any subsequent exposure to the same antigen, an allergic reaction is triggered.

● In all these subsequent exposures, the specific antigen causes cross-linking of the surface antigen-specific IgE molecules to mast cells and basophils; this in turn triggers degranulation and the release of vasoactive compounds from these cells (Chapel and Haeney 1993).

● Histamine is the most potent of these compounds, causing smooth muscle contraction and endothelial cell contraction (Seymour *et al.* 1995), leading to vascular permeability and oedema. Histamine causes increased secretions; for example, mucosal and gastric secretions, tears, contraction of bronchial smooth muscle, leading to bronchial constriction, and vasodilation, causing increased blood flow into the area.

● The most serious form of atopy is acute systematic anaphylaxis, which can be fatal if not treated immediately.

Anaphylaxis

Before reading any further you may find it helpful to return to Case Study 2 at the beginning of the chapter and relate the issues here to Thomas Worthington who was diagnosed as having a severe anaphylactic shock. Anaphylaxis is an acute multisystem severe type I hypersensitivity reaction. You will have read about hypersensitivities in this section of the chapter. This needs to be treated quickly; it is regarded as a medical emergency which may require resuscitation management, including ensuring that his airway is open, oxygen therapy and large volumes of intravenous fluids, and he will have to be closely monitored until his condition improves.

Anaphylaxis occurs in highly sensitive persons following injection of a specific antigen. Anaphylaxis rarely follows oral ingestion, although this is possible.

The reaction begins within minutes of exposure to the allergen and may be almost instantaneous. The release of histamine and other mediators causes vasodilation and increased capillary permeability, smooth muscle contraction and bronchial constriction. These chemical mediators cause the person to experience the typical manifestations of anaphylaxis. Initially, a sense of foreboding or uneasiness, light-headedness and itchy palms and scalp may be noted. Hives may develop, along with angioedema (localised tissue swelling) of the eyelids, lips, tongue, hands, feet and genitals. Swelling can also affect the uvula and larynx, impairing breathing and bronchial constriction. The person exhibits air hunger, stridor and wheezing, and a barking cough. These respiratory effects can be lethal if the reaction is severe and intervention is not immediately available. Vasodilation and fluid loss from the vascular system can lead to impaired tissue perfusion and hypotension, a condition known as anaphylactic shock.

Type II hypersensitivity – antibody-mediated hypersensitivity

Antibody-mediated hypersensitivity reactions normally manifest themselves as the destruction of a target cell through the

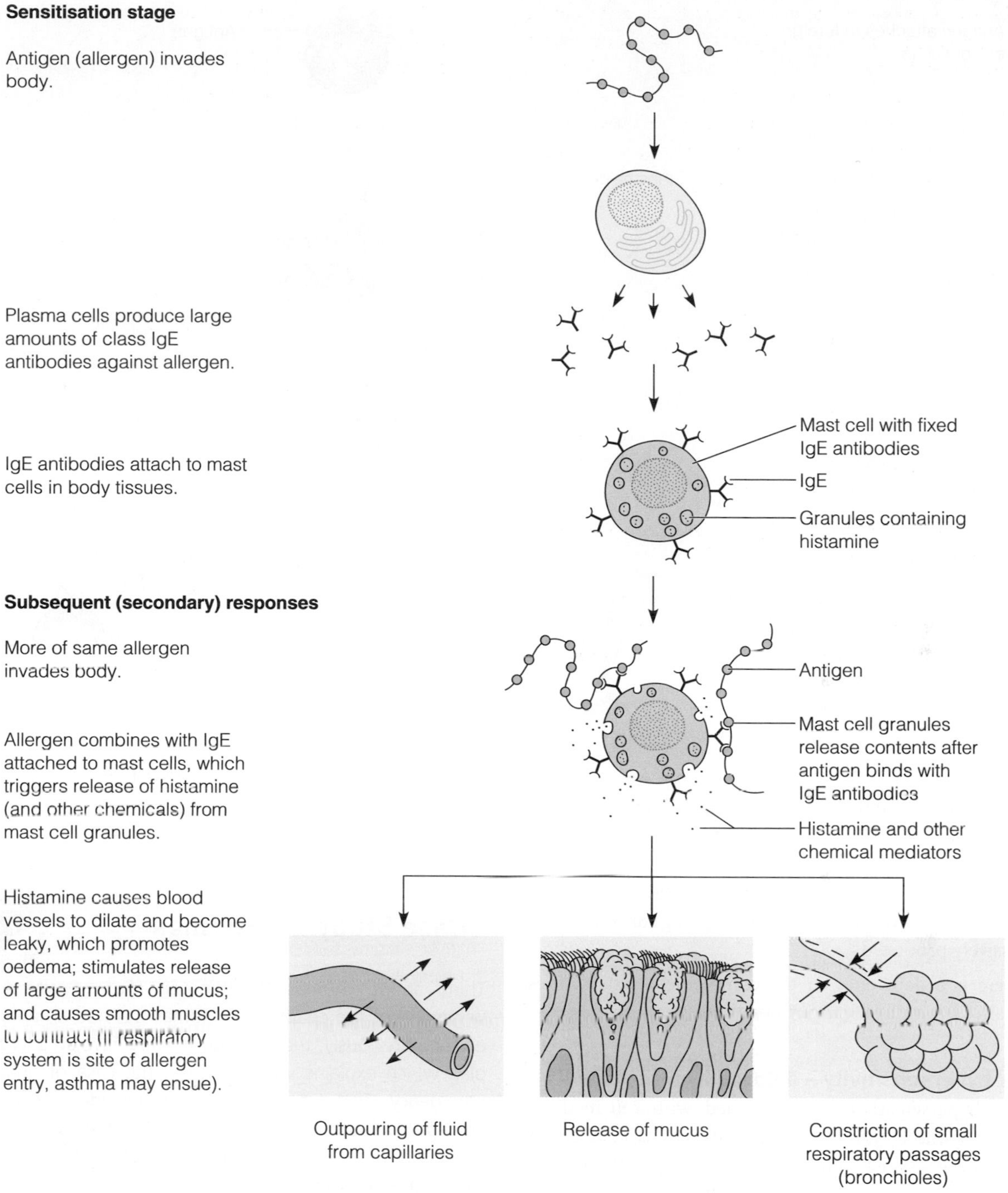

Sensitisation stage

Antigen (allergen) invades body.

Plasma cells produce large amounts of class IgE antibodies against allergen.

IgE antibodies attach to mast cells in body tissues.

Subsequent (secondary) responses

More of same allergen invades body.

Allergen combines with IgE attached to mast cells, which triggers release of histamine (and other chemicals) from mast cell granules.

Histamine causes blood vessels to dilate and become leaky, which promotes oedema; stimulates release of large amounts of mucus; and causes smooth muscles to contract (if respiratory system is site of allergen entry, asthma may ensue).

Mast cell with fixed IgE antibodies

IgE

Granules containing histamine

Antigen

Mast cell granules release contents after antigen binds with IgE antibodies

Histamine and other chemical mediators

Outpouring of fluid from capillaries

Release of mucus

Constriction of small respiratory passages (bronchioles)

Figure 4.11 Type I IgE-mediated hypersensitivity response.

antibody acting as an antigen in the cell's plasma membrane (Rote 2010a) (see Figure 4.12).

The reactions are caused, not by IgE, but by either IgG or IgM binding to the surface cells, and this binding frequently damages red blood cells and cells of solid tissue. There are four mechanisms by which type II hypersensitivity occurs (see Figure 4.12), although they all begin with either IgG or IgM binding to tissue-specific antigens.

Type III hypersensitivity – immune complex disease

When antigens combine with antibodies, antigen–antibody complexes are produced. These immune complexes are usually quickly cleared from the circulation (see Figure 4.13 on p. 125). In some people, however, these complexes persist in the blood circulation and can cause serious medical conditions, such as renal failure. This persistence of immune complexes can occur in one of two ways:

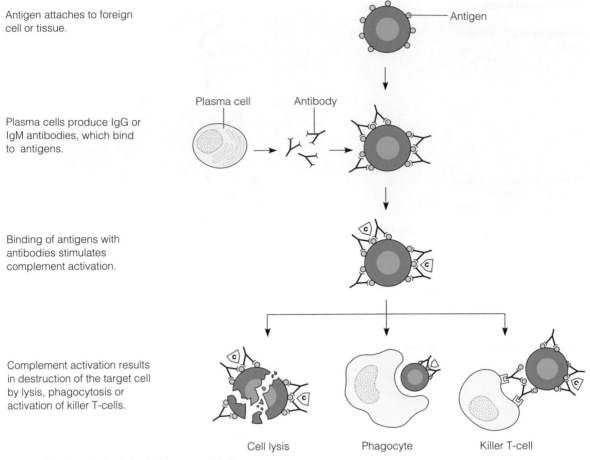

Antigen attaches to foreign cell or tissue.

Plasma cells produce IgG or IgM antibodies, which bind to antigens.

Binding of antigens with antibodies stimulates complement activation.

Complement activation results in destruction of the target cell by lysis, phagocytosis or activation of killer T-cells.

Antigen

Plasma cell   Antibody

Cell lysis   Phagocyte   Killer T-cell

Figure 4.12 Type II cytotoxic hypersensitivity response.

1. If the immune complex clearing processes are saturated because these immune complexes are being continually and excessively produced.

2. If there is a deficiency in the complement system, these clearance procedures cannot function.

Type IV hypersensitivity – delayed hypersensitivity

Type IV hypersensitivity is concerned with cell-mediated immune response. This hypersensitivity is characterised by T-helper 1 cells, which initiate, and drive, an inflammatory response (see Figure 4.14 on p. 126). This inflammatory response is also mediated by macrophages (Nairn and Helbert 2007). Delayed hypersensitivity reactions usually take place any time from 2–10 days after exposure to the antigen. It can be a reaction to a variety of antigens that are not easily destroyed, for example, hepatitis B virus. It can also be a reaction to environmental antigens such as plant extracts (contact dermatitis), or a reaction to autoantigens, for example type 1 diabetes, where the pancreatic islet cell antigens act as autoantigens.

Several autoimmune diseases are caused by delayed hypersensitivity, including:

Case Study 2 – Thomas

Think about Thomas Worthington (*Case Study 2* at the beginning of the chapter), if Thomas has had an anaphylactic episode previously, then he may already have an allergy action plan which explains what to do in the case of anaphylactic emergency. This action plan usually includes the use of an epinephrine auto-injector (an injection that is used to give measured doses of epinephrine intramuscularly), a medical alert bracelet to be worn at all times which states Thomas's condition and what to do if he goes into anaphylaxis. If, however, this is the first time that Thomas has had an anaphylactic reaction, then he will need to be taught about it, including how to avoid it and how to manage the situation another time, i.e. what to do in an emergency. He will also need much counselling and reassuring. Do not forget that Thomas's friend who came into the A & E department may also need support and reassurance.

Antigens invade body and bind to antibodies in circulation. Antigen–antibody complexes are formed.

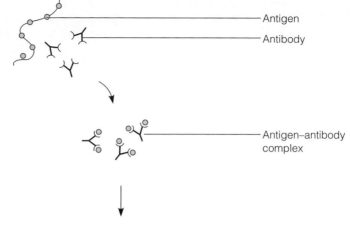

Antigen

Antibody

Antigen–antibody complex

Antigen–antibody complexes are deposited in the basement membrane of vessel walls and other body tissues, activating complement.

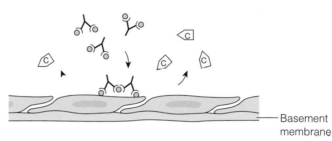

Basement membrane

Complement activation leads to release of inflammatory chemical mediators. Infiltration of polymorphonuclear leucocytes (PMNs) is followed by release of lysozymes. Tissue damage may be extensive.

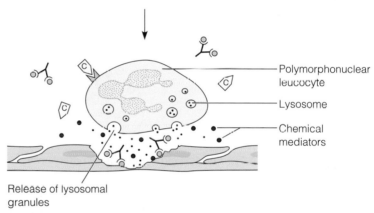

Polymorphonuclear leucocyte

Lysosome

Chemical mediators

Release of lysosomal granules

Figure 4.14 Type III immune complex-mediated hypersensitivity response.

- rheumatoid arthritis;
- type 1 diabetes;
- coeliac disease;
- multiple sclerosis.

Another reaction caused by type IV hypersensitivity is graft rejection (which is a form of autoimmunity).

Autoimmune disease

The last group of disorders linked to the immune system that we will discuss is that of autoimmunity. Autoimmune diseases occur as a result of an acquired immune response being mounted against the body's own cells, which act as self-antigens. They are caused by autoreactive T-cells which react against the host's own cells. The autoimmune response involves both T-cell lymphocytes and antibodies (autoantibodies).

Causes of autoimmune disease

We all produce some autoantibodies, usually at a very low level, and they also have a poor affinity for binding to auto-antigens. Although it is possible that the autoantibodies in healthy people could cause autoimmune diseases, the evidence appears to show that it is the T-cells which initiate an auto-immune disease (Nairn and Helbert 2007). Autoantigens, once established, are difficult to clear from the body so, once an autoimmune disease has been initiated, it tends to be present

Antigen-presenting cell
encounters cytotoxic
T-cell.

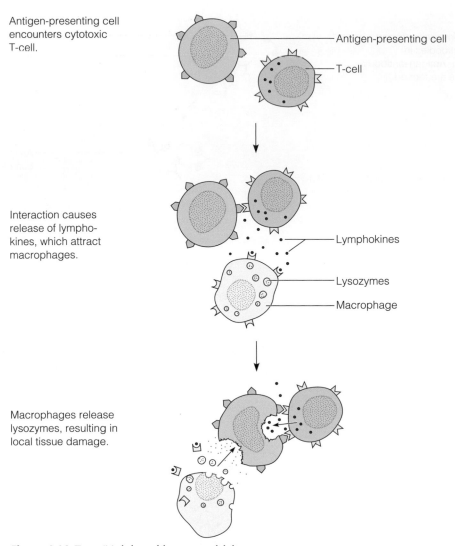

Antigen-presenting cell

T-cell

Interaction causes
release of lympho-
kines, which attract
macrophages.

Lymphokines

Lysozymes

Macrophage

Macrophages release
lysozymes, resulting in
local tissue damage.

Figure 4.14 Type IV delayed hypersensitivity response.

for a long time (even for life). Earlier in this chapter, we discussed the way in which potential autoreactive T-cells were eliminated in the thymus, so we need to ask how some T-cells can become autoreactive and provoke autoimmune disease. There may be a genetic susceptibility to autoimmunity in some people and several possible loci have been identified for susceptibility to multiple sclerosis, systemic lupus erythromatosus (SLE) and Crohn's disease (Kamradt and Mitchison 2001).

Isenberg and Morrow (1995) have proposed another theory surrounding autoantibody production, leading to autoimmune disease. They suggest that there is an imbalance in the immune regulatory functioning of T-cell immunity, with unregulated autoantibody production resulting from poor or inadequate T-cell immune suppressor functioning.

Another factor being investigated is complement deficiency. The *complement* system is activated following the formation of antigen–antibody *immune complexes*, which it then dissolves, and it is possible that a deficiency of some of

the complement factors may prevent this, leaving the complex to cause problems. We do know that C2 deficiency is a major risk factor for developing various autoimmune diseases, including SLE and myositis.

Other possibilities for the development of autoimmune disorders are hormones, particularly the sex hormones. Women are much more likely to have an autoimmune disease than men. Women's sex hormones fluctuate at times during their lives, for example during adolescence, during and after pregnancy and at the time of menstruation, and it is this fluctuation that seems to be the link. After pregnancy, when there is a fall in levels of oestrogen and progesterone, is associated with the start of several autoimmune disorders. Oral contraception containing oestrogen can exacerbate or induce relapses of autoimmune disease. During pregnancy, for example, rheumatoid arthritis improves but it always flares up again once pregnancy is over. SLE often becomes more active during pregnancy. Consider Kate Stable's condition, how might her condition be managed if she were pregnant?

Case Study 1 – Kate

At this point go back to Case Study 1 about Kate Stable and relate this section to Kate's condition. How might her condition be managed if she were pregnant? The next sections give some further information about how Kate may have been diagnosed and treated. Kate will need to be asked to return as an out-patient for ongoing monitoring and assessment of her condition. She may also be referred for counselling if she wishes to have children. The nurse should be ready to provide Kate with further resources that may help her managed her condition, for example, the UK Lupus group.

Diagnosis of SLE

- *Antibody tests.* Various antibody tests help to identify certain infections and some other disorders.
- *Other antibody tests (anti-Ro and antiphospholipid)* give information on the likelihood of skin rashes occurring and the risk of miscarriages in future pregnancies.

- *Complement level test.* 'Complement' is a chemical in the body that forms part of the immune system.
- *Erythrocyte sedimentation rate (ESR) test* can indicate inflammation.
- *Kidney and liver function tests* to look for problems caused either by SLE itself or as a side-effect of drug treatment.
- *Blood cell counts* to check the haemoglobin level, white and red blood cell numbers and platelets.

Treatment of SLE

It is important to be aware that SLE cannot be cured, but the symptoms can be controlled:

- Joint pains can be treated with corticosteroids to reduce inflammation.
- Skin rashes can be treated with creams containing steroids and hydroxychloroquinone tablets.
- More serious complications such as pleurisy (lung infection discussed in Chapter 11), pericarditis (infection of part of the heart discussed in Chapter 9), severe anaemia (discussed in Chapter 10) or severe inflammation of the kidneys can be treated with steroids or with immunosuppressive drugs.

INFECTION

Infectious diseases

Modern medicine, antibiotic therapy, immunisations and other public health measures to protect food and water supplies have significantly reduced the prevalence of infectious diseases in many parts of the world. In spite of these advances, many infections, including malaria, typhoid and tuberculosis, remain prevalent in developing nations. STIs are present worldwide. In addition, there is always the threat that new varieties and strains of pathogens, such as HIV and swine flu, will evolve to cause disease.

To a certain extent, modern medicine has contributed to the development of infectious diseases caused by antibiotic-resistant strains of micro-organisms. For example, tuberculosis, whilst always being a problem in developing countries, is now on the rise again in developed countries, partly because organisms have become resistant to standard therapies, and partly because of the immune deficiencies that arise as a result of the growth of HIV. People who receive immunosuppressive therapy following transplantation or in the treatment of neoplasms are more susceptible to infection. It has also become apparent that diseases long considered unrelated to micro-organisms may actually be infectious; for example, colonisation of the gastric mucosa with *Helicobacter pylori* is the

COMMUNITY-BASED CARE

Swine flu presents particular challenges for some care home providers. In care homes infections and diseases can spread very rapidly because they are closed communities. Those aged 65 years and over are defined as a high-risk group by the Department of Health. It is important that care home providers have in place robust plans to deal with an outbreak of the virus.

Older people may be more likely to experience a more severe illness when they get flu and they may deteriorate more rapidly because of underlying disease, ageing of their immune system, reduced mobility and debility.

Many care home providers are prepared for an outbreak of swine flu, as they already have measures in place to deal with diseases such as MRSA. Good cleaning regimes will help manage the spread of swine flu, and fundamentals such as hand washing are essential. There are other common-sense measures that should also be implemented, and these include ensuring that laundry is not left lying in corridors and taking time to clean items such as light switches and door handles. Sometimes these may be missed by cleaners and in communal settings like care homes they are touched by a large number of people.

predominant cause of peptic ulcer disease (see Chapter 7), and oncogenic viruses have the ability to transform normal cells into malignant cells. In this section, we will consider the pathogenesis of infections, the different types of infectious organisms and the infective process before looking at nursing care for people with infections.

Pathogenesis of infectious diseases

Infection occurs when an organism is able to colonise and multiply within a host. The host can be any organism capable of supporting the nutritional and physical growth requirements of the micro-organism, for example humans. When the host experiences injury, pathogenic changes, inflammation or organ dysfunction in response to an infection or from intoxication by cellular poisons produced by a pathogen, the host is said to have an infectious disease.

For a micro-organism to cause infection, it must have disease-causing potential (virulence), be transmitted from its reservoir and gain entry into a susceptible host. This is known as the chain of infection (Figure 4.15).

To cause disease, most pathogenic organisms need to:

● gain access to the host;

● adhere to host tissues;

● penetrate or evade host defences;

● damage the host tissues.

However, some microbes do not cause disease themselves by directly damaging the host tissue; instead it is the accumulation

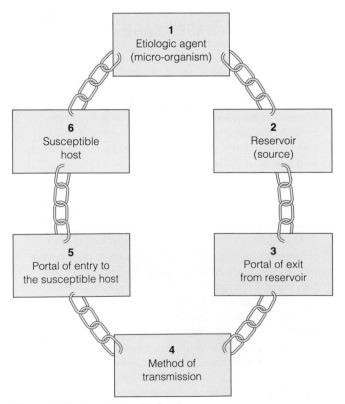

Figure 4.15 The chain of infection.

of their waste products that causes the disease. Although some microbes can cause disease without penetrating the body – think of tooth decay and acne – most pathogenic organisms do gain entrance into the human body. They do this through 'portals of entry' (see Figure 4.15).

Portals of entry

The portals of entry to pathogenic organisms are:

● mucous membranes;

● skin;

● the parenteral route (inoculation).

See Chapter 5 for discussion of the skin and below for inoculation.

Many bacteria and viruses gain access to the body by penetrating the mucous membranes:

● the respiratory tract;

● the gastrointestinal tract;

● the genitourinary tract;

● the conjunctiva.

The most favoured tracts for pathogens to enter through the mucous membranes are the gastrointestinal and respiratory tracts. As regards the respiratory tract, pathogenic microbes are inhaled via the nose or mouth in drops of moisture and dust particles. Diseases commonly contracted via this route include:

● the common cold;

● pneumonia;

● tuberculosis;

● influenza;

● measles.

Pathogenic micro-organisms can gain access to the gastro-intestinal tract in food and water, as well as by means of contaminated fingers. Most infecting organisms that enter the gastrointestinal tract from the mouth are destroyed by hydrochloric acid and enzymes in the stomach or, if they survive the stomach, they are destroyed by bile and enzymes in the small intestine. Any that survive these two hazards are able then to cause disease, including:

● poliomyelitis;

● hepatitis A;

● typhoid fever;

● amoebic dysentery;

● cholera.

These pathogenic micro-organisms will then be eliminated within the faeces, from where they can be transmitted to other hosts via:

● water;

● food;

● fingers.

The genitourinary tract is also a portal of entry for pathogenic organisms that are contracted sexually. Some pathogens that cause STIs may penetrate unbroken mucous membranes, whilst others require a cut or abrasion of some sort:

- HIV
- genital warts
- chlamydia
- herpes
- syphilis
- gonorrhoea

Once the infectious micro-organism has gained entry into the body, it then has to be able to evade the immune system otherwise it will be killed before it can cause problems.

Evading the immune system

Viruses have a variety of mechanisms that enable them to evade the host's immune defences. They gain access to cells because of the attachment sites that they have for receptors on target cells, so that the virus is able to bind to the cell and penetrate it.

Some viruses have attachment receptors that mimic substances that are useful to those cells, and this is how they are able to gain access to the target cells. The attachment sites of the rabies virus, for example, can mimic the neurotransmitter acetylcholine, and this allows the virus to enter the target cell along with the acetylcholine (Tortora *et al.* 2004).

Pathogenic organisms

There are numerous types of pathogenic organisms that can cause infections in humans. These include bacteria and viruses as the main ones, although, there are many more that our immune systems have to deal with.

Bacteria

Bacteria are single-celled and relatively small, simple organisms, containing a single chromosome. A flexible cell membrane and rigid cell wall surround their cytoplasm, giving them a distinctive shape; some also have an extracellular capsule for additional protection. Bacteria have different characteristics and growth requirements: aerobes require oxygen for survival, whereas anaerobes die in the presence of oxygen; gram-positive bacteria stain purple when subjected to crystal violet stain, whereas gram-negative bacteria do not stain with crystal violet but turn red when subjected to safranin stain; the colonies formed by replicating bacteria differ from one another.

Viruses

Viruses are obligate intracellular parasites (they can only reproduce inside a living cell). Viruses consist of a protein coat around a core of either DNA or RNA. Some viruses are shed continuously from infected cell surfaces; others, after inserting their genetic material into that of the infected cell, remain latent until they are stimulated to replicate. Viruses may or may not cause lysis and death of the host cell during replication. Oncogenic viruses are able to transform normal cells into malignant cells.

Mycoplasma

Although similar to bacteria, mycoplasma are smaller, and they have no cell wall, making them resistant to antibiotics that inhibit cell wall synthesis (for example, penicillins).

Rickettsia and *Chlamydia*

As obligate intracellular parasites with a rigid cell wall, *Rickettsia* and *Chlamydia* have some features of both bacteria and viruses. Rather than depending on the host cell for reproduction, they use vitamins, nutrients or products of metabolism (for example, ATP) from the host. *Chlamydia* are transmitted by direct contact, whereas many *Rickettsia* infect the cells of arthropods (for example, fleas, ticks and lice) and are transmitted from these vectors to humans.

Fungi

Fungi are prevalent throughout the world, but few are capable of causing disease in humans. Most fungal infections are self-limited, affecting the skin and subcutaneous tissue. Some fungi, such as *Pneumocystis jiroveci*, can cause life-threatening opportunistic infections in the immunocompromised host.

Parasites

The term *parasite* is typically applied to members of the animal kingdom that infect and cause disease in other animals. Protozoa are single-celled organisms transmitted via direct or indirect contact or an arthropod vector. Helminths are worm-like parasites (roundworms and tapeworms are examples); they gain entry into humans primarily through ingestion of fertilised eggs or penetration of larvae through the skin or mucous membranes. Arthropod parasites typically infest external body surfaces, causing localised tissue damage and inflammation; transmission is by direct contact with the arthropod or its eggs (Porth 2009).

Stages of the infectious process

When infectious disease develops in the host, it typically follows a predictable course with four stages based on the progression and intensity of manifestations.

1. The *initial stage*. The incubation period, during which the pathogen begins active replication but does not yet cause symptoms, may last from hours, as with salmonella, to years, as with HIV infection.

2. The *prodromal stage* follows, during which symptoms first begin to appear; for example, general malaise, fever, myalgia (muscle aches and pains), headache and fatigue.

3. The *acute stage*. Maximal impact of the infectious process is felt during the acute phase as the pathogen proliferates and disseminates rapidly. Toxic by-products of micro-organism

metabolism and cell lysis, along with the immune response, produce tissue damage and inflammation during this stage (Porth 2009). Manifestations are more pronounced and specific to the infecting organism and site during the acute stage, and fever and chills may be significant. The person is often tachycardic (rapid heart rate) and tachypnoeic (rapid breathing). Localised manifestations include redness, heat, swelling, pain and impaired function. When the infectious disease affects an internal organ, manifestations are related to inflammatory changes in that organ and surrounding tissue. The person may experience tenderness to palpation over the site or show signs of impaired function, such as the haematuria (blood in the urine) and proteinuria (protein in the urine) which are characteristic of renal infections.

If the infectious process is prolonged, manifestations of the continuing immune response may become apparent. Catabolic (breakdown of large molecules) and anorexic effects of the infection can lead to loss of body fat and muscle wasting. Immune complexes may be deposited at sites other than the primary infection, resulting in an inflammatory process.

4. As the infection is contained and the pathogen eliminated, the *convalescent stage* of the disease occurs. During this stage, affected tissues are repaired and manifestations resolve. A carrier state develops when host defences eliminate the infectious disease but the organism continues to multiply on mucosal sites (Fauci *et al.* 1998).

NURSING CARE FOR INFECTION

Nursing management related to infectious disease has two foci:

1. prevention;
2. health promotion and maintenance.

Prevention

Prevention focuses on assessing the person's risk for infection based on underlying conditions, immune response and prophylactic measures such as immunisations.

Health promotion

Preventing infection requires education for healthcare professionals and the general public and includes understanding:

- the importance of immunisations;
- guidelines for using antibiotics to prevent drug-resistant micro-organisms;
- the risk of diarrhoea with the taking of broad-spectrum antibiotics;
- ways to prevent the spread of infection.

Check immunisation records for all family members and encourage them to keep their immunisations up to date.

Increase public awareness and education regarding appropriate antibiotic use.

Guidelines for preventing the spread of infection to others include the following:

- Avoid crowds and contact with susceptible persons, especially the immunosuppressed (for example, persons who are undergoing therapy for cancer).
- Use disposable tissues to contain respiratory secretions when coughing or sneezing.
- Use appropriate food-handling precautions for diseases spread via the faecal–oral route.
- Avoid contact with or sharing of body fluids.

Assessment

If a person has an infection, it is important to make a full assessment of the individual and the environment. The following data are collected through a health history and physical examination.

Health history: age, medications, nutrition, exposure to infectious persons, immunisations, invasive procedures and therapies and chronic diseases such as diabetes mellitus or cancer.

Physical assessment: vital signs, body system(s) where infection is suspected, lymph node enlargement and tenderness.

Nursing diagnoses and interventions

Those with an infection may be cared for in hospital or at home. During the acute phase, nursing care includes administering prescribed antibiotics, implementing and maintaining aseptic technique and infection control measures together with encouraging a balance of rest and activity, good nutritional intake and other general health measures to support immunologic function and healing.

Risk for spread of infection

Spread of infection is a risk in any facility that houses many people. It is a particular risk in hospitals, where many people have at least some degree of immunosuppression and many drug-resistant strains of pathogens are prevalent. It is vital that nurses use good hand hygiene techniques at all times, employ standard precautions with all people and use category-specific isolation techniques as indicated to prevent infectious spread to other people, themselves and their families.

+ Admit those with known or suspected infections to a private room.

+ Utilise appropriate hand hygiene techniques on entering and leaving the person's room.

+ Use standard precautions and personal protective devices to reduce the risk of transmission. Gloves, gowns and masks are to be worn whenever there is a risk of skin or mucous membrane contamination by direct contact with infectious material, airborne spread of organisms or droplet nuclei.

Table 4.1 Transmission-based precautions

Category	Infectious diseases	Purpose	Precautions
Airborne precautions	Pulmonary tuberculosis, chickenpox (with contact precautions), measles, respiratory infections (pneumonia).	Reduce risk of airborne transmission of infectious agents. Airborne transmission occurs by dissemination of either airborne droplet nuclei or dust particles containing the infectious agent.	Private room with hand washing and toilet facilities, and special ventilation that does not allow air to circulate to general hospital ventilation system; mask or special filter respirator for everyone entering room.
Droplet precautions	Meningitis, pertussis.	Reduce risk of droplet transmission of infectious agents. Droplet transmission involves contact of conjunctivae of the eyes or mucous membranes of the nose or mouth with large-particle droplets generated during coughing, sneezing, talking or procedures such as suctioning.	Private room with hand washing and toilet facilities; mask, eye protection and/or face shields worn by everyone entering room.
Contact precautions	Acute diarrhoea, chickenpox (with airborne precautions), respiratory syncytial virus (RSV); skin, wound or urinary tract infection with multidrug-resistant organisms; *S. aureus* infections.	Reduce risk of transmission by direct or indirect contact. Direct contact transmission involves skin-to-skin contact and physical transfer of organisms. It may occur between people or during direct care activities such as bathing or turning. Indirect contact involves contact with a contaminated object.	Private room with hand washing and toilet facilities; gowns and protective apparel to provide barrier protection; disposable supplies or decontamination of all articles leaving room.

+ Explain the reasons for and importance of isolation procedures during hospitalisation.

+ Place a mask on the person and/or cover all infectious lesions or wounds completely when transporting the person to other parts of the facility for diagnostic or treatment procedures.

+ Collect a culture and sensitivity (C&S) specimen as ordered or indicated by purulent drainage, pyuria, or other manifestations of infection.

Precautions which can be taken to prevent transmission of infection are listed in Table 4.1.

Antibiotics and infection

It is essential that all aspects of nursing care have a sound evidence base. The administration of antibiotics is often seen as a routine activity; however, the nurse must remember that failure to administer antibiotics as per prescription as well as providing education can have a detrimental effect on the care of the person.

Nurses discharging those from out-patient and acute care settings frequently teach people to take a complete prescribed dose of oral antibiotics to manage acute infections. Ingesting less than complete doses exposes people being cared for to the risk of resistant infections and poor therapeutic outcomes. There are many potential restraining forces to the completion of antibiotic dosing: cost of purchase; difficulty swallowing the pills; multiple, frequent doses; and the potential for adverse, unpleasant side-effects.

Because adherence is so important and nurses are healthcare educators, Aronson (2005) studied in depth the experience of 11 people who had just completed a short-term antibiotic regimen to treat a variety of acute infectious illnesses with various antibiotic regimens. The 11 subjects represent diverse gender and cultural backgrounds. They participated in 30-minute audiotaped interviews within two weeks of completing their antibiotics. This qualitative study is the first part of a research programme to evaluate an intervention to promote adherence to taking antibiotics for a short-term period. The descriptions, views and experiences of those being cared for gave an insight into adherence to antibiotic self-administration.

Aronson (2005) analysed these descriptions of the experience of taking antibiotics by organising the responses into categories of consistent themes; the data were independently analysed and the results compared until the categories were agreed on by both. The central theme that emerged was just how successful antibiotic self-administration was. Those being cared for integrated the antibiotic administration into their daily schedules and adapted to any unplanned circumstances. The primary categories involved in self-administration were (1) medication-taking behaviours, (2) factors influencing adherence and (3) attitudes and beliefs about the medication and the value of completing the prescribed dose. Subcategories were identified for each of these main categories.

Individuals described methods for remembering to take the medication, methods of dealing with anticipated or experienced side-effects and factors that build trust in their relationship with the prescriber. The severity of the symptoms that led to antibiotic prescription made them more likely to report intention to adhere to the dosing regimen.

Implications for nursing

The findings from this study can be used to guide educational interactions. Based on the findings in this study, encourage involvement in the decision to take short-term antibiotic medications in order to strengthen the relationship between the prescriber and those taking the antibiotics. Ask those being cared for to identify the method they will use to remind themselves of each dose; enquire about their knowledge of and plans to manage side-effects from the medication.

Primary and secondary response to infection

Having looked at defects in the immune system, we turn our attention to the role for which the immune system is best known – fighting infections. When we first encounter an infectious micro-organism, there are two processes that we go through, starting with the primary response. Subsequent infection by the same micro-organism leads directly to the secondary response, assuming that we do not have an immune deficiency.

Primary immune response

What is so distinct about the acquired immune system is its ability to 'remember' previous encounters with a particular antigen. If our immune system did not have this ability, then each time we came into contact with a particular antigen, we would be at risk of a serious, if not fatal, illness. This ability to remember a previous infecting antigen allows the body to subsequently make an immediate immune response against the antigen, rather than having to wait for the immune system to work out each time how to defeat it.

This primary immune response lag time can take anything from five to 10 days, before there has been sufficient production of antibodies to destroy the infecting antigen; during this period, we can become very ill, and may even die. If we do not die, but recover from the infection, from then on we will possess immunity to that particular antigen, and will be able to respond to subsequent infections much quicker.

A secondary immunological response to that specific antigen will occur without the need for a further primary immune response (but only to that pathogen – not to different pathogens, each of which will need an initial primary response from our acquired immune system when it first infects us).

Secondary immune response

In a secondary immune response to infection, the immune system is immediately aware when an infecting antigen is present and also aware of how it can be destroyed. When a particular infectious micro-organism (a pathogen), which has already once infected us, enters our bodies, the memory lymphocytes that carry a 'blueprint' of that particular antigen spring into action.

You will probably encounter the same antigen frequently throughout your life, and these subsequent encounters with the same infectious micro-organisms serve to reinforce the immune response. However, sometimes there can be a long gap between the first encounter and subsequent ones. To deal with this, the immune system also has long-term memory (see Figure 4.16).

This immunological memory and the primary and secondary immune responses to infection are the basis for the success of immunisations and vaccinations, which we will now explore.

Immunisations

More than 70 bacteria, viruses, fungi and parasites have been identified as pathogenic infectious organisms that are capable of causing serious diseases in humans (Ada and Ramsey 1997). Vaccines are available against some of these, and work is in progress to find vaccines for almost all these bacteria and viruses, and about half of the parasites (Ada 2001).

Immunisation, or vaccination, is either the process of transferring antibodies to an individual who is lacking them, or the process of inducing an immune reaction in an individual. The second process is possible because of the primary and secondary responses to infection.

Immunisations induce a primary response by exposing the immune system to an infectious organism. This infectious organism is either killed or attenuated (weakened) so that it is no longer infectious, but it still possesses the antigenic receptors that stimulate the immune system.

If a vaccine is effective, it provides herd immunity to a population. In other words, by reducing the number of people in a population who are susceptible to a particular disease-causing organism, there is a reduction in the natural reservoir of infected people in that population. This then reduces the risk of transmission of the infectious organism, so that even individuals in that population who have not been vaccinated are also protected against that organism (Janeway *et al.* 2005).

Types of immunisation

There are two types of immunisation – passive and active.

Passive immunisation

In passive immunisation, the individual is actually injected with the antibodies:

1. The mother transfers IgG antibodies across the placenta to the foetus, so that whatever organisms the mother is immune to, the baby will also be immune to them.
2. The second form of passive immunisation takes place during breastfeeding when the mother passes IgA antibodies to the baby in her colostrum and milk.

IgG has a short half-life and IgA has an even shorter half-life, so it can be seen that passive immunisation is also short

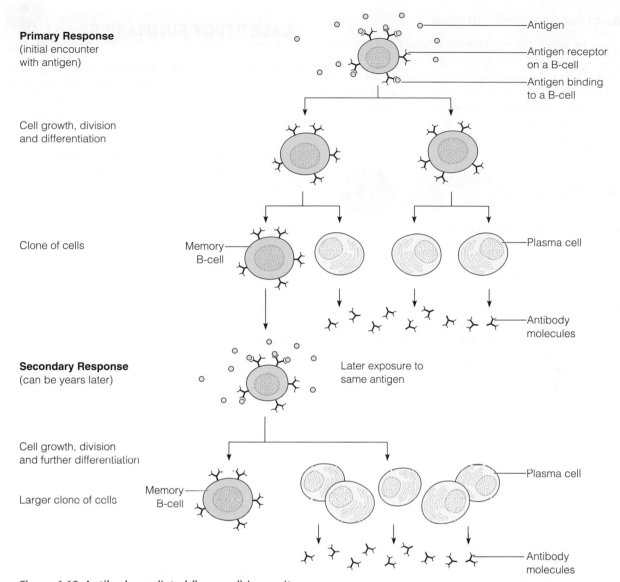

Figure 4.16 Antibody-mediated (humoral) immunity.

lived, and lasts only as long as it takes for these antibodies to be cleared from the body. This type of immunisation will not normally provoke an immune response in the recipient's body, and therefore there will be no immunological cover for subsequent exposure to that particular antigen.

In addition, passive immunisation is often given in the form of gammaglobulin infusions, when a person is immunocompromised in some way, such as following cytotoxic chemotherapy, radiation therapy or bone marrow transplantation, or when the person has a primary or secondary immunodeficiency.

Passive immunity occurs when injecting a mother with antibodies against rhesus antigens to prevent rhesus incompatibility in future pregnancies.

Active immunisation

Active immunity is the process of presenting antigens to the immune system to induce an immune response against them, for example by means of vaccines. This is the type of

immunity that takes advantage of the primary and secondary responses to immunity.

In a vaccine, the antigen presented to the immune system is made as safe as possible by either using a whole micro-organism and making it weaker whilst keeping it alive (live-attenuated vaccine), or killing it and possibly just using part of the micro-organism (inactivated vaccine).

Another approach to making safe and effective vaccines is by adding adjuvants to purified antigen. On their own, purified antigens are not normally very immunogenic. Adjuvants are substances that enhance the immunogenicity of antigens, improving the effectiveness of many antigens. Adjuvants often retain the antigen at the site of injection, and release it slowly. Alum (aluminium phosphate or aluminium hydroxide) is one such chemical that has been approved as an adjuvant for human use. Tetanus toxoids are not immunogenic but, once linked to aluminium hydroxide (alum), they become effectively immunogenic.

Route of vaccine administration

The route by which the vaccines are administered is important. Currently, most vaccines are given by intramuscular injection. There is, however, an immunological problem with this method, because it does not mimic the usual route of entry of many important pathogens, which infect either mucosal surfaces or enter the body through the mucosa and include respiratory and enteric pathogens.

FAST FACTS

Vaccine for whooping cough

- Before the vaccination against whooping cough was introduced in the 1950s, there were more than 100 000 reported cases in England and Wales per year.

- Three out of four children caught the disease and some died every year.

- Today only a few get whooping cough, with less than 150 cases being reported in children aged four and under during 2007.

Source: NHS Choices 2010b.

CASE STUDY SUMMARIES

The two case studies at the beginning of the chapter have discussed conditions associated with the immune system. These case studies demonstrate the role of the nurse in assessment, planning, implementation and evaluation of nursing care.

Case Study 1. Ms Stable returns to the immunology department at the hospital every six months as part of follow-up and her condition is monitored by the nurse consultant.

Case Study 2. Thomas Worthington now carries an EpiPen® with him at all times, he has just undertaken the London to Paris bike ride raising funds for the charity Allergy UK.

The immune system is a complex system, with each of the many components interacting with others. The immune system plays a major role, that of keeping us safe. Immunology is a dynamic subject. Continually research is bringing us new knowledge, not only of the anatomy and physiology of the immune system, but also of disorders affected by it, and, of course, new therapies. There is now so much progress being made in immunology that it is impossible to predict the future.

CHAPTER HIGHLIGHTS

- The immune system is a crucial part of health – so much so that without it, we would not survive more than a few days outside of the womb.

- Because it impacts upon the whole body, the immune system is linked to almost every disease and disorder to which we are vulnerable. This chapter examined the causes, treatment and nursing care of just a few of them as examples of how to nurse people who have a disease/disorder of altered immunity.

- Systemic lupus erythematosus (SLE) is an autoimmune disorder that affects women between the menarche and the menopause, and can have profound effects on many of the organs of the body, particularly as a result of inflammation.

- Inflammation is a necessary part of our immune defence against disease and injury, and a lack of wound healing can lead to the development of chronic wounds including pressure ulcers.

- Primary immunodeficiencies are a little-known group of diseases, but they can have profound effects on the lives of those who have them. Some of them can be severe, and require life long drug therapy; others are very severe and require a bone marrow transplant to cure; whilst others are very mild, and rarely affect the lives of those who have them.

- Secondary immunodeficiencies are very common, and we all, at some stage of our lives, have had, and recovered from without any problems, a secondary immunodeficiency.

- Another common disease that is underpinned by the immune system is that of allergies such as asthma and eczema. As with many immune disorders, there is rarely a cure and people have to live with them for all their lives – leading to medical, physical and psychosocial problems.

- This chapter has introduced you to the problems that can be caused by altered immunity. There is not enough space in the chapter to discuss all the disorders linked to it – for that you will have to look at other textbooks – but after reading this chapter you will at least be able to make sense of what you read elsewhere.

TEST YOURSELF

1. Which blood cell is the odd one out here?
   a. lymphocyte
   b. eosinophil
   c. neutrophil
   d. macrophage

2. Which three excretions are useful as important parts of our innate immune system?
   a. breast milk
   b. urine
   c. semen
   d. sweat

3. Phagocytosis is:
   a. the production of cytokines
   b. the opsonisation of bacteria
   c. the movement of cells of the immune system to a site of infection
   d. the act of engulfing and destroying non-self matter

4. Which of these are signs of an inflammation?
   a. swelling
   b. pain
   c. heat
   d. pallor

5. Which of these plasma protein systems are activated in inflammation?
   a. clotting
   b. creatinine
   c. complement
   d. coping

6. What causes the redness in inflammation?
   a. cellular infiltration
   b. vasodilation
   c. stimulation of nerve endings
   d. vascular permeability

7. Cytokines are:
   a. cell membranes
   b. the result of cellular respiration
   c. chemical alterations to the cell
   d. chemical messengers sent from the cell

8. Which of these are the result of Interleukin-α (IL-α)?
   a. they activate T-cell lymphocytes
   b. they provide antiviral protection
   c. they activate phagocytes
   d. they induce a pyrexia

9. The classical pathway of the complement system is activated by which of the following processes?
   a. the recognition–activation complex
   b. the antigen–antibody complex
   c. the mannan–lectin complex
   d. the inflammation–opsonin complex

10. Which of these describes one of the roles of opsonins
    a. they provide nutrients for the bacteria
    b. they prepare the bacteria for phagocytosis
    c. they increase vascular permeability
    d. they facilitate the movement of lymphocytes to sites of infection.

Further resources

UK Lupus
http://www.uklupus.co.uk/
A guide for people with SLE and their families. Provides practical information and advice.

Arthritis Research UK
http://www.arthritisresearchUK.org
A charity working to take the pain away for sufferers of all forms of arthritis and helping people to remain active. The charity funds high-class research, providing information and campaigning.

Tissue Viability Society (TVS)
http://www.tvs.org.uk/
Aims to provide expertise in wound management to all healthcare professionals. Formed 30 years ago, disseminates information, promotes research and increases awareness of all aspects of good clinical practice in wound prevention and management.

National Institute for Health and Clinical Excellence (NICE)
http://www.nice.org.uk/
Provides guidance, sets quality standards and manages a national database to improve people's health and prevent and treat ill health.

UK NHS Immunisations
http://www.nhs.uk/chq/Pages/1039.aspx?CategoryID=62&SubCategoryID=63
Provides information about a number of health-related conditions.

UK Department of Health (DoH)
http://www.dh.gov.uk/en/Publichealth/Immunisation/index.htm
Government department advising the public and healthcare professionals.

UK Resuscitation Council – Emergency Treatment of Anaphylactic Reactions
http://www.resus.org.uk/pages/reaction.pdf
Up-to-date information regarding the emergency treatment of anaphylaxis.

Allergy UK
http://www.allergyuk.org/
Provides advice, information and support to people with allergies, food intolerance and chemical sensitivity.

UK Primary Immunodeficiency Network (PIN) – UK doctors and nurses
http://www.ukpin.org.uk/
Site for healthcare professionals, produces updates concerning immunodeficiency.

Primary Immunodeficiency Association (PIA) – UK patients
http://www.pia.org.uk/
Site for healthcare for the public, provides updates concerning immunodeficiency, offers practical advice and help.

Medline Plus – Autoimmune Diseases
http://www.nlm.nih.gov/medlineplus/autoimmunediseases.html
A free American site for patients, their families and friends. Providing information about diseases, conditions and wellness.

Bibliography

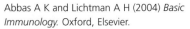

Abbas A K and Lichtman A H (2004) *Basic Immunology*. Oxford, Elsevier.

Ada G L (2001) Vaccines and vaccination. *New England Journal of Medicine*, **345**(14), 1042–1053.

Ada G L and Ramsey A J (1997) *Vaccines, Vaccination and the Immune Response*. Philadelphia, PA, Lippincott-Raven.

Aronson B (2005) Medication management behaviors of adherent short-term antibiotic users. *Clinical Excellence for Nurse Practitioners*, **9**(1), 23–30.

Buckley R H (2000) Primary immunodeficiency diseases due to defects in lymphocytes. *New England Journal of Medicine*, **343**(18), 1313–1324.

Candy D, Davies G and Ross P (2001) *Clinical Paediatrics and Child Health*. Edinburgh, WB Saunders.

Chapel H and Haeney M (1993) *Essentials of Clinical Immunology* (3rd edn). Oxford, Blackwell Scientific Publications.

Cochran S (1994) A mark of approval: Patient satisfaction with an IV self-infusion teaching programme. *Professional Nurse*, **10**(2), 106–111.

Crew R J, Radhakrishnan J and Appel G (2004) Complications of the nephrotic syndrome and their treatment. *Clinical Nephrology*, **62**, 245.

Davey B and Hart G (2002) HIV and AIDS. In Davey B and Seale C (eds), *Experiencing and Explaining Disease* (3rd edn). Buckingham, Open University Press, 83–117.

Delves P J and Roitt I M (2000) The immune system: part 1. *New England Journal of Medicine*, **343**(1), 37–49.

DeMeyer E S and Buchsel P C (2005) A dendritic cell primer for oncology nurses. *Clinical Journal of Oncology Nursing*, **9**(4), 460–464.

Fauci A S, Braunwald E, Isselbacher H J, *et al.* (1998) *Harrison's Principles of Internal Medicine* (14th edn). New York, McGraw-Hill.

Feary J, Venn A, Brown A *et al.* (2009) Safety of hookworm infection in individuals with measurable airway responsiveness: a randomized placebo-controlled feasibility study. *Clinical & Experimental Allergy*, **39**, 1060–1068.

Flanagan M (2000) The physiology of wound healing. *Journal of Wound Care*, **9**(6), 299–300.

Gardulf A, Nicolay U, Math D *et al.* (2004) Children and adults with primary antibody deficiencies gain quality of life by subcutaneous IgG self-infusions at home. *Journal of Allergy and Clinical Immunology*, **114**(4), 936–942.

Gell P G H and Coombs R R A (1968) *Clinical Aspects of Immunology* (2nd edn). Philadelphia, PA, FA Davis.

Grubeck-Loebenstein B and Wick G (2002) The aging of the immune system. *Advances in Immunology*, **80**, 243–284.

Hansen S, Gustafson R, Smith C I E *et al.* (2002) Express subcutaneous IgG infusions: decreased time of delivery with maintained safety. *Clinical Immunology*, **104**(3), 237–241.

Henderson K (2003) Training and support to enable home immunoglobulin therapy. *Nursing Times*, **99**, 45.

HPA (2010) *HIV in the United Kingdom: 2010 Report*. London, Health Protection Agency.

Isenberg D and Morrow J (1995) *Friendly Fire: Explaining auto-immune disease*. Oxford, Oxford Medical Publications.

Janeway C A, Travers P, Walport M and Shlomchik M J (2005) Immunobiology. *The Immune System in Health and Disease* (6th edn). New York, Churchill Livingstone.

Kamradt T and Mitchison N A (2001) Tolerance and autoimmunity. *New England Journal of Medicine*, **344**(9), 655–664.

Kay A B (2001) Allergy and allergic diseases: part 1. *New England Journal of Medicine*, **344**(1), 30–37.

Khan F H (2009) *The Elements of Immunology*. Delhi, Pearson Education.

Klein J and Sato A (2000) The HLA System: part 1. *New England Journal of Medicine*, **343**(10), 702–709.

Male D (2004) *Immunology: An Illustrated Outline* (4th edn). Edinburgh, Mosby.

Misbah S A, and Chapel H M (1993) Adverse effects of intravenous immunoglobulin. *Drug Safety*, **9**(4), 254–262.

Mosby's Medical Dictionary (8th edn). (2009) St Louis, MO, Mosby Elsevier.

Murphy K, Travers P, and Walport M (2008) *Janeway's Immunobiology* (7th edn). New York, Garland Science.

Nairn R and Helbert M (2007) *Immunology for Medical Students* (2nd edn). St Louis, MO, Mosby.

NHS Choices (2010a) *Pressure Ulcers*. Available at: http://www.nhs.uk/conditions/Pressure-ulcers/Pages/Introduction.aspx (accessed September 2011).

NHS Choices (2010b) *Whooping Cough*. Available at: http://www.nhs.uk/conditions/Whooping-cough/Pages/Introduction.aspx (accessed September 2011).

Pacifici G (2005) Transfer of antivirals across the human placenta. *Early Human Development*, **81**(8), 647–654.

Porth C (2009) *Pathophysiology: Concepts of altered health states* (9th edn). Philadelphia, PA, Lippincott.

RCN (2005) *The Management of Pressure Ulcers in Primary and Secondary Care: A Clinical Practice Guideline*. London, Royal College of Nursing, available at: http://www.rcn.org.uk/__data/assets/pdf_file/0017/65015/management_pressure_ulcers.pdf (accessed August 2011).

Rezaei N, Bonilla F A, Sullivan K E *et al.* (2008) An introduction to primary immunodeficiency diseases. In Rezaei N, Aghamohammadi A and Notarangelo L D (eds), *Primary Immunodeficiency Diseases*. Berlin, Springer, 1–38.

Rink L and Gabriel P (2000) Zinc and the immune system. *Proceedings of the Nutrition Society*, **59**(4), 541–552.

Roitt I M (2001) *Roitt's Essential Immunology* (10th edn). Oxford, Blackwell Scientific Publications.

Rote N S (2010a) Alterations in immunity and inflammation. In McCance K L, Huether S E, Brashers, V L and Rote N S (eds), *Pathophysiology: The biologic basis for disease in adults and children* (6th edn). St Louis, MO, Mosby, 256–293.

Rote N S (2010b) Adaptive immunity. In McCance K L, Huether S E, Brashers V L and Rote N S (eds), *Pathophysiology: The biologic basis for disease in adults and children* (6th edn). St Louis, MO, Mosby, 217–255.

Rote N S and Huether S E (2010) Innate immunity: inflammation. In McCance K L, Huether S E, Brashers V L and Rote N S (eds), *Pathophysiology: The biologic basis for disease in adults and children* (6th edn). St Louis, MO, Mosby, 183–216.

Seymour G J, Savage N E and Walsh L J (1995) *Immunology: An Introduction for the Health Sciences*. Roseville, McGraw-Hill.

Sherrif A, Golding J and ALSPAC Study Team (2002a) Factors associated with different hygiene practices in the homes of 15 month old infants. *Archives of Disease in Children*, **86**, 30–35.

Sherrif A, Golding J, and ALSPAC Study Team (2002b) Hygiene levels in a contemporary population cohort are associated with wheezing and atopic eczema in preschool infants. *Archives of Disease in Children*, **87**, 26–29.

Strachen D P (1989) Hay fever, hygiene and household size. *British Medical Journal*, **299**, 1258–1259.

Tierney L, McPhee S and Papadakis M (eds) (2005) *Current Medical Diagnosis & Treatment* (44th edn). New York, Lange Medical Books/McGraw-Hill.

Toolan J (2006) Common Variable Immunodeficiency (CVID). In Vickers P S, Toolan J, Salomé-Bentley N and Cochrane S (eds), *Immunology/Immunodeficiencies – antibody deficiency. Nurse Education Module* (CD-Rom). Baxter's/RCN Immunology & Allergy Nurses Group, 137–164.

Tortora G J, Funke B R and Case C L (2004) *Microbiology: An Introduction* (8th edn). San Francisco, CA, Pearson Benjamin Cummings.

Vickers P S (2005) Acquired defences. In Montague S E, Watson R and Herbert R A (eds), *Physiology for Nursing Practice* (3rd edn). Edinburgh, Elsevier, 685–724.

Vickers P S (2006) Anatomy and physiology of the immune system. In Vickers P S, Toolan J, Salomé-Bentley N and Cochrane S (eds), *Immunology/Immunodeficiencies – Antibody Deficiency. Nurse Education Module* (CD-Rom). Baxter's/RCN Immunology & Allergy Nurses Group, 3–51.

Vickers P S (2009a) Inflammation, immune response and healing. In Nair M and Peate I (eds), *Fundamentals of Applied Pathophysiology: An essential guide for nursing students*. Chichester, Wiley-Blackwell, 61–85.

Vickers P S (2009b) *Severe Combined Immune Deficiency: Early hospitalisation and isolation*. Chichester, Wiley-Blackwell.

Von Mutius E, Martinez F D, Fritzsch C *et al.* (1994) Prevalence of asthma and atopy in two areas of West and East Germany. *American Journal of Respiratory Critical Care Medicine*, **149**, 358–364.

Walport M J (2001) Complement; part 1. *New England Journal of Medicine*, **344**(14), 1058–1066.

Weinberg E D (1987) Pregnancy-associated immune suppression: Risks and mechanisms. *Microbial Pathogenesis*, **3**, 393.

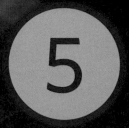

5

Caring for people with altered skin function

Learning outcomes

- Describe, identify and relate the anatomy and physiology of the skin, hair and nails, explaining the pathophysiological processes to wound healing.

- Identify factors affecting wound healing and skin breakdown to be considered during the assessment process and describe methods and management used to promote wound healing.

- Identify common altered skin function conditions.

- Explain the importance of skin/wound assessment, identifying the tools, diagnostic tests and factors that should be considered during the assessment process.

- Review professional issues that occur in the management of altered skin function.

Clinical competencies

- Assess the health status of individuals and the effects pathologies have on the function of the skin.

- Plan and implement individualised nursing care, promote wound healing and/or prevention of skin breakdown in people at risk, or altered skin function.

- Plan and provide appropriate teaching for health promotion.

- Identify members of the interdisciplinary team who will assist in the care of patients with altered skin function.

CASE STUDIES

Below are three case studies that you may wish to consider before, during or after you have read this chapter. There are no right or wrong answers to these case studies but you should think about the physical, psychological and social implications. Think about these anatomical structures of the skin, hair and nails as well as the nursing assessment needed to assess patients with altered skin function.

Case Study 1 – John

Mr John Tyson, aged 48, has had arthritis since he was a child. He is married and both he and his wife Jenny (48) have moderate learning disabilities. John was admitted after a fall at home, when Jenny could not get him back into his wheelchair. His BMI is 18.5, he looks grey, emaciated and frail. On further examination, John is found to have a grade 4 pressure ulcer to his left trochanter (hip) which tracks to his perineum.

Case Study 2 – Bernard

Mr Bernard Farmer is 64 and was admitted as an emergency with a ruptured colon due to untreated diverticulitis. He had formation of a colostomy in theatre and was given prophylactic antibiotics. On return to the ward his wound dehisced (broke down); he returned to theatre for insertion of a Teflon graft to keep peritoneal contents in place, but the rest of his wound was left to heal by secondary intention.

Case Study 3 – Simon

Mr Simon Dawson is 20, in his final year at university. He has attended the walk-in centre as a rash has developed on his hands. He admits to being obsessive about hand washing, on examination he has a raised red rash to both hands that is very itchy and burns, and this is now spreading to his abdomen and back. He is worried about the rash worsening as he has exams to revise for.

INTRODUCTION

The development of the management of skin conditions has a long-documented history. The earliest recording is from Edwin Smith Papyrus from Luxor 1700BC, an ancient medical text on surgical trauma. The papyrus includes 48 cases of injury with each case detailing the type of the injury, examination of the patient, diagnosis, prognosis and treatment.

Famous scholars and medics such as Hippocrates (460–377BC), Sushruta (800BC), Celsus (50–25BC) and Galen (199–129BC) all developed extensive work on their observations of the skin, wounds and wound healing and their responses to topical treatments, diet and surgery. Hippocrates was the first to document the importance of cleanliness in wound care and hand washing and documented that wounds that healed by primary intention (edges brought together) healed quicker than those laid open.

In modern healthcare practices, the management of the skin has never been more important, as the launch of the High Impact Actions for Nursing and Midwifery (NHSIII 2009), in particular the 'Your Skin Matters' document, has had nurses exploring and developing novel and innovative ways of reducing cost, but improving care in pressure ulcer management. The aim is to eliminate all avoidable pressure ulcers, reducing treatment costs locally (DoH 2009). Care bundles, a set of evidence-based practices, have been developed to improve patient outcomes (Health Protection Scotland 2008) – these currently concern prevention of surgical site infections and have been created to enhance patient outcomes.

Other documents concerning skin and wound management include the Essence of Care document (DoH 2010b), a benchmark for prevention and management of pressure ulcers, National Institute for Health and Clinical Excellence (NICE) guidance and appraisals of practices in wound debridement, negative pressure, hydrosurgery, pressure ulcer prevention and treatment and surgical site infections too (NICE 2001a,b, 2004b, 2008, 2009). These initiatives have led to developments within skin and wound care, based not only on personal choice of the practitioner, but also on cost-effectiveness, efficiency and a sound evidence base. The management of all altered skin conditions should ensure patient safety, patient experience and effectiveness of care (DoH 2008), ensuring quality and appropriate treatment.

The threat of litigation is real and, as the Nursing and Midwifery Council hold nurses to account for their actions (NMC 2008) and the cost of wound care management rises (estimated at £2.3–£3.1 billion per year, Posnett and Franks 2007), it is essential that the right thing is done to the right person at the right time.

ANATOMY, PHYSIOLOGY AND FUNCTION OF THE SKIN, HAIR AND NAILS

The skin, the hair and the nails make up the integumentary system. The skin, the largest organ of the body, provides an external covering, separating and protecting the organs and tissues from the external environment. Functions of the skin, hair and nails are summarised in Table 5.1. Disorders of the skin, hair and nails may be caused by a variety of factors, including pressure, shear, friction, cardiovascular conditions, allergies, infection, infestation, cancer and genetic influences.

THE SKIN

The epidermis

This is the surface or outermost part of the skin, consisting of epithelial cells. It has either four or five layers, depending on location; there are five layers over the palms of the hands and soles of the feet, and four layers over the rest of the body.

The stratum basale is the deepest layer of the epidermis, containing melanocytes, cells producing the pigment melanin, and keratinocytes, which produce keratin. Melanin forms a protective shield, protecting the keratinocytes and nerve endings in the dermis from the damaging effects of ultraviolet light. Melanocyte activity probably accounts for the difference in skin colour. Keratin is a fibrous, water-repellent protein giving the epidermis its tough, protective quality. As keratinocytes mature, they move upward through the epidermal layers, eventually becoming dead cells at the surface of the skin. Millions of these cells are worn off by abrasion daily, for example when rubbing skin with a towel or removing clothing, but millions are simultaneously produced in the stratum basale. The next layer is the stratum spinosum 8–10 cells thick, containing abundant cells arising from the bone marrow, migrating to the epidermis. Mitosis occurs at this layer, although not as abundantly as in the stratum basale.

The stratum granulosum is only two to three cells thick. Cells of the stratum granulosum contain a glycolipid, slowing water loss across the epidermis. Keratinisation, thickening of

FAST FACTS

The skin

- The skin has an average surface area of 1.9 m², weighing about 2.7–3.6 kg.
- It is estimated that each 2.54 cm² of skin contains 4.57 m of blood vessels, 3.66 m of nerves, 650 sweat **glands**, 100 oil glands, 1500 sensory receptors and more than three million cells, constantly dying and being replaced.
- The ph of skin is 4.5–6 (slightly acidic).
- The skin is composed of three regions: the **epidermis**, the **dermis** and the **subcutaneous** tissue (Figure 5.1).

Table 5.1 Function of the skin

Structure	Function
Epidermis	• Protects tissues from physical, chemical and biological damage. • Prevents water loss, serves as a water-repellent layer. • Stores melanin, protecting tissues from harmful effects of the ultraviolet radiation in sunlight. • Converts cholesterol molecules to vitamin D when exposed to sunlight. • Contains phagocytes, preventing bacteria from penetrating the skin.
Dermis	• Regulates body temperature by dilating and constricting capillaries. • Transmits messages via nerve endings to the central nervous system: touch, pain, heat, cold. • Communication, for example flushing of the skin when embarrassed, pallor when frightened or ill.
Sebaceous (oil) glands	• Secrete sebum, lubricating skin and hair, play a role in killing bacteria.
Eccrine sweat glands	• Regulate body heat, excretion of perspiration.
Apocrine sweat glands	• Remains of sexual scent gland.
Hair	• Cushions the scalp. • Eyelashes and cilia protect the body from foreign particles. • Provides insulation in cold weather.
Nails	• Protect the fingers and toes, aid in grasping and allow for various other activities, such as scratching the skin, picking up small items.

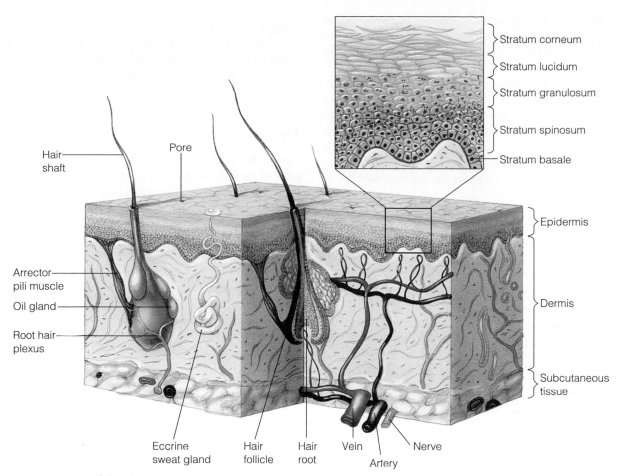

Figure 5.1 Anatomy of the skin.

the cells' plasma membranes, begins in the stratum granulosum. The stratum lucidum is present only in areas of thick skin and is made up of flattened, dead keratinocytes.

The outermost layer of the epidermis, the stratum corneum, is also the thickest, making up about 75% of the epidermis's total thickness. It consists of about 20–30 sheets of dead cells filled with keratin fragments arranged in 'shingles' that flake off as dry skin.

The dermis

The second, deeper layer of skin is made of a flexible connective tissue, richly supplied with blood cells, nerve fibres and lymphatic vessels. Most of the hair follicles, sebaceous glands (glands secreting an oil called sebum) and sweat glands are located in the dermis, which consists of a papillary and a reticular layer. The papillary layer contains ridges indenting the overlying epidermis, capillaries and receptors for pain and touch. The deeper, reticular layer contains blood vessels, sweat and sebaceous glands, deep pressure receptors and dense bundles of collagen fibres. The regions between these bundles form lines of cleavage in the skin, ridges of the skin that run downward, forward and almost horizontally around the body. Surgical incisions parallel to these lines of cleavage heal more easily and with less scarring than incisions or traumatic wounds across cleavage lines.

Subcutaneous tissue

A layer of subcutaneous tissue called the superficial fascia lies under the dermis. Consisting primarily of adipose (fat) tissue, it helps the skin adhere to underlying structures.

Glands of the skin

The skin contains sebaceous (oil) glands, sudoriferous (sweat) glands and ceruminous (earwax) glands. Each one has a different function.

Sebaceous glands are found all over the body except on the palms and soles and secrete an oily substance called sebum, which usually is ducted into hair follicles. Sebum softens and lubricates the skin and hair and decreases water loss from the skin in low humidity. Sebum protects from infection by killing bacteria and is stimulated by hormones, especially androgens (sex hormones). Acne vulgaris is an inflammation of the sebaceous glands.

There are two types of sweat glands: eccrine and apocrine. Eccrine sweat glands are more numerous on the forehead, palms and soles. The gland is located in the dermis; the duct to the skin rises through the epidermis to open in a pore at the surface. Sweat, the secretion of the eccrine glands, is composed mostly of water and contains sodium, antibodies, small amounts of metabolic waste, lactic acid and vitamin C. Sweat production is regulated by the sympathetic nervous system; it serves to maintain normal body temperature and occurs in response to emotions.

Most apocrine sweat glands are located in the axillary (armpit), anal and genital areas. Secretions are similar to those of sweat glands, and they contain fatty acids and proteins. Apocrine glands are remnants of mammalian sexual scent glands. Ceruminous glands are modified apocrine sweat glands. Located in the skin of the external ear canal, they secrete yellow-brown waxy cerumen, providing a sticky trap for foreign materials.

Skin colour

Skin colour varies, ranging from a pinkish white to various shades of brown and black. Special care must be taken when assessing changes in skin colour in people with dark skin, such as Africans, Afro-Caribbeans, Asians, people of Mediterranean descent and Caucasians who are deeply suntanned.

The colour of the skin is the result of varying levels of pigmentation. Melanin, a yellow-to-brown pigment, is darker and produced in greater amounts in persons with dark skin colour than in those with light skin. Exposure to the sun causes a buildup of melanin and a darkening or tanning of the skin in people with light skin. Carotene, a yellow-to-orange pigment, is found most in areas of the body where the stratum corneum is thickest, such as the palms of the hands. Carotene is more abundant in the skins of persons of Asian ancestry and, together with melanin, accounts for their golden skin tone. The epidermis in Caucasian skin has very little melanin and is almost transparent. Thus, the colour of the haemoglobin found in red blood cells (RBCs) circulating through the dermis shows through, lending Caucasians a pinkish skin tone.

Skin colour is influenced by emotions and illnesses. A reddening of the skin may occur with embarrassment (blushing), fever, hypertension or inflammation. It may also result from a drug reaction, sunburn, acne rosacea (characterised by facial redness and pimples) or other factors. A bluish discoloration of the skin and mucous membranes (cyanosis) results from poor oxygenation of haemoglobin. Pallor, or paleness, may occur with shock, fear or anger or in anaemia and hypoxia. Jaundice (increased bilirubin in the blood) is a yellow-to-orange colour visible in the skin and mucous membranes, often the result of a liver disorder. As wounds heal, the colour of the new epidermal layer regardless of the ethnic origin of the person, is pink in colour and, if the scar tissue covers a large surface area, this may lead to altered body image, requiring a referral to a cosmetic camouflage nurse for further support and advice.

> ### *Consider this . . .*
>
> It is often difficult to assess **erythema** (reddening of the skin), **hyperaemia** (increased blood flow to the skin), carbon monoxide poisoning, **venous stasis** (slow blood flow of the veins), jaundice and uraemia (accumulation of urea in the blood) in patients with dark or Asian skin tones. Skin may appear dull, have a yellow, ashen grey or dark red cast. Skin may be painful, firm, soft, warmer or cooler to touch as compared to adjacent tissue or you may have to assess the nail bed, oral mucosa and conjunctivae to help aid diagnosis.

THE HAIR

Hair is distributed all over the body, except the lips, nipples, parts of the external genitals, palms of the hands and soles of the feet. Hair is produced by a hair bulb and its root is enclosed in a hair follicle (see Figure 5.2). The exposed part – the shaft – consists mainly of dead cells. Hair follicles extend into the dermis and in some places, such as the scalp, below the dermis. Many factors, including nutrition and hormones, influence hair growth. Hair in various parts of the body has protective functions: the eyebrows and eyelashes protect the eyes; hair in the nose helps keep foreign materials out of the upper respiratory tract; and hair on the head protects the scalp from heat loss and sunlight.

THE NAILS

These are modified scale-like epidermal structures; nails consist mainly of dead cells, arising from the stratum germinativum of the epidermis. The body of the nail rests on the nail bed (see Figure 5.3). The nail matrix is the active, growing part of the nail. The visible end, near the skin, has a white crescent, called a lunula. The sides are overlapped by skin, called nail folds. The proximal nail fold is thickened and is called the eponychium or cuticle. Nails form a protective coating over the dorsum of each digit.

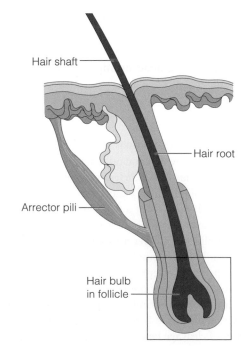

Hair shaft

Hair root

Arrector pili

Hair bulb in follicle

Figure 5.2 Anatomy of a hair follicle.

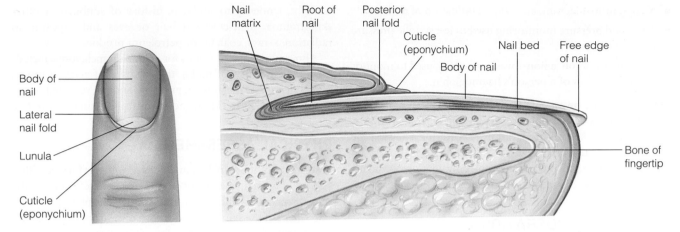

Figure 5.3 Anatomy of a nail (frontal and side views).

Types of altered skin function

Alteration in skin integrity is an issue in clinical practice for all nurses. Damage to the skin may be due to many factors such as mechanical, chemical, vascular, infectious, allergic and thermal, each of which results in a different response within the skin. For example, an ulcer, lesion, fistulae (an abnormal connection or passageway), papule or erosion may go on to develop into more serious secondary lesions.

It is important to understand the causes and types of altered skin problems, which may present in practice, so that assessment can occur and appropriate care be provided. Altered skin function can also be classified according to the depth of tissue damage and morphology (form and structure of wounds).

Assessing skin function

The functions of skin are assessed by findings from diagnostic tests, a health assessment interview to collect subjective data and a physical assessment to collect objective data.

DIAGNOSTIC TESTS

Results of diagnostic tests of the structure and function of skin are used to support the diagnosis of a specific injury or disease, providing information to identify or modify the appropriate medication or treatments used to treat disease, and to help nurses monitor the person's responses to nursing interventions. Diagnostic tests include:

- Skin biopsy to differentiate a benign skin lesion from a skin cancer or to determine infection that is not obtained by wound swabbing. Can be obtained by using a punch technique, incision, excision or shaving.

- Cultures to identify infections may be conducted on tissue samples, drainage and exudate from lesions and, if an illness is generalised, serum.

- Tests used to identify infections include immunofluorescent studies, Wood's lamp, potassium hydroxide and the Tzanck test.

- Allergies may be determined through patch tests or scratch tests.

- X-rays to determine osteomyelitis.

- Doppler ultrasonography to determine systolic pressure in arteries of arms and legs calculating the ankle brachial pressure index (ABPI).

- Colour Duplex Scan to provide information on the flow of blood, width and wall of arteries using Doppler ultrasonography.

- Photoplethysmography, a non-invasive test, used to measure venous reflux and filling times using infrared light source and transducer light probe.

- Phlebography to highlight the venous system by injecting radio-opaque dye into the veins of the lower limbs.

- Sonography using reflections of high-frequency sound waves to construct an image of a body organ.

- Computed tomography, an x-ray used to produce an image of a body structure.

- Magnetic resonance scan, a non-invasive medical diagnostic technique.

- Blood tests to assess for anaemia, liver function, renal function, white cell count, platelets.

- Body mass index to assess the height and weight range of the individual.

- Blood sugar to determine the plasma glucose level in diabetics. This may be followed up by a haemoglobin A1C test to determine blood glucose levels from the previous three months.

- Urinalysis used as a screening and/or diagnostic tool to detect different metabolic and kidney disorders.

- Sinogram/fistulagram, an x-ray examination of a wound.
- Toe blood pressure monitoring used to test systolic pressure levels in the toes.
- Oxygen saturation, a non-invasive method, used to monitor the oxygenation of a person's haemoglobin.

Other diagnostic investigations may be carried out.

The nurse is responsible for explaining all tests, the procedure and any special preparation needed, for assessing for medication use that may affect test outcomes, for supporting the person before, during and after the examination, for documenting the procedures and for monitoring test results.

GENETIC CONSIDERATIONS

It is important to consider genetic influences on the health of the adult. During the health assessment interview, ask about skin disorders or abnormalities in immediate family members and also inquire about their gender. During the physical assessment, assess for any manifestations that indicate a genetic disorder. If data are found that indicate genetic risk factors or alterations, ask about genetic testing and refer for appropriate genetic counselling and evaluation.

HEALTH ASSESSMENT INTERVIEW

This may be conducted during health screening, may focus on a chief complaint, or may be part of a total health assessment. If the person has a skin problem, analyse onset, characteristics and course, severity, precipitating and relieving factors, noting the timing and circumstances of any associated symptoms. Ask the person:

- What type of itching have you experienced?
- When did you first notice a change in this mole?
- Did you change to any different kinds of shampoo or other hair products just before you started to lose your hair?
- How did you injure yourself?

Ask about changes in health, rashes, itching, colour changes, dryness or oiliness, growth of or changes in warts or moles and the presence of lesions. Precipitating causes, such as medications, use of new soaps, skin care agents, cosmetics, pets, travel, stress or dietary changes, must also be explored. In assessing hair problems, ask about any thinning or baldness, excessive hair loss, change in distribution of hair, use of hair care products, diet, and dieting. When assessing nail problems, ask about nail splitting or breakage, discoloration, infection, diet, and exposure to chemicals.

The medical history is important. Questions focus on previous problems, allergies and lesions. Skin problems may be manifestations of other disorders, such as cardiovascular disease, endocrine disorders, hepatic disease and haematological disorders. Occupational and social history may provide clues to skin problems; ask about travel, exposure to toxic substances at work, use of alcohol and responses to stress.

Assess the presence of risk factors for skin cancer carefully including gender, age, family history, extended exposure to sunlight, tendency to sunburn, history of sunburn or other skin trauma, light-coloured hair or eyes and exposure to radiation, x-rays, coal, tar or petroleum products.

Also explore the risk factors for malignant melanoma, including a large number of moles, the presence of atypical moles, family history of melanoma, prior melanoma, repeated severe sunburns, ease of freckling and sunburning or inability to tan.

PHYSICAL ASSESSMENT

Assessment of the skin, hair and nails may be performed either as part of a total assessment or a focussed assessment of the skin for people with known or suspected problems. Physical assessment of the skin, hair and nails is conducted by inspection and palpation. Assess the skin for colour, presence of lesions (observable changes from normal skin structure), temperature, texture, moisture, turgor and presence of oedema. Characteristics of lesions/wounds to note include site, location and distribution, colour and type of tissue at the wound bed, pattern, edges, size (measure with a ruler in centimetres), elevation and type of exudates, odour and pain (if present) and peri wound area. Examine hair for colour, texture, quality and scalp lesions. Determine shape, colour, contour and condition of the nails.

The examination should be conducted in a warm, private room. The person removes all clothing and puts on a gown. Areas to be examined should be fully exposed, but protect modesty by keeping other areas covered. The person may stand, sit or lie down at various times of the examination. Don disposable gloves when palpating open lesions, if skin surfaces are indicative of infections or infestations, or if there is discharge from lesions/ wounds of the skin and mucous membranes. Standard precautions should be adhered to when conducting a skin assessment. A ruler, grid or photography is used to measure the lesions and wounds. A tape measure is used to measure leg circumference. A torch allows better visualisation of lesions. Depending on the lesion or wound, classification tools are used to document the assessment, for example pressure ulcers and diabetic foot ulcers.

IN PRACTICE

PUSH tool

The PUSH (Pressure Ulcer Scale for Healing) Tool was developed by the National Pressure Ulcer Advisory Panel (NPUAP) (1997) based upon a critical review of the literature to be used as a tool to monitor the change in pressure ulcer status over time.

The nurse needs to examine and measure the pressure ulcer and classify it in relation to the surface area, exudate and type of wound tissue at the wound bed. A sub-score is recorded for each of the ulcer features; once completed, add the sub-scores to obtain the total score. Over time the recordings can be compared, providing an indication of improvement or deterioration in pressure ulcer healing.

COMMON SKIN PROBLEMS AND LESIONS

There are many disorders of the skin. They are often treated in out-patient settings, in the community or by self-care from discussions with and over-the-counter prescriptions and purchases from the pharmacist.

The person with pruritus

Pruritus is a subjective itching sensation, producing an urge to scratch, which may occur in a small, circumscribed area, or may involve a widespread area. It may or may not be associated with a rash. Pruritus is believed to result from either stimulation of itch receptors in the skin or as a response to the stimulation of skin receptors for pain and touch.

Almost anything in the internal or external environment can cause pruritus. Insects, animals, plants, fabrics, metals, medications, allergies and even emotional distress are the most common causes. Pruritus can occur as a secondary manifestation of systemic disorders, such as certain types of cancer, diabetes mellitus, hepatic disease and renal failure. The exact physiology is unknown, but it is known that heat and prostaglandins (messenger molecules) trigger pruritus and that histamine and morphine increase it.

Secondary effects of pruritus include skin excoriation, erythema (redness), wheals (a small raised bump of the skin that swells), changes in pigmentation and infections. Sleep patterns may be interrupted, because the itching sensation is often more intense at night when heat causes blood vessels in the skin to vasodilate. Long-term pruritus may be debilitating and increases the risk of infection as excoriation occurs.

The person with dry skin (xerosis)

Dry skin (xerosis) is most often a problem in the older adult. Xerosis commonly results from a decrease in the activity of sebaceous and sweat glands, reducing the skin's lubrication and moisture retention. Dry skin may occur at any age from exposure to environmental heat and low humidity, sunlight, excessive bathing and a decreased intake of liquids.

The person with a benign skin lesion

The skin is subject to many different types and kinds of benign skin lesions, including cysts, keloid scars, naevi, angiomas, skin tags and keratoses. These benign lesions are often considered more of a nuisance than an illness; they do require monitoring for an increase in size, interfering with the skin's appearance or function.

Most benign lesions do not require treatment, although excision or laser surgery may sometimes be desired or necessary. Cysts may enlarge, skin tags may become irritated and bleed, naevi may change in appearance, or they may cause discomfort with appearance.

Cysts

Cysts of the skin are benign closed sacs in or under the skin surface lined with epithelium, containing fluid or a semi-solid material. Epidermal inclusion cysts and pilar cysts are the most common types and may occur anywhere on the body, although most often found on the head and trunk. Although they are painless, they may grow so large that they become irritated by contact with clothing (e.g., if located on the back of the neck) or cause obstruction (e.g., if located on the nose). They contain a semi-solid material composed mainly of keratin. Pilar cysts are found on the scalp originating from sebaceous glands. They are also painless. These cysts rarely require treatment unless they become large and bothersome.

Keloid scars

Keloid scars are elevated, irregularly shaped, progressively enlarging scars, arising from excessive amounts of collagen in the stratum corneum during scar formation in connective tissue repair. They are more common in young adults and appear within one year of the initial trauma.

This abnormal response most often occurs in people of African and Asian descent who sustain burns of the skin, but even seemingly minor trauma can result in keloid formation. There is a familial tendency to develop keloid scars. Other risk factors include excessive tension on a wound and poor alignment of skin edges following accidental or intentional skin trauma. Certain skin surfaces, the chin, ears, shoulders, back and lower legs, are more likely to develop keloid scars.

The excessive scar formation is associated with increased metabolic activity of fibroblasts and increased type III collagen. The swollen appearance of the keloid scar is the result of an excess of extracellular material. Scars first appear as red, firm, rubbery plaques persisting for several months after the initial trauma. Uncontrolled overgrowth over time causes the keloid scars to extend beyond the original scar. Eventually, the scar becomes smooth and hyperpigmented.

Naevi

Naevi, commonly called moles, are flat or raised macules or papules with rounded, well-defined borders. They arise from melanocytes during early childhood, with the cells initially accumulating at the junction of the dermis and epidermis.

Over time, the cluster of cells moves into the dermis, and the lesion becomes visible. Most adults have naevi.

Naevi range from flesh-coloured to black and occasionally contain hair. They can occur on any skin surface of the body and may arise as single lesions or in groups. Some pigmented naevi can transform into malignant lesions. The average adult has about 20 naevi, but only four people out of 100 000 develop a malignant melanoma. However, it is important to monitor naevi for changes in size, thickness, colour, bleeding or itching. If these occur, the person should seek immediate professional assessment.

Angiomas

Angiomas, also called haemangiomas, are benign vascular tumours, appearing in the adult in different forms:

- Naevus flammeus (port-wine stain) is a congenital vascular lesion involving the capillaries. The lesions tend to occur on the upper body or face as macular patches ranging from light red to dark purple. They are present at birth and grow proportionately with the child into adulthood.
- Cherry angiomas are small, rounded papules that may occur at any age, but they most commonly arise in the 40s and gradually increase in number. They range in colour from bright red to purple and are often found on the trunk.
- Spider angiomas are dilated superficial arteries, common in pregnant women and in persons with hepatic disease. They occur most often on the face, neck and upper chest and are usually small, bright red papules with radiating lines.
- Telangiectases are single dilated capillaries or terminal arteries often appearing on the cheeks and nose. They are most common in older adults and result from photoaged skin. The lesions look like broken veins.
- Venous lakes are small, flat, blue blood vessels. They are seen on the exposed skin of the older adult: the ears, lips and backs of the hands.

Skin tags

Skin tags are soft papules on a pedicle (stalk). They can be as small as a pinhead or as large as a pea and are most often found on the front or side of the neck and in the axillae, as well as in areas where clothing (such as underwear) rubs the skin. They have normal skin colour and texture.

Keratoses

A keratosis is any skin condition in which there is a benign overgrowth and thickening of the outer layers of the skin. These lesions most often appear in adults after age 50.

Seborrhoeic keratoses appear as superficial flat, smooth or warty-surfaced growths, 5–20 mm in diameter, most often on the face and trunk. The lesions may be tan, waxy yellow, dark brown or flesh-coloured, and appear greasy. They are most often seen in the older adult and do not appear to be related to damage from sun exposure.

The person with psoriasis

Psoriasis is a chronic immune skin disorder characterised by raised, reddened, round circumscribed plaques (solid elevation of skin) covered by silvery white scales of varying size. They may appear anywhere on the body but are most commonly found on the scalp, extensor surfaces of the arms and legs (elbows, knees) sacrum (base of the spine) and around the nails. As with any chronic illness, the skin manifestations may occur and disappear throughout life, with no discernible pattern to the recurrence.

The incidence of psoriasis is lower in warm, sunny climates. Onset usually occurs in the 20s, but it may occur at any age. Psoriasis occurs more often in Caucasians; men and women are affected equally. Sunlight, stress, seasonal changes, hormone fluctuations, steroid withdrawal and certain drugs (such as alcohol, corticosteroids, lithium and chloroquine) appear to exacerbate the disorder. About one-third of people have a family history of psoriasis. Trauma to the skin from such events as surgery, sunburn or excoriation is also a common precipitating factor; lesions that result from trauma are called Köbner's reaction.

INFECTIONS AND INFESTATIONS OF THE SKIN

The skin's resistance to infections and infestations is provided by protective mechanisms, including skin flora, sebum and the immune response. The skin is normally resistant to infections and infestations. These disorders may occur as a result of a break in the skin surface, a virulent agent and/or decreased resistance due to a compromised immune system. This section discusses skin disorders resulting from bacterial infections, fungal infections, parasitic infestations and viral infections.

The person with a bacterial infection of the skin

A number of bacteria normally inhabit the skin and do not cause an infection. When a break in the skin allows invasion by pathogenic bacteria, an infection, called a pyoderma, may occur. The most common bacterial infections are caused by gram-positive *Staphylococcus aureus* and beta-haemolytic streptococci (gram-positive bacteria retain the colour of the crystal violet stain in the Gram stain).

Bacterial infections of the skin may be primary or secondary. Primary infections are caused by a single pathogen arising from normal skin; secondary infections develop in traumatised or diseased skin.

Most bacterial infections are treated by a primary care provider, and the person remains at home for care. If the infection becomes more serious, in-patient care may be required. In addition, hospital-acquired infections of wounds or open lesions in people are often the result of bacterial infections, especially by methicillin-resistant *Staphylococcus aureus* (MRSA).

PRACTICE ALERT

- Remember to apply standard precautions.
- Avoid contact with bodily fluids, by means of the wearing of non-porous items such as medical gloves, goggles and face shields.
- For those who have MRSA, hand washing is the most successful preventative method of reducing the spread of bacteria from one person to another.

Pathophysiology of bacterial infections of the skin

Bacterial infections of the skin arise from the hair follicle, where bacteria accumulate and grow causing a localised infection. The bacteria can also invade deeper tissues causing a systemic infection, a potentially life-threatening disorder. Many bacterial infections involve the skin, including folliculitis, furuncles, carbuncles, cellulitis and erysipelas.

Folliculitis

Folliculitis is a bacterial infection of the hair follicle, commonly caused by *Staphylococcus aureus*. The infection begins at the follicle opening and extends down into the follicle. Bacteria release enzymes and chemical agents causing inflammation. Lesions appear as pustules surrounded by an area of erythema on the surface of the skin. They are accompanied by discomfort ranging from slight burning to intense itching. A major complication is abscess formation. Folliculitis is found most often on the scalp and extremities and is also seen on the face of bearded men (called sycosis-barbae), on the legs of women who shave and on the eyelids (called a stye).

Folliculitis may appear without any apparent cause. Contributing factors include poor hygiene, poor nutrition, prolonged skin moisture, tight heavy fabrics on the upper legs and trauma to the skin.

PRACTICE ALERT

A specific type of folliculitis, called 'hot tub folliculitis,' is caused by *Pseudomonas aeruginosa* bacteria, and is characterised by follicular or pustular lesions occurring one to four days after being in a hot tub, whirlpool or public swimming pool. Treatment may not be necessary, but in severe cases antibiotics may be prescribed. Abscess formation can occur.

Furuncles

Furuncles (boils) are also inflammations of the hair follicle. Beginning as folliculitis, the infection spreads down the hair shaft, through the wall of the follicle and into the dermis. The causative organism is commonly *Staphylococcus aureus*. A furuncle is initially a deep, firm, red, painful nodule 1–5 cm in diameter. After a few days, the nodule changes into a large, painful cystic nodule. The cysts may drain substantial amounts of purulent drainage (infected, malodorous pus).

Furuncles may occur on any part of the body that has hair. Contributing factors include poor hygiene, trauma to the skin, areas of excessive moisture (including perspiration) and systemic diseases such as diabetes mellitus and haematologic malignancies.

Carbuncles

A carbuncle is a group of infected hair follicles and begins as a firm mass located in the subcutaneous tissue and the lower dermis. This mass becomes swollen and painful and has multiple openings to the skin surface. They are most frequently found on the back of the neck, the upper back and the lateral thighs. In addition to the local manifestations, the person may experience chills, fever and malaise. Contributing factors for carbuncles are the same as for furuncles.

Cellulitis

Cellulitis is a localised infection of the dermis and subcutaneous tissue and can occur following a wound or skin ulcer or as an extension of furuncles or carbuncles. Infection spreads as a result of a substance produced by the causative organism, called spreading factor (hyaluronidase). This breaks down the fibrin network and other barriers that normally localise the infection. The area of cellulitis is red, swollen and painful. Vesicles (fluid-filled eruptions on the skin) may form over the area of cellulitis. There may be fever, chills, malaise, headache and swollen lymph glands.

Erysipelas

Erysipelas is an infection of the skin most often caused by group A streptococci bacteria. Chills, fever and malaise are warning signs and symptoms, occurring from four hours to 20 days before the skin lesion appears. Initially infection appears as firm red spots enlarging and joining to form a circumscribed, bright red, raised, hot lesion. Vesicles may form over the surface of the lesion. The area usually is painful, itches and burns. Erysipelas most commonly appears on the face, ears and lower legs.

THE PERSON WITH A FUNGAL INFECTION OF THE SKIN

Fungi are free-living plant-like organisms living in the soil, on animals and humans. The fungi causing superficial skin infections are called dermatophytes. In humans, the dermatophytes live on keratin in the stratum corneum, hair and nails. Fungal disorders are also called mycoses.

Pathophysiology of fungal infections of the skin

Fungal infections include dermatophytoses (tinea or ringworm) and candidiasis (yeast) infections.

Dermatophytoses (tinea / ringworm)

Superficial fungal infections of the skin are called dermatophytoses or, more commonly, ringworm, and occur when a susceptible host comes in contact with the organism. The organism may be transmitted by direct contact with animals or other infected persons or by inanimate objects such as combs, pillowcases and towels. The most important factor in the development of the infection is moisture; the onset and spread of the infection is greatest in areas where moisture content is high, such as within skin folds, between the toes and in the mouth. Other factors increasing the risk of a fungal infection include the use of broad-spectrum antibiotics that kill off normal flora allowing the fungi to grow, diabetes mellitus, immunodeficiencies, nutritional deficiencies, pregnancy, increasing age and iron deficiency. The dermatophyte infections are named by the body part affected, as follows:

- *Tineapedis* – infection of the soles of the feet, the space between the toes and/or the toenails, often called athlete's foot, the most common tinea infection. Lesions vary from mild scaliness to painful fissures with drainage, usually accompanied by pruritus and a foul odour. The infection is often chronic, absent in winter but reappearing in hot weather when perspiring feet are encased in shoes.

- *Tineacapitis* – infection of the scalp. The primary lesions are grey, round, bald spots, often accompanied by erythema and crusting. Hair loss is usually temporary. Tineacapitis is seen more often in children than in adults.

- *Tineacorporis* – infection of the body. It can be caused by various fungi; the lesions vary according to the causative organism. Most common lesions are large circular patches with raised red borders of vesicles, papules or pustules with pruritus and erythema.

- *Tineaversicolour* – infection of the upper chest, back and sometimes the arms. Lesions are yellow, pink or brown sheets of scaling skin. The patches do not have pigment and do not tan when exposed to ultraviolet light.

- *Tineacruris* – infection of the groin that may extend to the inner thighs and buttocks. Often associated with tinea pedis and more common in people who are physically active, are obese and/or wear tight underclothing.

Candidiasis

Candidiasis infections are caused by *Candida albicans*, a yeast-like fungus, normally found on mucous membranes, on the skin, in the vagina and in the gastrointestinal tract (Figure 5.4). The fungus becomes a pathogen when the following encourage its growth:

- a local environment of moisture, warmth or altered skin integrity;
- the administration of systemic antibiotics;
- pregnancy;
- the use of birth control pills;
- poor nutrition;
- the presence of diabetes mellitus, Cushing's disease or other chronic debilitating illnesses;
- immunosuppression;
- some malignancies of the blood.

Candidiasis affects the outer layers of the skin and mucous membranes of the mouth, vagina, uncircumcised penis, nails and deep skin folds. The first sign of infection is a pustule that extends under the stratum corneum. The pustule has an inflamed base and often burns and itches. As infection spreads, the accumulation of inflammatory cells and shedding of surface cells produce a white-to-yellow curd-like substance covering the infected area. Satellite lesions (maculopapular areas found outside the clearly demarcated border of the original infection) are characteristic of candidiasis. The appearance of the infection differs by location.

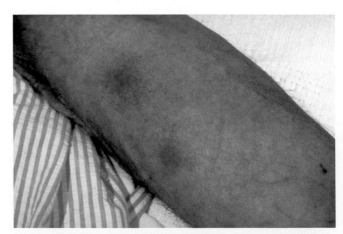

Figure 5.4 *Candida albicans*, a fungus. Causes a skin infection characterised by erythema, pustules and a typical white substance covering the area.
Source: Stuart M. Levitz, M. D.

The person with a parasitic infestation of the skin

Parasitic infections are more common in developing countries but may occur in any geographic area of the world. They affect people of all social classes but are associated with crowded or unsanitary living conditions.

Pathophysiology of parasitic infestations of the skin

Two of the more common parasitic infestations of the skin are caused by lice and mites. These parasites do not normally live on the skin, but infest the skin through contact with an infested person or contact with clothing, linens or objects infested with the parasites.

Pediculosis

Pediculosis is an infestation with lice, parasites that live on the blood of an animal or human host. The louse is a 2–4 mm oval organism with a stylet that pierces the skin; an anticoagulant in its saliva prevents host blood from clotting while it eats. The female louse lays its eggs (small pearl-grey or brown eggs, called nits) on hair shafts. The louse within the egg hatches, reaches the adult reproductive stage, and dies in 30–50 days.

There are three types of human pediculosis:

- *pediculosiscorporis* – an infestation with body lice;
- *pediculosis pubis* – an infestation with pubic lice (often called crabs);
- *pediculosiscapitis* – an infestation with head lice.

Scabies

Scabies is a parasitic infestation caused by a mite (*Sarcoptesscabiei*). The pregnant female mite burrows into the skin and lays two to three eggs each day for about a month. The eggs hatch in

FAST FACTS

Head lice

- Head lice do not mind if hair is clean or dirty; they cannot live away from the human head; home hygiene has nothing to do with infection.
- Lice have neither the right sort of legs for jumping nor wings, so they cannot jump, fly or crawl across clothing; they only move directly from one person's hair to hair on another head. Sometimes when combing or brushing the hair, the electrostatic charge can make lice appear to leap away from the head.
- Lice will happily live in 1 cm of hair; the only advantage of short hair is that detection and treatment can be easier.

three to five days, the larvae migrate to the surface but burrow into the skin for food or protection, larvae develop and the cycle repeats. Scabies infestation affects people of all socioeconomic classes. The infestation is found in webs between the fingers, the inner surfaces of the wrist and elbow, the axillae, the female nipple, the penis, the belt line and the gluteal crease. Lesions are a small red–brown burrow, about 2 mm in length, sometimes covered with vesicles, appearing as a rash. Pruritus in response to the mite or its faeces is common, especially at night, and excoriations may develop, predisposing the person to secondary bacterial infections.

The person with a viral infection of the skin

Viruses are pathogens that consist of an RNA or DNA core surrounded by a protein coat. They depend on live cells for reproduction and so are classified as intracellular pathogens. Viruses that cause skin lesions invade the keratinocyte, reproduce and either increase cellular growth or cause cellular death.

An increase in the incidence of viral skin disorders has been attributed to a variety of causes. Some commonly used drugs, such as birth control medications and corticosteroids, are known to have immunosuppressive properties allowing the viruses to multiply. Other drugs, such as antibiotics, kill off normal skin bacteria that would otherwise serve as defence against viral infections.

Pathophysiology of viral infections of the skin

Viral infections cause warts, herpes simplex infections and herpes zoster infections.

Warts

Warts, or verrucae, are lesions of the skin caused by the human papillomavirus (HPV). More than 60 types of HPVs have been found on the human skin and mucous membranes. Warts may be found on non-genital or genital skin and mucous membranes. Non-genital warts are benign lesions; genital warts may be pre-cancerous. Warts are transmitted through skin contact; they may be flat, fusiform (tapered at both ends) or round; most are round and raised and have a rough, grey surface. Location and appearance of the warts depend on the causative virus. Those most common are:

- A common wart (*verruca vulgaris*) may appear anywhere on the skin and mucous membranes, but most commonly appears on the fingers. They grow above the skin surface and may be dome-shaped with ragged borders.
- Plantar warts occur at pressure points on the soles of the feet. The pressure of shoes and walking prevents these warts from growing outward; they tend to extend deeper beneath the skin surface than do common warts. Plantar warts are often painful.

- A flat wart (*verruca plana*) is a small flat lesion, usually seen on the forehead or back of the hand.
- Condylomata acuminata, also called HPV or venereal warts, occur in moist areas, along the glans of the penis, in the anal region and on the vulva and cervix. They are usually cauliflower-like in appearance and have a pink or purple colour.

Warts resolve spontaneously when immunity to the virus develops. This response may take up to five years.

Herpes simplex

Herpes simplex (also called a cold sore) virus infections of the skin and mucous membranes are caused by two types of herpes virus: HSV-1 and HSV-2. Most infections above the waist are caused by HSV-1, with herpes simplex lesions most often found on the lips, face and mouth. The virus may be transmitted by physical contact, oral sex or kissing.

Infection begins with a burning or tingling sensation, followed by the development of erythema, vesicle formation and pain. Vesicles progress through pustules, ulcers and crusting until healing occurs in 10–14 days.

Initial infection is often severe and accompanied by systemic manifestations, such as fever and sore throat; recurrences are more localised and less severe. The virus lives in nerve ganglia (swellings that stick out from the lining of a joint or tendon) and may cause recurrent lesions in response to sunlight, menstruation, injury or stress.

Herpes zoster

Herpes zoster, (shingles) is a viral infection of a dermatome section of the skin caused by varicella zoster (the herpes virus that also causes chickenpox). Infection is believed to result from reactivation of a varicella virus remaining in the sensory dorsal ganglia after a childhood infection of chickenpox. When reactivated, it travels from the ganglia to the corresponding skin dermatome area.

Herpes zoster usually affects adults over 60 years. People with Hodgkin's disease, certain types of leukaemia and lymphomas are more susceptible to an outbreak of the disease. Herpes zoster is more prevalent in immune compromised people, such as those with human immunodeficiency virus (HIV) infections, those receiving radiation therapy or chemotherapy and those who have had organ transplants. The appearance of the lesions in people with HIV infections may be one of the first manifestations of immune compromise. The herpes eruption lasts for about two to three weeks and usually does not recur.

Herpes zoster lesions are vesicles with a reddened base. The vesicles appear on the skin area supplied by the neurons of a single or associated group of dorsal root ganglia (although they may occur beyond this area in immune suppressed people). The lesions usually appear unilaterally on the face, trunk and thorax. New lesions continue to erupt for three to five days, crust and dry. Recovery occurs in two to three weeks. The person often experiences severe pain for up to 48 hours before and during eruption of the lesions. Pain may continue for weeks to months after the lesions have disappeared. The older adult is especially sensitive to the pain and often experiences more severe outbreaks of herpes zoster lesions.

Eruption of vesicles over a single dermatome (an area of the skin supplied by nerves from a single spinal root) usually only occurs one time. Generalised herpes zoster may indicate an associated immune compromised disease. Those with HIV are 20 times more likely to develop herpes zoster.

Complications include post-herpetic neuralgia (a sharp, spasmodic pain along the course of one or more nerves) and visual loss. The neuralgia, described as burning or stabbing, results from inflammation of the root ganglia. This complication is more common in those over 55 years. Permanent loss of vision may follow occurrence of lesions arising from the ophthalmic division of the trigeminal nerve. The disease may disseminate in immune compromised people, causing lesions beyond the dermatome, visceral lesions and encephalitis, and this may result in death.

INFLAMMATORY DISORDERS OF THE SKIN

Inflammatory skin disorders to be discussed include dermatitis, acne, pemphigus and lichen planus.

The person with dermatitis

Dermatitis is an inflammation of the skin characterised by erythema and pain or pruritus. Dermatitis may be acute or chronic.

Pathophysiology of dermatitis

In dermatitis, various internal and external agents cause an inflammatory response of the skin. Different types of skin eruptions occur, often specific to the causative allergen, infection or disease. Initial skin responses to these agents or illnesses include erythema, formation of vesicles and scales and pruritus. Subsequently, irritation from scratching promotes oedema, a serous discharge and crusting. Long-term irritation in chronic dermatitis causes skin to become thickened, leathery and darker in colour.

Contact dermatitis

Contact dermatitis is a type of dermatitis caused by a hypersensitivity response or chemical irritation. Major sources known to cause contact dermatitis are dyes, perfumes, poison plants, chemicals and metals. A contact dermatitis common in the healthcare field is latex (glove) dermatitis.

Allergic contact dermatitis is a cell-mediated or delayed hypersensitivity to a variety of allergens. Sensitising antigens include micro-organisms, plants, chemicals, drugs, metals or foreign proteins. On initial contact with the skin, the allergen binds to a carrier protein, forming a sensitising antigen. The first exposure is the sensitising contact, manifestations occurring only with subsequent exposures. These manifestations include erythema, swelling and pruritic vesicles in the area of allergen contact. A person hypersensitive to metal may have lesions under a ring or watch.

Irritant contact dermatitis is an inflammation of the skin from irritants; it is not a hypersensitivity response. Sources of irritant contact dermatitis include chemicals (such as acids), soaps and detergents. Skin lesions are similar to those seen in allergic contact dermatitis.

Atopic dermatitis

Atopic dermatitis is an inflammatory skin disorder also called *eczema,* the exact cause of which is unknown. Related factors include depressed cell-mediated immunity, elevated IgE levels (antibody) and increased histamine sensitivity. This is seen more often in children, but chronic forms persist throughout life.

There is usually a family history of hypersensitivity reactions, such as dry skin, eczema, asthma and allergic rhinitis (inflammation and irritation of the linings in the nose and eyes). Although up to one-third of people with atopic dermatitis also have food allergies, a positive correlation has not been found.

The dermatitis results when mast cells, T lymphocytes, monocytes and other inflammatory cells are activated and release histamine, lymphokines and other inflammatory mediators. The immune response is activated creating a chronic inflammatory condition. In the adult, characteristic lesions include chronic lichenification (thickened and leathery skin), erythema and scaling, caused by pruritus and scratching. Lesions are usually found on the hands, feet or flexor surfaces of the arms and legs (folds of skin). Secondary infection is caused by scratching and excoriation, as well as invasion of the skin by viruses such as herpes simplex.

Seborrhoeic dermatitis

Seborrhoeic dermatitis is a chronic inflammatory disorder of the skin involving the scalp, eyebrows, eyelids, ear canals, nasolabial folds, axillae and trunk – cause unknown. This disorder is seen in all ages, from the very young to the very old. People taking methyldopa (Aldomet) for hypertension occasionally develop this disorder, and it is a component of Parkinson's disease.

The lesions are yellow or white plaques with scales and crusts. Scales are often yellow or orange with a greasy appearance. Mild pruritus is also present. Diffuse dandruff with erythema of the scalp often accompanies lesions.

Exfoliative dermatitis

Exfoliative dermatitis is an inflammatory skin disorder characterised by excessive peeling or shedding of skin. In half of cases cause is unknown, but a pre-existing skin disorder is found in most cases. Reactions to medications, such as sulfonamides (sulfa-related antibiotics), account for 20–40% of cases. Certain cancers (such as lymphoma) may cause exfoliative dermatitis.

Systemic and localised manifestations may appear. Systemic manifestations include weakness, malaise, fever, chills and weight loss. Scaling, erythema and pruritus may be localised or involve the entire body. In addition to peeling of skin, the person may lose the hair and nails. Generalised exfoliative dermatitis may cause debility and dehydration. The impairment of skin integrity increases the risk for local and systemic infections.

The person with acne

Acne is a disorder of the pilosebaceous (hair and sebaceous gland) structure, which opens to the skin surface through pores. Sebaceous glands empty directly into the hair follicle, producing sebum, a lipid substance. They are present all over the skin except the soles and the palms, the largest glands being on the face, scalp and scrotum. Sebum production is associated with hormonal stimulation by androgens.

Pathophysiology of acne

Acne may be non-inflammatory or inflammatory. Non-inflammatory lesions are primarily comedones, commonly called pimples, whiteheads (closed comedones) and blackheads (open comedones). The colour is the result of the movement of melanin into the plug from surrounding epidermal cells. Inflammatory acne lesions include comedones, erythematous pustules and cysts. Inflammation close to the skin surface results in pustules; deeper inflammation results in cysts. The inflammation is believed to result from irritation from fatty acid constituents of the sebum and from substances produced by *Propionibacterium acnes* bacteria, which escape into the dermis when closed comedones rupture.

The most common forms of acne are acne vulgaris, acne rosacea and acne conglobata.

Acne vulgaris

Acne vulgaris is common in adolescents and young to middle adults. The cause of acne vulgaris is unknown, but possible causes include androgenic influence on the sebaceous glands, increased sebum production and proliferation of the organism *Propionibacterium acnes*. High-fat diets, chocolate, infections and cosmetics do not cause acne vulgaris.

Mild cases may involve only a few scattered comedones; severe cases are manifested by multiple lesions of all types. Most lesions form on the face and neck, but they also occur on the back, chest and shoulders. Women in their 30s and 40s, often with no prior acne, may develop papular lesions on the chin and around the mouth, and these are usually mildly painful and itchy. Complications of acne vulgaris, especially in severe cases, are formation of cysts, pigment changes in persons with dark skin, severe scarring and lowered self-esteem from the skin eruptions.

Acne rosacea

Acne rosacea is a chronic type of facial acne occurring more often in middle and older adults – cause unknown. Lesions begin with erythema over cheeks and nose. Over the years, skin colour changes to dark red, and pores over the area become enlarged. The soft tissue of the nose may exhibit rhinophyma, an irregular bullous thickening.

Acne conglobata

Acne conglobata is a chronic type of acne, cause unknown, beginning in middle adulthood. This type causes serious skin lesions. Comedones, papules, pustules, nodules, cysts and scars occur primarily on the back, buttocks and chest and may occur elsewhere. The comedones have multiple openings and a discharge that ranges from serous to purulent with a foul odour.

The person with pemphigus vulgaris

Pemphigus vulgaris is a chronic disorder of the skin and oral mucous membranes characterised by blister formation which can be serious. It is caused by autoantibodies that cause acantholysis (the separation of epidermal cells from one another). Septicaemia from an infection of *Staphylococcus aureus* is the most common cause of death. It occurs in middle and older adults and is associated with other autoimmune disorders and with the administration of certain drugs, such as antirheumatic drugs and angiotensin-converting enzyme inhibitors.

The blisters usually appear first in the mouth and scalp, spreading in crops or waves (new groups) to involve large areas of the body. Blisters in the mouth ulcerate. The blisters form in the epidermis and cause the epidermal cells to separate above the basal layer; they rupture, leaving denuded skin, crusting, and oozing of fluid with a musty odour; lesions are painful. Pressure on a blister causes it to spread to adjacent skin and exfoliate (Nikolsky's sign). The loss of fluid from the blisters may result in fluid and electrolyte imbalances. Secondary bacterial infections are a serious risk.

The person with lichen planus

Lichen planus is an inflammatory disorder of the mucous membranes and skin. There is no known cause, but it is associated with exposure to some drugs and chemicals and affects those aged 30 to 70 years.

Lesions first appear as violet papules, 2–10 mm in size, occurring on the wrists, ankles, lower legs and genitals, and itching intensely. Persistent lesions thicken becoming dark red and forming hypertrophic lichen planus. Lesions on the oral mucous membranes appear as white lacy rings; lesions may also appear on the mucous membranes of the vagina and the penis. Nails become thin and may shed.

Lichen planus lesions are self-limiting, lasting for an average of 12–18 months. Diagnosis is based on clinical manifestations. Corticosteroids can control the inflammation, and antihistamines help control the pruritus.

Case Study 3 – Simon
NURSING CARE PLAN Contact dermatitis

Simon, aged 20, attended the walk-in centre as a rash has developed on his hands, spreading to his abdomen and back. We now consider his care in the community.

Assessment

The advanced nurse practitioner noticed Simon had a red, itchy, scaly rash on both hands. During the consultation it was noted:

+ Simon had admitted to being obsessive about hand washing.
+ He had recently bought a new type of hand wash.
+ He was so uncomfortable, he was losing sleep and was distracted from studying.
+ His skin was painful.
+ He had tried using some of his partner's handcream.
+ He thinks the stress of studying is worsening the rash.

Case Study 3 – Simon

Diagnosis

A diagnosis of contact dermatitis was made after a full medical history, information gained about exposure to irritants and the effect on Simon's work and social life.

Medication

The advanced nurse practitioner prescribed:

+ antihistamines to reduce the itching and to aid sleep;
+ a barrier cream to protect the skin and retain moisture.

Nursing care

Dermatitis relies on an irritant or an allergen to initiate the reaction, it is important for the patient to identify the responsible agent and avoid it. Specific care included:

NURSING CARE PLAN   Contact dermatitis

+ to avoid the new hand wash;
+ to use the cream and antihistamines on a regular basis for one week;
+ to seek help from his personal tutor, student support and academic supervisor in relation to his university examinations;
+ to return if the problem did not improve over the next 7–14 days.

Evaluation

After Simon's consultation the nurse documented the meeting on the computer-held records.

MALIGNANT SKIN DISORDERS

The skin is a common site for malignant lesions. Many lesions are found on skin surfaces that have undergone long-term exposure to the sun or the environment. Malignant skin tumours are the most common of all cancers.

The person with actinic keratosis

Actinic keratosis, also called senile or solar keratosis, is an epidermal skin lesion directly related to chronic sun exposure and photodamage. Prevalence is highest in people with light-coloured skin; lesions are rare in people with dark skin. Actinic keratosis may progress to squamous cell carcinoma. Fewer than 1% of early lesions become malignant, but many of those that persist progress to malignancy (BAD 2010). The lesions are classified as premalignant.

Lesions are erythematous rough macules a few millimetres in diameter. They are often shiny but may be scaly; if scales are removed, underlying skin bleeds. They occur in multiple patches, primarily on the face, dorsa of the hands, the forearms and sometimes on the upper trunk. Enlargement or ulceration of the lesions suggests transformation to malignancy.

The person with non-melanoma skin cancer

Non-melanoma skin cancer is the most common malignant neoplasm found in fair-skinned, blue-eyed patients. Cancer Research UK estimates that around 100 000 new cases of non-melanoma skin cancer occur each year, and that the majority can be cured if detected and treated early (Cancer Research UK 2011). Men develop non-melanoma skin cancer more than women do, probably because of occupational exposures. Non-melanoma skin cancer can occur at any age, but the incidence increases with each decade of life. Adults aged 30–60 years have the majority of these cancers.

FAST FACTS

Risk factors for non-melanoma skin cancer

● Fair skin, freckles, blue or green eyes, blond or red hair.
● Family history of skin cancer – genetic dispostion or Gorlins syndrome (genetic disposition to nevoid basal cell carcinoma).
● Unprotected and/or excessive exposure to UV radiation (natural or artificial).
● Radiation treatment.
● Occupational exposures to coal, tar, pitch (resin), creosote, asphalt, arsenic compounds, petroleum derivatives or radium.
● Severe sunburns as a child.
● Lowered immunity due to medication.

Source: Macmillan Cancer Support 2009.

Pathophysiology of non-melanoma skin cancer

Basal cell cancer

Basal cell cancer is an epithelial tumour believed to originate either from the basal layer of the epidermis or from cells in the surrounding dermal structures. They are characterised by an impaired ability of the basal cells of the epidermis to mature into keratinocytes, with mitotic division beyond the basal layer, resulting in a bulky neoplasm that grows by direct expansion, destroying surrounding tissue, including healthy skin, nerves, blood vessels, lymphatic tissue, cartilage and bone. Basal cell cancer is the most common but least aggressive type of skin cancer, rarely spreading to other organs.

Basal cell cancers tend to recur. Tumours greater than 2 cm in diameter have a high recurrence rate. Predisposing factors for metastasis are the size of the tumour and the person's resistance to treatment with surgery or chemotherapy. Even though they rarely metastasise, untreated basal cell cancers invade surrounding tissue and may destroy body parts, such as the nose or eyelid.

Basal cell cancer is classified into different types: nodular, superficial, pigmented, morpheaform and keratotic.

Nodular basal cell cancer, the most common type of basal cell cancer, often appears on the face, neck and head. The tumour is made up of masses of cells resembling epidermal basal cells and grows in a bulky, nodular form from a lack of keratinisation, not progressing through the normal process to become stratum corneum. In early stages, the tumour is a papule similar to a smooth pimple. It is often pruritic, continuing to grow at a steady rate, doubling in size every 6–12 months. As the tumour grows, the epidermis thins, but it remains intact. The skin over the tumour is shiny, and either pearly white, pink or flesh-coloured. Telangiectasis may be visible over the area of the tumour. As the tumour increases in size, the centre or periphery may ulcerate, and the tumour develops well-circumscribed borders, bleeding easily from mild injury.

Superficial basal cell cancer, often on the trunk and extremities, is the second most common type of basal cell cancer. This tumour is a proliferating tissue attached to the undersurface of the epithelium. The tumour is a flat papule or plaque, often erythematous, with well-defined borders. It may ulcerate and be covered with crusts or shallow erosions.

Pigmented basal cell cancer, on the head, neck and face, is less common. This tumour concentrates melanin pigment in the centre of the basal cancer cells, giving it a dark brown, blue or black appearance. The border of the tumour is shiny and well defined.

Morpheaform basal cell cancer, the rarest form of basal cell cancer, usually develops on the head and neck. The tumour forms finger-like projections that extend in any direction along dermal tissue planes, resembling a flat ivory- or flesh-coloured scar.

Keratotic basal cell cancer (basosquamous) is found on the pre-auricular and post-auricular groove (in front of and behind the ear) containing basal cells and square-like-appearing cells that keratinise.

Squamous cell cancer

Squamous cell cancer is a malignant tumour of the squamous epithelium of the skin or mucous membranes, occurring most often on areas of skin exposed to ultraviolet rays and weather. Squamous cell cancer may also arise on skin that has been burned or has chronic inflammation. This is a more aggressive cancer than basal cell cancer, with a faster growth rate and a greater potential for metastasis if untreated.

Tumours arise when the keratinising cells of the squamous epithelium proliferate, producing a growth eventually filling the epidermis and invading the dermal tissue planes. Keratinisation of some cells is present, and the formation of keratin 'pearls' is common. The keratin formation diminishes as the tumour grows, and as it grows the tumour cells and rate of mitosis increase forming odd shapes.

Squamous cell cancer begins as a small, firm red nodule. The tumour may be crusted with keratin products. As it grows, it may ulcerate, bleed and become painful; it extends into the surrounding tissue becoming a nodule, and the surrounding area becomes indurated (hardened).

Invasive squamous cell cancer may arise from pre-existing skin lesions, such as scars and actinic keratosis, and extend into the dermis (called intraepidermal squamous cell cancer). This form appears as a slightly raised erythematous plaque with well-defined borders. Metastasis usually occurs via the lymphatics. The degree of risk for metastasis depends on the size and depth of penetration of the tumour.

The person with malignant melanoma

Malignant melanoma arises from melanocytes. This serious skin cancer is increasing in incidence each year. Melanoma in 2008 accounted for about 10% of skin cancers, but it causes about 79% of skin cancer deaths (ONS 2010).

Incidence of malignant melanoma

This disease is 10 times more common in fair-skinned people than in dark-skinned people. As with the non-melanoma skin cancers, an increase in the incidence of malignant melanoma is believed to be related to the thinning ozone layer and increased exposure to ultraviolet rays. Incidence is highest in Caucasian upper-middle-class professionals who work indoors. This group of people often had severe sunburn with blistering during childhood and often holiday in areas of intense sun exposure. Malignant melanoma is more common in people who live in sunny climates, burn easily and use tanning shops. However, malignant melanoma may arise from already present lesions or from skin normally covered with clothing.

Risk factors for malignant melanoma

The exact cause of melanoma is unknown, but certain risk factors are associated with the disease. The risk factors are a high number of moles or large moles, fair skin, freckling, blond hair and blue eyes, a close relative with the disease, men with genetic changes and coming from a family with a familial history of ovarian or breast cancer, treatment with medications that suppress the immune system, excessive exposure to UV radiations, women over 50, xerodermapigmentosus (a rare inherited disease in which people are less able to repair damage caused by sunlight), a past history of melanoma or lack of the use of sunscreen.

Pathophysiology of malignant melanoma

Malignant melanomas arise from melanocytes – cells located at or near the basal layer (the deepest epidermal layer), which produce melanin, the dark skin pigment. Melanin is made in granules and transferred to keratinocytes, where it accumulates on the exterior side of each keratinocyte forming a shield of pigment over the nucleus as protection against ultraviolet rays. Malignant melanomas can develop wherever there is pigment, and about one-third of them originate in existing moles.

Most malignant melanomas are more than 6 mm in diameter, asymmetric and initially develop within the epidermis over a long period. While they are still confined to the epidermis, the lesions (called malignant melanoma *in situ*) are flat and relatively benign. However, when they penetrate the dermis, they mingle with blood and lymph vessels and are able to metastasise at this stage. The tumours develop a raised or nodular appearance and often have smaller nodules, called satellite lesions, around the periphery.

Prognosis for survival with malignant melanoma is determined by several variables, including tumour thickness, ulceration, metastasis, site, age and gender. Younger people and women have a better chance of survival. Tumours on the hands, feet and scalp have a poorer prognosis; tumours of the feet and scalp are less visible and may not be diagnosed until they grow into the dermis.

Precursor lesions

Three specific precursor lesions for the development of malignant melanoma are congenital naevi, dysplastic naevi and lentigomaligna. A precursor lesion is also called a pre-malignant lesion, a name that indicates that the lesion's risk of becoming malignant is greater than normal.

Classification

Malignant melanomas are classified into different types. The major types are superficial spreading melanoma, lentigomaligna melanoma, nodular melanoma and acrallentiginous melanoma, each characterised by a radial and/or vertical growth phase. During the initial radial phase, which may last from 1–25 years (depending on the type), the melanoma grows parallel to the skin surface. During this phase, the tumour rarely metastasises and is often curable by excision. However, during the vertical growth phase, atypical melanocytes rapidly penetrate into the dermis and subcutaneous tissue, greatly increasing the risk for metastasis and death. Figure 5.5 illustrates Clark's levels for staging melanomas.

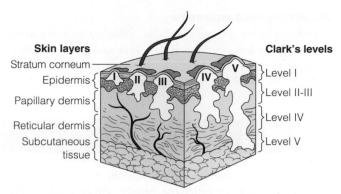

Figure 5.5 Clark's levels for staging measure the invasion of a melanoma from the epidermis to the subcutaneous tissue.

Superficial spreading melanoma

Superficial spreading melanoma is the most common type, comprising about 70% of all melanomas. Lesions are usually flat and scaly or crusty and about 2 cm in diameter. They often arise from a pre-existing naevus, found on the trunk and back of men and on the legs of women. Superficial spreading melanomas occur more often in women. The median age of occurrence is the 50s.

The radial growth phase lasts from one to five or more years. When the lesion enters the vertical growth phase, it grows rapidly and its colour changes from a mixture of tan, brown and black to a characteristic red, white and blue. The lesion develops irregular borders and often has raised nodules and ulcerations

Lentigomaligna melanoma

Lentigomaligna melanoma often arises from the precursor lesion, lentigomaligna. The lesions are large and tan with different shades of brown. This type makes up 4–10% of malignant melanomas and is the least serious form. It occurs on skin that has had long-term sun exposure. Lentigomaligna melanoma affects more women, typically diagnosed in those aged between 60 and 70 years. It is characterised by a proliferation of atypical melanocytes parallel to the basal layer of the epidermis; the radial growth phase may last from 10–25 years, with the lesion growing to as large as 10 cm. The lesion becomes malignant as soon as the melanocytes invade the dermis. In the vertical growth phase, raised nodules may appear on the surface of the lesion, and it tends to acquire a freckled or mottled appearance.

Nodular melanoma

Nodular melanoma lesions are raised, dome-shaped, blue-black or red nodules on areas of the head, neck and trunk. The lesions may look like a blood blister, and they may ulcerate and bleed. They arise from unaffected skin rather than from a pre-existing lesion. This type makes up 15–30% of malignant melanomas and is often diagnosed in people in their 50s.

Nodular melanoma has only a vertical growth phase, growing aggressively during that phase. The absence of a radial growth phase makes this type more difficult to diagnose before it metastasises.

Acrallentiginous melanoma

Acrallentiginous melanoma, also called mucocutaneous melanoma, is less common in fair skin and more common in dark skin. Lesions progress from tan, brown or black flat lesions to elevated nodules and are about 3 cm in diameter. The radial phase lasts from two to five years. They are found on the palms and soles, mucous membranes and nail beds. Acrallentiginous melanoma affects men and women equally, most often diagnosed in people in their 50s and 60s.

WOUNDS

A wound occurs when the skin or another external surface is torn, pierced, cut, or otherwise broken, either intentionally or through trauma, causing the loss of skin integrity. Other altered skin function causes are due to wounding of the skin; these types of skin damage include pressure ulcers, leg ulcers and surgical wounds. These types of wounds are classified according to depth and colour. Collier (2002) classifies these wounds into four main categories:

- *mechanical* – traumatic or surgical wounds;
- *chronic* – leg ulcers and pressure ulcers;
- *burns* – chemical or thermal;
- *malignant* – fungating wounds.

Wounds can also be classified as:

- *Superficial.* These involve only the epidermal layer of the skin.
- *Partial-thickness.* These involve the entire epidermis, extending into the dermis, but not through it.
- *Full-thickness.* These involve all layers of the skin, including the epidermis, the dermis and the epidermal appendages. The wound may extend into the subcutaneous fat, connective tissue, muscle, and bone or expose these body tissues and structures.

Some wounds are self-inflicted, and these are classified as factitious wounds.

This section of the chapter looks at wound healing in general before considering care for persons with minor injuries, surgical wounds and burns and moving on to chronic conditions such pressure and leg ulcers, finishing with a look at wound care options.

Wound healing

Wounds occur when the skin or another external surface, such as a mucous membrane, is torn, pierced, cut or otherwise broken, either intentionally or through trauma, causing the loss of skin integrity. The rate of wound healing is affected by the type of injury, the general health and wellbeing of the patient and the extent of damage to skin. Small superficial wounds heal quicker than wounds that are complex, deep, cover a larger surface area and when there is damage to underlying tissues. Regardless of wound type all pass through a complex sequence of events enabling full healing and scar formation to occur. The process of wound healing is continuous; cells biologically modify to assist in aiding haemostasis, inflammation, proliferation and maturation. The time for which these four stages last is affected by the amount of tissue loss. Wounds can heal by primary, secondary or tertiary intention (see Table 5.2 and Figure 5.6). Through understanding and then being able to recognise the wound healing process, nurses can make informed decisions in the care of a patient with a wound.

Primary intention

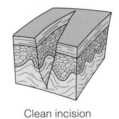

Clean incision   Early suture   'Hairline' scar

Secondary intention

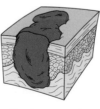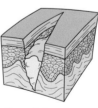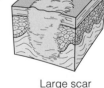

Gaping wound with blood clot   Granulation tissue fills in wound   Large scar

Tertiary intention

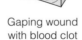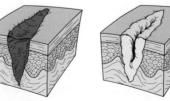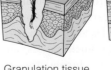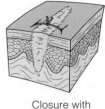

Contaminated wound   Granulation tissue   Closure with wide scar

Figure 5.6 Wound healing by primary, secondary and tertiary intention.

Table 5.2 Healing intention

Primary intention	Secondary intention	Tertiary intention
Primary intention wound healing occurs when there is no tissue loss, skin edges are brought together to be sutured, stapled or glued. These wounds are usually surgical or traumatic in nature.	With wound edges that are too far apart to be brought together, with a greater degree of tissue loss or undermining of deeper layers of the skin, the wound has to heal by secondary intention. The wound has to fill with granulation tissue (new connective tissue and tiny blood vessels) and contract to a scar which is 10% of the original deficit width. This takes longer to heal, with more scar tissue and has a higher risk of complications than primary intention.	Tertiary intention or delayed primary closure is when a wound is left open for four to five days before being closed with sutures, staples, glue or a skin graft. The purpose is to allow the wound to drain as it may be infected, oedematous or have excessive **exudate**.

The healing process

Wound healing is a normal biological process, responding to injury of the skin and its layers, whether the cause is mechanical, chemical or thermal. The process commences with a cascade of events which in a healthy adult results in skin repair (lasting days) and includes four main phases or stages: haemostasis, inflammation, proliferation and maturation.

Haemostasis

When the skin is damaged or injured, initial reaction at the site is bleeding, filling the wound with blood. Circulating platelets adhere to collagen that is exposed in the walls of the damaged vessels. They then flatten and release substances which activate proteins and factor XII (Hageman factor), making the platelets sticky. Fibrin, an elastic insoluble protein derived from fibrinogen, combines with the platelets and any red blood cells that are caught in the area, resulting in the formation of a blood clot and haemostasis (the process in which bleeding stops), protecting the circulatory system from blood loss, acting as a primary environment where cells that assist in wound healing can migrate. After the clot has formed, fibrinolysis takes place when plasmin cells start to break down the clot to allow further cells such as platelets and white blood cells to enter the wound area, allowing the next stage of wound healing to take place.

Inflammation

Platelets release growth factors – platelet-derived growth factors and epidermal growth factors – which are some of the essential proteins involved in wound healing, providing cell communication. Platelet-derived growth factor supports the inflammatory stage of wound healing, with formation of granulation tissue, ground substance (an amorphous gel-like substance) and collagen. Epidermal growth factor has a role in epithelialisation and granulation. Growth factors are chemoattractant (chemically attractive) signalling the migration of white blood cells such as neutrophils to the wound area. Monocytes and neutrophils are found at the wound in the first 24–72 hours of tissue injury. Their role is wound cleansing, removing bacteria, devitalised tissue and debris by phagocytosis and ensuring the wound is ready for the next phase. Other cytokines, such as tumour necrosing factor, interleukins (proteins and signalling molecules) and interferons, are stimulated at the wound bed due to pathogens, endotoxins, tissue degradation products and hypoxia. They regulate repair processes such as cell proliferation, migration, inflammation, synthesis and degradation. These processes can be synergistic, additive or inhibitory (stops the effects of cell activities).

During the inflammatory stage, the release of histamine and serotonin causes vasodilation and permeability of the blood vessels, allowing plasma to leak into the wound bed, which is rich in growth factors and promotes wound repair. Visually, this is often seen as erythema, heat, oedema and pain at the wound site and should not to be confused with infection.

IN PRACTICE

Diagnosing wound infection

- Signs and symptoms of local infection include increasing pain in the wound, erythema, oedema, heat of the periwound area, foul odour and purulent drainage. These are localised signs and symptoms of infection, not systemic signs of infection.

- In addition to the localised signs above, elevated white blood cell count and body temperature are signs of systemic infection, such as **cellulitis**, osteomyelitis and bacteraemia. When localised infection is present always assess for signs of systemic infection.

- It is necessary to obtain a wound swab, a piece of wound tissue or fluid to send for culture and sensitivity.

Neutrophils decay at the end of the acute inflammatory stage of wound healing and are phagocytosed by macrophages (once monocytes), which continue to perform autolytic debridement of the wound.

Proliferation

The formation of granulation tissue is the major distinctive feature of this phase of wound healing. This occurs through the secretion by macrophages of growth factors that aid the growth of new blood vessels (angiogenesis), cell migration and proliferation resulting in new tissue being created, which contains a matrix of fibrin, fibronectin, collagens, proteoglycans, glycosaminoglycans and other glycoproteins (proteins and carbohydrate protein complexes creating adherence to the wound surface). Oxygen from a good blood supply is essential during the proliferation stage as reduced oxygen concentration at the wound bed halts macrophage activity. Macrophages release fibroblast growth factors, essential for new blood vessel and granulation tissue production.

Endothelial cells that make up new blood vessels and fibroblasts also require wound exudate to stimulate cell activity. Fibroblasts supply the wound bed with collagen and ground substance which they have secreted, forming a temporary wound bed environment or extra cellular matrix for wound repair. The extracellular matrix is made up of proteins and polysaccharides, the two main proteins being fibrous (elastin and collagen) and adhesive (fibronectin and laminin). Their functions are to maintain tissue shape and to offer structural and metabolic support to other cells. New capillaries grow from small blood vessels at the wound edges, fusing to form loops, and these loops penetrate the extracellular matrix to enable the supply of oxygen and nutrients to the wound bed.

The appearance of the wound at this stage of wound healing is red and granular (resembling or consisting of small grains or particles) and is noted as granulation tissue. Macrophages and fibroblasts reduce in number and the wound contracts, usually occurring five to six days post-injury. Fibroblasts and myofibroblasts (muscle fibres) are thought to be responsible for wound contraction, using cellular mechanisms to bring the wound edges closer, by as much as 40–80% of the wound surface area. Basal cells normally attached to the dermis become less adhesive and leapfrog or travel in a train-like fashion horizontally across the extracellular matrix, only stopping when they meet another basal cell (contact inhibition).

Maturation

Collagen fibres are restructured during the maturation phase, as they become thicker and stronger, due to the extracellular matrix initial fibre network, a network of proteins which is made up of fibronectin, hyaluronic acid and proteoglycans, allowing for cell migration, cell growth and collagen deposition. Collagen is constantly being degraded and new fibres synthesised, and this remodelling can take months or even years. The wound's tensile strength (the strength a scar can withhold) increases and within three weeks 20% strength is restored. Final tensile strength of the scar tissue will only reach 70–80% of that of normal skin.

During maturation, cellular activity and blood supply decreases and the resultant final product of wound healing is scar formation. Scars tend to soften, flatten and fade. Abnormal scarring occurs if collagen is produced faster than it is destroyed and can lead to hypertrophic and keloid scarring.

Keloid scars are the consequence of excess growth of dense fibrous tissue occurring after wound healing. The scar develops further than the margins of the original wound site and commonly does not revert spontaneously, tending to recur after excision. Keloid scars are often found in patients aged 10–30 years from Afro-Caribbean, Polynesian or Chinese backgrounds.

Hypertrophic scars are distinguished by their red, itchy, raised fibrous wound that characteristically does not develop beyond the margins of the initial wound and may undergo partial spontaneous resolution. Hypertrophic scars are common after burns injuries or those involving the deep dermis.

Moist wound healing

Historically wounds were allowed to dry out to form a scab. It was believed this was the best method in which the skin would repair itself, the scab offering protection from the external environment. In 1962 George Winter undertook research on pigs, as their skin is considered similar in characteristics to human skin. He created superficial wounds on the backs of two groups of pigs; one experiment group whose wounds were covered in polymer and one control group whose wounds were left to dry out and scab over. Winter determined that those pigs covered in polymer healed nearly twice as quickly as those who were left to dry and scab over, demonstrating that the polythene kept the wound moist, supporting cell migration.

Many researchers were concerned that the polythene would increase infection in the wound as bacteria like to develop in a moist environment. However, these anxieties were dispelled when Hutchinson and Lawrence (1991) demonstrated that occlusive (air- and watertight) dressings had a lower infection rate. The advantages of a moist wound healing include:

- less pain at the wound bed as nerve endings are bathed in exudate;
- reduction in infections as host defences are more viable, there is less dry dead tissue to harbour bacteria and less risk of bacteria transferring via airborne dispersal;
- less injury to the wound bed on removal of dressings;
- clinical and cost-effective in surgical wounds, **chronic wounds** and burns wounds;
- assists in autolytic debridement.

There are many dressings available that provide a moist wound healing setting so that wounds have the optimal environment to progress and these will be explored on pages 175–176.

PRACTICE ALERT

Some caution should be observed with a moist wound environment, particularly in the management of ischaemic and neuroischaemic (reduced nerve and blood supply) foot ulcers and wounds infected with anaerobic bacteria. Work closely with diabetic foot clinic team members such as podiatry and tissue viability nurses for these types of patients, to enable evidence-based wound management.

Acute, chronic and palliative wounds

Wounds that result in restoration of anatomical and functional integrity from a healing process that is timely and without complication are considered **acute wounds**; these are new or relatively new in injury, occurring suddenly. Acute wounds include surgical incisions, traumatic injuries such as lacerations, bites, abrasions, burns and avulsions.

A chronic wound digresses from the normal order of repair in terms of length of time (may develop over time, lasting more than six weeks), appearance and reaction to management, or restoration of anatomical and functional effect. These wounds start as an acute wound and then get trapped in the inflammatory and proliferative stages of wound healing. Overproduction of matrix molecules, scavenging of growth factors and blocking of proliferation cells slow the wound healing process down. Factors inducing chronicity include repeated trauma, ischaemic reperfusion injury (refers to tissue damage caused when blood supply returns to the tissue after a period of reduced blood supply), bacterial contamination and foreign bodies, leading to full thickness tissue loss. Types of chronic wounds include pressure ulcers, leg ulcers, burns and dehisced (ruptured or burst open) surgical wounds.

A **palliative wound** is one that cannot be classified as acute or chronic and whose outcome of wound healing is considered both challenging and unattainable. Causes of these types of wound are complex or not resolvable; therefore, management is palliative, not curative. Common practices (moist wound healing and wound bed preparation) cannot be easily applied to the management of fungating wounds and therefore quality of life, symptom management and safeguarding of dignity and privacy take precedent. Types of palliative wounds are malignant lesions of the skin, epidermylosis bullosa (an inherited connective tissue disease causing blisters in the skin and mucosal membranes) and progressive arterial disease.

Consider this . . .

Consider the case studies in relation to the anatomical structures affected by their altered skin function and what stage of wound healing they might be at in relation to wound age and healing intention. How might this information affect choice of management and what information might you further need to assist in assessment?

Factors affecting skin breakdown and repair

Reduced oxygen supply and hypoxia

Wounds or lesions with a poor blood supply heal slowly and therefore if nutrients and oxygen take time to reach the wound bed, healing is delayed. Some areas, such as the face, have a rich blood supply; however, poorly supplied areas, such as the pretibial area of the leg or heel, take longer to heal and require minimum trauma to cause a large wound. Cell division does not occur where there are low oxygen levels; this can lead to macrophages not being able to destroy ingested material, and therefore not releasing factors to stimulate angiogenesis, and a lack of collagen linking. Patients who are bleeding heavily, are anaemic, have atherosclerosis, atheroma or respiratory conditions may have lower oxygen levels, and this may further compound factors. Hypoxia can also be caused by unrelieved pressure.

Dehydration

If a wound is left exposed to the air it will dry out and desiccation of the surface layers occurs with long-term results of pronounced tissue loss, scarring and delayed healing. Epithelial cells need a moist wound bed to migrate and divide across the wound. Systemic dehydration causes a decrease in the circulating blood volume and cell turgidity, which can increase the risk of damage from pressure and lack of oxygen to the skin or wound bed.

Excess exudate

Symmetry is required between a moist wound bed and removal of excess exudates. Exotoxins and cell debris in exudate delay wound healing by maintaining the inflammatory stage of wound healing.

Fall in body and wound temperature

Phagocytic and mitotic activity requires wound temperature to be above 28°C. When body temperature or wound temperature falls, natural homeostatic response is vasoconstriction of the blood vessels in the dermis and wound bed with delayed recovery for several hours once warming begins (Lock 1979). This can be caused through lack of adequate clothing prior to surgery or during hospitalisation, inappropriate removal of dressings for ward rounds and appointments.

Necrotic tissue, excess slough and foreign bodies

The presence of foreign bodies, excess slough and necrosis increases risk of infection and delays wound healing. It is important to remove these sources as soon as possible with minimal trauma to the wound bed.

PRACTICE ALERT

Patients with impaired blood supply and/or diabetes, who have necrotic tissue present, especially the feet and hands, must have further investigations and referral for vascular/diabetologist opinion before any debridement, as it may be safer to allow autolytic debridement to occur to reduce the risk of infection and osteomyelitis.

Haematoma

The development of a **haematoma** due to surgery or trauma can delay healing as it will provide a culture medium for micro-organisms, increase wound tension and act as a foreign body, preventing vascular link up in grafts and flaps.

Recurrent trauma

Mechanical forces such as pressure, shear, friction and careless removal of dressings can traumatise fragile skin or cause deterioration at the wound bed.

Malnutrition

Malnutrition is one of the major causes of skin breakdown and delayed wound healing, it lowers the ability of tissue to regenerate and is damaging to the immune response.

- Protein is required for collagen formation, to provide fuel for macrophages, lymphocytes and fibroblasts and to mediate the inflammatory response.
- Protein and nucleic synthesis requires zinc, and vitamin C is essential for collagen production.
- Glucose is essential for cell metabolism – the larger the wound the larger the energy consumption.
- Polyunsaturated fatty acids are fundamental to cell membrane structure and function. They produce eicosanoids which effect cellular defence, inflammatory response and vascular tone.

Immunosuppression

Immunosuppression by cortisol is an essential part of the body's response to injury. Diabetes, chronic infection and immune disorders delay wound healing because of the reduced efficiency of the immune system – catabolism and depletion of the protein pool occur.

Age

Over the age of 30 years, a significant decline in body system function occurs and therefore affects skin breakdown and wound healing. Skin also ages with time, and reactions such as inflammatory response to injury, sensory perception, epidermal replacement rate, mechanical protection barrier functions are affected.

Psychosocial factors

Patients who are less anxious are physiologically more able to deal with pathological disturbances and have a more effective immune system.

Medication

Medications can affect skin breakdown and repair. Cytotoxic drugs, radiotherapy and steroids can affect wound activities such as cell proliferation and neutropaenia, suppress multiplication of fibroblasts, collagen synthesis and capillary budding, retard wound healing and cause long-term damage.

Inappropriate management

Neglecting to identify the cause of altered skin function or local problems at the lesion or wound site, inappropriate preparations and cleansing agents are avoidable causes of skin breakdown and delayed wound healing.

Immobility

Immobility is a significant factor in the development and non-healing of some lesions and wounds. Immobility reduces blood flow due to stasis oedema and the delay in the removal of waste products.

Sleeping

During sleep the body enters a state of anabolism, promoting the secretion of somatrophin, testosterone and prolactin which repairs cells and wounds. Lack of sleep causes the body to remains in a catabolic state, releasing hormones such as catecholamine and cortisol which stimulate tissue degradation.

Elimination

Maceration, moisture lesions, excoriation and infection can occur due to problems with elimination of urine, faeces, gastric contents and exudate, soiling dressings or contaminating wounds and the skin.

Personal cleansing and dressing

Wound infection risks increase if poor standards of hygiene are not addressed.

Education

Patient involvement and education in management of altered skin function can improve outcomes and healing rates.

Age of the wound

Chronic long-term altered skin function takes longer to heal. Proteases can have a damaging effect on growth factors causing delays in healing.

Smoking

Nicotine and carbon monoxide inhaled during smoking reduce oxygen content. Peripheral blood flow is reduced by 50% for up to one hour after smoking. Smoking inhibits epithelialisation and in scarring.

Genetic disorders

If one component is missing from the sequence of events that repair and heal the skin, then altered skin function and wound healing can be impaired. This can include hereditary disorders such as clotting disorders, namely Christmas disease and haemophilia, chronic granulomatous, a defective bone marrow disorder affecting the functioning of neutrophils, and thrombocytopaenia, a condition that decreases the number of platelets.

Jaundice

Jaundice caused by a malignant disease increases wound **dehiscence**. Vitamin K and antibiotic prophylaxis is recommended for this group of patients.

Malignancy

The link between malignancy and altered skin function and healing is reduced nutritional status, caused by altered eating habits, altered taste and diminished appetite.

Type of lesion

Certain types of wounds and lesions do not heal, for example malignant lesions and wounds. Whereas in a healthy wound healing occurs in a timely manner, lesions and wounds with a multifaceted underlying pathology take longer to heal.

Shape of lesion

Deep and irregular-shaped wounds and lesions are left to heal by secondary intention and take longer to heal than healing by primary closure.

Extent of damage

The larger the wound and the greater extent of damage the longer the wound will take to heal.

Poor surgical technique

This includes rough handling of tissues, excessive use of diathermy and leaving too much dead space between the wound margins which can lead to haematoma formation, infection and wound dehiscence.

Tissue at the wound bed

Recognition of tissue at the wound bed assists the practitioner in being able to ascertain how quickly a wound will heal. Bone, parenchymal cells (liver) and epithelium heal well, but cartilage heals more slowly.

The colour of the tissue at the wound bed affects wound healing rates. The colour of tissue is defined as black – necrotic tissue, green / yellow – sloughy tissue, red – granulation tissue and pink – epithelial tissue. The colour of tissue will also determine the dressing choice.

Infection

The skin is host to a multitude of bacteria. Contamination of a wound is usually due to the bacteria living on the skin and also because the body's immune response is weak. Infection affects skin function and healing because abscesses may form. It increases the demand in the inflammatory response and detracts from the action of cells at the wound bed, discourages fibroblast activity and encourages lysosome activity, weakening collagen and wound strength, and infecting organisms take vital oxygen and nutrients from cells of the skin.

The person with a minor injury

Minor injuries to the skin made up approximately 1.5 million visits to accident and emergency units across England in 2009/10 (NHS Information Centre 2011). These types of wounds frequently heal by primary intention devoid of difficulties or incident. In A&E, minor wounds are prioritorised on the basis of the severity of injury and clinical urgency, with consideration given to description of the wound, mechanism of injury, tetanus status, current medication and allergies and first aid measures used prior to hospitalisation.

Classification of minor injuries

Types of wounds often seen in A/E include the following.

- *A cut* is a break in the skin usually caused by a sharp instrument. On assessment the break in the skin is usually straight with well-defined edges and with little bruising of the soft tissue. These wounds are usually repaired with sutures, steri-strips or tissue adhesive (glue for skin) depending on location.

- *Lacerations* are caused by blunt appliances or force causing a break or split in the natural skin integrity over a bony prominence. Lacerations usually follow falls, crushing injuries or blows to the skin. They have irregular wound edges, take longer to heal and often heal by secondary intention.

- *Skin tears* are types of lacerations occurring in the older person due to the fragility of the skin from ageing, medication or altered skin function. The main cause is shearing and friction forces to the skin which separate the epidermis from the dermis or dermis from the subcutaneous layers. These wounds take longer to heal due to altered vascular supply and also further skin stripping as the surrounding skin may be equally as friable and fragile as the wound bed.

- *Abrasions* are caused by friction and shear between a blunt item and the skin, for example falling on gravel and developing an abrasion to the skin over the patella. Abrasions often dry out, form a scab and heal without scarring. Care must be taken not to leave gravel in a wound as this may cause permanent tattooing of the skin.

- *Contusions / bruises* occur after trauma to the skin, causing bleeding into the tissue spaces. Bruises can be scored on a scale of 0–5, 0 being a light bruise with little damage and 5 being a critical bruise with risk of death, for example bleeding into the brain or compartment syndrome of muscle tissue (bleeding into the muscle compartment, leading to muscle and tissue death). In a simple bruise the fluid constituent is reabsorbed. It is important with bruises to exclude gripping injuries that can cause wheals or discrete bruises from physical abuse or bruising from an underlying medical condition such as platelet or coagulation problems, leukaemia or meningococcal infection.

- *Bites* can lead to heavily contaminated wounds with debris. Prior to assessing a bite wound it is important to determine the basis of the bite – human or animal – allowing assessment of the type of toxins and bacteria that might be present in the wound. Often bite wounds heal through tertiary wound healing.

- *Avulsions* of the skin occur where the skin has been pulled off from an abrasion injury, with or without bone. These include fingers with rings caught on a fixed object when the ring pulls the skin off, fingers caught in doors and hands and fingers caught in machinery. Often these injuries require plastic surgery.

Some of these are illustrated in Figure 5.7.

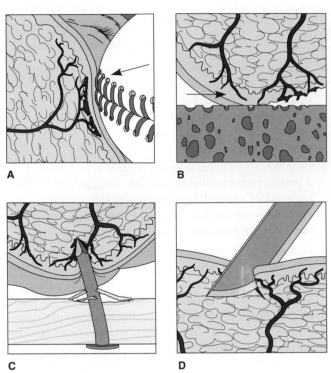

A

B

C

D

Figure 5.7 Traumatic injuries to the skin include (A) contusion; (B) abrasion; (C) puncture wound; (D) laceration.

The person with a surgical wound

In order to perform a surgical procedure it is often necessary to make a deliberate breach of skin integrity, directly where access to the underlying structures is needed. Over 2 270 000 operations occurred in 2004/5 and most healed with minimal skin loss by primary intention. However, surgical site infections account for 15% of all hospital-acquired infections, not only doubling the length of stay in hospital for a person but also increasing mortality (Health Protection Agency 2009). Surgical wound infections range from a simple wound discharge to a life-threatening post-operative complication.

A surgical wound can be described as an intentional break in the skin as a result of surgery. Many factors can affect the healing of a surgical wound, including the person's age, body size, nutritional status, underlying medical conditions and also skin preparation, body temperature during the operation, surgical technique and materials used when cleansing and closing the wound. In many hospitals, skin care bundles (evidence-based practices) are used to ensure staff minimise the risk of surgical site infections by ensuring best practice.

Classification of surgical wounds

Surgical wounds are audited and classified post-operatively as:

- Clean: an incision in which no inflammation is encountered in a surgical procedure, without a break in sterile technique, and during which the respiratory tract, alimentary or genitourinary tracts are not entered.

- Clean-contaminated: an incision through which the respiratory, alimentary or genitourinary tract is entered under controlled conditions but with no contamination encountered.

- Contaminated: an incision in which there is a major break in sterile technique, or gross spillage from the gastrointestinal tract, or an incision in which acute, non-purulent inflammation is encountered, as well as open traumatic wounds that are more than 12–24 hours old.

- Dirty or infected: an incision in which the viscera (internal organs) are perforated or when acute inflammation with pus is encountered (for example, emergency surgery for faecal peritonitis), and for traumatic wounds where treatment is delayed, there is faecal contamination, or devitalised tissue is present. (NICE 2008, 9)

> **Consider this . . .**
>
> Hair removal at the surgical site is not considered routine practice. If hair removal is necessary, use electric clippers with a single head on the day of surgery only. Do not use razors as this increases the risk of surgical site infection.

Wound closure

Wound closure material choice is based upon patient history, type of surgery, severity of the incision and personal choice. Materials often used include sutures, staples, adhesive skin closures strips and tissue adhesive.

- *Sutures* are either naturally or synthetically made and are passed through both sides of the wound and then securely tied with a knot. They can be non-dissolvable or dissolvable. Sutures maintain scar formation by reducing mobility of the wound, providing strength, preventing the wound edges from moving and causing irritation, and they also minimise scarring. Sutures are often removed 5–10 days post-operatively.

- *Staples* are titanium strips of metal used in conjunction with a staple gun allowing the joining of tissue edges with little tissue destruction and a patent scar. The benefits of staples over sutures are reduced rates of infection and faster recovery times. Staples are removed with a staple remover.

- *Tissue adhesive* is a glue used to bring wound edges together, often used in A&E departments with little pain on closure of the wound edges, reducing bruising, oedema and bleeding. Tissue adhesive is used in head trauma and in children, but is not used where a wound has occurred over a joint.

- *Adhesive skin closure strips* or butterfly sutures are used to bring wound edges together in superficial small wounds or after suture/staple removal for extra scar site support. Space must be left between each strip to allow exudate drainage.

Wound complications

- *Dehiscence* (Figure 5.8A) is when the opposite edges of a surgical wound open spontaneously, possible causes include surgical technique, inadequate number or knotting of sutures, haematoma formation, infection, age, diabetes and trauma to the wound post-surgery. Many patients will return to theatre for resuturing of their wound; others may have insertion of supporting Teflon grafts and have the wound heal by secondary or tertiary intention.

- *Evisceration* (Figure 5.8B) is when wound dehiscence occurs and internal organs such as the gastrointestinal tract protrude through the opening. This can be quite a frightening experience for both patients and staff, but a calm nurse who can organise pain management, medical assistance and maintaining the viscera moist and in position with a sterile moist towel is essential. Lie the person down and elevate the foot of the bed by 20 degrees. Keep the individual nil by mouth as a return to theatre is necessary. Regularly observe vital signs for the presence of shock. Thirty per cent of viscerated wounds will herniate once healed. A Teflon graft may be inserted underneath the subcutaneous layers at a later date.

- A *sinus* is an epithelial cell-lined, blind-ended tube leading from the outside of the body to the inside forming a cavity or bursa. Three mechanisms that can cause a sinus include an underlying infection, liquefaction (breakdown) of dead tissue or a foreign body (hair, splinters, glass). Significant factors that increase a patient's susceptibility to sinus formation are: sedentary lifestyle or job, previous abscess formation (there is a high rate of recurrence), previous surgery at the site (there may be retained material), recent blunt trauma causing haematomas and recent immobility. Assessment of the sinus includes extent, direction and duration of the sinus and then, if the sinus persists after

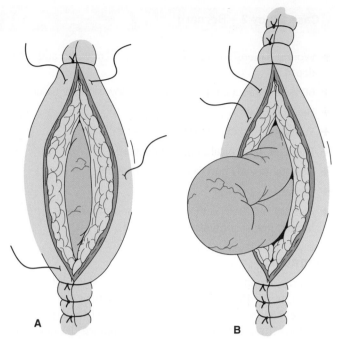

Figure 5.8 Wound complications. **(A)** Dehiscence is a disruption in the incision resulting in a separation of the layers of the wound. **(B)** Evisceration is a protrusion of a body organ through a surgical incision.

conservative treatment, referral for underlying cause and surgical removal and healing by primary or secondary intention.

- A *fistula* is the formation of a passage between two organs of the body; for example, a common fistula is an enterocutaneous fistula between the bowel and the skin. In this instance, the output from the fistula can be bile, digestive contents, faeces and blood; however, this will vary dependent on where the fistula occurs (biliary, recto-vaginal). Fistulae can occur post-operatively or of their own accord, may be single or multiple tract. Causative factors can include malignancy, inflammatory bowel disease or unknown, and treatment will depend upon the cause.

Case Study 2 – Bernard
NURSING CARE PLAN Surgical wound

Return now to Case Study 2 at the beginning of the chapter, Bernard is 64, admitted as an emergency with a ruptured colon due to untreated diverticulitis, formation of a colostomy in theatre occurred and prophylactic antibiotics given. Returning to the ward his wound dehisced (broke down) and he went back to theatre for insertion of a Teflon graft. The rest of his wound was left to heal by secondary intention.

Let us now consider his nursing care.

Assessment

Bernard is five days post-operative and his wound dressings are leaking profusely and are being changed every four to six hours. His surrounding skin is becoming sore and he is feeling very low in mood. His wife is worried he is becoming withdrawn. During the assessment the surgical nurse notes the following:

✚ Wound dimensions 22 cm length, 17.5 cm width and 4 cm depth.

✚ 60% red granulating tissue, 40% yellow sloughy tissue.

✚ Heavy exudate.

✚ Surrounding skin red and excoriated.

✚ There are no clinical signs of infection.

✚ Hospital Anxiety and Depression Score 11.

✚ Bernard is apyrexial.

✚ Bernard is scared to move around and mobilise as he feels his abdominal contents will 'pop' out.

Diagnosis

Bernard's wound is in the inflammatory stage of wound healing, but requires a dressing that will manage the exudates and allow Bernard to mobilise and not require dressing changes so often. The dressing will also need to reduce the odour as, even though the wound does not smell to others, Bernard can smell the wound all the time.

Nursing care

The nurse uses a wound manager or fistula bag to manage Bernard's wound. This includes:

✚ Preparation of the surrounding skin with a skin protectant.

✚ Application of the wound manager.

✚ Recording the wound assessment at each dressing change.

✚ Monitoring of vital signs to observe for signs of infection.

✚ Referral to the dietician for nutritional support.

✚ Discussion with the consultant regarding an abdominal support so that Bernard feels comfortable and supported when mobilising. A hole will be made to allow for the stoma.

✚ Referral to the physiotherapist for exercise.

Evaluation

At the end of the shift the nurse notes that Bernard seems happier in mood. He has asked for something to eat and he has walked to and from the bathroom with the aid of a nurse.

The person with a burn or a scald

Each year in the United Kingdom 250 000 people experience a burn injury (DoH 2010a). The severity of a burn is dependent on two factors: contact and duration of exposure to the causative factor. Most burns are accidental in nature and two groups of individuals are more at risk of burn injuries: the elderly and children. However, adults with epilepsy, neurological or cardiovascular conditions and those who are obese are similarly at risk.

> **Consider this . . .**
> What physiological changes are occurring in both the elderly and the child to make them more at risk of burns and scalds?

Types of burns

● *Thermal burns* are the most common cause of burn injuries and are often caused by fire, combustible products, fireworks and exposure to excessive heat, cold, steam, hot liquids or surfaces. They result in charring of vascular, bony, muscle and nervous tissue.

● *Electrical burns* are often difficult to find externally on the skin, but frequently the damage is internal, due to the high voltage of electricity that has passed through the body, known as the path of least resistance, which in the human body tends to lie along muscles, bone, blood vessels and nerves. Entry and exit wounds tend to be small, masking widespread tissue damage underneath. Tissue necrosis results from impaired blood flow, secondary to blood coagulation at the site of the electrical injury. Because electrical burn wounds of the extremities often cause severe tissue necrosis, they frequently develop gangrene that necessitates amputation. Those who have suffered an electrical burn should be cardiac monitored.

● *Chemical burns* occur when corrosive substances, acids or alkalis, have had direct contact with the skin or have been inhaled. Vital organs can easily become damaged if the chemical is absorbed into the bloodstream. Burns caused by alkalis are more difficult to neutralise than those caused by acids.

The severity of the chemical burn is related to type of agent, the concentration of the agent, mechanism of action, duration of contact and amount of body surface area exposed.

● *Radiation burns* are most commonly known as sunburn, but patients undergoing radiotherapy can often experience radiation burns. These burns tend to be superficial, involving only the outermost layers of the epidermis. All functions of the skin remain intact. Symptoms are limited to mild systemic reactions: headache, chills, local discomfort, nausea and vomiting.

Classification of burns

Burns are frequently classified in accordance with the depth of tissue damage, for example superficial, partial thickness or full thickness.

- A *superficial burn* involves only the epidermis. This type of burn most often results from damage from sunburn, ultraviolet light, minor flash injury (from a sudden ignition or explosion), or mild radiation burn associated with cancer treatment. Because the skin remains intact, this degree of burn is not calculated into the estimates of burn injury. Skin colour ranges from pink to bright red, with slight oedema over the burned area. Superficial burns involving large body surface areas may be manifested by chills, headache, nausea and vomiting. The injury usually heals in three to six days, with dryness and peeling of the outer layer of skin. There is no scar formation. Superficial burns are treated with mild analgesics and the application of water-soluble lotions. Extensive superficial burns, especially in older adults, may require intravenous fluid treatment.

- *Partial-thickness burns* may be subdivided into superficial partial-thickness and deep partial-thickness burns, classification depending on the depth of the burn.

- A *superficial partial-thickness burn* involves the entire dermis and the papillae of the dermis. Causes may include such injuries as brief exposure to a flash flame or dilute chemical agents, or contact with a hot surface. This burn is often bright red, with a moist, glistening appearance with blister formation. The burned area will blanch on pressure, and touch and pain sensation remain intact. Pain in response to temperature and air is usually severe. These injuries heal within 21 days with minimal or no scarring, but pigment changes are common. Analgesics are administered and, if large blistered areas are disrupted, skin substitutes may be used.

- A *deep partial-thickness burn* involves the entire dermis, extending further into the dermis than a superficial partial-thickness burn. Hair follicles, sebaceous glands and epidermal sweat glands remain intact. Hot liquids or solids, flash flame, direct flame, intense radiant energy or chemical agents may cause this level of wound. The surface of the wound appears pale and waxy and may be moist or dry. Large, easily ruptured blisters may occur, and the blisters may look like flat, dry tissue paper. Capillary refill is decreased, and sensation to deep pressure is present. The wound is less painful than a superficial partial-thickness burn, and areas of pain and areas of decreased sensation may be present. Deep partial-thickness burn wounds often require more than 21 days for healing and may convert to a full-thickness injury if necrosis extends the depth of the wound. Contractures are possible, as are hypertrophic scarring and functional impairment. Excision and grafting may be necessary to decrease scarring and loss of function.

- A *full-thickness burn* involves all layers of the skin, including the epidermis, the dermis and the epidermal appendages.

The burn wound may extend into the subcutaneous fat, connective tissue, muscle and bone. Full-thickness burns are caused by prolonged contact with flames, steam, chemicals or high-voltage electric current.

Depending on cause of injury, the burn wound may appear pale, waxy, yellow, brown, mottled, charred or non-blanching red. The wound surface is dry, leathery and firm to the touch. Thrombosed blood vessels may be visible under the surface of the wound. There is no sensation of pain or light touch, because pain and touch receptors have been destroyed. Full-thickness burns require skin grafting to heal.

Assessment of burns

Nursing assessment for a burns patient is continuous from the initial contact. Staff must act quickly to obtain the person's history of the burn injury, including time of injury, causative agents, early treatment, medical history, age and body weight. In most cases, the person is awake and oriented and able to provide information during the emergent phase of care. Changes in sensorium will become evident within the first few hours after a major burn; the nurse obtains as much information as possible immediately on the person's arrival.

Assessment of burns includes the Rule of Nines (Figure 5.9). In adult burns care, the body is divided into five surface areas – head, trunk, arms, legs and perineum – and percentages that equal or total a sum of nines are assigned to each body area. For example, a person with burns of the face, anterior right arm and anterior trunk has burn injury involving 27% of the total body surface area (TBSA) (in this example, face 4.5%, arm 4.5% and trunk 18% to total 27%). Only partial- and full-thickness burns are included in the estimation.

The Lund and Browder tool (Figure 5.10 on p. 167) is used in children. This determines surface area measurements for each body part according to age. These tools assist the nurse in determining the extent of damage. In A&E departments, guidance is available to enable decisions to be made on the management and treatment of those with burns. If in doubt, if a patient meets any of the following criteria once assessed (National Burn Care Review 2001) they should be transferred to a specialist burns centre:

- burns to the face, hands or feet;
- burns to a person aged 5 years and under or 60 years and over;
- burns that occur circumferential to a joint;
- chemical and electrical burns;
- inhalation injuries;
- more than 5% total body surface area in a child;
- more than 10% TBSA in an adult;
- any burn not healed in 14 days.

IN PRACTICE

Burn care

- Chemical burns require irrigation with sterile water or saline. If eyes are affected irrigation with 0.9% saline is recommended for 30 minutes, followed by application of an eye pad. The patient should be assessed by an ophthalmologist.

- Electrical burns can cause ventricular fibrillation and cardiac/respiratory arrest. It is important to know the voltage involved as this will aid with assessment and management.

- A patient can lose function if the burn affects an area such as the hands, feet, face or genitalia.

- Healing of a burn may be affected by co-morbidities.

- Check the patient's nostrils, eyebrows and facial hair. If there is loss of hair to these areas and soot is present the patient may have suffered an inhalation injury. This can have serious consequences; there may be heat damage to the respiratory tract, further complicating the burn injury.

- Mortality rates are higher in the elderly and very young burns patients.

- Post-traumatic stress, depression and reduced self-esteem are common mental health problems suffered by burns patients as a consequence of injury.

- Circumferential burns can lead to compartment syndrome in the limbs or depressed respiratory function. In these instances, escharotomy or fasciotomy may be performed to release pressure and prevent skin from splitting.

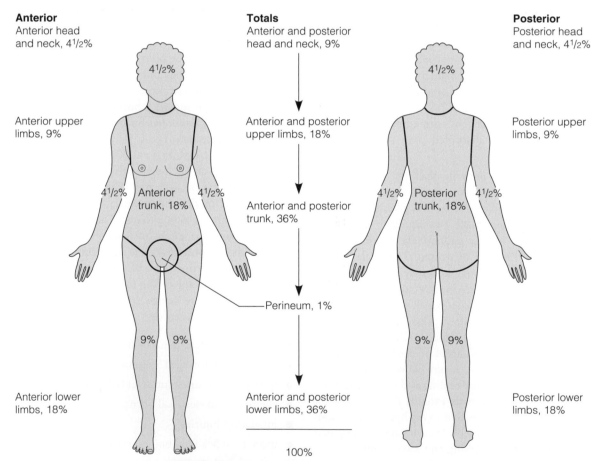

Figure 5.9 The 'rule of nines'. One method for quickly estimating the percentage of TBSA affected by a burn injury. Although useful in emergency care situations, the rule of nines is not accurate for estimating TBSA for adults who are short, obese or very thin.

Area	Age (years)					% 1°	% 2°	% 3°	% Total
	0–1	1–4	5–9	10–15	Adult				
Head	19	17	13	10	7				
Neck	2	2	2	2	2				
Ant. trunk	13	13	13	13	13				
Post. trunk	13	13	13	13	13				
R. buttock	$2\frac{1}{2}$	$2\frac{1}{2}$	$2\frac{1}{2}$	$2\frac{1}{2}$	$2\frac{1}{2}$				
L. buttock	$2\frac{1}{2}$	$2\frac{1}{2}$	$2\frac{1}{2}$	$2\frac{1}{2}$	$2\frac{1}{2}$				
Genitalia	1	1	1	1	1				
R.U. arm	4	4	4	4	4				
L.U. arm	4	4	4	4	4				
R.L. arm	3	3	3	3	3				
L.L. arm	3	3	3	3	3				
R. hand	$2\frac{1}{2}$	$2\frac{1}{2}$	$2\frac{1}{2}$	$2\frac{1}{2}$	$2\frac{1}{2}$				
L. hand	$2\frac{1}{2}$	$2\frac{1}{2}$	$2\frac{1}{2}$	$2\frac{1}{2}$	$2\frac{1}{2}$				
R. thigh	$5\frac{1}{2}$	$6\frac{1}{2}$	$8\frac{1}{2}$	$8\frac{1}{2}$	$9\frac{1}{2}$				
L. thigh	$5\frac{1}{2}$	$6\frac{1}{2}$	$8\frac{1}{2}$	$8\frac{1}{2}$	$9\frac{1}{2}$				
R. leg	5	5	$5\frac{1}{2}$	6	7				
L. leg	5	5	$5\frac{1}{2}$	6	7				
R. foot	$3\frac{1}{2}$	$3\frac{1}{2}$	$3\frac{1}{2}$	$3\frac{1}{2}$	$3\frac{1}{2}$				
L. foot	$3\frac{1}{2}$	$3\frac{1}{2}$	$3\frac{1}{2}$	$3\frac{1}{2}$	$3\frac{1}{2}$				
					Total				

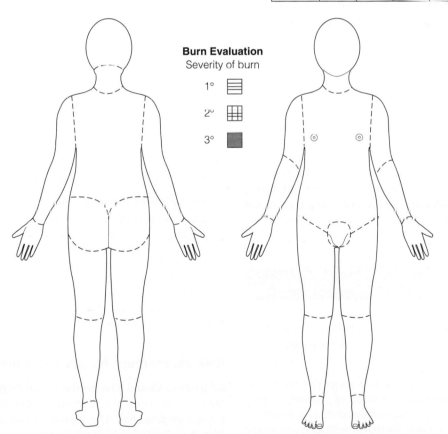

Burn Evaluation
Severity of burn

1°
2°
3°

Figure 5.10 The Lund and Browder burn assessment chart. This method of estimating TBSA affected by a burn injury is more accurate than the 'rule of nines' because it accounts for changes in body surface area across the lifespan.

COMMUNITY-BASED CARE

Understanding the causes of burns can help the nurse help others, particularly in the home care setting. Working with health visitors and other professional groups such as fire fighters can reduce the number of burns accidents. Burns are a commonly experienced injury in the UK. For instance, in 2008/09, burns caused over 87 000 emergency attendances and over 11 000 hospital episodes in England and Wales alone. Most cases are accidental, but small percentages are known to be self-inflicted or intentional forms of abuse. While any individual can experience a burn, certain people appear to be more at risk, including males, young children and older people and those living in deprived areas. While minor burns can be relatively easy to manage and quick to heal, the impacts of experiencing a severe burn can be problematic and even fatal. Physical impacts can include scarring, disability and restriction in motion. Adjusting to life following a burn can also be difficult, causing depression and anxiety, worries over appearance, sleep disruption and stress. For some, the injuries

sustained can hinder employment, requiring a change in job status.

The majority of burn injuries are preventable, and a number of strategies have been used to reduce the accidents that cause them, particularly among young children and the elderly. Community-based programmes have been devised to prevent the commonest accidents associated with burn injuries, such as home fires and contact with hot water and hot surfaces. Nurses working in residential care homes should make themselves aware of hazards that may put residents at risk of burn injuries as well as fire hazards. Safety education programmes provided in community settings, using a range of different strategies, can prevent burn injuries. Similarly, home fire risk checks combined with safety advice and the provision and installation of safety equipment can prevent fires, casualties and deaths.

Source: Wood *et al.* 2010.

Factitious wounds

Factitious wounds are caused through self-harm. Dermatology patients have the highest prevalence of factitious disorders, considered by Harth *et al.* (2010) as self-harming behaviours that directly or indirectly cause harm without link to suicidal intent. NICE (2004a) provides guidance for the management of patients with self-harm wounds, suggesting agents such as tissue adhesive, surgical assessment and exploration, depending on the depth and severity of the wound created. Patients who self-harm and are wounded require referrals that are timely and appropriate to ensure both the physical and mental health needs of the person who is self-harming are met (Ousey 2010).

The person with a pressure ulcer

According to the National Pressure Ulcer Advisory Panel and the European Pressure Ulcer Advisory Panel, a pressure ulcer is defined as:

> . . . localized injury to the skin and/or underlying tissue usually over a bony prominence, as a result of pressure, or pressure in combination with shear. A number of contributing or confounding factors are also associated with pressure ulcers; the significance of these factors is yet to be elucidated. (EPUAP and NPUAP 2009, 7)

Pressure ulcers in hospitals in the UK affect 10.2–10.3% of all in-patients with half being hospital acquired (Phillips and Buttery 2009). Not only do pressure ulcers represent a significant

cost to the NHS due to the cost of management and treatment, £1.4–2.1 billion per annum (Bennett *et al.* 2004), but they also cost patients in relation to their morbidity, mortality, sickness and quality of life.

The Office for Public Management on behalf of the NHS Institute for Improvement and Innovation (2010) explored current literature surrounding cost-effective methods of preventing pressure ulcers. The review team looked at the following four key areas:

1. introducing pressure ulcer prevention protocols;
2. use of pressure-relieving surfaces;
3. use of pressure ulcer risk assessments;
4. access to a specialist tissue viability nurse.

The introduction of pressure ulcer prevention protocols, the use of pressure-relieving surfaces and access to a specialist tissue viability nurse were found to be cost-effective ways of preventing pressure ulcers. However, no conclusions could be reached on the use of a pressure ulcer risk assessment in relation to cost-effectiveness.

Risk assessment for pressure ulcers

All patients should have an initial and ongoing assessment of their risk of developing pressure ulcers, by an appropriately trained professional. The choice of risk assessment tools – Waterlow, Braden or Norton – is based upon local policy guidance and should be relevant to the clinical setting, the clinical areas that should complete the assessment, the timing of the assessment/reassessment and documentation and communication of risk status. The assessment tool should be used alongside clinical judgement to identify risk status. However,

NICE (2005) recommend that pressure ulcer risk assessment should include exploration of the following risk factors:

- Current health status – does the person have an acute, chronic or terminal illness that may precipitate skin breakdown or affect pressure ulcer healing rates. For example diabetes, cardiovascular problems or malnutrition.
- What is the current mobility status of the person? Is the person able to change position, walk, move independently on a regular basis or is assistance required?
- What is the person's posture like? Does the person suffer from pelvic obliquity and posterior pelvic tilt (tilting and misalignment of the pelvis – this may show as one hip bone may be higher than the other)?
- Does the person suffer from any sensory impairment?
- Does the person have a reduced level of consciousness?
- Are there signs of a systemic infection?
- What is the person's current nutritional status?
- Are there any signs of previous pressure damage? Where is the site, location, category and previous interventions?
- Is the person currently experiencing any pain?
- Does the person suffer from any psychological issues – what are their mood, motivation and aptitude like?
- What is the person's socioeconomic status?
- What is their current continence status? Are they urinary, faecally or doubly incontinent? What is currently used to manage continence?
- Are they on any medication and what impact may this have on the skin?
- How is their cognitive status?
- What is the current blood flow to the skin like?

EPUAP and NPUAP (2009) also add body temperature of the patient, skin moisture and positioning of medical devices as risk factors, suggesting that skin inspection should also include looking for signs of oedema, induration and heat as warning signs for pressure ulcer development.

PRACTICE ALERT

Remember that in darkly pigmented skin these are not easily visible. Do not rub the skin at risk of pressure ulcer development, this may cause tissue destruction or rouse an inflammatory response.

The purpose of collecting these data and reviewing it on an ongoing basis is to ascertain the severity of skin damage, create a personal plan of care surrounding the skin integrity of the patient, initiate treatment, evaluate the intervention and consider any potential complications. This should be communicated to other members of the interdisciplinary team as necessary.

Causes of pressure ulcers

Pressure ulcers can be classified as either extrinsic or intrinsic.

Extrinsic causes

The three main extrinsic causes of pressure ulcers are pressure, shear and friction. These three mechanical causes affect the flow of blood to the skin over a bony prominence. This subsequently leads to lack of oxygen to the tissues and tissue death.

Pressure

Pressure damage occurs where the skin and underlying tissues are compressed between a hard surface and a bony prominence, either from a low pressure over a long period of time or a high pressure over a short period of time. Pressure obstructs normal blood flow, resulting in an absence of oxygen and nutrients and a buildup of toxins and carbon dioxide. Ischaemia causes cell death and the result is pressure damage. The depth and severity of damage to the skin and underlying tissues is difficult to assess, because the damage takes place at bone level and it may be several days before the extent of harm is exposed. Ulcers formed due to pressure are usually circular in shape and often have deep cavities.

The tolerance of the skin and underlying tissue to pressure depends on capillary closing pressures. Tissue tolerance is the ability of the skin and its underlying structures to endure the effects of pressure without adverse effects. Current thinking is that capillaries fill at 32 mmHg in healthy individuals, so if external pressure is more than this then blood flow will be obstructed and problems will occur. However, a review of the literature pertinent to capillary closing pressure by Lutz (2008) suggests that this does not take into account other factors, such as shear, moisture and time of compression, and underlying issues such as age, mobility, neurological damage and response to pain.

In a healthy individual, a person will move position in response to high pressures exerted on the skin; however, in a frail, elderly chronically ill person this ability is impaired and risk of damage is increased.

Shear

Shearing forces occur when a part of the body attempts to move, but the surface of the skin remains fixed and resists. Structures and blood vessels under the skin become distorted, stretched and compressed, whilst externally the skin puckers. Shearing occurs during moving and handling and repositioning or if the patient slides down the bed whilst in a sitting position. Pressure ulcers that are formed due to pressure and shear are usually tear drop shaped and have deep cavities.

Friction

Friction occurs as the skin's surface rubs across another surface, for example a shoe rubbing the heel or bedclothes rubbing the skin at the elbow. The result is an abrasion or blister over a bony prominence, increasing the risk of further damage. The skin is five times more susceptible to damage by friction if moist (Sciarra 2003).

Intrinsic causes

Intrinsic factors include mobility, age and general health and have been explored in more depth on page 159.

Classification of pressure ulcers

The classification of pressures ulcers has led to much debate and during 2009 there was a consensus decision made in relation to developing a common classification system. Within this was discussion around the words used to classify pressure ulcers such as grade, stage or category and also that pressure ulcers do not always progress from grade 1 to 4 or heal from grade 4 to 1. Therefore, across Europe the guidance suggests the following classifications should be used:

Category/Stage I: Non-blanchable erythema

Intact skin with non-blanchable redness of a localised area usually over a bony prominence. Darkly pigmented skin may not have visible blanching; colour may differ from the surrounding area. The area may be painful, firm, soft, warmer or cooler as compared to adjacent tissue. Category I may be difficult to detect in individuals with dark skin tones. May indicate 'at risk' persons.

Category/Stage II: Partial thickness

Partial thickness loss of dermis presenting as a shallow open ulcer with a red-pink wound bed, without slough. May also present as an intact or open/ruptured serum-filled or serosanginous filled blister. Presents as a shiny or dry shallow ulcer without slough or bruising*. This category should not be used to describe skin tears, tape burns, incontinence associated dermatitis, maceration or excoriation.

*Bruising indicates deep tissue injury.

Category/Stage III: Full thickness skin loss

Subcutaneous fat may be visible but bone, tendon or muscle are *not* exposed. Slough may be present but does not obscure the depth of tissue loss. *May* include undermining and tunnelling. The depth of a category/stage III pressure ulcer varies by anatomical location. The bridge of the nose, ear, occiput and malleolus do not have (adipose) subcutaneous tissue and category/stage III ulcers can be shallow. In contrast, areas of significant adiposity can develop extremely deep category/stage III pressure ulcers. Bone/tendon is not visible or directly palpable.

Category/Stage IV: Full thickness tissue loss

Full thickness tissue loss with exposed bone, tendon or muscle. Slough or eschar may be present. Often includes undermining and tunnelling. The depth of a category/stage IV pressure ulcer varies by anatomical location. The bridge of the nose, ear, occiput and malleolus do not have (adipose) subcutaneous tissue and these ulcers can be shallow. Category/stage IV ulcers can extend into muscle and/or supporting structures (for example, fascia, tendon or joint capsule) making osteomyelitis or osteitis likely to occur. Exposed bone/muscle is visible or directly palpable.

Additional Categories/Stages for the USA

Unstageable/Unclassified: Full thickness skin or tissue loss – depth unknown

Full thickness tissue loss in which actual depth of the ulcer is completely obscured by slough (yellow, tan, grey, green or brown) and/or eschar (tan, brown or black) in the wound bed. Until enough slough and/or eschar are removed to expose the base of the wound, the true depth cannot be determined; but it will be either a category/stage III or IV. Stable (dry, adherent, intact without erythema or fluctuance) eschar on the heels serves as 'the body's natural (biological) cover' and should not be removed.

Suspected Deep Tissue Injury – depth unknown

Purple or maroon localised area of discoloured intact skin or blood-filled blister due to damage of underlying soft tissue from pressure and/or *shear*. The area may be preceded by tissue that is painful, firm, mushy, boggy, warmer or cooler as compared to adjacent tissue. Deep tissue injury may be difficult to detect in individuals with dark skin tones. Evolution may include a thin blister over a dark wound bed. The wound may further evolve and become covered by thin eschar. Evolution may be rapid exposing additional layers of tissue even with optimal treatment (EPUAP and NPUAP 2009, 8–9).

Diagnostic issues

The National Patient Safety Agency (NPSA) (2009) found that of all the pressure ulcers reported to the national Reporting and Learning System (RLS), 13% were grade 1, 47% grade 2, 23% grade 3 and 17% were grade 4 (NPSA, 2009). NICE (2005) highlight that all pressure ulcers category 2 and above should be reported as a clinical incidence.

Care must be taken to distinguish between pressure ulcers and moisture lesions and reactive hyperaemia.

Assessment of the skin should be carried out by an appropriately trained member of staff.

Moisture lesions

Diagnosis of a pressure ulcer can be difficult, especially if this is in an area where moisture can cause problems, such as the anal cleft. In 2005 EPUAP published a position statement on the definition of a moisture lesion. The following should be taken into account when assessing whether a person has a moisture lesion:

- Is there moisture present and is the skin shiny and wet? Is the wet skin caused by incontinence?

- Is the moisture lesion over a bony prominence? Has shear and pressure been excluded as a causative factor? Is the lesion linear, in a cleft of skin or around the peri-anal area?

- Is the shape of the lesion diffuse, for example lots of spots in the area, irregular edging? Is the lesion a copy or kissing lesion and is a replica of the other cleft?

- Is the depth superficial, the lesion is red, not uniformly distributed and there is no necrosis?
- Is there maceration around the edges?
- Does the lesion improve with skin barrier products designed to manage incontinence issues?

If the answer is yes to all of these questions, then the ulcer is a moisture lesion and not a pressure ulcer.

Reactive hyperaemia

Reactive hyperaemia is the characteristically bright flush of the skin associated with the release of pressure as a direct response to incoming blood and is detected by applying light finger tip pressure to the area of discoloration for 10 seconds, release the pressure and if the area is white and returns to its original colour then the area has a good blood supply, the skin is healthy and this is reactive hyperaemia. If the skin does not react, remaining the same colour, then this demonstrates the development of a pressure ulcer and the need for care.

Prevention of pressure ulcers

Prevention is the key to pressure ulcer management and once a full skin and risk assessment is completed, the appropriate plan of care can be developed, implemented, regularly reassessed and evaluated. Management includes the use of support surfaces, turning charts, dressings, continence aids and referral to other members of the interdisciplinary team for advice and further management.

The person with a leg ulcer

According to the NHS CRD (1997) a leg ulcer is 'the loss of skin below the knee on the leg or foot, which takes more than 6 weeks to heal'. Leg ulcers will affect 1% of the population at some time in their lives (Callam 1992, p. 6).

Classification of leg ulcers

The main causative factors predisposing patients to leg ulceration are:

- venous hypertension;
- peripheral vascular disease;
- diabetes;
- rheumatoid arthritis and systemic vasculitis.

Venous hypertension

Venous hypertension occurs where there is impaired venous drainage due to damage to the veins in the valves from a deep vein thrombosis or sustained venous hypertension from pregnancy or obesity.

Between 60 and 80% of leg ulcers are venous in nature, occurring when the superficial, deep and perforator veins cease to work effectively, creating a backflow of blood. This leads to varicose veins and lipodermatosclerosis (woody induration or fibrosis of the skin and tissues), venous stasis and oedema. Immobility of calf muscle further compounds this, as usually when walking the calf muscle pump would aid venous return and prevent the backflow of blood into the tissues. There is usually pitting oedema, brown staining in the gaiter region of the leg, ankle flare (dilatation of superficial veins on the inside of the leg, near the ankle), heaviness, itchiness, pain and tenderness. Some patients have atrophie blanche (painful spots of white plaque on the skin).

Risk factors include family history, occupation where people stand for long periods, gender (more common in women than men), pregnancy, low-fibre diet, obesity, intravenous drug use, malnutrition and reduced mobility.

Peripheral vascular disease (PVD)

PVD impairs the arterial supply to the lower limb. It is a form of atheroma and atherosclerosis (hardening and narrowing of the arteries, due to the deposition of fat plaques). PVD affects 22% of people with leg ulceration and is common with people who are smokers, have a history or family history of cardiovascular disease, high alcohol intake, high cholesterol, sedentary lifestyle, are older than 50 years of age, male, diabetic, suffer with hypertension, an autoimmune disease or high homocystine levels (an amino acid linked with cardiovascular disease). PVD leads to a lack of nutrients and oxygen to the lower limb causing ischaemia and tissue death. Thrombosis and total occlusion of blood vessels can also occur with gangrene of the tissues and mummification of toes of the foot.

Symptoms of PVD include: intermittent claudication (means limping in Latin) and is caused by a cramping pain in the calf muscles, hips, thighs or buttocks on exercise triggered by an insufficient supply of oxygenated blood. Rest pain is pain experienced at night when the person attempts to lie flat in bed and is relieved when the legs are dangled out of bed or the person sleeps in a sitting position. There may be an absence of pulses in the foot, coldness and paleness of the leg and foot, a blue/red discoloration, fragile shiny skin and numbness or tingling in the leg, foot or toes. People usually have brittle toenails, ulcers that do not heal and worsen and sunset rubra (skin changes to a reddish colour on dependence).

> #### Consider this . . .
> Do not confuse pain in the lower leg with sciatica, deep vein thrombosis or muscle injury.

Diabetes

Approximately 5% of people with leg ulcer will have diabetes combined with a venous or arterial component.

Rheumatoid arthritis and systemic vasculitis

Around 9% of people with leg ulcer have rheumatoid arthritis. Ulcers may be venous, arterial or vasculitic. Table 5.3 illustrates the characteristics of arterial and venous leg ulcers.

Table 5.3 Indications for arterial and venous disease leg ulcers

	Arterial disease	Venous disease
Site	Common on the foot, can occur anywhere.	Medial malleolus and gaiter region.
Pain	Increased at night, with rest or when legs elevated.	Dull, aching and relieved by elevation.
Skin colour	Pale and hairless.	Brown staining, atrophie blanche and ankle flare.
Oedema	Often seen in dependent leg.	Reduces with elevation, increases through the day.
Toes	Poor capillary refill / cyanosed.	
Veins		Often distended, varicosities seen and spider veins.
Ulcer	Punched out, deep with extensive tissue loss.	Shallow, flat and high levels of exudates.
Eczema		Wet, dry or localised.
Pulses	ABPI ≤ 0.8	ABPI ≤ 0.9 – 1.2
History	Smoking, atherosclerosis.	DVT, phlebitis, varicose veins, surgery, multiple pregnancy.

Table 5.4 Differences in leg ulceration treatment options

Treatment options	Venous ulcer	Arterial ulcer
Dressing	Non-adhesive dressing and compression therapy	Dependent on whether for debridement via rehydration with hydrogels or autolytic debridement
Management of underlying condition	Medication or surgery – varicose veins, weight reduction	Medication, pain management, surgery such as angiogram, angioplasty, stents, bypass surgery or amputation, weight reduction, smoking cessation
Oedema	Exercise and elevation	Exercise and elevation only if tolerated
Skin care	50% white and liquid paraffin, avoid sensitisers, remove skin scales during washing	Keep hydrated
Limb elevation	To the level of the heart	Only if tolerated; patients with severe PVD will have leg dependency
Prevention of infection	Clean wound dressing technique, regular dressing changes	Aseptic technique, may require topical antiseptics, antimicrobials and antibiotics; this must be under the supervision of qualified staff

Assessment of a leg ulcer

Assessment of a leg ulcer should include a complete medical and nursing history, exploration of risk factors, the person's attitude to the ulceration, identification of signs and symptoms, swabs, urinalysis, blood sugar test, leg measurements (calf and ankle circumference) and a Doppler assessment (a hand-held ultrasonograph that determines the flow of blood in the arteries of the leg) to determine the ankle brachial pressure index (ABPI). Only when this diagnostic intervention is completed can appropriate treatment be planned. Table 5.4 illustrates the differences in leg ulcer treatment options for venous and arterial leg ulcers.

The person with diabetic foot

This is a foot with a collection of pathologic changes involving the lower extremity (foot) in diabetics which can lead to amputation and/or death due to complications. A non-healing skin ulcer is the major cause, and this can be aggravated and worsened by lack of sensation (neuropathy), increase in

FAST FACTS

Diabetic foot

- 2.6 million people in the UK have diabetes, and the incidence of diabetic foot ulcers is rising (Diabetes UK 2010).

- Diabetes accounts for the most common cause of lower limb amputations (NHS Scotland 2009).

- The rate of amputation is 15 times higher in persons with diabetes than in those without (Williams and Pickup 2004).

- 70% of diabetics live for only five years after having an amputation resulting from complications of their diabetes (Schofield et al. 2006).

- 100 patients a week lose a toe, foot or lower limb due to their diabetes (National Diabetes Support Team 2006).

pressure on the ulcer, deformities of the foot, ulcer infection and tissue necrosis.

A diabetic foot ulcer is a 'full-thickness lesion of the skin, i.e. a wound penetrating through the dermis; lesions such as blisters or skin mycosis (infection) are not included'. (International Working Group on the Diabetic Foot 2003).

People with diabetic foot ulcers may experience changes associated with neuropathy (disease or malfunction of the nerves) or ischaemia (depleted blood flow) or both. The most common cause is peripheral neuropathy, caused by excess of fructose and sorbitol, or linked to diminishing blood flow as a result of disease of the microcirculation (thrombosis, plaque formation and calcification). Nerves affected may be part of the autonomic, sensory or motor network, usually affecting both feet. Signs and symptoms can include:

- Loss of sensation, leading to damage to the skin of the foot. The patient may not feel heat or cold, their shoes rubbing, trauma when cutting toe nails.

- Dry skin caused by autonomic neuropathy reducing blood flow to the foot and in turn causing cracks, fissures and callus formation. These camouflage the true extent of damage to the foot.

- Infection and osteomyelitis are not always easily noticeable. However, some patients may have a gangrenous infected foot, mummified toes or a purulent discharge from the ulcer bed.

- Foot deformities such as Charcot's foot (a disease leading to destruction of joints and soft tissue), claw toes and prominent metatarsal heads, caused by motor neuropathy, altered gait and muscle atrophy.

Assessment and diagnosis of diabetic foot

People with diabetic foot ulcers will normally be assessed in a diabetic foot clinic, where a multidisciplinary team approach to care is provided. The cause of the ulcer is investigated as well as assessment of any underlying pathology, local wound problems, past medical history, current medications, tobacco and alcohol intake, glycaemic control, pain and social history.

The examination of the foot will be based on the Pedis system (International Working Group on the Diabetic Foot 2003) taking into consideration:

- **Perfusion**
- **Extent/size**
- **Depth/tissue loss**
- **Infection** and
- **Sensation**

Inspection provides a visual assessment of the foot, and include assessment of gait, mobility, posture, balance, reflexes, sensory function, foot pulses, Doppler (ABPI) and toe pressures (a monitor used to test systolic pressure levels in the toes). Other tests include vibration perception, using a tuning fork to test the protective pain sensation and a Semmes–Weinstein monofilament test touching various areas on the base of the foot to test for neuropathy.

Management of diabetic foot

Diabetic foot ulcer management requires a team approach ranging from education about good glycaemic control, to correct foot wear, including socks and stockings, foot screening, regular foot inspection and foot care, exercise and smoking cessation. Consideration has to be given to appropriate dressing choice for the ulcer, temporary casts to redistribute the pressure away from bony prominences, vascular surgery if necessary and regular reassessment.

Case Study 1 – John
NURSING CARE PLAN Pressure ulcer

John, aged 48, was admitted through A&E. On further examination, John is found to have a grade 4 pressure ulcer to his left trochanter (hip) which tracks to his perineum.

Assessment

John has a pressure ulcer from his left hip tracking to his perineum. The nurse practitioner contacts the surgical team for an opinion as he would like further advice concerning John's left hip bone and extent of damage.

During assessment the nurse notes that:

+ John's pressure ulcer risk status is very high.

+ The wound dimensions are 15 cm in length, 10 cm in width, depth is right through to the perineum.

+ The wound contains 100% green sloughy tissue, with exposed left hip bone which looks dry and stringy.

+ The exudate levels are high and green in colour.

+ There is an offensive odour.

+ The surrounding skin is excoriated.

+ John states his pain score is 8.

+ His wheelchair does not have any pressure-relieving cushion and he sleeps in a chair at home.

+ His body mass index is 18.5.

John is cannulated and prescribed fluids.

Diagnosis

John has a category 4 pressure ulcer and, due to the extent of tissue damage, he will require a full assessment, including investigations such as full blood count, urea and electrolytes and liver and bone function. Other tests will include:

+ x-ray of his left hip;

+ wound swabs or biopsy;

+ examination of wound under anaesthetic;

+ blood cultures.

Nursing care

The following management will be planned:

+ Dressings to the wound bed to control exudate, malodour, pain, the excoriated skin and infection. Cavity dressings that can be packed into the wound will be used with skin protectants and secondary dressings.

+ Pressure-relieving mattress that alternates underneath John, providing pressure relief and therapeutic management.

+ Total parenteral nutrition to increase nutritional intake until appetite returns.

+ A turning regimen, based on reactive hyperaemia response, that prevents further development of pressure ulcers on other parts of his body.

+ Regular observations of vital signs, four hourly monitoring for signs of infection.

+ Weekly weighting to ensure he is putting weight on.

+ Education of John and his wife regarding pressure relief, dietary intake and equipment.

+ Referral to other members of the interdisciplinary team to ensure a package of care and assessment.

+ Care pre- and post-operatively for examination of wound in theatre.

+ Documentation of care using nursing notes, wound care charts, turning charts, food diary and fluid balance charts.

+ Prescribing of analgesia and antibiotics.

+ Liaise with housekeeping for an air freshener machine to reduce the malodour.

Evaluation

At the end of the shift, the nurse evaluates the effectiveness of the care and continues all diagnoses and interventions. John underwent a 'hind quarter' operation (removal of whole of his left leg). Returning from theatre, his observations were stable and the wound drain contained 50 ml of old blood. He remained on a pressure-alternating mattress, turned between one and four hourly, and began to take sips of water.

INTERDISCIPLINARY CARE FOR ALTERED SKIN FUNCTION

Wound bed preparation

By definition, wound bed preparation is 'the management of a wound in order to accelerate endogenous healing or to facilitate the effectiveness of other therapeutic measures' (Falanga, 2001, p. 1). The intention is to produce an optimal wound-healing environment by creating a well-vascularised, constant wound bed with nominal exudate. The nurse needs to ensure that:

● The bacterial load of the wound does not interfere with the wound healing process and, if necessary, treat any infection with local or systemic therapy.

● Necrotic tissue is removed via a choice of debridement methods, noting some may take longer than others.

● Exudate is managed and the wound bed is neither too dry nor too wet.

● He/she understands the process of wound healing so as to determine if cellular processes or underlying pathologies are delaying wound healing, due to wound chronicity.

TIME

As stated earlier wound bed preparation removes local barriers which then facilitate healing and help determine efficient

wound management. The TIME principle (Schultz *et al.* 2003) is a systematic approach to the management of wound bed preparation, allowing the nurse to concentrate on each stage of wound healing, so barriers can be removed and healing of the wound facilitated. TIME theory is established upon intervention in four clinical areas, leading to an optimal well-vascularised wound bed. The acronym stands for:

● **T**issue non-viable or deficient, does the wound contain necrotic or sloughy tissue? Does this require debridement?

● **I**nfection or Inflammation, are there signs of infection, inflammation or increasing bacterial contamination? Does this require treatment?

● **M**oisture imbalance, is the wound too wet or dry, how should exudates be managed?

● **E**dge of the wound non-advancing or undermined, is the wound improving with epithelial cell migration or deteriorating with undermining?

Wound cleansing

This is the process in which foreign material, loose surface debris and previous dressings are removed from the wound bed (Dealey 2005); however, bacteria are just redistributed (Thomlinson 1987) and not removed from the surface of the wound as previously thought. The two preferred agents for cleansing of wounds are 0.9% sterile saline and water. In hospitals sterile saline is the preferred agent of choice, but this is based upon physiological arguments rather than conclusive evidence (Gannon 2007). The saline should be warmed, reducing thermal shock; when removing dressings and cleansing with room temperature or cold saline, wound temperature falls and hinders cell activity at the wound bed (Lock 1979). The pressure of the saline should be 8lb / inch squared (psi) so irrigation of the wound can occur. This is considered the safest and gentlest method, protecting wound environment.

In the community, patients may wish to have a shower or bathe and have wounds cleaned with water (Hollingworth and Kingston 1998).

Consider this . . .

Does the wound really need to be cleaned? Will wound cleansing cool the wound and remove vital cells, cytokines and growth factors?

Wound dressing selection

The main purposes of wound dressings are to produce speedy and cosmetically acceptable healing, remove or control odour, control exudate, reduce pain, cover the wound, manage infection and cause the minimum of distress (Thomas 1997).

Selection should be made taking into consideration a full wound assessment, detailed knowledge of the characteristics of the dressing, its uses, cautions and contraindications (some dressings are contraindicated, i.e. iodine-based products and patients with thyroid function problems, pregnancy or breast-feeding mothers), the evidence base, professional opinion, the person's choice, known allergies and medical history and cost. Manufacturers' guidelines on application, wear time and removal should be followed with each dressing used.

Products can be ordered via prescription in the community or through supplies in the hospital. Dressings are categorised by their properties and actions. Many hospitals and community services have wound care formularies, a guide for clinicians in the selection of advanced wound care products that are clinically and cost effective. It is important to know what dressings are available on the wound care formulary where you work.

Primary dressings

These dressings have low adherence that can be placed directly on the wound, usually with low exudates, and are covered or secured with tape or a secondary dressing. Some contain hydrogels, antiseptics and antimicrobials.

Consider this . . .

Check the past medical history of patients to assess thyroid function status before considering topical antiseptics.

Film dressings

Films consist of a polyurethane membrane coated with acrylic adhesive and are permeable to water vapour, but impermeable to bacteria. They are used as a primary or secondary dressing for non-infected, low exuding and shallow wounds, helping reduce pain, and providing an occlusive environment, and they are transparent so the wound can be seen through the dressing. Removal is via a stretch and relax method in the direction of hair growth. These dressing can be left on for five to seven days, depending on exudate levels.

Hydrogels

Hydrogels donate fluid to a wound when in contact with it. The main use is to rehydrate necrotic or sloughy tissue, and a secondary dressing is always needed. Hydrogels can be left on for up to three days depending on wound exudate levels.

Hydrocolloids

These groups of interactive dressing are made of cellulose, gelatine and pectin and are backed with polyurethane film or foam. They do not need a secondary dressing and are self-adhesive. They are for low to medium exuding wounds and can absorb and hold exudates, rehydrate and promote debridement of necrosis and slough and are water permeable. Like films, pain is reduced when in place and removal is stretch and relax technique. Patients can bathe and shower with hydrocolloid dressing in place. Weartime is up to seven days. Hydrocolloids are available as flat sheets or ribbon dressings which turn into a gel on absorption of exudates, acting as primary dressings, requiring a secondary dressing and are suitable for moderate to heavily exuding wounds.

Alginates

Derived from seaweed, alginates are fibrous dressings absorbing exudate when in contact with the wound bed, suitable for moderate to heavily exuding wounds and contain moisture and aid autolysis. They require a secondary dressing and can stay in place for up to seven days in a non-infected wound.

Foam dressings

Made of polyurethane or silicone, these are either flat to lie on top of a wound or fillers to place in a cavity, and they can be adhesive or non-adhesive. Their purpose is to absorb large amounts of exudate and provide a barrier to bacteria. On a clean, non-infected wound, the foam can be left in place up to four to five days. Foams can be primary or secondary dressings, dependent on the level of exudates and, due to their varied shapes and sizes, can be used on a variety of body areas, i.e. heels, elbows.

Charcoal dressings

Composed of activated charcoal cloth, these work by absorbing chemicals released from malodorous wounds. Some have silver included so as to attract bacteria away from the wound and into the dressing.

Antibacterial / antimicrobial dressings

These contain agents that are effective against a wide range of bacteria and contain either honey, silver or iodine. If a wound is infected it is correct to use systemic antibiotics. Nevertheless, where critical colonisation is identified, healing is delayed or infection is present but there is a poor blood supply, a topical antimicrobial agent may be used. This can be used alone or in combination with systemic therapy (Vowden and Cooper 2006). Secondary dressing may be necessary. Manufacturers' instructions for these dressings must be followed.

Skin protectants

These are liquid film dressings that can be applied to the periwound to prevent maceration and damage to surrounding skin. They can also be applied to skin before the application of dressings, to places susceptible to excoriation, dribbling and leaking stomas. The product is applied and left to dry for 30–90 seconds and reapplied if necessary. One application lasts two to three days according to the level of moisture present. Creams are also available.

Paste bandages

These are cotton bandages impregnated with medicated pastes, widely used on leg ulcers, cellulitic and eczematous legs. Some patients can be allergic to the contents. A secondary bandage is required.

Bandages

These are pieces of material used either to support a medical device such as a dressing or splint, or on its own to provide support to the body. They can also be used to restrict a part of the body. Bandages are classified into three categories which have clinical indications:

- Type 1. Retention bandages that are lightweight and made of conforming and stretching products whose main purpose is to retain a dressing, without restricting movement.
- Type 2. Light support bandages, often known as short stretch to minimal stretch bandages, made of heavily twisted yarns whose purposes are to prevent oedema and provide support, enhancing the action of the calf muscle pump.
- Type 3. Compression therapy bandages containing rubber or polyurethane yarns, which are used to treat venous ulcers, oedema, varices and varicosis and lymphoedema. Type 3 bandages have a further four categories 3a, b, c and d. These bandages may only be applied by appropriately qualified nurses and members of healthcare staff and only after a thorough assessment of the patient and an assessment of the patient's ABPI.

When selecting a bandage take into consideration the classification of a bandage and also the technique of application, the level of skill and frequency of application.

Having considered issues surrounding wounds, we will now finish with a look at some alternative therapies which can be helpful for persons with skin problems.

COMMUNITY-BASED CARE

When preparing patients with wounds for discharge home, plan in advance. Nurses should check whether dressings and equipment accessible in the hospital are available in the community. Often formularies and product selection varies or is inaccessible and other options need to be explored. There is also a need to ensure that the patient and their carer are aware of the dressing and equipment to be used. It may be an idea to liaise with the community nurse, practice nurse and local pharmacist to ensure that continuity of care is as seamless as possible. All of this should be done prior to discharge and in conjunction with the patient and their carer. Always ensure you provide detailed documentation of care regimens so that these can (if appropriate) be undertaken in the home setting.

Other therapies for persons with altered skin function

Therapeutic baths

Therapeutic baths have a variety of uses in treating skin disorders. Depending on the agent, the bath will soothe the skin, lower the bacterial count, clean and hydrate the skin and relieve itching. Agents used include saline or tap water and antibacterial agents such as potassium permanganate, acetic acid, hexachlorophene, colloid substances such as oatmeal, cornstarch and sodium bicarbonate, coal tar derivatives such as Balnetar, Zetar and Polytar, and emollients.

Medications

Medications used to treat skin disorders are listed in Table 5.5.

Leeches

Medicinal leeches evacuate haematomas, reduce venous congestion in reimplanted digits or myocutaneous flap reconstruction and can be used to treat cauliflower ear. They are single use and feed for 30–60 minutes, and treatment usually lasts five days. Observations are made regarding patient comfort, acceptance, leech feeding and movement and signs of bleeding and infection. Leeches are used with prophylactic antibiotics and are only used when prescribed.

Larvae

Larvae or maggot therapy is used to treat infected, sloughy or necrotic wounds that have been resistant to other debridement attempts. The larvae liquefy and breakdown necrotic tissue and stimulate granulation tissue. A consequence of their action is a reduction in wound odour and exudates in infected wounds.

Table 5.5 Medications used to treat skin disorders

Type	Use	Examples
Creams	Moisturise the skin	Aquacare Curel Nutraderm
Ointments	Lubricate the skin Retard water loss	Aquaphor Vaseline
Lotions	Moisturise the skin Lubricate the skin	Alpha-Keri Dermassage Lubriderm
Anaesthetics	Relieve itching	Xylocaine
Antibiotics	Treat infection	Bacitracin Polysporin Gentamicin Silvadene
Corticosteroids	Suppress inflammation Relieve itching	Dexamethasone Hydrocortisone Clocortolone Desonide

Hyperbaric oxygen

Treatment chambers that deliver 100% oxygen at a pressure greater than sea level are classed as hyperbaric oxygen chambers. It is standard treatment for decompression illness in divers, gas gangrene and gas and air embolism; however, it has been an adjuvant therapy for non-healing wounds in diabetics, necrotising fasciitis, Fournier's gangrene, post-radiation tissue damage and preparation for surgery of previous irradiated tissue.

Wound managers

Wound drainage bags have been designed to cope with varying amounts of liquids or semi-solid matter, when traditional dressings have failed. These include post-operative draining wounds, fistulae, sinuses, dehisced or eviscerated wounds and heavily infected wounds. Wound managers are similar to large stoma bags, effectively draining excess liquid away, but in the meantime protecting the surrounding skin, reducing odour, itching, excoriation and pain.

Pressure-relieving and pressure-reducing devices

These are an essential component in the management of pressure ulcer prevention and treatment. Cullum *et al.* (2001) suggests there are two main approaches to preventing and managing pressure ulcers using pressure-relieving devices:

1. The use of conforming support surfaces such as mattresses and cushions to redistribute the body weight over a larger surface area – named low-tech devices.

2. Use of alternating support mattresses and total bed frames, where cells inflate and deflate alternately – named high-tech devices.

As mattresses, beds and cushions can be classified in different ways, it is important that you familiarise yourself with the products used in clinical practice, seeking advice on how equipment is selected and processes you must follow to access equipment.

Repositioning

Regular repositioning of patients who are unable to move themselves and are at a high risk of pressure ulcer formation is essential. Repositioning can range from small shifts in position undertaken by the patient with encouragement, to full lateral repositioning/turning on behalf of the patient. There are various positions that have been recommended including the 90° laterally inclined, prone and the 30°tilt (Colin *et al.* 1996). Repositioning and turning of patients should be regularly documented, and patients at risk of pressure ulcer damage should not be sat out for more than two hours (NICE 2001c). Physiotherapists can help with developing correct repositioning routines and schedules for patients, ensuring correct posture, seating and lying positions and support of carriage.

Ultraviolet light therapy

Ultraviolet-B (UVB) light is the treatment of choice for generalised psoriasis; this decreases the growth rate of epidermal cells, decreasing hyperkeratosis. Mercury vapour lights or fluorescent UV tubes provide the UVB light; the latter are often arranged in a cabinet, exposing psoriatic lesions more easily.

Light therapy is administered in gradually increasing exposure times, until the person experiences a mild erythema, like mild sunburn. Treatments are given three times a week and are measured in seconds of exposure; eyes are shielded during the treatment. The erythema response occurs in about eight hours. Careful assessment is necessary to prevent more severe burning, which could exacerbate the psoriasis.

Photochemotherapy

In photochemotherapy, a light-activated form of the drug methoxsalen is used. This is an antimetabolite inhibiting DNA synthesis preventing cell mitosis, decreasing hyperkeratosis. Exposure to ultraviolet-A (UVA) rays activates methoxsalen; it is administered orally, and the person is exposed to UVA two hours later. The eyes are covered by dark glasses during the treatment. Treatments are administered two to three times a week; usually 10–20 total treatments are given over one to two months. Treatment causes tanning, and direct sunlight must be avoided for 8–12 hours thereafter. If the person exhibits erythema, treatments are stopped until the redness and swelling resolve.

Photochemotherapy has had a high success rate in achieving remission of psoriasis, but it can accelerate ageing of exposed skin, induce cataract development, alter immune function and increase the risk of melanoma.

Plasmapheresis

Plasmapheresis is occasionally used to treat pemphigus; the plasma is selectively removed from whole blood and reinfused into the person. This decreases the serum level of antibodies for a period of time.

Surgical excision

This may be minor or major, depending on the size and location of tumour, lesion or ulcer. Small-scale surgery is most often performed as an out-patient. Surgical excision allows rapid healing and yields good cosmetic results but, as with any surgery, carries the risk of infection.

The goal is to remove the tumour or lesion or ulcer completely, so some surrounding tissue is also excised. If the surgery is to the face, the incision is made along normal wrinkle or anatomical lines so that the scars will be less obvious. The incision is closed in layers leaving the smallest possible scar. A pressure dressing is usually applied providing support. If a large area is removed, a skin graft or skin flap may be performed to cover the excised area.

Fusiform excision is the removal of a full thickness of the epidermis and dermis, usually with a thin layer of subcutaneous tissue. It is used to remove tissue for biopsies and for complete removal of benign and malignant lesions of the skin.

Excision of small, superficial lesions is performed under a local anaesthetic, and care is taken to place the incision in a way that will provide good cosmetic results.

Electrosurgery involves the destruction or removal of tissue with high-frequency alternating current. A variety of surgical procedures may be performed, including *electrodesiccation* (which produces superficial skin destruction), *electrocoagulation* (which produces deeper tissue destruction) and *electrosection* (which can cut through skin and tissue). Electrodesiccation is used to remove benign surface lesions, such as skin tags, keratoses, warts and angiomas. It is also used to produce haemostasis for capillary bleeding. Electrocoagulation removes telangiectases, warts and superficial non-melanoma skin cancers. Electrosection is used to make incisions, excise tissue and perform biopsies.

Cryosurgery is the destruction of tissue by cold or freezing with special chemicals and is used to treat skin lesions. The freezing agents are applied topically to the lesion. The effects of freezing depend on the degree of freeze. Light freezing causes damage to the epidermis with blistering or crusting that heals without scarring. Deeper freezes, used to treat malignant cells, cause oedema, necrosis and tissue slough. The effects of cryosurgery may not be obvious until 24 hours following treatment. Post-operatively, infection is prevented by applying a topical antibiotic and keeping the treated areas clean. Healing occurs in two to three weeks.

Curettage is the removal of lesions with a curette (a semi-sharp cutting instrument). The curette cuts through soft or weak tissue, but not through normal tissue. It is used primarily to remove benign and malignant superficial epidermal lesions. Benign lesions removed by curettage include keratoses, naevi and angiomas. Non-melanoma skin lesions are removed by curettage if they are small, well-defined, primary tumours. Curettage is used to remove specimens of tissue for biopsy.

Following curettage, the wound may be treated with electrodesiccation to destroy any remaining malignant cells and to provide haemostasis. These wounds are not closed; they are left open to heal by secondary intention. Topical antibiotic ointments and dressings may be used in the post-operative period.

Laser surgery is used to treat a wide variety of skin disorders, including port-wine stains, telangiectases and venous lakes. A laser is an intense light producing a thermal injury on contact with tissue, causing coagulation, vapourisation, excision and ablation (removal of a growth). A local anaesthetic may be used.

Response differs by type of laser. Following treatment with the argon laser, the lesion changes from white to black in colour, a blister forms and the skin may peel. The area weeps, and an eschar forms; in 10–14 days, the eschar separates, revealing an underlying red area. The redness fades over a period of up to one year. However, pulsed dye laser treatment does not result in blistering or weeping; only rarely does it result in eschar.

Chemical destruction is the application of a specific chemical to produce destruction of skin lesions. Chemical destruction is used to treat both benign and pre-malignant lesions. After application, the treated area forms a thin crust that sloughs off in about a week.

Sclerotherapy is the removal of benign skin lesions with a sclerosing agent causing inflammation with fibrosis of tissue. Agents causing therapeutic sclerosis include aethoxysclerol (Sclerodex) and hypertonic sodium chloride. This type of treatment is used for telangiectases and superficial spider veins of the lower extremities. The solution is injected into the affected veins, causing a reaction closing the lumen of the vein.

Plastic surgery is the alteration, replacement or restoration of visible portions of the body, performed to correct a structural or cosmetic defect.

Many skin disorders discussed cause changes in appearance. For example, acne may leave deep pitting scars, naevi and keloids are often disfiguring and skin cancers may require wide excision and skin grafting. These scars, lesions and wounds often cause embarrassment and alterations in body image. In addition, the removal of lesions may leave unsightly scars or areas of obviously missing tissue.

Cosmetic surgery (aesthetic surgery) is one of two fields within plastic surgery. Cosmetic surgery enhances the attractiveness of normal features. The top five procedures are liposuction, breast augmentation, eyelid surgery, rhinoplasty and 'tummy tuck' (Keynote 2010). The other field, reconstructive surgery, uses similar techniques; however, its purpose is to improve the function or appearance of parts of the body damaged by trauma, disease or birth defects. Many of the plastic surgeries permanently alter body image.

Skin grafts and flaps restore function while also maintaining an acceptable appearance. Both procedures involve the movement of skin from one part of the body to another. A skin graft is a surgical method of detaching skin from a donor site and placing it in a recipient site, where a new blood supply from the base of the wound develops. Skin grafting is an effective way to cover wounds that have a good blood supply, are not infected and in which bleeding can be controlled.

Skin grafts may be either split-thickness or full-thickness. A *split-thickness graft* contains epidermis and only a portion of dermis of the donor site and ranges in thickness from 0.010 inch to greater than 0.015 inch. A common donor site is the anterior thigh. Skin is removed in sheets from the donor site with a dermatome. Donor sites of split-thickness grafts heal by re-epithelialisation. A meshed graft is a type of split-thickness graft that is rolled under a special cutting machine to form a mesh pattern with perforations to allow drainage of serum and blood from under the graft. After healing, however, the skin has a rough appearance. A *full–thickness graft* contains both epidermis and dermis. These layers contain the greatest number of skin elements (sweat glands, sebaceous glands or hair follicles) and are best able to withstand trauma. Areas of thin skin are the best donor sites for full-thickness skin grafts. The donor site must be surgically closed and will scar.

Other types of grafts are composite grafts and cultured epithelial grafts. Composite grafts are usually used on the face, containing skin, subcutaneous tissue, cartilage or other tissue. Cultured epithelial grafts are made from epithelial cells cultured *in vivo*, coalesced into sheets and used to cover full-thickness wounds. They are primarily used to treat burns.

A *skin flap* is a piece of tissue whose free end is moved from a donor site to a recipient site while maintaining a continuous blood supply through its connection at the base or pedicle. Flaps carry their own blood supply and are used to cover recipient sites that have a poor blood supply or have sustained a major tissue loss. They are often used for reconstruction or closure of large wounds. Microsurgical techniques, with anastomosis of small blood vessels and nerves, allow reconstruction with free flaps (in which the flap is completely removed from its donor site and moved to the recipient site).

Cultured epithelial autografting is a technique in which skin cells are removed from unburned sites on the person's body, then minced and placed in a culture medium for growth. Over a five- to seven-day period, the cells expand 50–70 times the size of the initial biopsies. The cells are again separated out and placed in a new culture medium for continued growth. With this technique, enough skin can be grown over a period of three to four weeks to cover the entire body. The cells are prepared in sheets and attached to petroleum jelly gauze backing, which is applied to the burn wound site. Problems with infection and lack of attachment have occurred.

Chemical peeling is the application of a chemical to produce a controlled and predictable injury altering the anatomy of the epidermis and superficial dermis. The result is skin that appears firmer, smoother and less wrinkled. This form of cos-

metic surgery is more useful in people who have fair, thin skin with fine wrinkling.

Chemical agents used for peeling include phenol, trichloroacetic acid (TCA) and alpha-hydroxy acids (AHAs). Phenol, a keratocoagulant, penetrates the epidermis and dermis; regeneration of the epithelium produces the desired results. After treatment, the entire surface of the face except the eyelids is covered with adhesive tape for one to two days. The adhesive is then removed, and the treated area forms a crust that heals in about a week. TCA has been used for years to obtain the desired effect. A light peel causes mild erythema followed by peeling (as from a mild sunburn) in three to five days. AHAs are organic acids used to produce light to moderate peeling to remove acne, fine lines, seborrhoeic keratosis, warts and mild scarring. Both TCA and AHA treatments may be repeated weekly. One complication of chemical peeling is bleaching of the skin (due to removal of melanocytes).

Liposuction is a method of changing the contours of the body by aspirating fat from the subcutaneous layer of tissue. It is not a cure for obesity and should not be used as a substitute for weight loss. The procedure is usually done for younger people because their skin is more elastic. Liposuction may be performed on either an out-patient or in-patient basis.

To aspirate fat, a small incision is made close to the area, and a suction cannula or curette is inserted and attached to the suction apparatus. The high vacuum pressure causes fat cells to emulsify, and they are aspirated out of the body. A pressure dressing is applied to help the skin conform to the new tissue size.

Dermabrasion is a method of removing facial scars, severe acne and pigment from unwanted tattoos. The area is sprayed with a chemical to cause light freezing and is then abraded with sandpaper or a revolving wire brush to remove the epidermis and a portion of the dermis.

Radiation therapy is most often used for reducing lesions that are inoperable because of their location (such as tumours on the corner of the nose, the eyelid, the canthus and the lip) or size (between 1 and 8 cm). Radiotherapy is also used for people who are older or of poor surgical risk. Radiation is painless and can be used to treat areas surrounding the tumour if necessary. The treatment is given over three to four weeks, does not allow control of tumour margins and may itself cause skin cancer. Radiation is used for palliation of symptoms resulting from metastasis to the brain, bone, lymph nodes, gastrointestinal tract, skin or subcutaneous tissue.

Biological and biosynthetic dressings

The terms *biological dressing* and *biosynthetic dressing* refer to any temporary material that rapidly adheres to the wound bed, promotes healing and/or prepares the burn wound for permanent autograft coverage. Ideally, these kinds of dressings should be easy to apply and remove, inexpensive, non-antigenic, elastic, reduce pain, serve as a bacterial barrier and to enhance the natural healing process. The dressings are applied to the burn wound as soon as possible. Covering the wound eliminates the loss of water through evaporation, reduces infection and promotes wound healing. Biologic and biosynthetic dressings that are currently in use include homograft (allograft), heterograft (xenograft), amnionic membranes and synthetic materials.

Homograft, or *allograft*, is human skin that has been harvested from cadavers. It is stored in skin banks. The development of methods to achieve prolonged storage of frozen, viable skin has increased the use of this dressing; however, its short supply and expense still pose problems. It is manufactured as strips cut to the pattern of the burn and applied using sterile technique. Usually a homograft is rejected within 14–21 days following application.

Heterograft, or *xenograft*, is skin obtained from an animal, usually a pig. Although fresh porcine heterograft is available at some centres, frozen heterograft is much more commonly used. Once applied, heterograft appears to undergo early softening and lysis from enzymatic action from the wound. As a result, frequent changes of the heterograft dressing are necessary. Because of the high infection rates associated with this dressing, silver-nitrate-treated porcine heterograft has been developed to retard microbial growth.

Positioning, *splints*, and *exercise contractures* are common problems for persons with burns and extensive traumatic injuries.

During therapy, the person must be maintained in positions preventing contractures from forming. Because flexion is the natural resting position of joints and extremities, early physical therapy includes maintaining antideformity positions. Splints immobilise body parts and prevent contractures of the joints. They are applied as soon as possible after the injury and removed according to schedules established by the physiotherapist and occupational therapist.

Support garments enable application of uniform pressure which can prevent or reduce hypertrophic scarring. Tubular support bandages are applied five to seven days post skin graft to maintain a tension ranging from 10–20 mmHg to control scarring. The person wears custom-made elastic pressure garments for six months to a year post graft. Occupational therapists and prosthetic and orthotic staff will help with the assessment, measurement and fitting of support garments.

Cosmetic camouflage

Cosmetic camouflage was developed to support people with a disfigurement to cope in their everyday lives, with the aid of simple cosmetic camouflage techniques. This service is provided by some NHS hospitals and the British Red Cross.

 CASE STUDY SUMMARIES

Case Study 1. John has developed a pressure sore as a result of a combination of factors as is often the case. The nurse has to ensure that all physical and psychological factors are taken into account when providing holistic care. The formation of pressure sores causes discomfort for the patient and their family; they lead to extended stays in hospital and they cost the nation a considerable amount of money. Prior to discharge, a full home assessment will need to be undertaken to ensure that John can be cared for safely at home. This will include an assessment of the physical environment, and attention should be paid to additional health and social care resources that John and his wife may need in order to provide John and Jenny with as much independence as possible.

Case Study 2. Bernard has undergone major emergency surgery. The surgery was carried out in an attempt to save Bernard's life and is not in itself free of risk. Infection

post-operatively can also be a risk to life. Swift action and skilled nursing care were required to detect the surgical complication (dehiscence), and prompt action was required by the whole surgical team on the ward and in the operating theatre. In order to care for Bernard safely the nurse must have an understanding of the pathophysiological changes that are associated with wound healing and the skills required to offer high-quality wound care.

Case Study 3. Simon's condition was diagnosed by the advanced nurse practitioner and treatment commenced immediately. The result was instantaneous, providing Simon with relief from the itchiness and soreness. Simon was seen in the out-patients department for follow-up care. With Simon's permission the nurse also referred Simon for cognitive behavioural therapy to help him cope with the anxieties that may have been responsible for the rash on his hands; the cognitive behavioural therapy also helped Simon prepare for his university examinations. Simon's condition could be classified as psychosomatic – a disease that involves both the mind and the body.

CHAPTER HIGHLIGHTS

- The skin is the largest organ of the body, providing an external covering, separating and protecting the organs and tissues from the external environment.

- The functions of the skin are protection from physical, chemical and biological damage, prevention of water loss, storing of melanin, conversion of vitamin D, regulation of body temperature, communication, insulation and lubrication.

- The skin is made up of three layers, the epidermis, dermis and subcutaneous tissue.

- Wounds occur when the skin or another external surface, such as a mucous membrane, is torn, pierced, cut or otherwise broken, either intentionally or through trauma, causing the loss of skin integrity. The rate of wound healing is affected by the type of injury, the general health and wellbeing of the patient and the extent of damage to skin. Small superficial wounds heal quicker than wounds that are complex, deep, cover a larger surface area and when there is damage to underlying tissues. Regardless of wound type, all pass through a complex sequence of events enabling full healing and scar formation to occur. The process of wound healing is continuous; cells biologically modify to assist in aiding haemostasis, inflammation, proliferation and maturation.

- Wounds can heal by primary, secondary or tertiary intention.

- The advantages of a moist wound healing include: less pain at the wound bed as nerve endings are bathed in exudate; reduction in infections as host defences are more viable; less dry dead tissue to harbour bacteria and less risk of bacteria transferring via airborne dispersal; less injury to the wound bed on removal of dressings; clinical and cost-effectiveness in the management of surgical wounds, chronic wounds and burns wounds; assist in autolytic debridement of necrotic tissue.

- Wounds that result in restoration of anatomical and functional integrity from a healing process that is timely and without complication are considered acute wounds. These are new or relatively new in injury, occurring suddenly. Acute wounds include surgical incisions, traumatic injuries such as lacerations, bites, abrasions, burns and avulsions.

- A chronic wound digresses from the normal order of repair in terms of length of time (may develop over time, lasting more than six weeks), appearance and reaction to management, or restoration of anatomical and functional effect.

- A palliative wound is one that cannot be classified as acute or chronic and whose outcome of wound healing is considered both challenging and unattainable. Causes of these types of wound are complex or not resolvable; therefore, management is palliative, not curative.

- There are many factors that can delay wound healing; these can be classified as intrinsic (reduced oxygen supply, patient's general medical condition, malnutrition) or extrinsic (pressure, shear and friction).

- Alteration in skin integrity is an issue in clinical practice for all nurses. Damage to the skin may be due to many factors such as mechanical, chemical, vascular, infectious, allergic and thermal. Each results in a different response within the skin; for example, an ulcer, lesion, fistula (an abnormal connection or passageway), papule or erosion may go on to develop into a more serious secondary lesion. It is important to understand the causes and types of altered skin problems, which may present in practice, so that assessment can occur and appropriate care be provided. Altered skin function can also be classified according to the depth of tissue damage and morphology (form and structure of wounds).

- The functions of skin are assessed by findings from diagnostic tests, a health assessment interview to collect subjective data and a physical assessment to collect objective data.

- Management of altered skin function is often via a variety of treatments and interdisciplinary working. Health promotion and education are key to the success of management.

TEST YOURSELF

1. Name the three layers of the skin
   a. epidermis, dermis and subcutaneous layer
   b. epidermis, dermis and stratum corneum
   c. epidermis, dermis and glands of the skin

2. What healing intention is initially left open and then closed 4–5 days later?
   a. primary
   b. secondary
   c. tertiary

3. In which stage of wound healing does angiogenesis occur?
   a. inflammation
   b. proliferation
   c. maturation
   d. contraction

4. What percentage of all hospital-acquired infections are related to a surgical site?
   a. 5%   b. 10%   c. 15%   d. 20%

5. True or false, head lice like clean hair.

6. List four risk factors for non-melanoma skin cancer.

7. What are the four main categories of wounds?
   a. mechanical, chronic, burn and malignant
   b. superficial, partial thickness, partial full thickness and full thickness
   c. pressure ulcers, leg ulcers, burns and fungating wounds

8. How are surgical wounds classified post-operatively?

9. Which common type of burn is caused by radiation?
   a. thermal
   b. electrical
   c. chemical
   d. sunburn

10. What are the three main extrinsic causes of pressure ulcers?

Further resources

World Wide Wounds
http://www.worldwidewounds.com
An electronic online journal providing peer-reviewed information on dressing materials.

National Pressure Ulcer Advisory Panel (NPUAP)
http://www.npuap.org/
NPUAP is an independent not-for-profit professional organisation dedicated to the prevention and management of pressure ulcers.

European Wound Management Association (EWMA)
http://ewma.org/english/about-ewma.html
EWMA is an organisation that links wound management associations across Europe and is made up of a multidisciplinary group who bring together individuals and organisations interested in wound management.

National Institute for Health and Clinical Excellence (NICE)
http://www.nice.org.uk/
NICE is an independent organisation responsible for providing national guidance on promoting good health and preventing and treating ill health. The NICE guideline on pressure ulcer management is available at http://www.nice.org.uk/nicemedia/pdf/CG029fullguideline.pdf.

Wounds International
http://www.woundsinternational.com/page.php?name=about-us
A free online practice-based journal for healthcare staff with an interest in wound care.

Bibliography

BAD (2010) *Actinic Keratoses*. London, British Association of Dermatology, available at: http://www.bad.org.uk/site/794/default.aspx (accessed September 2011).

Bennett G, Dealey C and Posnett J (2004) The cost of pressure ulcers in the UK, *Age and Ageing*, **33** 230–235.

Callam N (1992) Prevalence of chronic leg ulceration and severe chronic venous disease in western countries. *Phlebology*, **7**(Suppl 1), 6–12.

Cancer Research UK (2011) *Skin Cancer – UK incidence statistics*. London, available at: http://info.cancerresearchuk.org/cancerstats/types/skin/incidence/ (accessed September 2011).

Cohen V, Jellinek S P and Schwartz R A (2009) *Toxic Epidermal Necrolysis*. Available at: http://emedicine.medscape.com/article/229698-overview (accessed September 2011).

Colin D, Abraham P, Preault L, Bregeon C and Saumet J-L (1996) Comparison of 90° and 30° laterally inclined positions in the prevention of pressure ulcers using transcutaneous oxygen and carbon dioxide pressures. *Advances in Wound Care*, **9**(3), 35–38.

Collier M (2002) A ten-point assessment plan for wound management. *Journal of Community Nursing*, **16**(6), 22–26.

Cullum N, Nelson E A, Flemming K and Sheldon T (2001) Systematic reviews of wound care management: (5) beds; (6) compression; (7) laser therapy, therapeutic ultrasound, electrotherapy and electromagnetic therapy. *Health Technology Assessment*, **5**(9), 1–221.

Dealey C (2005) *The Care of Wounds* (3rd edn). Oxford, Wiley-Blackwell.

Diabetes UK (2010) *Diabetes in the UK 2010: Key statistics on diabetes*. London, Diabetes UK.

DiSanti L B S (2005) Pathophysiology and current management of burn injury. *Advances in Skin and Wound Care*, **18**(6), 323–332.

DoH (2008) *High Quality Care for All: NHS next stage review. Final Report*. London, Department of Health.

DoH (2009) *NHS 2010–2015: From good to great. Preventative, people, central and productive*. London, Department of Health.

DoH (2010a) *Accident and Emergency Attendances*. London, The Stationery Office.

DoH (2010b) *The Essence of Care*. London, Department of Health.

EPUAP and NPUAP (2009) *Prevention and Treatment of Pressure Ulcers: Quick reference guide*. Washington DC: National Pressure Ulcer Advisory Panel.

EPUAP (2005) *Pressure Ulcer Classification Differentiation Between Pressure Ulcers and Moisture Lesions*. Available at: https://uhra.herts.ac.uk/dspace/bitstream/2299/190/1/100614.pdf (accessed September 2011).

Falanga V (2001) Introducing the concept of wound bed preparation. *International Forum Wound Care*, **16**(1), 1–4.

Gannon R (2007) Wound cleansing: sterile water or saline? *Nursing Times*, **103**(9), 44–46.

Harth W, Taube M K and Gieler U (2010) Factitious disorders in dermatology. *Journal of Dutch Dermatology Ges*, **8**, 361–373.

Hollingworth H and Kingston J E (1998) Using a non sterile technique in wound care. *Professional Nurse*, **13**, 2269.

HPA (2009) *Healthcare-associated Infections in England: 2008–2009 Report*. London, Health Protection Agency.

HPS (2008) *Surgical Site Infection Bundle*. Glasgow, Health Protection Scotland, available at: http://www.hps.scot.nhs.uk/haiic/ic/bundles.aspx (accessed September 2011).

Hutchinson J J and Lawrence J C (1991) Wound infection under occlusive dressings. *Journal of Hospital Infection*, **17**(2), 83–94.

International Working Group on the Diabetic Foot (2003) *International Consensus: Ulcer classification*. Available at: http://www.iwgdf.org/index.php?option=com_content&task=view&id=84&Itemid=116 (accessed September 2011).

Keynote (2010) *Market Report Update, Cosmetic Surgery, Analyses the Market for Cosmetic Surgery and Cosmetic Procedures in the UK*. London, Keynote.

Lock P M (1979) *The Effects of Temperature on Mitotic Activity at the Edges of Experimental Wounds*. Kent, Lock Laboratories Research.

Lutz J (2008) *A Review of the Literature Pertinent to Capillary Closing Pressure of the Human Dermis*. New York, Gaymar Industries.

Macmillan Cancer Support (2009) *Risk Factors and Causes of Skin Cancer*. Available at: http://www.macmillan.org.uk/Cancerinformation/Cancertypes/Skin/Aboutskincancer/Causes.aspx (accessed September 2011).

National Burn Care Review (2001) *Standards and Strategy for Burn Care: A Review of Burn Care in the British Isles*. Available at: http://www.specialisedservices.nhs.uk/document/national-burn-care-review-2001 (accessed September 2011).

National Diabetes Support Team (2006) *Diabetic Foot Guide*. Available at: http://www.diabetes.

nhs.uk/document.php?o=196 (accessed September 2011).

NHS CRD (1997) Compression therapy for venous leg ulcers. *Effective Health Care*, **3**(4), 1–12.

NHSIII (2009) *High Impact Actions: Your skin matters*. London, National Health Service Institute for Innovation and Improvement, available at: http://www.institute.nhs.uk/building_capability/hia_supporting_info/your_skin_matters.html (accessed September 2011).

NHS Information Centre (2011) *Accident and Emergency Attendances in England (Experimental Statistics) 2009/10*. London, The Health and Social Care Information Centre.

NICE (2001a) *Wound Care Debriding Agents*. London, National Institute for Health and Clinical Excellence.

NICE (2001b) *Pressure Ulcer Risk Assessment and Prevention*. London, National Institute for Health and Clinical Excellence.

NICE (2001c) *Pressure Relieving Devices*. London, National Institute for Health and Clinical Excellence.

NICE (2004a) *Self-harm. The Short-term Physical and Psychological Management and Secondary Prevention of Self-harm in Primary and Secondary Care*. London, National Institute for Health and Clinical Excellence.

NICE (2004b) *Wound and Burn Debridement by a Hydrosurgery System*. London, National Institute for Health and Clinical Excellence.

NICE (2005) *Pressure Ulcers: The management of pressure ulcers in primary and secondary care*, CG29. London, National Institute for Health and Clinical Excellence.

NICE (2008) *Surgical Site Infection*. London, National Institute for Health and Clinical Excellence.

NICE (2009) *Negative Pressure Wound Therapy for the Open Abdomen*, IPG322. London, National Institute for Health and Clinical Excellence.

NMC (2008) *The Code*. London, Nursing and Midwifery Council.

Northern Burn Care Network (2003) *International Burn Care Standards*. Available at: http://www.nbcn.nhs.uk/international-burn-care-standards.htm (accessed September 2011).

NPSA (2009) *Pressure Ulcers: An analysis of RLS data, Quarterly Data*. Summary Issue 11. London, National Patient Safety Agency.

National Pressure Ulcer Advisory Panel (1997) PUSH Tool. Available at: http://www.npuap.org/pushins.htm (accessed September 2011).

NHS Scotland (2009) *Amputee Statistical Database for the United Kingdom*, Report 2006–07. Edinburgh, ISD Publications.

Office for National Statistics (2010) *Mortality Statistics: Cause. England and Wales 2008*. London, The Stationery Office.

Office for Public Management (2010) *Literature Review: Your skin matters*. London, NHS III.

Ousey K (2010) Intervention strategies for people who self harm. *Wounds UK*, **6**(4), 34–40.

Phillips L and Buttery J (2009) Exploring pressure ulcer prevalence and preventative care. *Nursing Times*, **105**, 16.

Posnett J and Franks P J (2007) *The Costs of Skin Breakdown and Ulceration in the UK. The Silent Epidemic*. Hull, Smith and Nephew.

RCN (2005) *The Management of Pressure Ulcers in Primary and Secondary Care: A Clinical Practice guideline*. Available at: http://www.rcn.org.uk/__data/assets/pdf_file/0017/65015/management_pressure_ulcers.pdf (accessed September 2011).

RCP (2008) *Latex Allergy: Occupational aspects of management*. London, Royal College of Physicians.

Schofield C J, Libby G, Brennan G M, *et al.* (2006) Mortality and hospitalization in patients, after amputation: a comparison between patients with and without diabetes. *Diabetes Care*, **29**(10), 2252–2256.

Schultz G S, Sibbald R G, Fallanga V, *et al.* (2003) Wound bed preparation: a systematic approach to wound management. *Wound Repair and Regeneration*, **11**, 1–28.

Sciarra J (2003) *Wound Care Made Incredibly Easy*. London, Lippincott, Williams and Wilkins.

Thomas S (1997) A structured approach to the selection of dressings. Available at: http://www.worldwidewounds.com/1997/July/Thomas-Guide/Dress-Select.html (accessed September 2011).

Thomlinson D (1987) To clean or not to clean? *Nursing Times*, **83** (9), 71–75.

Vowden P and Cooper R A (2006) An integrated approach to managing wound infection. In *European Wound Management Association Position Document. Management of Wound Infection*. London, MEP, 2–6.

Williams G and Pickup J C (2004) *Handbook of Diabetes*. Oxford, Blackwell.

Wood S, Bellis M A and Atherton J (2010) *Burns: A review of evidence for prevention from the UK Focal point for violence and injury prevention*. Liverpool, Centre for Public Health, Liverpool John Moores University.

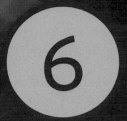

6

Caring for people with endocrine problems

Learning outcomes

- Describe the anatomy, physiology and functions of the **endocrine** glands.
- Explain the functions of the **hormones** secreted by the endocrine glands.
- Describe techniques for assessing the thyroid gland and the effects of altered endocrine function.
- Describe normal variations in assessment findings for the elderly.
- Identify abnormal findings that may indicate malfunction of the glands of the endocrine system.
- Use the nursing process as a framework for providing individualised care to persons with endocrine disorders.

Clinical competencies

- Carry out and document a health history for persons who have or are at risk for alterations in the structure or function of the endocrine glands.
- Carry out and document a physical assessment of the structure of the thyroid gland and the effects of altered endocrine function on other body structures and functions.
- Determine priority nursing diagnoses, based on assessed data, to select and implement individualised nursing interventions for persons with type 1 and type 2 diabetes mellitus.
- Administer medications used to treat type 1 and type 2 diabetes mellitus safely.
- Provide appropriate teaching to facilitate blood glucose monitoring, administration of oral **hypoglycaemic** medications, diabetic diet, appropriate exercise and foot care.

CASE STUDIES

Below are three case studies that you may wish to consider before, during or after you have read the chapter. There are no right or wrong answers to these case studies, but you should think about the physical, psychological and social implications. Also consider what questions you would ask the person so that you can help alleviate their anxieties.

Case Study 1 – Paulette

Mrs Paulette Jones, a 34-year-old woman, is admitted with a swollen neck and protruding eyeballs. She says to the nurse that she eats like a horse but is losing weight, suffers from blurred vision, cannot stand bright light and feels sick. Mrs Jones has lost 6.8 kg over two weeks. She says that she finds it difficult to sleep and is very restless. She also states that she is embarrassed to go out because of her looks and is conscious that people are staring at her. She has difficulty in swallowing and breathing, palpitations and heat intolerance and all this is getting her very depressed. The nurse noticed her skin is moist and warm, her hair thin and brittle. Mrs Jones has visible tremors in her hands. Her eyeballs protrude and she is unable to close her eyelids completely.

Case Study 2 – Veronica

Mrs Veronica Patel is a 32-year-old second-year student nurse. She went to see her GP as she was feeling unwell and gets tired very quickly. Mrs Patel indicated to her GP, 'Lately I have noticed that I have become intolerant to certain foods like milk, tea, coffee, cereals and bread. Regardless of what I ate I was tired and felt cold a lot of the time.' Mrs Patel also stated that she now suffers from constipation, stomach pains and bloating. She is frightened that she might have cancer because her father was diagnosed with stomach cancer and he passed away five years ago. She states, 'I am terrified that I will fall back in my studies and won't be able to attend my placement due to my ill health. I am also frightened that the university will throw me off the course.'

Case Study 3 – Kwan

Mr Lee Kwan is a third-year nursing student at the university. He was diagnosed with type 1 diabetes mellitus at age 12. Mr Lee also works 8 hours a week as a campus student security guard. His working hours are 8 p.m. to midnight, two nights a week. He lives with his girlfriend, who is also a student. Neither of them like to cook, and they usually eat 'whatever is handy'. He is worried about having repeated severe hypoglycaemic attacks during the night for the last three weeks. He tells you that when this happens his blood glucose levels have been around 2.0–3.0 mmol/L. He is concerned, as he is not having any warning signs prior to the attack. He no longer feels confident travelling on his own. He also mentions that over the last couple of months he has put on weight despite not changing his diet at all and requests some orlistat (which he read about in the *Daily Mail*).

INTRODUCTION

This chapter will discuss the physiology of the endocrine system and the disordered endocrine function (producing health problems such as diabetes and Graves' disease) and subsequent treatment. The endocrine system has an important role in maintaining homeostasis. Hormones released by the endocrine glands, such as the thyroid gland, pancreas and the pituitary gland, have a physiological control over the function of cells and organs elsewhere in the body. The role of each hormone varies, but the primary function of the hormones is to regulate the body's internal environment. The endocrine system regulates such varied functions as growth, reproduction, metabolism, fluid and electrolyte balance, and gender differentiation. It also helps the body adapt to constant alterations in the internal and external environment.

ANATOMY, PHYSIOLOGY AND FUNCTIONS OF THE ENDOCRINE SYSTEM

In order to care for persons with endocrine disorders, you need to know what the endocrine organs are and their role in regulating body functions. Through hormones secreted by these glands, the endocrine system regulates functions such as growth, reproduction, metabolism and fluid and electrolyte balance.

The major endocrine organs are the hypothalamus, pituitary gland, thyroid gland, thymus, parathyroid glands, adrenal glands, pancreas and gonads (reproductive glands). The locations of these glands are illustrated in Figure 6.1. Table 6.1 summarises the functions of the endocrine organs and their hormones.

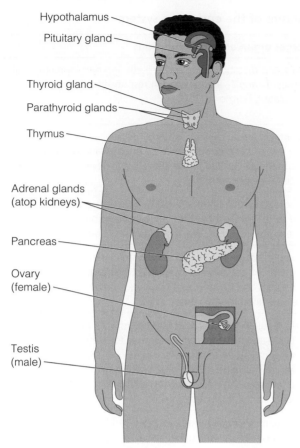

Figure 6.1 The locations of the major endocrine glands.

PITUITARY GLAND

The pituitary gland (**hypophysis**) is located in the skull beneath the hypothalamus of the brain. It is often called the 'master gland' because its hormones regulate many body functions. The pituitary gland has two parts: the anterior pituitary (or adenohypophysis) and the posterior pituitary (or **neurohypophysis**). The anterior pituitary is glandular tissue, whereas the posterior pituitary is actually an extension of the hypothalamus.

Anterior pituitary

The anterior pituitary has several types of endocrine cells and secretes at least six major hormones (see Figure 6.2):

- Somatotropic cells secrete growth hormone (GH) (also called somatotropin). GH stimulates growth of the body by signalling cells to increase protein production and by stimulating the epiphyseal plates of the long bones.
- Lactotropic cells secrete prolactin (PRL). Prolactin stimulates the production of breast milk.
- Thyrotropic cells secrete thyroid-stimulating hormone (TSH).
- Corticotropic cells secrete adrenocorticotropic hormone (ACTH).
- Gonadotropic cells secrete the gonadotropin hormones, follicle-stimulating hormone (FSH) and luteinising hormone (LH).

Posterior pituitary

The posterior pituitary is made of nervous tissue. Its primary function is to store and release antidiuretic hormone (ADH) and oxytocin, produced in the hypothalamus:

- ADH, also called vasopressin, decreases urine production by causing the renal tubules to reabsorb water from the urine and return it to the circulating blood.

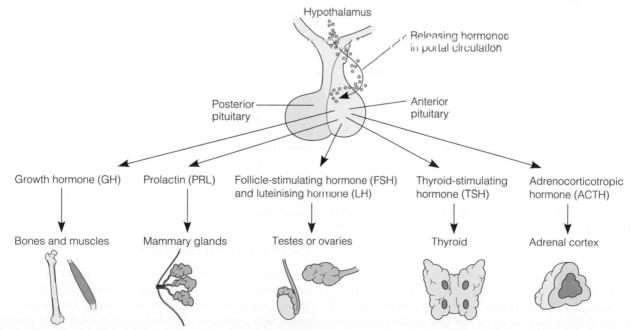

Figure 6.2 Actions of the major hormones of the anterior pituitary.

Table 6.1 Organs, hormones, functions and feedback mechanisms of the endocrine system

Endocrine organ	Hormone secreted	Target organ and their functions
Thyroid gland	Thyroid hormone (TH): thyroxin (T$_4$) is the major hormone secreted by the thyroid gland. It is converted to tri-iodothyronine (T$_3$) at the target tissues.	Maintains metabolic rate and growth and development of all tissues. T$_3$ and T$_4$ are secreted in response to thyroid-stimulating hormone (TSH).
	Calcitonin	Maintains serum calcium levels by decreasing bone resorption (the loss of bone or substance by disease) and decreasing resorption of calcium in the kidneys whenever levels of plasma calcium are elevated.
Parathyroid gland	Parathyroid hormone (PTH)	Maintains serum calcium levels by stimulating bone resorption and formation and by stimulating kidney resorption of calcium in response to falling levels of plasma calcium.
Adrenal cortex	Mineralocorticoids (e.g., aldosterone)	Promote kidney tubule reabsorption of sodium and water and excretion of potassium in response to elevated levels of potassium and low levels of sodium, thereby increasing blood pressure and blood volume.
	Glucocorticoids (e.g., cortisol)	Help regulate metabolism of carbohydrates, fats and proteins. Activate anti-inflammatory responses to stressors. Low cortisol levels stimulate hypothalamic secretion of corticotropin-releasing hormone (CRH), which stimulates the anterior pituitary gland to release ACTH, which in turn stimulates the adrenal cortex to secrete cortisol.
	Gonadocorticoids (androgens and small amounts of oestrogen and progesterone)	The quantity of sex hormones produced here is small, and the mechanism is not well understood.
Adrenal medulla	Catecholamine (epinephrine and norepinephrine)	Stimulate the heart, constrict blood vessels, inhibit visceral muscles, dilate bronchioles, increase respiration and metabolism and promote hyperglycaemia. Secreted in response to physical or psychological stress.
Anterior pituitary (adenohypophysis)	Growth hormone (GH)	Promotes growth of body tissues by enhancing protein synthesis and promoting use of fat for energy and thus conserving glucose. Release is stimulated by growth hormone releasing hormone (GHRH) in response to low GH levels, **hypoglycaemia**, increased amino acids, low fatty acids and stress.

● Oxytocin induces contraction of the smooth muscles in the reproductive organs. In women, oxytocin stimulates the myometrium of the uterus to contract during labour. It also induces milk ejection from the breasts.

THYROID GLAND

The thyroid gland is anterior (in the front) to the upper part of the trachea and just inferior (below) to the larynx. This butterfly-shaped gland has two lobes connected by a structure called the isthmus.

The glandular tissue consists of follicles filled with a jelly-like colloid substance called thyroglobin, a glycoprotein–iodine complex. Cells within the follicles secrete thyroid hormone (TH), a general name for two similar hormones: thyroxin (T$_4$) and tri-iodothyronine (T$_3$). The primary role of

thyroid hormones in adults is to increase metabolism. TH secretion is initiated by the release of TSH by the pituitary gland and is dependent on an adequate supply of iodine. The thyroid gland also secretes calcitonin, a hormone that decreases excessive levels of calcium in the blood by slowing the calcium-releasing activity of bone cells, serves as a marker for sepsis (infection) and is believed to be a mediator of inflammatory responses.

PARATHYROID GLANDS

The parathyroid glands (usually four to six in number) are embedded on the posterior surface of the lobes of the thyroid gland. They secrete parathyroid hormone (PTH), or parathormone. When calcium levels in the plasma fall, PTH secretion increases. PTH also controls phosphate metabolism. It acts primarily by increasing renal excretion of phosphate in the urine, by decreasing the excretion of calcium, and by increasing bone reabsorption to cause the release of calcium from bones. Normal levels of vitamin D are necessary for PTH to exert these effects on bone and kidneys.

ADRENAL GLANDS

The two adrenal glands are pyramid-shaped organs that sit on top of the kidneys. Each gland consists of two parts, which are distinct organs: an inner medulla and an outer cortex.

The adrenal medulla produces two hormones (also called catecholamine): epinephrine (adrenaline) and norepinephrine (noradrenaline). These hormones are similar to substances released by the sympathetic nervous system and thus are not essential to life. Epinephrine increases blood glucose levels and stimulates the release of ACTH from the pituitary; ACTH, in turn, stimulates the adrenal cortex to release glucocorticoids. Epinephrine also increases the rate and force of cardiac contractions; constricts blood vessels in the skin, mucous membranes and kidneys; and dilates blood vessels in the skeletal muscles, coronary arteries and pulmonary arteries. Norepinephrine increases both heart rate and the force of cardiac contractions and vasoconstricts throughout the body.

The adrenal cortex secretes several hormones, all corticosteroids. They are classified into two groups: mineralocorticoids and glucocorticoids. These hormones are essential to life. The release of the mineralocorticoids is controlled primarily by an enzyme called renin. When a decrease in blood pressure or sodium is detected, specialised kidney cells release renin to act on a substance called angiotensinogen (plasma protein produced by the liver). Angiotensinogen is modified by renin and other enzymes to become angiotensin II, which stimulates the release of aldosterone from the adrenal cortex. Aldosterone prompts the distal tubules and the collecting ducts of the nephron to reabsorb increased amounts of water and sodium back into the circulating blood to increase circulating blood volume and pressure.

The glucocorticoids include cortisol and cortisone. These hormones affect carbohydrate metabolism by regulating glucose use in body tissues, mobilising fatty acids from fatty tissue and shifting the source of energy for muscle cells from glucose to fatty acids. Glucocorticoids are released in times of stress. An excess of glucocorticoids in the body depresses the inflammatory response and inhibits the effectiveness of the immune system.

PANCREAS

The pancreas, located behind the stomach between the spleen and the duodenum, is both an endocrine gland (producing hormones) and an **exocrine** gland (producing digestive enzymes). The endocrine cells of the pancreas produce hormones that regulate carbohydrate metabolism. They are clustered in bodies called pancreatic islets (or islets of Langerhans) scattered throughout the gland. Pancreatic islets have at least four different cell types:

- Alpha cells produce glucagon.
- Beta cells produce insulin.
- Delta cells secrete somatostatin.
- F cells secrete pancreatic polypeptide.

GONADS

The gonads are the testes in men and the ovaries in women. These organs are the primary source of steroid sex hormones in the body. The hormones of the gonads are important in regulating body growth and promoting the onset of puberty. In men, androgens (primarily testosterone) produced by the testes maintain reproductive functioning and secondary sex characteristics and promote the production of sperm. In women, the ovaries secrete oestrogens and progesterone to maintain reproductive functioning and secondary sex characteristics. Progesterone also promotes the growth of the lining of the uterus to prepare for implantation of a fertilised ovum.

An overview of hormones

Although we rarely think about the glands of the endocrine system, the hormones they release influence almost every cell, organ and function of our bodies. The endocrine system is instrumental in regulating mood, growth and development, tissue function and metabolism, as well as sexual function and reproductive processes. So what are hormones?

Hormones are chemical messengers secreted by the endocrine organs and transported throughout the body, where they exert their action on specific cells called target cells. Hormones do not cause reactions directly but rather regulate tissue responses. They may produce either generalised effects or local effects.

Hormones are transported from endocrine gland cells to target cells in the body in one of four ways.

- Endocrine glands release most hormones, including TH and insulin, into the bloodstream.
- Neurons release some hormones, such as epinephrine, into the bloodstream.
- The hypothalamus releases its hormones directly to target cells in the posterior pituitary by nerve cell extension.
- With the paracrine ('para' = near; group of local hormones that work on nearby cells) method, released messengers diffuse through the interstitial fluid. This method of transport involves a number of hormonal peptides that are released throughout various organs and cells and act locally. An example is endorphins, which act to relieve pain.

Hormones that are released into the bloodstream circulate as either free, unbound molecules or as hormones attached to transport carriers. Peptide and protein hormones (such as insulin) circulate unbound, while steroid and thyroid hormones are carried by specific transport carriers **synthesised** by the liver. Hormone receptors are complex molecular structures, located on or inside target cells. They act by binding to specific receptor sites located on the surfaces of the target cells. These receptors recognise a specific hormone and translate the message into a cellular response. The receptor sites are structured so that they respond only to a specific hormone; for example, receptors in the thyroid gland are responsive to TSH but not to LH.

Hormone levels are controlled by the pituitary gland and by feedback mechanisms. Although most feedback mechanisms are negative, a few are positive. Negative feedback is controlled much as the thermostat in a house regulates temperature. Sensors in the endocrine system detect changes in hormone levels and adjust hormone secretion to maintain normal body levels. When the sensors detect a decrease in hormone levels, they begin actions to cause an increase in hormone levels; when hormone levels rise above normal, the sensors cause a decrease in hormone production and release. For example, when the hypothalamus or anterior pituitary gland senses increased blood levels of TH, it releases hormones, causing a reduction in the secretion of TSH, which in turn prompts a decrease in the output of TH by the thyroid gland (see Figure 6.3).

In positive feedback mechanisms, increasing levels of one hormone cause another gland to release a hormone. For example, the increased production of oestradiol (a female ovarian hormone) during the follicular stage of the menstrual cycle in turn stimulates increased FSH production by the anterior pituitary gland. Oestradiol levels continue to increase until the ovarian follicle disappears, eliminating the source of the stimulation for FSH, which then decreases.

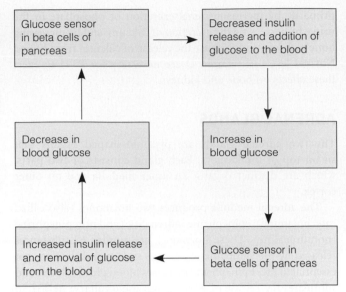

Figure 6.3 Negative feedback.

Stimuli for hormone release may also be classified as hormonal, **humoral** or neural (Figure 6.4 A, B, C). In hormonal release, hypothalamic hormones stimulate the anterior pituitary to release hormones. Fluctuations in the serum (fluid portion of the blood) level of these hormones in turn prompt other endocrine glands to release hormones. In the case of humoral release, changes in the serum levels of certain electrolytes and nutrients stimulate specific endocrine glands to release hormones to bring these levels back to normal. However, in neural release, nerve fibres stimulate the release of hormones.

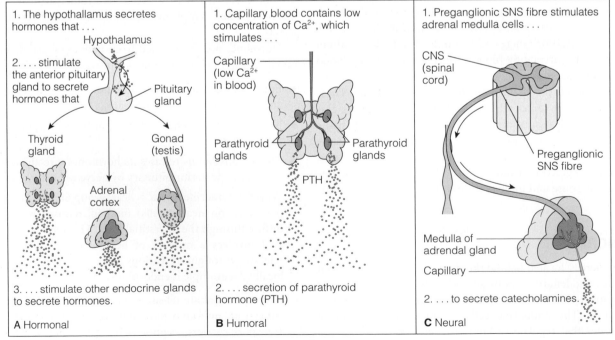

Figure 6.4 Examples of three mechanisms of hormone release.

DISORDERS OF THE ENDOCRINE SYSTEM

Now that we have looked at the anatomy and physiology of the endocrine system, let us consider some of the disorders that you might come across in practice such as hyper- and **hypothyroidism**, diabetes mellitus and disorders of the pituitary gland.

FAST FACTS

Hyperthyroidism

About 2 in 100 women and 2 in 1000 men develop **hyperthyroidism** at some stage of their life and it can occur at any age.

Source: Patient UK 2010.

The person with hyperthyroidism

Hyperthyroidism (also called thyrotoxicosis) is a disorder caused by excessive secretion of TH. Because the primary function of TH is to increase metabolism and protein synthesis, hyperthyroidism affects all major organ systems of the body. The increase in metabolic rate and the alterations in cardiac output, peripheral blood flow, oxygen consumption and body temperature are similar to those found in increased sympathetic nervous system activity. The effects of hyperthyroidism are the result of increased circulating levels of TH. This hormonal excess increases the metabolic rate and heightens the sympathetic nervous system's physiologic response to stimulation.

Pathophysiology of hyperthyroidism

Hyperthyroidism results from many different factors, including autoimmune stimulation (as in Graves' disease), excess secretion of TSH by the pituitary gland, thyroiditis, neoplasm (such as toxic multinodular goitre) and an excessive intake of iodine-containing drugs such as amiodarone. The most common aetiologies of hyperthyroidism are Graves' disease and toxic multinodular **goitre**.

Signs and symptoms of hyperthyroidism

Signs and symptoms of hyperthyroidism include:

- increased appetite yet with weight loss as a result of increased metabolism;
- increased **peristalsis** and diarrhoea;
- heat intolerance;
- insomnia;
- palpitations;
- increased sweating;

- skin is smooth and warm;
- hair becomes fine;
- hair loss in the scalp, eyebrow, axilla.

For multisystem effects of hyperthyroidism see Figure 6.5.

Graves' disease

Graves' disease results from overactivity of the thyroid gland. It is thought to be an autoimmune disease, where the immune system produces an antibody that stimulates the cells of the thyroid gland to secrete an excessive amount of thyroid hormones. The disease is seen five times more often in women than in men and occurs most frequently between the ages of 20 and 40. It has a strong hereditary component; when one identical twin has Graves' disease, the other twin will have it 25% of the time. Factors that can trigger the onset of Graves' disease include stress, smoking, radiation to the neck and infectious organisms such as viruses.

The ophthalmopathy (disease of the eye) of Graves' disease is manifested as **proptosis** and visual dysfunction. Proptosis (forward displacement) of the eye occurs in about one-third of cases. The forward protrusion of the eyeballs (exophthalmoses) results from an accumulation of inflammation byproducts in the retro-orbital tissues. Often the sclera is visible above the iris. The upper lids are often retracted, and the person has a characteristic unblinking stare. Graves' disease can have an effect on many parts of the body such as the nervous system, eyes, skin, hair/nails, lungs, digestive system, muscles/bones and reproductive system.

Toxic multinodular goitre

Toxic multinodular goitre is a tumour characterised by small, discrete, independently functioning nodules in the thyroid gland tissue that secrete excessive amounts of TH. It is not known how these nodules grow or become independent, but a genetic mutation of follicle cells is suspected. Elevated TH levels result in signs and symptoms of hyperthyroidism; however, they are slower to develop and neither ophthalmopathy nor dermopathy develop. The person with this type of hyperthyroidism is usually a woman in her 60s or 70s who has had goitre for a number of years.

INTERDISCIPLINARY CARE FOR HYPERTHYROIDISM

Hyperthyroidism results from a raised level of thyroid hormone (TH). The treatment of hyperthyroidism focuses on reducing the production of TH by the thyroid gland. Treatment is usually effective. The treatment to reduce the thyroxine level include: medicines, radioiodine and surgery. Long-term follow-up is important, even after successful treatment.

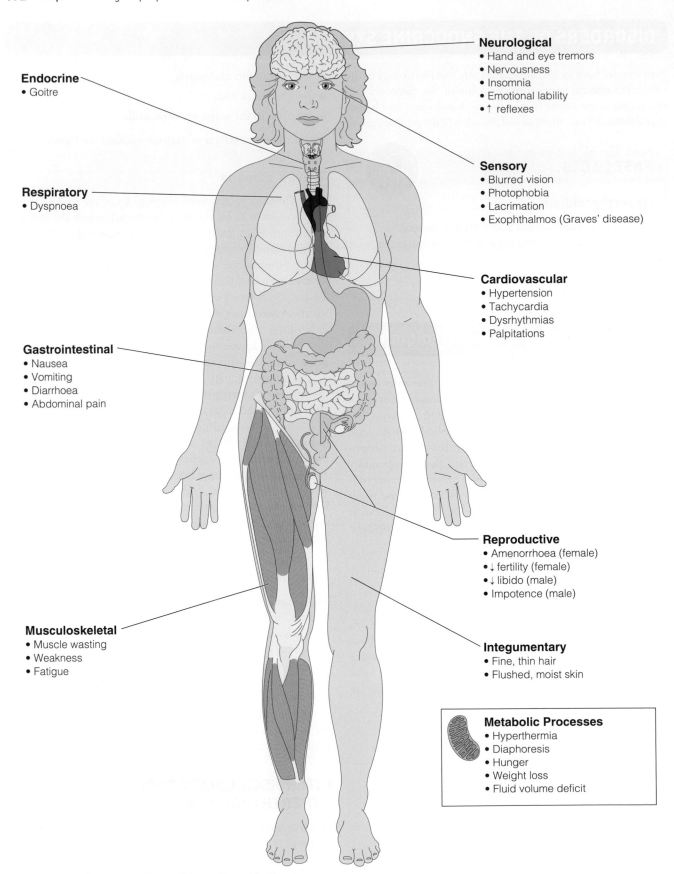

Endocrine
• Goitre

Respiratory
• Dyspnoea

Gastrointestinal
• Nausea
• Vomiting
• Diarrhoea
• Abdominal pain

Musculoskeletal
• Muscle wasting
• Weakness
• Fatigue

Neurological
• Hand and eye tremors
• Nervousness
• Insomnia
• Emotional lability
• ↑ reflexes

Sensory
• Blurred vision
• Photophobia
• Lacrimation
• Exophthalmos (Graves' disease)

Cardiovascular
• Hypertension
• Tachycardia
• Dysrhythmias
• Palpitations

Reproductive
• Amenorrhoea (female)
• ↓ fertility (female)
• ↓ libido (male)
• Impotence (male)

Integumentary
• Fine, thin hair
• Flushed, moist skin

Metabolic Processes
• Hyperthermia
• Diaphoresis
• Hunger
• Weight loss
• Fluid volume deficit

Figure 6.5 Multisystem effects of hyperthyroidism.

Medication

Hyperthyroidism is treated by administering antithyroid medications, such as carbimazole 30–40 mg/day, which reduce TH production. Because antithyroid drugs do not affect the release or activity of hormone that is already formed, therapeutic effects may not be seen for several weeks. The person will continue to take the medication until euthyroid state is achieved. To rapidly decrease the cardiovascular symptoms such as **hypertension** associated with hyperthyroidism, propanolol (Inderal), a beta blocker, may form part of initial treatment.

Surgery

Some hyperthyroid persons have such enlarged thyroid glands that pressure on the oesophagus or trachea causes swallowing or breathing problems respectively. In these cases, removal of all or part of the gland is indicated. In partial **thyroidectomy** enough of the gland is left in place to produce an adequate amount of TH. However, in total thyroidectomy the person then requires lifelong hormone replacement therapy.

Radioactive therapy

Radioactive iodine-131 (^{131}I) is absorbed and is concentrated in the thyroid gland. Iodine-131 damages or destroys thyroid cells resulting in less production of the thyroid hormone. The drug is administered as a single capsule and the patient is advised not to eat for approximately four hours in order for the effective absorption of the iodine. Patients are also advised to drink approximately 2–3 L of fluid over the 24-hour period and to urinate frequently to get rid of the filtrated radioactive iodine promptly. This treatment is offered to patients who may not be suitable for surgery.

NURSING CARE PLAN The person having a partial thyroidectomy

Review Chapter 1 for routine pre- and post-operative care.

Pre-operative care

+ Persons are prepared in accordance with the local policy and guidelines.

+ Teach the person to support the neck by placing both hands behind the neck when sitting up in bed, while moving about and while coughing. *Placing the hands behind the neck provides support for the suture line.*

+ Answer questions and allow time for the person to verbalise concerns. *Because the incision is made at the base of the throat, persons (especially women) are often concerned about their appearance after surgery.* Explain that the scar will eventually be only a thin line and that jewellery or scarves may be used to cover the scar.

+ Teach the person to expect hoarseness due to generalised swelling at the suture line. *This is expected to diminish with healing and is not caused by laryngeal nerve damage.*

+ Provide information about pain control post-operatively *to lessen the person's anxiety about pain control.*

+ Check with local protocols with regard to safe preparation of a person for partial thyroidectomy.

+ Document all care in accordance with the NMC guidelines for records and record keeping.

Post-operative care

+ Nurses should monitor the person's airway half hourly as a result of surgery to the neck area. Ensure that the airway is not obstructed and that the person is sitting in an upright position with the neck supported by pillows. *The support should provide comfort for the person, reduce the strain on the suture line and minimise the pain level.*

+ Monitor the wound site for any haemorrhage following surgery. Record blood pressure, respiration and heart rate half hourly and report any changes in the vital signs immediately to facilitate prompt action. *An increase in heart rate and a drop in blood pressure may indicate a haemorrhaging wound which should be reported immediately for prompt action.*

+ Observe for signs such as **stridor**, difficulty in swallowing, noisy breathing which could indicate laryngeal nerve damage from surgery. *One of the possible complications of thyroidectomy is damage to the laryngeal nerve during surgery. This nerve damage could result in vocal cord spasm and paralysis of the larynx which could suppress respiration.*

+ Observe for signs of tetany resulting from accidental removal of the parathyroid glands: tingling of toes, fingers and lips; muscular twitches; positive **Chvostek's sign** and **Trousseau's sign**. *A sudden decrease in calcium level could result in tetany and if untreated could be fatal for the person.*

+ Document all care provided in accordance with the Nursing and Midwifery Guidelines for records and record keeping.

NURSING CARE FOR HYPERTHYROIDISM

Nursing diagnoses and interventions

Nursing diagnoses and interventions for hyperthyroidism focus on cardiac output, sensory perception and body image.

Risk for decreased cardiac output

The person with hyperthyroidism is at risk for alterations in cardiac output. Excess TH directly affects the heart, resulting in increased rate and stroke volume. Increases in the metabolic demands and oxygen requirements of peripheral tissues increase the demands on the heart, and systolic hypertension, angina, arrhythmias or cardiac failure may occur. The person often has palpitations and shortness of breath and is easily fatigued. The risk of complications is greater in persons with pre-existing cardiovascular disorders.

✚ Monitor blood pressure, pulse rate and rhythm and respiratory rate and sounds. Assess for peripheral oedema, jugular vein distention and increased activity intolerance. Increased TH increases cardiac rate, stroke volume and tissue demand

COMMUNITY-BASED CARE

Persons with hyperthyroidism primarily provide self-care at home. Teaching is individualised to meet the person's needs. Nurses need to address the following topics:

● The person taking oral medications must understand the need for lifelong treatment.

● The person who has a thyroidectomy requires information about post-operative wound care.

● The person having radioactive iodine therapy needs to know the symptoms of hypothyroidism.

● Depending on the age of the person and the support systems available, referral to community healthcare agencies may be necessary.

● In addition, suggest the following resources which are accessible via the Internet:
  – British Thyroid Foundation (www.btf-thyroid.org);
  – Thyroid Eye Disease Charitable Trust (www.tedct.co.uk)

for oxygen, causing stress on the heart. This may result in hypertension, arrhythmias, tachycardia and congestive heart failure.

✚ Suggest keeping the environment as cool and free of distraction as possible. Decrease stress by explaining interventions and teaching relaxation procedures. A physically comfortable and psychologically calm environment can reduce stimuli and stressors. Stress increases circulating catecholamine, which further increases cardiac workload.

Disturbed sensory perception

Visual changes that occur in clients with hyperthyroidism include difficulty in focusing, diplopia (double vision) or visual loss. If the patient is unable to close the eyelids because of exophthalmos, the risk of corneal dryness with resultant infection or injury increases. Visual deficits may also result from pressure on the optic nerve from retro-orbital oedema and the shortening of eye muscles. Therefore nurses need to:

✚ Monitor visual acuity, photophobia, integrity of the cornea and lid closure. *The cornea is at risk for dryness, injury, conjunctivitis, and corneal infections. Injury and infection of the cornea can result in further loss of visual acuity.*

✚ Teach measures for protecting the eye from injury and maintaining visual acuity:
  a. Use tinted glasses or shields as protection.
  b. Use appropriate eye drops to moisten the eyes.
  c. Use cool, moist compresses to relieve irritation.
  d. Cover or tape eyelids shut at night if they do not close.
  e. Elevate the head of the bed to 45 degrees to promote periorbital fluid decrease.
  f. Promptly report any pain or changes in vision.

Disturbed body image

Physical changes common in hyperthyroidism include exophthalmos, goitre, tremors, hair loss, weight loss and changes in sexual function such as amenorrhoea in women and impotence in men. In addition, the patient may have mood changes and insomnia. The changes are of concern to the patient and their family.

✚ Nurses need to establish a trusting relationship. Encourage the patient to verbalise their worries about their condition and ask questions. *Establishing a trust facilitates open sharing of feelings and promotes recovery.*

Case Study 1 – Paulette
NURSING CARE PLAN Hyperthyroidism

Remember in planning care, you should utilise the four key aspects of the nursing process (NP): that is, assessment, planning, implementation and evaluation. These four elements of the NP can be used with any models of care, such as Roper, Logan and

Tierney's 12 activities of living. Remember that Mrs Paulette Jones was admitted with swollen neck and protruding eyeballs, eats like a horse but is losing weight. What is her diagnosis? Explain with rationale the presenting signs and symptoms.

Case Study 1 – Paulette

NURSING CARE PLAN Hyperthyroidism

Actual/potential problems from her assessment

✚ Mrs Jones is losing weight even though she has a good appetite. This may be due to increased metabolism.

✚ Risk for disturbed sensory perception: she is unable to close the eyelids completely. This may be due to conjunctival oedema or exophthalmos. This may cause visual loss.

✚ Anxiety related to a lack of knowledge about disease process.

Objectives/goals–planning process

✚ We know that Mrs Jones has not lost her appetite and is eating well. The aim here is to ensure that Mrs Jones gains at least 0.45 kg every two weeks.

✚ Maintain normal vision (with no evidence of corneal damage) and verbalise measures to protect her eyes.

✚ Mrs Jones will verbalise self-care needs.

✚ Mrs Jones will verbalise a decrease in anxiety after gaining information about the illness.

Nursing interventions – implementation of care

✚ Request that she keeps a record of daily weight. Inform the person to weigh herself the same time of the day before breakfast and preferably wearing the same clothing.

✚ Discuss eating a high-kilocalorie diet. Identify food she likes and dislikes, as well as foods that increase diarrhoea, before instituting a plan to increase food intake.

✚ Advise on the correct method of applying eye drops.

✚ Explain the need to elevate the head of the bed to 45 degrees at night, and tape eye shields over eyes before sleep.

✚ Give information about the disease, the medication's effects and side-effects and the need for continued nursing care.

Evaluation

Mrs Jones has gained 0.45 kg and has discussed her dietary needs with the nurse and her husband. She is having diarrhoea less often. She has safely applied the eye drops and states that she uses the eye shields and elevates the head of her bed at night. The practice nurse reviewed the written and verbal information about Graves' disease and the medication prescribed. Mrs Jones verbalises her understanding, stating, *'I'll always take my medicine – I never want to feel like that again!'* She also says that she feels less anxious now that she understands her illness.

Consider this . . .

● What is the rationale for Mrs Jones' abnormal vital signs?

● What is the rationale for having the person with exophthalmos elevate the head of the bed at night?

● Discuss the health promotion/education for a person following a partial thyroidectomy.

PRACTICE ALERT

Teach the person to cover or tape the eyelids shut at night if they do not close and to sleep with the head of the bed elevated.

IN PRACTICE

Radioactive iodine therapy

Before commencing radioactive iodine therapy, the person will have stopped taking any thyroid hormones for approximately three to six weeks. This is to ensure that the level of TSH rises in the bloodstream, which improves the uptake of radioactive iodine. Before radioactive iodine treatment the person may be asked to start eating a low-iodine diet, avoiding foods such as fish or sea-food and also vitamin supplements that contain iodine, as too much iodine in the body will make the treatment less effective. Nursing responsibilities include:

● Assessing the person for hypersensitivity to radioactive iodine before giving the medication; for example, ask the person if they are allergic to shellfish.

● The person and their relatives should be given clear explanation on the effects of iodine and the reason why the

person is nursed in a single room and why the visitors are restricted. Nurses should take every precaution when handling the person's body fluid, such as wearing gloves, wearing film badges by nurses to indicate radiation exposure.

● Measures should be taken to prevent constipation, as this prevents the excretion of the radioactive material. Encourage the person to take 2.5–3 L of fluid to promote good urinary output. Where possible disposable crockery should be used.

● Commodes or bedpans should be designated for the person's exclusive use as all body fluid will be highly radioactive.

● Encourage the person to shower or bathe regularly to remove contaminated perspiration.

● Document the outcome of the treatment in the patient's notes.

Now let us look at hypothyroidism. Hypothyroidism means that the thyroid gland does not make enough thyroxine (hormone). It is often called an underactive thyroid. This causes many of the body's functions to slow down. In contrast, if you have hyperthyroidism, you make too much thyroxine. This causes many of the body's functions to speed up.

The person with hypothyroidism

Hypothyroidism is a disorder that results when the thyroid gland produces an insufficient amount of TH. Low levels of TH decreases metabolic rate and heat production, and hypothyroidism can affect all systems of the body (see Figure 6.6). Hypothyroidism is more common in women than men and most common between the ages of 30 and 60 years. However, the disorder can occur at any stage of life. Careful evaluation of symptoms is important in the older adult because signs and symptoms of hypothyroidism are often thought to be the result of ageing instead of a pathological process.

FAST FACTS

Hypothyroidism

About 1 in 50 women and about 1 in 1000 men develop hypothyroidism at some time in their life.

It most commonly develops in adult women, and becomes more common with increasing age.

Source: Patient UK 2011.

The hypothyroid state in adults is sometimes called myxoedema. The term reflects the characteristic accumulation of non-pitting (no indentation mark on the skin when pressed) oedema in the connective tissues throughout the body. The oedema is the result of water retention in mucoprotein (hydrophilic proteoglycans) deposits in the interstitial spaces (space surrounding a cell). The face of a person with myxoedema appears puffy, the tongue is enlarged and the voice is hoarse and husky.

Pathophysiology of hypothyroidism

Hypothyroidism may be either primary or secondary. Primary hypothyroidism (which is more common) may be caused by congenital defects in the gland, loss of thyroid tissue following treatment for hyperthyroidism with surgery or radiation, antithyroid medications, thyroiditis or endemic iodine deficiency. Secondary hypothyroidism may result from pituitary TSH deficiency or peripheral resistance to thyroid hormones.

Hypothyroidism has a slow onset, with signs and symptoms occurring over months or even years. With treatment, the mental and physical symptoms rapidly improve in persons of all ages.

When TH production decreases, the thyroid gland enlarges in a compensatory attempt to produce more hormones. The goitre that results is usually a simple or non-toxic form. People living in certain areas of the world where the soil is deficient in iodine, the substance necessary for TH synthesis and secretion, are more prone to become hypothyroid and develop simple goitre.

Signs and symptoms of hypothyroidism

Signs and symptoms of hypothyroidism include:

- fluid retention;
- oedema (swelling as a result of accumulation of serous fluid);
- decreased appetite;
- weight gain;
- constipation;
- dry skin;
- dyspnoea (shortness of breath);
- pallor;
- hoarseness
- muscle stiffness;
- low basal metabolic rate;
- sleep apnoea (absence of spontaneous breathing);
- bradycardia (low pulse rate).

INTERDISCIPLINARY CARE FOR HYPOTHYROIDISM

Medication

Hypothyroidism is treated with medications that replace TH. Levothyroxine (thyroxin, T_4) is the treatment of choice. In elderly persons, an age-related decrease in serum albumin and renal excretion can increase the amount of available drug and cause an exaggerated pharmacologic effect. Therefore, the elderly may require less thyroid medication than a younger person.

NURSING CARE FOR HYPOTHYROIDISM

The nursing management of the person with hypothyroidism focuses on diagnosis, prevention or treatment of complications and replacement of the deficient TH. With early and continued treatment, both appearance and mental function return to normal. In planning and implementing care for persons with hypothyroidism, the nurse must take into account that the disorder affects all organ systems.

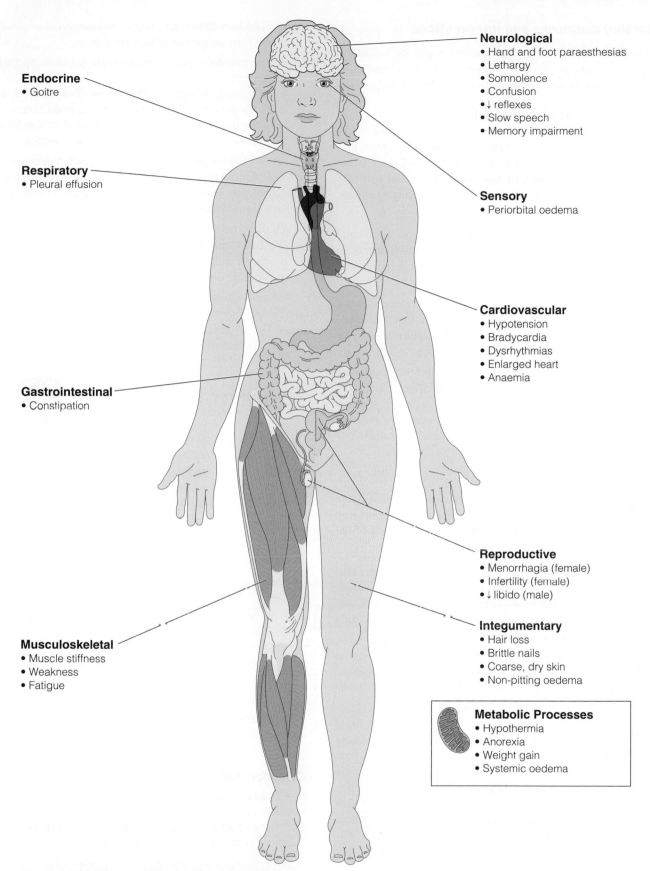

Endocrine
• Goitre

Respiratory
• Pleural effusion

Gastrointestinal
• Constipation

Musculoskeletal
• Muscle stiffness
• Weakness
• Fatigue

Neurological
• Hand and foot paraesthesias
• Lethargy
• Somnolence
• Confusion
• ↓ reflexes
• Slow speech
• Memory impairment

Sensory
• Periorbital oedema

Cardiovascular
• Hypotension
• Bradycardia
• Dysrhythmias
• Enlarged heart
• Anaemia

Reproductive
• Menorrhagia (female)
• Infertility (female)
• ↓ libido (male)

Integumentary
• Hair loss
• Brittle nails
• Coarse, dry skin
• Non-pitting oedema

Metabolic Processes
• Hypothermia
• Anorexia
• Weight gain
• Systemic oedema

Figure 6.6 Multisystem effects of hypothyroidism.

Nursing diagnoses and interventions

Although many nursing interventions might be valid, this section focuses on specific person needs with regards to cardiovascular function, elimination and skin integrity.

Risk for decreased cardiac output

A TH deficit causes a reduction in heart rate and stroke volume, resulting in decreased cardiac output. There may also be an accumulation of fluid in the pericardial sac (from the oedema characteristic of hypothyroidism), and coronary artery disease may be present, further compromising cardiac function.

✚ Monitor blood pressure, rate and rhythm of apical and peripheral pulses, respiratory rate, and sounds. *Hypotension indicates decreasing peripheral blood. Fluid in the pericardial sac restricts cardiac function.*

✚ Suggest the person avoid cold room temperature; increase room temperature, use additional bed covers and avoid drafts. *Chilling of the body increases metabolic rate and puts increased stress on the heart.*

✚ Explain the need to alternate activity with rest periods. Ask the person to report any breathing difficulties, chest pain, heart palpitations or dizziness. *Activity increases demands on the heart and should be balanced with rest. Symptoms of cardiac stress include dyspnoea, chest pain, palpitations and dizziness.*

Risk for constipation

The hypothyroid person is likely to have a reduced appetite and decreased food intake, a diminished activity level because of muscle aches and weakness and reduced peristalsis of the intestine to the point that faecal impactions may occur.

✚ Encourage a fluid intake of up to 2500–3000 mL per day. Discuss preferred liquids and the best times of day to drink fluids. If kilocalorie intake is restricted, ensure that liquids have no kilocalorie or are low in kilocalories. *Sufficient fluid intake is necessary to promote proper stool consistency.*

✚ Discuss ways to maintain a high-fibre diet. *Diets high in fibre and fluid produce soft stools. Fibre that is not digested absorbs water, which adds bulk to the stool and assists in the movement of faecal material through the intestines.*

✚ Encourage activity as tolerated. *Activity influences bowel elimination by improving muscle tone and stimulating peristalsis.*

Risk for impaired skin integrity

The person with hypothyroidism is at risk for impaired skin integrity related to the accumulation of fluid in the interstitial spaces and to dry, rough skin. Decreased peripheral circulation, decreased activity levels and slow wound healing further increase the risk.

✚ Monitor skin surfaces for redness or lesions, especially if the person's activity is greatly reduced. Use a pressure ulcer risk assessment scale to identify persons at risk.

Hypothyroidism causes dry, rough, oedematous skin conditions that increase the risk of skin breakdown.

✚ Teach the immobile person measures to promote optimal circulation:
  – use a turning schedule if the person is on bedrest, or teach the person to change position every two hours;
  – limit the time for sitting in one position; shift weight or lift the body using arm rests every 20–30 minutes;

✚ Teach and implement a schedule of range-of-motion exercises. *Prolonged pressure, especially in persons with oedema and circulatory impairment, can occlude capillaries and cause hypoxic tissue damage.*

✚ Teach the person measures to maintain skin integrity:
  – take baths only as necessary; use warm (not hot) water;
  – use gentle motions when washing and drying skin;
  – use suitable ointments or lotions.

Dry skin and oedema increase the risk of skin breakdown. Hot water, rough massage and alcohol-based preparations may increase skin dryness, further impairing the body's ability to maintain skin integrity.

COMMUNITY-BASED CARE

Persons with hypothyroidism require lifelong care, primarily at home. The community nursing team should reinforce the explanations given by the nurses in the hospital, such as the need to continue treatment at home. Nurses need to address the following topics:

● the need to take medications (thyroxine replacement therapy) for the rest of the person's life;

● the need for periodic dosage reassessments;

● the importance of attending regular checkups to ensure that a euthyroid state is achieved and maintained;

● if the persons suffers any unwanted side-effects from the hormone therapy, to report to his/her GP or practice immediately;

● if the person is older or does not have a support system, helpful community resources;

● additional resources: British Thyroid Foundation (www.btf-thyroid.org).

Consider this . . .

Persons who suffer from hypo/hyperthyroidism require careful monitoring of their vital signs. What is the reason for this? Think about the thyroid gland and what hormone it secretes and the function of the hormone.

How is hypothyroidism related to osteoporosis? What specific pathophysiological processes increase the risk of osteoporosis? How does a calcium supplement prevent the development of osteoporosis?

Case Study 2 – Veronica
NURSING CARE PLAN Hypothyroidism

You now have some knowledge about hypothyroidism and the problems associated with it, so let us now return to Mrs Veronica Patel. Here we have a second-year student nurse who is generally feeling unwell, feels cold most of the time and has become intolerant to certain foodstuff. What do think her diagnosis is and can you list some of the signs and symptoms related to the condition?

Actual/potential problems from her assessment

✚ *Constipation* related to decreased peristalsis, as evidenced by hard, formed stools every four days.

✚ *Feeling cold as a result of low metabolism.*

✚ *Low self-esteem* related to tiredness and depression.

Objectives/goals – planning process

✚ Regain normal bowel elimination patterns, having a soft, formed stool at least every other day.

✚ Mrs Patel to verbalise that she is not feeling cold as a result of increased metabolism.

✚ Regain positive self-esteem as medication reduces tiredness and depression.

Nursing interventions – implementations of care

✚ Educate Mrs Patel to increase fluids, bulk and fibre in the diet to help regain a normal bowel elimination pattern of a soft, formed stool every other day.

✚ Take medication as prescribed and do not expect immediate reversal of symptoms.

✚ Plan activities around rest periods. Encourage her husband to help with housecleaning and cooking.

✚ Encourage Mrs Patel to rest between activities.

✚ Teach Mrs Patel to weigh herself once a week, at the same time and wearing the same clothing.

Evaluation

On return to the health centre two months later, Mrs Patel reports that she is no longer constipated but that she is continuing to drink six glasses of water and eating oatmeal every day. She no longer feels cold, is regaining her normal energy and even feels well enough to do some gardening. Her speech is clear and easy to understand. As she leaves the health centre, Mrs Patel says, 'It's hard to believe that I have changed so much–now I look and feel like the "old" me!'

> ### Consider this . . .
> - What physical changes that normally occur with ageing are similar to the signs and symptoms of hypothyroidism?
> - Describe the factors that put Mrs Patel's safety at risk.
> - What alterations in her home environment would you suggest to promote safety until the prescribed medications take effect?

The person with cancer of the thyroid

Each year in England and Wales there are an estimated 1200 new cases of thyroid cancer (NHS Choices 2011). It is more common in women than men and can occur at any age. The risk of thyroid cancer goes up with age in men until 75 years of age. For women, the risk stays fairly constant between the ages of 30 and 55 and then falls. Of the several types of thyroid cancer, the most common types are:

- Papillary thyroid carcinoma is the most common thyroid malignancy. It is usually detected as a single nodule, but may arise from a multinodular goitre. The average age of diagnosis is 42, with 70% of cases occurring in women. Risks for the development of this form are exposure to external x-ray treatments to the head or neck as a child, childhood exposure to radioactive isotopes of iodine in nuclear fallout and a family history. Papillary thyroid carcinoma is the least aggressive type, but does metastasise to the local and regional lymph nodes and lungs.

- Follicular thyroid cancer is the second most common thyroid malignancy. The average age of diagnosis is 50, with 73% of cases occurring in women. This form is more aggressive, with potential for vascular invasion and spread to lung and bone.

- People exposed to high levels of radiation are much more likely than others to develop papillary or follicular thyroid cancer.

FAST FACTS

Thyroid cancer

- Carcinoma of the thyroid gland is rare, comprising approximately 1% of all cancers.

- It is three times more common in women than men and can occur at any age.

Source: http://www.nhsdirect.wales.nhs.uk/encyclopaedia/c/article/cancerofthethyroid/ (accessed September 2011).

Thyroid cancer is manifested by a palpable, firm non-tender nodule in the thyroid. If undetected, the tumour may grow and impinge on the oesophagus or trachea, causing difficulty in swallowing or breathing. Most people with thyroid cancer do not have elevated thyroid hormone levels. The diagnosis is made by measuring thyroid hormones, performing thyroid scans and by fine-needle biopsy of the nodule. The usual treatment is subtotal or total thyroidectomy. TSH suppression therapy with levothyroxine may be conducted prior to surgery. Radioactive iodine therapy (^{131}I) and chemotherapy are additional therapeutic options.

The nursing care should include:

- person/relatives education about treatment and condition;
- health promotion – altered body image; compliance to treatment;
- counselling;
- financial support.

Persons diagnosed with cancer will need a lot of support from doctors, specialist nurses and other organisations.

Consider this . . .

Why are persons encouraged to drink large volumes of fluid during radioactive iodine (131) therapy? Think about the effect the iodine will have on the bladder wall.

DISORDERS OF THE PITUITARY GLAND

The pituitary gland produces hormones that affect multiple body systems through regulation of endocrine function. Target tissues include the thyroid, adrenal cortex, ovary, uterus, mammary glands, testes and kidneys. Disorders result from an excess or deficiency of one or more of the pituitary hormones due to a pathological condition within the gland itself or to hypothalamic dysfunction (abnormal function of the thalamus which is located in the brain). Although disorders of the pituitary cause diverse and serious problems, they are not as common as disorders of other endocrine glands. As you are aware, the pituitary gland is divided into anterior and posterior pituitary gland. Thus the following section will discuss disorders related to these two parts of the pituitary.

The person with a disorder of the anterior pituitary gland

Hyperfunction of the anterior pituitary gland, characterised by excess production and secretion of one or more tropic hormones, is usually the result of a pituitary tumour or pituitary hyperplasia (an increase in the number of cells). The most common cause of hyperpituitarism is a benign tumour. The signs and symptoms result from pressure on the optic nerve causing visual changes or an excess of GH, PRL, ACTH or TSH. Typically, 70–90% of the anterior pituitary is damaged before clinical signs and symptoms develop.

Hypofunction of the anterior pituitary gland results in a deficiency of one or more of the gland's hormones. Conditions causing hypopituitarism include pituitary tumours, surgical removal of the pituitary gland, radiation, infection or trauma.

Pathophysiology of disorders of the anterior pituitary gland

GH (also called somatotropin) is produced by cells in the anterior pituitary throughout life. It is necessary for growth and also contributes to metabolic regulation. GH stimulates all aspects of cartilage growth, and one of its major effects is to stimulate the growth of the epiphyseal cartilage plates of long bones. In addition, other body tissues respond to the metabolic effect of GH with increases in bone width and the growth of visceral and endocrine organs, skeletal and cardiac muscle, skin and connective tissue. Gigantism and acromegaly result from overstimulation. Growth retardation and short stature result from deficient production of GH.

Hypersecretion of PRL affects reproductive and sexual function. Women may have irregular or absent menstruation (periods), difficulty becoming pregnant and decreased libido. Men may be impotent and have decreased libido. PRL deficiency in post-partum women causes a failure to lactate. An excess secretion of ACTH overstimulates the adrenal cortex, which in turn increases secretion of adrenal hormones. The result is **Cushing's syndrome**. Deficiencies of TSH are uncommon, but cause hypothyroidism.

Signs and symptoms of disorders of the anterior pituitary gland

The signs and symptoms of the disorders of the anterior pituitary gland depend on the hypersecretion or **hyposecretion** of the hormones from the anterior pituitary. It will be difficult to list all the signs and symptoms in this section.

INTERDISCIPLINARY CARE FOR DISORDERS OF THE ANTERIOR PITUITARY GLAND

The treatment involves treating the diseases of the anterior pituitary gland such as treating the cause of gigantism, Cushing's disease and other diseases associated with the anterior pituitary.

The person with a disorder of the posterior pituitary gland

Disorders of the posterior pituitary are related primarily to excessive or deficient ADH secretion. The disorders discussed here are the syndrome of inappropriate ADH secretion (SIADH) and **diabetes insipidus** (DI).

Pathophysiology of disorders of the posterior pituitary gland

ADH is secreted in response to serum osmolality, which is monitored by osmoreceptors in the hypothalamus. When a condition of hyperosmolality occurs, ADH secretion increases, and water is reabsorbed from the renal tubules. Hypo-osmolality causes the suppression of ADH, and water excretion increases from the renal tubules.

Syndrome of inappropriate ADH secretion (SIADH)

Pathophysiology

SIADH is characterised by high levels of ADH in the absence of serum hypo-osmolality (decrease in the solute concentration of the body fluids). This disorder is most often caused by the ectopic (displaced) production of ADH by malignant tumours (for example, oat cell carcinoma of the lung, pancreatic carcinoma, leukaemia and Hodgkin's disease). A transient (lasting for a short time) form of the disorder may follow a head injury, pituitary surgery or the use of medications such as barbiturates, anaesthetics or diuretics.

Signs and symptoms
- Hyponatraemia (low sodium).
- Fluid retention.
- Swelling of the brain.
- Headache.
- Lethargy.
- Irritability.
- Seizures.
- Coma.

Treatment
Treatment addresses the low sodium and intracellular swelling. Besides keeping the person safe, nursing care involves

teaching the person about restricting fluids to 1 L/day. Fluid restriction continues for 3–10 days until the malignant source of ADH is successfully removed.

Diabetes insipidus (DI)
DI is a rare disorder where the system the body uses to regulate its water levels becomes disrupted. This disruption leads to the two most common symptoms of diabetes insipidus:

- excessive and prolonged thirst;
- passing large amounts of urine and needing to urinate frequently.

There are two main types of diabetes insipidus and they are:

- cranial diabetes insipidus, a disorder due to a deficiency of hypothalamic secretion of ADH;
- nephrogenic diabetes insipidus, a disorder in which the renal tubules are not sensitive to ADH.

Diabetes insipidus may result from brain tumours or infections, pituitary surgery, cerebral vascular accidents and renal and organ failure. It is also a complication of closed-head trauma with increased intracranial pressure. A deficit of ADH causes excretion of large amounts of dilute urine (polyuria), in some instances as much as 12 L/day. The person has extreme thirst and drinks large volumes of water (polydipsia). If unable to replace the water loss, the person becomes dehydrated and hypernatraemic (high levels of sodium). Even though hyperosmolality is present, the urine is dilute and has a low specific gravity. If this disorder is caused by cerebral injury, symptoms commonly appear three to six days after the initial injury and last for 7–10 days. If the increased intracranial pressure is relieved, symptoms of diabetes insipidus usually disappear. However, diabetes insipidus may also be a chronic illness requiring lifelong treatment and care.

FAST FACTS

Diabetes insipidus

The condition 'diabetes insipidus' (DI) is characterised by the passage of large volumes of urine (> 3 L/24hrs), and persistent thirst.

NURSING CARE FOR DIABETES INSIPIDUS AND SIADH

Nursing care for the person with SIADH and DI focuses on the person's problems with fluid and electrolyte balance. SIADH is treated by correcting underlying causes, treating the hyponatraemia with intravenous hypertonic saline and restricting oral fluids to less than 800 mL/day.

DI is also treated by correcting underlying causes, if possible. Other medical interventions include administering intravenous hypotonic fluids, increasing oral fluids and replacing ADH hormone. You need to be aware that DI is very different from diabetes mellitus, which is often just referred to as diabetes.

Diabetes mellitus is far more common and occurs when there is too much glucose in the blood. However, it is possible for someone with diabetes mellitus to also develop DI although this is extremely rare. The next section will concentrate on the care of a person with diabetes mellitus.

DIABETES MELLITUS (DM)

Diabetes was first mentioned in approximately 1550 BC in an Egyptian papyrus which talked of a rare disease that causes the person to lose weight rapidly and urinate frequently. This is thought to be the first reference to the disease. Diabetes was given its name by the Greek physician Aretaeus. He recorded a disease with symptoms such as constant thirst (polydipsia), excessive urination (polyuria) and loss of weight. He named the condition 'diabetes', meaning 'a flowing through'. Later, Galen noted the rarity of this condition and theorised that it was an affliction of the kidneys. Throughout the 20th century, treatment and understanding of the disease has advanced significantly. Although prevention and management remain difficult, the life of an average diabetic is becoming both longer and easier all the time.

Diabetes mellitus has been recognised as a disease for centuries. *Diabetes* derives from a Greek word meaning 'to siphon', referring to the increased output of urine. *Mellitus* derives from a Latin word meaning 'sweet'. The two words together identify the disease as an outpouring of sweet urine. It was not until 1921 that techniques were developed for extracting insulin from pancreatic tissue and for measuring blood glucose. At the same time, researchers discovered that insulin, when injected, produces a dramatic drop in blood glucose. This meant that diabetes was no longer a terminal illness because **hyperglycaemia** (excess amount of blood glucose) could be controlled. Since that time, oral hypoglycaemic drugs, human insulin products, insulin pumps, home blood glucose monitoring and transplantation of the pancreas or of pancreatic islet or beta cells have advanced the treatment and care of people with diabetes.

ENDOCRINE HORMONES OF THE PANCREAS AND GLUCOSE HOMEOSTASIS

Hormones

The endocrine pancreas produces hormones necessary for the metabolism and cellular utilisation of carbohydrates, proteins and fats. The cells that produce these hormones are clustered in groups of cells called the islets of Langerhans. These islets have three different types of cells—alpha, beta and delta cells:

- Alpha cells produce the hormone *glucagon*, which stimulates the breakdown of glycogen in the liver, the formation of carbohydrates in the liver and the breakdown of lipids in both the liver and adipose tissue. The primary function of glucagon is to decrease glucose oxidation and to increase blood glucose levels. Through glycogenolysis (the breakdown of liver glycogen) and gluconeogenesis (the formation of glucose from fats and proteins), glucagon prevents blood glucose from decreasing below a certain level when the body is fasting or in between meals.

- Beta cells secrete the hormone insulin, which facilitates the movement of glucose across cell membranes into cells, decreasing blood glucose levels. Insulin prevents the excessive breakdown of glycogen in the liver and in muscle, facilitates lipid formation while inhibiting the breakdown of stored fats, and helps move amino acids into cells for protein synthesis. After secretion by the beta cells, insulin enters the portal circulation, travels directly to the liver and is then released into the general circulation. Circulating insulin is rapidly bound to receptor sites on peripheral tissues (especially muscle and fat cells) or is destroyed by the liver or kidneys. Insulin release is regulated by blood glucose; it increases when blood glucose levels increase, and it decreases when blood glucose levels decrease. When a person eats food, insulin levels begin to rise in minutes, peak in 30–60 minutes and return to baseline in two to three hours.

- Delta cells produce *somatostatin*, which is believed to be a neurotransmitter that inhibits the production of both glucagon and insulin.

Blood glucose homeostasis

All body tissues and organs require a constant supply of glucose; however, not all tissues require insulin for glucose

FAST FACTS

Diabetes

After his victory in the rowing at the Sydney Olympic Games in 2000, Sir Steve Redgrave became the only British athlete ever to have won gold medals at five consecutive Olympic Games. What many people don't realise is that Sir Steve achieved this final triumph against all the odds because just three years before competing in the Sydney Olympics he discovered he had diabetes.

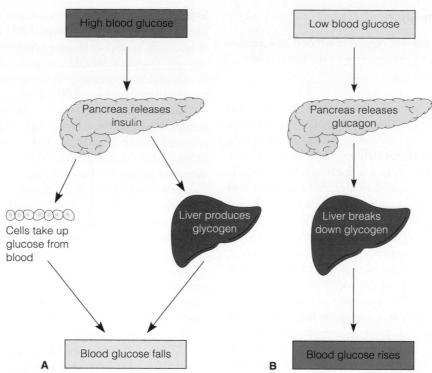

Figure 6.7 Regulation (homeostasis) of blood glucose levels by insulin and glucagon. **(A)** High blood glucose is lowered by insulin release. **(B)** Low blood glucose is raised by glucagon release.

uptake. The brain, liver, intestines and renal tubules do not require insulin to transfer glucose into their cells. Skeletal muscle, cardiac muscle and adipose tissue do require insulin for glucose movement into the cells.

Normal blood glucose is maintained primarily through the actions of insulin and glucagon. Increased blood glucose levels, amino acids and fatty acids stimulate pancreatic beta cells to produce insulin. As cells of cardiac muscle, skeletal muscle and adipose tissue take up glucose, plasma levels of nutrients decrease, suppressing the stimulus to produce insulin. If blood glucose falls, glucagon is released to raise hepatic glucose output, raising glucose levels. Epinephrine, growth hormone, thyroxin and glucocorticoids (often referred to as glucose counter-regulatory hormones) also stimulate an increase in glucose in times of hypoglycaemia, stress, growth or increased metabolic demand. The regulation of blood glucose levels by insulin and glucagon is illustrated in Figure 6.7 A and B.

The person with DM

DM is a chronic and progressive illness that affects all ages. It can affect children, young people and adults and is becoming more common. There are 1.8 million people with diagnosed diabetes and this figure is increasing every year, and the estimated cost to the NHS is £5 million per day for treatment. With an ageing population, the number of males and females

with diagnosed diabetes is projected to rise by 37% for males and 24% for females by 2023 (Newnham *et al.* 2002).

There are two main types of DM. Type 1 accounts for 15% of all diagnosed cases, while type 2 accounts for 85% of persons with DM (Patient UK 2009). In addition to type 1 and type 2, there are other types of diabetes, such as gestational diabetes, diabetes due to side-effects of steroid therapy and diabetes associated with hormonal disorders, such as maturity-onset diabetes of the young, cystic fibrosis-related diabetes and Cushing's syndrome, caused by prolonged exposure of the body tissues to high levels of the hormone cortisol.

FAST FACTS

Diabetes mellitus

- Over 5% of men and 4% of women in England have diagnosed diabetes.
- It has been estimated that 3.1% of men and 1.5% of women aged 35 and over have undiagnosed diabetes.

Source: Patient UK 2009.

Persons with DM face lifelong changes in lifestyle and health status. Nursing care is provided in many settings for the diagnosis and care of the disease and treatment of complications. The role of the nurse is to provide health promotion/education in both hospital and community settings to persons with DM.

Type 1 diabetes mellitus

Type 1 diabetes most often occurs in childhood and adolescence, but it may occur at any age, even in the 80s and 90s.

Pathophysiology

This disorder is characterised by hyperglycaemia (elevated blood glucose levels), a breakdown of body fats and proteins, and the development of ketosis (an accumulation of ketone bodies produced during the oxidation of fatty acids). Type 1 DM is the result of the destruction of the beta cells of the islets of Langerhans in the pancreas, the only cells in the body that make insulin. When beta cells are destroyed, insulin is no longer produced. Although type 1 DM may be classified as either an autoimmune (immune system mistakenly attacks and destroys healthy body tissue) or idiopathic (unknown cause) disorder, 90% of the cases are immune mediated (conditions which result from abnormal activity of the body's immune system).

The disorder begins with insulinitis, a chronic inflammatory process that occurs in response to the autoimmune destruction of islet cells. This process slowly destroys beta cell production of insulin, with the onset of hyperglycaemia occurring when 80–90% of beta cell function is lost. This process usually occurs over a long preclinical period. It is believed that both alpha cell and beta cell functions are abnormal, with a lack of insulin and a relative excess of glucagon resulting in hyperglycaemia.

Risk factors

Genetic predisposition plays a role in the development of type 1 DM. Although the risk in the general population ranges from one in 400 to one in 1000, the child of a person with diabetes has a one in 20 to one in 50 risk. Genetic markers that determine immune responses – specifically, DR3 and DR4 antigens on chromosome 6 of the human leucocyte antigen (HLA) system – have been found in 95% of people diagnosed with type 1 DM. (HLAs are cell surface proteins, controlled by genes on chromosome 6.) Although the presence of these markers does not guarantee that the person will develop type 1 DM, they do indicate increased susceptibility.

Environmental factors are believed to trigger the development of type 1 DM. The trigger can be a viral infection (mumps, rubella or coxsackievirus B4) or a chemical toxin, such as those found in smoked and cured meats. As a result of exposure to the virus or chemical, an abnormal autoimmune response occurs in which antibodies respond to normal islet beta cells as though they were foreign substances, destroying them. The signs and symptoms of type 1 DM appear when approximately 90% of the beta cells are destroyed. However, signs and symptoms may appear at any time during the loss of beta cells if an acute illness or stress increases the demand for insulin beyond the reserves of the damaged cells. The actual cause and exact sequence are not completely understood, but research continues to identify the genetic markers of this disorder and to investigate ways of altering the immune response to prevent or cure type 1 DM.

Signs and symptoms

The signs and symptoms of type 1 DM are the result of a lack of insulin to transport glucose across the cell membrane into the cells (Figure 6.8). Glucose molecules accumulate in the circulating blood, resulting in hyperglycaemia. Hyperglycaemia causes serum hyperosmolality, drawing water from the intracellular spaces into the general circulation. The increased blood volume increases renal blood flow, and the hyperglycaemia acts as an osmotic diuretic. The resulting osmotic diuresis increases urine output. This condition is called polyuria. When the blood glucose level exceeds the renal threshold for glucose – usually about 10 mmol/L – glucose is excreted in the urine, a condition called glucosuria. The decrease in intracellular volume and the increased urinary output cause dehydration. The mouth becomes dry and thirst sensors are activated, causing the person to drink increased amounts of fluid (polydipsia).

Because glucose cannot enter the cell without insulin, energy production decreases. This decrease in energy stimulates hunger, and the person eats more food (polyphagia). Despite increased food intake, the person loses weight as the body loses water and breaks down proteins and fats in an attempt to restore energy sources. Malaise and fatigue accompany the decrease in energy. Blurred vision is also common, resulting from osmotic effects that cause swelling of the lenses of the eyes.

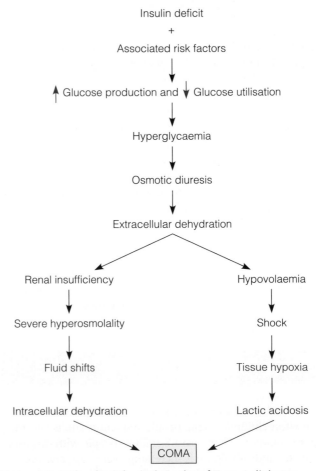

Figure 6.8 Pathophysiological results of Type 1 diabetes mellitus.

Thus, the classic signs and symptoms are polyuria, polydipsia and polyphagia, accompanied by weight loss, malaise and fatigue. Depending on the degree of insulin lack, the signs and symptoms vary from slight to severe. People with type 1 DM require exogenous insulin to maintain life.

Type 2 diabetes mellitus

Pathophysiology

Type 2 diabetes is caused by the body not producing enough insulin or not using what it produces effectively. Type 2 DM can occur at any age, but it is usually seen in middle-age and older people. Heredity plays a role in its transmission. The level of insulin produced varies in type 2 diabetes, and despite its availability, its function is impaired by insulin resistance. Insulin resistance forces the pancreas to work harder and produce more insulin, but when demand exceeds supply, diabetes results. Whatever the cause, there is sufficient insulin production to prevent the breakdown of fats with resultant ketosis; thus, type 2 diabetes is characterised as a non-ketotic form of diabetes (no ketones in the urine). However, the amount of insulin available is not sufficient to lower blood glucose levels through the uptake of glucose by muscle and fat cells.

FAST FACTS

Ethnicity and DM

People of South Asian, African, African-Caribbean, Polynesian, Middle-Eastern and American-Indian descent are at greater risk of type 2 diabetes, compared with the white population.

A major factor in the development of type 2 DM is cellular resistance to the effect of insulin. This resistance is increased by obesity, inactivity, illnesses, medications and increasing age. In obesity, insulin has a decreased ability to influence glucose metabolism and uptake by the liver, skeletal muscles and adipose tissue. Although the exact reason for this is not clear, it is known that weight loss and exercise may improve the mechanism responsible for insulin receptor binding or post-receptor activity. Hyperglycaemia increases gradually and may exist over a long time before diabetes is diagnosed; thus, approximately half the newly diagnosed type 2 diabetics already have complications. Treatment usually begins with prescriptions for weight loss and increased activity. If these changes can be sustained, no further treatment will be necessary for many individuals. Hypoglycaemic medications are begun when lifestyle changes are insufficient. Often, a combination of insulin and hypoglycaemic medication is used to achieve the best glycaemic control in the person with type 2 DM.

Risk factors

The major risk factors for type 2 diabetes are as follows:

● History of diabetes in parents or siblings. The children of a person with type 2 diabetes have a 15% chance of developing type 2 diabetes and a 30% risk of developing glucose intolerance (the inability to metabolise carbohydrate normally).

● Obesity, defined as being at least 20% over desired body weight or having a body mass index of at least 27 kg/m^2. Obesity, especially of the upper body, decreases the number of available insulin receptor sites in cells of skeletal muscles and adipose tissues, a process called *peripheral insulin resistance*. In addition, obesity impairs the ability of the beta cells to release insulin in response to increasing glucose levels.

● Physical inactivity.

● In women, a history of gestational diabetes, polycystic ovary syndrome or delivering a baby weighing approximately more than 4 kg.

● Hypertension.

Signs and symptoms

The person with type 2 diabetes experiences a slow onset of signs and symptoms and is often unaware of the disease until seeking healthcare for some other problem. The hyperglycaemia in type 2 is usually not as severe as in type 1, but similar symptoms occur, especially polyuria and polydipsia. Polyphagia is not often seen, and weight loss is uncommon. Other signs and symptoms are also the result of hyperglycaemia: blurred vision, fatigue, paraesthesias and skin infections. If available insulin decreases, especially in times of physical or emotional stress, the person with type 2 diabetes may develop diabetic ketoacidosis (DKA), but this occurrence is uncommon.

INTERDISCIPLINARY CARE FOR DM

Medication

The pharmacological treatment for diabetes mellitus depends on the type of diabetes. People with type 1 diabetes must have insulin and diet therapy; those with type 2 diabetes are usually able to control glucose levels with an oral hypoglycaemic medication, with diet and exercise, but they may require insulin if control is inadequate.

Insulin

The person with type 1 diabetes requires a lifelong exogenous source of the insulin hormone to maintain life. Insulin is not a cure for diabetes; rather, it is a means of controlling hyperglycaemia. Insulin is also necessary in other situations, such as these:

● People with diabetes who are unable to control glucose levels with oral antidiabetic drugs and/or diet. Introduced when beta cell function declines, insulin maintains blood glucose level and prevents complications.

- People with diabetes who are experiencing physical stress (such as an infection or surgery) or who are taking corticoid-steroid drugs.
- Women with gestational diabetes who are unable to control glucose with diet.
- People with DKA or hyperosmolar hyperglycaemic state (HHS).
- People who are receiving high-calorie tube feedings or total parenteral nutrition (TPN).

Insulin preparations are derived from animal (pork pancreas) or synthesised in the laboratory from either an alteration of pork insulin or recombinant DNA technology, using strains of *E. coli* to form biosynthetic human insulin. Insulin analogues have been developed by modifying the amino acid sequence of the insulin molecule. Although different types are prescribed on an individualised basis, it is standard practice to prescribe human insulin.

Insulin preparations

Insulin is available in rapid-acting, short-acting, intermediate-acting and long-acting preparations. The trade names and times of onset, peak and duration of action are listed in Table 6.2.

Insulin lispro (Humalog) is a human insulin analogue that is derived from genetically altered *E. coli* that includes the gene for insulin lispro. It is classified as rapid-acting or ultra-short-acting insulin. Compared to regular insulin, insulin lispro has a more rapid onset (< 15 minutes), an earlier peak of glucose lowering (30–60 minutes) and a shorter duration of activity (three to four hours). This means that lispro should be administered 15 minutes before a meal, rather than 30–60 minutes before as recommended for regular insulin. Persons with type 1 DM usually also require concurrent use of a longer-acting insulin product. Lispro is much less likely than regular insulin to cause tissue changes and may lower the risk of nocturnal hypoglycaemia in persons with type 1 DM.

Regular insulin is unmodified crystalline insulin, classified as short-acting insulin. Regular insulin is clear in appearance and is the only insulin preparation that can be given by the intravenous route; the other types are suspensions and could be harmful if given by this route. Regular insulin is also used to treat DKA, to initiate treatment for newly diagnosed type 1 DM and, in combination with intermediate-acting insulin, to provide better glucose control.

The onset and peak and duration of action of insulin can be changed by adding acetate buffers and protamine. Zinc and protamine are added to NPH insulin to prolong their action, and they are classified as intermediate- or long-acting insulin. These preparations appear cloudy when properly mixed prior to injection. Protamine and zinc are foreign substances and may cause hypersensitivity reactions.

PRACTICE ALERT

Insulin glargine is clear unlike other intermediate- or long-acting insulins. Do not mistake this for regular insulin. Do not mix with any other insulins. Do not inject intravenously, only subcutaneously.

Hypoglycaemic medications

Hypoglycaemic drugs are used to treat people with type 2 DM. These medications lower blood glucose by stimulating or increasing insulin secretion, preventing breakdown of glycogen to glucose by the liver and increasing peripheral uptake of glucose by making cells less resistant to insulin. Peripheral uptake refers to uptake by muscles and fat in the arms and legs rather than in the trunk. Some hypoglycaemic medications keep blood glucose low by blocking absorption of carbohydrates in the intestines.

Nutrition

The management of diabetes requires a careful balance between the intake of nutrients, the expenditure of energy and the dose and timing of insulin or oral antidiabetic agents. Although everyone has the same need for basic nutrition, the person with diabetes must eat a more structured diet to prevent hyperglycaemia.

Table 6.2 Insulin preparations

Preparation	Name	Onset (H)	Peak (H)	Duration (H)
Rapid-acting	Lispro	0–15 minutes	1–1.5	3–4
	Aspart (NovoLog)	0–15 minutes	40–50 minutes	3–5
	Glulisine (Apidra)	0–15 minutes	1–1.5	3–5
Short-acting	Regular (Novolin-R, Humulin-R)	0.5–1.0	2–3	4–6
Intermediate-acting	NPH Humulin (N)	2	6.8	12–16
Long-acting	Lantus	2 (Onset and peak not defined)	16–20	24+ 24
Combinations	Humulin 50/50	0.5	3	22–24
	Humulin 70/30	0.5	4–8	24
	Novolin 70/30	0.5	4–8	24

IN PRACTICE

Insulin therapy

The overall aim in administration of insulin therapy is to achieve the best control of blood glucose over the 24-hour period. Insulin dose will vary from person to person. Insulin is give by subcutaneous injections, and the most common sites for insulin injections are the upper thighs and the abdominal wall. See Figure 6.9 for sites of insulin injections.

Injection technique:

● Insulin is injected at room temperature.

● There is no need to cleanse the skin prior to injection.

● Make sure that there are no air bubbles in the syringe.

● Pinch a mound of skin gently.

● The syringe or pen is inserted into the subcutaneous layer of the skin at 90° angle.

● Insulin is injected steadily and the needle is held in position for a further six seconds and then removed steadily.

● Do not change the direction of the needle during insertion or withdrawal.

● Do not re-sheath the needle.

● Make the patient comfortable.

● Dispose of the needle and the syringe into a sharps box.

● Wash your hands.

● Document the outcome of the procedure in the nurses notes.

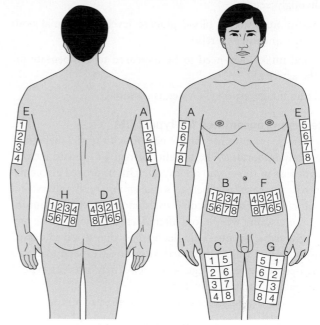

Figure 6.9 Sites of insulin injection.

● Maintain as near normal blood glucose levels as possible by balancing food intake with insulin or oral glucose.

● Achieve normal serum lipid levels.

● Provide adequate calories to maintain or attain reasonable weights, and to recover from catabolic illness (illness as a result of the breakdown of protein and fat).

● Prevent and treat the acute complications of DM, short-term illnesses and exercise-related problems; or the long-term complications of diabetes.

Exercise

The third component of diabetes management is a regular exercise programme. The benefits of exercise are the same for everyone, with or without diabetes: improved physical fitness, improved emotional state, weight control and improved work capacity. In people with diabetes, exercise increases the uptake of glucose by muscle cells, potentially reducing the need for insulin. Exercise also decreases cholesterol and triglycerides, reducing the risk of cardiovascular disorders. People with diabetes should consult the practice nurse before beginning or changing an exercise programme. The ability to maintain an exercise programme is affected by many different factors, including fatigue and glucose levels. It is as important to assess the

person's usual lifestyle before establishing an exercise programme as it is before planning a diet. Factors to consider include the person's usual exercise habits, living environment and community programmes. The exercise that the person enjoys most is probably the one that he or she will continue throughout life.

Exercise programmes for type 1 DM

In the person with type 1 diabetes, glycaemic responses to exercise vary according to the type, intensity and duration of the exercise. Other factors that influence responses include the timing of exercise in relation to meals and insulin injections, and the time of day of the activity. Unless these factors are integrated into the exercise programme, the person with type 1 diabetes has an increased risk of hypoglycaemia and hyperglycaemia. The following are general guidelines for an exercise programme:

● People who have frequent hyperglycaemia or hypoglycaemia should avoid prolonged exercise until glucose control improves.

● The risk of exercise-induced hypoglycaemia is lowest before breakfast, when free-insulin levels tend to be lower than they are before meals later in the day or at bedtime.

● Low-impact aerobic exercises are encouraged.

- Exercise should be moderate and regular; brief, intense exercise tends to cause mild hyperglycaemia, and prolonged exercise can lead to hypoglycaemia.

- Exercising at a peak insulin action time may lead to hypoglycaemia.

- Self-monitoring of blood glucose levels is essential both before and after exercise.

- Food intake may need to be increased to compensate for the activity.

- Fluid intake, especially water, is essential.

Exercise programmes for type 2 DM

An exercise programme for the person with type 2 diabetes is especially important. The benefits of regular exercise include weight loss in those who are overweight, improved glycaemic control, increased wellbeing, socialisation with others and a reduction of cardiovascular risk factors. A combination of diet, exercise and weight loss often decreases the need for oral hypoglycaemic agents. This decrease is due to an increased sensitivity to insulin, increased kilocalorie expenditure and increased self-esteem. Regular exercise may prevent type 2 diabetes in high-risk individuals.

The following are general guidelines for an exercise programme:

- Before beginning the programme, have a medical screening for previously undiagnosed hypertension, neuropathy, retinopathy and nephropathy.

- Begin the programme with mild exercises, and gradually increase intensity and duration.

- Self-monitor blood glucose before and after exercise.

- Exercise at least three times a week or every other day, for at least 20–30 minutes.

- Include muscle-strengthening and low-impact aerobic exercises in the programme.

Complications of DM

The person with diabetes mellitus, regardless of type, is at increased risk for complications involving many different body systems. Alterations in blood glucose levels, alterations in the cardiovascular system, neuropathies (inflammation of the peripheral nerves), an increased susceptibility to infection and periodontal disease are common. In addition, the interaction of several complications can cause problems of the feet. For the multisystem effects of diabetes mellitus see Figure 6.10. A discussion of each of these complications follows; related interdisciplinary care and nursing care are discussed later in the chapter.

Diabetic ketoacidosis (DKA)

As the pathophysiology of untreated type 1 DM continues, the insulin deficit causes fat stores to break down, resulting in continued hyperglycaemia and mobilisation of fatty acids with a subsequent ketosis. DKA develops when there is an absolute deficiency of insulin and an increase in the insulin counter-regulatory hormones. Glucose production by the liver increases, peripheral glucose use decreases, fat mobilisation increases and ketogenesis (ketone formation) is stimulated. Increased glucagon levels activate the gluconeogenic and ketogenic pathways in the liver. In the presence of insulin deficiency, hepatic overproduction of beta-hydroxybutyrate and acetoacetic acids (ketone bodies) causes increased ketone concentrations and an increased release of free fatty acids. As a result of a loss of bicarbonate (which occurs when the ketone is formed), bicarbonate buffering does not occur, and a metabolic acidosis occurs, called DKA. Depression of the central nervous system from the accumulation of ketones and the resulting acidosis may cause coma and death if left untreated (See Figure 6.11 A, B, C).

So why is DKA dangerous? When blood glucose levels are higher than about 15 mmol/l and the person is ill, the body may start to produce ketones. Ketones are poisonous and make the blood very acidic, hence the term ketoacidosis. Ketoacidosis usually takes at least 24 hours to develop, but once it starts it will get worse until action as taken.

DKA may also occur in a person with diagnosed diabetes when energy requirements increase during physical or emotional stress. Stress states initiate the release of gluconeogenic hormones, resulting in the formation of carbohydrates from protein or fat. The person who is sick, has an infection or who decreases or omits insulin doses is at a greatly increased risk for developing DKA.

Signs and symptoms

Signs and symptoms of DKA result from severe dehydration and acidosis. Other signs and symptoms include:

- thirst;
- warm dry skin with poor turgor;
- weakness;
- malaise;
- nausea and vomiting;
- rapid weak pulse;
- hypotension;
- ketone breath (fruity, alcohol-like);
- lethargy;
- soft eyeballs;
- coma;
- Kussmaul's respiration (increased rate and depth of breathing, with a longer expiration).

Treatment

DKA requires immediate medical attention. Admission to the hospital is appropriate when the person has blood glucose of greater than 13.9 mmol/L, a decreasing pH and ketones in the urine. If the person is alert and conscious, fluids may be replaced orally. In the first 12 hours of treatment, adults usually require 8–10 L of fluid to replace losses from polyuria and vomiting. However, alterations in level of consciousness, vomiting and acidosis are common, necessitating intravenous fluid

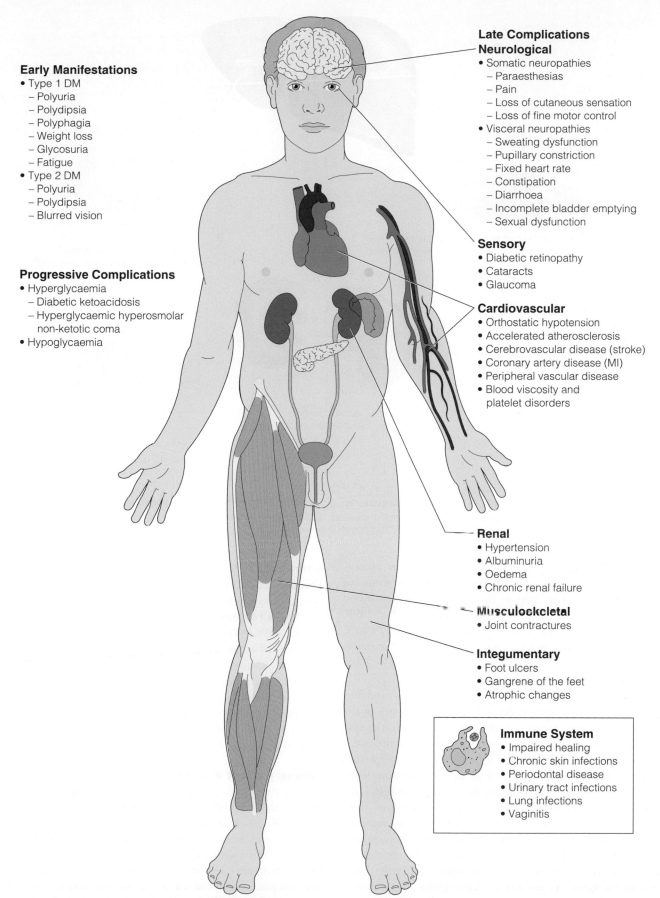

Figure 6.10 Multisystem effects of diabetes mellitus.

Early Manifestations
- Type 1 DM
  – Polyuria
  – Polydipsia
  – Polyphagia
  – Weight loss
  – Glycosuria
  – Fatigue
- Type 2 DM
  – Polyuria
  – Polydipsia
  – Blurred vision

Progressive Complications
- Hyperglycaemia
  – Diabetic ketoacidosis
  – Hyperglycaemic hyperosmolar non-ketotic coma
- Hypoglycaemia

Late Complications
Neurological
- Somatic neuropathies
  – Paraesthesias
  – Pain
  – Loss of cutaneous sensation
  – Loss of fine motor control
- Visceral neuropathies
  – Sweating dysfunction
  – Pupillary constriction
  – Fixed heart rate
  – Constipation
  – Diarrhoea
  – Incomplete bladder emptying
  – Sexual dysfunction

Sensory
- Diabetic retinopathy
- Cataracts
- Glaucoma

Cardiovascular
- Orthostatic hypotension
- Accelerated atherosclerosis
- Cerebrovascular disease (stroke)
- Coronary artery disease (MI)
- Peripheral vascular disease
- Blood viscosity and platelet disorders

Renal
- Hypertension
- Albuminuria
- Oedema
- Chronic renal failure

Musculoskeletal
- Joint contractures

Integumentary
- Foot ulcers
- Gangrene of the feet
- Atrophic changes

Immune System
- Impaired healing
- Chronic skin infections
- Periodontal disease
- Urinary tract infections
- Lung infections
- Vaginitis

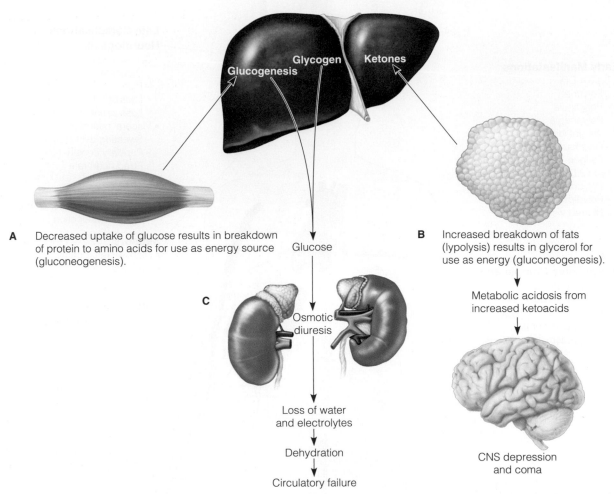

A Decreased uptake of glucose results in breakdown of protein to amino acids for use as energy source (gluconeogenesis).

Glucose

B Increased breakdown of fats (lypolysis) results in glycerol for use as energy (gluconeogenesis).

C

Osmotic diuresis

Metabolic acidosis from increased ketoacids

Loss of water and electrolytes

Dehydration

CNS depression and coma

Circulatory failure

Figure 6.11 In type 1 diabetes mellitus, without adequate insulin, muscle (A) and fat (B) cells are metabolised to provide sources of energy. Increased glucose (C) causes osmotic diuresis leading to dehydration and decreased circulatory volume.

replacement. The initial fluid replacement may be accomplished by administering 0.9% saline solution at a rate of 500–1000 mL/h. After two to three hours (or when blood pressure is returning to normal), the administration of 0.45% saline at 200–500 mL/h may continue for several more hours. When the blood glucose levels reach 13.9 mmol/L, dextrose is added to prevent rapid decreases in glucose as hypoglycaemia could result in fatal cerebral oedema.

Regular insulin is used in the management of DKA and may be given by various routes, depending on the severity of the condition. Mild ketosis may be treated with subcutaneous insulin, whereas severe ketosis requires intravenous insulin infusion.

The electrolyte imbalance of primary concern is depletion of body stores of potassium. Initially, serum potassium levels may be normal, but they decrease during treatment. In DKA (and from rehydration), the body loses potassium from increased urinary output, acidosis, catabolic state and vomiting or diarrhoea. Potassium replacement is begun early in the course of treatment, usually by adding potassium to the rehydration fluids. Replacement is essential for preventing cardiac dysrhythmias secondary to hypokalemia. Cardiac rhythms and potassium levels must be monitored every two to four hours.

Alterations in the cardiovascular system

The macrocirculation (large blood vessels) in people with diabetes undergoes changes due to atherosclerosis, abnormalities in platelets, red blood cells and clotting factors, and changes in arterial walls. It has been established that atherosclerosis has an increased incidence and earlier age of onset in people with diabetes (although the reason is unknown). Other risk factors that contribute to the development of macrovascular disease of diabetes are hypertension, **hyperlipidemia**, cigarette smoking and obesity. Alterations in the vascular system increase the risk of the long-term complications of coronary artery disease, cerebrovascular disease and peripheral vascular disease.

Coronary artery disease

Coronary artery disease is a major risk factor in the development of myocardial infarction in people with diabetes, especially in the middle to older adult with type 2 DM. Coronary artery disease is the most common cause of death in people with diabetes. People with diabetes who have myocardial infarction (heart attack) are more prone to develop congestive heart failure as a complication of the infarction and are also less likely to survive in the period immediately following the infarction.

Hypertension

Hypertension (blood pressure $\geq$ 140/90 mmHg) is a common complication of diabetes. It affects 20–60% of all people with diabetes, and is a major risk factor for cardiovascular disease and microvascular complications such as retinopathy and nephropathy. Hypertension may be reduced by weight loss, exercise and decreasing sodium intake and alcohol consumption. If these methods are not effective, treatment with antihypertensive medications is necessary.

Stroke (cerebrovascular accident)

People with diabetes, especially the elderly with type 2 diabetes, are two to six times more likely to have a stroke. Although the exact relationship between diabetes and cerebral vascular disease is unknown, hypertension (a risk factor for stroke) is a common health problem in those who have diabetes. In addition, atherosclerosis of the cerebral vessels develops at an earlier age and is more extensive in people with diabetes.

The signs and symptoms of impaired cerebral circulation are often similar to those of hypoglycaemia or HHS: blurred vision, slurred speech, weakness and dizziness. People with these signs and symptoms have potentially life-threatening health problems and require constant medical attention.

Peripheral vascular disease

Peripheral vascular disease of the lower extremities accompanies both types of DM, but the incidence is greater in people with type 2 DM. Atherosclerosis of vessels in the legs of people with diabetes begins at an earlier age, advances more rapidly and is equally common in both men and women. Impaired peripheral vascular circulation leads to peripheral vascular insufficiency with intermittent claudication (pain) in the lower legs and ulcerations of the feet. Occlusion and thrombosis of large vessels and small arteries and arterioles, as well as alterations in neurologic function and infection, result in gangrene (necrosis, or the death of tissue). Gangrene from diabetes is the most common cause of non-traumatic amputations of the lower leg. In people with diabetes, dry gangrene is most common, manifested by cold, dry, shrivelled and black tissues of the toes and feet. The gangrene usually begins in the toes and moves proximally into the foot.

Complications involving the feet

The high incidence of both amputations and problems with the feet in people with diabetes is the result of diseased blood vessels (angiopathy), damage to the nerves (neuropathy) and infection. People with diabetes are at high risk for amputation of a lower extremity, with increased risk in those who have had DM for more than 10 years, are male, have poor glucose control or have cardiovascular, retinal or renal complications.

Vascular changes in the lower extremities of the person with diabetes result in arteriosclerosis. Diabetes-induced arteriosclerosis tends to occur at an earlier age, occurs equally in men and women, is usually bilateral and progresses more rapidly. The blood vessels most often affected are located below the knee. Blockages form in the large, medium and small arteries of the lower legs and feet. Multiple occlusions with decreased blood flow result in the signs and symptoms of peripheral vascular disease.

Diabetic neuropathy of the foot produces multiple problems. Because the sense of touch and perception of pain are absent, the person with diabetes may have some type of foot trauma without being aware of it. The person is thus at increased risk for trauma to tissues of the feet, leading to ulcer development. Infections commonly occur in traumatised or ulcerated tissue.

Despite the many potential sources of foot trauma in the person with diabetes, the most common are cracks and fissures caused by dry skin or infections such as athlete's foot, blisters caused by improperly fitting shoes, pressure from stockings or shoes, in-growing toenails and direct injury (cuts, bruises or burns). It is important to remember that the person with diabetic neuropathy who has lost the perception of pain may not be aware that these injuries have occurred. In addition, when a part of the body loses sensation, the person tends to dissociate from or ignore the part, so that an injury may go unattended for days or weeks. The injury may even be forgotten entirely.

Diabetic neuropathy

Neuropathy is a medical term which refers to a nerve disorder. Diabetic neuropathy is nerve disorder caused by either type 1 or type 2 diabetes. Over time, diabetics who do not strictly control their diabetes may develop damage to the nerves around the body. Incidences are more common in persons with poor control, who are overweight, have higher levels of blood fat and blood pressure and are over the age of 40. The longer a person has diabetes, the greater the risk becomes of developing neuropathies.

Neuropathies are manifested as a numbness or pain in the hands, feet, arms or legs. However, they may also affect the organs, including the heart and sex organs. The scale of the complication is immense, with an estimated half of all diabetics suffering from some form of neuropathy.

Diabetic retinopathy

Diabetic retinopathy is the name for the changes in the retina that occur in the person with diabetes. The retinal capillary structure undergoes alterations in blood flow, leading to retinal ischaemia (decreased blood supply resulting in severe pain) and a breakdown in the blood–retinal barrier (consists of cells that are joined tightly together in order to prevent certain substances from entering the tissue of the retina). In some people with diabetic retinopathy, blood vessels may swell and leak fluid. In other people, abnormal new blood vessels grow on the surface of the retina. The retina is the light-sensitive tissue at the back of the eye. A healthy retina is necessary for good vision.

Diabetic retinopathy is a common complication of diabetes and is the leading cause of blindness in adults under the age of 65. It is estimated that 25% of people with type 1 diabetes will have some degree of diabetic retinopathy five years after their symptoms first develop. In cases of type 2 diabetes, five years after the onset of symptoms, 25% of people who do not require insulin will have some degree of diabetic retinopathy.

The figure is higher for people who require insulin, at an estimated 40%.

Diabetic nephropathy

Diabetic nephropathy is the kidney disease that occurs as a result of diabetes. It is a leading cause of kidney failure in Europe. After many years of diabetes, the delicate filtering system in the kidney becomes destroyed, initially becoming leaky to large blood proteins such as albumin which are then lost in urine. This is more likely to occur if the blood glucose is poorly controlled.

Diabetic nephropathy is a disease of the kidneys characterised by the presence of albumin in the urine, hypertension, oedema and progressive renal insufficiency. Despite research, the exact pathological origin of diabetic nephropathy is unknown; it has been established, however, that thickening of the basement membrane of the glomeruli eventually impairs renal function. It has been suggested that an increased intracellular concentration of glucose supports the formation of abnormal glycoproteins in the basement membrane and mesangium. The accumulation of these large proteins stimulates glomerulosclerosis (fibrosis of the glomerular tissue).

The first indication of nephropathy is microalbuminuria (a low but abnormal level of albumin in the urine). Without specific interventions, people with type 1 diabetes with sustained microalbuminuria will develop overt nephropathy, accompanied by hypertension, over a period of 10–15 years. People with type 2 diabetes often have microalbuminuria and overt nephropathy shortly after diagnosis, because the diabetes has often been present but undiagnosed for many years. Because the hypertension accelerates the progress of diabetic nephropathy, the person should be treated with antihypertensive. Management should include control of hypertension with ACE inhibitors such as captopril (Capoten), weight loss, reduced salt intake and exercise.

Increased susceptibility to infection

The person with diabetes has an increased risk of developing infections. The exact relationship between infection and diabetes is not clear, but many dysfunctions that result from diabetic complications predispose the person to develop an infection. Vascular and neurologic impairments, hyperglycaemia and altered **neutrophil** (a type of white blood cell) function are believed to be responsible.

The person with diabetes may have sensory deficits resulting in inattention to trauma and vascular deficits that decrease circulation to the injured area; as a result, the normal inflammatory response is diminished and healing is slowed. Nephrosclerosis (kidney disorder where small blood vessels of the kidney are damaged) and inadequate bladder emptying with retention of urine predispose the person with diabetes to pyelonephritis (infection of the renal pelvis of the kidney) and urinary tract infections. Bacterial and fungal infections of the skin, nails and mucous membranes are common. Tuberculosis is more prevalent in people with diabetes than in the general population.

Periodontal disease

Although periodontal disease does not occur more often in people with diabetes, it does progress more rapidly, especially if the diabetes is poorly controlled. It is believed to be caused by microangiopathy, with changes in vascularisation of the gums. As a result, gingivitis (inflammation of the gums) and periodontitis (inflammation of the bone underlying the gums) occur.

Hypoglycaemia

Hypoglycaemia (low blood glucose levels) is common in people with type 1 DM and occasionally occurs in people with type 2 DM who are treated with oral hypoglycaemic agents. This condition is often called insulin shock, insulin reaction or 'the lows' in person with type 1 DM. Hypoglycaemia results primarily from a mismatch between insulin intake (for example, an error in insulin dose), physical activity and carbohydrate availability (for example, omitting a meal). The intake of alcohol and drugs such as chloramphenicol (Chloromycetin), warfarin (Coumadin), monoamine oxidase inhibitors, probenecid (Benemid), salicylates and sulphonamides can also cause hypoglycaemia.

The signs and symptoms of hypoglycaemia (see below) result from a compensatory autonomic nervous system (ANS) response and from impaired cerebral function due to a decrease in glucose available for use by the brain. The signs and symptoms vary, particularly in elderly. The onset is sudden, and blood glucose is usually less than 3.5 mmol/L. Severe hypoglycaemia may cause death.

Signs and symptoms

Symptoms caused by responses of the autonomic nervous system:

- hunger;
- shakiness;
- nausea;
- irritability;
- anxiety;
- rapid pulse;
- pale, cool skin;
- hypotension;
- sweating.

Symptoms caused by impaired cerebral function:

- strange or unusual feelings;
- slurred speech;
- blurred vision;
- headache;
- decreasing levels of consciousness;
- difficulty in thinking;
- inability to concentrate;
- seizures;
- change in emotional behaviour;
- coma.

Treatment of mild hypoglycaemia

When mild hypoglycaemia occurs, immediate treatment is necessary. People experiencing hypoglycaemia should take about 15 g of a rapid-acting sugar. This amount of sugar is found, for example, in three glucose tablets, 1/2 cup of fruit juice, 8 oz of skimmed milk, three large marshmallows or 3 tsp of sugar or honey. Sugar should not be added to fruit juice. Adding sugar to the fruit sugar already in the juice could cause a rapid rise in blood glucose, with persistent hyperglycaemia.

Treatment of severe hypoglycaemia

People with diabetes who have severe hypoglycaemia are often hospitalised. The criteria for hospitalisation are one or more of the following:

- blood glucose is less than 2.6 mmol/L, and the prompt treatment of hypoglycaemia has not resulted in recovery;
- the person has coma, seizures or altered behaviour;
- the hypoglycaemia has been treated, but a responsible adult cannot be with the person for the following 12 hours;
- the hypoglycaemia was caused by a sulphonylurea drug (antidiabetic drug).

If the person is conscious and alert, 10–15 g of an oral carbohydrate may be given. If the person has altered levels of consciousness, parenteral glucose or glucagon is administered. Glucagon is an antihypoglycaemic hormone that raises blood glucose by promoting the conversion of hepatic glycogen to glucose. It is used in severe insulin-induced hypoglycaemia and may be given in the recommended dose of 1 mg by the subcutaneous, intramuscular or intravenous route. Glucagon has a short period of action; an oral (if the person is conscious) or intravenous carbohydrate should be administered following the glucagon to prevent a recurrence of hypoglycaemia. If the person has been unconscious, glucagon may cause vomiting when consciousness returns.

NURSING CARE FOR DM

The responses of the person with diabetes to the illness are often complex and individual, involving multiple body systems. Assessments, planning and implementation differ for the person with newly diagnosed diabetes, the person with long-term diabetes and the person with acute complications of diabetes. The plan of care and content of teaching also differ according to the type of diabetes, the person's age and culture and the person's intellectual, psychological and social resources. However, nursing care often focuses on teaching the person to manage the illness.

Health promotion

Health promotion activities primarily focus on preventing the complications of diabetes. The prevention of the disease has not been determined, although it is recommended that all people should prevent or decrease excess weight, follow a sensible and well-balanced diet and maintain a regular physical exercise programme. Blood glucose screening at three-year intervals beginning at age 45 is recommended for those in the high-risk groups. These same activities, when combined with medications and self-monitoring, are also beneficial in reducing the onset of complications.

- Advice on the cessation of smoking and the use of cessation smoking devices, such as nicotine patches, should be offered as smoking is an established risk factor for cardiovascular and other related diseases.
- An individual dietary plan to meet the person's needs. This should take into account the person's cultural, ethnic and social values.

Assessment

The data should be collected through nursing and health history and physical examination. When assessing the elderly person, be aware of normal ageing changes in all body systems that may alter interpretation of findings.

- *Health history*: family history of diabetes; history of hypertension or other cardiovascular problems; history of any change in vision (for example, blurring) or speech, dizziness, numbness or tingling in hands or feet; pain when walking; frequent voiding; change in weight, appetite, infections and healing; problems with gastrointestinal function or urination; or altered sexual function.
- *Physical assessment*: height/weight ratio, vital signs, visual acuity, cranial nerves, sensory ability (touch, hot/cold, vibration) of extremities, peripheral pulses, skin and mucous membranes (hair loss, appearance, lesions, rash, itching, vaginal discharge).

Nursing diagnoses and interventions

Risk for impaired skin integrity

The person with diabetes is at increased risk for altered skin integrity as a result of decreased or absent sensation from neuropathies, decreased tissue perfusion from cardiovascular complications and infection. In addition, poor vision increases the risk of trauma, and an open lesion is more prone to infection and delayed healing. Impaired skin and tissue integrity, with resultant gangrene, is especially common in the feet and lower extremities.

Conduct baseline and ongoing assessments of the feet, including:

- Musculoskeletal assessment that includes foot and ankle joint range of motion, bone abnormalities (bunions, hammertoes, overlapping digits), gait patterns, use of assistive devices for walking and abnormal wear patterns on shoes.
- Neurologic assessment that includes sensations of touch and position, pain and temperature.
- Vascular examination that includes assessment of lower-extremity pulses, capillary refill, colour and temperature of skin, lesions and oedema.

+ Hydration status, including dryness or excessive perspiration.
+ Lesions, fissures between toes, corns, calluses, plantar warts, ingrown or overgrown toenails, redness over pressure points, blisters, cellulitis or gangrene. *People with diabetes are at significant risk for lower-extremity gangrene. Peripheral neuropathies may result in alterations in the perception of pain, loss of deep tendon reflexes, loss of cutaneous pressure and position sensation, foot drop, changes in the shape of the foot and changes in bones and joints. Peripheral vascular disease may cause intermittent claudication, absent pulses, delayed venous filling on elevation and gangrene. Injuries, lesions and changes in skin hydration potentiate infections, delayed healing and tissue loss in the person with DM.*

> ## PRACTICE ALERT
>
> Teach the person with diabetes to always test the water temperature in the shower or bath before stepping in.

+ Teach foot hygiene. Wash the feet daily with lukewarm water and mild hand soap; pat dry and dry well between the toes. Apply a very thin coat of lubricating cream if dryness is present (but not between the toes). *Proper hygiene decreases the chance of infection. Temperature receptors may be impaired, so the water should always be tested before use.*
+ Discuss the importance of not smoking if the person smokes. *Nicotine in tobacco causes vasoconstriction, further decreasing the blood supply to the feet.*
+ Discuss the importance of maintaining blood glucose levels through prescribed diet, medication and exercise. *Hyperglycaemia promotes the growth of micro-organisms.*
+ Advise person in the care of the feet. Include information about proper shoe fit and composition, avoiding clothing or activities that decrease circulation to the feet, foot inspections, the care of toenails and the importance of obtaining medical care for lesions. If the person has visual deficits, is obese or cannot reach the feet, teach the caregiver how to inspect and care for the feet. Feet should be inspected daily. *Foot care is a priority in diabetes management to prevent serious problems. Many people with diabetes are unaware of lesions or injury until infection and compromised circulation are far advanced. The hows and whys of each component must be included in teaching. A variety of methods may be used, including demonstration, return demonstration, audiovisual aids and written lists. If the person is wearing shoes and socks, ask him or her to remove them to practise foot care effectively.*

> ## PRACTICE ALERT
>
> Suggest the use of a hand mirror to check the bottom of the feet and the back of the heel.

Risk for infection

The person with diabetes is at increased risk for infection. The risk of infection is believed to be due to vascular insufficiency that limits the inflammatory response, neurologic abnormalities that limit the awareness of trauma, and a predisposition to bacterial and fungal infections.

+ Advise the person on hand washing technique and the importance of it. *Hand washing is the single most effective method for preventing the spread of infection.*
+ Monitor for signs and symptoms of infection: increased temperature, pain, malaise, swelling, redness, discharge and cough. *Early diagnosis and treatment of infections can control their severity and decrease complications.*
+ Discuss the importance of skin care. Keep the skin clean and dry, using lukewarm water and mild soap. *People with diabetes are more prone to develop furuncles and carbuncles; the infection often increases the need for insulin. Clean, intact skin and mucous membranes are the first line of defence against infection.*
+ Advise the person on dental healthcare measures:
   a. Maintain careful oral hygiene, which includes brushing the teeth with a soft toothbrush and fluoridated toothpaste at least twice a day and flossing as recommended.
   b. Be aware of the symptoms requiring dental care: bad breath, unpleasant taste in the mouth, bleeding, red or sore gums, and tooth pain.
   c. If dental surgery is necessary, monitor for need to make adjustments in insulin.

   All people with diabetes need to be taught proper oral hygiene, the risk of periodontal disease and the importance of obtaining dental care for symptoms of oral or dental problems.
+ Advise women with diabetes about the symptoms and preventive measures for vaginitis caused by *Candida albicans*. Symptoms include an odourless, white or yellow cheese-like discharge and itching. Sexual transmission is unlikely, but discomfort may cause the person to avoid sexual activity. *Diabetes is a predisposing factor for* Candida albicans *vaginitis, the most common form of vaginitis. Poor personal hygiene and wearing clothing that keeps the vaginal area warm and moist increase the risk of vaginitis. The infection may spread to the urinary tract, resulting in urinary tract infections; preventing and treating vaginitis decreases this risk.*

> ## PRACTICE ALERT
>
> Teach women with diabetes to take preventive measures by maintaining good personal hygiene, wiping front to back after voiding, wearing cotton underwear, avoiding tight jeans and nylon tights and avoiding douching.

COMMUNITY-BASED CARE

Teaching the person and family to self-manage diabetes is a nursing responsibility. Even if a formal teaching plan is developed and implemented by advanced practice nurses, all nurses must be able to reinforce knowledge and answer questions. Teaching is necessary for both the person who is newly diagnosed and for the person who has had diabetes for years. In fact, the latter may need almost as much teaching as the newly diagnosed person. Products for diabetes care, especially insulins, have changed dramatically, and knowledge about risk reduction to prevent complications has increased.

For the hospitalised persons with diabetes, teaching should begin on admission. Prior to designing the teaching plan, the nurse makes an initial assessment of the person's and family's knowledge and learning needs, outlining past diabetes management practices and identifying physical, emotional and sociocultural needs. Educational level, preferred learning methods and style, life experiences and support systems are also assessed.

The following should be included in teaching the person and family about care at home:

● Information about normal metabolism, diabetes mellitus and how diabetes changes metabolism.

● Diet plan: how diet helps keep blood glucose in normal range; number of kcal required and why; amount of carbohydrates, meats and fats allowed and why; and how to calculate the diet, integrating personal food preferences.

● Exercise: how it helps lower blood glucose; the importance of a regular programme; types of exercise; integrating personal exercise preferences; how to handle increased activity.

● Self-monitoring of blood glucose: how to perform the tests accurately; how to care for equipment; what to do for high or low blood glucose.

● Medications:
  – insulin: type, dosage, mixing instructions (if necessary), times of onset and peak actions, how to get and care for equipment, how to give injections, where to give injections;
  – oral medications: type, dosage, side-effects, interaction with other drugs.

● signs and symptoms of acute complications of hypoglycaemia and hyperglycaemia; what to do when they occur.

● Hygiene: skin care, dental care, foot care.

● Sick days: what to do about food, fluids and medications.

Consider this . . .

Research studies have identified that diabetes doubles the risk of developing serious blood vessel diseases and life-threatening events such as strokes and heart attacks. Therefore when nurses provide health education for persons with diabetes, they need to make the person aware of these risks. NICE has recommended that all people with diabetes should be offered structured education, provided by a trained specialist team of healthcare professionals. NICE considers the team should include a diabetes specialist nurse (or a GP practice nurse who has experience in diabetes) and a dietitian (someone who can give specialist advice on diet). Other health professionals should join the team if needed. Therefore a multidisciplinary approach should form part of the care.

Case Study 3 – Kwan
NURSING CARE PLAN Type 1 diabetes mellitus

If you remember Mr Lee Kwan was diagnosed with type 1 diabetes mellitus at age 12 and probably takes insulin to control his diabetes. In the first instance, you will need a full assessment of Mr Lee. The aim of the nursing assessment is to:

✚ assess any problems in glycaemic control and address them to improve it.

✚ detect any complications of diabetes and treat them appropriately.

✚ Educate and reinforce healthy lifestyle advice.

✚ assess the person's overall health and treat any associated or coincidental illness, physical or mental.

✚ provide support and advice to the person on how to cope with living with a chronic illness, and how they can best alter their lifestyle to maintain their health.

What are the symptoms of type 1 diabetes mellitus? How does type 1 differ from type 2 diabetes mellitus?

Assessment

The assessment should include a full nursing assessment of the person. A comprehensive nursing assessment is essential in order to plan nursing care. On admission to the ward, Mr Lee's blood glucose level is measured and it is 15.5 mmol/L. Urinalysis

Case Study 3 – Kwan | **NURSING CARE PLAN Type 1 diabetes mellitus**

showed that he has glucose (glycosuria) and ketones (ketonuria) in his urine. His urine specific gravity (SG) is 1030. What does the high SG value indicate? Can you also list other tests that may be done to confirm Mr Lee's diagnosis of diabetes? Give rationale for the tests that may be done.

The priority in this case is to bring down the blood glucose level to normal or near-normal level. Hourly to two hourly BM stick is done to monitor his blood glucose levels and insulin is administered accordingly. Remember that his specific gravity is 1030 which may indicate that he is dehydrated. Therefore Mr Lee needs to be hydrated with an intravenous infusion of normal saline (0.9%).

Investigations

A simple urine test using multistick can detect glucose in a sample of urine. This may suggest the diagnosis of diabetes. However, the only way to confirm the diagnosis is to have a blood test to look at the level of glucose in the blood. If this is high then it will confirm that Mr Lee has diabetes. The blood test is known as 'fasting blood test' (have nothing to eat or drink, other than water, from midnight before the blood test is performed).

Diagnoses

+ Powerlessness related to a perceived lack of control of diabetes due to present demands on time.

+ Deficient knowledge of self-management of diabetes.

+ Lack of knowledge in any other risk factors which may increase the risk of developing complications.

Expected outcomes

+ Identify those aspects of diabetes that can be controlled and participate in making decisions about self-managing care.

+ Demonstrate an understanding of diabetes self-management through planned medication, diet, exercise and blood glucose self-monitoring activities.

+ Explore Mr Lee's level of understanding of the possible complications related to diabetes and the importance of maintaining a healthy lifestyle.

Planning and implementation

+ Mutually establish specific and individualised short-term and long-term goals for self-management to control blood glucose.

+ Provide opportunities for Mr Lee to express his feelings about himself and his illness.

+ Explore perceptions of his own ability to control his illness and his future, and clarify these perceptions by providing information about resources and support groups.

+ Facilitate decision-making abilities in self-managing his prescribed treatment regimen.

+ Provide positive reinforcement for increasing involvement in self-care activities.

+ Provide relevant learning activities about insulin administration, dietary management, exercise, self-monitoring of blood glucose and healthy lifestyle.

Evalution

After taking an active part in the weekly educational meetings for two months, Mr Lee has greatly enhanced his understanding of and compliance with self-management of his diabetes. He states that he finally understands how insulin, food and exercise affect his body, having previously thought they were 'just things I should do when I wanted to'. He decides to perform self-management activities one week at a time, rather than think too far into (and thereby feel overwhelmed by) the future. Mr Lee and his girlfriend have developed a workable meal schedule and weekly grocery list, and they have begun eating breakfast and dinner together. They both go for walks of two to three miles three times a week on a community hiking trail. To gain a sense of control over his illness, he has also worked out a schedule that allows time for school, healthcare and himself.

> *Consider this ...*
> ● How can smoking and poor self-management of diabetes increase the risk of long-term complications?
> ● Discuss the nurse's role in health education/promotion of persons with diabetes.
> ● Discuss any differences and similarities in the nursing management of persons with type 1 and type 2 diabetes.

CASE STUDY SUMMARIES

Case Study 1. Mrs Jones before she is discharged home will need information about her condition and what she can do to minimise complications. The inability to close the eyelids

completely over the protruding eyeballs increases the risk of corneal dryness, irritation, infection and ulceration. Mrs Jones should be shown how to tape her eyelids during the night to prevent these complications.

She will need information about any medications that she may be discharged with and the importance of taking the medications as prescribed. Regular checks are recommended, even after Mrs Jones completes a successful treatment. It is very important to have a regular blood test (at least every year) to check that she has the right level of thyroid hormone (thyroxine) in her blood.

Case Study 2. Mrs Patel will have a review with her GP approximately two months after she has been discharged from hospital. She will need regular blood tests through her GP to ensure the thyroid hormone is at the normal level. Mrs Patel will need information about any medication she is sent home with.

The practice nurse will keep a close eye on the blood pressure. She will need information on foodstuff that may interact with the thyroid hormone therapy. Excessive intake of foodstuff such as carrots, spinach, turnips and peaches may inhibit the utilisation of thyroid hormone.

Case Study 3. Mr Lee is typical of young adults who do not take their illness seriously. This may be through lack of knowledge or just being complacent. Before discharge from the hospital, Mr Lee had health education with regard to his condition and the importance of taking his medications regularly and maintaining a healthy diet. He has had information on how and when to check his blood glucose levels.

An out-patient appointment with the practice nurse to monitor his progress has been made and he has been informed of the importance of keeping his appointment. He now feels confident to travel alone to university for his studies.

CHAPTER HIGHLIGHTS

- Hormones regulate growth, development and metabolism. Homeostasis is dependent on a balanced level of each type of hormone. Not only do hormones affect organ function, they interact and, when excesses or deficits occur, signs and symptoms are manifested.

- Thyroid disorders are the most common endocrine disorders. Occurring mainly among women, these diseases change body image and impose upsets to energy levels creating fatigue and exhaustion.

- Diabetes mellitus (DM) is a chronic and progressive illness affecting people of all age groups. There are 1.8 million people in the UK with diagnosed diabetes, and this figure is increasing every year. The estimated cost to the NHS is £5 million per day for treatment. With an ageing population, the number of males and females with diagnosed diabetes is projected to rise by 37% for males and 24% for females by 2023.

- Type 2 DM has a hereditary link and is characterised by obesity and sedentary lifestyles. Unlike type 1 DM, in which the onset is often sudden, the development of symptoms that bring persons to their healthcare providers for evaluation is slow.

- Tighter, more intensive blood glucose control is increasingly the focus of care for hospitalised persons with hyperglycaemia.

- Treatment for persons with DM includes insulin, non-insulin hypoglycaemics and blood glucose monitoring devices. Nurses must be familiar with these products and help persons become proficient in their use.

TEST YOURSELF

1. What physiologic response is expected if the pituitary produces an increased amount of ADH?

   a. increased output of urine
   b. decreased output of urine
   c. increased facial hair growth in women
   d. decreased production of testosterone

2. Which of the following hormones does the hypothalamus release?

   a. aldosterone
   b. renin
   c. thyroid releasing hormone
   d. cortisol

3. Excessive amounts of glucocorticoids, produced by the adrenal cortex, result in what pathophysiologic health problem?

   a. inhibited immune response
   b. increased response to glucagon
   c. delayed onset of puberty
   d. decreased metabolic rate

4. ACTH stimulates which gland(s)?

   a. pancreas
   b. spleen
   c. adrenal glands
   d. thyroid gland

5. Oxytocin is produced by the:
   a. anterior pituitary gland
   b. posterior pituitary gland
   c. thyroid gland
   d. ovary

6. The beta cells of the pancreas produce:
   a. glucagon
   b. insulin
   c. somatostatin
   d. androgens

7. Which of the following tests is the most accurate indicator of thyroid function?
   a. GH
   b. FBS
   c. aldosterone
   d. TSH

8. Which is the only endocrine organ that can be palpated during physical assessment?
   a. pancreas
   b. liver
   c. thyroid
   d. pituitary

9. You are caring for a person with newly diagnosed hypothyroidism. What skin assessment might you find?
   a. increased hair growth
   b. rough, dry skin
   c. smooth, flushed skin
   d. cold and clammy skin

10. Which of the following persons would be most at risk for the development of type 2 diabetes?
    a. young adult who is a professional football player
    b. middle-aged man who maintains normal weight
    c. middle-aged woman who is the sole caretaker of her parents
    d. woman over age 70 who is overweight and sedentary

Further resources

Diabetes UK
www.diabetes.org.uk/
Diabetes UK is a useful link for all students to browse through. It is the largest organisation in the UK working for people with diabetes, funding research, campaigning and helping people live with the condition. It provides a quick guide on diabetes for both adults and children.

National Institute for Health and Clinical Excellence (NICE)
www.nice.org.uk/CG66
This is a National Institute for Health and Clinical Excellence website. We think that you will find this link valuable as NICE gives guidance on type 2 diabetes. We think that this link is a must for both students and qualified nurses.

Department of Health (DoH)
www.dh.gov.uk/en/Healthcare/Diabetes/index.htm
This is a Department of Health (DH) website. It is useful because you will find the 12 standards of the Diabetes National Service Framework and all aspects of diabetes care and prevention. This site also provides links to other publications and recommendations by DoH.

Simon's Graves' Disease
simonwaters.technocool.net/mygraves.html
In this link you will find one person's personal story about Graves' disease. It is called Simon's Graves' Disease. We think it will be useful when you provide advice to people with Graves' disease and health promotion. You will also find others bringing their personal experience about their illness, which makes it a rich discussion forum for students.

Cancer Research UK
www.cancerhelp.org.uk/type/thyroid-cancer/treatment/index.htm
Cancer Research UK is a useful site for students to look at the work of cancer support groups, again a site you may recommend in health promotion, because it improves the lives of people affected by cancer. This particular link tells you about the treatment for thyroid cancer. It includes information about surgery, radiotherapy and chemotherapy as well as information about follow-up and research into treatments for thyroid cancer.

Macmillan
www.macmillan.org.uk/Cancerinformation/Cancertypes/Thyroid/Aboutthyroidcancer/Thyroidcancer.aspx
Another support group site, this site is managed by Macmillan. This link provides information about thyroid: symptoms, causes, treatments – provides further links to other resources which you may find useful.

Bibliography

Alexander M F, Fawcett J and Runciman P J (2007) *Nursing Practice – Hospitals and Home*. Edinburgh, Churchill Livingstone.

Capriotti T (2005) Type 2 diabetes epidemic increases use of oral anti-diabetic agents. *MEDSURG Nursing,* **14**(5), 341–347.

Department of Health (2005) *Improving Diabetes Services – The NSF two years on*. London, HMSO.

Health Statistics Quarterly (2002) *Prevalence of Diagnosed Diabetes Mellitus in General Practice in England and Wales 1994–1998*. London, HMSO.

Kumar P and Clark M (2009) *Clinical Medicine* (7th edn). Edinburgh, WB Saunders.

Lehne RA (2010) *Pharmacology for Nursing Care* (7th edn). St Louis, MO, Saunders/Elsevier.

McCance K L, Huether S E, Brashers V L and Rote N S (2010) *Pathophysiology: The biologic basis for disease in adults and children* (6th edn). St Louis, MO, Mosby.

Newnham A, Ryan R, Khunti K and Majeed A (2002) Prevalence of diagnosed diabetes mellitus in general practice in England and Wales. *Health Statistics Quarterly*, Summer, 5–13.

NHS Choices (2011) *Thyroid Cancer*. Available at: http://www.nhs.uk/Conditions/Cancer-of-the-thyroid/Pages/Introduction.aspx (accessed September 2011).

NICE (2003) *Person-education Models for Diabetes: Understanding NICE Guidance – Information for People with Diabetes, and the Public*. London, National Institute for Health and Clinical Excellence.

NICE (2004) *Type 1 Diabetes: Diagnosis and management of Type 1 diabetes in adults,* CG15. London, National Institute for Health and Clinical Excellence.

NICE (2009) *Type 2 Diabetes* – Newer Agents (partial update of CG66), CG87. London, National Institute for Health and Clinical Excellence.

NMC (2010) *Guidelines for Record and Record Keeping*. London, Nursing and Midwifery Council.

Patient UK (2009) *Diabetes Mellitus*. Available at: http://www.patient.co.uk/doctor/Diabetes-Mellitus.htm (accessed September 2011).

Patient UK (2010) *Hyperthyroidism (Overactive Thyroid)*. Available at: http://www.patient.co.uk/health/Hyperthyroidism-Overactive-Thyroid.htm (accessed September 2011).

Patient UK (2011) *Hypothyroidism – Underactive Thyroid*. Available at: http://www.patient.co.uk/health/Hypothyroidism-Underactive-Thyroid.htm (accessed September 2011).

Porth C (2009) *Pathophysiology: Concepts of altered health states* (9th edn). Philadelphia, PA, Lippincott.

Roberts C K and Barnard R J (2005) Effects of exercise and diet on chronic disease. *Journal of Applied Physiology,* **98**, 3–30.

Saudek C D and Margolis S (2005) *Diabetes. The Johns Hopkins White Papers*. Baltimore, MD, Johns Hopkins Medicine.

SIGN (2001) *Management of Diabetes*. Edinburgh, Scottish Intercollegiate Guidelines Network.

Tierney L M, McPhee S J and Papadakis M A (eds) (2005) *Current Medical Diagnosis and Treatment* (44th edn). New York, McGraw Hill.

Caring for people with gastrointestinal problems

CASE STUDIES

Below are three case studies that you may wish to consider before, during or after you have read the chapter. There are no right or wrong answers to these case studies, but you should think about the physical, psychological and social implications. Also consider what questions you would ask the person so that you can help alleviate their anxieties.

Case Study 1 – Mary

Ms Mary Peters, a 30-year-old woman, went to see her practice nurse with depression, breathlessness and generally feeling unwell. Ms Peters is 18 stone and has tried every diet to lose weight. She has even thought of having gastric surgery, but the cost has put her off as she could not afford it. Ms Peters smokes 25 cigarettes a day. She said to the nurse, 'I am aware that my weight has health implications and it was desperation that made me think about having surgery. The problem is that the unhealthy food is everywhere. There are three fast food shops near my house and it is so convenient – no need to cook. You go to the supermarket, these foods are within easy reach and even in the petrol station there are sweets. You can't run away from it.' She said to the nurse that she wanted to be a size 12 but with all these temptations she is finding it difficult to diet and keep her weight down.

Case Study 2 – Monica

Mrs Monica Stone is a 47-year-old police officer who lives and works in a metropolitan area. Mrs Stone has had 'heartburn' and abdominal discomfort for years, but thought it went along with the stress of her job. Last year she went to see her GP, after becoming weak, light-headed and short of breath. Mrs Stone was found to be anaemic and was diagnosed as having a duodenal ulcer. She took omeprazole and ferrous sulphate for three months before stopping both medications, saying she had 'never felt better in her life'. Mrs Stone has now been admitted to the hospital with pain in her stomach and vomiting blood.

Case Study 3 – Sunita

Mrs Sunita Chowdrey, a 37-year-old woman, went to see her GP for abdominal pain and vomiting. She also tells her GP that her appetite is poor and she has no energy to do any housework. She tells the doctor, 'I don't smoke or drink any alcohol but I seem to burp a lot.' Her GP suspects that Sunita may have gastritis and puts her on a course of tablets and asks her to come back and see him in two weeks. Mrs Chowdrey feels relieved and gets the medications from the chemist and takes them as she was told. After a week on tablets, Sunita is still not feeling well. So she decides to visit her GP again. This time, the doctor decides to refer her to the local hospital for tests and investigations.

INTRODUCTION

For every physical activity the body requires energy, and the amount depends on the duration and type of activity we do. Energy is measured in calories and is obtained from the body stores or the food we eat. Glycogen (excess glucose is converted into glycogen and stored in the liver and muscles) is the main source of fuel used by the muscles to enable us to undertake both aerobic (with oxygen) and anaerobic (without oxygen) exercise. If you train with low glycogen stores, you will feel constantly tired, training performance will be lower and you will be more prone to injury and illness. Nutrition is the process by which the body ingests, absorbs, transports, uses and eliminates nutrients in food. The digestive organs responsible for these processes are the gastrointestinal tract (also called the alimentary canal) and the accessory digestive organs. The gastrointestinal tract consists of the mouth, pharynx, oesophagus, stomach, small intestine and large intestine. The accessory digestive organs include the liver, gall bladder and pancreas (Figure 7.1). The chapter begins with a review of the nutrients essential for cellular function, an overview of the anatomy and physiology of the gastrointestinal (GI) tract and some common nutritional disorders.

Nutrients

Nutrition is a vital component for human existence. An adequate intake of nutrients is essential for the survival of the body systems. Nutrients are substances found in food and are used by the body to promote growth, maintenance and repair. Organic (any chemical compound that contains carbon) nutrients include carbohydrates, fats, proteins and vitamins. Inorganic (any chemical compound that does not contain

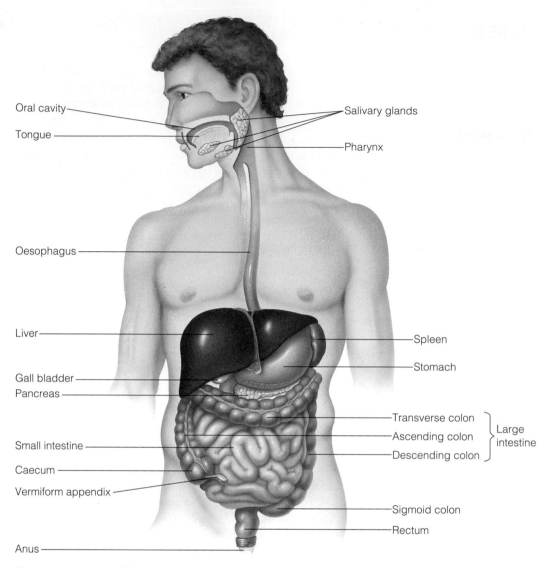

Figure 7.1 Organs of the gastrointestinal tract and accessory digestive organs.

carbon) chemical compounds such as dietary minerals, water and oxygen may also be considered nutrients. A nutrient is essential to an organism; if it cannot be synthesised by the organism in sufficient quantities it must be obtained from an external source. Nutrients needed in large quantities are called macronutrients; micronutrients are required in only small quantities. The categories of nutrients are carbohydrates, proteins, fats, vitamins, minerals and water. Nurses have a clear responsibility to ensure that persons' nutritional needs are met whilst the persons are under their care. Let us now look at them in a bit more detail.

CARBOHYDRATES

The primary sources of carbohydrates (which include sugars and starches) are plant foods. Monosaccharide and disaccharides come from milk, sugar cane, sugar beets, honey and fruits. Polysaccharide starch is found in grains, legumes and root vegetables. Following ingestion, digestion and metabolism, carbohydrates are converted primarily to glucose, the molecule body cells use to make adenosine triphosphate (ATP). Excess glucose in the healthy person is converted to glycogen or fat. Glycogen is stored in the liver and muscles; fat is stored as adipose tissue. Regardless of the source, all carbohydrates supply 4 kcal per gram of energy.

PROTEINS

Proteins are classified as either complete or incomplete. Complete proteins are found in animal products such as eggs, milk, milk products and meat. They contain the greatest amount of amino acids and meet the body's amino acid requirements for tissue growth and maintenance. Incomplete proteins are found in legumes, nuts, grains, cereals and vegetables. These sources are low in or lack one or more of the amino acids essential for building complete proteins.

The body uses proteins to build many different structures, including skin keratin, the collagen and elastin in connective tissues, and muscles. They are also used to make enzymes, haemoglobin, plasma proteins, and some hormones. Proteins provide 4 kcal per gram of energy.

FATS (LIPIDS)

Fats, or lipids, include phospholipids; steroids, such as cholesterol; and neutral fats, more commonly known as triglycerides. Neutral fats are the most abundant fats in the diet. They may be either saturated or unsaturated. Saturated fats are found in animal products (milk and meats) and in some plant products (such as coconut). Unsaturated fats are found in seeds, nuts and most vegetable oils. Sources of cholesterol include meats, milk products and egg yolks. Fats supply 9 kcal per gram of energy.

Fats are a necessary part of the structure and function of the body. For example:

- Phospholipids are a part of all cell membranes.
- Triglycerides are the major energy source for hepatocytes and skeletal muscle cells.
- Dietary fats facilitate absorption of fat-soluble vitamins.
- Cholesterol is the essential component of **bile** salts, steroid hormones and vitamin D.
- Adipose tissue serves as a protection around body organs, as a layer of insulation under the skin and as a concentrated source of fuel for cellular energy.

VITAMINS

Vitamins are organic compounds that facilitate the body's use of carbohydrates, proteins and fats. All of the vitamins except vitamins D and K must be ingested in foods or taken as supplements. Vitamin D is made by ultraviolet irradiation of cholesterol molecules in the skin, and vitamin K is synthesised by bacteria in the intestine.

Vitamins are categorised as either fat soluble or water soluble. The fat-soluble vitamins (A, D, E and K) bind to ingested fats and are absorbed as the fats are absorbed. Water-soluble vitamins (the B complex and C) are absorbed with water in the GI tract; however, vitamin B_{12} must become attached to intrinsic factor (a substance that is secreted by the gastric mucous membrane and is essential for the absorption of vitamin B_{12} in the intestines) to be absorbed. Fat-soluble vitamins are stored in the body, and excesses may cause toxicity; water-soluble vitamins in excess of body requirements are excreted in the urine.

MINERALS

Minerals are essential nutrients that your body needs in small amounts to work properly. We need them in the form they are found in food. Minerals can be found in varying amounts in a variety of foods such as meat, cereals (including cereal products such as bread), fish, milk and dairy foods, vegetables, fruit (especially dried fruit) and nuts.

Minerals are necessary for three main reasons:

- building strong bones and teeth;
- controlling body fluids inside and outside cells;
- turning the food we eat into energy.

These are all essential minerals:

- calcium;
- iron;
- magnesium;
- phosphorus;
- potassium;
- sodium;
- sulphur.

ANATOMY, PHYSIOLOGY AND FUNCTIONS OF THE GASTROINTESTINAL (GI) SYSTEM

The study of the GI system is essential for nursing practice as the digestive processes are the means by which foods and liquids are digested and absorbed and transported by the blood to cells for cellular metabolism. The GI system consists of a variety of organs with important functions; disorders to any of these organs can produce distressing and embarrassing symptoms which may impact on a person's social life. This section will describe the structure and function of the different components of the GI tract and the accessory organs of digestion such as the liver, pancreas and the gall bladder in order to help you understand the diseases of this system.

The GI tract is a continuous hollow tube, extending from the mouth to the anus. Once foods are placed in the mouth, they are subjected to a variety of processes that move them and break them down into end products that can be absorbed from the lumen of the small intestine into the blood or lymph. These digestive processes are as follows:

- ingestion of food;
- movement of food and wastes;
- secretion of mucus, water and enzymes;
- mechanical digestion of food;

- chemical digestion of food;
- absorption of digested food.

THE MOUTH

The mouth, also called the oral or buccal cavity, is lined with mucous membranes and is enclosed by the lips, cheeks, palate and tongue (Figure 7.2).

The lips and cheeks are skeletal muscle covered externally by skin. Their function is to keep food in the mouth during chewing. The palate consists of two regions: the hard palate and the soft palate. The hard palate covers bone in the roof of the mouth and provides a hard surface against which the tongue forces food. The soft palate, extending from the hard palate and ending at the back of the mouth as a fold called the uvula, is primarily muscle. When food is swallowed, the soft palate rises as a reflex to close off the oropharynx.

The tongue, composed of skeletal muscle and connective tissue, is located in the floor of the mouth. It contains mucous and serous glands, taste buds and papillae. The tongue mixes food with saliva during chewing, forms the food into a mass (called a *bolus*) and initiates swallowing. Some papillae provide surface roughness to facilitate licking and moving food; other papillae house the taste buds.

Saliva moistens food so it can be made into a bolus, dissolves food chemicals so they can be tasted and provides enzymes (such as amylase) that begin the chemical breakdown of starches. Saliva is produced by salivary glands, most of which lie superior or inferior to the mouth and drain into it. The salivary glands include the parotid, the submaxillary and the sublingual glands.

The teeth chew (masticate) and grind food to break it down into smaller parts. As the food is masticated, it is mixed with saliva. Adults have 32 permanent teeth. The teeth are embedded in the gingiva (gums), with the crown of each tooth visible above the gingiva.

THE PHARYNX

The pharynx consists of the oropharynx and the laryngopharynx (see Figure 7.2). Both structures provide passageways for food, fluids and air. The pharynx is made of skeletal muscles and is lined with mucous membranes. The skeletal muscles move food to the oesophagus via the pharynx through **peristalsis** (alternating waves of contraction and relaxation of involuntary muscle). The mucosa of the pharynx contains mucous-producing glands that provide fluid to facilitate the passage of the bolus of food as it is swallowed.

THE OESOPHAGUS

The oesophagus, a muscular tube about 10 inches (25 cm) long, serves as a passageway for food from the pharynx to the stomach (see Figures 7.1 and 7.2). The epiglottis, a flap of cartilage over the top of the larynx, keeps food out of the larynx during swallowing. The oesophagus descends through the thorax and diaphragm, entering the stomach at the cardiac orifice. The gastro-oesophageal sphincter surrounds this opening. This sphincter, along with the diaphragm, keeps the orifice closed when food is not being swallowed.

For most of its length, the oesophagus is lined with stratified squamous epithelium; simple columnar epithelium (see Figure 7.3) lines the oesophagus where it joins the stomach. The mucosa and submucosa of the oesophagus lie in longitudinal folds when the oesophagus is empty.

THE STOMACH

The stomach, located high on the left side of the abdominal cavity, is connected to the oesophagus at the upper end and to the small intestine at the lower end (Figure 7.4). Normally about 10 inches (25 cm) long, the stomach is a distensible organ that

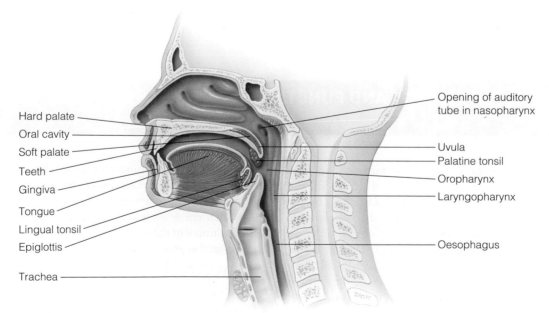

Figure 7.2 Structures of the mouth, the pharynx and the oesophagus.

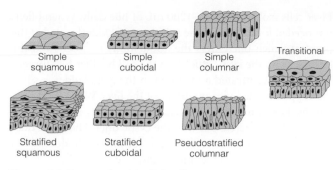

Figure 7.3 Types of epithelial cells.

can expand to hold up to 4 L of food and fluid. The concave surface of the stomach is called the lesser curvature; the convex surface is called the greater curvature. The stomach may be divided into regions extending from the distal end of the oesophagus to the opening into the small intestine. These regions are the cardiac region, fundus body and pylorus (see Figure 7.4). The pyloric sphincter controls emptying of the stomach into the duodenal portion of the small intestine. The stomach is a storage reservoir for food, which continues the mechanical breakdown of food, begins the process of protein digestion and mixes the food with gastric juices into a thick fluid called **chyme**.

The stomach is lined with columnar epithelial, mucous-producing cells. Millions of openings in the lining lead to gastric glands that can produce 4–5 L of gastric juice each day. The gastric glands contain a variety of secretory cells, including the following:

- Mucous cells produce alkaline mucus that clings to the lining of the stomach and protects it from being digested by gastric juice.

- Zymogenic cells produce pepsinogen (an inactive form of pepsin, a protein-digesting enzyme).

- Parietal cells secrete hydrochloric acid and intrinsic factor. Hydrochloric acid activates and increases the activity of

protein-digesting cells and also is bactericidal. Intrinsic factor is necessary for the absorption of vitamin B_{12} in the small intestine.

- Enteroendocrine cells secrete gastrin, histamine, endorphins, serotonin and somatostatin. These hormones or hormone-like substances diffuse into the blood. Gastrin is important in regulating secretion and motility of the stomach.

The secretion of gastric juice is under both neural and **endocrine** control. Stimulation of the **parasympathetic** vagus nerve increases secretory activity; in contrast, stimulation of **sympathetic** nerves decreases secretions. The three phases of secretory activity are the cephalic phase, the gastric phase and the intestinal phase.

1. The *cephalic phase* prepares for digestion and is triggered by the sight, odour, taste or thought of food. During this initial phase, motor impulses are transmitted via the vagus nerve to the stomach.

2. The *gastric phase* begins when food enters the stomach. Stomach distention (stimulating stretch receptors) and chemical stimuli from partially digested proteins initiate this phase. Gastrin-secreting cells produce gastrin, which in turn stimulates the gastric glands (especially the parietal cells) to produce more gastric juice. Histamine also stimulates hydrochloric acid secretion.

3. The *intestinal phase* is initiated when partially digested food begins to enter the small intestine, stimulating mucous cells of the intestine to release a hormone that promotes continued gastric secretion.

Mechanical digestion in the stomach is accomplished by peristaltic movements that churn and mix the food with the gastric juices to form chyme. Gastric motility is enhanced or retarded by the same factors that affect secretion, namely, distention and the effect of gastrin. After a person eats a well-balanced meal, the stomach empties completely in approximately four to six hours. Gastric emptying depends on the volume, chemical composition and osmotic pressure of the gastric contents. The stomach empties large volumes of liquid content more rapidly, while gastric emptying is slowed by solids and fats.

THE SMALL INTESTINE

The small intestine begins at the pyloric sphincter and ends at the ileocaecal junction at the entrance of the large intestine (see Figure 7.1). The small intestine is about 6 m long but only about 2.5 cm in diameter. This long tube hangs in coils in the abdominal cavity, suspended by the mesentery and surrounded by the large intestine. The small intestine has three regions: the duodenum, the jejunum and the ileum. The duodenum begins at the pyloric sphincter and extends around the head of the pancreas for about 25 cm. Both pancreatic enzymes and bile from the liver enter the small intestine at the duodenum. The jejunum, the middle region of the small intestine, extends for about 2.4 m. The ileum, the terminal end of the small intestine, is approximately 3.6 m long and meets the large intestine at the ileocaecal valve.

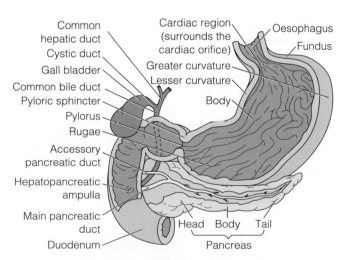

Figure 7.4 The internal anatomical structures of the stomach, including the pancreatic, cystic and hepatic ducts, the pancreas and the gall bladder.

THE LARGE INTESTINE

The large intestine, also known as the colon, commences from the ileocaecal valve and terminates at the rectum (see Figure 7.5). The large intestine is approximately 2 m in length and 6 cm in diameter. The large intestine consists of the caecum, ascending, transverse, descending and sigmoid colons; the rectum and the anus (see Figure 7.5). The functions of the large intestine include:

- absorption of nutrients and water;
- production of vitamin K and some B complexes such as B_1, B_2 and folic acid;
- secretion of mucus for lubrication of faeces;
- storage of indigestible food substances such as cellulose;
- defecation.

THE ACCESSORY DIGESTIVE ORGANS

The liver, gall bladder and exocrine pancreas secrete substances necessary for the digestion of chyme. The liver produces bile, necessary for fat digestion and absorption, and stores it in the gall bladder. The liver also receives nutrients absorbed by the small intestine and metabolises or synthesises these nutrients so they are in a form that can be used by the cells of the body. The exocrine pancreas produces enzymes necessary for digestion of fats, proteins and carbohydrates.

The liver and gall bladder

The liver weighs about 1.4 kg in the average-size adult. It is located in the right side of the abdomen, inferior to the diaphragm and anterior to the stomach (see Figure 7.1). The liver has four lobes: right, left, caudate and quadrate. A mesenteric ligament separates the right and left lobes and suspends the liver from the diaphragm and anterior abdominal wall. Liver tissue consists of units called lobules, which are composed of plates of hepatocytes (liver cells).

Bile production is the liver's primary digestive function. Bile is a greenish, watery solution containing bile salts, cholesterol, bilirubin, electrolytes, water and phospholipids. These substances are necessary to emulsify and promote the absorption of fats.

Liver cells make from 700–1200 mL of bile daily. When bile is not needed for digestion, the sphincter of Oddi (located at the point at which bile enters the duodenum) is closed, and the bile backs up the cystic **duct** into the gall bladder for storage.

Bile is concentrated and stored in the gall bladder, a small sac cupped in the inferior surface of the liver. When food containing fats enters the duodenum, hormones stimulate the gall bladder to secrete bile into the cystic duct. The cystic duct joins the hepatic duct to form the common bile duct, from which bile enters into the duodenum (see Figure 7.4).

The exocrine pancreas

The pancreas, a gland located between the stomach and small intestine, is the primary enzyme-producing organ of the digestive system. It is a triangular gland extending across the abdomen, with its tail next to the spleen and its head next to the duodenum (see Figure 7.4). The body and tail of the pancreas are retroperitoneal, lying behind the greater curvature of the stomach. The pancreas is actually two organs in one, having both exocrine and endocrine structures and functions. The exocrine portion of the pancreas, through secretory units called acini, secretes alkaline pancreatic juice containing many different enzymes. The acini, clusters of secretory cells surrounding ducts, drain into the pancreatic duct. The pancreatic duct joins with the common bile duct just before it enters the duodenum (so that pancreatic juice and bile from the liver enter the small intestine together). The pancreas also has endocrine functions (see Chapter 6).

The pancreas produces from 1–1.5 L of pancreatic juice daily. Pancreatic juice is clear and has high bicarbonate content. This alkaline fluid neutralises the acidic chyme as it enters the duodenum, optimising the pH for intestinal and pancreatic enzyme activity. The secretion of pancreatic juice is controlled by the vagus nerve and the intestinal hormones secretin and cholecystokinin.

The person with obesity

Obesity is one of the biggest health challenges we face. The government is committed to taking action to prevent more

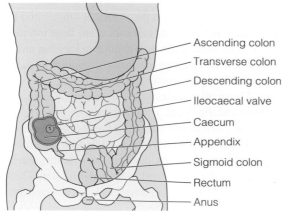

Figure 7.5 Anatomy of the large intestine.

- Ascending colon
- Transverse colon
- Descending colon
- Ileocaecal valve
- Caecum
- Appendix
- Sigmoid colon
- Rectum
- Anus

FAST FACTS

Overweight

- In the UK an estimated 60.8% of adults and 31.1% of children are overweight.
- According to figures from 2009, almost a quarter of adults (22% of men and 24% of women) in England were classified as obese (BMI 30 kg/m² or over).

Source: http://www.bbc.co.uk/health/physical_health/conditions/obesity. shtml (accessed September 2011).

serious illness and much bigger costs to the health service and the country in years to come. The government's ambition is to be the first major nation to reverse the rising tide of obesity and overweight in the population, by enabling everyone to achieve and maintain a healthy weight. The government's initial focus is on children: by 2020, they aim to reduce the proportion of overweight and obese children to 2000 levels.

Given the impact on individual health, obese and overweight individuals also place a significant burden on the NHS. Direct costs are estimated to be £4.2 billion and Foresight have forecasted that this will more than double by 2050 if we continue as we are. But there are also costs to society and the economy more broadly – for example, sickness absence reduces productivity. Foresight estimated that weight problems already cost the wider economy in the region of £16 billion, and that this will rise to £50 billion per year by 2050 if left unchecked (DoH 2011).

The term obesity is used when a person has excess amount of adipose tissue (connective tissue for storage of fats) where the fat may settle on the abdominal region (apple-shaped), hips or thighs (pear-shaped). Overweight refers to an increase in weight in relation to the individual's height and when the body mass index (BMI) is 25–29.9 kg/m². The overweight may be due to an increase in adipose tissue or due to an increase in muscle mass. For example, a bodybuilder may be very lean and muscular but weigh more than others of same height. Thus a bodybuilder may be considered as overweight as a result of an increased muscle mass but not fat.

Obesity and overweight are very common and affect most parts of the world, despite numerous health education and interventions. Obesity rates increase in the older population; obesity is much more common among the lower socioeconomic groups; and the number is escalating. The estimated cost of obesity to the nation is £3.3–3.7 billion per year and the cost of obesity plus those who are overweight is £6.6–7.4 billion. Obesity is an excessive accumulation of fat cells (adipose tissue) for an individual's height, weight, gender and ethnicity to such an extent that obesity could lead to health problems. One useful tool for calculating obesity is BMI. The formula for BMI is as follows:

$$\text{BMI} = \text{weight (kg)/(height (m))}^2$$

An individual with a BMI between 19 and 24.9 kg/m² is of normal weight; 25–29.9 kg/m² is considered overweight and people with a BMI of over 30 kg/m² are considered obese.

Aetiology of obesity

Both hereditary and environmental factors have been associated with obesity which includes physiological, psychological and cultural influences. Some of the causes include:

- Endocrine disorders such as hypothyroidism (underactive thyroid) and Cushing's syndrome (a hormonal disorder caused by prolonged exposure of the body's tissues to high levels of the hormone cortisol).
- Familial history – if one or both parents are obese, this increases the chance of the children getting obese.

- Depression as a result of bereavement, low self-esteem.
- High consumption of alcohol, eating unhealthy food, lack of exercise and comfort eating as a result of painful life events such as bereavement in the family.
- Stress which may result in the person overeating.
- Steroid therapy.
- Women as a result of hormonal changes after having a baby.
- South Asian and Afro-Caribbean people are particularly at risk.
- Men and women are most likely to put on weight between the ages of 20 and 40.
- The changes in levels of hormones during the menopause can make it easier to put on weight.

Assessment tools used to identify obesity

Although body weight may be used to identify obesity, measures of body fat are more accurate. Males at ideal body weight have 10–20% body fat, whereas females at ideal body weight have 20–30% body fat.

- BMI is calculated by dividing the weight (in kilograms) by the height in metres squared (m²). BMI calculations may not as accurately reflect the extent of adipose tissue in people who are highly muscular (for example, bodybuilders) or in those who have lost muscle mass (for example, the elderly). Figure 7.6 shows how to calculate BMI.
- Anthropometry includes measurements of height, weight, bone size and skinfold measurement to estimate subcutaneous (just under the skin) fat.
- Underwater weighing (hydrodensitometry) is considered the most accurate way to determine body fat. This technique involves submerging the whole body and then measuring the amount of displaced water.
- Waist circumference is measured to determine body fat distribution. Men with a waist measurement of 102 cm or greater and women with a waist measurement of 88 cm or greater have a higher risk for complications of obesity.
- Malnutrition Universal Screening Tool (MUST) is used to determine nutritional status (to determine if the person is obese or undernourished).

FAST FACTS

Calculating body mass index (BMI)

$$\text{BMI} = \text{weight (kg)/(height(m))}^2$$

Normal = BMI 18.5–24.9 kg/m²
Overweight = BMI 25–29.9 kg/m²
Obese = BMI > 30 kg/m²
Extremely obese = BMI > 40 kg/m²

Body Mass Index (BMI) Chart of Adults

■ Obese (>30)　□ Overweight (25–30)　▨ Normal (18.5–25)　▫ Underweight (<18.5)

HEIGHT in feet/inches and centimeters

WEIGHT lbs	(kg)	4'8" 142cm	4'9" 147	4'10" 150	4'11" 152	5'0" 155	5'1" 157	5'2" 160	5'3" 163	5'4" 165	5'5" 168	5'6" 170	5'7" 173	5'8" 175	5'9" 178	5'10" 180	5'11" 183	6'0" 185	6'1" 188	6'2" 191	6'3" 193	6'4" 196	6'5"
260	(117.9)	58	56	54	53	51	49	48	46	45	43	42	41	40	38	37	36	35	34	33	32	32	31
255	(115.7)	57	55	53	51	50	48	47	45	44	42	41	40	39	38	37	36	35	34	33	32	32	31
250	(113.4)	56	54	52	50	49	47	46	44	43	42	40	39	38	37	36	35	34	33	32	31	30	30
245	(111.1)	55	53	51	49	48	46	45	43	42	41	40	38	37	36	35	34	33	32	31	31	30	29
240	(108.9)	54	52	50	48	47	45	44	43	41	40	39	38	36	35	34	33	33	32	31	30	29	28
235	(106.6)	53	51	49	47	46	44	43	42	40	39	38	37	36	35	34	33	32	31	30	29	29	28
230	(104.3)	52	50	48	46	45	43	42	41	39	38	37	36	35	34	33	32	31	30	30	29	28	27
225	(102.1)	50	49	47	45	44	43	41	40	39	37	36	35	34	33	32	31	31	30	29	28	27	27
220	(99.8)	49	48	46	44	43	42	40	39	38	37	36	34	33	32	32	31	30	29	28	27	27	26
215	(97.5)	48	47	45	43	42	41	39	38	37	36	35	33	32	31	31	30	29	28	28	27	26	25
210	(95.3)	47	45	44	42	41	40	38	37	36	35	34	33	32	31	30	29	28	28	27	26	26	25
205	(93.0)	46	44	43	41	40	39	37	36	35	34	33	32	31	30	29	29	28	27	26	26	25	24
200	(90.7)	45	43	42	40	39	38	37	35	34	33	32	31	30	30	29	28	27	26	26	25	24	24
195	(88.5)	44	42	41	39	38	37	36	35	33	32	31	31	30	29	28	27	26	26	25	24	24	23
190	(86.2)	43	41	40	38	37	36	35	34	33	32	31	30	29	28	27	26	26	25	24	24	23	23
185	(83.9)	41	40	39	37	36	35	34	33	32	31	30	29	28	27	27	26	25	24	24	23	23	22
180	(81.6)	40	39	38	36	35	34	33	32	31	30	29	28	27	27	26	25	25	24	23	22	22	21
175	(79.4)	39	38	37	35	34	33	32	31	30	29	28	27	27	26	25	24	24	23	22	22	21	21
170	(77.1)	38	37	36	34	33	32	31	30	29	28	27	27	26	25	24	24	23	22	22	21	21	20
165	(74.8)	37	36	34	33	32	31	30	29	28	27	27	26	25	24	24	23	22	22	21	21	20	20
160	(72.6)	36	35	33	32	31	30	29	28	27	27	26	25	24	24	23	22	22	21	21	20	19	19
155	(70.3)	35	34	32	31	30	29	28	27	27	26	25	24	24	23	22	22	21	20	20	19	19	18
150	(68.0)	34	32	31	30	29	28	27	27	26	25	24	23	23	22	22	21	20	20	19	19	18	18
145	(65.8)	33	31	30	29	28	27	27	26	25	24	23	23	22	21	21	20	20	19	19	18	18	17
140	(63.5)	31	30	29	28	27	26	26	25	24	23	23	22	21	21	20	20	19	18	18	17	17	17
135	(61.2)	30	29	28	27	26	26	25	24	23	22	22	21	21	20	19	19	18	18	17	17	16	16
130	(59.0)	29	28	27	26	25	25	24	23	22	22	21	20	20	19	19	18	18	17	17	16	16	15
125	(56.7)	28	27	26	25	24	24	23	22	21	21	20	20	19	18	18	17	17	16	16	15	15	15
120	(54.4)	27	26	25	24	23	23	22	21	21	20	19	19	18	18	17	17	16	16	15	15	15	14
115	(52.2)	26	25	24	23	22	22	21	20	20	19	19	18	17	17	16	16	16	15	15	14	14	14
110	(49.9)	25	24	23	22	21	21	20	19	19	18	18	17	17	16	16	15	15	15	14	14	13	13
105	(47.6)	24	23	22	21	21	20	19	19	18	17	17	16	16	15	16	14	14	13	13	13	13	12
100	(45.4)	22	22	21	20	20	19	18	18	17	17	16	16	15	15	14	14	14	13	13	12	12	12
95	(43.1)	21	21	20	19	19	18	17	17	16	16	15	15	14	14	13	13	13	12	12	12	11	11
90	(40.8)	20	19	19	18	18	17	16	16	15	15	15	14	14	13	13	13	12	12	12	11	11	11
85	(38.6)	19	18	18	17	17	16	16	15	15	14	14	13	13	13	12	12	12	11	11	11	10	10
80	(36.3)	18	17	17	16	16	15	15	14	14	13	13	13	12	12	11	11	11	11	10	10	10	9

Note: BMI values rounded to the nearest whole number. BMI categories based on CDC (Centers for Disease Control and Prevention) criteria.
www.vertex42.com　BMI = Weight[kg] / (Height[m] × Height[m]) = 703 × Weight[lb] / (Height[in] × Height[in])　© 2009 Vertex42 LLC

Figure 7.6 BMI chart.

INTERDISCIPLINARY CARE FOR OBESITY

Interventions to reduce weight instigated or maintained by the nurse include healthy eating and lifestyle changes. There are number of approaches to the treatment of obesity and they are:

- medications for the treatment of obesity;
- exercise;
- dietary change;
- behaviour modification;
- surgery.

Now let us consider the above points in a little more detail.

Medication

Currently two medicines have been recommended by National Institute for Health and Clinical Excellence (NICE) and they are:

- *Orlistat* reduces gastrointestinal absorption of fatty acids, cholesterol and fat-soluble vitamins and increasing faecal fat **elimination**.
- *Sibutramine* blocks the re-uptake of serotonin and noradrenaline in the brain.

These medicines are not recommended for all obese persons, only for persons with a BMI of 35 kg/m² and above and should be prescribed in concurrence with advice on diet, physical activity and lifestyle changes.

Exercise

The person should be encouraged to take regular exercise for weight reduction. Unless contraindicated, the British Nutrition Foundation Task Force recommends 30 minutes exercise such as walking, cycling or swimming at least five times per week under the supervision of the practice nurse. The level of activity should be gradually increased to the level the person can tolerate. The person should be encouraged to participate in group activities such as WeightWatchers Club which could help them to lose weight. The aim is to ensure that energy output is greater than energy intake, and this may be achieved through exercise and dieting. An individual may put on weight if the energy intake is more than energy expenditure.

Dietary change

The diet is planned to create a daily 500–1000 kcal deficit. Ideally, the diet should be low in kilocalories and fat and contain adequate nutrients, minerals and fibre. The person should eat regular meals with small servings. A gradual, slow weight loss of no more than 1–2 lb per week is recommended. Do not lower the calorie intake by more than 500 calories below the daily body needs. Doing so may cause an opposite response. Fewer than 1200 kcal each day may lead to loss of lean tissue and nutritional deficiencies. The recommended diet generally is low in fat and high in dietary fibre. Excessive calorie restrictions can lead to failure to follow the prescribed diet, feelings of guilt and overeating. 'Yo-yo' dieting (repeated cycles of weight loss and gain) may lead to a metabolic deficiency that makes subsequent weight loss efforts increasingly difficult. Therefore, it is critical that dieters take any weight loss effort seriously and include plans for long-term maintenance.

Behaviour modification

Behaviour modification is a critical component of successful weight management. Strategies such as keeping food records, eliminating cues that precipitate eating and changing the act of eating are often helpful. Recording food intake, amount, location of eating and situations that induce eating often help the dieter gain self-control. These strategies are often most effective when used in combination with other behaviour modification approaches. Other behaviour modification approaches focus on helping persons examine factors that affect eating behaviours. Social support and group programmes, such as Weight Watchers and Overeaters Anonymous, promote weight loss success through peer support. Most organised programmes require participants to pay a fee, which may improve compliance.

Surgery

Obesity can be treated with surgery if other interventions are not successful. Surgery may be offered to some persons when dieting and exercise have not been successful in reducing their weight. Surgical procedures such as gastric bypass may be carried out to limit the quantity of food the individual can eat each time (see Figure 7.7).

NURSING CARE FOR OBESITY

Nursing care for the person who has undergone bariatric surgery (weight loss surgery) is substantially the same as for a person who has undergone a gastric resection, but there are some additional nursing care needs related to the effects of the surgery on GI function such as dietary modification. As a nurse you need to be aware that the persons may be at risk of malnutrition after surgery if dietary intake is not carefully monitored.

Health promotion

Maintaining a healthy weight throughout the lifespan begins in childhood. Obese children and teenagers become obese adults. A nurse should promote healthy eating, including a diet rich in whole grains, fruits and vegetables and low in fat. Encourage all children and adults to maintain an active lifestyle, engaging in at least 30 minutes of aerobic activity daily. Encourage parents to limit time children spend watching television, using the computer and playing video games. Discuss the effects of smoking and excess alcohol use on nutrition and activity. When providing health promotion, nurses need to consider the health history of the person and ensure that a physical examination is done.

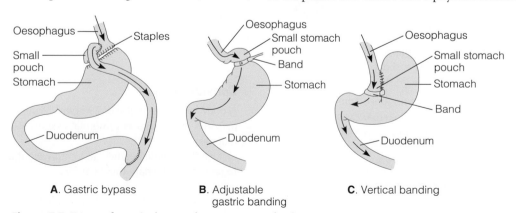

A. Gastric bypass **B**. Adjustable gastric banding **C**. Vertical banding

Figure 7.7 Types of surgical procedures to treat obesity.

COMMUNITY-BASED CARE

Weight reduction usually occurs in community-based settings. Weight loss and maintenance require a long-term commitment by the person, family and support systems. Nurses should address the following topics with the person and family prior to discharge:

- Lifestyle changes are more effective than diets. Weight loss diet (FAD) diets promote rapid weight loss but often are not nutritionally sound or may be difficult to maintain for a lifetime.
- All household members should consume a diet that is nutritionally sound, low in fat and high in fibre.

- Establish realistic weight loss goals and a system of non-food rewards for achieving each goal.
- Identify an 'exercise buddy' or support system to promote continued physical activity.
- Expect occasional failures. Resume prescribed diet and exercise routine as soon as possible; the goal is long-term weight management.
- Community resources such as Weight Watchers or healthcare-based programmes provide information, strategies and support for successful weight management.

Case Study 1 – Mary
NURSING CARE PLAN Obesity

Obesity is considered a major world health problem and the number of obese persons is rapidly increasing. The government is concerned about the levels of obesity in this country. Ms Mary Peters is 18 stone and is very keen to lose weight. She is finding it difficult to keep to a dietary plan.

Assessment

Can you list the possible causes of obesity?

In the first instance, you will need to take a full nursing and medical history from Ms Peters. Does Ms Peters suffer from any illness such as depression and eating disorders? Find out about Ms Peters' eating habits and lifestyle. Occasionally medical conditions and medication may cause obesity.

BMI, biochemical tests and anthropometry measurements are some of the assessment tools that are being used to determine if the person is overweight. Also consider visual assessment. Look at Ms Peters' skin condition. Are there any signs that Ms Peters may be suffering from any skin condition that may result in depression?

Treatment

There are a number of treatments available for Ms Peters, including modification of her diet, programmed physical activity, behavioural changes to dietary habits, medications and surgery. The nurse will need to discuss these treatments and allow Ms Peters to make an informed choice.

In the UK there are two types of medications recommended by NICE. Both these medications have been shown to help reduce weight, but there are side-effects associated with these medications.

Surgery may be the last resort and Ms Peters will need to be informed that any surgery will carry an element of risk and that currently only a few hospitals in the UK offer this kind of surgery.

FAST FACTS

Obesity

- The latest Health Survey for England (HSE) data shows that nearly one in four adults and over one in 10 children aged 2–10 are obese.
- In 2007, the government-commissioned Foresight report predicted that if no action was taken, 60% of men, 50% of women and 25% of children would be obese by 2050.

Source: DoH 2011.

Consider this . . .

A bodybuilder has a BMI of 29 kg/m². Would you say the person is overweight or of normal weight? What is your rationale?

Identify potential barriers to losing weight and strategies to reduce or eliminate these barriers.

The person with malnutrition

Malnutrition is a general term used to define undernutrition as a result of inadequate intake, dietary imbalance or over-nutrition from excess consumption of food. In clinical practice, malnutrition is regarded as undernutrition and overnutrition.

Undernutrition refers to the inability to meet the body's need for nutrition and energy. It could result from low intake of nutrients, high calorie demand of the body and poor absorption of nutrients from the GI tract, for example as a result of stomach cancer. Undernutrition can be detrimental to health and, if untreated, could result in severe complications such as infection, severe weight loss, multisystem failure (see Figure 7.8) and death.

FAST FACT

Undernutrition

Undernutrition is becoming increasingly prevalent in the ever-growing elderly population.

Carbohydrates and fats are the main energy source of the body. When dietary intake is not sufficient to meet the energy requirements of the body, stored glycogen, body protein and fats are used to produce energy. In a severe state of undernutrition the body uses fat reserve and converts it into fatty acid and ketones, which provide energy for the brain. As the disease process progresses, body mass is reduced and there is a reduction in energy expenditure.

Risk factors for undernutrition

Possible risk factors for undernutrition include:

- stress as a result of hospital admission;
- pain as a result of surgery or chronic disease may reduce appetite;
- presentation and the taste of hospital food may not be to the person's taste;
- unfamiliar environment;
- hospital mealtimes may not be suitable for the person.

Other risk factors related to undernutrition include:

- age – older adults are at greater risk for malnutrition due to a variety of factors;
- oral or GI problems that affect food intake, digestion and absorption;
- inability to eat for five or more days as a result of illness;
- chronic pain or chronic diseases such as pulmonary, cardio-vascular, renal or endocrine disorders, or cancer;

- dementia, mental health disorders;
- medications or treatments that affect appetite;
- alcohol or drug addiction;
- acute problems such as infection, surgery, or trauma.

Signs and symptoms of undernutrition

Signs and symptoms associated with undernutrition include:

- BMI between 17 and 18.5 kg/m^2 – mild undernutrition;
- BMI between 16 and 17 kg/m^2 – moderate undernutrition;
- BMI less than 16 kg/m^2 – severe malnutrition;
- severe muscle wasting;
- wrinkled skin observed in persons with marasmus;
- distended abdomen observed in persons with kwashiorkor;
- swollen ankles observed in persons with kwashiorkor;
- dry and brittle hair;
- fatigue/exhaustion.

Screening tools for undernutrition

Several tools can be used to assess for undernutrition:

- clinical assessment of the person;
- Malnutrition Universal Screening Tool (MUST) to determine nutritional status;
- BMI;
- anthropometry measurements.

INTERDISCIPLINARY CARE FOR UNDERNUTRITION

Medication

Malnourished persons generally require supplemental vitamins and minerals to restore these essential micronutrients. A multivitamin and mineral supplement may be given, or therapy may be tailored to correct specific deficiencies.

Nutrition

The person should be encouraged to keep a food diary of the quantity of food and fluids consumed each day. Weigh the person daily (same time and wearing the same clothing) to ensure that the person is gaining weight. The weight should be recorded and documented. Offer advice on the type of food to purchase that is nutritious and healthy. When giving advice, the nurse needs to consider the person's preferences and their cultural and religious beliefs. For persons who may find Ensure drinks unacceptable due to high milk content, they may prefer fruit flavoured-supplements such as Enlive or Fortijuice. The dietitian will be able to give advice on the appropriate supplement for the person to take. Advice on supplements should be

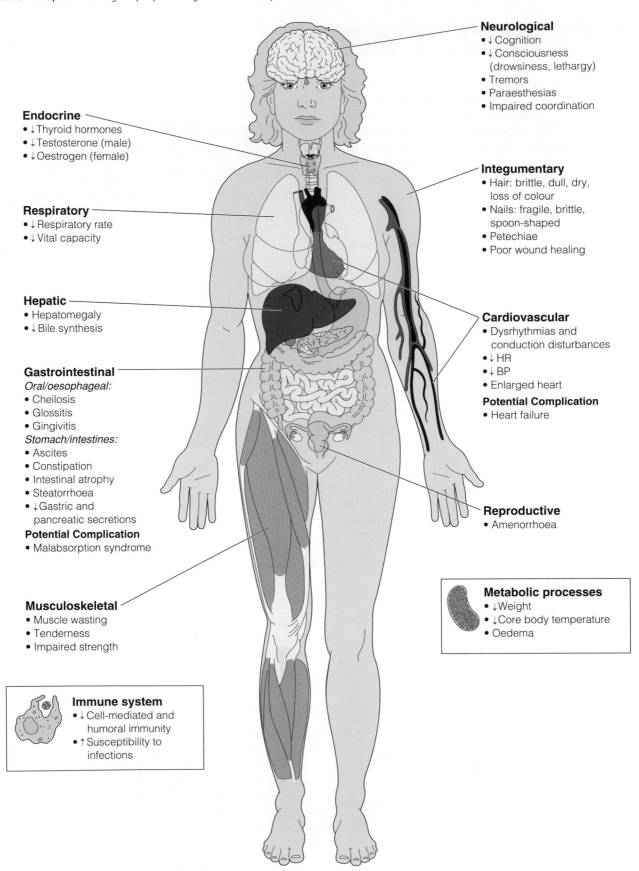

Neurological
- ↓Cognition
- ↓Consciousness (drowsiness, lethargy)
- Tremors
- Paraesthesias
- Impaired coordination

Endocrine
- ↓Thyroid hormones
- ↓Testosterone (male)
- ↓Oestrogen (female)

Integumentary
- Hair: brittle, dull, dry, loss of colour
- Nails: fragile, brittle, spoon-shaped
- Petechiae
- Poor wound healing

Respiratory
- ↓Respiratory rate
- ↓Vital capacity

Hepatic
- Hepatomegaly
- ↓Bile synthesis

Cardiovascular
- Dysrhythmias and conduction disturbances
- ↓HR
- ↓BP
- Enlarged heart

Potential Complication
- Heart failure

Gastrointestinal
Oral/oesophageal:
- Cheilosis
- Glossitis
- Gingivitis

Stomach/intestines:
- Ascites
- Constipation
- Intestinal atrophy
- Steatorrhoea
- ↓Gastric and pancreatic secretions

Potential Complication
- Malabsorption syndrome

Reproductive
- Amenorrhoea

Metabolic processes
- ↓Weight
- ↓Core body temperature
- Oedema

Musculoskeletal
- Muscle wasting
- Tenderness
- Impaired strength

Immune system
- ↓Cell-mediated and humoral immunity
- ↑Susceptibility to infections

Figure 7.8 Multisystem effects of malnutrition.

offered in accordance with the NICE recommendations and guidelines on nutritional support in adults.

Enternal nutrition

Enteral nutrition, or tube feeding, may be used to meet calorie and protein requirements in persons unable to consume adequate food. Indications for tube feedings include difficulty swallowing, unresponsiveness, oral or neck surgery or trauma, anorexia or serious illness. Tube feedings may provide part or all of a person's nutritional needs. Recent evidence supports using the enteral route for nutritional support whenever possible. Enteral feedings provide nutrients directly to the gut and other digestive organs, reduce the incidence of enteric pathogens, promote blood flow to the gut and support other functions of the GI tract such as the release of hormones and epidermal growth factor.

There are three types of enteral feeding:

- *Nasogastric (NG) tube feeding.* This involves the insertion of a nasogastric tube via the nasopharynx into the stomach. The procedure is normally carried out by a registered nurse or medical staff.

- *Nasojejunal (NJ) tube feeding.* This involves the insertion of a tube via the nasopharynx and the stomach into the jejunum. Insertion of the NJ tube is carried out by medical staff using endoscopy and is confirmed in place radiologically.

- *Percutaneous endoscopic gastrostomy (PEG) or jejunostomy (PEJ).* This involves the insertion of a tube into the stomach

through the abdominal wall. The procedure is carried out by the medical staff surgically.

Parenteral nutrition

Total parenteral nutrition (TPN), also known as *hyperalimentation*, is the intravenous administration of carbohydrates (high concentrations of dextrose), protein (amino acids), electrolytes, vitamins, minerals and fat emulsions. These hypertonic solutions are usually administered through a central vein, such as the subclavian vein (Figure 7.9). A peripherally inserted central catheter line may be used for short-term TPN. Partial parenteral nutrition (used to support the person who is able to consume some nutrients or in conjunction with enteral feeding) may be given through a peripheral vein.

TPN is initiated when a person's nutritional requirements cannot be met through diet, enteral feedings or peripheral vein infusions. Persons who have undergone major surgery or trauma or are seriously undernourished are often candidates for TPN. TPN is used for both short- and long-term management of nutritional deficiencies, and many persons are discharged to home with TPN and monitored by district nurses.

Disruption of the skin barrier and administration of a solution high in glucose presents a risk for infection in persons receiving TPN. Infection may be local, limited to the exit site or surrounding a tunnelled catheter, or may lead to sepsis (blood infection). The temperature and other manifestations of infection are carefully monitored. Strict sterile technique is used for site and

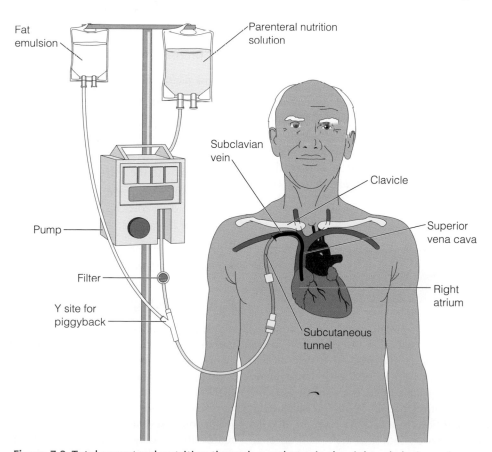

Figure 7.9 Total parenteral nutrition through a catheter in the right subclavian vein.

COMMUNITY-BASED CARE

Persons with malnutrition may be cared for at home or in the hospital with diet, enteral or parenteral therapy. It is more common to see persons managing tube feeding or TPN at home with the help of the family and the nurses in the community. Teaching for the person and family includes the following topics:

● Diet recommendations and use of nutritional supplements.

● Where to obtain recommended foods and nutritional supplements.

● If continuing enteral or parenteral nutrition, how to (1) prepare and/or handle solutions, (2) add them to either the feeding tube or central line, (3) manage infusion pumps, (4) care for the feeding tube or central catheter, (5) recognise and manage problems and complications and (6) how and when to notify the GP or the district nurse of problems.

catheter care and bag and tubing changes. For further in-depth discussion regarding the special care of persons receiving parenteral nutrition look at *The Royal Marsden Hospital Manual of Clinical Nursing Procedures* (Dougherty and Lister 2008).

IN PRACTICE

Nasogastric feeding

Nasogastric (NG) tube insertion is normally carried out by a qualified nurse or a doctor. In some surgical cases, the NG tube is inserted in theatre. Nurses need to adhere to local policies and guidelines for the insertion and checking its position after insertion.

The NG tube position is checked before feeding a person via the NG tube, giving medication via the NG tube and if the person complains of discomfort. If you suspect that the NG tube may have moved, you must report it immediately to the registered nurse, doctor, dietitian or the nutritional nurse specialist. Do not start a feed or give anything via the NG tube until the position of the tube is confirmed.

DISORDERS OF THE STOMACH AND DUODENUM

Disorders of the stomach and the duodenum are the most common sites for problems associated with the GI tract. The major disorders that affect digestion are nausea and vomiting, gastritis, peptic ulcer disease and cancer of the stomach. It is estimated that in the UK, 103 per 100 000 adults per year suffer from GI disorders and the incidence rises with age. Nursing roles in managing these disorders include both acute care for the hospitalised person and teaching to give the person the skills and knowledge to manage these conditions at home.

The person with peptic ulcer disease (PUD)

The term peptic ulcer refers to both gastric and duodenal ulcers. *Helicobacter pylori* infection is associated with about 95% of duodenal ulcers and 80% of gastric ulcers. PUD, a break in the mucous lining of the GI tract where it comes in contact with gastric juice, is a chronic health-care problem. PUD can affect people of any age, including children, but the condition is most common in people who are 60 years of age, or over. Both sexes are equally affected by PUD.

Risk factors for PUD

The risk factors for PUD include:

● infection with *H. pylori*;

● non-steroidal anti-inflammatory drugs (NSAIDs), including aspirin, ibuprofen and many painkillers used for conditions such as arthritis – ulcers and haemorrhage are a common problem with these drugs;

● use of other medications, such as the anticoagulant warfarin (Coumadin), corticosteroids or the osteoporosis drug alendronate (Fosamax);

● smoking and excessive alcohol consumption;

● family history of ulcers.

Pathophysiology of PUD

An ulcer, or break in the GI mucosa, develops when the mucosal barrier is unable to protect the mucosa from damage by hydrochloric acid and pepsin, the gastric digestive juices.

H. pylori infection, found in about 70% of people who have PUD, is unique in colonising the stomach. It is spread person to person (oral–oral or faecal–oral), and contributes to ulcer formation in several ways. The bacteria produce enzymes that reduce the efficacy of mucous gel in protecting the gastric mucosa. In addition, the host's inflammatory response to

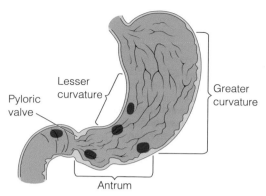

Figure 7.10 Common sites affected by peptic ulcer disease.

H. pylori contributes to gastric epithelial cell damage without producing immunity to the infection. Although the gastric mucosa is the usual site for *H. pylori* infection, this infection also contributes to duodenal ulcers. This is possibly related to increased gastric acid production associated with *H. pylori* infection.

The ulcers of PUD may affect the oesophagus, stomach or duodenum. They may be superficial or deep, affecting all layers of the mucosa. Duodenal ulcers, the most common, usually develop in the proximal portion of the duodenum, close to the pylorus (Figure 7.10). They are sharply demarcated and usually less than 1 cm in diameter. Gastric ulcers are often found on the lesser curvature and the area immediately proximal to the pylorus. Gastric ulcers are associated with an increased incidence of gastric cancer. Peptic ulcer disease may

be chronic, with spontaneous remissions and exacerbations. Exacerbations of the disease may be associated with trauma, infection or other physical or psychological stressors. See Figures 7.11–7.14 for pathophysiology illustrated.

Signs and symptoms of PUD

Symptoms of dyspepsia are very non-specific and diagnosis is unreliable on history alone:

- Epigastric pain usually one to three hours postprandial (after eating a meal) – it may sometimes wake the person in the night and be relieved by food.
- Oral flatulence, bloating, distension and intolerance of fatty food – the last is also associated with gallstones.
- Heartburn sometimes occurs although it is more typically associated with gastro-oesophageal reflux.
- A posterior ulcer may cause pain radiating to the back.
- Symptoms are relieved by antacids (very non-specific).
- Occult or obvious blood in the stool.
- Haematemesis (vomiting blood).
- Fatigue, weakness, dizziness.
- Hypovolaemic shock.

Complications of PUD

The complications associated with peptic ulcers include haemorrhage, obstruction and perforation. Approximately

In the stomach and duodenum, the mucosal barrier protects the gastric mucosa (including the epithelial, vascular, and smooth muscle layers) from damage. Specialised mucous cells throughout the gastric mucosa produce a mucus (a mixture of water, lipids and glycoproteins) that serves as a barrier to the diffusion of ions (such as hydrogen ion) and molecules (such as pepsin). A thin layer of bicarbonate, secreted by surface epithelial cells, forms between the mucus and cell membranes. Blood flow to the gastric mucosa is vital to maintain this barrier. Prostaglandins and nitric oxide stimulate mucus and bicarbonate production, helping maintain it as well. The mucosal barrier constantly bathes surfaces of the gastric epithelial lining.

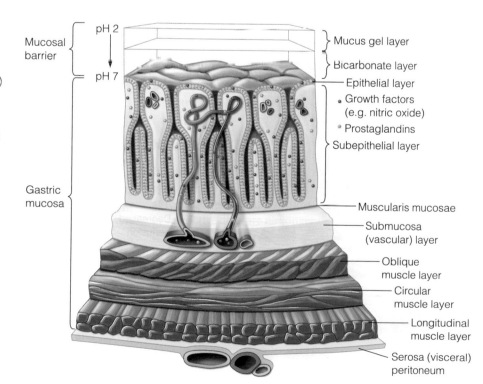

Figure 7.11 Normal gastric mucosa.

- recurrence of PUD;
- failure of drug treatment;
- complications of PUD such as perforation of the stomach lining or haemorrhage.

NURSING CARE FOR PUD

A full medical and nursing history should be obtained in order to formulate a care plan to meet the specific needs of the person. The care should include dietary advice, altering lifestyle, avoiding stressful situations and compliance to the medications prescribed.

Health promotion

Although it is difficult to predict which persons will develop PUD, nurses should attempt to promote health by advising persons to avoid risk factors such as excessive aspirin or NSAID use and cigarette smoking. In addition, encourage persons to seek treatment for manifestations of Gerd (acid reflux) or chronic gastritis, both of which are also associated with *H. pylori* infection.

Nursing diagnoses and interventions

Nursing diagnoses and interventions focus on pre- and post-operative care for persons undergoing surgery and on pain control.

Pre- and post-operative care

Persons who undergo surgery for PUD require full pre-operative preparation prior to surgery. Nurses need to follow local and NMC polices and guidelines in the safe preparation of persons for surgery. Review Chapter 1 for routine pre- and post-operative care. Immediate post-operative care on return to the ward should include the following:

- care of airway, breathing and circulation. Recording of vital signs two to four hourly depending on the person's condition;
- management of wound drains, NG tube (if inserted) and wound site;
- management of pain control;
- care of intravenous infusion and management of intravenous site;
- management of urinary output and catheter if inserted;
- prevention of DVT;
- personal and oral hygiene;
- management of fluid balance chart;
- psychological care.

Risk for pain

The pain of PUD is often predictable and preventable. Pain is typically experienced two to four hours after eating, as high levels of gastric acid and pepsin irritate the exposed mucosa. Measures to neutralise the acid, minimise its production or protect the mucosa often relieve this pain, minimising the

need for analgesics. For detailed advice on pain management refer to Chapter 2. Nurses should:

- Assess pain, including location, type, severity, frequency and duration, and its relationship to food intake or other contributing factors.

PRACTICE ALERT

Avoid making assumptions about pain. Acute pain may indicate a complication, such as perforation (often heralded by sudden, severe epigastric pain and a rigid, board-like abdomen), or it may be totally unrelated to PUD (for example, angina, gall bladder disease or **pancreatitis**).

- Administer PPIs, H$_2$-receptor antagonists, antacids or mucosal protective agents as prescribed. Monitor for effectiveness and side-effects or adverse reactions. *The pain associated with PUD is generally caused by the effect of gastric juices on exposed mucosal tissue. These medications reduce pain and promote healing by reducing acid production, neutralising acid or providing a barrier for the damaged mucosa.*

- Advise regarding relaxation, stress reduction and lifestyle management techniques. Refer for stress management counselling or classes as indicated. *Although there is no clear relationship between stress and PUD, measures to relieve stress and promote physical and emotional rest help reduce the perception of pain and may reduce ulcer genesis.*

COMMUNITY-BASED CARE

Peptic ulcer disease is managed in home- and community-based settings; only its complications typically require treatment in an acute care setting. Nurses should provide the following information when preparing the person for discharge:

- Prescribed medication regimen, including desired and potential side-effects.
- Importance of continuing therapy even when symptoms are relieved.
- Relationship between peptic ulcers and factors such as NSAID use and smoking. If indicated, refer to a smoking cessation clinic or programme.
- Importance of avoiding aspirin and other NSAIDs; stress the necessity of reading the labels of over-the-counter medications for possible aspirin content.
- Symptoms of complications that should be reported to the practice nurse, including increased abdominal pain or distention, vomiting, black or tarry stools, light-headedness or fainting.
- Stress and lifestyle management techniques that may help prevent exacerbation. Refer to resources for stress management, such as classes, counselling and formal or informal groups.

CASE STUDY 2 – Monica
NURSING CARE PLAN The patient with PUD

Now let us recall Mrs Monica Stone. Before working though this case study, revise the anatomy and physiology of the stomach.

Assessment

On initial assessment, Mrs Stone is alert and oriented, though very apprehensive about her condition. Skin pale and cool; BP 136/78 mmHg, P 98 beats per minute; abdomen distended and tender with hyperactive bowel sounds; 200 mL bright red blood was obtained on insertion of nasogastric tube. Haemoglobin 8.2 g/dL and haematocrit 23% on admission. Mrs Stone is taken to the endoscopy unit where her bleeding is controlled using laser surgery. On her return to the ward, she receives two units of packed red blood cells and intravenous fluids to restore blood volume. A five-day course of oral omeprazole (40 mg) is prescribed and Mrs Stone is allowed to begin a soft diet 24 hours after her endoscopy. Tissue biopsy obtained during endoscopy confirms the presence of *H. pylori* infection.

How does the organism *H. pylori* get into the stomach? What is role of the medication omeprazole? List the investigations that may be carried out to confirm the diagnosis of PUD.

Diagnoses

Mrs Stone completed the blood transfusion without any complications. Her haemoglobin level is now within safe limits after her blood transfusion. She is also put on a course of antibiotics to treat the *H. pylori* infection and advised on taking her meals regularly and healthy eating. Mrs Stone is also advised on other risk factors such as stress, alcohol and smoking that could contribute to PUD.

Evaluation

Mrs Stone is discharged 48 hours after admission. She has had no further evidence of bleeding, and has resumed a regular diet. Her haemoglobin and haematocrit remain slightly low, and she has a prescription for ferrous sulphate. She will complete the prescribed high-dose omeprazole regimen at home, then begin treatment with omeprazole, amoxicillin and metroniadzole to eradicate the *H. pylori* infection detected during endoscopy. After two weeks of this regimen, she will continue taking omeprazole at bedtime for four to eight weeks. She verbalises a good understanding of her treatment and the importance of completing the entire regimen. Mrs Stone expresses concern about her ability to 'keep her cool on the inside' when under stress. The nurse gives her the contact details of several support groups to help with stress management in case she wants help.

> ### Consider this . . .
> Researchers are not certain how people contract *H. pylori*, but they think it may be through food or water. Researchers have found *H. pylori* in the saliva of some infected people, so the bacteria may also spread through mouth-to-mouth contact such as kissing.

The person with cancer of the stomach

FAST FACTS

Gastric cancer

- Gastric cancer is the second most common cause of cancer-related death in the world.
- It is more common in men than women and is usually found in 50–75-year-olds.
- About 8000 people get stomach (gastric) cancer each year in the UK.

Source: http://www.macmillan.org.uk/Cancerinformation/Cancertypes/Stomach/Stomachcancer.aspx (accessed September 2011).

Worldwide, cancer of the stomach is the most common cancer (after skin cancer). Each year, about 8000 people in the UK develop stomach cancer. The elderly are more likely to develop gastric cancer; however, it is more common in men than women. In the UK, stomach cancer is much less common than it used to be – the number of new persons each year has halved over the past 30 years.

Risk factors for stomach cancer

Risk factors include:

- Ageing – stomach cancer is more common in older people; most cases are in people over the age of 60.
- People who suffer from pernicious anaemia, which causes a lack of vitamin B_{12}, are slightly at risk of developing stomach cancer.
- Diet is probably a factor: countries such as Japan where people eat a lot of salt, pickled and smoked foods have a

high rate of stomach cancer. Eating a lot of fruit and green vegetables can reduce the risk.

- Long-term infection of the stomach lining with a bacterium called *H. pylori* seems to lead to a slightly higher risk of stomach cancer.
- Gender – stomach cancer is twice as common in men than women.
- Family history – for some cases, stomach cancer may run in the family.
- Smoking and alcohol may increase the risk of developing stomach cancer.

Pathophysiology of stomach cancer

Adenocarcinoma, which involves the mucus-producing cells of the stomach, is the most common form of gastric cancer. These carcinomas may arise anywhere on the mucosal surface of the stomach but are most frequently found in the distal portion. Half of all gastric cancers occur in the antrum or pyloric region. Gastric cancer begins as a localised lesion (*in situ*), then progresses to involve the mucosa or submucosa (early gastric carcinoma). Lesions may spread by direct extension to tissues surrounding the stomach, the liver in particular. The lesion may ulcerate or appear as a polypoid (polyp-like) mass. Lymph node involvement and metastasis (spread of the disease to other parts of the body) occur early due to the rich blood and lymphatic supply to the stomach. Metastatic lesions are often found in the liver, lungs, ovaries and peritoneum.

Signs and symptoms of stomach cancer

Signs and symptoms can include:

- indigestion, acidity and burping;
- feeling full;
- bleeding or tiredness and breathlessness as a result of blood loss;
- anorexia;
- epigastric pain;
- feeling or being sick;
- difficulty in swallowing;
- loss of appetite or weight loss (usually symptoms of a more advanced cancer);
- vomiting.

INTERDISCIPLINARY CARE FOR STOMACH CANCER

Surgery

If the cancer is diagnosed at an early stage, an operation may be all that is needed to cure it. This may involve removing part of the stomach (a partial gastrectomy) or all of the stomach (a total gastrectomy). The type of operation needed depends on

the size of the tumour and where it is located, in the stomach. See Figure 7.15 A–C for partial and total gastrectomy.

Complications of gastric surgery

Dumping syndrome is a complication following gastric surgery. This condition may develop after eating a meal and the person may complain of symptoms such as epigastric fullness, discomfort, excessive sweating and feeling unwell. Early symptoms of dumping syndrome may occur within 5–30 minutes after eating.

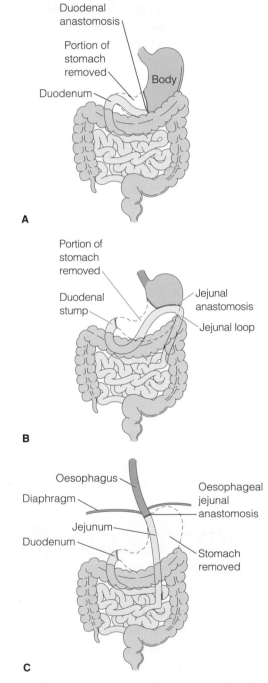

Figure 7.15 Partial and total gastrectomy procedures.
(A) Partial gastrectomy with anastomosis to the duodenum.
(B) Partial gastrectomy with anastomosis to the jejunum. **(C)** Total gastrectomy with anastomosis of the oesophagus and jejunum.

The amount of proteins and fats in the diet is increased, because they leave the stomach more slowly than carbohydrates. Carbohydrates, especially simple sugars, should be reduced. The person is instructed to rest in a recumbent (reclining) or semi-recumbent position for 30–60 minutes after meals.

Anaemia may be a chronic problem after a major gastric resection. Iron is absorbed primarily in the duodenum and proximal jejunum; rapid gastric emptying may interfere with adequate absorption.

The cells of the stomach produce intrinsic factor, required for the absorption of vitamin B_{12}. Vitamin B_{12} deficiency leads to pernicious anaemia. Because of hepatic stores of vitamin B_{12}, symptoms of anaemia may not be seen for one to two years after surgery. Vitamin B_{12} levels are routinely monitored following extensive gastric resections.

Other nutritional problems seen following surgery include folic acid deficiency and decreased absorption of calcium and vitamin D. Poor absorption of nutrients, combined with the inability to eat large meals, puts the person at risk for weight loss in addition to the more specific nutrient deficiencies.

Other treatments

Radiation or chemotherapy may be used to eliminate any lymphatic or metastatic spread. For the person with more advanced disease, treatment is palliative and may include surgery and chemotherapy. These persons may require a gastrostomy or jejunostomy feeding tube (Figures 7.16A and B). Because gastric cancer is generally advanced by the time of diagnosis, the prognosis is poor. The five-year survival rate of all persons treated for gastric carcinoma is 10%.

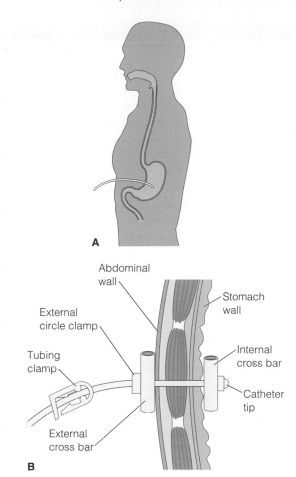

Figure 7.16 Gastrostomy. (A) Gastrostomy tube placement. **(B)** The tube is fixed against both the abdomen and the stomach walls by cross bars.

NURSING CARE PLAN The person having gastric surgery

Review Chapter 1 for routine pre- and post-operative care.

Pre-operative care

+ Nurses should adhere to local and NMC policies and guidelines for the safe preparation of the person for gastric surgery.
+ Insert a NG tube if requested pre-operatively. *Although it is often inserted in the surgical suite just prior to surgery, the NG tube may be placed pre-operatively to remove secretions and empty stomach contents.*
+ Nurses should allow time for the person to ask questions that they may have about their surgery and recovery.

Post-operative care

+ On return to the ward, the first nursing priority is to obtain and record vital signs. These will give the nurses an indication as to the condition of the person. Any changes in the vital signs should be reported immediately in order to take prompt action.

+ Assess position and patency of NG tube, connecting it to low suction. Gently irrigate with sterile normal saline if tube becomes clogged. *The NG tube will be placed in surgery to avoid disruption of the gastric suture lines and should be well secured. If repositioning or tube replacement is needed, notify the surgeon. Patency must be maintained to keep the stomach decompressed, reducing pressure on sutures.*

+ Assess colour, amount and odour of gastric drainage, noting any changes in these parameters or the presence of clots or bright bleeding. *Initial drainage is bright red. It becomes dark, then clear or greenish-yellow over the first two to three days. A change in the colour, amount or odour may indicate a complication such as haemorrhage, intestinal obstruction or infection.*

+ Maintain intravenous fluids while nasogastric suction is in place. *The person on nasogastric suction is not only unable to take oral food and fluids but also is losing electrolyte-rich fluid through the nasogastric tube. If replacement fluid and electrolytes are not maintained, the person is at risk for*

NURSING CARE PLAN The person having gastric surgery (continued)

dehydration; imbalances of sodium, potassium and chloride; and metabolic alkalosis.

✚ Administer medications as prescribed. *Medications may be prescribed for the post-operative person, depending on the procedure performed. Antibiotic therapy is a common preventive measure for infection that may result from contamination of the abdominal cavity with gastric contents.*

✚ Monitor bowel sounds and abdominal distension. Bowel sounds indicate resumption of peristalsis. *Increasing distension may indicate third spacing, obstruction or infection.*

✚ Commence oral food and fluids once bowel sounds are establised. Initial feedings are clear liquids, progressing to full liquids and then frequent small meals of regular foods. Monitor bowel sounds and for abdominal distension frequently during this period. *Oral feedings are reintroduced slowly to minimise trauma to the suture lines by possible gastric distension.*

✚ Encourage mobilisation. *Mobilisation stimulates peristalsis and helps avoid post-operative complications such as deep vein thrombosis.*

NURSING CARE FOR STOMACH CANCER

Health promotion

Although the exact causes of gastric cancer are unknown, contributing factors such as *H. pylori* infection and consumption of foods preserved with nitrates have been identified. To reduce their risk of developing gastric cancer, encourage persons with known *H. pylori* infection to complete the prescribed course of treatment and verify that it has eradicated the infection. With all persons, discuss the relationship between gastric cancer and consumption of foods preserved with nitrates (such as bacon and other processed meats), and encourage limited consumption of these products.

Nursing diagnoses and interventions

Risk for imbalanced nutrition: less than body requirements

The person with gastric cancer may be malnourished because of anorexia, early satiety and increased metabolic needs related to the tumour. Extensive gastric resection also makes it difficult to consume an adequate diet. Malnourishment, in turn, impairs healing and the person's ability to tolerate cancer treatment.

✚ Consult with dietitian for a complete nutrition assessment and diet planning. *The person is at risk for protein–calorie malnutrition, which impairs the ability to heal and recover from extensive surgery.*

✚ Weigh daily. Monitor laboratory values such as haemoglobin, haematocrit and serum albumin levels. *Daily weights are a valuable measurement of both fluid and nutritional status. Laboratory values provide further evidence of nutritional status.*

✚ Provide preferred foods; have family prepare meals when possible. Provide supplemental feedings between meals. *Small, frequent feedings and preferred foods encourage intake of nutrients.*

PRACTICE ALERT

Advise the person to report increasing or persistent symptoms of anorexia, nausea and vomiting, or fullness to the nurse.

COMMUNITY-BASED CARE

Although the person with gastric cancer may be hospitalised for surgery, most care is provided in the home and community-based settings such as hospice care. When preparing the person and family for home care, the nurse should provide information on the following topics:

● Care of incision and feeding tube (if present)

● Maintaining nutrition and preventing complications of surgery such as dumping syndrome

● Pain management

● Provide referrals to home care agencies, hospice and cancer support groups as appropriate.

● Provide information about services available in the community such as:
  – primary care teams, working in the community;
  – cancer units in district hospitals;
  – palliative care services;
  – hospice care if needed.

Case Study 3 – Sunita
NURSING CARE PLAN Carcinoma of the stomach

Now let us consider a person with stomach cancer. If you remember, Mrs Sunita Chowdrey went to see her GP as a result of abdominal pain and vomiting. She was treated with some tablets which did not help her problem and her GP decides to refer her to the local hospital.

Can you list the investigations that the doctors in the hospital may carry out to confirm her diagnosis? List the symptoms that Mrs Chowdrey may experience as a result of carcinoma of the stomach.

Assessment

You will need to take a detail nursing and medical history. The history should include her symptoms such as epigastric pain, any weight loss and her eating habits. How long Mrs Chowdrey has been complaining of abdominal pain and what her eating habits are like. Changes in her bowel habits, for example, are her bowels regular; any blood identified in her stool or any discomfort when going to toilet. Physical assessment should include general appearance, height, weight and abdominal distension. Mrs Chowdrey will then be prepared for surgery.

Diagnosis

+ *Imbalanced nutrition: less than body requirements* related to anorexia and difficulty in eating.

+ *Acute pain* following surgery.

+ *Risk for ineffective airway clearance* related to upper abdominal surgery.

+ *Anticipatory grieving* related to recent diagnosis of cancer.

Expected outcomes

+ Maintain present weight during hospitalisation.

+ Resume a high-calorie, high-protein diet by time of discharge.

+ Verbalise effective pain management, maintaining a reported pain level of 3 or less on a scale of 1 to 10.

+ Maintain a patent airway and clear breath sounds.

+ Verbalise feelings regarding diagnosis and participate in decision-making.

Planning and implementation

+ Weigh weekly.

+ Maintain NG tube, patency and suction as requested.

+ Maintain intravenous fluid regimen as prescribed until oral food intake is resumed.

+ Offer dietary advice, including strategies to prevent dumping syndrome, before discharge.

+ Maintain person-controlled analgesia until able to take oral analgesics.

+ Assess respiratory status including rate, depth, and breath sounds hourly, then every four hours.

+ Assist to cough, deep breathe every two to four hours. Encourage Sunita to support her abdomen during coughing.

+ Encourage verbalisation of feelings about diagnosis and perceived losses.

+ Encourage participation in decision-making.

Evaluation

Mrs Chowdrey's weight remained stable throughout her stay in hospital. On discharge she is taking a high-protein, high-calorie diet in six small feedings per day. She and her husband have reviewed her diet with the dietitian and are planning on using some dietary supplements at home to meet protein needs. She verbalises an understanding of measures to prevent dumping syndrome, including separating her intake of solid foods and liquids. Mrs Chowdrey is using oral analgesia in the morning and at bedtime to control her pain. She and her husband have begun to discuss the meaning of her diagnosis. Her husband tells the nurse, 'We are going to go to a support group called "Coping with Cancer" when my wife is stronger.'

Consider this . . .

● What is the rationale for maintaining NG aspiration after gastrojejunostomy?

● Develop a pre-operative teaching plan for a person undergoing a partial gastrectomy.

● Mrs Chowdrey calls you just before the initial dose of chemotherapy and says, '*Everyone tells me that chemotherapy will cause vomiting, and I don't think I can take being sick again.*' How would you respond?

● Plan interventions to ensure adequate nutrition for people with advanced gastric cancer.

PRACTICE ALERT

Assess ability to consume adequate nutrients.
Nausea and feelings of early satiety may impair nutrient consumption, indicating a need to institute enteral or parenteral feedings.

In the above section we have considered disorders related to the stomach and care of the person with gastritis and stomach cancer. Now let us consider the disorders associated with the liver and the pancreas.

The person with hepatitis

Hepatitis is inflammation of the liver. It is usually caused by a virus, although it may result from exposure to alcohol, drugs and toxins or other pathogens. Hepatitis may be acute or chronic in nature. Chronic hepatitis also increases the risk for developing liver cancer.

Pathophysiology and signs and symptoms of hepatitis

The inflammatory process of hepatitis, whether caused by a virus, toxin or other mechanism, damages hepatic cells and disrupts liver function. Cell-mediated immune responses damage hepatocytes and Kupffer cells, leading to hyperplasia, necrosis and cellular regeneration. The flow of bile through bile canaliculi and into the biliary system can be impaired by the inflammatory process, leading to jaundice. When the inflammatory process is mild (for example, hepatitis A), the liver parenchyma is not significantly damaged. The inflammatory processes associated with hepatitis B and hepatitis C, however, can lead to severe liver damage. The metabolism of nutrients, drugs, alcohol and toxins and the process of bile elimination are disrupted by the inflammation of hepatitis.

Viral hepatitis

At least five viruses are known to cause hepatitis: hepatitis A virus (HAV), hepatitis B virus (HBV), hepatitis C virus (HCV), the hepatitis B-associated delta virus (HDV) and hepatitis E virus (HEV). Hepatitis viruses replicate in the liver, damaging liver cells (hepatocytes). The viruses provoke an immune response that causes inflammation and necrosis of hepatocytes as well. Although the extent of damage and the immune response vary among the different hepatitis viruses, the disease itself usually follows a predictable pattern.

No symptoms are present during the incubation period after exposure to the virus. The *prodromal* or *preicteric* (before jaundice) *phase* may begin abruptly or insidiously, with general malaise, anorexia, fatigue and muscle and body aches. These signs and symptoms of nausea, vomiting, diarrhoea or constipation may develop, as well as mild right upper quadrant abdominal pain. Chills and fever may be present.

The *icteric* (jaundiced) *phase* usually begins 5–10 days after the onset of symptoms. It is heralded by jaundice of the sclera, skin and mucous membranes. Inflammation of the liver and bile ducts prevents bilirubin from being excreted into the small intestine. As a result, the serum bilirubin levels are elevated, causing yellowing of the skin and mucous membranes. Pruritus may develop due to deposition of bile salts on the skin. The stools are light brown or clay coloured because bile pigment is not excreted through the normal faecal pathway. Instead, the pigment is excreted by the kidneys, causing the urine to turn brown. Whereas persons with acute hepatitis A or B are likely to develop jaundice, many people with hepatitis C do not develop jaundice. As a result, the infection may go undiagnosed for an extended period of time.

Hepatitis A

Hepatitis A, or *infectious hepatitis*, often occurs in either sporadic attacks or mild epidemics. It is transmitted by the faecal–oral route via contaminated food, water, shellfish and direct contact with an infected person. The virus is in the stool of infected persons up to two weeks before symptoms develop. Once jaundice develops, the amount of virus in the stool and the risk of spreading the disease decrease significantly. Although hepatitis A usually has an abrupt onset, it is typically a benign and self-limited disease with few long-term consequences. Symptoms could last up to two months.

Hepatitis B

Hepatitis B can cause acute hepatitis, chronic hepatitis, *fulminant* (rapidly progressive) hepatitis or a carrier state. In a *carrier state*, the person harbours the active virus and is capable of spreading it to others, even though there are no discernible manifestations of the disease. This virus is spread through contact with infected blood and body fluids. Healthcare workers are at risk through exposure to blood and needle-stick injuries. Other high-risk groups for hepatitis B include injection drug users, people with multiple sex partners, men who have sex with other men and people frequently exposed to blood products (such as people on haemodialysis). Hepatitis B is a major risk factor for primary liver cancer.

Hepatitis C

Hepatitis C, formerly known as non-A, non-B hepatitis, is the primary worldwide cause of chronic hepatitis, cirrhosis and liver cancer. It is transmitted through infected blood and body fluids. Injection drug use is the primary risk factor for HCV infection. Acute hepatitis C usually is asymptomatic; if symptoms do develop, they often are mild and non-specific. The disease is often recognised long after exposure occurred, when secondary effects of the disease (such as chronic hepatitis or cirrhosis) develop. Hepatitis C is unique, in that it does not produce lasting immunity to reinfection. Only about 15% of acute infections completely resolve; most progress to chronic active hepatitis.

Chronic hepatitis

Chronic hepatitis is chronic infection of the liver. Although it may cause few symptoms, it is the primary cause of liver damage leading to cirrhosis, liver cancer and liver transplantation. Three of the known hepatitis viruses cause chronic hepatitis: HBV, HCV and HDV. Symptoms of chronic hepatitis include malaise, fatigue and hepatomegaly. Occasional icteric (jaundiced) periods may occur. Liver enzymes, particularly serum aminotransferase levels, typically are elevated. In *chronic active hepatitis*, inflammation extends to involve entire hepatic lobules. Chronic active hepatitis usually leads to cirrhosis of the liver and end-stage liver failure.

INTERDISCIPLINARY CARE FOR HEPATITIS

Medication

There are a number of drugs available to treat hepatitis:

Interferon alfa:

- used to treat chronic hepatitis B and C as well as some lymphomas and tumours;
- used with ribavirin;
- side-effects include nausea, loss of appetite, flu-like symptoms, lethargy, cardiovascular, hepatic and renal toxicity;
- used in the treatment of HBV;
- usage in chronic hepatitis C is subject to NICE guidelines.

Peginterferon alfa:

- used since 2000.
- causes the interferon to persist longer in the blood by reducing rate of clearance by the kidneys.

Lamivudine:

- indicated in chronic hepatitis B;
- inhibits virus replication by inhibiting a reverse transcriptase enzyme;
- has minimal side-effects;
- some persons may develop drug resistance in the first year of therapy;

Adefovir dipivoxil:

- used for chronic hepatitis B;
- inhibits viral replication and is given orally as a once-daily dosage;
- resistance is very low, but it is about three times the cost of lamivudine.

Ribavirin:

- used in combination with peginterferon alfa and interferon alfa for chronic hepatitis C;
- inhibits a wide range of DNA and RNA viruses;
- can produce haemolytic anaemia and rashes;
- ribavirin (and interferon)-induced retinopathy can also occur.

Entecavir:

- used for lamivudine-resistant chronic hepatitis B.

NURSING CARE FOR HEPATITIS

Health promotion

Nurses play an important role in preventing the spread of hepatitis. Emphasis on personal hygiene measures such as hand washing after toileting and before all food handling is important. Discuss the dangers of injection drug use and, with drug users, of sharing needles or other equipment. Encourage all sexually active persons to use safer sexual practices such as abstinence, mutual monogamy and barrier protection (such as male or female condoms).

Discuss recommendations for hepatitis A and hepatitis B vaccine with people in high or moderate risk groups for these infections. Ensure that nurses and other healthcare workers at risk for exposure to blood and body fluids are effectively vaccinated against hepatitis A and B.

Nursing diagnoses and interventions

Risk for infection (transmission)

An important goal when caring for persons with acute viral hepatitis is preventing spread of the infection.

- ✚ Use standard precautions. Practise meticulous hand washing. The hepatitis viruses are spread by direct contact with faeces or blood and body fluids. *Standard precautions and good hand washing protect both healthcare workers and other persons from exposure to the virus.*
- ✚ For persons with HAV or HEV, use standard precautions and contact isolation if faecal incontinence is present. *The faecal–oral route is the primary mode of transmission of these viruses. Other hepatitis viruses are transmitted through blood and other body fluids.*
- ✚ Encourage prophylactic treatment of all members of household and intimate sexual contacts. *Prophylactic treatment of people in close contact with the person decreases their risk of contracting the disease or, if already infected, the severity of the disease.*

PRACTICE ALERT

If the person diagnosed with hepatitis A is employed as a food handler or child care worker, contact the local health department to report possible exposure of patrons. Maintain confidentiality. Prophylactic treatment of people who have possibly been exposed to the virus can prevent a local epidemic of the disease.

Risk for fatigue

Fatigue and possible weakness are common in acute hepatitis. Although bedrest is rarely indicated, adequate rest periods and limitation of activities may be necessary. Many persons with acute hepatitis may be unable to resume normal activity levels for four or more weeks.

- ✚ Encourage planned rest periods throughout the day. *Adequate rest is necessary for optimal immune function.*
- ✚ Assist to identify essential activities and those that can be deferred or delegated to others. *Identifying essential and non-essential activities promotes the person's sense of control.*

✚ Suggest using level of fatigue to determine activity level, with gradual resumption of activities as fatigue and sense of well-being improve. *Fatigue associated with activity is an indicator of appropriate and inappropriate activity levels. As recovery progresses, increasing activity levels are tolerated with less fatigue.*

Risk for impaired nutrition

Adequate nutrition is important for immune function and healing in persons with acute or chronic hepatitis.

✚ Help plan a diet of appealing foods that provides a high-kilocalorie intake of approximately 16 carbohydrate kilocalories per kilogram of ideal body weight. *Sufficient energy is required for healing; adequate carbohydrate intake can spare protein.*

✚ Encourage planning food intake according to symptoms of the disease. Discuss eating smaller meals and using between-meal snacks to maintain nutrient and calorie intake. *Persons with acute hepatitis are often more anorexic and nauseated in the afternoon and evening; planning the majority of calorie intake in the morning helps maintain adequate intake. Limiting fat intake and the size of meals may reduce the incidence of nausea.*

✚ Instruct to avoid alcohol intake and diet drinks. *Alcohol avoidance is vital to prevent further liver damage and promote healing. Diet drinks (for example, diet sodas or juice drinks) provide few calories when an increased calorie intake is needed for healing.*

✚ Encourage use of nutritional supplements such as Ensure or instant breakfast drinks to maintain calorie and nutrient intake. *Nutritional supplement drinks are an additional source of concentrated calories and nutrients.*

The above section has given you some information with regards to hepatitis and care of the person with hepatitis, now let us consider the person with pancreatitis.

The person with pancreatitis

FAST FACTS

Pancreatitis

● Approximately, five in 100 000 people have acute pancreatitis each year in the UK.

● Acute pancreatitis has become more common in recent years. One of the reasons for this is that there has been an increase in alcohol consumption recently – in particular, binge drinking.

Source: http://www.patient.co.uk/health/Pancreatitis-Acute.htm (accessed September 2011).

Pancreatitis means inflammation of the pancreas. There are two types:

● acute pancreatitis;
● chronic pancreatitis.

Acute pancreatitis

Pathophysiology

Acute pancreatitis means inflammation of the pancreas that develops quickly. The main symptom is abdominal pain. It usually settles in a few days, but sometimes it becomes severe and very serious. Acute pancreatitis is more common in adults; its incidence is higher in men than in women. Acute pancreatitis is usually associated with gallstones in women and with alcoholism in men. Some persons recover completely, others experience recurring attacks, and still others develop chronic pancreatitis. The mortality and symptoms depend on the severity and type of pancreatitis: With mild pancreatic oedema, mortality is low (6%); with severe necrotic pancreatitis, the mortality rate is high (23%).

Although the exact cause of pancreatitis is not known, the following factors may activate pancreatic enzymes within the pancreas, leading to autodigestion, inflammation, oedema and/or necrosis.

● Gallstones may obstruct the pancreatic duct or cause bile reflux, activating pancreatic enzymes in the pancreatic duct system.

● Alcohol causes duodenal oedema, and may increase pressure and spasm in the sphincter of Oddi, obstructing pancreatic outflow. It also stimulates pancreatic enzyme production, thus raising pressure within the pancreas.

Other factors associated with acute pancreatitis include tissue ischaemia or anoxia, trauma or surgery, pancreatic tumours, third-trimester pregnancy, infectious agents (viral, bacterial or parasitic), elevated calcium levels and hyperlipidaemia. Some medications have been linked with this disorder, including thiazide diuretics, oestrogen, steroids, salicylates and NSAIDs.

Signs and symptoms

● Severe epigastric and abdominal pain radiating to the back, often felt after a fatty meal or excessive alcohol intake.
● Nausea and vomiting.
● Abdominal distension and rigidity.
● Decreased bowel sounds.
● Tachycardia.
● Hypotension.
● Pyrexia.
● Cold and clammy skin.
● Mild jaundice.

Chronic pancreatitis

Pathophysiology

Chronic pancreatitis is characterised by gradual destruction of functional pancreatic tissue. In contrast to acute pancreatitis, which may completely resolve with no long-term effects, chronic pancreatitis is an irreversible process that eventually leads to pancreatic insufficiency. Alcoholism is the primary risk factor for chronic pancreatitis. Malnutrition is a major worldwide risk factor. About 10–20% of chronic pancreatitis is idiopathic, with no identified cause. A genetic mutation on a gene associated with cystic fibrosis may play a role in these cases.

In chronic pancreatitis related to alcoholism, pancreatic secretions have an increased concentration of insoluble proteins. These proteins calcify, forming plugs that block pancreatic ducts and the flow of pancreatic juices. This blockage leads to inflammation and fibrosis of pancreatic tissue. In other cases, a stricture or stone may block pancreatic outflow, causing chronic obstructive pancreatitis. In chronic pancreatitis, recurrent episodes of inflammation eventually lead to fibrotic changes in the parenchyma of the pancreas, with loss of exocrine function. This leads to malabsorption from pancreatic insufficiency. If endocrine function is disrupted as well, clinical diabetes mellitus may develop.

Signs and symptoms
- Epigastric and upper abdominal pain radiating to the back.
- Anorexia.
- Nausea and vomiting.
- Weight loss.
- Flatulence.
- Constipation.
- Steatorrhoea (fatty, frothy foul-smelling stool caused by a decrease in pancreatic enzyme secretion).

INTERDISCIPLINARY CARE FOR PANCREATITIS

Medication

The treatment of acute pancreatitis is largely supportive. Narcotic analgesics such as morphine sulphate are used to control pain. Antibiotics are often prescribed to prevent or treat infection. Persons with chronic pancreatitis also require analgesics, but are closely monitored to prevent drug dependence. Narcotics are avoided when possible. Pancreatic enzyme supplements are given to reduce steatorrhoea. Persons with chronic pancreatitis may need to remain on pancreatic enzyme supplements for life. H_2 blockers such as cimetidine (Tagamet) and ranitidine (Zantac) and PPIs such as omeprazole (Prilosec) may be given to decrease gastric acid secretions. Octreotide (Sandostatin), a synthetic hormone, suppresses pancreatic enzyme secretion and may be used to relieve pain in chronic pancreatitis.

Nutrition

Oral food and fluids are withheld during acute episodes of pancreatitis to reduce pancreatic secretions and promote rest of the organ. A NG tube may be inserted and connected to suction. Intravenous fluids are administered to maintain vascular volume, and TPN is initiated. Oral food and fluids are begun once the serum amylase levels have returned to normal, bowel sounds are present and pain disappears. A low-fat diet is ordered, and alcohol intake is strictly prohibited.

NURSING CARE FOR PANCREATITIS

The nurse should monitor persons regularly for signs of tachycardia, pyrexia, hypotension and maintain a strict fluid balance chart and record hourly urine output (the optimum being on or above 30 ml/hour) to observe haemodynamic status, as hypovolaemia, shock, sepsis or renal failure may develop.

Nursing diagnoses and interventions

Nursing care for the person with acute pancreatitis focuses on managing pain, nutrition and maintaining fluid balance.

Risk for pain

Nurses should use an effective pain scale to assess the person and liaise with the pain management team for suitable pain relief. Obstruction of pancreatic ducts and inflammation, oedema and swelling cause severe epigastric, left upper abdominal or mid-scapular back pain. The pain is often accompanied by nausea and vomiting, abdominal tenderness and muscle guarding.

- Using a standard pain scale assess pain, including location, radiation, duration and character. Note non-verbal clues of pain: restlessness or remaining rigidly still; tense facial features; clenched fists; rapid, shallow respirations; tachycardia; and diaphoresis.

- Administer analgesics on a regular schedule. Pain assessment before and after analgesic administration measures its effectiveness. *Administering analgesics on a regular schedule prevents pain from becoming established, severe and difficult to control. Unrelieved pain has negative consequences; for example, pain, anxiety and restlessness may increase pancreatic enzyme secretion.*

- Maintain nil by mouth and NG tube patency as ordered. *Gastric secretions stimulate hormones that stimulate pancreatic secretion, aggravating pain. Eliminating oral intake and maintaining gastric suction reduce gastric secretions. Nasogastric suction also decreases nausea, vomiting and intestinal distention.*

- Maintain bedrest in a calm, quiet environment. Encourage use of non-pharmacological pain management techniques such as meditation and guided imagery. *Decreasing physical movement and mental stimulation decreases metabolic rate, GI secretion, pancreatic secretions and resulting pain.*

Adjunctive pain relief measures enhance the effectiveness of analgesics.

✚ Assist to a comfortable position, such as a side-lying position with knees flexed and head elevated 45 degrees. *Sitting up, leaning forward or lying in a foetal position tends to decrease pain caused by stretching of the peritoneum by oedema and swelling.*

✚ Remind family and visitors to avoid bringing food into the person's room. *The sight or smell of food may stimulate secretory activity of the pancreas through the cephalic phase of digestion.*

PRACTICE ALERT

Regularly assess respiratory status (at least every four to eight hours), including respiratory rate, depth and pattern; breath sounds; oxygen saturation and arterial blood gas results. Report tachypnea, adventitious or absent breath sounds, oxygen saturation levels below 92%, $PaO_2 < 70$ mmHg or $PaCO_2 > 45$ mmHg. Severe abdominal pain causes shallow respirations and hypoventilation, and suppresses cough effectiveness, which can lead to pooling of secretions, atelectasis and pneumonia.

Risk for imbalanced nutrition

The nurse and dietitian should work together to determine the person's nutritional needs. TPN is often used when food intake is restricted for long periods.

Nurses should follow local policy and guidelines when administering TPN and ensure persons eat a well-balanced diet once their condition allows, usually when abdominal pain has subsided and on doctors' instruction.

✚ Weigh daily or every other day. *Short-term weight changes (over hours to days) accurately reflect fluid balance, whereas weight changes over days to weeks reflect nutritional status.*

✚ Maintain stool chart; note frequency, colour, odour and consistency of stools. *Protein and fat metabolism are impaired in pancreatitis; undigested fats are excreted in the stool. Steatorrhoea indicates impaired digestion and, possibly, an increase in the severity of pancreatitis.*

✚ Monitor bowel sounds. *The return of bowel sounds indicates return of peristalsis; NG suction is usually discontinued within 24–48 hours thereafter.*

✚ Provide oral and nasal hygiene every one to two hours. *Fasting and NG suction increase the risk for mucous membrane irritation and breakdown.*

✚ When oral intake resumes, offer small, frequent feedings. Provide oral hygiene before and after meals. *Oral hygiene decreases oral micro-organisms that can cause foul odour and taste, decreasing appetite. Small, frequent feedings reduce pancreatic enzyme secretion and are more easily digested and absorbed.*

COMMUNITY-BASED CARE

The person with pancreatitis is often acutely ill and, along with family members, needs information about both hospital procedures and self-care at home following discharge. During the acute stage, keep explanations brief and simple.

Prior to discharge, teach the person and family about the disease and how to prevent further attacks of inflammation. Include the following topics as appropriate:

● Alcohol can cause stones to form, blocking pancreatic ducts and the outflow of pancreatic juice. Continued alcohol intake is likely to cause further inflammation and destruction of the pancreas. Avoid alcohol entirely.

● Smoking and stress may contribute to pancreatitis and should be avoided.

● If pancreatic function has been severely impaired, discuss appropriate use of pancreatic enzymes, including timing, dose, potential side-effects and monitoring of effectiveness.

● A low-fat diet is recommended. Provide a list of high-fat foods to avoid. Crash dieting and binge eating should also be avoided as they may sometimes precipitate attacks. Spicy foods, coffee, tea or colas, and gas-forming foods stimulate gastric and pancreatic secretions and may precipitate pain. Avoid them if this occurs.

● Report symptoms of infection (fever of 38 °C or more, pain, rapid pulse, malaise) because a pancreatic abscess can develop after initial recovery.

● Refer to a dietitian for diet teaching and nutritional advice. If appropriate, refer to community agencies, such as Alcoholics Anonymous, or to an alcohol treatment programme. Provide referrals to community or home health agencies as needed for continued monitoring and teaching at home.

The person with pancreatic cancer

FAST FACTS

Pancreatic cancer

● Pancreatic cancer is the fifth most common cause of death from cancer, accounting for 5% of all cancer cases.

● Around 7800 people are diagnosed with it each year.

Source: http://www.nhs.uk/conditions/Cancer-of-the-pancreas/Pages/Introduction.aspx (accessed September 2011).

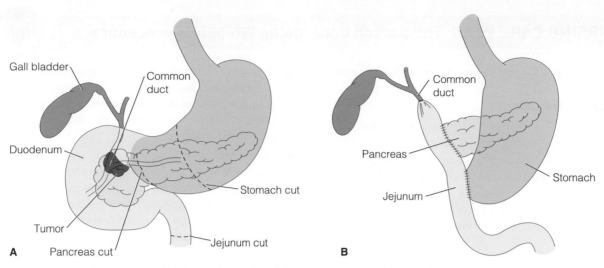

Figure 7.17 Pancreatoduodectomy. (A) Areas of resection. **(B)** Appearance following resection.

Cancer of the pancreas (also known as 'pancreatic cancer') is a relatively rare form of cancer. Pancreatic cancer tends to affect people between 60 and 80 years of age. Around 63% of people diagnosed with cancer of the pancreas are over 70 years of age and men tend to be slightly more at risk than women. Pancreatic cancer is the eleventh most common cancer in men, with around 3700 new cases diagnosed in 2006. Persons with pancreatic cancer will undergo a surgery called Whipple's procedure (see Figures 7.17 A and B).

FAST FACTS

Identified risk factors for pancreatic cancer

- Cigarette smoking – the incidence is twice as high in smokers as in non-smokers.
- Exposure to industrial chemicals or environmental toxins.
- Chronic pancreatitis.
- Diabetes mellitus.
- Obesity, high-fat diet.

In contrast to acute and chronic pancreatitis, alcohol abuse and gallstones are not identified risk factors for pancreatic cancer.

Pathophysiology and signs and symptoms of pancreatic cancer

Most cancers of the pancreas occur in the exocrine pancreas, are adenocarcinomas and cause death within one to three years after diagnosis. Cancer of the pancreas has a slow onset, with signs and symptoms of anorexia, nausea, weight loss, flatulence and dull epigastric pain. The pain increases in severity as the tumour grows. Other manifestations depend on the location of the tumour. Cancer of the head of the pancreas, which is the most common site, often obstructs bile flow through the common bile duct and the ampulla of Vater, resulting in jaundice, clay-coloured stools, dark urine and pruritus (itching). Cancer of the body of the pancreas presses on the coeliac ganglion, causing pain that increases when the person eats or lies supine. Cancer of the tail of the pancreas often causes no symptoms until it has metastasised. Other late manifestations include a palpable abdominal mass and ascites. Because the signs and symptoms are non-specific, up to 85% of persons with cancer of the pancreas do not see their GP until the cancer becomes too far advanced for a cure.

INTERDISCIPLINARY CARE FOR PANCREATIC CANCER

The Whipple procedure is the most common operation used to treat pancreatic cancer. It involves removing the head of the pancreas. The first part of the small intestine (bowel), the muscular sac that stores bile (gall bladder) and part of the bile duct are removed. Sometimes part of the stomach also has to be removed. The end of the bile duct and the remaining part of the pancreas is then connected to the small intestine. This ensures that the bile and pancreatic enzymes (chemicals that speed up chemical reactions in the body) can still be released into the digestive system.

NURSING CARE PLAN The person undergoing Whipple's procedure

Review Chapter 1 for routine pre- and post-operative care.

Pre-operative care

✛ Nurses need to adhere to local policies and guidelines in the safe preparation of persons for surgery.

✛ Extensive discussion and teaching as needed. Provide psychological support for person and family. *The person and family faced with a diagnosis of pancreatic cancer may require reinforcement of teaching as anxiety, fear and possible denial can interfere with learning.*

Post-operative care

Nurses need to adhere to local policies and guidelines in post-operative care of persons after surgery.

✛ Maintain in semi-Fowler's position. *Semi-Fowler's position facilitates lung expansion and reduces stress on the anastomosis and suture line.*

✛ Maintain low GI suction. If drainage is not adequate, obtain an order to irrigate, using minimal pressure. Do not reposition NG. *Pressure within the operative area from retained secretions increases intraluminal pressure and places stress on the suture line. Forceful irrigations and repositioning of the NG tube may disrupt the suture line.*

✛ Maintain pain control using analgesics as prescribed (patient-controlled analgesia – PCA, infusion or given on a regular basis). Assess effectiveness of pain management. *Doses higher than normal may be required if narcotic analgesics have been used prior to surgery to manage pain.*

✛ Increased pain may indicate complications such as disruption of suture line, leakage from anastomosis or peritonitis. *Adequate pain management increases resistance to stress, facilitates healing and increases the ability to cough, deep breathe and change position.*

✛ Assist with coughing, deep breathing and changing position every one to two hours. Splint incision during coughing and deep breathing. *The location of the incision makes coughing and deep breathing more painful. The prolonged surgical procedure, anaesthesia, location of incision and immobility increase the risk of retained secretions, atelectasis and pneumonia. Changing position facilitates drainage of secretions; effective coughing and deep breathing remove secretions and open distal alveoli.*

✛ Monitor for complications:

a. Take vital signs every two to four hours or as indicated; immediately report changes (such as elevated temperature; hypotension; weak, thready pulse; increased or difficult respirations).
b. Assess skin colour, temperature, moisture and turgor.
c. Measure urinary output, gastrointestinal output and drainage from any other tubes; monitor amount and type of wound drainage.
d. Assess level of consciousness.
e. Monitor results of laboratory tests, especially arterial blood gases, haemoglobin and haematocrit.

The major complications following Whipple's procedure are haemorrhage, hypovolaemic shock and hepatorenal failure. The assessments listed provide information about the person's status and alert the nurse to abnormal findings that signal the onset of these complications.

Now let us consider a common bowel condition that affects people of all ages. The severity of constipation can vary greatly. Many people only experience constipation for a short period of time with no lasting effects on their health. It may be a result of diet, medications or diseases.

The person with constipation

Constipation is defined as the infrequent (two or fewer bowel movements weekly) or difficult passage of stools. Constipation affects older adults more frequently than younger people. Although faecal transit in the large intestine slows with ageing, the increased incidence of constipation is thought to relate more to impaired general health status, increased medication use and decreased physical activity in the elderly.

FAST FACTS

Constipation

Constipation is a very common condition that affects people of all ages.

Pathophysiology of constipation

Constipation may be a primary problem or a manifestation of another disease or condition. Acute constipation, a definite change in the bowel elimination pattern, is often caused by an organic process. A change in bowel patterns that persists or becomes more frequent or severe may be due to a tumour or other partial bowel obstruction. With chronic constipation, functional causes that impair storage, transport and evacuation mechanisms impede the normal passage of stools. Common causes of constipation are listed in Table 7.1.

Table 7.1 Selected causes of constipation

Factors	Related cause
Activity	Lack of exercise: bedrest
Dietary	Highly refined, low-fibre foods; inadequate fluid intake
Drugs	Antacids containing aluminium or calcium salts; narcotic analgesics; anticholinergics; many antidepressants, tranquillisers and sedatives; antihypertensives, such as ganglionic blockers, calcium-channel blockers, beta-adrenergic blockers and diuretics; iron salts
Large bowel	Diverticular disease, inflammatory disease, tumour, obstruction; changes in rectal or anal structure or function
Psychogenical	Voluntary suppression of urge; perceived need to defecate on schedule; depression
Systemic	Advanced age; pregnancy; neurologic conditions (trauma, multiple sclerosis, tumours, cerebrovascular accident, Parkinsonism); endocrine and metabolic disorders (hypothyroidism, hypercalcaemia, uraemia, porphyria)
Other	Chronic laxative or enema use

Signs and symptoms of constipation

The symptoms of constipation include having bowel movements less often than the usual pattern, frequent flatus, abdominal discomfort, anorexia, straining to have a bowel movement and the passage of hard, dry stools. With significant constipation or long-term dependence on laxatives or enemas, faecal impaction may develop. Impaction may also occur following barium administration for radiologic exam. The impaction is felt as a rock-hard or putty-like mass of faeces in the rectum. Abdominal cramping and a full sensation in the rectal area may be manifestations of impaction. Watery mucus or foul-smelling liquid stool may be passed around the impaction, causing the person to complain of diarrhoea.

INTERDISCIPLINARY CARE FOR CONSTIPATION

Medication

Laxative and cathartic preparations are used to promote stool evacuation. Milder preparations are generally known as laxatives; cathartics have a stronger effect. Most laxatives are appropriate only for short-term use. Cathartics and enemas interfere with normal bowel reflexes and should not be used for simple constipation. Laxatives should never be given if a person has an undiagnosed intestinal obstruction, abdominal pain, faecal impaction, rectal fissures, ulcerated haemorrhoids, Crohn's disease, ulcerative colitis or chronic inflammatory bowel disease. When the bowel is obstructed, laxatives or cathartics may cause serious mechanical damage and perforate the bowel.

NURSING CARE FOR CONSTIPATION

Health promotion

Education can prevent constipation. Teach the person the importance of maintaining a diet high in natural fibre. Foods such as fresh fruits, vegetables, whole-grain products and bran provide natural fibre. Encourage reducing consumption of meats and refined foods, which are low in fibre and can be constipating. Emphasise the need to maintain a high fluid intake every day, particularly during hot weather and exercise. Discuss the relationship between exercise and bowel regularity. Encourage the person to engage in some form of exercise, such as walking daily.

Discuss normal bowel habits, and explain that a daily bowel movement is not the norm for all people. Encourage the person to respond to the urge to defecate when it occurs. Suggest setting aside a time, usually following a meal, for elimination.

Nutrition

Foods that have a high fibre content are recommended. Vegetable fibre is largely indigestible and unabsorbable, so it increases stool bulk. Fibre also helps draw water into the faecal mass,

COMMUNITY-BASED CARE

Include the following topics when teaching self-care measures to prevent and treat constipation:

- Increasing dietary fibre intake by including fresh fruits and vegetables, whole grains, high-fibre breakfast cereals and unprocessed bran in the diet. (Bran can be sprinkled on cereals, mixed into bread or muffin recipes or mixed with fruit juice to increase its palatability.)
- Maintaining fluid intake of six to eight glasses of water per day (unless contraindicated).
- Suggestions for remaining physically active to promote bowel function and maintain muscle tone
- Responding to the urge to defecate when perceived.
- Appropriate use of laxatives:
  - do not use laxatives, suppositories or enemas on a regular basis;
  - bulk-forming agents provide insoluble fibre and are safe for long-term use – it is important to drink at least six to eight glasses of water daily when using these (or any) laxatives;
  - other laxatives such as milk of magnesia, docusate (Colace, DSS), bisacodyl (Dulcolax), cascara or castor oil should be used only occasionally to relieve constipation.
- Reporting any change in bowel habits such as new or persistent constipation or diarrhoea, abdominal pain, black or bloody stools, nausea or anorexia, weakness or unexplained weight loss to the GP or practice nurse.

softening the stool and making defecation easier. Raw fruits and vegetables are good sources of dietary fibre, as is cereal bran. Use two to three teaspoons of unprocessed bran with meals (sprinkled on fruit or cereal) or up to the recommended intake of 18g of fibre a day.

Fluids are also important to maintain bowel motility and soft stools. The person should drink six to eight glasses of fluid per day. It is important to advise the person to increase fluid intake when dietary fibre is initially increased to decrease flatus and help maintain softer stools.

IN PRACTICE

Administering an enema

An enema is the insertion of liquid into the colon or rectum. There are various types of enemas available, including cleansing and retention enemas. Enemas must be prescribed before administration. Nurses must always:

- Explain the procedure to the person.
- Ensure that the bed is screened in order to provide privacy.
- If possible ask the person to empty their bladder because this may reduce discomfort during the procedure.
- Prepare the enema according the manufacturer's recommendation.
- Lie the person on the left side.
- Wash hands, don gloves and observe infection control procedure as indicated by local policy and procedure.
- Lubricate the tip of the enema.
- Gently insert the enema into the rectum and squeeze the bag to insert the fluid.
- Observe the person all the time during the procedure.
- On completion gently remove the bag from the rectum while at the same time keeping the bag squeezed.
- Wipe the person's anal area and encourage the person to retain the enema for 5–15 minutes.
- Ensure that the person is comfortable.
- Dispose of used equipments and wash your hands.
- When the person is ready to defecate, assist them to the toilet or give a bedpan or bedside commode.
- Document the outcome of the procedure.

The person with inflammatory bowel disease (IBD)

Inflammatory bowel disease (IBD) isn't a single disease. The term IBD is used mainly to describe two diseases, Crohn's disease and ulcerative colitis. Both these diseases are chronic conditions which involve inflammation of the GI tract. IBD affects other systems of the body (see Figure 7.18).

FAST FACT

Inflammatory bowel disease

Ulcerative colitis and Crohn's disease affect about one person in every 250 in the UK population.

Source: http://www.nacc.org.uk/content/ibd.asp (accessed September 2011).

Ulcerative colitis (UC)

Ulcerative colitis (UC) is a long-term (chronic) condition affecting the colon. Conditions that cause inflammation of the intestines, such as ulcerative colitis or Crohn's disease, are known as IBD. IBD should not be confused with irritable bowel syndrome (IBS), which is a different condition and requires different treatment. Around 100 000 people in the UK have ulcerative colitis. The condition normally appears between the ages of 15 and 30. The condition is more common in people of European descent, especially those people descended from Ashkenazi Jewish communities (Jews who lived in Eastern Europe and Russia).

Pathophysiology

UC is a disease that causes inflammation and sores, called ulcers, in the lining of the rectum and colon. Ulcers form where inflammation has killed the cells that usually line the colon, then bleed and produce pus. Inflammation in the colon also causes the colon to empty frequently, causing diarrhoea. In ulcerative colitis, inflammatory changes occur in the mucosa and the submucosa of the colon. These inflammatory changes are diffuse with widespread superficial ulceration. Ulcerative colitis always affects the rectum – that part of the large bowel which lies just inside the anus. Sometimes, the inflammation is limited just to the rectum – this is known as proctitis. However, the inflammation can involve a variable length of the colon. When the whole colon is affected, this is called pan-colitis or total colitis.

Initially, there is reddening and oedema of the mucosa and this is followed by ulceration. Ulcerative colitis usually does not affect the full thickness of the wall of the large intestine and hardly ever affects the small intestine. The disease usually begins in the rectum or the rectum and the sigmoid colon (the lower end of the large intestine) but may eventually spread along part or all of the large intestine.

Signs and symptoms

- Diarrhoea with blood and mucus.
- Anaemia.

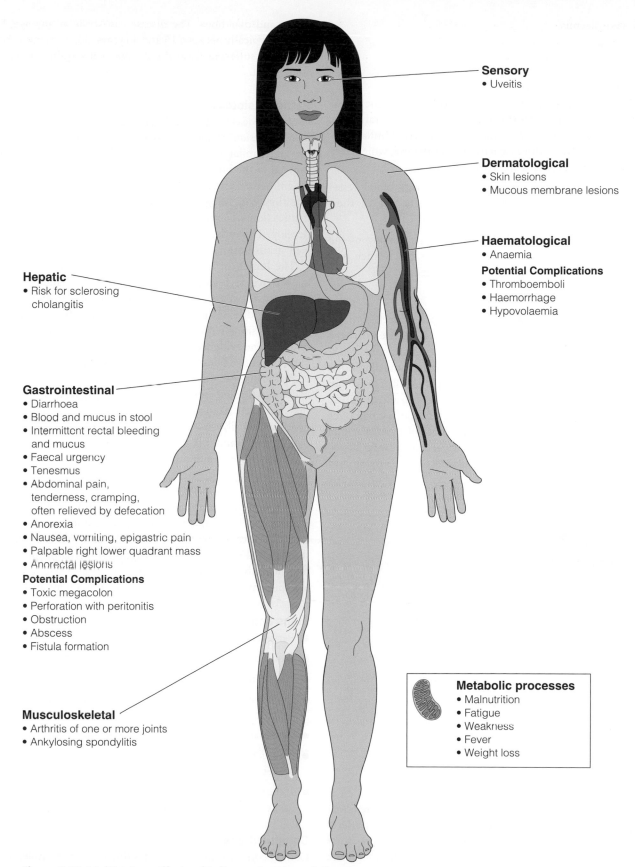

Sensory
- Uveitis

Dermatological
- Skin lesions
- Mucous membrane lesions

Haematological
- Anaemia

Potential Complications
- Thromboemboli
- Haemorrhage
- Hypovolaemia

Hepatic
- Risk for sclerosing cholangitis

Gastrointestinal
- Diarrhoea
- Blood and mucus in stool
- Intermittent rectal bleeding and mucus
- Faecal urgency
- Tenesmus
- Abdominal pain, tenderness, cramping, often relieved by defecation
- Anorexia
- Nausea, vomiting, epigastric pain
- Palpable right lower quadrant mass
- Anorectal lesions

Potential Complications
- Toxic megacolon
- Perforation with peritonitis
- Obstruction
- Abscess
- Fistula formation

Musculoskeletal
- Arthritis of one or more joints
- Ankylosing spondylitis

Metabolic processes
- Malnutrition
- Fatigue
- Weakness
- Fever
- Weight loss

Figure 7.18 Multisystem effects of inflammatory bowel disease.

- Hypovolaemia.
- Fatigue.
- Anorexia.
- Weakness.
- Persons with severe disease may also have systemic manifestations such as arthritis involving one or several joints, skin and mucous membrane lesions or *uveitis* (inflammation of the uvea, the vascular layer of the eye, which may also involve the sclera and cornea).
- Some persons develop thromboemboli, with blood vessel obstruction due to clots carried from the site of their formation.
- Sclerosing cholangitis (inflammation and scarring of the bile ducts) may occur, more often in men than women, and most commonly in the third to fifth decade of life.

Complications

Acute complications of ulcerative colitis include haemorrhage, toxic megacolon and colon perforation. Massive haemorrhage may occur with severe attacks of the disease. *Toxic megacolon*, a condition characterised by acute motor paralysis and dilation of the colon to greater than 6 cm, may affect part or all of the colon. The transverse segment of the bowel is most often affected. Toxic megacolon may be triggered by the use of laxatives, narcotics and anticholinergic drugs and the presence of hypokalaemia. Symptoms of toxic megacolon include fever, tachycardia, hypotension, dehydration, abdominal tenderness and cramping, and a change in the number of stools per day. Perforation is rare, but the risk of this dangerous complication is increased with toxic megacolon. Perforation leads to peritonitis.

> **Consider this . . .**
>
> Studies in America have shown that drinking tapeworm eggs does help in the symptoms of ulcerative colitis. Other researchers have used eggs from hookworms, threadworms, whipworms and roundworms. Crohn's disease, ulcerative colitis and other forms of IBD appear to be caused by an overactive immune system, which causes inflammation in the digestive system. These parasites downregulate the immune system for its own benefit. Studies have shown that parasite secretions can manipulate the immune system, alleviating lung inflammation, Crohn's disease and rheumatoid arthritis in animal models of disease.

Crohn's disease

Like ulcerative colitis, Crohn's disease, also known as regional enteritis, is a chronic, relapsing inflammatory disorder affecting the GI tract. Crohn's disease can affect any portion of the GI tract from the mouth to the anus, but usually affects the terminal ileum and ascending colon. Crohn's disease affects between one in 500 and one in 1000 people within the UK, causing inflammation of the GI tract and leading to pain,

ulcers and diarrhoea. The disease can strike at any age, but onset is typically between 15 and 40 years old. As many as 80% of people suffering from the disease will require surgery at some point.

Pathophysiology

Crohn's disease typically begins as a small inflammatory *aphthoid lesion* (shallow ulcers with a white base and elevated margin, similar to a canker sore) of the mucosa and submucosa of the bowel. These initial lesions may regress, or the inflammatory process can progress to involve all layers of the intestinal wall. Deeper ulcerations, granulomatous lesions and fissures (knife-like clefts that extend deeply into the bowel wall) develop. The inflammatory process involves the entire bowel wall (transmural).

The lumen of the affected bowel assumes a 'cobblestone appearance' as fissures and ulcers surround islands of intact mucosa over oedematous submucosa. The inflammatory lesions of Crohn's disease are not continuous; rather, they often occur as 'skip' lesions with intervening areas of normal-appearing bowel. Some evidence suggests that despite its normal appearance, the entire bowel is affected by this disorder.

As the disease progresses, fibrotic changes in the bowel wall cause it to thicken and lose flexibility, taking on an appearance that has been likened to a rubber hose. The inflammation, oedema and fibrosis can lead to local obstruction, abscess development and the formation of fistulas between loops of bowel or bowel and other organs (Figure 7.19). Depending on the severity and extent of the disease, malabsorption and malnutrition may develop as the ulcers prevent absorption of nutrients. When the jejunum and ileum are affected, the absorption of multiple nutrients may be impaired, including carbohydrates, proteins, fats, vitamins and folate. Disease in the terminal ileum can lead to vitamin B_{12} malabsorption and bile salt reabsorption. The ulcerations can also lead to protein loss and chronic, slow blood loss with consequent anaemia.

Signs and symptoms

- Persistent diarrhoea.
- Stools are liquid or semi-formed and do not contain blood.
- Abdominal pain and tenderness are also common.
- Pain may be located in the right lower quadrant and relieved by defecation.
- Fever, fatigue, malaise, weight loss and anaemia are common.
- Anorectal lesions such as fissures, ulcers, fistulas and abscesses are also common.
- If the stomach and duodenum are involved, nausea, vomiting and epigastric pain may occur.

Complications

Certain complications of Crohn's disease (for example, intestinal obstruction, abscess and fistula) are so common that they are considered part of the disease process. For many persons, the disease initially presents with one of these complications.

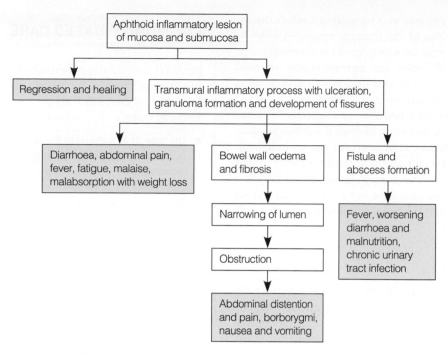

Figure 7.19 The progression of Crohn's disease.

Intestinal obstruction is a common complication caused by repeated inflammation and scarring of the bowel that leads to fibrosis and stricture. Obstruction of the bowel lumen causes abdominal distention, cramping pain and borborygmi (rumbling sound of the stomach). Nausea and vomiting may occur.

Fistulas may be asymptomatic, particularly if they occur between loops of small bowel. When fistulisation causes an abscess, chills and fever, a tender abdominal mass and leukocytosis develop. A fistula between the small bowel and colon may exacerbate diarrhoea, weight loss and malnutrition. When the bladder is involved, recurrent urinary tract infections occur.

INTERDISCIPLINARY CARE FOR IBD

Medication

The ultimate goal of care is to terminate acute attacks as quickly as possible and reduce the incidence of relapse. Drug therapy plays a key role in achieving this goal. Locally acting and systemic anti-inflammatory drugs are the primary medications used to manage mild to moderate IBD. Drugs to suppress the immune response may be used to treat persons with severe disease.

Steroids are a type of hormone medication. Hormones are groups of powerful chemicals that have a wide range of effects on the body. One such effect is to reduce inflammation. Steroids are usually only used to treat the active disease because their long-term use is associated with a range of adverse side-effects. Budesonide and prednisolone are two steroids that are often used to treat Crohn's disease. Side-effects of budesonide include:

- acne;
- swelling of the face;

- swelling of the hands, arms, feet and legs due to a build-up of fluids (oedema);
- mood changes, such as feeling irritable or anxious;
- insomnia;
- indigestion.

Prednisolone has the same type of short-term and long-term side-effects as budesonide. In addition, prednisolone has been known to cause mental health problems in an estimated 5% of people. These include:

- feeling depressed and thinking about suicide;
- feeling very excited and happy;
- experiencing sudden and severe mood changes (happy one minute, very depressed the next);
- feeling anxious;
- having problems thinking clearly and feeling particularly confused;
- memory loss;
- hallucinations (seeing and hearing things that are not real).

Sulfasalazine belongs to a group of medicines called aminosalicylates. Aminosalicylates are known to reduce inflammation inside the colon. Sulfasalazine can be used as an alternative to steroids to treat mild cases of Crohn's disease. Common side-effects of sulfasalazine include:

- headache;
- nausea;
- abdominal pain;
- diarrhoea.

Immunosuppressants may also be used in Crohn's disease to suppress the activities of the immune system in order to help reduce inflammation on a long-term basis. Immunosuppressants such as azathioprine and mercaptopurine are used in maintenance therapy and in combination with steroids when a person has a relapse of symptoms.

Biological therapies are a new type of medication that are created using naturally occurring biological substances, such as antibodies and enzymes. At present, in England, infliximab is the only biological therapy that is licensed for the treatment of Crohn's disease. The drug is only recommended in severe cases of Crohn's disease that have not responded to steroid and immunosuppressant treatments, and where the person is unsuitable for surgery.

Nutrition

Antigens in the diet may stimulate the immune response in the bowel, exacerbating IBD. As a result, dietary management for inflammatory bowel disease is individualised. Some persons benefit from eliminating all milk and milk products from the diet. Increased dietary fibre may help reduce diarrhoea and relieve rectal manifestations, but is contraindicated for persons with intestinal strictures caused by repeated inflammation and scarring.

All food may be withheld to promote bowel rest during an acute exacerbation of Crohn's disease. Nutritional status is maintained using enteral nutrition or TPN. TPN carries a higher risk of complications than does enteral nutrition. An elemental diet such as Ensure, which contains all essential nutrients in a residue-free formula, may be prescribed. Enteral diets provide essential nutrients to the small intestine to support cell growth, but are not always palatable.

Surgery

Surgery is often required when the symptoms of Crohn's disease cannot be controlled using medication alone. An estimated 80% of people with Crohn's disease do require surgery at some point in their life. Surgery cannot cure Crohn's disease, but it can provide long periods of remission, often lasting several years. During surgery, the inflamed section of the digestive system is removed and the remaining part is reattached.

Ileostomy

An ileostomy is a surgically created opening between the intestine and the abdominal wall that allows the passage of faecal material. The surface opening is called a stoma. The precise name of the colostomy depends on the location of the stoma. An ileostomy is a colostomy made in the ileum of the small intestine. In an

ileostomy, the colon, rectum and anus are usually completely removed (*total proctocolectomy with permanent ileostomy*). The anal canal is closed, and the end of the terminal ileum is brought to the body surface through the right abdominal wall to form the stoma. A temporary or *loop ileostomy* may be formed to eliminate faeces and allow tissue healing for two to three months. A loop of ileum is brought to the body surface to form a stoma and allow stool drainage into an external pouch. When the ileostomy is no longer necessary, a second surgery is performed to close the stoma and repair the bowel, restoring faecal elimination through the anus.

COMMUNITY-BASED CARE

IBD is a chronic condition for which the person provides daily self-management. For this reason, teaching is a vital component of care. Teach the person and family about the following topics:

- The type of IBD affecting the person, including the disease process, short- and long-term effects, the relationship of stress to disease exacerbations and the manifestations of complications.
- Prescribed medications, including drug names, desired effects, schedules for tapering the doses if ordered (as with corticosteroids) and possible side-effects or adverse reactions and their management.
- The recommended diet and the rationale for any specific restrictions.
- Use of nutritional supplements such as Ensure to maintain weight and nutritional status.
- Indicators of malabsorption and impaired nutrition; recommendations for self-care and when to seek medical intervention.
- If discharged with a central catheter and home parenteral nutrition, written and verbal instructions on catheter care, troubleshooting and TPN administration. (Have the person and a family member demonstrate catheter care and TPN maintenance.)
- The importance of maintaining a fluid intake of at least 2–3 L per day, increasing fluid intake during warm weather, exercise or strenuous work, and when fever is present.
- The increased risk for colorectal cancer and importance of regular bowel exams.
- Risks and benefits of various treatment options.

NURSING CARE PLAN The person having an ileostomy

Review Chapter 1 for routine pre- and post-operative care.

Pre-operative care

+ Nurses need to adhere to local policies and guidelines in the safe preparation of the person for ileostomy.

+ Refer to a stoma therapist for marking and teaching about the stoma location, ileostomy care, and options for stoma appliances. *It is important to begin teaching prior to surgery to facilitate learning and acceptance of the ileostomy post-operatively.*

+ Discuss the availability of support groups or associations, and provide a referral as necessary or desired. *People from support groups may help with information and support with regards to living with a stoma.*

+ Provide pre-operative bowel preparation as ordered. *Cathartics, enemas and pre-operative antibiotics are often prescribed to reduce the risk of abdominal contamination and infection after surgery.*

Post-operative care

+ Nurses must adhere to local policies and guidelines in post-operative care.

+ Apply an ileostomy pouch over the stoma. *Stool from an ileostomy is expressed continuously or irregularly, and it is liquid in nature; continuous use of a pouch to collect the drainage is necessary.*

+ Assess frequently for bleeding, stoma viability and function. In the early post-operative period, small amounts of blood in the pouch are expected. A healthy stoma appears pink or red and moist as a result of mucous production. It should protrude approximately 2 cm from the abdominal wall. *Frequent assessment is particularly important in the initial post-operative period to ensure stoma health and monitor for possible complications. A dusky, brown, black or white stoma indicates circulatory compromise. Other possible stoma complications include retraction (indentation or loss of the external portion of the stoma) or prolapse (outward telescoping of the stoma, that is, an abnormally long stoma).*

+ As the stoma starts to function, empty the pouch, explaining the procedure to the person. Initial drainage is dark green, viscid and usually odourless. Drainage gradually thickens and becomes yellow-brown. Empty the pouch when it is one-third full. Measure drainage, and include it as output on intake and output records. Rinse the pouch and reapply the clamp. *Emptying the pouch when it is no more than one-third full helps prevent the skin seal from breaking as a result of the weight of the pouch. Because of the potential for excess fluid loss through ileostomy drainage, it is important to include it as fluid output.*

+ Assess the peristomal skin. Skin around the stoma should remain clean and pink and free of irritation, rashes, inflammation or excoriation. *Skin complications may arise from appliance irritation or hypersensitivity, excoriation from a leaking appliance or* Candida albicans, *a yeast infection.*

+ Protect peristomal skin from enzymes and bile salts in the ileostomy effluent. Using a skin barrier on the pouch is essential. Change the pouch if leakage occurs or if the person complains of burning or itching skin. *Enzymes and bile salts normally reabsorbed in the large intestine are irritating to the skin. Excoriation of skin surrounding the stoma impairs the first line of defence against micro-organisms and can interfere with the ability to achieve a tight skin seal and prevent pouch leakage.*

+ Report the following abnormal assessment findings to the doctor:
  a. Allergic or contact dermatitis. *A rash may result from contact with faecal drainage or indicate sensitivity to pouch, paste, tape or sealant.*
  b. Purulent ulcerated areas surrounding the stoma. *Disruption of the protective barrier of the skin allows bacterial entry.*
  c. A red, bumpy, itchy rash or white-coated area. *This is a manifestation of* Candida albicans, *a yeast infection.*
  d. Bulging around the stoma. *This finding may indicate herniation, caused by loops of intestine protruding through the abdominal wall.*

+ Apply protective ointments to the perirectal area of persons with newly functioning ileoanal reservoirs and anatomises. *This helps protect the skin from the initial stools. As stools thicken and become fewer per day, the person experiences less perirectal irritation.*

Health education for the person and family

+ While caring for the ileostomy, explain procedures to the person. *Teaching is immediate and ongoing to facilitate acceptance of the ileostomy and self-care.*

+ Teach to manage the stoma bag. *Self-care is vital to independence and self-esteem.*

+ Instruct now to use an electric razor to shave the peristomal hair if necessary. *An electric razor prevents accidental cutting of the stoma with a razor blade.*

+ Teach to check the stoma and peristomal skin with each stoma bag change. *Ongoing assessment is important for optimal health and function of the stoma and surrounding skin. Stripping of tape or excessively frequent pouch removal may cause mechanical trauma to peristomal skin. Chronic skin irritation by ileostomy effluent may lead to pseudoveracous lesions, or wart-like nodules.*

+ Advise the person to report abnormal appearance of the stoma or surrounding skin (as noted previously and below) to the stoma nurse:
  a. Narrowing of the stoma lumen. *This indicates stenosis and may interfere with faecal elimination.*

> ### NURSING CARE PLAN The person having an ileostomy (continued)

b. Lacerations or cuts in the stoma. *The stoma contains no nerves, so trauma may occur without pain.*

c. Separation of the stoma from the abdominal surface. *This potential complication may require surgical repair.*

+ Emphasise the importance of adequate fluid and salt intake; the risk for dehydration and hyponatremia is increased particularly during hot weather, when fluid is lost through perspiration as well as ileostomy drainage. Water intake should be sufficient to maintain good urine output. When exercising in hot weather, the person should consume extra water and salt. High-potassium foods, such as bananas and oranges, may also be recommended. *Loss of the reabsorptive surface of the large bowel increases the amount of water and sodium loss in the stool. If the ileostomy is high (more proximal in the ileum), additional potassium losses may also occur.*

+ Discuss symptoms of fluid and electrolyte imbalances such as:
  a. Extreme thirst
  b. Dry skin and oral mucous membrane
  c. Decreased urine output
  d. Weakness, fatigue
  e. Muscle cramps
  f. Abdominal cramps, nausea, vomiting
  g. Shortness of breath
  h. Orthostatic hypotension (feeling faint when suddenly changing positions).

+ Discuss dietary concerns. Foods that may cause excessive odour or gas are typically avoided as well. *Because food blockage is a potential problem, high-fibre foods are limited, and foods that may cause blockage, such as popcorn, corn, nuts, cucumbers, celery, fresh tomatoes, figs, strawberries, blackberries and caraway seeds, are avoided. Symptoms of food blockage include abdominal cramping, swelling of the stoma, and absence of ileostomy output for over four to six hours.*

+ Teach self-care measures to relieve food blockage:
  a. Take a warm shower or bath. *This can help relax the abdominal muscles.*
  b. Assume a knee–chest position. *The knee–chest position reduces intra-abdominal pressure.*
  c. Drink warm fluids or grape juice if not vomiting. *This provides a mild cathartic effect.*
  d. Massage peristomal area. *Massage may stimulate peristalsis and faecal elimination.*
  e. Remove stoma bag if the stoma is swollen, and apply a bag with a larger opening. *If the stoma swells, the pouch may create a mechanical obstruction to output.*

+ Notify the GP or stoma nurse if:
  a. The above measures fail to relieve the obstruction.
  b. Signs of a partial obstruction persist including high-volume odorous fluid output, abdominal cramps, nausea, and vomiting.
  c. There is no ileostomy output for four to six hours.
  d. Signs of fluid and electrolyte imbalance occur, such as weakness, dizziness, light-headedness or headache.

The person with colorectal cancer

Colorectal cancer (also known as bowel cancer) affects the lower part of the digestive system – the large bowel and the rectum. It affects men and women equally, and is the third most common type of cancer in men and the second most common in women. One in 20 people in the UK will develop bowel cancer in their lifetime.

The condition is rare in people under 40, and almost 85% of cases are diagnosed in the over 65 year olds. Each year, more than 35 000 people are diagnosed with bowel cancer and about 16 000 die as a result of the disease. If caught early, this cancer can be treated effectively, and survival has doubled over the last 30 years because of early diagnosis. The exact cause of bowel cancer isn't known, but a family history of the condition can increase the risk. If a member of your immediate family is diagnosed with colorectal cancer before the age of 45 or two immediate family members are affected by the disease, then you should consult your GP about genetic screening to see if you're at risk. The risk of developing colorectal cancer increases with age; however, younger people can develop the disease.

Risk factors for colorectal cancer

Risk factors for colorectal cancer include:

- age over 50 years;
- polyps of the colon and/or rectum;
- family history of colorectal cancer;
- inflammatory bowel disease;
- exposure to radiation;
- diet: high animal fat and kilocalorie intake.

Diet plays a role in the development of colorectal cancer. The disease is prevalent in economically prosperous countries where people consume diets high in calories, meat proteins and fats. This dietary regime may increase the population of anaerobic bacteria in the gut. These anaerobes convert bile acids into carcinogens. Diets high in fruits and vegetables, folic acid and calcium appear to reduce the risk of colorectal cancer. Cereal fibre, once thought to reduce colorectal cancer risk, does not now appear to play a role either way in its development. Other factors that may reduce the risk of colorectal cancer include regular exercise, taking a daily multivitamin and the use of aspirin and other NSAIDs.

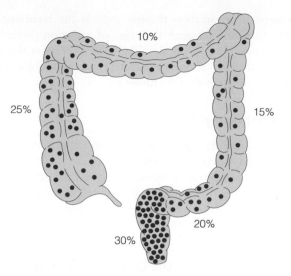

Figure 7.20 The distribution and frequency of cancer of the colon and rectum.

Pathophysiology of colorectal cancer

Nearly all colorectal cancers are adenocarcinomas that begin as adenomatous polyps. Most tumours develop in the rectum and sigmoid colon, although any portion of the colon may be affected (Figure 7.20). The tumour typically grows undetected, producing few symptoms. By the time symptoms occur, the disease may have spread into deeper layers of the bowel tissue and adjacent organs. Colorectal cancer spreads by direct extension to involve the entire bowel circumference, the submucosa and outer bowel wall layers. Neighbouring organs such as the liver, greater curvature of the stomach, duodenum, small intestine, pancreas, spleen, genitourinary tract and abdominal wall may also be involved by direct extension. Metastasis to regional lymph nodes is the most common form of tumour spread. This is not always an orderly process; distal nodes may contain cancer cells while regional nodes remain normal. Cancerous cells from the primary tumour may also spread by way of the lymphatic system or circulatory system to secondary sites such as the liver, lungs, brain, bones and kidneys. The spread of the tumour to other areas of the peritoneal cavity can occur when the tumour extends through the serosa or during surgical resection.

Signs and symptoms of colorectal cancer

Signs and symptoms of colorectal cancer include:

- rectal bleeding;
- change of bowel habits;
- diarrhoea or constipation;
- pain;
- anorexia;
- weight loss;
- anaemia from occult bleeding.

Complications of colorectal cancer

The primary complications associated with colorectal cancer are (1) bowel obstruction due to narrowing of the bowel lumen by the lesion; (2) perforation of the bowel wall by the tumour, allowing contamination of the peritoneal cavity by bowel contents; and (3) direct extension of the tumour to involve adjacent organs.

Most recurrences of colorectal cancer after tumour removal occur within the first four years. The size of the primary tumour does not necessarily relate to long-term survival. The number of involved lymph nodes, penetration of the tumour through the bowel wall and tumour adherence to adjacent organs are better predictors of the prognosis for the disease.

INTERDISCIPLINARY CARE FOR COLORECTAL CANCER

Surgery

Surgical resection of the tumour, adjacent colon and regional lymph nodes is the treatment of choice for colorectal cancer. Options for surgical treatment vary from destruction of the tumour by laser photocoagulation performed during endoscopy to abdominoperineal resection with permanent colostomy. When possible, the anal sphincter is preserved and colostomy avoided.

Most persons with colorectal cancer undergo surgical resection of the colon with anastomosis of remaining bowel as a curative procedure. The distribution of regional lymph nodes determines the extent of resection because these may contain metastatic lesions. Most tumours of the ascending, transverse, descending and sigmoid colon can be resected.

Tumours of the rectum usually are treated with an abdominoperineal resection in which the sigmoid colon, rectum and anus are removed through both abdominal and perineal incisions. A permanent sigmoid colostomy is performed to provide for elimination of faeces.

Surgical resection of the bowel may be accompanied by a colostomy for diversion of faecal contents. A colostomy is an ostomy (surgically created opening) made in the colon. It may be created if the bowel is obstructed by the tumour, as a temporary measure to promote healing of anastomises or as a permanent means of faecal evacuation when the distal colon and rectum are removed. Colostomies take the name of the portion of the colon from which they are formed: ascending colostomy, transverse colostomy, descending colostomy and sigmoid colostomy (Figure 7.21).

A *sigmoid colostomy* is the most common permanent colostomy performed, particularly for cancer of the rectum. It is usually created during an abdominoperineal resection. This procedure involves the removal of the sigmoid colon, rectum and anus through abdominal and perineal incisions. The anal canal is closed, and a stoma formed from the proximal sigmoid colon. The stoma is usually located on the lower left quadrant of the abdomen.

When a *double-barrel colostomy* is performed, two separate stomas are created (Figure 7.22). The distal colon is not removed,

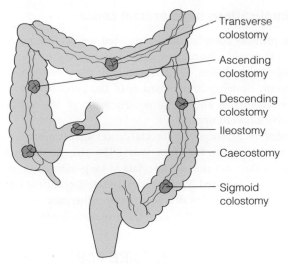

Figure 7.21 Various colostomy levels and sites.

but bypassed. The proximal stoma, which is functional, diverts faeces to the abdominal wall. The distal stoma, also called the mucous fistula, expels mucus from the distal colon. It may be pouched or dressed with a gauge dressing. A double-barrel colostomy may be created for cases of trauma, tumour or inflammation, and it may be temporary or permanent.

An emergency procedure used to relieve an intestinal obstruction or perforation is called a *transverse loop colostomy*. During this procedure, a loop of the transverse colon is brought out from the abdominal wall and suspended over a plastic rod or bridge, which prevents the loop from slipping back into the abdominal cavity.

Radiation therapy

Although radiation therapy is not used as a primary treatment for colon cancer, it is used with surgical resection for treating rectal tumours. Small rectal cancers may be treated with intra-cavitary, external or implantation radiation. Rectal cancer has a high rate of regional recurrence following complete surgical resection, particularly when the tumour has invaded tissues outside the bowel wall or regional lymph nodes. Pre- or

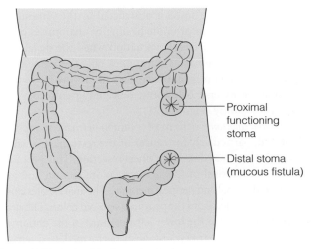

Figure 7.22 A double-barrel colostomy.

post-operative radiation therapy reduces the recurrence of pelvic tumours, although the effect of radiation therapy on long-term survival is less clear. Radiation therapy is also used pre-operatively to shrink large rectal tumours enough to permit surgical removal of the tumour.

Chemotherapy

Chemotherapeutic agents, such as intravenous fluorouracil (5-FU) and folinic acid (leucovorin), are also used post-operatively as adjunctive therapy for colorectal cancer. When combined with radiation therapy, chemotherapy reduces the rate of tumour recurrence and prolongs survival for persons with stage II and stage III rectal tumours.

NURSING CARE FOR COLORECTAL CANCER

Health promotion

Primary prevention of colorectal cancer is a significant nursing care issue. Nurses should teach persons about dietary intake. Advice should include decreasing the amount of fat, refined sugar and red meats in the diet while increasing intake of dietary fibre. Foods that contain high amounts of fibre include raw fruits and vegetables, legumes and whole-grain products.

Stress the importance of regular health examinations, including digital rectal exams. Discuss recommendations for regular haemoccult (test for occult blood in the stool) testing of stool after age 40. Include the importance of seeking medical treatment if blood is noted in or on the stool. Teach persons the warning signs for cancer, including those specific to bowel cancer, such as a change in bowel habits.

Nursing diagnoses and interventions

In planning and implementing care, consider both physical care needs and emotional response to the diagnosis. Because colorectal cancer is often advanced at the time of diagnosis, the prognosis, even with treatment, may be poor. Denial and anger are common. Extensive abdominal surgery and potentially a colostomy may be necessary, and the effects of chemotherapy and radiation therapy can leave the person fatigued and discouraged.

Nursing care includes providing emotional support, teaching and direct care before and after diagnostic procedures and surgery and during adjunctive treatments. Priority nursing diagnoses include acute pain, imbalanced nutrition and anticipatory grieving. Risk for sexual dysfunction should be considered as a priority diagnosis if a colostomy has been created.

PRACTICE ALERT

If an abdominoperineal resection has been performed, alert all care personnel to avoid rectal temperatures, suppository use or other procedures that could damage sutures.

NURSING CARE PLAN The person having a colostomy

Review Chapter 1 for routine pre- and post-operative care.

Pre-operative care

+ Ensure that the patient understands diagnosis and the post-operative care. *To reduce anxiety and promote uneventful post-operative recovery.*

+ Teach deep breathing exercises. *Deep breathing exercises improves circulation and prevents chest infection post-operatively.*

+ Teach leg exercises. *Passive movement of limbs prevents deep vein thrombosis and improves circulation.*

+ Bowel preparation as per local policy.

+ Complete checklist such as patient is wearing correct identification bracelet, valuables are safely locked away, patient has signed consent form, the patient has fasted as per local trust policy, prior to administration of premedication.

Post-operative care

+ Assess the location of the stoma and the type of colostomy performed. *Stoma location is an indicator of the section of bowel in which it is located and a predictor of the type of faecal drainage to expect.*

+ Assess stoma appearance and surrounding skin condition frequently. *Assessment of stoma and skin condition is particularly important in the early post-operative period, when complications are most likely to occur and most treatable.*

+ Position a collection bag or drainable pouch over the stoma. *Initial drainage may contain more mucus and serosan-guineous fluid than faecal material. As the bowel starts to resume function, drainage becomes faecal in nature. The consistency of drainage depends on the stoma location in the bowel.*

+ Empty a drainable pouch or replace the colostomy bag as needed or when it is no more than one-third full. *If the pouch is allowed to overfill, its weight may impair the seal and cause leakage.*

+ Provide stomal and skin care for the person with a colostomy as for the person with an ileostomy. *Good skin and stoma care is important to maintain skin integrity and function as the first line of defence against infection. The contents of the bag should be observed and any changes such as retraction of the stoma reported immediately.*

+ Use stomahesive or karaya paste, and a skin barrier wafer as needed to maintain a secure colostomy pouch. *This may be particularly important for the person with a loop colostomy. The main challenge for a person with a transverse loop*

colostomy is to maintain a secure colostomy pouch over the plastic bridge.*

Health education for the person and family

+ Prior to discharge, provide written, verbal and psychomotor instruction on colostomy care, pouch management, skin care and irrigation for the person. *Whether the colostomy is temporary or permanent, the person will be responsible for its management. Good understanding of procedures and care enhances the ability to provide self-care, as well as self-esteem and control.*

+ Allow ample time for the person (and family, if necessary) to practise changing the pouch, either on the person or a model. *Practice of psychomotor skills improves learning and confidence.*

+ If an abdominoperineal resection has been performed, emphasise the importance of using no rectal suppositories, rectal temperatures or enemas. Suggest that the person carry medical identification or a Medic-Alert tag or bracelet. *These measures are important to prevent trauma to the tissues when the rectum has been removed.*

+ The diet for a person with a colostomy is individualised and may require no alteration from that consumed pre-operatively. Dietary teaching should, however, include information on foods that cause stool odour and gas and foods that thicken and loosen stools. Foods that cause these effects on colostomy output are listed below.

Foods that increase stool odour:
- asparagus
- fish
- beans
- garlic
- cabbage
- onions
- eggs
- some spices

Foods that increase intestinal gas:
- beer
- cucumbers
- broccoli
- dairy products
- brussels sprouts
- dried beans
- cabbage
- peas
- carbonated drinks
- radishes
- cauliflower
- spinach
- corn

Foods that thicken stools:
- applesauce
- pasta
- bananas
- pretzels
- bread
- rice
- cheese
- tapioca
- yogurt
- creamy peanut butter

Foods that loosen stools:
- chocolate
- highly spiced foods
- dried beans
- leafy green vegetables
- raw fruits and juices
- fried foods
- greasy foods
- raw vegetables

Foods that colour stools:
- beets
- red gelatine

Risk for acute pain

The person with colorectal cancer may experience pain related to preparatory procedures, diagnostic examinations and surgery. Following an abdominoperineal resection, 'phantom' rectal pain related to the severing of nerves during the wide excision of the rectum may develop. Finally, the primary tumour itself and, potentially, metastatic tumours may impinge on nerves and other organs, causing pain. In the early post-operative period, an epidural infusion or PCA often is used to manage pain. PCA, routine administration of ordered analgesics or a continuous analgesia delivery (CAD) system may also be used for pain management when the tumour is far enough advanced to preclude surgical resection.

Monitor for adequate pain relief. Use subjective and objective information, including the location, intensity and character of the pain, as well as non-verbal signs, such as grimacing, muscle tension, apparent dozing, changes in pulse or blood pressure or rapid, shallow respirations. The person may assume that pain is to be expected or tolerated or may fear becoming addicted to analgesic medications. Careful questioning and assessment can provide accurate information about pain status, allowing better control of discomfort.

Ask the person to rate pain using a 0–10 pain scale chart. Document the level of pain. Pain is a subjective experience. Persons perceive and respond to pain differently. Religion and ethnic background may affect the response to pain. Monitor analgesic effectiveness 30 minutes after administration. Monitor for pain relief and adverse effects. The method of delivery, dosage or medication itself may need to be adjusted to provide adequate pain relief.

+ Assess the incision for inflammation or swelling; assess drainage catheters and tubes for patency. *Poorly controlled pain or pain that changes may be related to organ distention from an obstructed NG tube, urinary catheter or wound drain, or may indicate an infection.*

+ Assess the abdomen for distention, tenderness and bowel sounds. *Intra-abdominal bleeding, peritonitis or paralytic ileus can cause pain that may be confused with incisional pain.*

+ Assist with adjunctive comfort measures, such as positioning, diversional activities, management of environmental stimuli, guided imagery and teaching relaxation techniques. *These measures enhance the effects of analgesia by reducing muscle tension.*

+ Splint incision with a pillow, and teach the person how to self-splint when coughing and deep breathing *to prevent respiratory complications related to fear of pain.*

Consider this . . .

- What is the cause of phantom rectal pain?
- Why is it important to discuss dietary concerns with a person with a colostomy, especially odour- and gas-forming foods?

Risk for impaired nutrition

Bowel preparation for diagnostic procedures, surgery, radiation therapy and chemotherapy place the person with colorectal cancer at risk for nutritional deficiencies. Fluid and electrolyte replacement is provided following surgery, along with possible TPN. Adequate kilocalorie and nutrient intake are necessary for healing after surgery. Additionally, if the tumour is advanced, metabolic needs may be increased and the appetite decreased.

+ Assess nutritional status, using data such as height and weight, skinfold measurements, BMI calculation and laboratory data including serum albumin level. Refer to dietitian or nutritionist for dietary management. *The person who is malnourished before beginning aggressive cancer treatment requires more vigorous nutrition management to promote healing.*

+ Assess readiness for resumption of oral intake after surgery or procedures using data such as statements of hunger, presence of bowel sounds, passage of flatus and minimal abdominal distention. *Manipulation of the bowel interrupts peristalsis of the GI tract. It is important to ensure that peristalsis has resumed prior to resumption of oral intake.*

+ Monitor and document food and fluid intake. *Documentation helps identify the adequacy of kilocalories and other nutrient intake.*

+ Weigh daily. *Weight fluctuation may indicate adequate or inadequate dietary intake.*

+ Maintain TPN and central intravenous lines as ordered. *Parenteral nutrition prevents tissue catabolism and promotes healing when food intake is disrupted for more than two to three days.*

+ When oral intake resumes, help the person develop a meal plan that incorporates food preferences and considers the person's schedule and environment. *Consideration of likes, dislikes and circumstances in meal planning promotes adequate intake.*

Risk for anticipatory grieving

When a bowel resection is performed for colorectal cancer, the person needs to adjust to the loss of a major body part as well as to the diagnosis of cancer. Even when the prognosis for recovery is good, many people perceive cancer as fatal. Supporting the person and family during the initial stages of grieving can improve physical recovery as well as psychological coping and eventual adaptation.

+ Work to develop a trusting relationship with the person and family. *This increases the nurse's effectiveness in helping them work through the grieving process.*

+ Listen actively, encouraging the person and family to express their fears and concerns. Assist to identify strengths, past experiences and support systems:
  a. Demonstrate respect for cultural, spiritual and religious values and beliefs; encourage use of these resources to cope with losses.

IN PRACTICE

Colorectal cancer care

For any person to be told that they have colorectal cancer is the most stressful news they can have. From the moment the person is admitted for surgery, nurses need to be sensitive and empathetic. Generally nurses find it difficult to talk to persons who have been diagnosed with cancer. The lack of knowledge and skills in communicating with cancer patients and providing psychological care are some of the anxieties nurses have in caring for cancer patients (see Chapter 2 for cancer care). The person's family or significant others need to be involved in any discussion regarding care and treatment. This

helps to promote a trusting relationship between the nurse and the person. All these should form part of the pre-operative preparation of the person for surgery. A multidisciplinary team approach by other healthcare professionals is paramount in the physical and psychological preparation of the person.

When the person is ready to be discharged, a comprehensive discharge plan should be put in place. This should take into account all support systems available in the community for the person and his/her family. Persons and their relatives will need information on services available in the community such as colostomy societies, counselling (if necessary), meals on wheels, stoma nurse to help them lead a normal life.

b. Encourage discussion of the potential impact of loss on individual family members, family structure and family function. Assist family members to share concerns with one another.

c. Refer to cancer support groups, social services or counselling as appropriate.

Risk for sexual dysfunction

Colorectal cancer and colostomy surgery increase the risk for sexual dysfunction, defined as a change in sexual function so that it becomes unsatisfying, unrewarding or inadequate. Physical factors that can lead to sexual dysfunction include disruption of nerves and blood vessels that supply the genitals, radiation therapy, chemotherapy and other medications prescribed after surgery.

Psychologically, the person with a colostomy experiences an altered body image and may develop low self-esteem. The person may feel undesirable and fear rejection. He or she may be concerned about odours or pouch leakage during sexual activity. This emotional stress can also contribute to sexual dysfunction.

✚ Provide opportunities for the person and family to express feelings about the cancer diagnosis, colostomy and effects of other treatments. *Encouraging verbalisation of feelings about the diagnosis, colostomy and treatments provides an opportunity to validate that feelings of anger and depression are normal responses to the diagnosis and change in body function.*

✚ Provide consistent colostomy care. *An accepting attitude and consistent care that provides a secure appliance and controls odour and leakage instil a sense of confidence in the person.*

COMMUNITY-BASED CARE

Once the surgery is done and the person is ready to go home, discuss the following topics (as appropriate) in teaching for home care:

● Pain management (refer to Chapter 2 for pain management).

● Skin care and management of potential adverse effects of radiation therapy and/or chemotherapy.

● Incision and colostomy care.

● Dietary advice.

● Follow-up appointments and care.

● Support systems available such as the Colostomy Association.

● Exercise: gentle exercise is recommended to strengthen the muscles around the stoma. Stoma specialist or practice

nurse should be able to advise on the type of exercises to do.

● Many people worry that their pouch will give off a smell that other people will notice. However, this is unlikely if an odour-resistant pouch system is used and emptied regularly. Special liquids and tablets that can be placed in the pouch to reduce any smell are also available. Eating yogurt and buttermilk can also help to reduce smell.

● Advise the person on complications such as rectal discharge, phantom rectum and parastomal hernia.

● If the tumour is inoperable or a cure is not anticipated, provide information about pain and symptom management. Discuss the hospice care and available services. Provide a referral to a local hospice or palliative care nurses.

✦ Encourage expression of sexual concerns. Provide privacy and caregivers who have established trust with the person and family and are comfortable with discussions about sexual concerns. *Sexuality is a very private concern to most people. The person and family are not likely to express their concerns openly unless trust has been established.*

✦ Reassure the person and significant other that the effect of physical illness and prescribed interventions on sexuality is usually temporary. *The person and partner may misinterpret*

an initial decrease in libido as evidence that sexual activity will not be possible or resume following recovery.

✦ Refer the person and partner to social services or for counselling so that they can discuss their fears and worries. *Ongoing counselling provides a continuing resource.*

✦ Arrange for a visit from a person who has had a positive outcome. *People who are living and coping with a colostomy can provide information and support, helping the person to overcome feelings of isolation and rejection.*

CASE STUDY SUMMARIES

Case Study 1. With a strict diet regimen and programmed exercise Ms Peters started to lose weight. The option of surgery is available to her; however, on the current treatment she feels confident that she will lose weight. She still gets the urge every now and then to eat fast food. With the help of the district nurse and her GP Ms Peters is managing to avoid these foodstuffs. Ms Peters is aware that the road to losing weight is not an easy one, but she is determined to give it a go.

Case Study 2. Mrs Stone made a good recovery from surgery and was discharged. She completed her course of antibiotics

to treat her *H. pylori* but still continues to take omeprazole to control her gastric acid secretions and ferrous sulphate for anaemia. Mrs Stone maintains that she will continue on the dietary advice given by the dietitian and is determined to attend stress reduction classes.

Case Study 3. Mrs Chowdrey made an uneventful recovery and is determined not to let the cancer take over her life. She now wants to enjoy her life, go on holidays and lead a normal life. Mrs Chowdrey is determined to attend to attend support groups for cancer persons. She and her husband want to raise funds for the hospital to show appreciation for the treatment and care she has received.

CHAPTER HIGHLIGHTS

● Nursing care for persons who are obese focuses on health promotion, education and support of the prescribed treatment plan.

● Exercise and reduced kilocalorie intake are the main way of treating obesity. Drugs that suppress the appetite or interfere with fat absorption in the gut may be used to facilitate weight loss in persons with multiple risk factors for obesity complications or people who have had difficulty achieving weight loss through diet and exercise.

● Nausea and vomiting, common GI symptoms, may be indicative of disorders affecting many organ systems, including the GI tract, inner ear, CNS or heart. Complications such as dehydration, electrolyte imbalance and aspiration of gastric contents are primary concerns in treating nausea and vomiting.

● *H. pylori* infection is also a major risk factor for peptic ulcer disease (PUD) and gastric cancer. Effectively treating the infection can reduce or eliminate the risk of future exacerbations of PUD.

● Hepatitis, inflammation of functional liver tissue, is usually a viral disease and therefore cannot be cured at this time. Preventing the spread of hepatitis through use of standard and body substance precautions is an important nursing responsibility.

● Hepatitis A, commonly transmitted via the faecal–oral route, is generally a self-limiting disease. Some types of viral hepatitis, most notably hepatitis B and C, can become chronic and ultimately lead to liver failure and an increased risk for liver cancer. Hepatitis B and C can result in a carrier state in which the infected person has no symptoms of the disease, but can spread it to others.

● Alcohol abuse is a significant risk factor for liver and pancreatic disorders. Prevention, early identification and treatment of alcohol abuse reduce the risk of these disorders. Absolute abstinence from alcohol is an important part of the treatment plan for persons with liver and pancreatic disorders.

TEST YOURSELF

1. What is the digestive function of the liver?

   a. to secrete bile
   b. to release glucose
   c. to synthesise plasma proteins
   d. to store iron as ferritin

2. The breakdown of carbohydrates to produce ATP is an example of:

   a. metabolism
   b. anabolism
   c. catabolism
   d. lipidism

3. A person asks you what type of foods are complete proteins. What would be your best response?

   a. none
   b. eggs and milk
   c. fruits and vegetables
   d. butter and oils

4. A person who is deficient in vitamin K may have what type of problem with minor surgery?

   a. infection
   b. blood clotting
   c. keloid formation
   d. slow peristalsis

5. During a health history for nutritional problems, it is important to ask the person to describe:

   a. the type, amount and character of pain experienced
   b. the odour and colour of urine
   c. the ability to put joints through full range of motion
   d. the usual food and fluid intake for a 24-hour period

6. On monitoring a person's lab results, you notice a greatly elevated serum amylase level. What disease does this indicate?

   a. cheilosis
   b. gastric reflux
   c. gallstones
   d. acute pancreatitis

7. When assessing the abdomen, what assessment technique is used last?

   a. observation
   b. auscultation
   c. palpation
   d. percussion

8. Which of the following is a high-priority nursing intervention to prevent malnutrition in the surgical person?

   a. aggressive pain management
   b. daily weights
   c. maintaining intravenous flow
   d. requesting early restoration of oral intake

9. The evening following a gastric resection, the nurse notes that there has been no drainage from the nasogastric tube for the past three hours. The nurse should:

   a. chart the finding
   b. reposition the nasogastric tube
   c. gently irrigate the tube with normal saline
   d. notify the doctor

10. A person has developed a paralytic ileus following a recent abdominal surgery. What is the most important nursing consideration when caring for this person?

    a. ensure that the person is able to eat a clear liquid diet
    b. maintain the person on strict bedrest
    c. monitor bowel sounds every hour
    d. ensure nasogastric tube is functioning

Further resources

British Obesity Surgery Person Association (BOSPA)
www.bospa.org
BOSPA has information on many types of weight-loss surgery. We think that you will find this website useful as it provides information on different types of surgery for obese people, information on support groups and patients' experiences after the surgery.

National Institute for Health and Clinical Excellence (NICE)
http://guidance.nice.org.uk/CG43/Guidance/Section
This link provides you with information on obesity from NICE. We think it is useful website for all nursing students and qualified nurses. As you are aware, obesity in the UK is alarmingly high and even in children this is a big problem. The government is committed to reducing obesity in children and adults as it has an impact on health and public resources.

NICE
http://guidance.nice.org.uk/CSGCC
This link provides information on NICE guidance on improving outcomes in colorectal cancer. We think this is a website that will give you some insight into NICE guidance on the outcome of the disease which you will find useful for your studies.

BUPA
http://www.bupa.co.uk/health-information/directory/s/stomach-cancer
This is a BUPA website. It has useful information about stomach cancer. We think that you will find this link very useful as it gives an overview of the causes, signs and symptoms, treatment and some preventative measures for stomach cancer. They also give a link to other websites which deal with cancer and references for journal articles which deal with cancer.

Cancer Research UK
http://cancerhelp.cancerresearchuk.org/type/bowel-cancer/
We think that this website gives some insight into colorectal cancer. The information on this website should give you some insight into colorectal cancer. They also provide some useful journal links on colorectal cancer. This site may be useful for your studies.

Department of Health (DoH)
http://www.dh.gov.uk/en/Publichealth/Obesity/index.htm
This is a Department of Health website on obesity. Here you will find the latest Health Survey for England (HSE). It is alarming to find that the data shows that nearly one in four adults and over one in 10 children aged 2–10 are obese. If you researching topics on nutrition, we think that this link will be a valuable resource for you. It also provides information on other topic areas relating to public health.

Bibliography

Alexander M F, Fawcett J N and Runciman P J (2007) *Nursing Practice: Hospital and Home – The Adult* (3rd edn). Edinburgh, Churchill Livingstone.

British Nutrition Foundation Task Force (1999) *Obesity*. Oxford, Blackwell Science.

DoH (2011) *Obesity General Information*. London, Department of Health, available at: http://www.dh.gov.uk/en/Publichealth/Obesity/DH_078098 (accessed September 2011).

Dougherty L and Lister S (2008) *The Royal Marsden Hospital Manual of Clinical Nursing Procedures*. Oxford, Blackwell Science.

House of Commons Health Committee (2004) *Obesity. Third report of session 2003–04 Volume 1*. London, The Stationery Office.

LeMone P and Burke K (2008) *Medical–Surgical Nursing: Critical Thinking in Person Care* (4th edn). Englewood Cliffs, NJ, Prentice Hall.

Malnutrition Advisory Group (2003) *The MUST report. Nutritional screening of adults: a multidisciplinary responsibility*. London, British Association for Parenteral and Enteral Nutrition.

MeReC Bulletin (1998) Oral nutritional support (part 2): nutritional supplements. *MeReC Bulletin*, 9, 33–36.

Nair M and Peate I (2009) *Fundamentals of Applied Pathophysiology: An essential guide for nursing students*. Chichester, Wiley-Blackwell.

NICE (2002) *Guidance on the Use of Surgery to Aid Weight Reduction for People with Morbid Obesity*, TAG 46. London, National Institute for Health and Clinical Excellence.

NICE (2004) *Technology Appraisal: Hepatitis C – pegylated interferons, ribavarin and alfa interferon, Interferon alfa and ribavirin for the treatment of chronic hepatitis C – part review of exisiting guidance no.14*, TA 75. London, National Institute for Health and Clinical Excellence.

NICE (2006a) *Treatment for People Who are Overweight or Obese*, CGG3. London, National Institute for Health and Clinical Excellence.

NICE (2006b) *Nutrition Support in Adults – Nutrition support in adults: oral nutrition support, enteral tube feeding parenteral nutrition*, CG 32. London, National Institute for Health and Clinical Excellence.

NMC (2010) *Standards for Medicine Management*. London, Nursing and Midwifery Council.

NMC (2010) *Guidelines for Record and Record Keeping*. London, Nursing and Midwifery Council.

Omari A and Caterson I D (2007) Overweight and obesity. In Mann J and Truswell A S (eds) *Essentials of Human Nutrition* (3rd edn). Oxford, Oxford University Press, 273–288.

Peate I (2007) *Men's Health – The Practice Nurse's Handbook*. Chichester, Wiley.

Say J (2010) Eating and drinking: nutrient and fluid replacement for health. In Peate I (ed.) *Nursing Care and the Activities of Living* (2nd edn). London, Wiley-Blackwell.

WHO (2003) *Nutrition. Controlling the Global Obesity Epidemic*. Geneva, World Health Organization.

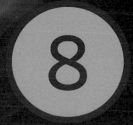

Caring for people with urinary elimination and kidney problems

Learning outcomes

- Describe the anatomy, physiology and functions of the urinary system.
- Explain the role of the urinary system in maintaining homeostasis.
- Explain the pathophysiology of common urinary tract disorders.
- Discuss the nursing implications of medications and treatments prescribed for persons with urinary tract disorders.
- Discuss risk factors for kidney disorders and nursing care to reduce these risks.

Clinical competencies

- Conduct and document a health history for persons who have or are at risk for alterations in urinary elimination.
- Assess the functional health status of persons with urinary tract disorders, using data to determine priority nursing diagnoses and select individualised nursing interventions.
- Use evidence-based research to plan and implement nursing care for persons with urinary tract disorders.
- Provide effective nursing care for persons undergoing surgery of the urinary tract.
- Plan and provide appropriate teaching for prevention of and self-care of urinary tract disorders.
- Evaluate person responses, revising plan of care as needed to promote, maintain or restore functional health of persons with urinary tract disorders.

CASE STUDIES

Below are three case studies that you may wish to consider before, during or after you have read the chapter. There are no right or wrong answers to these case studies, but you should think about the physical, psychological and social implications. Also consider what questions you would ask the person so that you can help alleviate their anxieties.

Case Study 1 – Suresh

Mr Suresh Tamwar, a 67-year-old man, went to see his GP complaining of poor stream, blood in the urine, dribbling and a burning feeling when passing urine. He complained to his GP that passing urine has become a painful experience and sometimes he feels like killing himself. He says, 'My wife does not know about my problem, doctor, because in my culture these are things you don't talk to other people about because of the shame. I am now wetting my pants and that is getting me down. I like to drink lots of water, but I am now frightened to drink because of my problem. I get up three or four times at night to pass urine. Is there anything you can do?'

Case Study 2 – Martin

Mr Martin Chapel is a 75-year-old man who went to see his GP with a 48-hour history of passing small amounts of urine and it hurts when he does. He also thinks he may have seen some blood in his urine but wasn't sure. He complained of difficulty in passing urine, cloudy urine and fever. Mr Chapel stated that, 'I have been suffering from a urine problem for about a week now and it is becoming more and more frequent. I tried all kind of remedies but nothing helped and it may have made things worse.' Mr Chapel stated that he was treated with antibiotics before, 'sometimes these work sometimes not. I am so sick of it and it's bringing me down, it is starting to control my life and I'm worried it is getting in the way of hobbies and my relationship. I feel I have put on weight and at times find it difficult to walk up the stairs'.

Case Study 3 – Steve

Mr Steve Take, a 55-year-old postman, has a history of diabetes mellitus which is controlled by diet and pills. He also suffers from frequent urinary tract infection. Steve noticed that he gets tired quickly and has lost his appetite. He also noticed some blood in his urine and that the amount of urine has been diminishing. Frightened, Mr Take decided to visit his GP. One of Mr Take's work colleagues drove him to the GP's surgery. He complained to the GP that his ankles seem swollen and that lately he has been suffering from fatigue. 'Can you help me doctor, I do not know what is happening with me.'

INTRODUCTION

The functions of the urinary system (also called the renal system) are to regulate body fluids, to filter metabolic wastes from the bloodstream, to reabsorb needed substances and water into the bloodstream and to eliminate metabolic wastes and water as urine. Any alteration in the structure or function of the urinary system affects the whole body. In turn, healthy urinary system function depends on the health of other body systems, especially the circulatory, endocrine and nervous systems.

ANATOMY, PHYSIOLOGY AND FUNCTIONS OF THE URINARY SYSTEM

The organs of the urinary system are the paired kidneys, the paired **ureters**, the urinary bladder and the **urethra** (Figure 8.1A and B). Each structure is essential to the total functioning of the urinary system.

THE KIDNEYS

The two kidneys are located outside the peritoneal cavity and on either side of the vertebral column at the levels of T_{12} through L_3. These highly vascular, bean-shaped organs are approximately 11.4 cm long and 6.4 cm wide. The lateral surface of the kidney is convex; the medial surface is concave and forms a vertical cleft, the **hilum**. The ureter, **renal artery**, **renal vein**, lymphatic vessels and nerves enter or exit the kidney at the level of the hilum.

The kidney is supported by three layers of connective tissue: the outer renal fascia, the middle adipose capsule and the inner renal capsule. The renal fascia, made up of dense

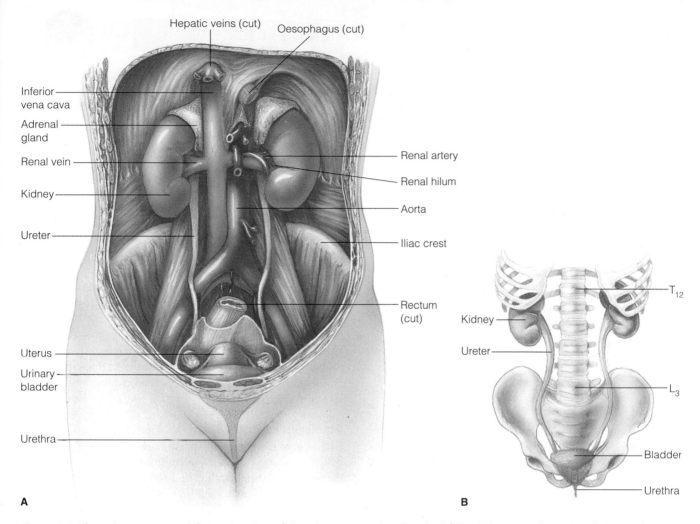

Figure 8.1 **The urinary system. (A)** Anterior view of the urinary system in a female. **(B)** The kidneys are shown in relation to the vertebrae and ribs.

connective tissue, surrounds the kidney (and the adrenal gland, a discrete organ that sits on top of each kidney) and anchors it to surrounding structures. The middle adipose capsule is a fatty mass that holds the kidney in place and also cushions it against trauma. The inner renal capsule provides a barrier against infection and helps protect the kidney from trauma.

Internally, each kidney has three distinct regions: the cortex, medulla and pelvis. The outer region, or **renal cortex**, is light in colour and has a granular appearance (Figure 8.2). This region of the kidney contains the **glomeruli**, small clusters of capillaries. The glomeruli bring blood to and carry waste products from the **nephrons**, the functional units of the kidney.

The **renal medulla**, just below the cortex, contains cone-shaped tissue masses called **renal pyramids**, formed almost entirely of bundles of collecting tubules. Areas of lighter coloured tissue called renal columns are extensions of the cortex and serve to separate the pyramids. The collecting tubules that make up the pyramids channel urine into the innermost region, the **renal pelvis**.

The renal pelvis is continuous with the ureter as it leaves the hilum. Branches of the pelvis known as the major and minor **calyces** extend toward the medulla and serve to collect

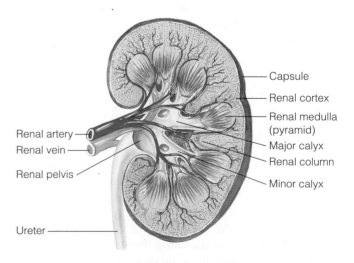

Figure 8.2 The internal anatomy of the kidney.

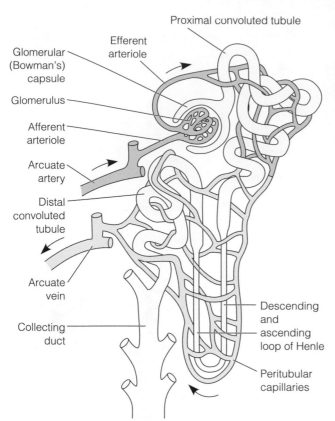

Figure 8.3 The structure of a nephrone, showing the glomerulus within the glomerular capsule.

Formation of urine

The complex structures of the kidneys process about 180 L of blood-derived fluid each day. Of this amount, only 1% is excreted as urine; the rest is returned to the circulation. (Normal and abnormal findings of urine on laboratory analysis are listed in Table 8.1.) Urine formation is accomplished entirely by the nephron through three processes: glomerular **filtration**, tubular reabsorption and tubular secretion (Figure 8.4).

Glomerular filtration

Glomerular filtration is a passive, non-selective process in which hydrostatic pressure forces fluid and solutes through a membrane. The amount of fluid filtered from the blood into

urine and empty it into the pelvis. From the pelvis, urine is channelled through the ureter and into the bladder for storage. The walls of the calyces, the renal pelvis and the ureter contain smooth muscle that moves urine along by peristalsis.

Each kidney contains approximately one million nephrons, which filter the blood to make urine (Figure 8.3). Each nephron contains a tuft of capillaries called the glomerulus, which is completely surrounded by the glomerular (Bowman's) capsule. Together, the glomerulus and its surrounding capsule are called the renal corpuscle. The endothelium of the glomerulus allows capillaries to be extremely porous. Thus, large amounts of solute-rich fluid pass from the capillaries into the capsule.

This fluid, called the filtrate, is the raw material of urine. Filtrate leaves the capsule and is channelled into the proximal convoluted tubule (PCT) of the nephron. About 70% of the water in the filtrate, as well as chloride and bicarbonate, are reabsorbed by passive transport.

The filtrate then moves into the U-shaped loop of Henle and is concentrated. The descending limb of the U is relatively thin and freely permeable to water, whereas the ascending segment is thick and thereby less permeable. The distal convoluted tubule (DCT) receives filtrate from the loop of Henle which then passes the urine into the collecting duct. The collecting duct receives the newly formed urine from many nephrons and channels urine through the minor and major calyces of the renal pelvis and into the ureter.

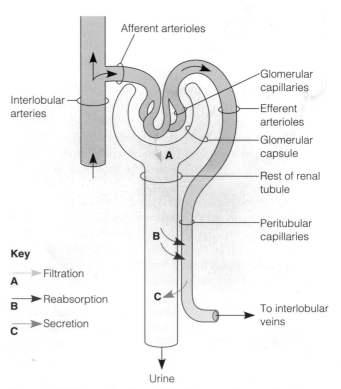

Figure 8.4 Schematic view of the three major mechanisms by which the kidneys adjust to the composition of plasma.

Table 8.1 Normal and abnormal findings: urinalysis

Characteristic or component	Normal results	Abnormal finding with possible cause
Colour	Light straw to amber yellow	• Red, dark, smoky colour may be the result of blood in the urine (**haematuria** or menstrual blood). • Cloudy urine occurs from infection. • Colourless urine indicates very dilute urine, such as in overhydration, kidney disease, alcohol ingestion or diabetes insipidus. • Very dark yellow urine indicates dehydration and/or fever. • Red or red brown urine may be caused by sulfisoxazole-phenazopyridine (Azo Gantrisin), phenytoin (Dilantin), cascara, chlorpromazine (Thorazine), docusate calcium and phenolphthalein (Doxidan); and by carrots, rhubarb and food colouring. • Orange urine is caused by fever, urobilin, phenazopyridine (Pyridium), amidopyrine, nitrofurantoin, sulfonamides, carrots, beetroot and food colouring. • Blue or green urine is caused by *Pseudomonas*, amitriptyline (Elavil), methylene blue, methocarbamol (Robaxin) and yeast concentrates. • Brown or black urine is caused by Lysol poisoning, melanin, bilirubin, methaemoglobin, porphyrin, cascara and injectable iron.
Appearance	Clear	• Hazy or cloudy urine indicates bacteria, pus, red blood cells (RBCs), white blood cells (WBCs), phosphates, prostatic fluid spermatozoa or urates. • Milky urine is the result of fats or **pyuria**. • Yellow foam results from bilirubin, bile or severe cirrhosis of the liver. • A dark yellow to brownish colour is seen with deficient fluid volume.
Odour	Aromatic	• Ammonia smell increases as urine stands outside the body. • Urinary tract infection (UTI) causes a foul or unpleasant odour, depending on the causative organism. • Asparagus causes a distinctive odour. • Mousy odours result from phenylketonuria. • Sweet or fruity odours occur in starvation and diabetic ketoacidosis.
pH	4.5–8.0	• < 4.5: metabolic acidosis, respiratory acidosis, diet high in meat protein, ammonium chloride and mandelic acid. • > 8.0: bacteriuria, UTI, antibiotics (neomycin, kanamycin), sulfonamides, sodium bicarbonate, acetazolamide (Diamox), potassium citrate.
Specific gravity	1.005–1.030	• < 1.005: diabetes insipidus, overhydration, renal disease, severe potassium deficit. • > 1.030: dehydration, fever, diabetes mellitus, vomiting, diarrhoea, contrast media.
Protein	2–8 mg/dL	• > 8 mg/dL: **proteinuria**, exercise, fever, stress, acute infection, kidney disease, lupus erythematosus, leukaemia, multiple myeloma, cardiac disease, toxaemia of pregnancy, septicaemia, lead, mercury, neomycin, barbiturates, sulfonamides.
Glucose	Negative	• > 15 mg/dL or 14: diabetes mellitus, stroke, Cushing's syndrome, anaesthesia, glucose infusions, severe stress, infections, ascorbic acid, aspirin, cephalosporins, epinephrine.
Ketones	Negative	• 11–13: ketoacidosis, starvation, high-protein diet.
RBCs	Rare	• > 2 per low-power field: kidney trauma, kidney diseases, renal **calculi**, cystitis, excess aspirin, anticoagulants, sulfonamides, menstrual contamination.
WBCs	3–4	• > 4 per low-power field: UTI, fever, strenuous exercise, kidney diseases.
Casts	Occasional hyaline	• Fever, kidney diseases, heart failure.

the capsule per minute is called the glomerular filtration rate (GFR). Three factors influence this rate: the total surface area available for filtration, the permeability of the filtration membrane and the net filtration pressure.

Net filtration pressure is responsible for the formation of filtrate and is determined by two forces: hydrostatic pressure ('push') and osmotic pressure ('pull'). The glomerular hydrostatic pressure pushes water and solutes across the membrane. This pressure is opposed by the osmotic pressure in the glomerulus (primarily the colloid osmotic pressure of plasma proteins in the glomerular blood) and the capsular hydrostatic pressure exerted by fluids within the glomerular capsule. The difference between these forces determines the net filtration pressure, which is directly proportional to the GFR. The normal GFR in both kidneys is 120–125 mL/min in adults.

Tubular reabsorption

Tubular reabsorption begins as the filtrate enters the proximal tubules. In healthy kidneys, virtually all organic nutrients such as glucose and amino acids are reabsorbed. However, the tubules constantly regulate and adjust the rate and degree of water and ion reabsorption in response to hormonal signals. Reabsorption may be active or passive. Substances reclaimed through active tubular reabsorption are usually moving against electrical and/or chemical gradients. These substances, including glucose, amino acids, lactate, vitamins and most ions, require an ATP-dependent carrier to be transported into the interstitial space. In passive tubular reabsorption, which includes diffusion and osmosis, substances move along their gradient without expenditure of energy.

Tubular secretion

The final process in urine formation is tubular secretion, which is essentially reabsorption in reverse. Substances such as hydrogen and potassium ions, creatinine, ammonia and organic acids move from the blood of the peritubular capillaries into the tubules themselves as filtrate. Thus, urine consists of both filtered and secreted substances. Tubular secretion is important for disposing of substances not already in the filtrate, such as medications. This process eliminates unwanted substances that have been reabsorbed by passive processes and rids the body of excessive potassium ions. It is also a vital force in the regulation of blood pH.

Clearing waste products

The kidneys excrete water-soluble waste products and other chemicals or substances from the body. This process is called renal plasma clearance, which refers to the ability of the kidneys to clear (cleanse) a given amount of plasma of a particular substance in a given time (usually one minute). The kidneys clear 25–30 g of urea (a nitrogenous waste product formed in the liver from the breakdown of amino acids) each day. They also clear creatinine (an end product of creatine phosphate, found in skeletal muscle), uric acid (a metabolite of nucleic acid metabolism) and ammonia, as well as bacterial toxins and water-soluble drugs. Tests of renal clearance are often used to determine the GFR and glomerular damage.

THE URETERS

The ureters are bilateral tubes approximately 26–30 cm long. They transport urine from the kidney to the bladder through peristaltic waves originating in the renal pelvis. The wall of the ureter has three layers: an inner epithelial mucosa, a middle layer of smooth muscle and an outer layer of fibrous connective tissue.

THE URINARY BLADDER

The urinary bladder is **posterior** to the symphysis pubis and serves as a storage site for urine. In males, the bladder lies immediately in front of the rectum; in females, the bladder lies in front of the vagina and the uterus. Openings for the ureters and the urethra are inside the bladder: The trigone is the smooth triangular portion of the base of the bladder outlined by these three openings (Figure 8.5).

The size of the bladder varies with the amount of urine it contains. In healthy adults, the bladder holds about 300–500 mL of urine before internal pressure rises and signals the need to empty the bladder through **micturition** (also called urination or voiding). However, the bladder can hold more than twice that amount if necessary. The bladder has an internal urethral **sphincter** that relaxes in response to a full bladder and signals the need to urinate. A second external urethral sphincter is formed by skeletal muscle and is under **voluntary** control.

THE URETHRA

The urethra is a thin-walled muscular tube that channels urine to the outside of the body. It extends from the base of the

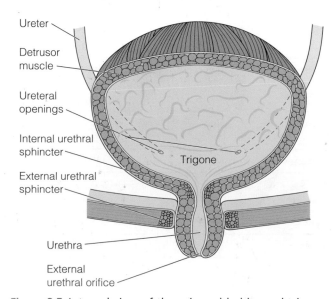

Figure 8.5 Internal view of the urinary bladder and trigone.

bladder to the external urinary meatus. In females, the urethra is approximately 3–5 cm long, and the urinary meatus is **anterior** to the vaginal orifice. In males, the urethra is approximately 20 cm long and serves as a channel for semen as well as urine. The prostate gland encircles the urethra at the base of the bladder in males. The male urinary meatus is located at the end of the glans penis.

The person with a urinary tract infection (UTI)

Bacterial infections of the urinary tract are a common reason for seeking health services, second only to upper respiratory infections. More than eight million people are treated annually for UTI. Community-acquired UTIs are common in young women, and unusual in men under the age of 50. UTI ranges from cystitis to pyelonephritis.

Most community-acquired UTIs are caused by *Escherichia coli*, common gram-negative enteral bacteria. About 10–15% of symptomatic UTIs are caused by *Staphylococcus saprophyticus*, a gram-positive organism. Catheter-associated UTIs often involve other gram-negative bacteria such as *Proteus*, *Klebsiella*, *Serratia* and *Pseudomonas*.

FAST FACTS

Urinary tract infection

- UTI is 50 times more common in women, with about 5% per year developing symptoms.
- UTI is uncommon in men below 60 years of age, but the frequency is similar in men and women in older age groups.

Source: Hackett 2011.

Risk factors for UTI

Female:

- short, straight urethra;
- proximity of urinary meatus to vagina and anus;
- sexual intercourse;
- use of diaphragm and spermicidal compounds for birth control;
- pregnancy.

Male:

- uncircumcised;
- prostatic hypertrophy;
- anal intercourse.

Both:

- ageing;
- urinary tract obstruction;
- neurogenic bladder dysfunction;
- vesicoureteral reflux;
- genetic factors;
- catheterisation.

Cystitis

Pathophysiology

Cystitis, inflammation of the urinary bladder, is the most common UTI. The infection tends to remain superficial, involving the bladder mucosa. The mucosa becomes hyperemic (red) and may haemorrhage. The inflammatory response causes pus to form. This process causes the classic signs and symptoms associated with cystitis.

Signs and symptoms

- **Dysuria**.
- **Urgency**.
- **Nocturia**.
- Pyuria.
- Haematuria.

Cystitis occurs most frequently in adult females, usually because of colonisation of the bladder by bacteria normally found in the lower gastrointestinal tract. These bacteria gain entry by ascending the short, straight female urethra. Elderly persons may not experience the classic symptoms of cystitis. Instead, they often present with non-specific symptoms such as nocturia, incontinence, confusion, behaviour change, lethargy, anorexia or 'just not feeling right.' Fever may be present; however, hypothermia may also develop in an older adult.

Although the bacteriostatic effect of prostatic fluid and a longer urethra provide an effective barrier to bladder infection for adult males, the prostatic hypertrophy commonly associated with ageing increases the risk of cystitis in elderly males. An enlarged prostate can impede urine flow, leading to incomplete bladder emptying and urinary stasis. Bacteria are not

FAST FACTS

UTI and gender

- Up to three UTIs annually is considered to be within normal limits for sexually active women and does not usually warrant additional diagnostic tests beyond urine culture.
- In healthy adult men, however, UTIs are unusual and may prompt additional diagnostic testing.

completely flushed with voiding, allowing colonisation of the bladder. Cystitis is usually uncomplicated and readily responds to treatment. When left untreated, the infection can ascend to involve the kidneys.

Pyelonephritis

Pyelonephritis is inflammation of the renal pelvis and **parenchyma**, the functional kidney tissue. Acute pyelonephritis is a bacterial infection of the kidney; chronic pyelonephritis is associated with non-bacterial infections and inflammatory processes that may be metabolic, chemical or immunologic in origin.

Acute pyelonephritis

Pathophysiology

Acute pyelonephritis usually results from an infection that ascends to the kidney from the lower urinary tract. Asymptomatic bacteriuria or cystitis can lead to acute pyelonephritis. Risk factors include pregnancy (leading to slow ureteral peristalsis), urinary tract obstruction and congenital malformation. Urinary tract trauma, scarring, calculi (stones), kidney disorders such as polycystic or hypertensive kidney disease and chronic diseases such as diabetes may also contribute to pyelonephritis. *Vesicoureteral reflux*, a condition in which urine moves from the bladder back toward the kidney, is a common risk factor in children who develop pyelonephritis and is also seen in adults when bladder outflow is obstructed.

The infection spreads from the renal pelvis to the renal cortex. The pelvis, calyces and medulla of the kidney are primarily affected, with WBC infiltration and inflammation. The kidney becomes grossly oedematous. Localised abscesses may develop on the cortical surface of the kidney. As with cystitis, *E. coli* is the organism responsible for 85% of the cases of acute pyelonephritis. Other organisms commonly found include *Proteus* and *Klebsiella*, bacteria that normally inhabit the intestinal tract.

The onset of acute pyelonephritis is typically rapid, with chills and fever, malaise, vomiting, flank pain, costovertebral tenderness, urinary frequency and dysuria (see below). Symptoms of cystitis also may be present. The older adult may present with a change in behaviour, acute confusion, incontinence or a general deterioration in condition.

Signs and symptoms

- Urinary frequency.
- Dysuria.
- Pyuria.
- Haematuria.
- Flank pain.
- Vomiting.
- Diarrhoea.

- Acute fever.
- Shaking chills.
- Malaise.

Chronic pyelonephritis

Chronic pyelonephritis involves chronic inflammation and scarring of the tubules and interstitial tissues of the kidney. It is a common cause of chronic renal failure. It may develop as a result of UTIs or other conditions that damage the kidneys, such as hypertension or vascular conditions, severe vesicoureteral reflux or obstruction of the urinary tract. The person with chronic pyelonephritis may be asymptomatic or have mild symptoms such as urinary frequency, dysuria, flank pain and hypertension.

> **FAST FACT**
>
> ### UTI route of entry
>
> The most common route of entry for a UTI is ascending, from colonisation of the perineal tissues by faecal bacteria (usually *E. coli*), through the urethra, into the bladder (cystitis) and possibly kidney tissue (pyelonephritis).

INTERDISCIPLINARY CARE FOR UTI

Medication

Most uncomplicated infections of the lower urinary tract can be treated with a short course of antibiotic therapy. Upper urinary tract infections, in contrast, usually require longer treatment (two or more weeks) to eradicate the infecting organism. Short-course therapy (either a single antibiotic dose or a three-day course of treatment) reduces treatment cost, increases compliance and has a lower rate of side-effects. Single-dose therapy is associated with a higher rate of recurrent infection and continued vaginal colonisation with *E. coli*, making a three-day course of treatment the preferred option for uncomplicated cystitis. Some of the antibiotics used to treat UTI include:

- trimethoprim (Trimpex);
- trimethoprim/sulfamethoxazole (Bactrim, Septra, Cotrim);
- amoxicillin (Amoxil, Trimox, Wymox);
- nitrofurantoin (Macrodantin, Furadantin; technically termed 'urinary tract antiseptics').

NURSING CARE FOR UTI

Health promotion

Nurses should teach measures to prevent UTI to all persons, particularly young adults and sexually active women.

Encourage persons to maintain a generous fluid intake of 2.5–3 L per day, increasing intake during hot weather or strenuous activity. Discuss the need to avoid voluntary urinary retention, emptying the bladder every three to four hours. Nurses should advise women to cleanse the perineal area from front to back after voiding and defecating. Teach to void before and after sexual intercourse to flush out bacteria introduced into the urethra and bladder. Teach measures to maintain the integrity of perineal tissues: avoid bubble baths, feminine hygiene sprays and vaginal douches; wear cotton briefs, avoid synthetic materials; if post-menopausal, use hormone replacement therapy or oestrogen cream. Unless contraindicated, suggest measures to maintain acid urine: drink two glasses of low-sugar cranberry juice daily; take ascorbic acid (vitamin C); and avoid excess intake of milk and milk products and other fruit juices.

Assessment

The assessment of the person with a UTI includes the following:

+ *Health history.* Current symptoms, including frequency, urgency, burning on urination, frequency per night; colour, clarity and odour of urine; other symptoms such as lower abdominal, back or flank pain, nausea or vomiting, fever; duration of symptoms and any treatment attempted; history of previous UTIs and their frequency; possibility of pregnancy and type of birth control used; chronic diseases such as diabetes; current medications and any known allergies.

> **PRACTICE ALERT**
>
> Follow-up urine culture is scheduled 10 days to two weeks following completion of antibiotic therapy for UTI to ensure that bacteria have been eradicated from the urinary tract.

Nursing diagnoses and interventions

Risk for pain

Pain is a common manifestation of both lower and upper UTI. Urinary tract pain is caused primarily by distention and increased pressure within the tract. The severity of the pain is related to the rate at which inflammation and distention develop, not their degree.

In cystitis, inflammation causes a sensation of fullness; dull, constant suprapubic pain; and possibly low back pain. The inflamed bladder wall and urethra cause dysuria (difficult or painful micturition), pain and burning on urination. Bladder spasms may develop, causing periodic severe, stabbing discomfort. Pain associated with pyelonephritis is often steady and dull, localised to the outer abdomen or flank region. Urologic disorders rarely cause central abdominal pain.

+ Assess pain: timing, quality, intensity, location, duration and aggravating and alleviating factors. *A change in the nature, location or intensity of the pain could indicate an extension of the infection or a related but separate problem.*

+ Advise the person on comfort measures such as warm baths and balanced rest and activity. A suitable analgesic or antispasmodic medication may be used as prescribed. *Warmth relaxes muscles, relieves spasms and increases local blood supply. Because pain can stimulate a stress response and delay healing, it should be relieved when possible.*

+ Increase fluid intake unless contraindicated. *Increased fluid dilutes urine, reducing irritation of the inflamed bladder and urethral mucosa.*

+ Advise the person to see his/her GP if pain and discomfort continue or intensify after therapy is initiated. *Pain and discomfort in voiding typically are relieved within 24 hours of the initiation of antibiotic therapy. Continued discomfort may indicate a complicated UTI or other urinary tract disorder.*

> **PRACTICE ALERT**
>
> The adult with a UTI may not complain of dysuria. Be alert for other symptoms of UTI such as incontinence or cloudy or malodorous urine. Inflammatory and immune responses tend to diminish with ageing, reducing the irritative symptoms of UTI.

Risk for impaired urinary elimination

Inflammation of the bladder and urethral mucosa affects the normal process and patterns of voiding, causing frequency, urgency and burning on urination, as well as nocturia (passing large volume of urine at night). Urine may be blood tinged, cloudy and malodorous. The person with short- or long-term urinary retention requires additional measures to assess for and prevent UTI.

+ Nurses should monitor (or advise the person to monitor) colour, clarity and odour of urine. *Urine should return to clear yellow within 48 hours, unless drug therapy causes a change in the colour of urine. If clarity does not return, further investigation may be necessary.*

+ Advise to avoid caffeinated drinks, including coffee, tea and cola; citrus juices; drinks containing artificial sweeteners; and alcoholic beverages. *Caffeine, citrus juices and artificial sweeteners irritate bladder mucosa and the detrusor muscle, and can increase urgency and bladder spasms.*

> **PRACTICE ALERT**
>
> Provide for easy access to a bedpan, urinal, commode or bathroom. Make sure that lighting is adequate and that pathways are free of obstacles. Frequency, urgency and nocturia increase the risk of urinary incontinence and of injury due to falls, particularly in the older or debilitated person.

+ When necessary, use intermittent straight catheterisation to relieve urinary retention. Remove indwelling urinary catheters as soon as possible. *Using intermittent straight catheterisation allows the bladder to fill and completely empty in a more normal manner, maintaining physiologic function. The risk of infection associated with an indwelling catheter is about 3–5% per day of catheterisation (Kasper et al. 2005).*

+ Provide perineal care on a regular basis and following defecation. Use antiseptic preparations only as ordered. *Regular cleansing of perineal tissues reduces the risk of colonisation by bowel or other bacteria. While antiseptic solutions may be ordered for catheter care, they can dry perineal tissues and reduce normal flora, increasing the risk of colonisation by pathogens, and should not routinely be used.*

COMMUNITY-BASED CARE

Because both upper and lower UTIs are usually managed in the community, teaching is the most important nursing intervention. Provide instruction on the following topics:

● Risk factors for UTI and how to minimise or eliminate these factors through increased fluid intake, regular elimination and personal hygiene measures.

● Early symptoms of UTI and the importance of seeking medical intervention promptly.

● Maintaining optimal immune system function by attending to physical and psychosocial stressors, such as lack of adequate rest, poor nutrition and high levels of emotional stress.

● The importance of completing the prescribed treatment and keeping follow-up appointments.

● Minimising the risk of UTI when an indwelling urinary catheter is necessary:
  – Use alternatives to an indwelling catheter when possible. For urinary incontinence, try scheduled toileting, incontinence pads or diapers, and external catheters if possible. For urinary retention, teach the person or a family member to perform straight catheterisation every three to four hours using clean technique.
  – Teach care measures such as perineal care, managing and emptying the collection chamber, maintaining a closed system and bladder irrigation or flushing if ordered when an indwelling catheter is necessary.

Recurrent UTI

If UTIs keep occurring, identification and treatment of the underlying cause is essential. Persons who have the same infection coming back can be managed successfully by attending to 'bladder toilet' (drinking 2–3 L of fluid daily and always passing urine at bedtime and after sex). Drinking

250–500 ml of cranberry juice daily and avoidance of bubble baths may also help.

IN PRACTICE

Acute pyelonephritis

The person with acute pyelonephritis will require a period of bedrest as the person will present with severe **pyrexia** alternating with chill and severe pain. The will require antibiotics for the infection and analgesia for the pain. Attention should be given to personal hygiene as these persons are not able to wash as a result of the severe pain.

Maintain strict fluid balance chart and encourage the person to take at least 3 L of fluid over 24 hours. Taking in a good volume of fluid encourages good urine production and decreases the growth of bacteria. As the person recovers, the nurse should concentrate on the health promotion with regards to fluid intake and teaching proper hygiene. Inform the person that failure to take good intake of fluid could result in complications such as kidney failure and/or blood infection.

The person with urinary calculi

Urinary calculi, stones in the urinary tract, are the most common cause of upper urinary tract obstruction. The term lithiasis means 'stone formation'; when the stones form in the kidney, it is known as *nephrolithiasis*; when they form elsewhere in the urinary tract (for example, the bladder), it is called *urolithiasis*. Stones may form and obstruct the urinary tract at any point. In the industrialised countries, renal or kidney stones are the most common. Although the majority of stones are idiopathic (having no demonstrable cause), a number of risk factors have been identified.

FAST FACTS

Renal stones

● Renal stones are common, being present at some time in one in ten of the population, although a significant proportion will remain asymptomatic.

● The annual incidence is about one to two cases per 1000 people and the average lifetime risk is around 5–10%.

● Men are more commonly affected than women with a male to female ratio of 3:1.

● The peak age for developing stones is between 30 and 50, and recurrence is common.

Source: Patient UK 2010a.

Risk factors for urinary calculi

Risk factors for urinary calculi include:

- family history of urinary calculi;
- dehydration;
- immobility;
- excess dietary intake of calcium, oxalate, proteins;
- gout;
- hyperthyroidism;
- urinary stasis;
- urinary tract infection.

Pathophysiology of urinary calculi

Three factors contribute to urolithiasis: supersaturation, nucleation and lack of inhibitory substances in the urine.

When the concentration of an insoluble salt in the urine is very high, that is, when the urine is supersaturated, crystals may form. Usually, these crystals disperse and are eliminated because the bonds holding them together are weak. However, a nucleus of crystals may develop stable bonds to form a stone. More often, crystals form around an organic matrix or mucoprotein nucleus to become a stone. The stimulus required to initiate crystallisation in supersaturated urine may be minimal. Ingesting a meal high in insoluble salt, or decreased fluid intake as occurs during sleep, allows the concentration to increase to the point where precipitation occurs and stones are formed and grow. When fluid intake is adequate, no stone growth occurs. The acidity or alkalinity of the urine and the presence or absence of calculus-inhibiting compounds also affects lithiasis.

Most (75–80%) kidney stones are calcium stones, composed of calcium oxalate and/or calcium phosphate. These stones are generally associated with high concentrations of calcium in the blood or urine. Uric acid stones develop when the urine concentration of uric acid is high. They are more common in men, and may be associated with gout. Genetic factors contribute to the development of uric acid stones and calcium stones. Struvite stones are associated with UTI caused by urease-producing bacteria such as *Proteus*. These stones can grow to become very large, filling the renal pelvis and calyces. They are often called staghorn stones because of their shape. Cystine stones are rare, and are associated with a genetic defect.

FAST FACTS

Course of renal stones

- Most urinary stones form in the renal pelvis and are composed primarily of calcium salts.
- Loss of calcium from the bones (for example, due to immobility) and dehydration are major risk factors for urinary stones.

Signs and symptoms of urinary calculi

Signs and symptoms of kidney, ureteral and bladder stones are:

Kidney stones:
- often asymptomatic;
- dull, aching flank pain;
- microscopic haematuria;
- symptoms of UTI.

Ureteral stones:
- renal colic;
- acute, severe flank pain on affected side;
- often radiates to suprapubic region, groin and external genitals;
- nausea, vomiting, pallor and cool, clammy skin.

Bladder stones:
- may be asymptomatic;
- dull suprapubic pain, possibly associated with exercise or voiding;
- gross or microscopic haematuria;
- symptoms of UTI.

Complications of urinary calculi

Urinary stones may obstruct urine flow at any point of the urinary tract, leading to complications such as hydronephrosis and urinary stasis with subsequent infection.

Obstruction

Stones can obstruct the urinary tract at any point from the calyces of the kidney to the distal urethra, impeding the outflow of urine. If the obstruction develops slowly, there may be few or no symptoms, whereas sudden obstruction (for example, blockage of a ureter by a passing stone) may cause severe symptoms. Urinary tract obstruction can ultimately lead to renal failure. The degree of obstruction, its location and the duration of impaired urine flow determine the effect on renal function.

Hydronephrosis

The kidneys continue to produce urine, causing increased pressure and distention of the urinary tract behind the obstruction. Hydronephrosis, distention of the renal pelvis and calyces, and hydroureter, distention of the ureter, are possible results. If the pressure is unrelieved, the collecting tubules, proximal tubules and glomeruli of the kidney are damaged, causing a gradual loss of renal function.

Acute hydronephrosis typically causes colicky pain on the affected side. The pain may radiate into the groin. Chronic hydronephrosis develops slowly, and may have few symptoms other than dull, aching back or flank pain. When hydronephrosis is significant, a palpable mass may be felt in the flank region. Haematuria and signs of UTI such as pyuria, fever and discomfort may occur. Gastrointestinal symptoms such as nausea, vomiting and abdominal pain may accompany hydronephrosis.

INTERDISCIPLINARY CARE FOR URINARY CALCULI

Medication

An acute episode of renal colic is treated with analgesia and hydration. A narcotic analgesic such as morphine sulphate is given, often intravenously, to relieve pain and reduce ureteral spasm. Indomethacin, a non-steroidal anti-inflammatory drug (NSAID), given as a suppository, may reduce the amount of narcotic analgesia required for acute renal colic. Oral or intravenous fluids reduce the risk of further stone formation and promote urine output.

After analysis of the calculus, various medications may be ordered to inhibit or prevent further lithiasis. A thiazide diuretic, frequently prescribed for calcium calculi, acts to reduce urinary calcium **excretion** and is very effective in preventing further stones. Potassium citrate raises the pH of urine and is often prescribed to prevent stones that tend to form in acidic urine (uric acid, cystine and some forms of calcium stones). Nursing responsibilities focus on teaching the person about the prescribed medication, its importance in preventing further stone formation and potential adverse effects.

Nutrition and fluid management

Diet modifications are often prescribed to change the character of the urine and prevent further lithiasis.

Increased fluid intake of 2.5–3.0 L per day is recommended, regardless of stone composition. A fluid intake to ensure the production of approximately 2.5–3.0 L of urine a day prevents the stone-forming salts from becoming concentrated enough to precipitate. Fluid intake should be spaced throughout the day and evening. Some authorities recommend that persons drink one to two glasses of water at night to prevent concentration of urine during sleep.

Recommended dietary changes may include reduced intake of the primary substance forming the calculi. For calcium stones, dietary calcium and vitamin D-enriched foods are limited. Limiting vitamin D inhibits the absorption of calcium from the gastrointestinal tract. Calcium stones may be either a calcium phosphate salt, calcium oxalate or a combination of both; therefore, phosphorus and/or oxalate may also be limited in the diet.

The person with uric acid stones requires a diet low in purines. Organ meats, sardines and other high-purine foods are eliminated from the diet. Foods with moderate levels of purines, such as red and white meats and some seafoods, may be limited.

In addition to limiting certain foods, the diet may be modified to maintain a urinary pH that does not promote lithiasis. Uric acid and cystine stones tend to form in acid urine. Foods that tend to alkalinise the urine may be recommended. Because alkaline urine promotes formation of calcium stones and UTIs, the diet may be modified to lower the pH of the urine.

Surgery

Treatment of existing calculi depends on the location of the stone, the extent of obstruction, renal function, the presence or absence of UTI and the person's general state of health. In general, the stone is removed if it is causing severe obstruction, infection, unrelieved pain or serious bleeding.

Lithotripsy, using sound or shock waves to crush a stone, is the preferred treatment for urinary calculi. Several techniques are available. Extracorporeal shock wave lithotripsy (ESWL) is a non-invasive technique for fragmenting kidney stones using shock waves generated outside the body. Acoustic shock waves are aimed under fluoroscopic guidance at the stone. These shock waves travel through soft tissue without causing damage, but shatter the stone as its greater density stops their progress. Repeated shock waves pulverise the stone into fragments small enough to be eliminated in the urine. The procedure may require 30 minutes to two hours to complete. Intravenous sedation is generally adequate to maintain comfort during the procedure.

Lithotripsy may also be performed using a percutaneous ultrasonic or laser technique. Percutaneous ultrasonic lithotripsy uses a nephroscope inserted into the kidney pelvis through a small flank incision (Figure 8.6). The stone is fragmented using a small ultrasonic transducer, and the fragments are

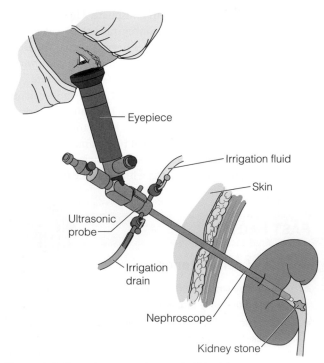

Figure 8.6 Percutaneous ultrasonic lithotripsy.

removed through the nephroscope. Laser lithotripsy is an alternative to ultrasonic lithotripsy. Laser beams are used to disintegrate the stone, without damaging soft tissue. A nephroscope or an ureteroscope (passed up the ureter from the bladder during cystoscopy) is used to guide the laser probe into direct contact with the stone.

NURSING CARE FOR URINARY CALCULI

Nursing care for the person with urolithiasis is directed at providing for comfort during acute renal colic, assisting with diagnostic procedures, ensuring adequate urinary output and teaching the person information necessary to prevent future stone formation.

Health promotion

Discuss the importance of maintaining an adequate fluid intake with all persons. Stress the need to increase fluid intake during warm weather and strenuous exercise or physical work. Discuss the relationship between weight-bearing activity and retention of calcium in the bones. Encourage all persons to remain as physically active as possible to prevent bone reabsorption (loss) and possible hypercalciuria.

Advise persons with known gout to maintain a good fluid intake of 2.5–3 L so as to produce at least 2 L of urine every day. Discuss the risk of lithiasis with persons who have frequent UTIs, and teach measures to reduce the incidence of UTI and the risk for lithiasis.

Assessment

Nurses should obtain subjective and objective assessment data specific to urolithiasis:

+ *Health history*: complaints of flank, back, or abdominal pain, radiation, characteristics and timing, aggravating or relieving factors; other symptoms such as nausea and vomiting; possible contributing factors such as dehydration; previous or family history of kidney stones; current or previous treatment measures.
+ *Physical examination*: general appearance including position, vital signs; skin colour, temperature, moisture, turgor; abdominal, flank or costovertebral tenderness; amount, colour and characteristics of urine (presence of haematuria, bacteria, pyuria, pH).

Nursing diagnoses and interventions

Risk for acute pain
Pain is the primary outward manifestation of urolithiasis, particularly when a stone lodges within a ureter, causing acute obstruction and distention. Invasive and non-invasive procedures to remove or crush stones also may be painful. Persons undergoing surgery also experience incision pain.

PRACTICE ALERT

The intensity of renal colic pain can cause a vasovagal response with resulting hypotension and syncope. Always provide for the person's safety.

+ Assess pain using a standard pain scale and its characteristics. Administer analgesia as ordered and monitor its effectiveness. *The intensity, type of pain and its responsiveness to analgesia provide valuable clues as to its cause. Regular administration of prescribed analgesics controls pain more effectively than waiting until pain becomes intolerable. Administering an ordered NSAID on a routine schedule may significantly reduce the need for narcotic analgesia in persons with renal colic.*

+ Unless contraindicated, encourage fluid intake and ambulation in the person with renal colic. *Increased fluids and ambulation increase urinary output, facilitating movement of the calculus through the ureter and decreasing pain.*

+ Use non-pharmacological measures such as positioning, relaxation techniques, guided imagery and diversion as adjunctive therapy for pain relief. *Adjunctive pain relief measures can enhance the effectiveness of analgesics and other prescribed treatment.*

+ If surgery has been performed, monitor urinary output, catheters, incision and wound drainage. *Pain may be a symptom of proximal distention due to a blocked catheter. Infection or haematoma at the surgical site can significantly increase perceived pain.*

Risk for impaired urinary elimination
Obstruction of the urinary tract is the primary problem associated with urolithiasis. Obstruction can ultimately lead to stasis, infection or irreversible renal damage.

+ Monitor amount and character of urine output. If catheterised, measure output hourly. Document any haematuria, dysuria, frequency, urgency and pyuria. Strain all urine for stones, saving any recovered stones for laboratory analysis. *The amount of urine output helps determine possible urinary tract obstruction and adequacy of hydration. Haematuria,*

PRACTICE ALERT

A stone that completely obstructs the ureter can lead to hydronephrosis and kidney damage on the affected side. Report symptoms of hydronephrosis such as dull flank pain or aching and changes in renal function studies [blood urea nitrogen (BUN) and serum creatinine]. Because the other kidney continues to function, urine output may not fall significantly with obstruction of one ureter. A rising BUN and serum creatinine may be early signs of renal failure.

gross or microscopic, is often associated with calculi and with procedures used to remove stones, such as cystoscopy or lithotripsy. A change in the amount of haematuria may indicate stone passage or a complication. Dysuria, frequency urgency and cloudy urine are symptoms of UTI, often associated with urolithiasis. Antibiotic therapy may be required. Analysis of stones recovered from the urine can direct measures to prevent further lithiasis.

+ Maintain patency and integrity of all catheter systems. Secure catheters well, label as indicated and use sterile technique for all ordered irrigations or other procedures. *A kinked or plugged catheter, particularly a ureteral catheter or nephrostomy tube, may damage the urinary system. Labelling catheters can prevent mistakes, such as inappropriate irrigation or clamping. Any catheter increases the risk of infection; aseptic technique in all procedures reduces this risk.*

COMMUNITY-BASED CARE

The person with urinary calculi needs to know how to manage existing stones and what to do to reduce the risk of future stone formation. Discuss the following topics to prepare the person and family for home care:

● Importance of maintaining a fluid intake adequate to produce 2 L of urine per day.

● Prescribed medications, their management and potential adverse effects.

● Dietary recommendations.

● Prevention, recognition and management of UTI.

● Any further diagnostic or treatment measures planned.

When the person is to be discharged with dressings, a nephrostomy tube or a catheter, educate the person and family about the following:

● How to change dressings, maintaining aseptic technique.

● Assessment of the wound and skin for healing and possible complications such as infection or skin breakdown.

● How to manage drainage systems and maintain their patency.

● Emptying drainage bags and assessing urine output.

● When to contact the doctor and recommendations for follow-up care.

IN PRACTICE

Renal stones – avoiding recurrence

Recurrence of renal stones is common and therefore persons who have had a renal stone should be advised to adapt several lifestyle measures which will help to prevent or delay recurrence:

● Increase fluid intake to maintain urine output at 2–3 L per day.

● Reduce salt intake.

● Reduce the amount of meat and animal protein eaten.

● Reduce oxalate intake (foods rich in oxalate include chocolate, rhubarb, nuts) and urate-rich foods (e.g. offal and certain fish).

● Drink regular cranberry juice: increases citrate excretion and reduces oxalate and phosphate excretion.

● Maintain calcium intake at normal levels (lowering intake increases excretion of calcium oxalate).

Nurses should advise the person to:

● Report visible haematuria and monitor vital signs.

● Keep a record of their intake and output.

● Report an absence of urine production.

● Observe for signs of infection such as frequency, burning sensation when voiding urine and cloudy urine.

Health education/prevention:

● A good fluid intake is important (2.5–3 L daily unless contraindicated).

● Dietary restrictions will be necessary (once the composition of the stone is determined) and gentle exercise is recommended.

The person with bladder cancer

Classification of bladder cancers

There are several different types of bladder cancer. They are named after the type of cells they first occur in:

● transitional cell carcinoma (TCC);

● squamous cell carcinoma (SCC);

● adenocarcinoma.

TCC is the most common type of bladder cancer in the UK. Some bladder cancers form small mushroom-like growths on the lining of the bladder. These are called papillary cancers.

Bladder cancer is also classified according to how far it has spread.

- Non-muscle invasive cancer – the cancer is only in the bladder lining.
- Muscle-invasive cancer – the cancer has spread to the muscle wall of the bladder.
- Advanced cancer – the cancer has spread through the bladder wall into nearby organs such as the prostate gland, vagina, bowel or lymph nodes. Further spread to other organs such as bones and liver is possible. Around eight out of 10 bladder cancers are non-muscle invasive.

Risk factors for bladder cancer

The causes of bladder cancer aren't fully understood; however, the following are some of the risk factors:

- smoking – smokers are three to four times more likely to develop bladder cancer and passive smoking may also increase the risk;
- exposure to certain industrial chemicals (e.g. in the rubber, paint, dye, printing and textile industries, gas and tar manufacturing, iron and aluminium processing);
- long-term infection with the tropical disease bilharzia;
- long-term or repeated bladder infection.

Pathophysiology of bladder cancer

Most urinary tract malignancies arise from epithelial tissue. Transitional epithelium lines the entire tract from the renal pelvis through the urethra. Carcinogenic breakdown products of certain chemicals and from cigarette smoke are excreted in the urine and stored in the bladder, possibly causing a local influence on abnormal cell development. Squamous cell carcinoma of the urinary tract occurs less frequently than transitional epithelial cell tumours.

Urinary tract tumours begin as non-specific cellular alterations that develop into either flat or papillary lesions. These lesions may be either superficial or invasive. About 75% of bladder tumours are papillary lesions (papillomas), a polyp-like structure attached by a stalk to the bladder mucosa. Papillomas are generally superficial, non-invasive tumours that bleed easily and frequently recur. They rarely progress to become invasive, and the prognosis for recovery is good.

Carcinoma *in situ* (CIS), which occurs less frequently, is a poorly differentiated flat tumour that invades directly and is associated with a poorer prognosis. Bladder tumours are rated by their cell type and grade. Grade I tumours are highly differentiated and rarely progress to become invasive, whereas grade III tumours are poorly differentiated and usually progress. The staging of bladder tumours is outlined in Table 8.2.

Signs and symptoms of bladder cancer

Signs and symptoms of bladder cancer include:

- painless haematuria is the presenting sign in 75% of urinary tract tumours;
- frequency;
- urgency;
- dysuria;
- may cause UTI.

PRACTICE ALERT

Intermittent painless haematuria is the most common presenting symptom of bladder cancer. Advise all persons with painless haematuria to contact their doctor for follow-up testing.

Table 8.2 Bladder tumour staging

Depth of involvement	TNM (tumour, node, metastasis) stage	Tumour involvement
Superficial	T_a	Limited to the bladder mucosa
	T_1	Involvement of the bladder mucosa and submucosal layers
Invasive	T_2	Invasion of superficial muscle of bladder wall
	T_{3a}	Deep muscle invasion
	T_{3b}	Involvement of perivesicular fat
	$T_{3-4}N_1$	Regional (pelvic) lymph node involvement
	$T_{3-4}M_1$	Metastasis to distant lymph nodes or organs

INTERDISCIPLINARY CARE FOR BLADDER CANCER

Radiation therapy

Radiation is adjunctive therapy used in the treatment of urinary tumours. Although radiation alone is not curative, it can reduce tumour size prior to surgery and is used as palliative treatment for inoperable tumours and persons who cannot tolerate surgery. Radiation therapy is also used in combination with systemic chemotherapy to improve local and distant relapse rates.

Surgery

A number of surgical procedures, ranging from simple resection of non-invasive tumours to removal of the bladder and surrounding structures, are used to treat urinary tract tumours.

Transurethral tumour resection may be performed by excision, *fulguration* (destruction of tissue using electric sparks generated by high-frequency current) or *laser photocoagulation* (use of light energy to destroy abnormal tissue). Laser surgery carries the lowest risk of bleeding and perforation of the bladder wall. Following cystoscopic tumour resection, persons are followed at three-month intervals for tumour recurrence. Recurrences may develop anywhere in the urinary tract, including the renal pelvis, ureter or urethra.

Cystectomy, surgical removal of the bladder, is necessary to treat invasive cancers. Partial cystectomy may be done to remove a solitary lesion; however, radical cystectomy is the standard treatment for invasive tumours. The bladder and adjacent muscles and tissues are removed. In men, the prostate and seminal vessels are also removed, resulting in impotence. In women, a total hysterectomy and bilateral salpingo-oophorectomy (removal of the uterus, fallopian tubes and ovaries) accompanies the procedure, causing sterility. At the time of surgery, a urinary diversion is created to provide for urine collection and drainage. Either an ileal conduit (Figure 8.7 A) or a continent urinary diversion (Figure 8.7 B) is created to collect and drain urine.

NURSING CARE FOR BLADDER CANCER

Health promotion

Encourage all persons not to smoke. Provide referral to smoking cessation programmes or clinics for persons who wish to quit smoking. Encourage persons at high risk for developing bladder cancer to have periodic examinations, including urinalysis and possible urine cytology.

Assessment

Nursing assessment related to urinary tract cancer includes both subjective and objective information. Nurses should obtain:

+ *Health history*: risk factors; history of haematuria or symptoms of UTI (dysuria, frequency, urgency, pyuria); lower abdominal discomfort or flank pain.
+ *Physical examination*: general health; abdominal tenderness; urine for analysis.

Nursing diagnoses and interventions

Risk for impaired urinary elimination

Whether the person has undergone transurethral resection of a bladder tumour or radical cystectomy with urinary diversion, urinary elimination is altered at least temporarily.

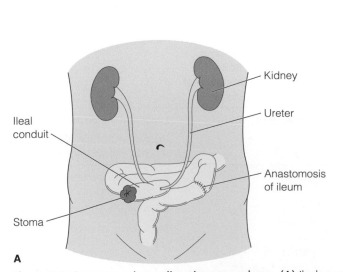

A

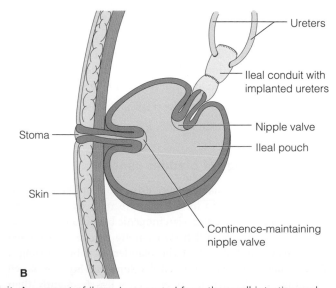

B

Figure 8.7 Common urinary diversion procedures. (A) Ileal conduit. A segment of ileum is separated from the small intestine and formed into a tubular pouch with the opening end brought to the skin surface to form a stoma. The ureters are then connected to the pouch. **(B)** A continent urinary diversion. A segment of the ileum is separated from the small intestine and formed into a pouch. Nipple valves are formed at each end of the pouch to prevent leakage.

+ Monitor urine output from all catheters, stents and tubes for amount, colour and clarity hourly for the first 24 hours post-operatively, then every four to eight hours. *Decreased urine output may indicate impaired catheter or drainage system patency. Prompt intervention is necessary to prevent hydronephrosis. A change in colour or clarity may indicate a complication such as haemorrhage or infection.*

PRACTICE ALERT

Promptly report urine output of less than 30 mL per hour, which may indicate low vascular volume or renal insufficiency. Prompt intervention is vital to restore cardiac output and prevent acute kidney injury.

+ Label all catheters, stents and their drainage containers. Maintain separate closed gravity drainage systems for each. *Clear identification of each tube can prevent errors in irrigating and calculating outputs. Separate closed systems minimise the risk and extent of potential bacterial contamination and resultant infection.*

+ Secure ureteral catheters and stents with tape; prevent kinking or occlusion; and maintain gravity flow by keeping drainage bag below level of kidneys. *Impaired urine flow can lead to urinary retention and distention of the bladder, a newly created reservoir or the renal pelvis (hydronephrosis).*

+ Encourage fluid intake of 2.5–3 L per day. *Increased fluid intake maintains a high urinary output, reducing the risk of infection. Dilute urine is less irritating to the skin surrounding the stoma site. Electrolyte reabsorption from reservoirs may increase risk of calculi; high fluid intake and urine output reduce this risk.*

+ Encourage tolerance to activity. *Ambulation promotes drainage of urine from reservoirs and helps prevent calcium loss from bones, which could precipitate calculus formation.*

PRACTICE ALERT

Monitor urine output closely for first 24 hours after stents or ureteral catheters are removed. Oedema or stricture of ureters may impede output, leading to hydronephrosis and kidney damage.

Risk for impaired skin integrity
The skin surrounding the stoma site of an ileal conduit is at risk for irritation and breakdown. Because urine is acidic and contains high concentrations of electrolytes, it has a corrosive effect on skin. In addition, adhesives and sealants used to prevent pouch leakage may irritate the skin.

+ Assess peristomal skin for redness, excoriation or signs of breakdown. Assess for urine leakage from catheters, stents or drains. Keep the skin clean and dry. Change wet dressings. *Intact skin is the first line of defence against infection. Impaired skin integrity may lead to local or systemic infection and impaired healing.*

+ Ensure gravity drainage of urine collection device or empty bag every two hours. *Overfilling of the collection bag may damage the seal, allowing leakage and contact of urine with skin.*

+ Change urine collection appliance as needed, removing any mucus from stoma. *Meticulous care and protection of skin surrounding stoma can maintain integrity and prevent breakdown.*

Risk for altered body image
A radical cystectomy and urinary diversion affect the person's body image. In most cases, an abdominal stoma is created, requiring either a drainage appliance or regular catheterisation of the stoma to drain urine. Removal of the prostate and seminal vesicles or the uterus and ovaries leaves the person sterile. If radiation or chemotherapy is planned as adjunctive therapy, the person may experience hair loss, stomatitis, nausea and vomiting or other disturbing side-effects of therapy. Nurses should:

+ Use therapeutic communication techniques, actively listening and responding to the person's and family's concerns. *Persons must know their feelings and concerns are respected and valued. Denial, anger, guilt, bargaining or depression are common during grieving and normal for a person undergoing a significant change in body image.*

+ Recognise and accept behaviours that indicate use of coping mechanisms, encouraging adaptive mechanisms. *The person may initially use defensive coping mechanisms such as denial, minimisation and dissociation from the immediate situation to reduce anxiety and maintain psychological integrity. Adaptive mechanisms include learning as much as possible about the surgery and its effects, practising procedures, setting realistic goals and rehearsing various alternative outcomes.*

+ Encourage looking at, touching and caring for the stoma and appliance as soon as possible. Allow the person to proceed gradually, providing support and encouragement. *Accepting the stoma as part of the self is vital to adapting to the changed body image and is indicated by a willingness to provide self-care.*

+ Discuss concerns about returning to usual activities, perceived relationship changes and resumption of sexual relations. Provide referral to support group or provide for contact with someone who has successfully adjusted to a urinary diversion. *Persons and families may be reluctant to discuss topics of concern. An atmosphere of openness and acceptance facilitates expression of concerns and anxieties related to the changed body image.*

Risk for infection

Diagnostic instrumentation procedures, surgical manipulation and disruption of normal urinary tract defence mechanisms increase the risk of ascending UTI. When an ileal conduit or artificial bladder is created using bowel tissue, the normal bacteriostatic activity of bladder mucosa is lost. In addition, the peristaltic action of the ureters may be disrupted, and the vesicoureteral junction no longer prevents urine reflux. Adjunctive chemotherapy or radiation treatments may impair normal immune function and further increase the risk of infection.

+ Maintain separate closed drainage systems, keeping drainage bags lower than the kidney, and prevent loops or kinks in drainage tubing, which impede urine flow. *Although urine is sterile when it leaves the kidney, bacteria grow rapidly in urine. Prevention of urine reflux is essential to preventing UTI.*

+ Monitor for signs of infection: elevated temperature, cloudy or foul-smelling urine, haematuria, general malaise, back or abdominal pain and nausea and vomiting. Infection undermines the healing process. *Early detection and treatment help prevent long-term consequences such as chronic pyelonephritis.*

PRACTICE ALERT

Impaired immune function (due to ageing or the effects of chemotherapy) and urine cloudiness (related to the effects of urine on ileal mucosa) can mask usual signs of UTI such as fever and altered urine clarity. Be alert for more generalised symptoms such as increased fatigue and malaise.

+ Teach signs and symptoms of infection and self-care measures to prevent UTI. *The person with a cystectomy and ileal diversion, urostomy or continent reservoir is at risk of UTI for life because of impaired urinary defence mechanisms. Using clean or aseptic technique in providing care, increasing fluid intake and using measures to acidify urine minimise this risk to a certain degree but do not eliminate it.*

COMMUNITY-BASED CARE

The need for individual and family teaching for the person who has had surgery to treat a urinary tract tumour is significant. For many persons, surgery means a lifelong change in urinary elimination. Even the person who has undergone transurethral excision of bladder tumours requires follow-up cystoscopy on a regular basis and needs to be alert for signs of tumour recurrence.

The person who has had a urinary diversion needs teaching about care of the stoma and surrounding skin, prevention of urine reflux and infection, signs and symptoms of UTI and renal calculi and, in some cases, self-catheterisation using clean technique.

The Urostomy Association is one area where support is offered specifically by members who are living with a urinary diversion. Joining a support group will provide the person with the opportunity to form new friendships and explore what it is like to live with a stoma.

IN PRACTICE

Urinary catheterisation

The person with a urinary catheter *in situ* should be encouraged to drink at least 2.5–3 L of fluid per day unless they suffer from cardiac problems. The person should be encouraged to undertake daily meatal hygiene to ensure that the person does not develop UTI. Where possible, nurses should encourage the person to take daily showers, instead of a bath. For uncircumcised males, nurses should instruct the person to gently retract the foreskin over the head of the penis away from the catheter. Using soap and water, cleanse around the head of the meatus.

Gently apply torsion to the catheter and clean away from the tip of the penis where the catheter enters the penis, wiping 7–10 cm down the tubing towards the catheter bag. Care should be taken not to introduce any infection when cleaning the head of the meatus. Wipe and dry with a clean towel.

NURSING CARE PLAN The person having a cystectomy and urinary diversion

Review Chapter 1 for routine pre- and post-operative care.

Pre-operative care

+ Provide routine pre-operative care. Nurses must adhere to local policies and guidelines in the safe preparation of a person for theatre.

+ Assess knowledge of the proposed surgery and its long-term implications, clarifying misunderstandings and discussing concerns. *Persons having surgery for cancer of the urinary tract are trying to cope with diagnosis of cancer and may not fully understand the surgery and its potential effects. Open discussion can facilitate post-operative recovery and adjustment.*

+ Begin teaching about post-operative tubes and drains, self-care of stoma and control of drainage and odour. *Post-operative physiologic and psychological stressors may interfere with learning. A basic understanding of what to expect in the way of tubes, drains and procedures reduces stress in the immediate post-operative period. Pre-operative teaching can enhance recall and post-operative learning.*

+ Assist in identifying stoma site, avoiding folds of skin, bones, scar tissue and the waistline or belt area. Be sure to consider the person's occupation and style of clothing. The site should be visible to the person and accessible for manipulation. *Stoma placement is a vital component of adjustment and self-care. Care is taken to place the stoma away from areas of constant irritation by clothing or movement. It should be located so that the person can cover and disguise the collecting device, maintain the seal to prevent leakage and effectively cleanse and maintain the site.*

+ Perform bowel-preparation activities as requested. *Bowel preparation is done to prevent faecal contamination of the peritoneal cavity and to decompress the bowel during surgery.*

Post-operative care

+ Post-operative care should include monitoring vital signs, pain management, risk assessment for deep vein thrombosis, pressure sores, personal hygiene, nutrition and other routine post-operative care.

+ Monitor intake and output carefully, assessing urine output every hour for the first 24 hours, then every four hours or as ordered. Inform the doctor if urine output is less than 30 mL per hour. *Tissue oedema and bleeding may interfere with urinary output from stoma, catheters or drains. Maintenance of urine outflow is vital to prevent* hydronephrosis and possible renal damage. A urine output of at least 30 mL per hour is necessary for effective renal function.

+ Assess colour and consistency of urine. Expect pink or bright red urine fading to pink and then clearing by the third post-operative day. Urine may be cloudy due to mucous production by bowel mucosa. *Bright red blood in the urine from a urinary diversion may indicate haemorrhage, necessitating further surgery. Excessive cloudiness or malodorous urine may indicate infection.*

+ Assess size, colour and condition of the stoma and surrounding skin every two hours for the first 24 hours, then every four hours for 48–72 hours. Expect the stoma to appear bright red and slightly oedematous initially. Slight bleeding during cleansing is normal. *Compromised circulation causes the stoma to appear pale, grey or cyanotic or blanch when touched. Other complications, such as infection or impaired healing, may be evidenced by a change in the appearance of the stoma or incision.*

+ Irrigate the ileal diversion catheter with 30–60 mL of normal saline every four hours or as requested. *Mucus produced by the bowel wall may accumulate in the newly devised reservoir or obstruct catheters.*

Health education for the person and family

+ Teach the person and family about stoma and urinary diversion care, including odour management, skin care, increased fluid intake, pouch application and leakage prevention, self-catheterisation for persons with continent reservoirs and signs of infection and other complications. *The ability to provide self-care is a significant factor in the adjustment to a changed body image. Teaching family members facilitates acceptance and adjustment. The family also needs this knowledge in case illness or disability interferes with the self-care capacity.*

IN PRACTICE

Urinary diversion – support issues

The person admitted for urinary diversion will need considerable psychological preparation to come to terms with the stoma. The person needs to come to terms with lifestyle changes and altered body image. The person will have concerns about pain after surgery and how to manage a urostomy bag. The information-giving should continue throughout the post-operative period. The aim is to help the person to lead a normal life in society, to adapt to changed body image, to reduce anxiety and to reassure the person that the support services will continue in the community after their discharge. The nurse needs to discuss some of the possible complications of the urinary diversion. They include:

● urine infection;
● mucus build up which may cause stones to form;
● leakage via stoma site;
● stenosis of the stoma.

The nurse should also discuss with the person the services available in the community to support him/her and their family.

Case Study 1 – Suresh
NURSING CARE PLAN Bladder tumour

If you remember, Mr Suresh Tamwar went to see his GP when he noticed blood in the urine and a burning sensation whenever he voids urine. List any other symptoms that Mr Tamwar may experience with his condition. List the investigations that may be carried out to confirm diagnosis. His GP decides to refer Mr Tamwar to the urologist. After further investigation and tests, the consultant urologist decides to admit Suresh for surgery.

Assessment

You will need to obtain a full nursing and medical history from Mr Tamwar. During the nursing assessment, Mr Tamwar indicates that he has lost 4–8 kg during the last few months. He smoked two to three packs of cigarettes per day for 40 years, but cut back to a pack a day about a year ago. He says he could not quit smoking entirely. He drinks five to six cups of coffee daily but does not drink any alcohol. Mr Tamwar says that he is 'a little nervous about surgery and what they're going to find.' You notice that he fidgets and talks rapidly throughout the interview. He also expresses concern about how he will handle the pain after surgery and wearing a bag.

Diagnoses

+ *Anxiety* related to undetermined extent of disease and fear of pain.

+ *Deficient knowledge* related to care and management of continent urinary diversion.

+ *Impaired urinary elimination* related to cystectomy and urinary diversion.

+ *Risk for impaired gas exchange* related to smoking history and effects of anaesthesia.

Expected outcomes

+ Verbalise decreased feelings of anxiety.

+ Demonstrate appropriate post-operative pain relief through subjective reports of pain severity and objective findings.

+ Be able to care for urinary diversion and surrounding skin, prior to discharge.

+ Maintain normal urine output with acceptable colour and clarity and no signs of infection.

+ Maintain adequate gas exchange as evidenced by good skin colour, O_2 saturation greater than 95% and clear lung sounds on auscultation.

Planning and implementation

+ Spend as much time as possible with Mr Tamwar and his family pre-operatively, answering questions fully and encouraging expression of fears.

+ Provide written and verbal explanations when needed.

+ Administer analgesia on a regular basis for the first 48–72 hours. Monitor for objective signs of unrelieved pain.

+ Explain all procedures related to stoma and diversion care as they are being performed.

+ Encourage Mr Tamwar to look at stoma and touch it when ready.

+ Teach stoma and skin care, as well as self-catheterisation, emphasising measures to prevent skin irritation and UTI.

+ Monitor urine output, colour, clarity and consistency every hour for first 24 hours, then every four hours for 24 hours, then every eight hours. Report output of less than 30 mL per hour, bright bleeding, excessively cloudy or malodorous urine.

+ Refer Mr Tamwar to the stoma care nurse.

Evaluation

On discharge, Mr Tamwar has performed self-catheterisation and stoma and skin care several times. His wife is also able to catheterise the stoma and demonstrate skin care technique. His urine is pale yellow and slightly cloudy. Mr Tamwar is mobilising independently and using oxycodone (Percocet) twice a day for pain relief. His lungs are clear, and he is very proud of having 'survived' seven days without a cigarette. He says, 'Now I'm going to stop smoking completely.' Mr Tamwar is discharged with all the relevant information and an appointment for the after care team.

Consider this . . .

● How does cigarette smoking contribute to the increased risk of urinary tract tumours?

● Suppose Mr Tamwar had become confused and disoriented and had begun to experience visual hallucinations two to three days post-operatively. What would you suspect the cause to be? What would be the appropriate response?

● Develop a care plan for Suresh for the nursing diagnosis 'risk for sexual dysfunction'.

The person with a renal tumour

Renal tumours may be either benign or malignant, primary or metastatic. Benign renal tumours are infrequent and are often found only on autopsy. Most primary renal tumours arise from renal cells; a primary tumour may also develop in the renal pelvis, although less frequently. Metastatic lesions to the kidney are associated with lung and breast cancer, melanoma and malignant lymphoma.

Males are affected by renal cancer more than females by a 2:1 ratio. The highest incidence is seen in people over the age of 55 years. Smoking and obesity are risk factors; chronic irritation associated with renal calculi may also contribute. Some renal cancers are associated with genetic factors.

Pathophysiology of renal tumour

Most (85–95%) primary renal tumours are renal cell carcinomas. These tumours arise from tubular epithelium and can occur anywhere in the kidney. The tumour, which can range in size up to several centimetres, has clearly defined margins and contains areas of ischaemia, necrosis and haemorrhage. Renal tumors tend to invade the renal vein, and have often metastasised when first identified. Metastases tend to occur in the lungs, bone, lymph nodes, liver and brain.

The tumour may produce hormones or hormone-like substances, including parathyroid hormone, prostaglandins, prolactin, **renin**, gonadotropins and glucocorticoids. These substances produce paraneoplastic syndromes, with additional symptoms such as hypercalcaemia, hypertension and hyperglycaemia. Paraneoplastic syndromes are rare disorders triggered by the immune system's response to cancer cells, or by remote effects of tumour-derived factors. These syndromes are believed to occur when cancer-fighting antibodies or white blood cells, known as T-cells, mistakenly attack normal body cells. The progression of renal cell carcinomas varies from prolonged periods of stable disease to very aggressive.

FAST FACTS

Kidney cancer

- Each year, about 7800 people in the UK are diagnosed with kidney cancer.
- It affects more men than women and becomes more common as people get older.

Source: http://www.macmillan.org.uk/Cancerinformation/Cancertypes/Kidney/Aboutkidneycancer/Typesofkidneycancer.aspx (accessed September 2011).

Signs and symptoms of renal tumour

Signs and symptoms of a renal tumour include:

- heavy haematuria;
- flank pain;
- palpable abdominal mass;
- fever without signs of infection;
- fatigue;
- weight loss;
- anaemia.

INTERDISCIPLINARY CARE FOR RENAL TUMOUR

Surgery

Radical nephrectomy is the treatment of choice for kidney tumours. In a radical nephrectomy, the adrenal gland, upper ureter, fat and fascia surrounding the kidney, as well as the entire kidney, are removed. Regional lymph nodes may also be resected. Although nephrectomy can be done using a laparoscopic approach, laparotomy primarily is used for radical nephrectomy.

NURSING CARE PLAN The person having a nephrectomy

Review Chapter 1 for routine pre- and post-operative care.

Pre-operative care

+ Nurses need to adhere to local policies and guidance in the safe pre-operative preparation of a person for theatre, including giving information and identifying any special needs.

+ Report abnormal laboratory values to the surgeon. *Bacteriuria, blood coagulation abnormalities or other significant abnormal values may affect surgery and post-operative care.*

+ Discuss operative and post-operative expectations as indicated, including the location of the incision (Figures 8.8 A, B and C) and anticipated tubes, stents and drains. *Pre-operative teaching about post-operative expectations reduces anxiety for the person and family during the early post-operative period.*

Post-operative care

+ Monitor vital signs such as temperature, blood pressure, heart rate and respiration rate.

+ Frequently assess urine colour, amount and character, noting any haematuria, pyuria or sediment. Promptly report **oliguria** or **anuria**, as well as changes in urine colour or clarity. *Preserving function of the remaining kidney is*

NURSING CARE PLAN **The person having a nephrectomy** (continued)

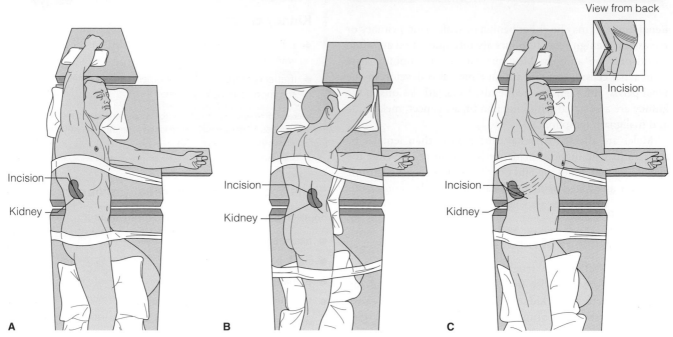

Figure 8.8 Incisions used for kidney surgery. **(A)** Flank. **(B)** Lumbar. **(C)** Thoracoabdominal.

critical; frequent assessment allows early intervention for potential problems.

+ Note the placement, status and drainage from ureteral catheters, stents, nephrostomy tubes or drains. Label each clearly. Maintain gravity drainage; irrigate only as ordered. *Maintaining drainage tube patency is vital to prevent potential hydronephrosis. Bright bleeding or unexpected drainage may indicate a surgical complication.*

+ Support the grieving process and adjustment to the loss of a kidney. *Loss of a major organ leads to a body image change and grief response. When renal cancer is the underlying diagnosis, the person may also grieve the loss of health and potential loss of life.*

Health education for the person and family

+ Nurses should provide the following home care instructions for the person and family:

   a. The importance of protecting the remaining kidney by preventing UTI, renal calculi and trauma. *Damage to the remaining kidney by UTI, renal calculi or trauma can lead to renal failure.*

   b. Maintain a fluid intake of 2500–3000 mL per day. *This important measure helps prevent dehydration and maintain good urine flow.*

   c. Gradually increase exercise tolerance, avoiding heavy lifting for a year after surgery. *Participation in contact sports is not recommended to reduce the risk of injury to the remaining kidney. Lifting is avoided to allow full tissue healing. Trauma to the remaining kidney could seriously jeopardise renal function.*

   d. Care of the incision and any remaining drainage tubes, catheters or stents. *This routine post-operative instruction is vital to prepare the person for self-care and prevent complications.*

   e. Report signs and symptoms to the doctor, including symptoms of UTI (dysuria, frequency, urgency, nocturia, cloudy, malodorous urine) or systemic infection (fever, general malaise, fatigue), redness, swelling, pain, or drainage from the incision or any catheter or drain tube site. *Prompt treatment of post-operative infection is vital to allow continued healing and prevent compromise of the remaining kidney.*

NURSING CARE FOR RENAL TUMOUR

Nurses should consider other aspects of care post-operatively. The care relates to diagnosis and to the surgical interventions. Post-operative pain is significant and the risk for respiratory complications is high. Nurses should also consider the psychological impact it may have on the patient.

Nursing diagnoses and interventions

Risk for pain

The size and location used for nephrectomy make pain management paramount. The patient may be prescribed patient-controlled analgesia (PCA), epidural or routine analgesia administration. Nursing care should focus on assessing pain relief using appropriate pain assessment tools such as visual analogue scale, administering prescribed analgesia at prescribed intervals and ensuring that the patient does not develop respiratory complications as a result of pain. Nurses should:

+ Assess pain hourly using pain score chart. Look out for non-verbal clues such as tachycardia, sweating, facial grimacing. *Controlling pain level in the patient promotes quick recovery.*

+ Check the wound site two hourly for swelling and drainage tubes for patency. *Swelling may indicate a haematoma as a result of internal bleeding. A haematoma can put pressure on the incision resulting in unnecessary pain.*

+ Use alternative pain relief measures such as positioning the patient comfortably and relaxation techniques through deep breathing exercises. *Alternative pain relief measures can enhance the effects of analgesia.*

Risk for ineffective breathing pattern

The location of the incision combined with the respiratory depressant effects of narcotic analgesics increases the risk for respiratory complications in the person who has had a nephrectomy.

+ Position the person, using semi-Fowler's position or side-lying positions as tolerated. *Lung expansion is improved in semi-Fowler's and Fowler's positions.*

PRACTICE ALERT

Assess respiratory status frequently, including rate and depth, cough, breath sounds, oxygen saturation and temperature. Pneumothorax on the operative side is common. Early identification and intervention can prevent major respiratory complications.

+ Change position frequently, mobilise as soon as possible. *These measures promote lung expansion and the movement of mucus out of airways.*

+ Encourage frequent (every one to two hours) deep breathing, spirometer use and coughing. Assist to splint the incision. *These measures promote alveolar ventilation, gas exchange and airway clearance.*

Risk for impaired urinary elimination

Surgery involving the urinary tract increases the risk for altered renal function and urine elimination. In addition, removal of one kidney dictates extra caution to maintain renal circulation, a sterile urinary tract and free urine flow. Nurses should:

+ Monitor vital signs and urine output every one to two hours initially, then every four hours. *Hypovolaemia due to haemorrhage,* **diuresis** *or fluid sequestering (third spacing)*

reduces blood flow to the kidney and increases the risk of renal ischaemia with possible acute tubular necrosis and acute kidney injury.

+ Frequently assess the amount and nature of drainage on surgical dressings and from wound drains and catheters. Measure and record output from the drain or catheter separately. *Frequent and accurate assessment of drainage helps to identify secondary bleeding, abnormal fluid loss, infection or other potential surgical complications.*

+ Maintain fluid intake with intravenous fluids until oral intake is resumed. Encourage an intake of 2500–3000 mL per day as soon as the person tolerates oral liquids. *A liberal fluid intake prevents dehydration, helps to dilute any nephrotoxic substances and promotes good urinary output.*

+ Nurses must adhere to strict aseptic technique in caring for all urinary catheters, drains and incisions. *Asepsis is vital to prevent infection and possible compromise of the remaining kidney.*

+ Following catheter removal, assess frequently for urinary retention. Notify the doctor if the person is unable to void within four to six hours or if symptoms of retention (distended bladder, discomfort, urinary dribbling) develop. *Maintenance of urine output is vital to prevent stasis and possible complications such as infection and hydronephrosis.*

+ Monitor laboratory results, including urinalysis, BUN, serum creatinine and serum electrolytes. Report abnormal findings to the doctor. *Abnormal values may indicate early acute kidney injury; prompt intervention is necessary to preserve renal function.*

Risk for anticipatory grieving

The person having a radical nephrectomy for renal cancer not only loses a major organ but also has to adjust to the diagnosis of cancer. Although the prognosis for recovery may be good, many people perceive cancer as always fatal. Providing support for the person and family during the initial stages of grieving can improve physical recovery, psychological coping and eventual adaptation.

+ Work to develop a trusting relationship with the person and family. *Trust increases the nurse's effectiveness in helping them work through the process of grieving.*

+ Listen actively, encouraging the person and family to express fears and concerns. *As they begin to express their concerns, the person and family can begin to deal more effectively with them.*

+ Assist the person and family to identify strengths, past experiences and support systems. *These resources can be employed in working through the grieving process.*

+ Demonstrate respect for cultural, spiritual and religious values and beliefs; encourage use of these resources to cope with losses. *Value and belief systems can provide a structure and form for dealing with the grieving process.*

✦ Encourage discussion of the potential impact of loss on the person and the family structure and function. Assist family members to share concerns with one another. *Sharing of fears and concerns among family members*

promotes involvement and support of the entire family unit so that the individual is not left to cope alone.

✦ Refer to cancer support groups, social services or counselling as appropriate. *Support groups and counselling services provide additional resources for coping.*

COMMUNITY-BASED CARE

If renal cancer was detected at an early stage and cure is anticipated, teaching for home care focuses on protecting the remaining kidney. Include the following measures to prevent infection, renal calculi, hydronephrosis and trauma:

● Maintain a fluid intake of 2000–2500 mL per day, increasing the amount during hot weather or strenuous exercise.

● Urinate when the urge is perceived, and before and after sexual intercourse.

● Properly clean the perineal area.

● Watch for symptoms of UTI, and understand the importance of early and appropriate evaluation and intervention.

● If the person is an older adult male, he should watch for symptoms of prostatic hypertrophy, a major cause of urinary tract obstruction. Stress the importance of routine screening examinations.

● Avoid contact sports such as football or hockey; use measures to prevent motor vehicle accidents and falls, which could damage the kidney.

RENAL FAILURE

Acute kidney injury (AKI), previously known as acute renal failure (ARF), is a condition in which the kidneys are unable to remove accumulated metabolites from the blood, leading to altered fluid, electrolyte and acid–base balance. The cause may be a primary kidney disorder, or renal failure may be secondary to a systemic disease or other urologic defects. AKI may be either acute or chronic. AKI has an abrupt onset and with prompt intervention is often reversible. Chronic kidney disease (CKD), previously chronic renal failure (CRF), is a silent disease, developing slowly and insidiously, with few symptoms until the kidneys are severely damaged and unable to meet the excretory needs of the body. Both forms are characterised by **azotemia**, increased levels of nitrogenous wastes in the blood.

The person with acute kidney injury (AKI)

AKI is a rapid decline in renal function with azotemia and fluid and electrolyte imbalances. The most common causes of acute kidney injury are ischaemia and nephrotoxins. The kidney is particularly vulnerable to both because of the amount of blood that passes through it. A fall in blood pressure or volume can cause ischaemia of kidney tissues. Nephrotoxins in the blood damage renal tissue directly.

FAST FACTS

Complications of AKI and CKD

● AKI is usually accompanied by oliguria or anuria, but polyuria may occur.

● People with any stage of CKD have an increased risk of developing heart disease or a stroke.

● Both AKI and CKD are characterised by azotemia, accumulation of nitrogenous (protein) waste products in the blood.

FAST FACTS

Acute kidney injury

● Recent studies have found an overall incidence of AKI of almost 500 per million per year and the incidence of AKI needing dialysis being more than 200 per million per year.

● Pre-renal AKI and ischaemic acute tubular necrosis (ATN) together account for 75% of the cases of AKI.

Source: Patient UK 2010b.

Risk factors for AKI

Risk factors of AKI include:

- elderly;
- hypertension;
- vascular disease;
- pre-existing renal impairment;
- congestive cardiac failure;
- diabetes;
- myeloma;
- chronic infection.

Pathophysiology of AKI

The causes and pathophysiology of AKI are commonly categorised as pre-renal, intrinsic and post-renal AKI. Pre-renal AKI is the most common, accounting for about 55% of the total. In pre-renal AKI, hypoperfusion leads to AKI without directly affecting the integrity of kidney tissues. Intrinsic (or intrarenal) AKI, due to direct damage to functional kidney tissue, is responsible for another 40%. Urinary tract obstruction with resulting kidney damage is the precipitating factor for post-renal AKI, the least common form.

Pre-renal conditions

Pre-renal AKI results from conditions that affect renal blood flow and perfusion. Any disorder that significantly decreases vascular volume, cardiac output or systemic vascular resistance can affect renal blood flow. The kidneys normally receive 20–25% of the cardiac output to maintain the GFR. A drop in renal blood flow to less than 20% of normal causes the GFR to fall. As the filtration of substances by the glomeruli is reduced, less reabsorption of substances in the tubule is required. As a result, kidney cells require less energy and oxygen, and their metabolism slows. Pre-renal AKI is rapidly reversed when blood flow is restored, and the renal parenchyma remains undamaged. Continued ischaemia can lead to tubular cell necrosis and significant nephron damage. Intrinsic AKI due to ischaemic injury may result.

Post-renal conditions

Obstructive causes of acute kidney injury are classified as post-renal. Any condition that prevents urine excretion can lead to post-renal AKI. Benign prostatic hypertrophy is the most common precipitating factor. Others include renal or urinary tract calculi and tumours.

Intrinsic (intrarenal) conditions

Intrinsic or intrarenal failure is characterised by acute damage to the renal parenchyma and nephrons. Intrarenal causes include diseases of the kidney itself and acute tubular necrosis, the most common intrarenal cause of AKI.

In acute glomerulonephritis, glomerular inflammation can reduce renal blood flow and cause AKI. Vascular disorders affecting the kidney, such as vasculitis (inflammation of the blood vessels), malignant hypertension and arterial or venous

occlusion, can damage nephrons sufficiently to result in acute kidney injury. See Figure 8.9 for pathophysiology of AKI.

Phases of AKI

The course of AKI due to ATN typically includes three phases: initiation, maintenance and recovery.

Initiation phase

The initiation phase may last hours to days. It begins with the initiating event (for example, haemorrhage) and ends when tubular injury occurs. If AKI is recognised and the initiating event is effectively treated during this phase, the prognosis is good. The initiation phase of AKI has few symptoms; in fact, it is often identified only when symptoms of the maintenance phase develop.

Maintenance phase

The maintenance phase of AKI is characterised by a significant fall in GFR and tubular necrosis. Oliguria may develop, although many persons continue to produce normal or near-normal amounts of urine (non-oliguric AKI). Even though urine may be produced, the kidney cannot efficiently eliminate metabolic wastes, water, electrolytes and acids from the body during the maintenance phase of AKI. Azotemia, fluid retention, electrolyte imbalances and metabolic acidosis develop. These abnormalities are more severe in the oliguric person than in the non-oliguric one, leading to a poorer prognosis with oliguria.

Other symptoms of the maintenance phase include:

- oedema and hypertension due to salt and water retention;
- confusion, disorientation, agitation or lethargy, hyper-reflexia and possible seizures or coma due to azotemia and electrolyte and acid–base imbalances;
- anorexia, nausea, vomiting, and decreased or absent bowel sounds.

Recovery phase

The recovery phase of AKI is characterised by a process of tubule cell repair and regeneration and gradual return of the GFR to normal or pre-AKI levels. Diuresis may occur as the nephrons and GFR recover, and retained salt, water and

FAST FACTS

Pre-renal AKI

- Pre-renal AKI is common, particularly in trauma, surgical and critically ill persons.
- Restoration of blood pressure and blood flow to the kidneys rapidly reverses pre-renal AKI.
- If not promptly identified and treated, pre-renal AKI leads to ischaemic acute tubular necrosis and intrarenal or intrinsic AKI.

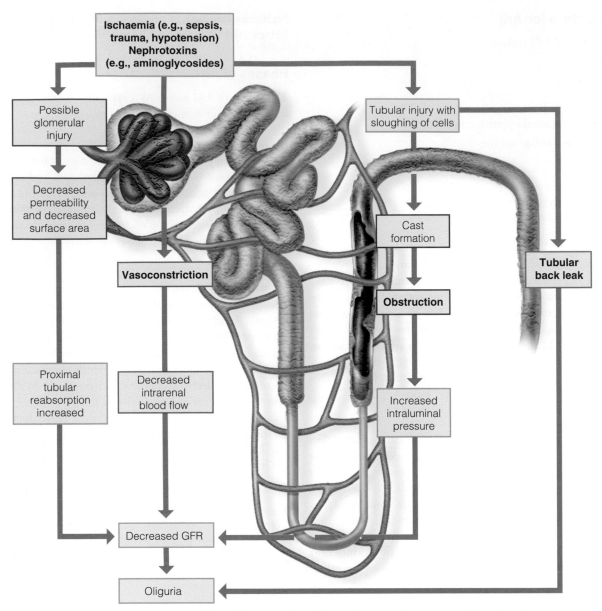

The initial kidney injury is usually associated with an acute condition such as sepsis, trauma and hypotension, or the result of treatment for an acute condition with a nephrotoxic medication. Injury to the kidney can occur because of glomerular injury, vasoconstriction of capillaries, or tubular injury. All consequences of injury lead to decreased glomerular filtration and oliguria.

Figure 8.9 Pathophysiology illustrated: acute renal failure.

solutes are excreted. Serum creatinine, BUN, potassium and phosphate levels remain high and may continue to rise in spite of increasing urine output. Renal function improves rapidly during the first 5–25 days of the recovery phase, and continues to improve for up to one year.

INTERDISCIPLINARY CARE FOR AKI

Medication

No drug treatment has been shown to limit the progression of, or speed up recovery from, AKI. The primary focus in drug

management for AKI is to restore and maintain renal perfusion and to eliminate drugs that are nephrotoxic from the treatment regimen. Nephrotoxic drugs, such as NSAIDs and aminoglycosides, should be avoided.

The person with AKI has an increased risk of gastrointestinal bleeding, probably related to the stress response and impaired platelet function. Regular doses of antacids, histamine H_2-receptor antagonists (for example, ranitidine) or a proton-pump inhibitor such as omeprazole (Prilosec) are often prescribed to prevent gastrointestinal haemorrhage.

Hyperkalaemia may require active intervention as well as restricted potassium intake. Serum levels of greater than

6.5 mmol/L are treated to prevent cardiac effects of **hyperkalaemia**. With significant hyperkalaemia, calcium chloride, bicarbonate and insulin and glucose may be given intravenously to reduce serum potassium levels by moving potassium into the cells. A potassium-binding exchange resin such as sodium polystyrene sulfonate (Kayexalate, SPS Suspension) may be given orally or by enema.

Fluid management

Once vascular volume and renal perfusion are restored, fluid intake is usually restricted. The allowed daily fluid intake is calculated by allowing 500 mL for insensible losses (respiration, perspiration, bowel losses) and adding the amount excreted as urine (or lost in vomit) during the previous 24 hours. For example, if a person with AKI excretes 325 mL of urine in 24 hours, the person is allowed a fluid intake (including oral and intravenous fluids) of 825 mL for the next 24 hours. Fluid balance is carefully monitored, using accurate weight measurements and the serum sodium as the primary indicators.

Nutrition

Renal insufficiency and the underlying disease process increase the rate of *catabolism* (the breakdown of body proteins) and decrease the rate of *anabolism* (body tissue repair). The person with AKI needs adequate nutrients and calories to prevent catabolism. Proteins are limited to 0.6 g per kilogram of body weight per day to minimise the degree of azotemia. Dietary proteins should be of high biologic value (rich in essential amino acids). Carbohydrates are increased to maintain adequate caloric intake and provide a protein-sparing effect.

Parenteral nutrition providing amino acids, concentrated carbohydrates and fats may be instituted when the person cannot consume an adequate diet (for example, due to nausea, vomiting or underlying critical illness). The disadvantages of parenteral nutrition in the person with AKI are the high volume of fluid required and the risk for infection through the venous line.

Dialysis for AKI

Some persons with AKI may need dialysis such as peritoneal dialysis to get rid of the waste products of metabolism such as urea, uric acid and fluid.

Peritoneal dialysis

In peritoneal dialysis, the highly vascular peritoneal membrane serves as the dialysing surface (Figure 8.10). Warmed sterile dialysate (special dialysis fluid) is instilled into the peritoneal cavity through a catheter inserted into the peritoneal cavity. Metabolic waste products and excess electrolytes diffuse into the dialysate while it remains in the abdomen. Water movement is controlled using dextrose as an osmotic agent to draw it into the dialysate. The fluid is then drained by gravity

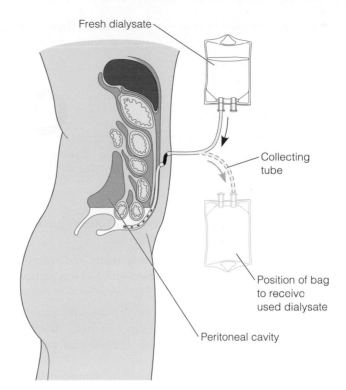

Figure 8.10 Peritoneal dialysis.

out of the peritoneal cavity into a sterile bag. This process of dialysate infusion, dwell time of the solution in the abdomen and drainage is repeated at prescribed intervals.

Because excess fluid and solutes are removed more gradually in peritoneal dialysis, it poses less risk for the unstable person; however, this slower rate of metabolite removal can be a disadvantage in AKI. Peritoneal dialysis increases the risk for developing peritonitis. It is contraindicated for persons who have had recent abdominal surgery, significant lung disease or peritonitis.

NURSING CARE FOR AKI

Nursing diagnoses and interventions

Risk for excess fluid volume

In AKI, the kidneys often cannot excrete adequate urine to maintain a normal extracellular fluid balance. Fluid retention is greater in oliguric renal failure than in non-oliguric failure. Rapid weight gain and oedema indicate fluid retention. In addition, heart failure and pulmonary oedema may develop. In the adult or severely debilitated person, fluid retention can present a significant management problem.

✛ Maintain hourly intake and output records. *Accurate intake and output records help guide therapy, especially fluid restrictions.*

✛ Weigh daily or more frequently, as ordered. Use standard technique (same scale, clothing or coverings) to ensure accuracy. *Rapid weight changes are an accurate indicator of fluid volume status, particularly in the oliguric person.*

✛ Assess vital signs at least every four hours. *Hypertension, tachycardia and tachypnoea may indicate excess fluid volume.*

PRACTICE ALERT

Frequently assess breath and heart sounds, neck veins for distention and back and extremities for oedema. Report abnormal findings immediately to the doctor.

✛ If not contraindicated, place in semi-Fowler's position *to enhance cardiac and respiratory function.*

✛ Report abnormal serum electrolyte values and symptoms of electrolyte imbalance. The person with AKI is at particular risk for the following electrolyte imbalances:

   a. *Hyperkalaemia* due to impaired potassium excretion. Symptoms include irritability, nausea, diarrhoea, abdominal cramping, cardiac dysrhythmias and ECG changes.

   b. *Hyponatraemia* due to water retention. Symptoms include nausea, vomiting and headache, with possible central nervous system (CNS) symptoms of lethargy, confusion, seizures and coma.

   c. *Hyperphosphataemia* due to decreased phosphate excretion. Symptoms include hyperreflexia, paraesthesias and possible tetany. *AKI impairs electrolyte and water excretion, causing multiple electrolyte imbalances*

✛ Restrict fluids as ordered. Provide frequent mouth care and encourage using hard candies to decrease thirst. If ice chips are allowed, include the water content (approximately one-half of the total volume) as intake. *Fluids are restricted to minimise fluid retention and complications of fluid volume excess.*

✛ Administer medications with meals. *Giving oral medications with meals minimises ingestion of excess fluids.*

✛ Turn frequently and provide good skin care. *Oedema decreases tissue perfusion and increases the risk of skin breakdown, especially in the elderly or debilitated person.*

Risk for imbalanced nutrition: less than body requirements

Anorexia and nausea associated with renal failure often interfere with food intake and nutrition. In addition, the disease process leading to AKI may contribute to increased nutritional needs for healing and decreased food intake.

✛ Monitor and record food intake, including the amount and type of food consumed. *A detailed intake record helps guide decisions about nutritional status and necessary supplements.*

✛ Weigh daily. *Weight changes over time (days to weeks) reflect nutritional status, while rapid weight changes are more reflective of fluid volume status. In AKI, weight may remain stable or increase due to fluid retention even though tissue mass is being lost.*

✛ Arrange for dietary consultation to plan meals within prescribed limitations that consider the person's food preferences. *Diets restricted in protein, salt and potassium can be unpalatable; intake and appetite improve when preferred foods are included as allowed.*

✛ Engage the person in planning daily menus. *Participation in meal planning increases the person's sense of control and autonomy.*

✛ Provide frequent, small meals or between-meal snacks. *These measures promote food intake in the fatigued or anorectic person.*

✛ Administer antiemetics as prescribed and provide mouth care prior to meals. *Nausea and a metallic taste in the mouth, common symptoms of uraemia, can decrease food intake.*

CASE STUDY 2 – Martin
NURSING CARE PLAN The person with AKI

If you remember, Mr Martin Chapel went to see his GP with a urinary problem which he had had for 48 hours. His GP examines Mr Chapel and decided to refer him to the urologist at the local hospital. After physical examination and some tests, the urologist decided to admit Mr Chapel with a provisional diagnosis of AKI.

Assessment

During the first few hours after admission, the nurse notes that Mr Chapel's hourly output has dropped from 55 mL to 45 to 28 mL of clear yellow urine. The doctor prescribes 500 mL intravenous fluid, which only produces a slight increase in urine output. Urinalysis results show a specific gravity of 1010 and the

presence of WBCs, red and white cell casts and tubular epithelial cells in the sediment. Mr Chapel's BUN is 28 mg/dL; his serum creatinine, 1.5 mg/dL. The doctor diagnoses probable AKI.

Investigations

The following investigations may be carried out for Mr Chapel:

✛ Urinalysis: blood and/or protein suggests a renal inflammatory process; microscopy for cells, casts, crystals; red cell casts diagnostic in glomerulonephritis; tubular cells or casts suggest acute tubular necrosis (ATN).

✛ Urine osmolality: osmolality of urine is over 500 mmol/kg if the cause is pre-renal and 300 mmol/kg or less if it is renal; patients

CASE STUDY 2 – Martin   **NURSING CARE PLAN The person with AKI**

with ATN lose the ability to concentrate and dilute the urine and will pass a constant volume with inappropriate osmolality.

✚ Full urea and electrolytes to determine urinary function and kidney injury.

✚ Full blood count to determine blood disorders.

✚ Kidney ultrasounds.

Nursing management

Mr Chapel will be very anxious about his illness. He should be reassured that most causes of AKI can be treated and the kidney function will return to normal with time. Replacement of the kidney function by dialysis may be necessary until kidney function has returned. Regardless of the cause, the same general treatment principles apply to all persons who develop AKI. Fluid and dietary management is paramount. A strict regimen should be adhered to in accordance with local policies and guidelines. A strict input and output chart should be maintained all the time until the patient has fully recovered.

Evaluation

After just over three days of oliguria, Mr Chapel's urine out-

put increases. By the end of the fourth day he is voiding 60–80 mL/h of urine. Although his BUN, serum creatinine and potassium levels remain high, they never reach a critical point, and dialysis is not required. When Mr Chapel is able to begin eating, he is placed on a low-potassium diet, restricted to 50 g of protein. His renal function gradually improves. By discharge, results of his renal function tests, including BUN and serum creatinine, are nearly normal. Mr Chapel verbalises an understanding of the need to avoid nephrotoxic medications such as NSAIDs until allowed by his doctor.

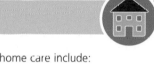

Consider this . . .

The National Kidney Foundation recommends three simple tests to detect kidney disease: a measure of blood pressure; protein or albumin in the urine (proteinuria) control; and a calculation of the GFR based on a measurement of serum creatinine. Urea nitrogen in the blood of measurement provides additional information. If these tests show a reduced kidney function, what other tests may be done to confirm Mr Chapel's diagnosis?

COMMUNITY-BASED CARE

Often the person is critically ill when AKI develops. Critical illness and the resulting state of person and family crisis can impair learning and retention of information. Include family members in teaching during the initial stages to promote understanding of what is happening and the reasons for specific treatment measures. Inclusion of the family reduces their anxiety, and provides a valuable resource for reinforcing person teaching about care after discharge.

Person teaching needs for home care include:

● avoiding exposure to nephrotoxins, particularly those in over-the-counter products;

● preventing infection and other major stressors that can slow healing;

● monitoring weight, blood pressure and pulse;

● continuing dietary restrictions;

● knowing when to contact the doctor.

The person with chronic kidney disease (CKD)

Although the kidneys usually recover from acute injury, many chronic conditions can lead to progressive renal tissue destruction and loss of function. Nephron units are lost and renal mass decreases, with progressive deterioration of glomerular filtration, tubular secretion and reabsorption. This process of CKD may progress slowly for many years without being recognised. Eventually, the kidneys are unable to excrete metabolic wastes and regulate fluid and electrolyte balance adequately, a condition known as end-stage renal disease (ESRD), the final stage of CKD.

FAST FACTS

Complications

● AKI develops abruptly and often can be reversed with appropriate treatment.

● CKD is the end stage of progressive destruction of the kidneys and cannot be reversed.

● Diabetes is the leading cause of chronic renal failure, followed by hypertension, glomerulonephritis, cystic kidney disease and all other causes.

Table 8.3 Pathophysiology of chronic kidney disease

Cause	Examples
Diabetic nephropathy	Changes in the glomerular basement membrane, chronic pyelonephritis and ischaemia lead to sclerosis of the glomerulus and gradual destruction of the nephron.
Hypertensive nephrosclerosis	Long-standing hypertension leads to renal arteriosclerosis and ischaemia resulting in glomerular destruction and tubular atrophy.
Chronic glomerulonephritis	Bilateral inflammatory process of the glomeruli leads to ischaemia, nephron loss and shrinkage of the kidney.
Chronic pyelonephritis	Chronic infection commonly associated with an obstructive or neurologic process and vesico-ureteral reflux leads to reflux nephropathy (renal scarring, atrophy and dilated calyces).
Polycystic kidney disease	Multiple bilateral cysts gradually destroy normal renal tissue by compression.
Systemic lupus erythematosus	Basement membrane damage by circulating immune complexes leads to focal, local or diffuse glomerulonephritis.

Pathophysiology of CKD

The pathophysiology of CKD involves a gradual loss of entire nephron units. In the early stages, as nephrons are destroyed, remaining functional nephrons hypertrophy. Glomerular capillary flow and pressure increase in these nephrons, and more solute particles are filtered to compensate for lost renal mass. This increased demand predisposes the remaining nephrons to glomerular sclerosis (scarring), resulting in their eventual destruction. This process of continued loss of nephron function may continue even after the initial disease process has resolved. Table 8.3 outlines common pathophysiogical processes leading to nephron destruction and ESRD.

The course of CKD is variable, progressing over a period of months to many years. In the early stage, known as *decreased renal reserve*, unaffected nephrons compensate for the lost nephrons. The GFR is about 50% of normal, and the person is asymptomatic with normal BUN and serum creatinine levels. As the disease progresses and the GFR falls to 20–50% of normal, azotemia and some symptoms of renal insufficiency may be seen. Any further insult to the kidneys at this stage (such as infection, dehydration or urinary tract obstruction) can further reduce function and precipitate the onset of renal failure.

Signs and symptoms of CKD

In the early stages of CKD, the person may be asymptomatic. Early symptoms of uraemia include nausea, apathy, weakness and fatigue, symptoms that are dismissed as a viral infection or influenza. As the condition progresses, frequent vomiting, increasing weakness, lethargy and confusion develop. For the multisystem effects of uraemia see Figure 8.11.

Complications of CKD

Fluid and electrolyte effects

Loss of functional kidney tissue impairs its ability to regulate fluid, electrolyte and acid–base balance. In the early stages of CKD, impaired filtration and reabsorption lead to proteinuria, haematuria and decreased urine-concentrating ability. Salt and water are poorly conserved, and risk for dehydration increases. Polyuria, nocturia and a fixed specific gravity of 1.008–1.012 are common. As the GFR decreases and renal function deteriorates further, sodium and water retention are common, necessitating salt and water restrictions.

As renal failure advances, hydrogen-ion excretion and buffer production are impaired, leading to metabolic acidosis. Respiratory rate and depth increase (Kussmaul's respirations) to compensate for metabolic acidosis. Although metabolic acidosis is often asymptomatic, other possible symptoms include general malaise, weakness, headache, nausea and vomiting and abdominal pain.

Cardiovascular effects

Cardiovascular disease is a common cause of death in ESRD, and results from accelerated atherosclerosis. Hypertension, hyperlipidaemia and glucose intolerance all contribute to the process. Cerebral and peripheral vascular symptoms of atherosclerosis are also seen.

Systemic hypertension is a common complication of ESRD. Hypertension results from excess fluid volume, increased renin–angiotensin activity, increased peripheral vascular resistance and decreased prostaglandins. Increased extracellular fluid volume also can lead to oedema and heart failure. Pulmonary oedema may result from heart failure and increased permeability of the alveolar capillary membrane.

Haematologic effects

Anaemia is common in uraemia, caused by multiple factors. The kidneys produce **erythropoietin**, a hormone that controls RBC production. In renal failure, erythropoietin production declines. Retained metabolic toxins further suppress RBC production, and contribute to a shortened RBC lifespan. Nutritional deficiencies (iron and folate) and increased risk for blood loss from the gastrointestinal tract also contribute to anaemia.

Anaemia contributes to symptoms such as fatigue, weakness, depression and impaired cognition. It also affects cardiovascular function, and may be a major contributing factor to coronary heart disease and heart failure associated with ESRD.

Renal failure impairs platelet function, increasing the risk of bleeding disorders such as epistaxis and gastrointestinal bleeding. The mechanism of impaired platelet function associated with renal failure is poorly understood.

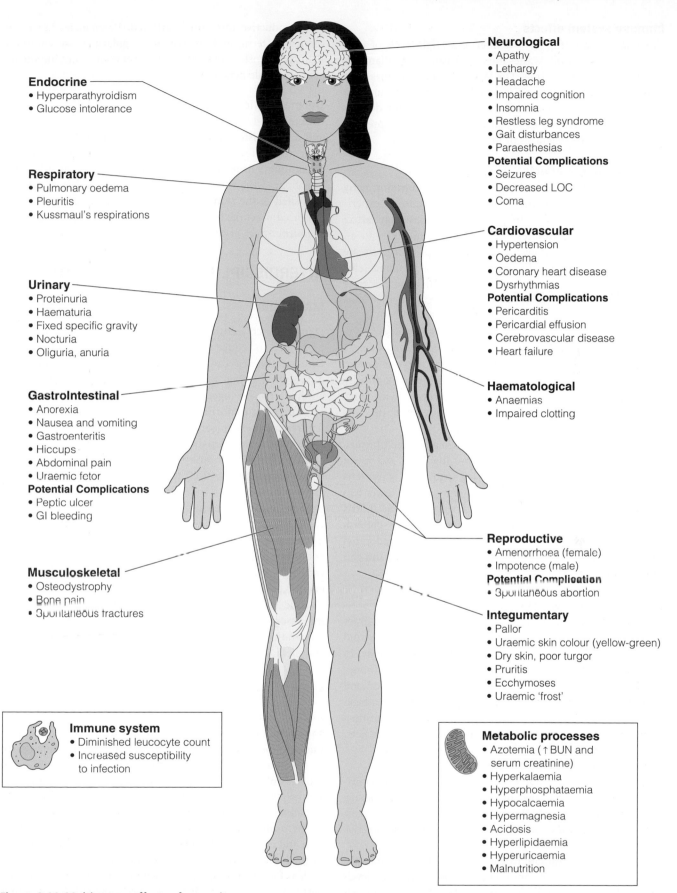

Neurological
- Apathy
- Lethargy
- Headache
- Impaired cognition
- Insomnia
- Restless leg syndrome
- Gait disturbances
- Paraesthesias

Potential Complications
- Seizures
- Decreased LOC
- Coma

Endocrine
- Hyperparathyroidism
- Glucose intolerance

Respiratory
- Pulmonary oedema
- Pleuritis
- Kussmaul's respirations

Cardiovascular
- Hypertension
- Oedema
- Coronary heart disease
- Dysrhythmias

Potential Complications
- Pericarditis
- Pericardial effusion
- Cerebrovascular disease
- Heart failure

Urinary
- Proteinuria
- Haematuria
- Fixed specific gravity
- Nocturia
- Oliguria, anuria

Haematological
- Anaemias
- Impaired clotting

GastroIntestinal
- Anorexia
- Nausea and vomiting
- Gastroenteritis
- Hiccups
- Abdominal pain
- Uraemic fetor

Potential Complications
- Peptic ulcer
- GI bleeding

Reproductive
- Amenorrhoea (female)
- Impotence (male)

Potential Complication
- Spontaneous abortion

Integumentary
- Pallor
- Uraemic skin colour (yellow-green)
- Dry skin, poor turgor
- Pruritis
- Ecchymoses
- Uraemic 'frost'

Musculoskeletal
- Osteodystrophy
- Bone pain
- Spontaneous fractures

Immune system
- Diminished leucocyte count
- Increased susceptibility to infection

Metabolic processes
- Azotemia (↑BUN and serum creatinine)
- Hyperkalaemia
- Hyperphosphataemia
- Hypocalcaemia
- Hypermagnesia
- Acidosis
- Hyperlipidaemia
- Hyperuricaemia
- Malnutrition

Figure 8.11 Multisystem effects of uraemia.

Immune system effects

Uraemia increases the risk for infection. High levels of urea and retained metabolic wastes impair all aspects of inflammation and immune function. The WBC declines, humoral and cell-mediated immunity are impaired and phagocyte function is defective. Both the acute inflammatory response and delayed hypersensitivity responses are affected. Fever is suppressed, often delaying the diagnosis of infection.

Gastrointestinal effects

Anorexia, nausea and vomiting are the most common early symptoms of uraemia. Hiccups also are commonly experienced. Gastroenteritis is frequent. Ulcerations may affect any level of the gastrointestinal tract and contribute to an increased risk of gastrointestinal bleeding. Peptic ulcer disease is particularly common in uraemic persons. Uraemic fetor (urine-like breath odour) often associated with a metallic taste in the mouth, may develop. Uraemic fetor can further contribute to anorexia.

Neurological effects

Uraemia alters both central and peripheral nervous system function. CNS symptoms occur early and include difficulty concentrating, fatigue and insomnia. Psychotic symptoms, seizures and coma are associated with advanced uraemic encephalopathy.

Peripheral neuropathy is also common in advanced uraemia. Both the sensory and motor tracts are involved. The lower limbs are initially affected. 'Restless leg syndrome', sensations of crawling or creeping, prickling or itching of the lower legs with frequent leg movement, increases during rest. Paraesthesias and sensory loss typically occur in a 'stocking-glove' pattern. As uraemia progresses, motor function is also impaired, causing muscle weakness, decreased deep tendon reflexes and gait disturbances.

Musculoskeletal effects

Hyperphosphatemia and hypocalcaemia associated with uraemia stimulate parathyroid hormone secretion. Parathyroid hormone causes increased calcium resorption from bone. In addition, osteoblast (bone-forming) and osteoclast (bone-destructing) cell activity is affected. This bone resorption and remodelling, combined with decreased vitamin D synthesis and decreased calcium absorption from the gastrointestinal tract, lead to *renal osteodystrophy*, also known as renal rickets.

Endocrine and metabolic effects

Accumulated waste products of protein metabolism are a primary factor involved in the effects and symptoms of uraemia. Serum creatinine and BUN levels are significantly elevated. Uric acid levels are increased, contributing to an increased risk of gout.

Tissues become resistant to the effects of insulin in uraemia, leading to glucose intolerance. High blood triglyceride levels and lower than normal high-density lipoprotein (HDL) levels contribute to the accelerated atherosclerotic process.

Reproductive function is affected. Pregnancies are rarely carried to term, and menstrual irregularities are common. Reduced testosterone levels, low sperm counts and impotence affect the male person with ESRD.

Dermatologic effects

Anaemia and retained pigmented metabolites cause pallor and a yellowish hue to the skin in uraemia. Dry skin with poor turgor, a result of dehydration and sweat gland atrophy, is common. Bruising and excoriations are frequently seen. Metabolic wastes not eliminated by the kidneys may be deposited in the skin, contributing to itching or pruritus. In advanced uraemia, high levels of urea in the sweat may result in *uraemic frost*, crystallised deposits of urea on the skin.

INTERDISCIPLINARY CARE FOR CKD

Medication

Diuretics such as furosemide or other loop diuretics may be prescribed to reduce extracellular fluid volume and oedema. Diuretic therapy can also reduce hypertension and cause potassium wasting, lowering serum potassium levels. Other antihypertensive agents are used to maintain the blood pressure within normal levels, slow the progress of renal failure and prevent complications of coronary heart disease and cerebral vascular disease. ACE inhibitors are preferred, although any class of antihypertensive agent may be prescribed. Other drugs may be used to manage electrolyte imbalances and acidosis.

If the serum potassium rises to dangerously high levels, a combination of bicarbonate, insulin and glucose may be given intravenously to promote potassium movement into the cells. Sodium polystyrene sulfonate (Kayexalate), a potassium-ion exchange resin, can be given either orally or rectally (as an enema).

Folic acid and iron supplements are given to combat anaemia associated with chronic renal failure. A multiple vitamin preparation is also often prescribed, because anorexia, nausea and dietary restrictions may limit nutrient intake.

Nutrition and fluid management

As renal function declines, the elimination of water, solutes and metabolic wastes is impaired. Accumulation of these wastes in the body leads to uraemic symptoms. Instituted early in the course of CKD, dietary modifications can slow the progress of nephron destruction, reduce uraemic symptoms and help prevent complications.

Unlike carbohydrates and fats, the body is unable to store excess proteins. Unused dietary proteins are degraded into urea and other nitrogenous wastes, which are then eliminated by the kidneys. Protein-rich foods also contain inorganic ions such as hydrogen ion, phosphate and sulphites that are eliminated by the kidneys. Research has shown that restricting dietary protein intake slows the progression of CKD and reduces uraemic symptoms. Water and sodium intake are regulated to maintain the extracellular fluid volume at normal levels. Stringent water and sodium restrictions may be necessary as renal failure progresses.

Dialysis

Chronic kidney damage is usually not reversible and, if extensive, the kidneys may eventually fail completely. Dialysis or kidney transplantation will then become necessary. Persons on long-term dialysis have a higher risk for complications and death than the general population. Many have other severe diseases along with ESRD. Infection and cardiovascular disease are common causes of illness and death.

Kidney transplant

Kidney transplant has become the treatment of choice for many persons with ESRD. Kidneys are the solid organ most commonly transplanted and, to date, kidney transplantation is the most successful of transplantation procedures. Kidney transplant as a treatment for ESRD is limited primarily by availability of organs.

NURSING CARE FOR CKD

Nursing care requires a strategy to help the person and family to live with the disease. Nursing interventions aim to help the person to maintain a good quality of life with support from healthcare professionals such as nurses, doctors and the pain control team.

Health promotion

Measures to reduce the risk of CKD focus on preventing kidney disease and appropriately managing diabetes and hypertension. Promote early and effective treatment of all infections, particularly skin and pharyngeal infections caused by streptococcal bacteria. Discuss measures to reduce the risk for UTI, and stress the importance of prompt treatment to eradicate the infecting organism. Discuss the relationship between diabetes, hypertension and kidney disease. Emphasise that maintaining blood glucose levels and the blood pressure within the recommended ranges reduces the risk of adverse effects on the kidneys. Ensure that all persons with less than optimal renal function are well hydrated, particularly when a nephrotoxic drug is prescribed or anticipated. Finally, encourage the person with ESRD to investigate options for early transplantation to avoid long-term dialysis.

Nursing diagnoses and interventions

Risk for ineffective tissue perfusion: renal

As renal perfusion and nephron function fall, the kidney is less able to maintain fluid and electrolyte balance and eliminate waste products from the body. Nurses should:

+ Monitor intake and output, vital signs, including orthostatic blood pressures, and weight. *These provide important data to identify changes in fluid volume.*

PRACTICE ALERT

Weight changes are a more accurate indicator of fluid volume status in the oliguric or anuric person than intake and output measurements.

+ Restrict fluids as ordered. *As renal function declines, the ability to eliminate excess fluid is impaired.*
+ Monitor respiratory status, including lung sounds, every four to eight hours. *Fluid volume overload may lead to heart failure and possible pulmonary oedema.*
+ Monitor BUN, serum creatinine, pH, electrolytes and CBC. Report significant changes. *As renal function declines, progressive azotemia with increasing BUN and serum creatinine is seen.*
+ Report symptoms of electrolyte imbalances, such as cardiac dysrhythmias and other ECG changes, muscle tremors and possible tetany, and Kussmaul's respirations. *Symptoms of electrolyte imbalance may indicate the need for intervention.*
+ Administer prescribed medications to treat electrolyte imbalances as ordered. *Medications may be prescribed to help maintain electrolyte and acid–base balance and prevent adverse effects of imbalances.*
+ Administer prescribed antihypertensive medications. *Hypertension management is an important factor in slowing the progression of CKD.*
+ Time activities and procedures to allow rest periods. *The anaemia associated with CKD may cause significant fatigue and activity intolerance.*

Risk for imbalanced nutrition: less than body requirements

Anorexia, nausea and vomiting are common symptoms of ESRD and uraemia. The person often has a metallic taste and bad breath, which also diminish appetite. A diet restricted in protein and sodium will compound these problems. Food intake may be insufficient to meet metabolic needs. Catabolism, the breakdown of body proteins to meet energy needs, exacerbates azotemia and uraemia. Nurses should:

+ Monitor food and nutrient intake as well as episodes of vomiting. *Careful monitoring helps determine the adequacy of intake.*
+ Weigh daily before breakfast. *This provides the most accurate measurement. Remember that a gain of half a kilogram or more over a 24-hour period is more likely to reflect fluid retention than a gain in body mass.*
+ Administer antiemetic agents 30–60 minutes before eating. *Antiemetics reduce nausea and the risk of vomiting with food intake.*

+ Assist with mouth care prior to meals and at bedtime. *Mouth care improves taste, stimulates the appetite and maintains the integrity of oral mucous membranes.*

+ Serve small meals and provide between-meal snacks. *Small meals are less likely to prompt nausea and help improve food intake.*

+ Arrange for a dietary consultation. Provide preferred foods to the extent possible, and involve the person in planning daily menus. Encourage family members to bring food as dietary restrictions allow. *Providing preferred foods within restrictions promotes intake.*

+ Monitor nutritional status by tracking weight, laboratory values, such as serum albumin and BUN, and anthropometric measurements. *Indicators of impaired nutrition develop gradually and may be subtle. Careful assessment is important.*

> ## PRACTICE ALERT
>
> Monitor carefully for desired and adverse effects of all medications. Impaired renal function affects drug elimination and increases the risk for toxic effects.

Risk for infection

Chronic kidney disease affects the immune system and leucocyte function, increasing susceptibility to infection. Invasive devices required for haemodialysis or peritoneal dialysis add to this risk. The person who has had a kidney transplant remains on immunosuppressive therapy for life, further depressing the immune system and increasing the risk for infection. Nurses should:

+ Use local policies, and guidelines on infection control and good hand washing technique at all times. *Hand washing is a primary means of preventing the transfer of organisms. Persons who are on haemodialysis or who have had multiple blood transfusions to treat anaemia have an increased risk for hepatitis B, hepatitis C and HIV infection.*

+ Monitor temperature and vital signs at least every four hours. *A low-grade fever or increased pulse rate may indicate an infection in the immunosuppressed person.*

+ Monitor WBC count and differential. *Increased WBCs may indicate a bacterial infection; decreased WBCs may indicate viral infection. A shift in the differential showing more immature WBCs (bands) in circulation is another indicator of infection.*

> ## PRACTICE ALERT
>
> Monitor clarity of dialysate return. Dialysate should return clear in the person undergoing peritoneal dialysis. Cloudy dialysate may indicate peritonitis, the most common complication of peritoneal dialysis, and should be reported and cultured.

+ Culture urine, peritoneal dialysis fluid and other drainage as indicated. *Culture is done to verify the presence of pathogens.*

+ Provide good respiratory hygiene including position changes, coughing and deep breathing. *These measures improve clearance of respiratory secretions, reducing the risk for infection.*

+ Restrict visits from relatives. Teach the person and family about the risk for infection and measures to reduce the spread of infection. *The person's resistance to infection is impaired, necessitating extra caution in preventing unnecessary exposures.*

Risk for disturbed body image

Chronic disease and impaired kidney function can affect the person's body image. Haemodialysis requires an arteriovenous fistula or shunt; a permanent peritoneal catheter is required for peritoneal dialysis. While kidney transplant can restore an image of wholeness, a visible scar remains and the organ may be perceived as 'foreign'. Nurses should:

+ Involve the person in care, including meal planning, dialysis and catheter, port or incision care to the extent possible. *Involvement improves acceptance and stimulates discussion about the effect of the disease and treatment measures on the person's life.*

+ Encourage expression of feelings and concerns, accepting perceptions and feelings without criticism. *Self-expression enhances the person's self-worth and acceptance.*

+ Include the person in decision-making and encourage self-care. *Increased autonomy enhances the person's sense of control, independence and confidence.*

+ Help the person develop and achieve realistic goals. *Realistic goals allow the person to see progress.*

+ Provide positive reinforcement and feedback. *These measures support growth and adaptation.*

+ Reinforce effective coping strategies. *Reinforcement helps the person develop positive versus negative strategies for coping.*

+ Facilitate contact with a support group or other community members affected by renal failure. *The person benefits by providing and receiving support in a group of people going through similar circumstances.*

+ Refer for counselling as indicated or desired. *Counselling can help the person develop effective coping and adaptation strategies.*

> ## FAST FACT
>
> ### Complications
>
> CKD is a potentially serious condition. People with CKD are known to have an increased risk of a stroke or heart attack because of the changes that occur to the circulation.

COMMUNITY-BASED CARE

Chronic renal failure and ESRD are long-term processes that require person management. No matter what treatment option is chosen (haemodialysis, peritoneal dialysis or renal transplantation), day-to-day management falls to the person and family. Teaching for home care includes the following topics:

- Nature of the kidney disease and renal failure, including expected progression and effects.
- Monitoring weight, vital signs and temperature.
- Prescribed dietary and fluid restrictions. (Involve the person, a dietitian and the family member usually responsible for cooking. Include strategies to manage nausea and relieve thirst within allowed fluid limits.)

- How to assess and protect a fistula or shunt for haemodialysis (or the extremity to be used if one is anticipated).
- Peritoneal catheter care and the procedure for peritoneal dialysis as indicated. (Include a family member or significant other, in case the person is unable to perform the procedure independently at some time.)
- Following kidney transplant, prescribed medications, adverse effects and their management, infection prevention, graft protection and symptoms of organ rejection.

Refer to a dietitian for diet planning and counselling. If home haemodialysis is planned, the carer should have support and advice in the care of a dialysis person.

CASE STUDY 3 – Steve
NURSING CARE PLAN The person with CKD

If you remember, Mr Steve Take had a history of diabetes mellitus which is diet and medication controlled. He was feeling unwell and his GP examined him, made a provisional diagnosis of CKD and decided to refer him to the urologist at the local hospital. The urologist, after some tests and an examination, concludes that Mr Take has CKD and decides to admit him for further investigations and treatment of his CKD.

Can you list the possible investigations that may be done to confirm diagnosis? Explain how complications of diabetes mellitus and urinary tract infection could cause CKD.

Assessment

On admission to the ward, the student nurse obtains a nursing assessment. Mr Take states that his diabetes has always been difficult to control. He has had numerous hypoglycaemic episodes and has been hospitalised 'four or five times' for ketoacidosis. Recently he has developed symptoms of peripheral neuropathy and increasing retinopathy. He attributed his lack of appetite, nausea, vomiting and fatigue over the past month to 'a touch of the flu'. His weight remained stable, so he did not worry about not eating much.

Physical assessment findings include T 36.5 °C, P 96 bpm, R 20 rpm and BP 178/100 mmHg. Skin cool and dry, with minor excoriations on forearms and lower legs. Bilateral pitting oedema of lower extremities to just below the knees; fingers and hands also oedematous. Abdominal assessment essentially normal, with hypoactive bowel sounds. Urinalysis shows a specific gravity of 1.011, gross proteinuria and multiple cell casts.

Diagnoses

- Excess fluid volume related to failure of kidneys to eliminate excess body fluid.
- Imbalanced nutrition: less than body requirements related to effects of uraemia.
- Impaired skin integrity of lower extremities related to dry skin and itching.
- Risk for infection related to invasive catheters and impaired immune function.

Expected outcomes

- Adhere to the prescribed fluid restriction of 750 mL per day.
- Demonstrate reduced extracellular fluid volume by weight loss, decreased peripheral oedema, clear lung sounds and normal heart sounds.
- Consume and retain 100% of prescribed diet, including snacks.
- Demonstrate healing of lower extremity skin lesions.
- Remain free of infection.
- Demonstrate appropriate peritoneal catheter care and continuous ambulatory peritoneal dialysis (CAPD).

Planning and implementation

- Space fluids, allowing 400 mL from 0700 to 1500, 200 mL from 1500 to 2300 and 100 mL from 2300 to 0700.
- Provide mouth care at least every four hours before and after every meal.

CASE STUDY 3 – Steve	NURSING CARE PLAN The person with CKD

+ Keep sugarless hard sweets and ice cubes at the bedside; include ice consumed as fluid intake.

+ Weigh daily before breakfast; monitor vital signs, and heart and lung sounds, every four hours.

+ Document intake and output every four hours.

+ Arrange dietary consultation for menu planning.

+ Administer prescribed antiemetic one hour before meals.

+ Monitor food intake, noting percentage and types of food consumed.

+ Clean lesions on lower extremities every eight hours and assess healing.

+ Teach CAPD procedure and peritoneal catheter care.

+ Assist to identify strengths and needs in health regimen management.

Evaluation

Mr Take was hospitalised for two weeks, undergoing four haemodialysis sessions to reduce uraemic symptoms. An arteriovenous fistula has been created in his left arm in case he should need haemodialysis in the future. He begins peritoneal dialysis the second week, and by discharge he is able to

manage the catheter care and dialysis runs with the help of his wife. His heart and lung sounds are normal, and he has minimal peripheral oedema on discharge. The excoriations on his legs have healed. His temperature is normal, and no evidence of infection is noted. Mr Take remains anorexic and slightly nauseated, but is eating most of his prescribed diet and snacks. He has lost 10 pounds with excess fluid removal by dialysis, but his weight remains stable during the second week. Mr Take and his wife have been introduced to another person who has been on CAPD for several years and promises to help them with problem-solving.

Consider this . . .

● How does diabetes mellitus damage the kidneys and lead to ESRD? Why is this more significant for a person with type 1 diabetes than for someone with type 2 diabetes?

● Why do high levels of urea in the blood often cause changes in cognition and mental status? What symptoms of encephalopathy would you expect to see?

● How might Mr Take's insulin dosage and diet need to be changed with the institution of peritoneal dialysis? Why?

CASE STUDY SUMMARIES

Case Study 1. Mr Tamwar should make a good recovery but he and his wife will need a lot of support from his GP, district nurse and community stoma nurse. The hospital staff should arrange for a district nurse to visit him when he first leaves hospital and is recovering. The nurse can help to sort out any problems he and wife may have with his urostomy. He should be encouraged to get in touch with a urostomy association or Macmillan nurses for guidance and support.

Case Study 2. Mr Chapel made a good recovery from his AKI. Prior to discharge the nurse should advise him to

maintain good fluid intake, eat a healthy diet and to keep any eye on his urine output. Once the cause has been identified, Mr Chapel needs to ensure that he does not have a reoccurrence of the problem. He should visit his GP on a regular basis who can keep an eye on his condition.

Case Study 3. Mr Take is managing his CKD at home with CAPD. He is visited by the district nurse once a week who keeps an eye on the peritoneal catheter to make sure that the catheter has not dislodged and that Mr Take does not have a UTI. Mr Take has been informed of the complications associated with CAPD and he is aware that he should get in touch with his GP if he develops any symptoms such as fluid overload, breathlessness and weight gain.

CHAPTER HIGHLIGHTS

● Urinary tract infections (UTIs) are very common and are a leading complication among hospitalised persons. Short-course antibiotic therapy is appropriate for uncomplicated infections of the lower urinary tract that are not associated with the presence of an indwelling urinary catheter.

● Urinary stones can obstruct the urinary tract at any level, and cause significant pain as they move from the kidney through the ureter. Advise persons who

have had a kidney stone to maintain a good fluid intake, particularly during exercise and warm weather, to reduce the risk of further stone formation.

● The risk for bladder cancer is greater among men than women, and cigarette smoking is the most significant risk factor for bladder cancer. Most tumours can be resected transurethrally if diagnosed early, before spreading to deeper layers of the bladder wall, the lymph nodes and adjacent tissue.

- Acute kidney injury (AKI) is a frequent complication of critical illnesses, typically occurring in people with no prior history of kidney disorders. Ischaemic and nephrotoxic damage to the kidney are the most common precipitating factors for AKI.

- Chronic kidney disease (CKD) is the end stage of numerous systemic and kidney disorders, such as diabetes mellitus, systemic lupus erythematosus and chronic glomerulonephritis.

TEST YOURSELF

1. What part of the kidney processes the blood to make urine?
   a. ureter
   b. medulla
   c. pyramids
   d. nephrons

2. A person has been vomiting for four hours. What hormone is increased as a result?
   a. thyroxine
   b. renin
   c. aldosterone
   d. ADH

3. What diagnostic test can be used to determine GFR as well as glomerular damage?
   a. routine urinalysis
   b. renal scan
   c. creatinine clearance
   d. renal biopsy

4. What gland encircles the male urethra at the base of the bladder?
   a. spleen
   b. pancreas
   c. prostate
   d. adrenal

5. A person tells you of having to get up to void several times a night. You record this finding as:
   a. polyuria
   b. nocturia
   c. dysuria
   d. haematuria

6. What question would you ask a person prior to an IVP?
   a. 'Are you allergic to shellfish?'
   b. 'Do you have burning on urination?'
   c. 'Have you ever had kidney stones?'
   d. 'Why are you having this test?'

7. Before beginning the physical assessment of the urinary system, you should ask the person to:
   a. empty the bladder
   b. take several deep breaths
   c. provide a urine specimen
   d. drink several glasses of water

8. Following surgery, a person has not voided for 12 hours. What assessment should you make?
   a. palpate for bladder distention
   b. listen for bowel sounds
   c. inspect for oedema of the urethra
   d. percuss for gastric tympany

9. Of the following health problems an older woman may have, which is not normally a part of ageing of the urinary system?
   a. increased risk for haematuria
   b. decreased risk for infection
   c. urine that is darker in colour
   d. urinary incontinence

10. What assessment would you use to assess the hydration status of a person?
    a. auscultation of renal arteries
    b. palpation for skin turgor
    c. percussion for dullness over bladder
    d. palpation of both kidneys

Further resources

Kidney Research UK
www.nkrf.org.uk
Kidney Research UK is the leading UK charity dedicated to funding research aimed at finding better treatments and, ultimately, a cure for kidney disease. We think you will find this site useful as it reports studies done on drug trials and other research material for kidney diseases.

Bladder and Bowel Foundation
www.bladderandbowelfoundation.org.uk
The Bladder and Bowel Foundation website is a valuable resource to give to people who suffer from bladder and bowel problems. They also provide information for health professionals and those people who may be looking after someone with a bladder and/or bowel problem, as well as family members and friends.

National Institute for Health and Clinical Excellence (NICE)
www.nice.org.uk/Guidance/CG40

This NICE guideline covers the care of women with urinary incontinence. Students should find this site useful in their studies dealing with people with urinary problems. It gives advice on treatments for several types of urinary incontinence and related conditions, including stress incontinence and overactive bladder syndrome, which may involve urge incontinence and stress.

Urostomy Association
www.urostomyassociation.org.uk

The Urostomy Association support group website deals with current research in UTIs and is a valuable source for students when they are providing health promotion to people who are undergoing urinary diversion.

British Journal of Primary Care Nursing
http://www.bjpcn-cardiovascular.com/issue/267/

The British Journal of Primary Care Nursing deals with many topical issues related to care. We think you will find it useful if you are researching information in primary care nursing. They store articles dated back to 2004.

NHS Evidence
http://www.evidence.nhs.uk/search?q=kidney%20disease

This is a good search engine from NHS Evidence for students who want more information on various health-related topics; however, you need to register onto this website. The registration is free. We think that this site is a must for all students undertaking nursing studies.

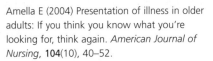

Bibliography

Amella E (2004) Presentation of illness in older adults: If you think you know what you're looking for, think again. *American Journal of Nursing*, **104**(10), 40–52.

Bland-Reid C (2004) Abdominal trauma: Dealing with the damage. *Nursing*, **34**(9), 36–42.

Consentino B (2004) Electrolyte imbalance: A matter of equilibrium. *Nursing Spectrum (New York/New Jersey Metro Edition)*, 4–6.

Cooper G and Watt E (2003) An exploration of acute care nurses' approach to assessment and management of people with urinary incontinence. *Journal of WOCN*, **30**(6), 305–313.

Dowling-Castronovo A (2004) Try this: Best practices in nursing care to older adults from the Hartford Institute for Geriatric Nursing. Urinary incontinence assessment. *Dermatology Nursing*, **16**(1), 97–98.

Eliopoulos C (2005) *Gerontological Nursing* (6th edn). Philadelphia, PA, Lippincott.

Enriquez E (2004) A nursing analysis of the causes of and approaches for urinary incontinence among elderly women in nursing homes. *Ostomy/Wound Management*, **50**(6), 24–26, 28, 30.

Hackett G (2011) *Urinary Tract Infection (UTI)*. Available at: http://www.netdoctor.co.uk/menshealth/facts/urinaryinfection.htm (accessed September 2011).

Hunt S (2002) Making sense of assessment data—continence charts. *ACCNS Journal for Community Nurses*, **7**(1), 17.

Jarvis C (2008) *Physical Examination & Health Assessment* (5th edn). St Louis, MO, Mosby.

Kasper D I, Braunwald E, Fauci A S, et al. (eds) (2005) *Harrison's Principles of Internal Medicine*. New York, McGraw Hill.

Kee J L F (2009) *Prentice Hall Handbook of Laboratory & Diagnostic Tests: With nursing implications*. Upper Saddle River, N.J, Pearson/Prentice Hall.

Kershen R and Appell R (2004) Voiding dysfunction: Evaluation and treatment after anti-incontinence surgery. *Contemporary Urology*, **16**(3), 31–32, 35–38, 41–43.

Lekan-Rutledge D (2004) Urinary incontinence strategies for frail elderly women. *Urologic Nursing*, **24**(4), 281–283, 287–302.

Mehta M (2003) Assessing the abdomen: Use sight, sound and touch to screen for abnormalities. *Nursing*, **33**(5), 54–55.

Midthun S (2004) Criteria for urinary tract infection in the elderly: Variables that challenge nursing assessment. *Urologic Nursing*, **24**(3), 157–162, 166–170, 186.

NICE (2006) *Urinary Incontinence: The management of urinary incontinence in women*, CG40. London, National Institute for Health and Clinical Excellence.

Norton P and Brubaker L (2006) Urinary incontinence. *Lancet*, Jan 7, **367**(9504), 57–67.

Palmer M (2004) Physiologic and psychologic age-related changes that affect urologic persons. *Urologic Nursing*, **24**(4), 247–252, 257.

Patient UK (2009) *Bladder Cancer*. Available at: http://www.patient.co.uk/health/Cancer-of-the-Bladder.htm (accessed September 2011).

Patient UK (2010a) *Urinary Tract Stones (Urolithiasis)*. Available at: http://www.patient.co.uk/doctor/Renal-Stones-%28Nephrolithiasis%29.htm (accessed September 2011).

Patient UK (2010b) *Acute Kidney Injury*. Available at: http://www.patient.co.uk/doctor/Acute-Renal-Failure-%28ARF%29.htm (accessed September 2011).

Perform abdominal assessment, or risk missing life-threatening trauma injury: Don't allow 'invisible' injuries to escape detection in your ED. (2004). *ED Nursing*, **7**(7), 73–75.

Porth C (2009) *Pathophysiology: Concepts of altered health states* (9th edn). Philadelphia, PA, Lippincott.

SIGN (2005a) *Management of Transitional Cell Carcinoma of the Bladder*. Edinburgh, Scottish Intercollegiate Guidelines Network.

SIGN (2005b) *Management of Urinary Incontinence in Primary Care*. Edinburgh, Scottish Intercollegiate Guidelines Network.

Welsh Cancer Intelligence and Surveillance Unit (2009) *Cancer Incidence in Wales*. Available at: http://www.wales.nhs.uk/sites3/home.cfm?orgid=242" (accessed August 2011).

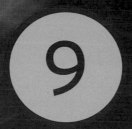

9

Caring for people with cardiovascular problems

Learning outcomes

- Describe the normal anatomy, physiology and functions of the heart and blood vessels comparing this with the disordered physiology in common cardiovascular problems.

- Discuss the coronary circulation and electrical properties of the heart to enable identification of common cardiac dysrhythmias.

- Compare and contrast the aetiology, pathophysiology and signs and symptoms of common cardiovascular problems.

- Describe the nursing care for people with cardiovascular problems.

- Discuss nursing implications for treatments used to prevent and treat **cardiovascular diseases**.

Clinical competencies

- Assess the person who presents with cardiac problems, identifying normal cardiac rhythm on an ECG.

- Monitor the individual with cardiovascular problems for expected and unexpected signs and symptoms, reporting and recording findings and results of diagnostic tests and apprising the appropriate team members of these.

- Use assessment data to plan nursing care, determine priorities of care and develop and implement individualised nursing interventions for these people.

- Provide appropriate teaching for prevention, health promotion and self-care related to cardiovascular diseases.

CASE STUDIES

Below are three case studies that you may wish to consider before, during or after you have read the chapter. There are no right or wrong answers to these case studies, but you should think about the physical, psychological and social implications.

Case Study 1 – Zahir

Mr Zahir Ahmed is a 48-year-old slightly overweight businessman who travels a great deal as part of his work, with chest pain that he describes as left-sided, sharp, stabbing pain. He has had a similar sensation before, but he was away from home at the time and did not seek medical help, dismissing the incident as stress-related as his main symptoms were breathlessness and diaphoresis (sweating). The pain presents more severely this time, just as he is preparing to go to work, and his wife urges him to go to the A & E department. He has refused to dial 999 and call the ambulance service but promises to call in to A & E on his way to work.

Case Study 2 – Mary

Mrs Mary Jones is a 58-year-old teacher who cycles to work, does not smoke and maintains a healthy lifestyle. Over the summer term, she notices that she has chest pains when cycling. Initially, she attributes this to stress, but the pains persist and her GP informs her that she is suffering from angina. Looking at Mary's family history, it would suggest that there is a genetic link as her father and uncle also had what has loosely been termed in the family as 'heart problems'.

Case Study 3 – John

Mr John Davis is a 61-year-old bus driver, who has woken up with chest pain and is feeling breathless. A week ago, he returned from a holiday in Bangkok. He and his wife were upgraded on their return flight and, as there was more leg room on the aeroplane, John opted not to put on his flight socks, claiming he had plenty of room to move. On boarding the flight, there was alcohol served and also more alcohol with the in-flight meal, which John had. On landing, John pulled up with cramp-like pain in his left leg, which eased slightly with rest. John is persuaded by his wife to see the GP. He was a cigarette smoker but gave up cigarettes 20 years ago, favouring the occasional cigar ever since.

INTRODUCTION

The heart is considered a key organ in the body; without a heart beat we are deemed to have died. It is also associated with emotions like love, being the key emblem on Valentine Day's cards, and if love is not reciprocated we claim to have had our hearts broken. In this chapter, the focus is on how the heart works and the problems that are encountered when heart function is impaired under the broad heading of cardiovascular disease (CVD); therefore, aspects of peripheral vascular diseases are included. The distinctions between acute and chronic diseases are blurred because few heart attacks occur in the absence of primary CVD which may have developed silently over the years.

The heart, a muscular pump, beats an average of 70 times per minute, or once every 0.86 second, every minute of a person's life. This continuous pumping moves blood through the body, nourishing tissue cells and removing waste products. Impaired blood flow to the heart muscle, called the myocardium, changes in the conduction of electrical impulses through the heart and structural changes in the heart itself affect the heart's ability to fulfil its major purpose: to pump enough blood to meet the body's demand for oxygen and nutrients. This affects the person's ability to participate in exercise and activities of daily living (ADLs). Disruptions in cardiac function affect other organ systems, potentially leading to organ system failure and death.

FAST FACTS

Heart disease

- Approximately 124 000 people in the UK have a 'heart attack' each year.

- CVD is the major cause of death in the UK; figures are greater than those for cancer, with about a quarter attributed to death from strokes and the rest due to heart disease.

- Men are more likely to die of heart disease than women, but this trend is changing, and the gap is narrowing.

- **Coronary heart disease** costs the NHS £3.2 billion a year.

Source: BHF 2010.

Heart disease is the main cause of death in the UK; one in five men and one in eight women die as a result of heart disease each year (British Heart Foundation Statistics Database, www.bhf.org.uk/heart-health/statistics.aspx).

The major contributing factors for all heart problems are (BHF 2010):

- smoking – 24% of men and 21% of women still smoke;
- obesity, which has increased 75% in men and 45% in women since 1994;
- diabetes, incidences of which have more than doubled in men and women over the last five years (see Chapter 6);
- lack of physical activity, with only 40% of women and 28% of men achieving recommended levels of exercise;
- living in socially deprived circumstances, which can increase risk of dying from heart disease by 60%;
- ethnicity – South Asians are the most vulnerable group in the UK.

ANATOMY, PHYSIOLOGY AND FUNCTIONS OF THE HEART

The heart is a hollow, conical organ approximately the size of an adult's fist, weighing between 230 and 340 g, located in the mediastinal cavity of the thorax, between the vertebral column and the sternum, flanked laterally by the lungs. Two-thirds of the heart mass lies to the left of the sternum; the top lies beneath the second rib, and the pointed end (apex) is approximate with the fifth intercostal space, midpoint to the clavicle.

LAYERS OF THE HEART WALL AND BLOOD VESSELS

The heart wall consists of three layers of tissue:

- the epicardium or pericardium;
- the myocardium;
- the endocardium.

The pericardium

This is a double layer of fibroserous membrane, which encases the heart and anchors it to surrounding structures, forming the pericardial sac. The snug fit prevents the heart from overfilling with blood. The outermost layer is the parietal pericardium, and the visceral pericardium (or epicardium) adheres to the heart surface. The small space between the visceral and parietal layers is called the pericardial cavity. A lubricating fluid produced in this space cushions the heart as it beats.

The myocardium

This middle layer of the heart wall consists of specialised cardiac muscle cells (cardiac myocytes) that provide the bulk of contractile heart muscle. These cells are specialised because they are interlocked and work as a single unit.

The endocardium

This inner covering is a membrane composed of three layers; the innermost layer is made up of smooth endothelial cells that line the inside of the heart's chambers and great vessels. The middle layers (inbetween the endothelial cells and the myocardium) are composed of connective and elastic tissue. The thickness of the endocardium alters depending on which part of the heart it is covering and it also forms the heart valves. The smooth endothelial cell lining continues from the heart and lines the blood vessels.

ARTERIES AND VEINS

These consist mainly of three layers:

- *tunica intima*, the inner layer called endothelium;
- *tunica media*, the middle layer of smooth muscle and elastic connective tissue;
- *tunica externa*, the outer connective tissue casing.

The thickness of each layer and its composition depends on the tasks particular vessels undertake. Blood vessels get smaller and smaller, ending in capillaries in the tissues which are made up of just the inner tunica intima, which allows the transfer of gases and nutrients to cross the barrier it presents.

CHAMBERS AND VALVES OF THE HEART

The heart has four hollow chambers, two upper atria and two lower ventricles separated longitudinally by the interventricular septum (see Figure 9.1).

The right atrium receives deoxygenated blood from the veins of the body: the superior vena cava returns blood from the body area above the diaphragm, the inferior vena cava returns blood from the body below and the coronary sinus drains blood from the heart. The left atrium receives freshly oxygenated blood from the lungs through the pulmonary veins.

The right ventricle receives deoxygenated blood from the right atrium and pumps it through the pulmonary artery to the pulmonary capillary bed for oxygenation in the lungs. The newly oxygenated blood then travels through the pulmonary veins to the left atrium, entering the left atrium and crossing the mitral (bicuspid) valve into the left ventricle. Blood is then pumped out of the aorta to the arterial circulation.

The atria are separated from the ventricles by the two atrioventricular (AV) valves; the tricuspid valve is on the right side, and the mitral valve is on the left. The flaps of each of these

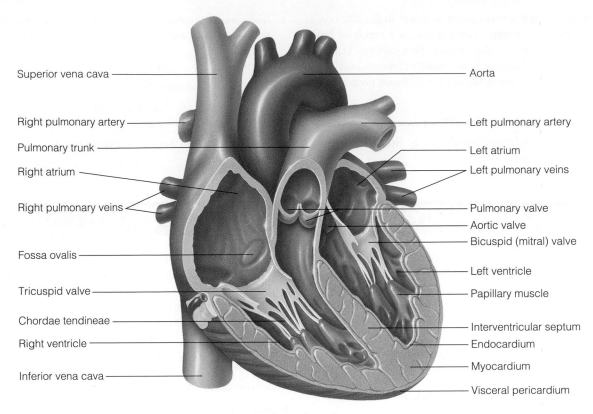

Figure 9.1 The internal anatomy of the heart – frontal section.

valves are anchored to the papillary muscles of the ventricles by the chordae tendineae, permitting blood to only flow in one direction, preventing backflow. The ventricles are connected to their great vessels by the semilunar valves. On the right, the pulmonary valve joins the right ventricle with the pulmonary artery. On the left, the aortic valve joins the left ventricle to the aorta.

Closure of the AV valves at the onset of contraction (systole) produces the first heart sound, or S_1 (characterised by the syllable 'lub'); closure of the semilunar valves at the onset of relaxation (diastole) produces the second heart sound, or S_2 (characterised by the syllable 'dub'), resulting in the characteristic sound of the heart of lub dub, lub dub for each cycle.

SYSTEMIC, PULMONARY AND CORONARY CIRCULATION

Each side of the heart both receives and ejects blood simultaneously, making the heart a double pump. Blood enters the right atrium and moves to the pulmonary bed at the same time that blood is entering the left atrium. The circulatory system has two parts: the pulmonary circulation and the systemic circulation. In addition, the heart muscle itself is supplied with blood via the coronary circulation (see Table 9.1 and Figure 9.2).

Blood flow through the coronary arteries is regulated by several factors:

Table 9.1 Blood circulation pathways

Systemic circulation	Pulmonary circulation	Coronary circulation
• Consists of the left atrium, ventricle, aorta, arteries and capillaries, the systemic venous system and venae cavae • Is a high-pressure system moving blood to the body's peripheries	• Consists of the right atrium, ventricle, pulmonary artery, capillaries and vein • Is a low-pressure system moving deoxygenated blood into the lungs for gaseous exchange and returning oxygenated blood to left atrium	• Consists of left and right coronary arteries originating from the base of the aorta and branching out over the myocardium • Coronary arteries fill during ventricular relaxation and veins drain deoxygenated blood into the coronary sinus which empties into the right side of the heart

contract and eject blood into the pulmonary and systemic circuits. Systole is followed by a relaxation phase or diastole, during which they refill, the atria contract and the myocardium is perfused. The cycle normally occurs 60–100 times per minute in adults, measured as the heart rate (HR).

During diastole, the volume in the ventricles increases to about 120 mL (the **end-diastolic volume**); at the end of systole, about 50 mL of blood remains in the ventricles (the **end-systolic volume**). The difference between the end-diastolic volume and the end-systolic volume is called the **stroke volume** (SV). SV ranges from 60–100 mL/beat and averages about 70 mL/beat in an adult. The **cardiac output** (CO) is the amount of blood pumped by the ventricles into the pulmonary and systemic circulations in 1 minute. Multiplying SV by HR determines the cardiac output: $SV \times HR = CO$.

The average adult cardiac output ranges from 4–8 L/min and is an indicator of how well the heart is functioning as a pump. If the heart cannot pump effectively, cardiac output and tissue perfusion are decreased; body tissues do not receive enough blood and oxygen (carried in the blood on haemoglobin) and become ischaemic (deprived of oxygen). If the tissues do not receive enough blood flow to maintain the functions of the cells, the cells die.

Cardiac output is influenced by:

- activity levels;
- metabolic rate;
- stress responses – both physiological and psychological;
- age;
- body size.

The heart's ability to respond to the body's changing need for cardiac output is called **cardiac reserve.**

Heart rate is affected by both direct (sympathetic and parasympathetic nerves) and indirect autonomic nervous system stimulation. The sympathetic nervous system acts like a car accelerator and increases the heart rate, whereas the parasympathetic vagal tone acts like car brakes and slows the heart rate. Reflex regulation of the heart rate in response to systemic blood pressure occurs through activation of sensory receptors known as baroreceptors or pressure receptors located in the carotid sinus, aortic arch, venae cavae and pulmonary veins.

If heart rate increases, cardiac output increases (up to a point) even if there is no change in stroke volume. Rapid heart rates can decrease the amount of time available for ventricular filling during diastole and cardiac output falls because of this, which limits the amount of blood entering the ventricles, thus decreasing stroke volume. Coronary artery perfusion decreases because the coronary arteries fill during diastole. Cardiac output decreases during bradycardia if stroke volume stays the same, because the number of cardiac cycles is decreased.

In diastole, the cardiac muscle stretches to accommodate the filling of the ventricles, and this tension is called **preload**. The greater the stretch, the greater the capacity of the ventricles when filling and a greater contraction is needed to empty the ventricles. This is known as Starling's Law of the Heart.

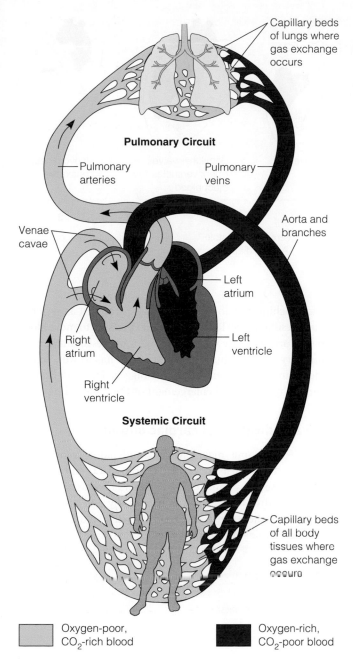

Figure 9.2 Pulmonary and systemic circulation.

- aortic pressure;
- heart rate – with most blood flowing when the heart is relaxed (diastole);
- metabolic activity of the heart;
- blood vessel tone (constriction or dilation).

THE CARDIAC CYCLE AND CARDIAC OUTPUT

The cardiac cycle (Figure 9.3) is one heart beat where the heart is relaxed whilst filling and then contracts. Ventricular filling is followed by ventricular systole, during which the ventricles

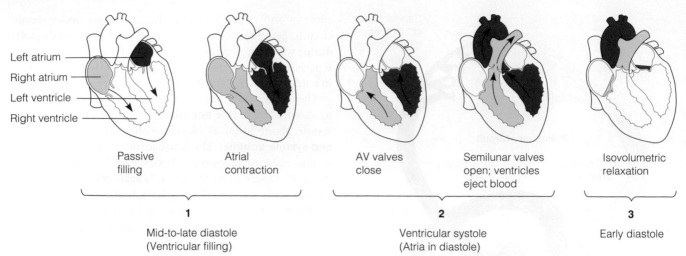

Left atrium				
Right atrium				
Left ventricle				
Right ventricle				

| Passive filling | Atrial contraction | AV valves close | Semilunar valves open; ventricles eject blood | Isovolumetric relaxation |

| **1** | | **2** | | **3** |
| Mid-to-late diastole (Ventricular filling) | | Ventricular systole (Atria in diastole) | | Early diastole |

Figure 9.3 The three events of the cardiac cycle.

Haemorrhage affects preload as there is a drop in the blood volume circulating, whereas renal disease and heart failure can increase the preload because of water retention in the circulatory system.

Preload affects contractility, the ability of the heart muscle to alter its tension. Poor contractility of the heart muscle reduces the forward flow of blood from the heart, increases the ventricular pressures from accumulation of blood volume and reduces cardiac output. Increased contractility may stress the heart.

Afterload is the force the ventricles must use to eject their blood volume into the arterial system ahead. The right ventricle must generate enough tension to open the pulmonary valve and eject its volume into the low-pressure pulmonary arteries; this is measured as pulmonary vascular resistance (PVR). The left ventricle, in contrast, ejects its load by overcoming the pressure behind the aortic valve and is measured as systemic vascular resistance (SVR). It takes greater pressure to move blood into the aorta, because it is thicker and more resistant than the pulmonary arteries; thus, the left ventricle has to work much harder than the right ventricle and is bigger; overwork leads to hypertrophy (abnormal enlargement of the myocardium).

Clinical indicators of cardiac output

Critically ill people may have haemodynamic monitoring catheters used to measure cardiac output (CO) and measure their response to treatment. The catheters measure atrial and venous pressures peripherally and centrally and blood gases and determine how well the heart is working. Figure 9.4 shows a haemodynamic monitoring system.

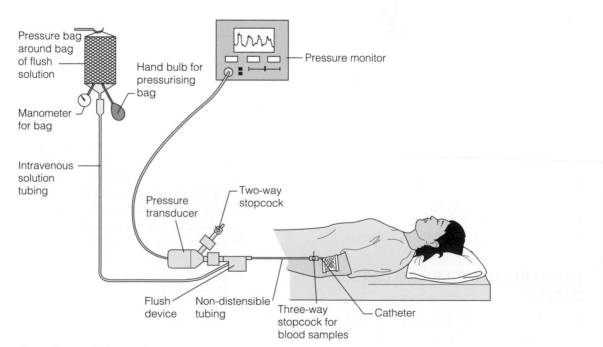

Figure 9.4 Haemodynamic monitoring system.

IN PRACTICE

Electrocardiogram (ECG)

The ECG is a graphic record of the heart's activity depicting the electrical impulses produced during a cardiac cycle and portraying them as a wave on graph paper through a heated stylus (Figure 9.5). The paper is marked at standard intervals that represent time and voltage or amplitude. Each small box is 1 mm^2. The recording speed of the standard ECG is 25 mm/second, so each small box represents 0.04 second. Five small boxes horizontally and vertically make one large box, equivalent to 0.20 second. Five large boxes represent one full second. Measured vertically, each small box represents 0.1 mV. Thus by counting the patterns occurring in the boxes it is possible to calculate heart beats per minute.

When the heart beats, the wave of electrical activity produced by the cells passes through the body; thus an electrode placed on an arm or leg can detect the signal of electrical activity from the heart beat. The ECG is based on the idea of an equilateral triangle, with the heart at the centre and the three points of the triangle being the right arm, left arm and left leg, which is where three electrodes are placed. The heart activity is then measured from three different approaches.

A standard ECG has 12 measurements referred to as leads (Figure 9.6):

- Lead 1 measures the electrical activity between the right and left arm.
- Lead 2 measures the electrical activity between the right arm and left leg.
- Lead 3 measures the electrical activity between the left leg and left arm.

These are called bipolar leads, i.e. between two points.

Leads 4 to 6 are unipolar, measuring between each point and the heart and are referred to as aV$_r$ (from the right arm), aV$_l$ (from the left arm) and aV$_f$ (from the left leg). A separate 4th electrode is placed on the chest wall at six specific points around the heart. The measurements are termed as the precordial leads and numbered V$_1$–V$_6$.

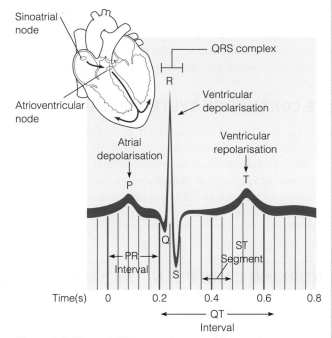

Figure 9.5 Normal ECG waveform and intervals.

The wave forms produced indicate if there is damage to the myocardium and any changes in heart rhythm. A normal wave would have P, Q, R, S, T waves and intervals demonstrating the wave of electrical activity passing through the heart with each cycle.

Looking at an ECG recording and counting the numbers of PQRS complexes in a six second strip and multiplying by 10 provides an estimate of the heart rate and its regularity. If the P wave is missing it would suggest that the rhythm does not originate from the sinus node. After every P wave a QRS complex should follow if it does not, then impulses are not spreading through from the atrial ventricular node. Extra (ectopic) beats can be seen as disrupting the pattern of electrical waves.

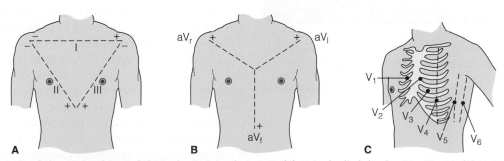

Figure 9.6 Leads of the 12-lead ECG. (A) Bipolar limb leads, I, II, III. **(B)** Unipolar limb leads, aV$_r$. aV$_l$, aV$_f$. (C) Unipolar precordial leads, V$_1$ to V$_6$.

Clinical indicators of low CO may be seen by changes in organ function that result from reduced blood flow; for example, a decrease in blood flow to the brain results in altered levels of consciousness; a decrease in blood flow to the kidneys results in a decreased urinary output.

CO varies with body size. By taking measurements of a person's weight and height, it is possible to work out the body surface area and cardiac index, which is the output required to perfuse the tissues of that person properly with blood.

THE CONDUCTION SYSTEM OF THE HEART

The main function of cardiac cells is to contract, and this is initiated by electrical changes across the cell membranes where ions, such as sodium, chlorine, potassium and calcium, move across and into and out of the cells acting as an ionic pump. Movement of ions across cell membranes causes the electrical impulse that stimulates muscle contraction. This electrical activity, called the *action potential*, produces the waveforms represented on **electrocardiogram** (ECG) strips.

Cardiac muscle cells possess an inherent characteristic of self-excitation, enabling them to initiate and transmit impulses independent of a stimulus. Specialised areas of myocardial cells exert a controlling influence in this electrical pathway. The sinoatrial node is called the pacemaker as this is where the wave of excitation starts and spreads down towards the atrial ventricular node and is seen on the ECG as the P wave. As the wave spreads from the atrial ventricular node, there is a slight pause on the ECG called the P–R interval. The wave of excitation or depolarisation then passes through the bundle of His into the Purkinje fibres in the ventricles causing the ventricles to contract, which is seen as the QRS complex on the ECG. The last electrical wave on the ECG is the T wave which is the ventricles repolarising or returning to the resting phase. Once stimulated, the cardiac muscle mass acts as one, and does not respond to additional stimuli until the contraction stops.

NURSING CARE PLAN The person having an ECG

Although taking an ECG recording is common practice in healthcare settings and seen frequently in TV medical drama programmes, not everyone has had a recording taken and, as the focus is on their heart, they may be anxious which will affect their heart rate and the recording will not reflect a true state. In all three case studies, the people may well be anxious. It is therefore important to check with them whether they have had this procedure before and to reassure those who have not that it is a painless procedure. The person may be lying down or semi-recumbent if they are breathless. They need to be comfortable and relaxed as they need to lie still whilst the recording is being made.

Electrodes will be placed on the right and left arms and the left leg, and the skin needs to be clean and intact before it is fixed to the skin. These are usually disposable and adhere to the skin easily. The leads are then attached to the electrodes before recording can take place. The chest area needs to be exposed for the chest electrode application and the person's modesty must be protected at all times.

Once the recording has been taken. The electrodes may be left on for further recordings but if they are not needed, they need to be removed and the area cleaned with a tissue as there is usually residual jelly from the electrode left on the skin. The jelly aids conduction of the electrical impulses from the skin.

Do not alarm the person by interpreting the findings at the bedside; take the recording away for consultation with the medical team out of the person's hearing and return to the person once the assessment has been completed.

Cardiovascular disease

Cardiovascular disease (CVD) is a generic term for disorders of the heart and blood vessels and can be divided into:

- coronary heart disease (CHD), which accounts for nearly 50% of deaths from cardiovascular disease;
- peripheral vascular diseases;
- strokes (see Chapter 13).

RISK FACTORS FOR DEVELOPING CVD

There are several risk factors for developing CVD, and these are mainly linked with lifestyle. *Hyperlipidaemia* is an abnormally high level of blood lipids and lipoproteins. Low-density lipoproteins (LDLs, memory cue: LDLs = **l**ess **d**esirable **l**ipoproteins) carry 70% of plasma cholesterol and promote **atherosclerosis**, a disease of the arteries, because LDLs are oxidised depositing cholesterol on artery walls. If cholesterol levels in the plasma rise over 6.2 mmol/L, it increases the risk of CVD. In contrast, high-density lipoproteins (HDLs or **h**ighly **d**esirable **l**ipoproteins) help clear cholesterol from the arteries, transporting it to the liver for excretion. HDL levels above 1.3 mmol/L have a protective effect, reducing the risk of CVD; in contrast, HDL levels lower than 1.3 mmol/L is associated with an increased risk for CVD. Triglycerides, compounds of fatty acids bound to glycerol and used for fat storage by the body, are carried on very low-density lipoprotein (VLDL) molecules. Elevated triglycerides also contribute to the risk for CVD.

Monounsaturated fats, found in olives, canola (rapeseed oil) and peanut oils, actually lower LDL and cholesterol levels. Certain cold-water fish, such as tuna, salmon and mackerel, contain high levels of omega-3 fatty acids, which help raise HDL levels and decrease serum triglycerides, total serum cholesterol and blood pressure.

Hypertension is consistent blood pressure readings greater than 140 mmHg systolic or 90 mmHg diastolic. Normally, adults have a blood pressure reading of 120/80 mmHg. Hypertensive people may also be overweight, consume high levels of sodium and alcohol and may also smoke. To lessen their risks of further complications, they would need to lose weight, reduce consumption of alcohol (women having no more than 175 ml of 13% strength wine (one glass) a day and men no more than one and half pints of beer) and salt, increase levels of exercise (walk for 30 minutes a day briskly) and increase consumption of fruit and vegetables.

Diabetes mellitus, a metabolic disease (see Chapter 6) involving a lack of or insufficient amount of insulin in the body to clear excess glucose from the body, contributes to CVD in several ways; it affects the endothelium of blood vessels, contributing to the process of atherosclerosis. Hyperglycaemia and hyperinsulinaemia, altered platelet function, elevated fibrinogen levels and inflammation also are thought to play a role. It is estimated that approximately 75% of diabetics (mainly those with non-insulin-dependent diabetes mellitus) will die of CVD (Aaronson and Ward 2007).

Cigarette smoking is a significant contributor to CVD, killing over half the people who indulge. Smoking:

- causes the development of atherosclerosis because it lowers HDLs;
- increases the potential of blood to clot;
- increases coronary artery spasm;
- raises the heart rate and blood pressure;
- reduces the ability of the blood cells to carry oxygen around the body, thus reducing the supply of oxygen to the heart muscle.

These risks are not reduced with the use of low-tar cigarettes.

Obesity (excess adipose tissue) and physical inactivity increases the risk for CVD because people have higher rates of hypertension, diabetes and hyperlipidaemia. The best indicator of central obesity is the waist circumference, where the waist circumference is larger than the hips. Sixty per cent of the world's population does not engage in 30 minutes of physical activity daily as recommended by the World Health Organization (WHO).

Diet is a risk factor for CVD, independent of fat and cholesterol intake. Diets high in fruits, vegetables, whole grains and unsaturated fatty acids appear to have a protective effect. The underlying factors are not clear, but probably relate to nutrients such as antioxidants, folic acid, other B vitamins, omega-3 fatty acids and other unidentified micronutrients.

Ethnicity is a significant factor in developing CVD and there is evidence that certain ethnic populations are more at risk. Asians are most severely affected, irrespective of where they live, because of their diet and lifestyle (Wachtel *et al.* 2010).

Gender issues

Researchers have focused more on men than women in cardiovascular trials and have assumed that men and women's disease presentation is similar; however, it would appear that women present more with atypical symptoms and are inclined to dismiss symptoms because they are intermittent or attributed to another cause. Women have different risk factors than men; they are less likely to engage in regular exercise and may have had oral contraceptives. In view of this, Albarran (2007) advocates that healthcare professionals take a more proactive approach when meeting women who may have CVD and that assessment should include gender-specific questions relating to use of contraceptives and exercise.

At menopause, serum HDL levels drop and LDL levels rise, increasing the risk of CVD. Early menopause (natural or surgically induced) increases the risk of CVD and myocardial infarction (MI). Women who have the ovaries removed before the age of 35 without hormone replacements are eight times more likely to have an MI than women experiencing natural menopause. Oestrogen replacement therapy reduces the risk of CVD in these women. Oral contraceptives increase the risk for myocardial infarction, particularly in women who also smoke, because they promote clotting, affect blood pressure and raise serum lipids.

Socioeconomic factors also place women at risk of CVD because women from lower socioeconomic groups tend to be unemployed, smoke more (smoking is perceived as a coping mechanism that also prevents weight gain) and engage less in physical activity. Walking in local parks seems to be considered unsafe in some deprived areas, thus limiting accessibility of this area of exercise.

Men are four times more at risk than premenopausal women of having an MI, and this is attributed to the protective nature of oestrogen and progesterone. Peate and Gault (2001) offer an interesting rationale for why men are more at risk of CVD, stating that men are generally risk-takers. Although not wishing to stereotype men, there are cultural and social pressures to behave in a typically 'male' role, to be strong, independent and act tough. They draw attention to statistics demonstrating that men do not access healthcare services as often as women and delay seeking advice until the condition requires either emergency treatment or is untreatable.

Consider this . . .
Looking at the three case studies and the risk factors of CVD listed above, which of the three people are the more serious contenders for developing CVD?

Risk factor management

Conservative management of CVD focuses on risk factor modification, including smoking, diet, exercise and management of contributing conditions. People who stop smoking reduce their risk by 50%, regardless of how long they smoked before this. For women, the risk becomes equivalent to a non-smoker within three to five years of smoking cessation.

IN PRACTICE

Cognitive behaviour therapy (CBT) and smoking cessation

People think and talk about giving up smoking; many try to give up and fail, sometimes doing this several times only to relapse again. CBT helps the smoker to examine their views and beliefs about all aspects of life and how they respond to stressful situations, and provides them with information regarding the consequences smoking has for their health and wellbeing.

The therapist and smoker devise an action plan of activities that will help them resist the urge to smoke and live without cigarettes and consider strategies or alternative behaviour patterns that replace the gratification given when smoking.

The smoker meets with the therapist regularly, once a week initially, for support and advice.

Source: Chummum 2009.

Alterations to diet by reducing intake of saturated fats such as those found in whole milk products, red meat and coconut oil lessens the risk of atheromatous plaque formation in the lining of the arteries. Increased intake of antioxidant nutrients (vitamin E, in particular) and foods rich in anti-oxidants (fruits and vegetables) appears to increase HDL levels and have a protective effect on CVD. A cardioprotective diet should include the following:

- two portions of fish a week, with one being oily fish like mackerel;
- five portions of fruit and vegetables a day, making up at least a third of the daily diet, with the exception of potatoes;
- low fat diet – fats used should be high in monounsaturated fatty acid, for example rapeseed or olive oil;
- limit salt intake;
- limit alcohol intake.

Regular physical exercise reduces the risk for CVD in several ways:

- It lowers VLDL, LDL and triglyceride levels and raises HDL levels.
- It reduces the blood pressure and insulin resistance.

Unless contraindicated, all people with CVD are encouraged to participate in at least 30 minutes of moderate intensity physical activity five to six days each week. To achieve weight loss and prevent weight gain, 60–90 minutes of moderate intensity exercise daily is recommended.

A short exercise programme for people with **chronic heart failure** undertaken over 12 weeks, where the person walks for six minutes a day, improves their sense of wellbeing and physical condition. Exercise does not have to be unduly strenuous to be beneficial and improve overall wellbeing.

DISORDERS OF MYOCARDIAL PERFUSION

The person with coronary heart disease (CHD)

Approximately 2.7 million people in the UK have CHD (BHF 2010). CHD is the major cause of premature death (i.e. people under the age of 75 years), although death rates in those aged under 65 years have fallen by 45%. However, the numbers of those living with CHD has risen because more people are living longer (Patient UK 2010). It usually results from atherosclerosis which occludes the coronary arteries and can result in people experiencing angina, myocardial ischaemia and **acute coronary syndrome** (ACS).

Research (Wrigley and Lathlean 2010) has established that CHD has a familial pattern. There are three key reasons for this:

- Families share their environment, especially in their formative stages.
- Lifestyle patterns are repeated in families, especially dietary patterns and obesity.
- Families share similar socioeconomic status, and CHD is more evident in families in lower socioeconomic groups.

Therefore, it is important that any assessment of people with suspected heart disease includes a full family history and assessment of lifestyle behaviours, which should include eating, drinking and smoking habits, employment history and psychological wellbeing.

Atherosclerosis

This is a progressive disease, and a major contributor to CHD, that can start early in life and is characterised by the formation of plaques, which are a collection of lipids collected between the intimal and medial layers of large and midsize arteries. Factors that affect the development of plaques are:

- age;
- gender;
- genetic makeup.

Pathophysiology

The formation of atheroma plaques is complex; when the endothelial lining of the vessels becomes damaged, macrophages attach themselves and infiltrate the damaged cell. LDLs also infiltrate and are digested by the macrophages resulting in the formation of foam cells, in which a collection of fats, cholesterol, platelets and cellular debris accumulates. These plaques can be covered with a protective fibrous cap. Problems occur when this fibrous capsule tears and the contents come into contact with the blood, because the small molecular weight glycoproteins in the cells initiate clotting. Plaques which are unlikely to rupture are called stable; they are usually calcified. Unstable plaques have a larger fatty core, and it is believed that macrophages in these plaques secrete proteolytic enzymes which break down the capsule. These plaques are more common in acute coronary syndrome (ACS) than in angina.

Dysfunction of the endothelial lining of the blood vessels is significant in various diseases:

- hypertension;
- coronary artery disease;
- peripheral artery disease;
- diabetes;
- chronic heart failure;
- chronic renal failure.

The endothelial lining of the blood vessels produces compounds that maintain the integrity of the lining and the health of the vessels, and these substances affect the contractility of the vessels and maintain homeostasis. Damage occurs as a result of infection or inflammation from substances being transported in the blood. This is known because various pathogens have been found within the plaques at post mortem. Plaques in the endothelial lining narrow the lumen of the vessels, thus affecting blood flow, which leads to ischaemia. Plaques also affect the elasticity of the vessels.

Plaque formation may be *eccentric*, located in a specific, asymmetric region of the vessel wall, or *concentric*, involving the entire vessel circumference. Signs of the process usually do not appear until about 75% of the arterial lumen has been occluded.

Men are more likely to be affected than women, probably because oestrogen and progesterone provide protection. After menopause, this no longer remains the case.

Myocardial ischaemia

Myocardial ischaemia occurs when the oxygen supply is inadequate to meet metabolic demands; this depends on coronary perfusion and myocardial workload. Perfusion of the heart muscle with oxygenated blood can be affected by several different mechanisms:

- One or more vessels may be partially occluded by large, stable areas of atheromatous plaque.
- Platelets can aggregate in narrowed vessels, forming a thrombus and blocking the artery.
- Normal or already narrowed vessels may go into spasm.
- A drop in blood pressure may lead to inadequate blood flow through coronary vessels.

Pathophysiology

The imbalance between myocardial blood supply and demand causes temporary and reversible myocardial ischaemia. Obstruction of a coronary artery deprives cells of oxygen and nutrients in that region of the heart. Reduced oxygen causes cells to switch from aerobic metabolism to anaerobic metabolism, causing lactic acid to build up. This affects cell membrane permeability, releasing substances such as histamine, kinins and specific enzymes that stimulate terminal nerve fibres in the cardiac muscle, sending pain impulses to the central nervous system. Pain radiates to the upper body because the heart shares the same dermatome (nerve supply). Return of adequate circulation (reperfusion) provides the nutrients needed by cells, and clears the waste products. If ischaemia lasts longer than 30 minutes, irreversible damage leading to necrosis of the heart muscle occurs in that area.

Silent myocardial ischaemia, or asymptomatic ischaemia, is thought to be common in people with CHD, precipitated by either activity or mental stress which increases the heart rate and blood pressure, increasing myocardial oxygen demand. Like symptomatic angina, silent myocardial ischaemia is associated with an increased chance of myocardial infarction; silent MI is more common in older people or those who are diabetic.

Signs and symptoms

- Nausea.
- Dizziness.
- Belching.
- Indigestion.

INTERDISCIPLINARY CARE FOR CHD

Diagnostic tests

The primary test used to identify the risk of coronary artery disease (CAD) is a measurement of lipid components of cholesterol, triglycerides and lipolipids in the blood. The ratio of HDLs to LDLs should be one to three.

Other tests include:

- Chest x-rays to determine size and position of the heart.
- Stress and exercise tests; for example, a treadmill exercise test to determine heart function.

- Myocardial perfusion scintigraphy (MPS); an imaging technique whereby a radioactive tracer (thallium – 201 or technetium – 99) is injected at rest and/or during exertion and the uptake is monitored on a gamma camera which rotates around the patient for 20 minutes. This procedure is currently reserved for those for whom a treadmill stress and exercise test is contraindicated.

- Coronary angiography (often called cardiac catheterisation, but this is a misnomer as catherterisation refers to the insertion of the catheter, whilst angiography is the test) evaluates the coronary arteries. A catheter introduced into the femoral or radial artery is threaded into the coronary artery. A radiopaque contrast medium allows visualisation of the main coronary branches, the efficacy with which the valves and ventricles are functioning and any abnormalities, such as stenosis or obstruction. The procedure is usually completed as a day case.

- Electron beam computed tomography (EBCT) creates a three-dimensional image of the heart and coronary arteries that can reveal plaque and other abnormalities.

Treatment

Statins (drugs that combine with bile salts in the intestine and prevent the absorption of cholesterol into the bloodstream) are used to counteract hyperlipidaemia as they lower LDL levels; they can cause myopathy (muscle weakness) so reporting muscle weakness is important, and pain and liver function tests are monitored as enzyme levels can increase. Statins on their own do not remove all the cholesterol from the atheromatous plaques; they should be combined with a low-fat diet.

The person with stable angina

Stable angina (or angina pectoris) is chest pain resulting from reduced coronary blood flow, causing a temporary imbalance between myocardial blood supply and demand. This may be due to CHD, atherosclerosis or vessel constriction. Hyper-metabolic conditions such as exercise, stimulant abuse (e.g., cocaine), hyperthyroidism and emotional stress can increase myocardial oxygen demand, precipitating angina. Anaemia, heart failure, ventricular hypertrophy or pulmonary diseases may affect blood and oxygen supplies as well, causing angina.

Pathophysiology and signs and symptoms of stable angina

Three types of angina have been identified:

- *Stable angina*, which is the most common form and is directly linked to increased activity or stress, exposure to cold and is relieved by rest and drugs.

- *Prinzmetal's (variant) angina*, which is not necessarily related to CHD and atherosclerosis, occurs unpredictably, unrelated to activity, often at night and is caused by coronary artery spasm; the exact mechanism is unknown.

- *Unstable angina*, where the pain is unpredictable and can occur at rest. The episodes increase in frequency, severity and duration and patients are at increased risk of myocardial infarction.

These last two are classified as ACS (see page 319).

The cardinal sign of angina is chest pain precipitated by an identifiable event, such as physical activity, strong emotion, stress, eating a heavy meal or exposure to cold. The classic sequence of angina is activity–pain, rest–relief. The person affected may describe the pain as a tight, squeezing, heavy pressure or as a constricting sensation. It characteristically begins beneath the sternum and may radiate to the jaw, neck, shoulder or arm; however, it may be felt in the epigastric region, or back. Anginal pain usually occurs in a *crescendo–decrescendo* pattern (increasing to a peak, then gradually decreasing), typically lasting two to five minutes. It is generally relieved by rest. ECG changes can be noted as depicted in Figure 9.7.

> **Consider this . . .**
>
> Chest pain can indicate other conditions besides myocardial infarction.
>
> - Pain that is worse on lying down could indicate pericarditis and retro-sternal pain with shortness of breath would indicate a pulmonary embolism.
> - Sometimes indigestion can be interpreted as chest pain.
>
> In all three case studies, the patients have chest pain; however, the pattern and degree of pain is different in each case. What questions would you ask to determine the different experiences?

Women frequently present with atypical symptoms of angina, including indigestion or nausea, vomiting and upper back pain.

The severity of angina can be graded by the degree to which it limits activities:

- Class I angina is prompted by strenuous, rapid or prolonged physical exertion, and not normal activity.
- Class II angina develops with rapid or prolonged walking or stair climbing.
- Class III angina severely limits ordinary physical activities.
- Class IV angina occurs at rest, as well as with any physical activity.

Case Study 2 – Mary
NURSING CARE PLAN Angina

When Mary presents at the GP's surgery, the decision is made to refer her to a specialist nurse-led rapid assessment clinic at the hospital where her assessment includes an exercise tolerance test. Depending on the severity of symptoms and a diagnosis of angina, she may be referred for angiography with a view to proceeding to percutaneous coronary intervention (PCI) or coronary artery bypass graft (CABG).

Early intervention and revascularisation (returning the blood to that area), following assessment at rapid assessment chest pain clinics improves patient outcomes and reduces healthcare costs, which complies with government guidelines (Tough and Morley 2008).

However, Mary's situation may be that she can be managed conservatively. If she has stable angina, her GP may refer her to undertake the angina plan. This is an education programme that is delivered over 12 weeks by a qualified facilitator, usually a nurse, which helps the person with angina to learn about their disease and develop a lifestyle that will minimise the risk of further problems.

It helps to dispel the myths that can be held, some of which are:

'Having angina means that I have had a small heart attack.'
'Exercise is dangerous and I should rest more.'
'There is nothing I can do about angina.'

It has been shown that regular exercise can reduce the number of angina attacks by 40%, and it also reduces the need for taking medication such as glyceryl trinitrate (GTN), a vasodilator which acts on the blood vessels so they widen and bring in more oxygenated blood to the heart muscle (Maclean *et al.* 2007).

Mary's family are very worried about her diagnosis of angina and put pressure on her to give up some of her activities, particularly cycling to work. Since Mary has attended the sessions and worked through the angina plan, she can now argue with some degree of certainty that to exercise will help maintain cardiac function rather than cause her problems. In fact a sedentary lifestyle will put her at more risk, and reduce her overall quality of life and may lead to her feeling depressed. Mary will continue to be monitored by the GP and practice nurses (Maclean *et al.* 2007).

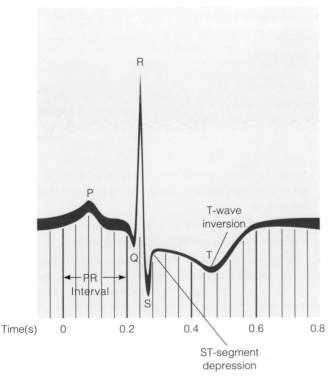

Figure 9.7 ECG changes during episode of angina.

INTERDISCIPLINARY CARE FOR STABLE ANGINA

Medication

Three main classes of drugs are used to treat angina:

- Glyceryl trinitrate (GTN) is used to treat acute attacks, and longer-acting nitrate preparations are used to prevent angina. Sublingually, GTN acts within one to two minutes, improving myocardial oxygen supply by dilating collateral blood vessels and reducing stenosis. It is available as an oral spray; some people find this easier to handle than small GTN tablets. Longer-acting preparations (oral tablets, ointment or transdermal patches) are used to prevent attacks of angina, not to treat an acute attack. Headache, nausea, dizziness and hypotension are common side-effects.

- Beta blockers are considered first-line drugs to treat stable angina (not Prinzmetal's angina as it may cause adverse side effects) as they interfere with the cardiac-stimulating effects of norepinephrine and epinephrine, and prevent anginal attacks by reducing heart rate, myocardial contractility and blood pressure. They may be used alone or with other medications but are contraindicated for people with asthma or severe COPD because they may cause severe broncho-spasm. Beta blockers are used as a long-term measure following aortic aneurysms.

● Calcium channel blockers reduce myocardial oxygen demand and increase myocardial blood and oxygen supply, lowering blood pressure and reducing myocardial contractility and heart rate. They are also potent coronary vasodilators which increases oxygen supply. Because they may actually increase ischaemia and mortality in those with heart failure or left ventricular dysfunction, these drugs are not usually prescribed in the initial treatment of angina. They are used cautiously in people with dysrhythmias, heart failure or hypotension.

Cardiac catheterisation

This is a generic term for a range of procedures such as angiography, ventriculography, atherectomy (the shaving off of atheromatous plaques from the artery wall) and PCI, which are performed under sterile conditions in a fluoroscopy suite to:

● diagnose CAD, heart abnormalities which may be congenital or have developed over time;

● assess whether it is possible to revascularise the heart by opening up the blocked artery;

● insert a stent;

● obtain a biopsy of the heart muscle;

● assess the heart's response to drug treatments.

Coronary artery bypass graft (CABG)

CABG involves using a section of a vein or an artery to create a connection (or bypass) between the aorta and the coronary artery beyond the obstruction, which allows blood to perfuse the ischaemic portion of the heart. The internal mammary artery in the chest and the saphenous vein from the leg are the vessels most commonly used. This procedure was used more frequently before treatment with PCI became common practice.

Bypass grafts are safe and effective; angina is totally relieved or significantly reduced in 90% of cases. While anginal pain may recur within three years, it rarely is as severe as before surgery. It is recommended for people who have multiple vessel disease and impaired left ventricular function or diabetes, and for those who have significant obstruction of the left main coronary artery. Over 30 000 operations are performed each year in the UK.

Newer techniques have been developed that allow surgeons to perform CABG without cardioplegia (stopping the heart) and using cardiopulmonary bypass. Off-pump coronary artery bypass (OPCAB) allows use of a smaller incision for access. Although cardiopulmonary bypass is used for the majority of coronary artery bypass procedures, OPCAB is a promising alternative. Controlled studies demonstrate lower mortality and morbidity rates and faster recovery for patients undergoing OPCAB as compared to CABG with cardiopulmonary bypass.

About 20–40% of people may develop atrial fibrillation after surgery and this has been attributed to haemodilution that occurs when the blood passes through the CPB pump: people can also develop hypokalaemia. Signs and symptoms of this complication include:

● low blood pressure;

● fast pulse;

● rapid respiration rate;

● dizziness;

● palpitations.

IN PRACTICE

Care following post-cardiac catheterisation

● Following cardiac catheterisation, these observations are recorded after the procedure:
  - blood pressure;
  - heart rate and rhythm;
  - respiration rate and pulse oximetry;
  - checking the wound site for seepage of blood;
  - checking the patient's colour, warmth and sensation in the extremities.

● Complications may develop up to several hours after the procedure; therefore, bedrest is recommended for three hours after the procedure if the femoral artery was used and for two hours if the radial artery was the insertion site.

● The person is advised to report if they experience shortness of breath, chest pain or discomfort and bleeding that may occur at the insertion site.

● The person needs to drink plenty of fluids to flush the dye out of their body and only have a light diet to avoid nausea and vomiting.

● If the person having the cardiac catheterisation was on anticoagulant therapy, this may be recommended.

● They are advised to avoid strenuous activity for 24 hours, which may dislodge the clot which has formed over the insertion site, and to have showers rather than hot baths, which would raise their blood pressure and increase peripheral dilatation of the capillaries, which may leave them feeling faint.

Source: Bowden 2009.

This needs reporting to the medical team immediately for further investigation and the person may be treated pharmacologically (beta blockers and anticoagulant therapy) with good effect.

NURSING CARE FOR STABLE ANGINA

Psychosocial issues

Denial may be strong in patients with angina pectoris, because many people think of the heart as the locus of life itself; problems such as angina remind people of their mortality, an uncomfortable fact. Denial may lead to 'forgetting' to take prescribed medications or to attempting activities that will precipitate angina. Some people, by contrast, may become 'cardiac cripples'; afraid to engage in activities because of anticipated chest pain and this may actually hasten the atherosclerotic process and inhibit collateral circulation development, worsening angina.

Health promotion

Many patients with stable angina manage their pain effectively, continuing to live active and productive lives. To do so, they need advice on the following:

✦ CHD, the processes that cause chest pain, including the relationship between the pain and reduced blood flow to the heart muscle.

✦ Use and effects (desired and adverse) of prescribed medications and the importance of not discontinuing medications abruptly, particularly those for hypertension.

✦ How to store and use GTN, that they should always carry some with them for use in emergency situations, and that it can be used prophylactically before activities that result in chest pain, and to seek medical advice immediately if three doses taken over 15–20 minutes do not relieve pain.

✦ The importance of calling 999 (in the UK) or going to the emergency department immediately for unrelieved chest pain.

Unstable angina

Unstable angina has been reclassified as NSTEMI as there is little difference between the two conditions. Unstable angina occurs more frequently than angina pectoris, the pain is more severe, lasts longer (more than 20 minutes) and there is only minimal relief from GTN. At least 30% of people with unstable angina progress to having a MI. It usually signifies that an atheromatous plaque has ruptured and a coronary artery has thrombosed. The main problem is that people presenting with this symptom may have normal troponin levels and can be discharged from hospital and their MI missed.

Variant angina

Variant angina is also called Prinzmetal's angina. People with this symptom usually experience chest pain at night and it represents coronary artery spasm rather than thrombosis. An ECG recording would show a raised ST segment.

The person with acute coronary syndrome (ACS)

ACS is an umbrella term for a group of conditions that result from CAD. It includes unstable and variant angina, together with acute myocardial ischaemia with or without significant injury of myocardial tissue (infarction). Myocardial infarction is dealt with in the next section. ACS occurs when the blood flow through the arteries is restricted or completely blocked, and it can range in the degree of severity depending on the size of the artery blocked and the area of myocardium affected. The main cause of ACS is atherosclerosis. Problems occur when:

● an atherosclerotic plaque ruptures and forms a blood clot that narrows or blocks the coronary artery;

● coronary arteries go into spasm as in Prinzmetal's angina;

● there is inflammation of a coronary artery;

● there is an increased myocardial oxygen demand and/or decreased supply (for example, acute blood loss or anaemia).

The main symptom of ACS is chest pain, usually substernal or epigastric, which often radiates to the neck, left shoulder and/or left arm and may occur at rest, typically lasting longer than 10–20 minutes. The pain is more severe and prolonged

IN PRACTICE

PQRST

PQRST is a useful mnemonic for assessing chest pain

P – Precipitating and palliative factors
- What was happening when the pain started?
- Is there anything that aggravates or alleviates the pain?
- Does taking a deep breath affect the pain?

Q – Quality
- What does the pain feel like? – descriptors such as sharp, tight, burning, heavy, deep

R – Region and radiation
- Exact location of pain
- Does it spread or travel to any other areas?

S – Severity
- On a scale of 1–10; rating pain where 10 is the worst pain ever experienced

T – Time
- When the pain started, is it transient?
- Has it occurred before?

than that previously experienced by the person; it may represent a pattern of increasing frequency and severity of anginal pain that does not diminish with rest or treatment with GTN, or it may be a new episode. The onset of pain is sudden and usually is not associated with activity. People with a history of angina may have more frequent anginal attacks in the days or weeks prior to the ACS event. However, up to 25% of patients may not feel any pain, or may complain of indigestion, heartburn, nausea with or without vomiting or feeling light-headed. Dyspnoea, diaphoresis (sweating), pallor and cool skin may be present with tachycardia (fast pulse rate) and hypotension (low blood pressure).

The person with myocardial infarction (MI)

MIs sometimes occur in patients without pre-existing coronary heart disease and are classified as either:

- STEMI (ST elevated myocardial infarction) – that is, there is an elevation of the ST segment on the ECG denoting muscle wall infarction. The ECG shows where the area of infarction has occurred and that is the full thickness of the heart muscle.

- NSTEMI (Non-ST elevated myocardial infarction) – where there are no specific changes to the ST part of the ECG, indicating that part of the heart muscle has been affected

but not the full thickness. As the ECG evidence is inconclusive, diagnosis depends on whether blood results contain increased levels of troponins.

ECG changes characteristic of MI are illustrated in Figure 9.8.

MIs can be a life-threatening event that occurs mostly in the morning which suggests that the circadian rhythm is partly implicated. The theory postulated is that during the night, the blood pressure falls, reaching its lowest point between 3 and 4am, and starts rising at 6am. At this point there is a surge in cardiac output and increased pressure on the ventricles. It is thought that this 'cardiac surge' dislodges an atherosclerotic plaque, which blocks a coronary artery, resulting in an MI. If circulation to the affected myocardium is not promptly restored, loss of functional myocardium affects the heart's ability to maintain an effective cardiac output which may ultimately lead to cardiogenic shock and death.

The majority of deaths from MI occur during the initial period after symptoms begin: approximately 60% occur within the first hour, and 40% prior to hospitalisation. Heightening public awareness of the signs of MI, the importance of seeking immediate medical assistance and training in cardiopulmonary resuscitation (CPR) techniques are vital to decrease deaths. The National Service Framework (DoH Heart Disease Policy Team 2006) has reported on the success of training community defibrillation officers who can respond quickly in emergency situations in public areas like restaurants and shopping malls and the placement of defibrillators in public areas.

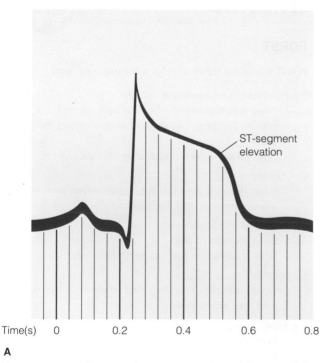

A

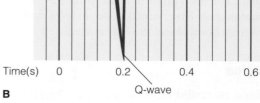

B

Figure 9.8 ECG changes characteristic of MI. **(A)** STEMI. **(B)** NSTEMI.

IN PRACTICE

The 'Chain of Survival'

The Resuscitation Council UK (2010) advocates a 'Chain of Survival' to improve patient outcomes which means:

- early recognition of deteriorating symptoms so that cardiac arrest can be prevented;
- early instigation of CPR;
- early defibrillation;
- effective post-resuscitation care.

Pathophysiology of MI

MIs occur more often in people with existing CHD. Blood flow to a portion of cardiac muscle is completely blocked, resulting in prolonged tissue ischaemia and irreversible cell damage. Coronary artery occlusion is usually caused by ulceration or rupture of a complicated atherosclerotic lesion. When ischaemia lasts more than 20–45 minutes, irreversible hypoxaemic damage causes cellular death and tissue necrosis. Oxygen, glycogen and adenosine triphosphate (ATP) stores of ischaemic cells are rapidly depleted. Cellular metabolism shifts to an anaerobic process, producing hydrogen ions and lactic acid. Cellular acidosis increases cells' vulnerability to further damage. Intracellular enzymes are released through damaged cell membranes into interstitial spaces. Cellular acidosis, electrolyte imbalances and hormones released in response to cellular ischaemia affect impulse conduction and myocardial contractility. This causes a risk for dysrhythmias, myocardial contractility decreases, reducing stroke volume, cardiac output, blood pressure and tissue perfusion. The subendocardium (inner lining of the heart) suffers the initial damage, within 20 minutes of injury, because this area is the most susceptible to changes in coronary blood flow.

Signs and symptoms of MI

Chest pain is the key symptom and it is more severe than anginal pain. The intensity distinguishes MI from angina, and the duration and its continuous nature are also significant. The pain may be described as:

- crushing,
- severe,
- heavy pressure,
- a squeezing sensation,
- chest tightness,
- burning.

The pain often begins in the centre of the chest (*substernal*), and may radiate to the shoulders, neck, jaw or arms. It is not relieved by rest or GTN.

Other symptoms present because the:

- Sympathetic nervous system is stimulated resulting in anxiety, tachycardia and vasoconstriction.
- Pain and blood chemistry changes affect the respiratory centre resulting in tachypnoea.
- Tissue necrosis (death) causes an inflammatory reaction resulting in an increased white blood cell count and pyrexia.
- Vagal stimulation causes nausea and vomiting, bradycardia and hypotension.
- Irritation of the diaphragm results in hiccupping.

The person often has a sense of impending doom and death and a cold and mottled skin.

Complications following an MI

Dysrhythmias

Dysrhythmias, disturbances or irregularities of heart rhythm, are the most frequent complication of MI; however, they can occur for many reasons in response to anxiety, fear, excitement and exercise as a result of stimulation of the sympathetic nervous system. Disruption to the heart rhythm can occur in varying degrees; the most severe result in cardiac arrest and are classified according to the area affected, for example:

- Supraventricular rhythms arise above the ventricles.
- Atrial ventricular blocks means impulses are not passing from atria to ventricles.
- Ventricular tachycardia is where the ventricles contract before the message has been transmitted from the atria and occurs in short bursts or runs.
- Ventricular fibrillation is extremely rapid, chaotic contraction of the ventricles where the heart fails to beat properly, resulting in cardiac arrest.

Infarcted tissue is *arrhythmogenic*, meaning the generation and conduction of electrical impulses in the heart are blocked. Premature ventricular contractions are common following an MI, developing in more than 90% of people having had a MI. While not dangerous in themselves, they may predispose to ventricular tachycardia or ventricular fibrillation. The risk of ventricular fibrillation is greatest the first hour after MI, and it is a frequent cause of sudden cardiac death. However, the incidence declines with time. Any degree of AV block may occur following MI, especially when the anterior wall is infarcted. Bradydysrhythmias (abnormal slow rhythms) also may develop, particularly when the inferior wall of the ventricle is affected.

PRACTICE ALERT

When checking pulses in people with dysrhythmias, it is essentially to do this manually as feeling the pulse gives more information about the quality and strength of the pulse.

Cardiogenic shock

Cardiogenic shock occurs when more than 40% of the heart function is reduced. Low cardiac output impairs perfusion of the coronary arteries and myocardium, further increasing tissue damage. Mortality from cardiogenic shock is greater than 70%, although this can be reduced by prompt intervention with revascularisation procedures.

Infarcts can extend or reinfarct in approximately 10% of people during the first 10–14 days after an MI because continued impairment of the blood flow results in further injury and necrosis of the tissues. This results in further chest pain and worsening heart failure.

Pericarditis

Pericarditis, inflammation of the pericardial tissue surrounding the heart, may complicate MI, usually within two to three days. Pericarditis causes chest pain that may be aching or sharp and stabbing, aggravated by movement or deep breathing. A *pericardial friction rub* may be heard when listening to heart sounds through a stethoscope.

INTERDISCIPLINARY CARE FOR MI

Following an MI, the immediate goals of care are to:

- relieve pain;
- reduce extent of myocardial damage;
- maintain cardiovascular stability;
- decrease cardiac workload;
- prevent further complications;
- attach a cardiac monitor to the patient and record an ECG;
- establish intravenous access to maintain fluid volume and enable easy collection of blood samples for further monitoring.

Investigations

When the heart muscle is damaged, cardiac enzymes are released. On their own, they do not provide conclusive evidence that a MI has occurred; they need to be considered along with the ECG. The blood is tested for the following enzymes:

- Cardiac muscle troponins, *cardiac-specific troponin T (cTnT)* and *cardiac-specific troponin I (cTnI)*, are sensitive indicators of myocardial damage, being elevated in ACS or within normal limits if chest pain is due to unstable angina. They remain in the blood from 10–14 days after an MI, making them a useful marker in diagnosing MIs when there has been a delay in seeking treatment.
- Creatine kinase (CK) and CK-MB (specific to myocardial muscle) levels are likely to be within normal limits or demonstrate transient elevation, returning to normal levels within 12–24 hours. In MI, these levels rise rapidly, peaking at 12–24 hours after the event and then declining. The rise depends on the amount of tissue damaged.

- Myoglobin is one of the first cardiac markers to be detectable in the blood after an MI. It is released within a few hours of symptom onset, but its lack of specificity to cardiac muscle and rapid excretion (blood levels return to normal within 24 hours) limit its use.

Assessment

Rapid assessment and early diagnosis is important in treating MI; within 15 minutes, 50% of the myocardium has died and in three hours 80% of the muscle is affected, hence the phrase 'time is muscle'. The evolution of an MI is dynamic: the quicker the artery is reopened (medically, surgically or spontaneously), the more myocardium can be salvaged. Survival and long-term outcomes following MI are improved by rapidly restoring blood flow to the 'stunned' myocardium surrounding the infarcted tissue, reducing myocardial oxygen demand and limiting the accumulation of toxic by-products of necrosis and reperfusion. The major problem interfering with timely reperfusion is delay in seeking medical care following the onset of symptoms. Up to 44% of people with symptoms of chest discomfort or pain wait more than four hours before seeking treatment. Many factors are cited as reasons for treatment delay, including advanced age, the misperception of the seriousness of symptoms, denial that this is happening, limited access to medical care, the availability of an emergency response system and in-hospital delays. Immediate evaluation of these symptoms of myocardial infarction is essential to early diagnosis and treatment.

Acute disease differs from chronic disease or chronic heart failure; when a patient presents with a MI, there is little time for lengthy assessments and the accompanying family or friends may be able to provide useful information. Whether the information is gleaned from the person or a family member, the key areas of interest are:

- current symptoms, when they started;
- previous medical history;
- current medication and drugs taken since the onset of chest pain;
- the usual coping mechanisms;
- the insight and understanding the person has of their symptoms;
- social and personal factors that may increase risk of CHD, such as levels of physical activity, diet, alcohol consumption, smoking.

Whilst the above are key areas of assessment, there are other associated factors that need to be ascertained. Is the person:

- breathless;
- nauseated;
- experiencing dizziness or light-headedness;
- sweating (diaphoresis)?

Treatment

The goals of treatment are to:

● restore blood to the damaged area of the heart as quickly as possible using reperfusion strategies such as percutaneous coronary interventions or thrombolysis (drugs that break down the blood clots);

● prevent further blood clots developing by giving antiplatelet therapy and anticoagulant therapy;

● monitor for risk factors and side-effects developing from the treatment.

Aspirin and clopidogrel

Aspirin therapy halves the rate of deaths for people who experience a non-fatal MI and unstable angina. As it does cause gastric bleeding, it is contraindicated for people who have had recent episodes of bleeding either in the brain or gastrointestinal tract, have active gastric or peptic ulcers or who are known to be allergic to the drug. The starting dose is 300 mg given orally, followed by a maintenance dose of 75 mg daily thereafter.

Clopidogrel 200 mg is usually given with aspirin because it enhances the blood thinning effect; however, it increases the risk of bleeding from the gastrointestinal tract. For people with a NSTEMI, the treatment continues for three months if there are no complications, and it is given for four weeks in those who have STEMI.

Managing pain and nausea

As well as using GTN to relieve pain, morphine is given as this helps to manage the anxiety as well as the pain. However, opioids such as morphine can make the people nauseous and an antiemetic is usually given at the same time. Metoclopramide

is the preferred antiemetic as it does not interfere with the heart rate unlike cyclizine (Chummum 2009).

Reperfusion using percutaneous coronary intervention (PCI)

PCI and stents (Figure 9.9) have become the primary treatment strategy for STEMI because it restores patency to the artery affected in 95% of cases (see section on cardiac catheterisation on page 318). One UK centre, Harefields Hospital, has negotiated with the local ambulance service to bring patients straight into the hospital, bypassing the local A & E unit. Patients are treated primarily with PCI (alternatively referred to as primary percutaneous coronary intervention – PPCI) without the use of thrombolytic drugs. Good outcomes have been reported, with fewer complications and cost savings to the NHS because people are discharged earlier.

The stents are fine metal mesh tubes that are inserted into the coronary arteries through a small sheath or catheter which has a deflated balloon in it. The introduction of the sheath is through a surface artery, either the radial or femoral artery, and its passage is monitored by a fluoroscope (continuous x-ray). Once the stent has reached the area of atherosclerosis which is blocking the coronary artery, the balloon is inflated pressing the stent into place and opening the artery by squeezing the atheromatous plague against the artery wall. The stent becomes covered with endothelial cells; however, these can later cause narrowing of the lumen. To prevent this, stents that are coated with drugs which affect cell reproduction can be used; these are called drug-eluting stents.

Research found 35.7% of patients reported complications following PCI procedure. In the main, these were oozing from the entry site and haematomas. As a result of the findings, monitoring of patients should extend to a year after the procedure; this can be, practically speaking, achieved through a simple telephone call (Higgins *et al.* 2008).

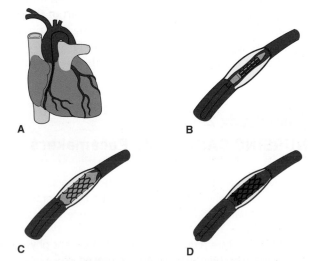

Figure 9.9 Percutaneous coronary intervention. (A) The balloon catheter with the stent is threaded into the affected coronary artery. **(B)** Balloon not inflated. **(C)** Balloon inflated. **(D)** Balloon removed leaving stent in place.

Case Study 1 – Zahir
NURSING CARE PLAN Coronary angioplasty

Zahir is to have coronary angioplasty, a surgical repair that will keep the coronary artery open and patent. Before the insertion of the stent (PCI) occurs, Zahir will be assessed to ensure that he has:

+ a full blood profile, which includes clotting times;
+ renal function tested as the dye used in the procedure can cause renal damage and he will need additional fluids to flush this out of his system;
+ a full medical history taken to exclude any conditions which might compromise his health status, such as gastrointestinal bleeds or strokes;
+ a drug allergy profile as he will have to take aspirin and clopidogrel after the stent insertion.

The medical team will also have to inform Zahir about the risks of the procedure:

+ 1:1000 people may have a stroke.
+ 3–4:100 people will have an MI and need coronary bypass surgery.
+ 1:100 people die.

Other risks are that he may bleed during the procedure, develop a haematoma or develop an aneurysm.

After the procedure, Zahir will need careful monitoring for bleeding at the puncture site or from the heart or from the anticoagulation or antiplatelet drugs that he has been given during the procedure, which means his pulse rate and blood pressure will need careful monitoring and an ECG recording should be taken regularly. Depending on whether the radial or femoral artery was used, the nurse would need to check the pulses below the point of insertion to ensure that these vessels have not shut down.

On discharge, Zahir will need to be given advice regarding medication; he will need to take aspirin for the rest of his life and not doing so would put him at risk of having a heart attack. Clopidogrel will have to be taken for 12 months.

Zahir will also require lifestyle advice. He would need to monitor his diet and, if a smoker, he would be advised to stop. Exercise is also an important part of his recovery programme.

If Zahir has a PCI inserted after an MI, he would be advised not to drive for four weeks; if this were an elective procedure, then he would be advised not to drive for at least a week. People who hold a Group 2 vehicle licence (category C – large lorries – and category D – buses) will be disqualified from driving for six weeks and may have to be retested by the DVLA before being permitted to regain this kind of work.

Source: adapted from Muggenthaler *et al.* 2008.

Thrombolysis (the breakdown of the blood clots blocking the coronary artery) was the standard treatment before the use of PCI became more widely available. Examples of thrombolytic agents are streptokinase and tissue plasma activators like altpase, reteplase and tenectoplase (NICE 2010), which are given intravenously up to 24 hours after the start of the chest pain for patients who have had a STEMI. Drugs like tirofiban stop platelets aggregating (gluing together to form a clot) and are used in NSTEMI, because they reduce the risk of death.

Pacemakers

Permanent pacemakers are small units that are inserted into the chest which sense dysrhythmias and provide an impulse which stimulates the heart to beat regularly. They are used to treat both acute and chronic conduction defects. When people with pacemakers die, the unit has to be removed, particularly prior to cremation.

Case Study 2 – Mary
NURSING CARE PLAN Pacemakers

Mary may manage her life well for a number of years. However, in older age, she may find that her condition deteriorates and it is possible that at some point she may require the insertion of a pacemaker.

Pre-operative care requires preparing the patient physically, psychologically and emotionally for the procedure.

Once the pacemaker is in place, it requires little in the way of aftercare. Mary may find that if she engages in strenuous exercise too quickly, she may experience breathlessness as there

has been insufficient time for the pacemaker to register the extra demand and respond by pacing the heart.

Pacemaker batteries last between six and 12 years and replacing the battery is a simple surgical procedure. Signs of pacemaker malfunction are:

- dizziness,
- fainting,
- fatigue,

Case Study 2 – Mary	NURSING CARE PLAN Pacemakers

- weakness,
- chest pain,
- palpitations.

Mary needs to carry a pacemaker identification card with her at all times, and be mindful that it can set off security alarms, for example at airports.

She can resume normal activity fairly quickly after insertion of a pacemaker but is advised not to engage in contact sport, which may be an unlikely pleasure pursuit in the older patients, but it is never safe to assume they do not participate in these sporting activities. Many octogenarians take part in the London Marathon.

NURSING CARE FOR MI

MOVE

The acronym MOVE highlights a framework nurses can use in caring for people who have experienced an MI (Chummum 2009):

✦ *Monitor*. The nurse needs to monitor the person closely for:
   a. further pain and maintain an accurate record on the pain chart;
   b. nausea and vomiting to minimise anxiety and physiological stress on the myocardium;
   c. heart rhythm through the use of ECG recordings;
   d. other vital signs like blood pressure, pulse and temperature;
   e. urine output as this may decrease as a result of shock.

✦ *Oxygen*. The nurse needs to ensure that the person's oxygen supply is not compromising the situation. This is monitored through pulse oximetry. If the nurse discovers early signs of breathlessness and low oxygen saturation, it must be reported immediately. High-flow oxygen of 15 L is usually given to people who are hypoxic.

✦ *Venous access*. Regular blood monitoring needs to be undertaken to monitor the effectiveness of treatment and whether fluid is being retained, which leads to pulmonary oedema, which in turn adds extra pressure on the damaged heart. Nurses need to ensure that the venous access site remains patent (by giving bolus injections of heparin) and free from infection as it is also used to administer drugs.

✦ *Expert advice*. ACS involves more than just the heart. Whilst healthcare professionals working specifically in coronary care units are expert in their field, people who have ACS may benefit from additional support and advice from nutritionists and psychologists after the event that has resulted in a hospital admission.

Psychosocial issues

When people have an MI, they report feelings of doom and foreboding. Dixon *et al.* (2000) conducted a study in Australia to ascertain the extent of reported psychosocial problems in patients who had suffered an MI. Their findings suggest that people who are married have fewer problems than those who live alone; however, over 50% reported having problems that affected their physical and emotional coping and their relationships with friends and family. Problems they highlighted were:

✦ frustration when unable to do what they had previously managed;
✦ lack of self-confidence;
✦ inability to return to usual social activities.

Approximately 17–27% of people who have cardiac problems experience depression, and this can persist for at least 12 months. Often the depression remains undiagnosed because:

✦ It is viewed as part of their condition.
✦ There is a general belief that having cardiac disease does make one depressed; it is understandable.
✦ It is masked by the person's anxiety.

By asking two simple questions, nurses would be able to ascertain whether people require further help:

✦ 'How are you feeling in yourself?'
✦ 'Have you been feeling down lately?'

Alternatively, assessment could be more thorough by using the Hospital Anxiety and Depression Scale (HADS) which consists of seven questions. Determining whether the person is suffering from depression is important because it can affect the outcome of their recovery.

IN PRACTICE

The Hospital Anxiety and Depression Scale (HADS)

The person is asked to give a score from 1–4 for each of the following statements, depending on the extent to which it describes their current state of mind.

1. I still enjoy the things I used to enjoy.
2. I can laugh and see the funny side of things.
3. Worrying thoughts go through my mind.
4. I get sudden feelings of panic.
5. I have lost interest in my appearance.
6. I have a feeling something awful is about to happen.
7. I feel restless and cannot read a book.

Now that we have looked at disorders of myocardial perfusion, we will go on to discuss sudden cardiac death.

Sudden cardiac death (SCD)

SCD occurs when the heart stops suddenly; more people in the world die this way than from strokes, lung and breast cancer and AIDs. It may occur if a person who is not usually active does something very strenuous. The main risk factor is a history of heart disease, especially if there are problems involving the left ventricle. SCD is more likely to happen in people's homes or when they are out and about. Two-thirds of those affected will probably have CHD, and people with congenital heart problems and chronic heart failure are more at risk than the general population.

FAST FACTS

Sudden cardiac death

- 74 000 people in the UK die this way every year
- 74% of SCD happens outside of hospitals
- A bystander giving CPR can triple the chance of survival

Source: Gregory and Quinn 2010.

- 84% of patients in hospital who have a cardiac arrest show signs of deterioration before the arrest.
- Early recognition of these signs could prevent arrests occurring, and helps to identify those for whom resuscitation is inappropriate.
- Less than 20% of hospitalised patients who have had a cardiac arrest survive to discharge.

Source: Oldroyd et al. 2010.

Basic life support (BLS)

Healthcare professionals and members of the public who have had the requisite training can undertake BLS. It involves the following (Resuscitation Council UK Guidelines 2010):

- Ensure that the person is in a safe place for care to be given and no-one is in any danger.
- Recognise that the person has had a cardiac arrest and check the airway is clear.
- Put out an emergency call for help and make a request for an automated external defibrillator – dialling 999 will secure emergency services outside of the hospital environment in the UK.
- Start CPR by compressing the chest 5–6 cm at a rate of 100–120 times in a minute, and not stopping unless the patient shows signs of life, for example coughing, regaining consciousness.
- If managing BLS singly, then undertake 30 chest compressions before giving two rescue breaths, then resume chest compressions as it is more important to carry out chest compressions than give rescue breaths.

Cardioversion and defibrillation

At cardiac arrest, the ventricles fibrillate (flutter rapidly), and this is a medical emergency requiring defibrillation to restore rhythm. It is achieved by delivering an electric shock to the heart; conductive gel pads are placed on the chest wall above and below the heart and the electric shock is transmitted through two paddles. Internal defibrillation can be given direct to the heart during surgery.

Cardioversion is similar to defibrillation. However, this is usually an elective procedure to treat supraventricular tachycardia, which occurs when extra beats are instigated in the atria outside of the normal process through the atrial ventricular node which trigger ventricular contractions (see section on dysrhythmias on page 321).

ACUTE AND CHRONIC HEART FAILURE

Heart failure maybe acute or chronic, resulting from the long-term effects of CHD, ACS, structural defects of the heart valves and hypertension. It costs the NHS £625 million pounds a year to care for people with heart failure (NHS Information Centre 2010). Previously regarded as a diagnosis, it is now considered a 'syndrome' because it is a constellation of associated problems mainly resulting from damage or abnormal function of the left ventricle (Crosbie et al. 2009).

The person with acute heart failure (AHF)

Surviving MIs, a history of chronic heart failure, COPD and an ageing population have resulted in AHF becoming a major health problem in the UK. There are also other reasons, such as anaemia, asthma and infection, for the condition developing. The main causative factors are:

- an acute coronary problem, for example STEMI or NSTEMI;
- hypertension that is no longer under control;
- infections, for example chest infections;
- disorders of the heart valves;
- cardiomyopathies;
- arrhythmias;
- chronic heart failure (CHF) that is no longer responding to treatment;
- non-concordance with treatment.

The condition is associated with a poor prognosis, and 30% of those diagnosed will die within a year. People with this condition face repeated hospital admissions for their last year of life.

Pathophysiology of AHF

The key problem in AHF is that the heart is failing as a pump and is no longer circulating fluid around the body efficiently, resulting in fluid overload, pulmonary oedema and a reduced cardiac output. The heart under pressure may stop and advanced life support is needed in this case. Atrial fibrillation may aggravate the situation and lead to ventricular fibrillation. This problem develops suddenly, and exerts strain on the heart muscle. The heart beats faster in an attempt to compensate for the fact that the ventricles are not ejecting the usual amount of blood. The fluid overload can be seen in the jugular veins which can become engorged. Fluid also accumulates in the ankles; if the person is sitting, fluid will be seen around the sacral area. Although the heart beats faster, the blood pressure drops which affects the movement of blood through the kidneys leading to renal failure (Whitlock 2010).

PRACTICE ALERT

- The person in AHF will feel cold and clammy; this is a classical sign.
- Their breathing will be laboured and short of breath, they will have a rapid pulse and a low blood pressure, and they may not be passing urine (oliguria).
- If the skin is pressed, it will blanch and take time to regain its colour, denoting poor peripheral circulation.
- They may also appear 'blue' (cyanotic) because the blood is not being oxygenated sufficiently due to the sluggish circulation.

INTERDISCIPLINARY CARE FOR AHF

Assessment

An ECG and chest x-ray are instigated as soon as the person is admitted. A useful mnemonic for covering all aspects of assessment is ABCDE, which stands for:

- airway,
- breathing,
- circulation,
- disability,
- exposure.

The respiration rate will be increased and oxygen saturation levels will be low; this could mean that the patient appears confused and unable to process information or respond to questions. The Glasgow Coma Scale is a useful way to measure the level of cerebral hypoxia.

The heart rate may be rapid, and it is important to check the pulse rate manually to determine its regularity and strength. A low blood pressure recording is associated with a poorer prognosis; it could be a high blood pressure that caused the AHF; however, a high blood pressure may result from the AHF.

The disability that the person experiences depends on the amount of fluid they are retaining. Besides monitoring their intake of fluid and measuring the amount of urine they are passing to assess this, weighing patients daily determines whether the person is responding to treatment and losing the excess fluid.

An echocardiograph depicts how well the heart is working and the extent to which the ventricles are emptying with each beat. It will also show how efficient the heart valves are.

A range of blood tests are performed:

- a full blood count because the person may be anaemic (15–55% of people with CHF are anaemic);
- c-reactive protein to ascertain if there is infection present;
- glomerular filtration rate to determine how well the kidneys are working;
- INR because there is a potential for the blood to clot and cause pulmonary emboli;
- arterial blood gases to determine how much oxygen is in the body and its ratio to carbon dioxide;
- cardiac markers, troponins to determine whether there has been an MI.

Nursing assessment should included checking the condition of the person's skin and assessing their risk for developing pressure sores, determining how far they can walk and what their exercise tolerance is, how well they have been sleeping, and is this in bed or sitting in an armchair. The National Heart Failure Audit undertaken in 2008–09 (as cited by Whitlock 2010) found that over a third of people with heart failure reported severe and prolonged depression; therefore, the nursing assessment should include questions focusing on this as previously stated on p. 325 in the discussion on psychosocial issues related to MIs.

Treatment

Medication

The aim of treatment is to reduce preload and afterload (see section on anatomy, physiology and functions on pages 309–310), and this is achieved through the use of diuretic and vasodilator drugs. An intravenous infusion containing a loop diuretic drug (affects the loop of Henle – see Chapter 8) such as furosemide is set up and a potassium sparing diuretic, for example spironolactone, is given orally to increase diuersis. To improve vasodilation, an angiotensin-converting enzyme (ACE) inhibitor, such as ramipril, or an angiotensin-receptor blocker, such as candesartan, is given as these block the mechanisms in the body that cause vasoconstriction. GTN is another vasodilator and this can be given intravenously; it acts on the renal arteries also and improves diuersis. The person's drug regime will need to be revised, especially if they have been taking drugs such as calcium channel blockers for their heart condition because these may have led to the development of AHF. Morphine is given because it relieves distress and is a vasodilator, although this treatment is currently under review as there has been some evidence that it delays recovery.

Ventricular assist devices (VADs)

VADs are pumps that can be fixed externally or inserted internally to the patient. External pumps tend to be used as an interim measure for people waiting for heart transplants. However, given the shortage of hearts being available for transplant, the devices can be fitted internally to provide a permanent solution for people who experience heart failure NYHA class 3 or 4 (see Practice box detailing NYHA classification). In left-sided heart failure, VADs take the blood from the left ventricle and transport it to a pump which then takes the blood to the aorta for circulation. In right-sided failure, blood is taken from the right ventricle into the pulmonary artery (see Figure 9.2 on page 309). Whilst these devices may prolong life, the person and their family and friends may consider that it adversely affects their quality of life and would prefer a palliative care approach to their symptom management. A great deal of psychological support is required, especially as people are very aware of the threat to their mortality that the condition brings (O'Donovan 2006).

Heart transplants

Heart transplants were pioneered in the mid 1960s by Doctor Christian Barnard, a South African doctor. These are now part of the standard care for end-stage heart disease and have a good success rate with 90% of people returning to normal functional abilities. The person needs preparing as for any surgical procedure. Post-operatively, complications can occur, the major concerns being:

- bleeding, chest drains are monitored every 15 minutes;
- cardiac tamponade (a buildup of fluid in the pericardium);
- atrial fibrillation;
- infection;
- rejection of the new heart, which can occur within weeks, months or years after surgery.

Acute rejection is treated with immunosuppressive therapy.

NURSING CARE FOR AHF

Nursing the person with AHF requires skill and attention to detail. Initial care demands a swift response to symptoms as the person's condition can deteriorate rapidly. Care involves more than the science of monitoring and measuring the physiological status; it demands the art of reassuring the person, communicating well to alleviate anxiety and fear that the condition causes and being attuned to the person's needs with personal hygiene. The person with AHF will find it more comfortable to be nursed upright and may prefer sitting in an armchair to lying in bed as being supine will make them feel more breathless. The person will require oxygen therapy which can be delivered by:

- non-invasive positive pressure ventilation (NIPPV);
- continuous positive airway pressure (CPAP);
- bi-level positive airway pressure (BiPAP).

Oxygen delivered this way reduces the effort the person has to make to breathe and causes them less fatigue. If these methods of oxygen administration are not effective, then it may be necessary to intubate the person.

As the person's mobility is compromised, they will require help with their personal care and the nurse will need to ensure that they do not develop pressure ulcers and other complications such as thromboembolisms, respiratory and urinary infections, and constipation.

The breathlessness will result in the person having a dry mouth, and they will require frequent mouth care to prevent infection. Sucking ice lollies or chilled pineapple chunks is very refreshing and reduces the risk of oral infection.

The person with chronic heart failure (CHF)

CHF is also referred to as congestive heart failure because the reduced cardiac output with each contraction leads to vascular congestion. CHF can be either right-sided (Figure 9.10), as a result of pulmonary disease, or left-sided (Figure 9.11), as a result of CHD and hypertension. The vascular congestion impacts on other organs in the body: the gaseous exchange in the lungs is sluggish, resulting in cyanosis (blue tinge to the skin colour because of the lack of oxygenated blood in the capillaries under the skin) and breathlessness at rest; the fall in cardiac output result in salt and water retention. CHF is a progressive disease which ultimately becomes a terminal condition unless the patient is fortunate enough to be offered a heart transplant. CHF is considered to have a worse prognosis than many cancers as many patients die within a year of the diagnosis being confirmed. It impacts on quality of life, affecting the person's abilities to do anything that is mildly strenuous because they get breathless; their exercise tolerance is greatly reduced. The severity of CHF is assessed using the New York Heart Association (NYHA) Functional Classification and this will influence treatment decisions.

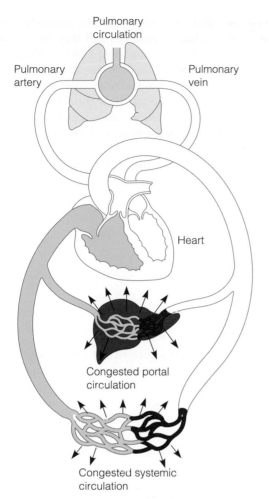

Figure 9.10 The haemodynamic effects of right-sided heart failure.

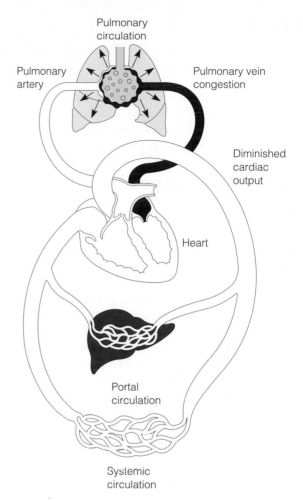

Figure 9.11 The haemodynamic effects of left-sided heart failure.

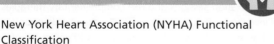

IN PRACTICE

New York Heart Association (NYHA) Functional Classification

Classification of chronic heart failure has been determined by the person's ability to function and is referred to as the NYHA Functional Classification.

NYHA 1	No symptoms interfering with normal activities, can walk upstairs without getting breathless
NYHA 2	Mild symptoms of breathlessness when undertaking some activities, experiences angina on exertion
NYHA 3	Has marked limitations, can only walk short distances before getting breathless and is only comfortable at rest
NYHA 4	Severe limitations with any physical activity and experiences symptoms at rest

INTERDISCIPLINARY CARE FOR CHF

Assessment

The National Institute for Health and Clinical Excellence (NICE 2010) published guidance on assessment of people with symptoms of CHF. Key points for assessment are:

- Determine the precipitating factors in the person's medical history such as previous MIs or hypertension.

- Check whether the person has any other comorbidities; are they obese, diabetic, do they have an infection?

- Determine their cardiac status by recording an ECG and performing transthoracic 2D Doppler echocardiography.

- Observe whether there is jugular vein distension, oedema in the ankles, liver enlargement.

- Check blood levels for serum electrolytes, urea, creatinine, estimated glomerular filtration rate and serum naturetic peptide levels [brain naturetic peptide (BNP), a hormone that accumulates in the ventricle's muscle, is released when the heart is under pressure, so levels rise – if these are normal then the symptoms are unlikely to be attributed to CHF, normal levels being 400 pg/ml].

Treatment

Initially, treatment for left ventricular systolic dysfunction should include ACE inhibitors and beta blockers and, if symptoms persist, then aldosterone antagonists should be prescribed. Besides medical treatment, the person with CHF needs to be advised on lifestyle changes that could modify the disease process, and this has already been covered in the discussion on risk management for CVD (see above).

NURSING CARE FOR CHF

Health promotion

NICE (2010) advocates that everyone with heart disease should undertake a rehabilitation programme; research evidence suggests that this can reduce mortality by 10–25%. Whilst the UK lags behind other European countries in this aspect of care, it forms part of care undertaken in the community. Most programmes are designed for groups, although South West Essex introduced a home-based rehabilitation programme which included education as well as an exercise programme. Findings from those who engage with the rehabilitation programmes is that their physical health improves as does their sense of wellbeing, and incidence of depression decreases. If mortality rates from CHF are to be addressed, then more effort is needed in recruiting people to these programmes (Riley 2010).

Psychosocial issues

It is not uncommon to find people with CHF are depressed to such an extent that it leads to insomnia and lack of concentration. Depression in CHF is worrying because the neurohormones it produces affect the heart rate, increase fluid retention and aggravate symptoms. People with depression and CHF are more likely to be readmitted to hospital and have a poorer prognosis. It is important to assess whether the person with CHF is at risk.

People with chronic heart failure find themselves socially isolated as their disease progresses and they are less able to leave the house and engage in normal social activities because of their breathlessness on exertion. Given that most people with CHF are elderly, they are not only coping with the losses that come with the disease and their shrinking social world, but also the loss of peers, siblings, friends and family. This can lead to feelings of low self-esteem and self-worth, low mood and depression.

Patients living with end-stage CHF experience:

- breathlessness,
- anorexia,
- insomnia,
- oedema,
- palpitations,
- fatigue,
- headaches,
- poor mobility.

These symptoms lead to increased fear and anxiety, especially if they experience sudden onset pulmonary oedema. They also lead to loss of independence, which is very frustrating and can be a cause of contention between the patient and their carers.

Carers also experience social isolation and feel very vulnerable. They report lack of sleep even if they are in separate rooms and increased anxiety over a sudden death occurring.

COMMUNITY-BASED CARE

Some healthcare trusts have invested in 'heart failure support programmes', where heart failure nurse specialists organise a multidisciplinary programme for people and their families, which includes education about the disease and offers attendees an opportunity to discuss their fears, access relaxation sessions and use complementary therapies to relieve stress. Programmes such as these enable people to verbalise their fears and anxieties and address issues of care, particularly in the later part of their illness trajectory.

Having discussed acute and chronic heart failure, we will now go on to look at structural problems of the heart and peripheral vascular disease before finishing with a consideration of end-of-life care.

The person with a structural problem of the heart

Structural defects occur when necrotic muscle is replaced by scar tissue which is thinner than the ventricular muscle mass,

IN PRACTICE

CHF and depression

Key questions to ask a person with CHF you suspect to be depressed:

- Would you say you are depressed?
- Would a close friend or a member of your family describe you as being depressed?
- What about the future, what will be happening to you in a year's time?

Source: adapted from Kirk and LeGeyt 2010.

leading to complications such as ventricular aneurysm, rupture of the interventricular septum or papillary muscle and myocardial rupture.

Ventricular aneurysm

A *ventricular aneurysm* is a ballooning of the ventricular wall which develops when a large section of the ventricle is replaced by scar tissue. As it does not contract during systole, stroke volume decreases with blood pooling within the aneurysm, causing clots to form. Ischaemia of the papillary muscle or chordae tendineae may cause structural damage leading to papillary muscle dysfunction or rupture. This affects AV valve function (usually the mitral valve), causing *regurgitation*, backflow of blood into the atria during systole. The interventricular septum may perforate or rupture due to ischaemia and infarction. Myocardial rupture is a risk between days four and seven after MI, when the injured tissue is soft and weak.

Structural problems can occur following infection, such as endocarditis and rheumatic fever which attack the heart valves, or may be congenital, present from birth but not giving rise to symptoms until adulthood. The valves can, as a result of scarring following infection, become stenotic; the flaps become fused together and fail to open and close properly, affecting cardiac output. The valves should be closed on ventricular contraction, but cannot, resulting in backflow into the atria. This is heard as a murmur; the usual lub dub sound is muffled by the back flow of blood. When the valves are stenosed, the ventricles have to work harder, leading to ventricular hypertrophy.

Valve replacements

Valves can be either mechanical or biological, made from either pig or calf pericardium, transplanted from a cadaver. Mechanical valves last longer, but patients require a lifetime of anticoagulant therapy. Biological valves have a low risk of thrombus formation, so do not require a lifetime on anticoagulant therapy, but they are less durable and need replacing after 15 years.

Cardiomyopathy

Cardiomyopathies are disorders of cardiac muscle; these can be primary, with an unknown cause, or secondary as a result of ischaemia, infections or from exposure to toxic substances such as chemotherapy. They are classified according to their pathophysiological presentation:

- *Dilated cardiomyopathy*, the most common presentation, where the heart chambers dilate, affecting contraction and cardiac output as a result of exposure to toxins. It is a progressive disease leading to heart failure(1:3 cases) and eventually death, which may be sudden.
- *Hypertrophic myopathy*, where the ventricular mass is significantly enlarged reducing ventricular filling and cardiac output. There is a genetic predisposition as over half of the

people who present with the condition have a family history of the disease. Young people with the disease may die suddenly after exercise, and it is the cause of death in approximately 36% of young athletes.

- Restrictive cardiomyopathy is the least common presentation, resulting from fibrosis of the myocardium and endocardium, restricting the movement of the ventricles and thus reducing cardiac output. Prognosis is poor with most patients dying within three years.

The person with peripheral vascular disease (PVD)

Peripheral vascular diseases occur as a result of damage to the circulatory system and they affect flow which interferes with blood pressure regulation. Arterial blood pressure depends on the force exerted during heart systole, and the cardiac output and the pressure wave from this action is felt as a peripheral pulse. In diastole, blood is prevented from flowing backwards by valves. Resistance is created when the arteries do not stretch as they should as a result of atherosclerosis, which has been explained earlier in the chapter. The main conditions are:

- hypertension,
- aneurysms,
- venous thrombosis.

Hypertension

Hypertension can be either primary (referred to as essential hypertension and the most common presentation) or secondary, resulting from an identifiable cause such as kidney disease or pregnancy. As seen above, it is a significant cause of CHD, strokes and renal failure. A genetic link has been identified in approximately 30% of people, and the incidence increases with age. It is believed that a quarter of the world's population has hypertension; the figures will rise because of lifestyle changes and each 20 mmHg increase above normal levels doubles the risk of death from CVD. It is usually controlled through a combination of medication: ACE inhibitors or low-dose thiazide diuretics.

Aneurysm

Aneurysm is an abnormal dilation of the blood vessel where the arterial wall has been weakened by arteriosclerosis or atherosclerosis and hypertension, occurring more commonly in men over the age of 50 years. They can occur in the thorax, abdomen or in the femoral and popliteal arteries. Most aneurysms are asymptomatic, but they can rupture resulting in hypovolaemic shock. A split in the inner lining of the aorta can result in a channel of blood forming between the layers of the aorta. When *dissection* occurs, the patient experiences excruciating pain in the chest or back. Blood pressure drops suddenly and immediate surgical intervention is required to repair the damage.

Venous thrombosis

Venous thrombosis can form in superficial or deep veins, and a deep vein thrombosis (DVT) is a common complication following surgery or prolonged bedrest. As seen in Case Study 3,

DVTs can occur during long flights: the blood becomes more viscous due to the altered cabin pressures in the aircraft, drinking alcohol can further dehydrate the person and thrombi can form. A clot fragment can break off and travel into the pulmonary circulation where it will occlude a pulmonary artery resulting in a pulmonary embolism. The patient experiences chest pain and breathlessness. The exact location and size of the thrombus is determined following a Doppler investigation.

Case Study 3 – John
NURSING CARE PLAN Deep vein thrombosis

Go back to Case Study 3 at the beginning of the chapter. John is convinced he has a bout of cramp, but this time the cramp pain is not getting better despite taking analgesia and resting his leg so he reluctantly visits the GP. The GP refers him to the acute admissions unit, especially as John tells him he woke up in the night with chest pain, where he has an x-ray, ECG recorded, a CT scan and an ultrasound investigation (Doppler test) to determine the extent of the DVT and whether he has had a pulmonary embolism.

John is started on subcutaneous injections of heparin (an anticoagulant) and, as he does not experience any adverse side-effects, is discharged to the care of the community nurses.

The community nurses arrive daily to give the heparin injections and take a blood sample for analysis of how readily his blood forms clots. Once his INR (international normalised ratio – which is a standardised test that measures how long it takes for blood plasma to clot when combined with tissue

factor) reaches between 2 and 3 (normally the INR range is between 0.8 and 1.2), he can start on oral medication of warfarin, and he then attends the local hospital for blood tests to monitor his INR. The warfarin dosage is adjusted to maintain a certain level of anticoagulation as overthinning the blood could result in haemorrhage.

As his DVT is below knee, John receives anticoagulant therapy for three months and is measured for an antithrombolytic stocking which he should wear for the next two years to prevent any further problems.

Certain foods, like broccoli, spinach, lettuce and liver, which have high concentrations of vitamin K can affect the INR levels, as they have natural clotting factors and should be avoided. John is advised of this and carries a card indicating that he is under treatment so that in the event of an accident, paramedics are aware that he may bleed for longer than normal.

End-of-life care

Patients with CHD and CHF deteriorate gradually, progressively finding that they do less and less before breathlessness takes over, limiting their activities (see NYHA classification cited on page 329). However, they are prone to a sudden exacerbation of their symptoms (referred to as heart failure decompensation) and approximately 50% of people may die; those that recover may see some improvement but not to their previous levels of activity. Recognising when the terminal phase is imminent is difficult; family and friends may prepare for death only to find that the person survives the latest illness episode. Research undertaken in the UK indicates that healthcare professionals, family and friends rarely discuss death and dying with the person involved. This may be in part due to the use of denial as a coping mechanism used by those with cardiac problems as discussed earlier. However, it is difficult to make plans for when and how one would wish to be cared for in the terminal phase when dying is sudden and unexpected.

People with chronic heart failure:

- have an uncertain disease trajectory;
- may die suddenly, without warning;
- do not have their symptoms controlled well;
- live with disability for much longer than cancer patients;
- are more likely to be socially isolated and rely on family members to care for them.

In comparison, people with cancer:

- have a predictable disease pathway and the end stage of disease is easily recognised;
- have their symptoms managed well;
- have the support of the huge investment made in palliative care by hospices and charities supporting cancer care.

For people with cancer, although the dying phase may take several days, there is no period of recovery.

The End of Life Care Strategy (DoH 2008) believes that everyone, irrespective of their disease, should be cared for appropriately when they are dying. This requires a degree of honesty on the part of healthcare professionals, skilled in the art of communicating sensitive information to the person with a poor prognosis and allowing them space and time to confront their situation and make decisions about the care they receive in the future. It may mean that the person with CHF makes a decision about active treatment.

COMMUNITY-BASED CARE

People with chronic heart disease are cared for in the community and specialist nurses monitor their progress and are on call for when there are acute exacerbations of the disease. These nurses ensure that people with heart disease are not admitted to acute care if they have decided that they no longer wish for this and they liaise with palliative care services for end-of-life care.

CASE STUDY SUMMARIES

Nursing patients with cardiovascular problems requires diligence, knowledge of the science and art of caring, skills in communication and an ability to respond quickly to emergency situations with dexterity and calmness. The three people used as case studies in this chapter experience chest pain, and it is the chest pain that motivates them to seek medical interventions. Chest pain can occur for a variety of reasons; it is not a single indicator of heart problems or indeed a cardiac arrest, other symptoms need to be considered. However, nurses should be ever vigilant when patients complain of chest pain.

Do not resuscitate orders (DNR)

As heart disease progresses, people may find themselves leading increasingly restrictive lives and the quality of life is deemed by them to be poor. They may wish to refuse further aggressive treatment of their symptoms when they relapse or present with yet another acute episode of illness. They may wish to state that in the event of cardiac or respiratory arrest, they do not wish for CPR. Making such a request does not mean that care stops; the person is still entitled to have pain relief, medications that treat infection and oxygen therapy. More specific requests regarding treatment can be made and documented in an Advanced Directive (formerly referred to as a living will).

Spirituality

It has been well-documented that people with heart problems experience depression that is often unrecognised. Sometimes this depression masks their spiritual distress; as they face their mortality, people may question their previously held values and beliefs, review their lives and question the legacy that they are about to leave behind. People in spiritual distress may express loss of hope, dignity and the will to live and feel that they are a burden to others. As stated above:

'It is frightening to think you might pop off at any moment.'

This type of statement requires further exploration by the nurse, to ascertain what is behind it. It is an opportunity to open up a discussion with the person, and discover if there are other aspects of need. Palliative care takes a holistic approach and relies on a multidisciplinary team to achieve its goals of meeting people's needs, whether they are physical, psychological, spiritual or social. Spirituality is expressed in diverse ways; for some, it is through religious observances and they may wish to observe particular customs as the end of life approaches. It is the nurse's role to facilitate this where possible (Ellis and Narayanasamy 2009).

All three will require hospitalisation and, although investigations such as ECG, x-rays and blood tests are the same, the outcomes are different. For example, cardiac markers are only present following a myocardial infarction and are not present in angina.

The risks factors for CVD are the same and lifestyle is a crucial factor that needs to be considered for all three. John needs to consider giving up smoking cigars; Zahir needs to consider his lifestyle pace, the travelling and other aspects that are part of a busy businessman's life; Mary needs to remain active and not become a 'cardiac cripple'. All three cases will benefit from a rehabilitation programme and advice regarding exercise and diet. All three could make a full recovery and live until old age.

CHAPTER HIGHLIGHTS

- Heart disease presents a challenge as it develops largely from lifestyle choices; the risk of developing heart disease increases in a society that is well fed, if not obese, and exercises less. Damage can be done while young and the consequences not realised until it is too late to change.

- Coronary heart disease is the UK's biggest killer, around one in five men and one in seven women die from the disease. Coronary heart disease is the term that describes what happens when the heart's blood supply is blocked or interrupted by a build up of fatty substances in the coronary arteries.

- There are several ways to help reduce the risk of developing coronary heart disease; these include reducing blood pressure and cholesterol levels. There are a number of ways this can be done, including eating a healthy, balanced diet, becoming more physically active and keep to a healthy weight.

- The acute coronary syndromes cover a spectrum of unstable coronary artery disease from unstable angina to transmural myocardial infarction. All have shared causes in the formation of thrombus on an inflamed and complicated atheromatous plaque. The principles behind the ways in which the patient presents, the various investigations and management of these syndromes are similar with important distinctions depending on the category of acute coronary syndrome.

- Sudden cardiac death is defined as an event that is non-traumatic, non-violent, unexpected, and resulting from sudden cardiac arrest within six hours of previously witnessed normal health. In 4% of sudden deaths in those aged between 16–64 years, post-mortem examination failed to identify any cause; these cases are diagnosed as having sudden arrhythmic death syndrome.

- Heart failure is a serious condition and describes what happens when the heart is having trouble pumping enough blood around the body and typically occurs as a result of the heart muscle becoming too weak or stiff to work effectively. Heart failure tends to affect older people, with an average age at diagnosis of 76 years; it is more common in men than women. The symptoms can happen quickly and this is known as acute heart failure. Usually the symptoms develop slowly over time, which is known as chronic heart failure.

- Patients with coronary heart disease and chronic heart failure deteriorate gradually, progressively finding that they do less and less before breathlessness takes over, reducing their activities. However, they are prone to a sudden exacerbation of their symptoms and approximately 50% of people may die; those that do recover may see some improvement but not to their previous levels of activity. Knowing when the terminal phase is imminent is difficult, family and friends may prepare for death only to find that the person survives the latest illness episode.

- Peripheral vascular disease happens when there is considerable narrowing of arteries distal to the arch of the aorta, usually due to atherosclerosis. Symptoms vary from calf pain on exercise to rest pain, skin ulceration and gangrene. Those diagnosed as having peripheral vascular disease, including those who have no symptoms, have an increased risk of mortality, myocardial infarction and stroke.

- In many cases life may continue after a major trauma such as a myocardial infarction and people may experience a reprieve.

- There are consequences to living with heart disease and the psychological impact that cardiovascular problems can cause should not be underestimated.

TEST YOURSELF

1. The heart consists of four chambers:

   a. blood from the pulmonary veins flows into the left atria

   b. blood from the pulmonary arteries flows into the left atria

   c. blood from the pulmonary veins flows into the right atria

   d. blood from the pulmonary arteries flows into the right atria

2. Pulmonary circulation takes the blood from:

   a. the heart to coronary arteries that supply the heart with oxygenated blood

   b. the heart to the lungs for oxygenation and then back to the heart

   c. the heart to the lungs for circulation of oxygenated blood to the body

   d. the heart to the body to supply it with oxygenated blood

3. Prinzmetal's angina occurs after:

   a. increased exercise, because of increased oxygen demand

   b. at night, due to coronary artery spasm

   c. following a large meal and increased metabolic activity

   d. the breakdown of an atheromatous plaque

4. When undertaking basic life support:

   a. it is more important to concentrate on the patient's breathing

   b. it is more important to concentrate on chest compressions and breathing at the same time

   c. it is more important to concentrate on chest compressions

   d. it is more important to summon help and concentrate on keeping the crowds away

5. The risk factors for developing CVD are:

   a. hypertension

   b. obesity

   c. smoking

   d. hypotension

6. From this list, which food would not be included in a cardioprotective diet?

   a. olive oil

   b. cod

   c. mackerel

   d. broccoli

7. Which of the following statements is not true about angina?

   a. 'Now I have angina I must exercise more.'

   b. 'Now I have angina I must have had a heart attack.'

   c. 'Now I have angina I must watch my salt intake.'

   d. 'Now I have angina I must carry pills at all times.'

8. The foods that can be eaten by a patient on anticoagulant therapy are:

   a. broccoli

   b. spinach

   c. runner beans

   d. cauliflower

9. Following cardiac catheterisation, a patient should rest for:

   a. 12 hours

   b. 24 hours

   c. 36 hours

   d. 48 hours

10. Of the following statements, which is not true about chronic heart disease?

    a. chronic heart disease has a typical, predictable disease progression

    b. chronic heart disease patients have poorer quality of life than cancer patients

    c. patients with chronic heart disease have similar symptoms to those with cancer

    d. patients with chronic heart disease are more likely to die suddenly

Further resources

British Heart Foundation (BHF)
http://www.bhf.org.uk
The BHF website offers information about heart disease and currently has dietary advice for people wishing to eat the right foods and lessen their risk of heart disease. The eat well plate educates us on the portion sizes we all should aim for to be healthy.

Patient UK
http://www.patient.co.uk/health/Myocardial-Infarction-(Heart-Attack).htm
This is another website with excellent explanations about myocardial infarction. There are links to other diseases, the explanations are supported with diagrams and it explains all the different drugs that may be prescribed and how they work.

WebMD
http://www.webmd.boots.com/heart-disease/default.htm
Boots The Chemist sponsor this website that provides useful information on all aspects of heart disease. There is patient

information which explains medical terms, sections to work through if you suspect you are a candidate for heart disease and advice on living with heart disease.

NHS Choices
http://www.nhs.uk/conditions/Cardiovascular-disease
This website gives detailed facts and figures about all aspects of heart disease and is a useful resource for healthcare professionals. It has all the relevant statistics. There are video clips and it is possible to analyse your own potential risk of developing heart disease.

Angina Plan
http://www.anginaplan.org.uk/index.htm
This website gives details about the 'angina plan', a cognitive behavioural approach that helps people learn to live with angina and improve their health status. The angina plan needs a facilitator, so this website is more appropriate for healthcare professionals. You can apply on-line and complete a distance learning course if you wish to develop further skills.

Bibliography

Aaronson P I and Ward J P T (2007) *The Cardiovascular System at a Glance* (3rd edn). Oxford, Blackwell Publishing.

Albarran J (2007) Women and coronary heart disease: new recommendations. *British Journal of Cardiac Care*, **2**(7), 314–316.

BHF (2010) *Coronary Heart Disease Statistics 2010*. London, British Heart Foundation.

Bowden T (2009) Evidence based care for patients undergoing angiography. *British Journal of Nursing*, **18**(13), 776–783.

Burgess J and Whitfield J (2009) Rehabilitation for patients with chronic heart failure: how do we deliver it to all? *British Journal of Cardiac Nursing*, **4**(1), 41–47.

Chummum H (2009) Reducing the incidence of coronary heart disease. *British Journal of Nursing*, **18**(14), 865–870.

Cortis J D and Williams A (2007) Palliative and supportive needs of older adults with heart failure. *International Council of Nurses*, **59**(3), 263–270.

Crosbie C, Coppinger T and Waywell C (2009) A practical guide to chronic heart failure. *Practice Nurse*, **20**(6), 288–294.

Daniels L (2002) Diet and coronary heart disease: advice on cardio protective diet. *British Journal of Community Nursing*, **7**(7), 346–350.

Dixon T, Lim L L Y, Powell H and Fisher J D (2000) Psychosocial experiences of cardiac patients in early recovery: a community based

study. *Journal of Advanced Nursing*, **31**(6), 1368–1375.

DoH (2008) *End of Life Care Strategy – Promoting high quality care for all adults at the end of life*. London, Department of Health.

DoH Heart Disease Policy Team (2006) *Shaping the Future: Progress Report for 2006. The Coronary Heart Disease National Service Framework*. Available at http://www.dh.gov.uk/prod_consum_dh/groups/dh_digitalassets/@dh/@en/documents/digitalasset/dh_063169.pdf (accessed September 2011).

Ellis H K and Narayanasamy A (2009) An investigation into the role of spirituality in nursing. *British Journal of Nursing*, **18**(14), 886–890.

Gibson T (2006) Factors determining diagnosis and admission of Bangladeshis with coronary symptoms. *British Journal of Cardiac Care*, **1**(1), 42–47.

Gray H H, Dawkins K D, Morgan J M and Simpson I A (2008) *Cardiology: Lecture Notes* (5th edn). Oxford, Blackwell Publishing.

Gregory P and Quinn T (2010) Out of hospital cardiac arrest and automated external defibrillation. In Kucia A M and Quinn T (eds), *Acute Cardiac Care: A practical guide for nurses*. Chichester, Wiley Blackwell, 145–151.

HDA (2001) *Coronary Heart Disease: Guidance for implementing the preventive aspects of the National Service Framework*. Health Development Agency.

Hemingway A (2007) Determinants of coronary heart disease risk for women on a low income: literature review. *Journal of Advanced Nursing*, **60**(4), 359–367.

Higgins M, Theobald K and Peters J (2008) Vascular access and cardiac complications after PCI: In and out of hospital outcome issues. *British Journal of Cardiac Nursing*, **3**(3), 111–116.

Jevon P and Hodgkins L (2010) Nurse led pharmacological stress testing: an overview. *British Journal of Nursing*, **19**(9), 569–574.

Keenan J (2010) Myocardial perfusion scintigraphy. *British Journal of Cardiac Nursing*, **5**(4), 173–177.

Kirk M and LeGeyt P (2010) Spotting early signs of depression in patients with chronic heart failure. *British Journal of Cardiac Nursing*, **5**(1), 13–18.

Kucia A M and Birchmore E (2010) Risk factors for cardiovascular disease. In Kucia A M and Quinn T (eds), *Acute Cardiac Care: A practical guide for nurses*. Chichester, Wiley Blackwell, 26–38.

Kucia A M and Horowitz J D (2010) Pathogenesis of acute coronary syndromes. In Kucia A M and Quinn T (eds), *Acute Cardiac Care: A practical guide for nurses*. Chichester, Wiley Blackwell, 161–166.

Kucia A M and Unger S A (2010) Cardiovascular assessment. In Kucia A M and Quinn T (eds), *Acute Cardiac Care: A practical guide for nurses*. Chichester, Wiley Blackwell, 67–80.

Maclean E, Patience F and Leslie S (2007) The Angina Plan: correcting misconceptions of patients with coronary heart disease. *British Journal of Cardiac Nursing*, **2**(8), 399–403.

Martin F (2010) The impact of depression on recovery and rehabilitation following STEMI. *British Journal of Cardiac Nursing*, **5**(2), 58–63.

Milerick Y (2008) Integrating palliative care recommendations into clinical practice for chronic heart failure. *British Journal of Cardiac Nursing*, **3**(12), 579–585.

Muggenthaler M, Sing A and Wilkinson P (2008) The role of coronary artery stents in PCI. *British Journal of Cardiac Nursing*, **3**(1), 24–30.

NHS Information Centre (2010) *National Heart Failure Audit*. Available at: http://www.ic.nhs.uk/ webfiles/publications/002_Audits/NHS_IC_ National_Heart_Failure_Audit_2010_04-01-11. pdf (accessed September 2011).

NICE (2010) *Chronic Heart Failure: Management of chronic heart failure in adults in primary and secondary care*, CG108. London, National Institute for Health and Clinical Excellence.

Nicholas M (2007) Setting up a primary percutaneous coronary intervention service. *British Journal of Cardiac Nursing*, **2**(9), 441–446.

O'Donovan K (2006) Ventricular assist devices: an overview. *British Journal of Cardiac Nursing*, **1**(8), 369–376.

O'Grady E (2007) *A Nurse's Guide to Cardiac Intervention Patients*. Chichester, Wiley.

Oldroyd C, Quinn T and Whiston P (2010) In-hospital resuscitation. In Kucia A M and Quinn T (eds), *Acute Cardiac Care: A practical guide for nurses*. Chichester, Wiley Blackwell, 243–256.

Patient UK (2010) *Epidemiology Coronary Heart Disease*. Available at: http://www.patient.co.uk/ doctor/Epidemiology-of-IHD.htm (accessed September 2011).

Peate I and Gault C (2001) Taking risks with coronary disease. *Practice Nurse*, **12**(3), 86–90.

Pierce-Hays I (2009) Heart attacks and circadian rhythms. *British Journal of Cardiac Nursing*, **4**(9), 416–423.

Prime K A (2006) The management of atrial fibrillation after coronary artery bypass surgery. *British Journal of Cardiac Nursing*, **1**(10), 462–469.

Resuscitation Council (UK) (2010) *2010 Resuscitation Guidelines*. London.

Riley J (2010) Updated NICE guidance on chronic heart failure. *British Journal of Cardiac Nursing*, **5**(11), 546–548.

Selman L, Harding R, Beynon T, *et al.* (2007) Improving end-of-life care for patients with chronic heart failure: 'Let's hope it'll get better, when I know in my heart of hearts it won't'. *Heart*, **93**, 963–967.

Stead C E (2009) Cardiac rehabilitation: benefits and low uptake, *Practice Nursing*, **20**(12), 596–600.

Thompson D R (2007) Improving end-of-life care for patients with chronic heart failure. *Heart*, **93**, 901–902.

Thorn M (2006) Cardiac tamponade in the immediate postoperative period following coronary artery bypass grafts. *British Journal of Cardiac Nursing*, **1**(12), 564–567.

Tough J and Morley R (2008) Service redesign of a rapid access chest pain clinic: reducing waiting times. *British Journal of Cardiac Nursing*, **3**(2), 71–77.

Wachtel T, Webster R and Smith J (2010) Populations at risk. In Kucia A M and Quinn T (eds), *Acute Cardiac Care: A practical guide for nurses*. Chichester, Wiley Blackwell, 39–49.

Whitlock A (2010) Acute heart failure: patient assessment and management. *British Journal of Cardiac Nursing*, **5**(11), 516–525.

Wrigley M and Lathlean J (2010) Family history of premature coronary heart disease: discussing the evidence. *British Journal of Cardiac Care*, **4**(12), 569–574.

Zeitz C J and Quinn T (2010) Reperfusion strategies. In Kucia A M and Quinn T (eds), *Acute Cardiac Care: A practical guide for nurses*. Chichester, Wiley Blackwell, 193–203.

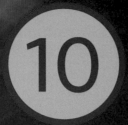

10

Caring for people with haematological problems

Learning outcomes

- Relate the physiology and assessment of the haematological system and related systems to commonly occurring haematological disorders.

- Describe the pathophysiology of common haematological disorders.

- Explain nursing implications for medications and other treatments prescribed for individuals with haematological disorders.

- Describe the major types of haematological cancers and nursing interventions.

- Compare and contrast the pathophysiology, signs and symptoms and management of bleeding disorders.

Clinical competencies

- Assess, monitor, document and deliver care related to the needs of people with haematological disorders taking into account the effects this may have on an individual's activities of living (ALs).

- Based on knowledge of pathophysiology, identify and prioritise nursing diagnoses for individuals with haematological disorders using up-to-date evidence-based knowledge.

- Safely and knowledgeably administer prescribed medications and treatments for individuals with haematological disorders.

- Work in a collaborative way with the multidisciplinary team to plan and provide coordinated, effective care.

- Provide appropriate teaching for individuals with haematological disorders, evaluating learning and the need for continued reinforcement of information.

CASE STUDIES

Below are three case studies that you may wish to consider before, during or after you have read the chapter. There are no right or wrong answers to these case studies, but you should think about the physical, psychological and social implications.

Case Study 1 – Malcolm

Mr Malcolm Donaldson is 30 years old, Caucasian, married to Sheila. He works as an accountant and they live in Manchester. Malcolm complained of feeling very tired with a chest cold which didn't seem to be getting better and prior to visiting the GP was sweating profusely at night. He was concerned that he had lost weight but usually had a good appetite.

The GP took a blood sample and telephoned Malcolm to attend the surgery for the results. He was advised his white cell count was high (40×10^9/L) and an urgent appointment had been made for Malcolm to attend the haematology clinic the next day. Sheila went with him to the clinic and, following further blood investigations by the haematologist, they were informed that Malcolm had acute lymphoblastic leukaemia (ALL).

Malcolm is admitted to the ward to commence chemotherapy the next day. Both Malcolm and Sheila are shocked and frightened. During assessment, Malcolm looks tired and informs the nurse he was scared of the diagnosis since his younger brother had the same diagnosis eight years earlier.

His height is 1.82 m and he weighs 88.2 kg. Vital sign monitoring highlights his temperature is 37.9 °C, pulse is 85 bpm and BP 120/80 mm/Hg, respiration is 20 breaths per minute. Malcolm informs you he has lost 1 kg in weight. He feels drained and finds he needs to rest quite a lot. In his words he describes himself as 'feeling old'.

He mentions he and Sheila were going to start a family – what actions should the nurse take?

Case Study 2 – Kirsty

Miss Kirsty James has just turned 17 years old and lives with her parents and two siblings, Monique, 20 years old and Carl, 14 years old, in Bristol. Kirsty was due to sit her mock GCSEs, but has been feeling very tired and has not been able to concentrate. Her parents have been very worried about her poor eating habits and loss of weight. On assessment, mum points out she had noticed Kirsty did not want to eat with the family, has been vomiting frequently and was quiet and withdrawn.

Her weight is 44.4 kg and her height is 1.52 m. These results raise concerns and following a clinical assessment Kirsty is diagnosed with anorexia nervosa. Blood investigations reveal Kirsty also has iron deficiency anaemia. During a conversation with Kirsty she has significant anxiety about gaining weight. She is referred to the mental health team and the dietician.

Case Study 3 – Marcia

Miss Marcia Anderson is 20 years old, an Afro-Caribbean, who was diagnosed with sickle cell anaemia when she was six months old. She lives in London with her parents and older sister, Carleen, who has sickle cell trait. She is in the second year of a business degree at a university 70 miles away from home. Marcia weighs 63.5 kg and her height is 1.52 m.

She arrived at the A&E department in an ambulance, with her sister, presenting with extreme pain in her right hip. Following triage, she was seen by the haematologist, and a physical assessment confirmed Marcia was having a vaso-occlusive sickling crisis. Her vital signs were recorded and her temperature raised concerns as it was 38 °C.

INTRODUCTION

Haematological disorders are diverse; many cause minor illnesses, but others can be life-threatening and life-shortening. Haematology is a fascinating subject, and this chapter will address the physiology of marrow cells, provide an overview of some haematological conditions and discuss general nursing principles in caring for patients with haematological conditions. The reader is guided to the further resources section at the end of the chapter for specialist books with more detailed information on haematology nursing and haematology disorders.

Haematological conditions can be myelodysplastic (poor production of myeloid marrow cells) or myeloproliferative, (excess production of marrow cells).

ANATOMY, PHYSIOLOGY AND FUNCTIONS OF THE HAEMATOLOGICAL SYSTEM

Blood is a transport system and is often referred to as 'the river of life'. It consists of fluid and cellular components. The fluid known as plasma makes up 55% of blood. The cellular components comprise 45% red blood cells (RBCs), platelets and white blood cells (WBCs).

The functions of blood include transporting oxygen, nutrients, hormones and metabolic waste; protecting against invasion of pathogens; maintaining blood coagulation; regulating fluids, electrolytes, acids–bases and body temperature.

Haemopoiesis is the production of marrow cells, which takes place within the bone marrow. In adults, the sternum, pelvis, cranium, upper epiphyses of the humeri, femuri and the vertebrae are the main sites of haemopoiesis. Marrow cells are red blood cells, white blood cells and platelets and they all originate from bone marrow cells known as **stem cells** or haemocytoblasts.

There is a fine balance in the bone marrow of supply and demand of marrow cells, and the production of any marrow cell is triggered by **growth factors**. Growth factors are glycoproteins which trigger stem cells to mature into marrow cells. Apart from platelets, all other marrow cells go through stages of **differentiation** to maturity (Figure 10.1).

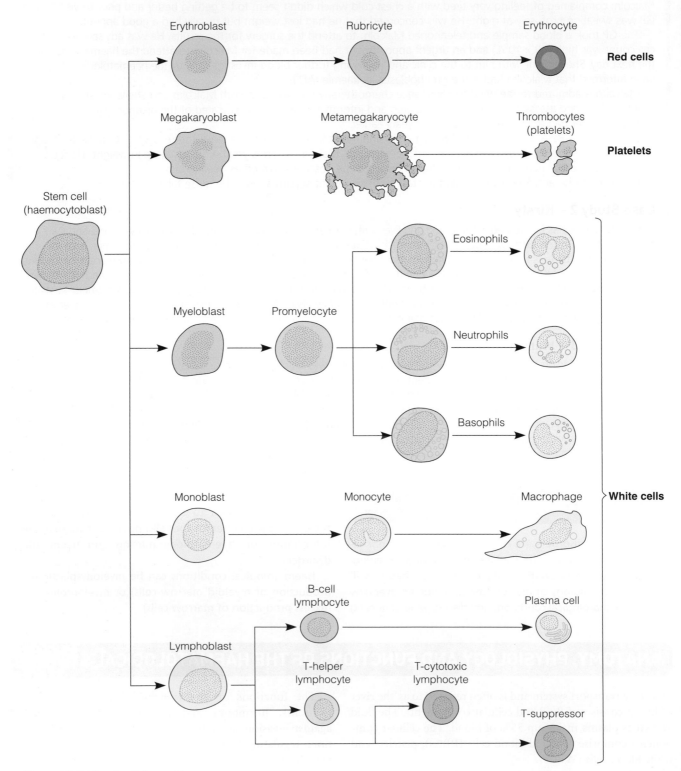

Figure 10.1 Blood cell formation.

Bone marrow ——————————————————————————————————————— → **Bloodstream** ——————→

Stem cell

Committed cell

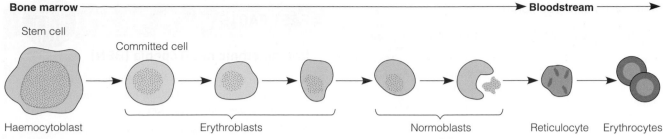

Haemocytoblast   Erythroblasts   Normoblasts   Reticulocyte   Erythrocytes

Figure 10.2 Erythropoiesis.

RED BLOOD CELLS (ERYTHROCYTES) (RBCs)

The stimulus for RBC production is tissue hypoxia. The hormone erythropoietin is released by the kidneys in response to hypoxia to stimulate the bone marrow to produce RBCs. Erythropoiesis is the name for the production of RBCs. There are several stages of differentiation from stem cell to erythrocyte (Figure 10.2). During differentiation the RBC starts out being very large and has a nucleus. Haemoglobin is formed in the proerythroblast stage and continues throughout the lifespan of the RBC. At the normoblast stage, the nucleus is ejected, leading to the characteristic biconcave shape of RBCs. The biconcave shape provides a greater surface area for gaseous exchange, and the structural and contractile muscles on the membrane of RBCs enable them to pass through very small capillaries (Figure 10.3).

The RBCs enter the bloodstream and circulate as reticulocytes (immature RBC) and fully mature in about 48 hours. From stem cell to RBC maturity takes approximately three to five days.

Consider this . . .

Did you know that, in order to compensate for excessive RBC destruction or during haemorrhage, the bone marrow responds by pushing out excessive reticulocytes into circulation? This is known as reticulocytosis.

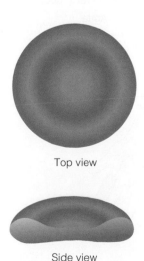

Top view

Side view

Figure 10.3 Top and side view of a red blood cell.

Haemoglobin molecules enable the RBCs to carry out their function of gaseous exchange. Haemoglobin carries oxygen (O_2) from the lungs to the tissues and is known as oxyhaemoglobin. There are approximately 300 million haemoglobin molecules in each RBC. Each haemoglobin molecule consists of a haem molecule, which holds an iron atom, and globin, a protein molecule. Globin is made of four polypeptide chains; two pairs of alpha chains (α) and two pairs of non-alpha chains. The iron atom binds reversibly with oxygen, allowing it to transport oxygen as oxyhaemoglobin. The amount of oxygen that reaches the tissues depends on a number of factors, including:

- available oxygen in the alveoli;
- the normal function of the lungs;
- the number of RBCs;
- the amount of haemoglobin in them;
- a normal functioning cardiovascular system.

The haemoglobin molecule also removes carbon dioxide (CO_2) (then known as carboxyhaemoglobin) from the tissues to the lungs for excretion. RBCs contain an enzyme called carbonic anhydrase, which converts CO_2 into hydrogen carbonate ions, reducing the acidity of RBCs.

The lifespan of RBCs is 120 days. Ageing and damaged RBCs are lysed (destroyed) by macrophages found in organs which make up the reticuloendothelial system (RES). Those organs are the spleen, liver, bone marrow and lymph nodes. Ageing RBCs undergo structural changes, becoming less efficient, and macrophages recognise these changes and destroy them. The process of RBC destruction is called haemolysis. When phagocytes engulf RBCs, the haemoglobin is split apart; the iron is separated from the haem, stored in the liver and reused for the production of new haemoglobin molecules. The haem is converted into bilirubin and stored in the gall bladder. The globin, being protein, is broken down into amino acids and is used in the making of new RBCs for its membrane and globin production.

Table 10.1 provides an example of normal blood values. Regionally these might vary slightly due to the demography of the local population. In the laboratory, the size, colour and shape of RBCs also may be analysed. RBCs may be normal size (normocytic), smaller than normal (microcytic) or larger than normal (macrocytic). Their colour may be normal (normochromic) or diminished (hypochromic) or increased (hyperchromic).

Abnormal numbers of RBCs, changes in their size and shape or altered haemoglobin content or structure can adversely affect health.

Table 10.1 Full blood count

Full blood count (FBC)	Normal values (indices)
RBC	Men: $4.5–5.5 \times 10^{12}$/L
	Women: $3.8–4.8 \times 10^{12}$/L
WBC	$4–11 \times 10^9$/L
Platelets	$150–400 \times 10^9$/L
Differential WBC	
Neutrophils	$2.0–7.0 \times 10^9$/L
Basophils	$0.05–0.1 \times 10^9$/L
Eosinophils	$0.02–0.5 \times 10^9$/L
Lymphocytes	$1.0–3.0 \times 10^9$/L
Monocytes	$0.2–1.0 \times 10^9$/L
Mean cell volume (MCV)	83–101 fl
Packed cell volume (PCV) (also known as haematocrit)	Men: 0.40–0.51
	Women: 0.36–0.48
Mean cell haemoglobin concentration (MCHC)	315–345 g/L
Mean cell haemoglobin (MCH)	27–32 pg*

* = picograms

THE LYMPHATIC SYSTEM

The structures of the lymphatic system include the lymphatic vessels and several lymphoid organs. The organs of the lymphatic system are the lymph nodes, the spleen, the thymus, the tonsils and the Peyer's patches of the small intestine. Lymph nodes are small aggregates of specialised cells that assist the immune system by removing foreign material, infectious organisms and tumour cells from lymph. Lymph nodes are distributed along the lymphatic vessels, forming clusters in certain body regions such as the neck, axilla and groin (see Figure 10.4).

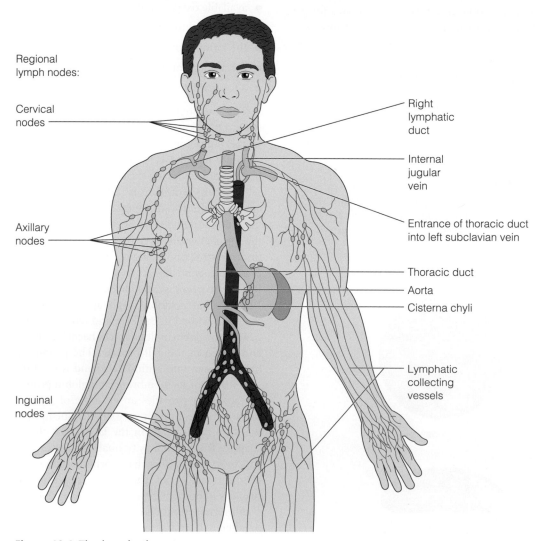

Figure 10.4 The lymphatic system.

The spleen, the largest lymphoid organ, is in the upper left quadrant of the abdomen under the thorax. The main function of the spleen is to filter the blood by breaking down old RBCs and storing or releasing to the liver their by-products (such as iron). The spleen also synthesises lymphocytes, stores platelets for blood clotting and serves as a reservoir of blood. The thymus gland is in the lower throat and is most active in childhood, producing hormones (such as thymosin) that facilitate the immune action of lymphocytes. The tonsils of the pharynx and Peyer's patches of the small intestine are lymphoid organs that protect the upper respiratory and digestive tracts respectively from foreign pathogens.

The lymphatic vessels or lymphatics form a network around the arterial and venous channels and interweave at the capillary beds. They collect and drain excess tissue fluid, called lymph, that 'leaks' from the cardiovascular system and accumulates at the venous end of the capillary bed. The lymphatics return this fluid to the heart through a one-way system of lymphatic venules and veins that eventually drain into the right lymphatic duct and left thoracic duct, both of which empty into their respective subclavian veins. Lymphatics are a low-pressure system without a pump; their fluid transport depends on the rhythmic contraction of their smooth muscle and the muscular and respiratory pumps that assist venous circulation.

DISORDERS OF THE RED BLOOD CELLS (ERYTHROCYTES)

The person with anaemia

Any dysfunction of an erythrocyte will compromise its ability to transport and distribute oxygen to tissues. The morphology (size and shape of red blood cells) tends to be altered in almost all erythrocyte disorders.

Anaemia is the most common problem of erythrocytes, which is defined as either a reduction in the number of circulating red blood cells or reduction in haemoglobin concentration or both.

Pathophysiology of anaemia

Anaemia can be classified into three categories as illustrated in Table 10.2. The type and severity of the anaemia will determine treatment interventions needed to manage it.

Table 10.2 Classification of anaemias

Anaemia due to reduced erythropoiesis	Anaemia due to excessive haemolysis	Anaemia due to blood loss
Aplastic anaemia	Sickle cell disease(H)	Gastric bleeding
Vitamin B$_{12}$ deficiency	Thalassaemia syndromes (H)	Menorrhagia
Folate deficiency	Hereditary sphercytosis (H)	Oesophageal varices
Iron deficiency	Glucose-6-phosphate-Dehydrogenase (G6PD)(H)	Inflammatory bowel disease
Crohn's disease	Disseminated intravascular coagulation (A)	Haemorrhoids
Myelodysplastic syndrome	Thrombotic thrombocytopenia purpura (A)	Uterine fibroids
	Burns (A)	
	Drugs – e.g. primaquine (A)	

A = acquired; H = hereditary.

Signs and symptoms of anaemia

General signs and symptoms of anaemia are:

- pallor;
- fatigue;
- general malaise;
- angina pectoris;
- dyspnoea;
- headaches;
- dizziness;
- oliguria;
- hypotension;
- tachycardia;
- jaundice;
- poor concentration;
- fainting;
- hyperplasia;
- cold, clammy skin;
- muscular weakness;
- pale-coloured stools;
- pica;
- paraesthesia;
- splenomegaly;
- altered levels of consciousness.

The multisystem effects of anaemia are illustrated in Figure 10.5.

Nutritional anaemias

There are a number of essential nutrients the lack of which compromises erythropoiesis. Iron is crucial for haemoglobin. Vitamin B$_{12}$ (cobalamin) is essential for nucleic synthesis in the pro-erythroblast stage. Folic acid aids in maturation of red blood cells and is also required for RNA synthesis. Copper acts

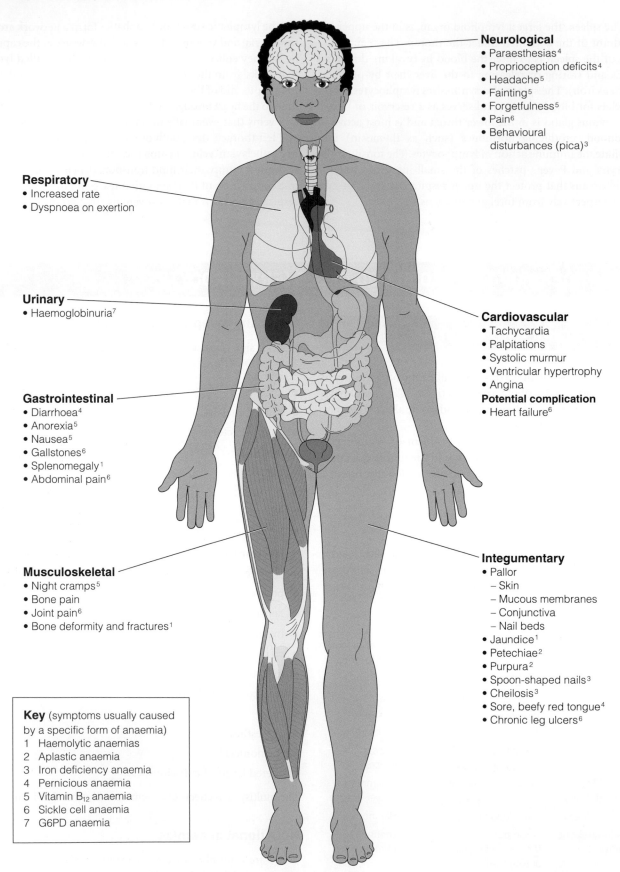

Neurological
- Paraesthesias[4]
- Proprioception deficits[4]
- Headache[5]
- Fainting[5]
- Forgetfulness[5]
- Pain[6]
- Behavioural disturbances (pica)[3]

Respiratory
- Increased rate
- Dyspnoea on exertion

Urinary
- Haemoglobinuria[7]

Cardiovascular
- Tachycardia
- Palpitations
- Systolic murmur
- Ventricular hypertrophy
- Angina
Potential complication
- Heart failure[6]

Gastrointestinal
- Diarrhoea[4]
- Anorexia[5]
- Nausea[5]
- Gallstones[6]
- Splenomegaly[1]
- Abdominal pain[6]

Musculoskeletal
- Night cramps[5]
- Bone pain
- Joint pain[6]
- Bone deformity and fractures[1]

Integumentary
- Pallor
  - Skin
  - Mucous membranes
  - Conjunctiva
  - Nail beds
- Jaundice[1]
- Petechiae[2]
- Purpura[2]
- Spoon-shaped nails[3]
- Cheilosis[3]
- Sore, beefy red tongue[4]
- Chronic leg ulcers[6]

Key (symptoms usually caused by a specific form of anaemia)
1 Haemolytic anaemias
2 Aplastic anaemia
3 Iron deficiency anaemia
4 Pernicious anaemia
5 Vitamin B_{12} anaemia
6 Sickle cell anaemia
7 G6PD anaemia

Figure 10.5 Multisystem effects of anaemia.

as a catalyst for iron to be utilised by haemoglobin. Protein is key for RBC membrane and globin manufacturing. Vitamin C aids in iron absorption and vitamin E, an antioxidant, helps to protect cells from damage and oxidation.

Iron deficiency anaemia (IDA)

IDA and pernicious anaemia (PA) are the most common nutritional anaemias in the UK. In IDA, the RBC are usually hypochromic, related to low haemoglobin and microcytic RBCs.

FAST FACT

IDA

Considering the variety of food available in the developed world, it could be considered surprising that 2–5% of men and post-menopausal women in the developed world have IDA.

Source: Goddard *et al.* 2005.

IDA occurs when demand outweighs supply, resulting in a reduction in RBC formation. Common causes of IDA are:

- chronic bleeding;
- gastric bleeding;
- menorrhagia;
- adolescent growth spurts;
- pregnancy;
- insufficient nutritional intake (less than 1 mg/day);
- malabsorption;
- schistosomiasis;
- Crohn's disease;
- ulcerative colitis;
- bowel cancer;
- stomach cancer;
- gastric ulcers;
- non-steroidal anti-inflammatory drugs (NSAIDs);
- vitamin C deficiency.

Signs and symptoms

General signs and symptoms are addressed on page 343, but there are particular manifestations seen in IDA, if severe, which are listed below:

- glossitis, (red swollen sore tongue);
- pica (craving–especially for ice);
- koilonychia (spoon-shaped finger nails);
- tinnitus;
- angular cheilitis (inflammatory lesions at the mouth's corners);
- restless leg syndrome (RLS);

- hair loss;
- twitching muscles;
- constipation;
- light-headedness.

Blood results which suggest IDA are *reduction* in:

- haemoglobin (Hb)
- mean cell volume (MCV)
- mean cell haemoglobin concentration (MCHC)
- mean cell haemoglobin (MCH)

and an *increase* in:

- total iron binding capacity (TIBC)
- Transferrin
- red cell distribution width (RDW).

Vitamin B$_{12}$ deficiency anaemia

Vitamin B$_{12}$ is essential for DNA synthesis in early RBC development, and the most common type of B$_{12}$ deficiency is known as pernicious anaemia (PA) (Addison's anaemia).

PA is caused by the lack of absorption of Vitamin B$_{12}$, known as the extrinsic factor. Its lack of absorption is due to the lack of the intrinsic factor (IF). The IF is found in hydrochloric acid (HCl) produced by the parietal cells in the stomach. PA is also known as megaloblasticanaemia because the RBCs are macrocytic (larger in size), hyperchromic (bright/deep in colour), but are reduced in number. Vitamin B$_{12}$ is stored in the liver and once the stores are depleted, the individual will exhibit signs of anaemia. Some of the causes of PA are total or partial gastrectomy and malabsorption disorders such as Crohn's disease. Evidence suggests that PA may have an autoimmune cause in which the individual produces antibodies directed against their parietal cells leading to atrophic gastritis. This would impair binding of vitamin B$_{12}$ to the IF. Dietary deficiencies of vitamin B$_{12}$ are rare, usually occurring only among strict vegetarians and vegans.

FAST FACTS

PA

- PA appears to be more common in people with blood group A, those who have a low level of IgA (immunoglobulin), hypoparathyroidism, carcinoma of the stomach, blue eyes and premature greying.
- Women are at a higher risk of developing PA.
- PA tends to occur in people who are over 40 years old.
- The incidence of PA is approximately 10 per 100 000 of people who are of Celtic (i.e. Scottish, English, Irish) and Scandinavian origins.

Source: Van Amsterdam *et al.* 2005.

Signs and symptoms

General signs and symptoms are as outlined in Table 10.2, but there are some specific ones that are associated with PA:

- degeneration of the myelin sheath leads to significant potential neurological problems including damage to the optic nerve, causing blurred vision and potential blindness, ataxia, hallucinations, depression;

- **orthopnoea**;

- hyperpigmentation in black people is quite common;

- weight loss may occur due to anorexia;

- constipation;

- diarrhoea.

Laboratory results confirming PA are outlined below:

- macrocytic red blood cells;

- MCV and MCH are increased;

- MCHC tends to be normal;

- the Schillings test may be conducted – the purpose of this test is to differentiate between B_{12} deficiency due to PA and an intestinal lesion causing malabsorption.

Folic acid deficiency anaemia

Folic acid is stored in the liver, and a deficiency is almost always due to insufficient amounts in the diet. It is quite common for folic acid deficiency and vitamin B_{12} deficiency to coexist, but a key difference in symptom presentation is the lack of neurological symptoms in folic acid deficiency.

Folic acid deficiency anaemia is more common among people who are chronically undernourished. This includes the elderly, alcoholics and drug users. Alcoholics are especially at risk because alcohol suppresses folate metabolism, which forms folic acid. Increased folic acid requirements such as in pregnancy, infants and adolescent growth spurts can lead to anaemia if not addressed. Chronic exfoliative dermatitis, intestinal diseases, liver and gastric cancers can also lead to folic acid deficiency. Drugs such as methotrexate and some anticonvulsants, for example phenytoin, can also lead to folate deficiency.

Haemolytic anaemias

Haemolytic anaemias relate to excessive destruction of RBCs leading to anaemia. In response to the excessive haemolysis, the haematopoietic activity of bone marrow increases, leading to increased reticulocytes (immature RBCs) in circulating blood, but they are ineffective in gaseous exchange.

Haemolytic anaemias are classified as hereditary (caused by an intrinsic fault) or acquired (caused by an extrinsic fault). Table 10.2 has examples of the different types of haemolytic anaemias. This section will discuss the pathophysiology and nursing interventions for sickle cell anaemia, thalassaemia and acquired anaemias.

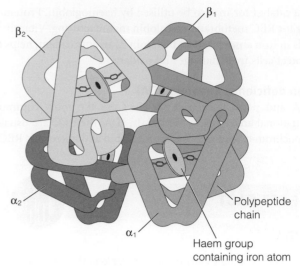

Figure 10.6 Haemoglobin molecule.

Sickle cell disease (SCD)

All individuals inherit their haemoglobin genotype. The normal haemoglobin genotype is known as HbAA. The globin structure is the portion of the haemoglobin which is inherited and determines the genotype. Haemoglobin A is composed of alpha amino acids (α) and beta amino acids (β) (Figure 10.6).

In SCD the genetic fault occurs on the 6th beta chain which leads to a substitution of the protein glutamic acid required for HbAA and is replaced by the protein valine, which produces HbSS.

The sickle gene originated in parts of the world where malaria is endemic. It is therefore found predominantly in West Africa (especially Nigeria), the Caribbean, the Mediterranean, the Middle East and the Indian subcontinent (particularly the Orissa state). The incidence of carrier status is illustrated in Table 10.3.

People with sickle cell trait (HbAS) are healthy unaffected individuals who carry one gene for sickle haemoglobin and one gene for normal haemoglobin. It has been well recognised that HbAS offers protection against *Plasmodium falciparum*, a type of malaria infection.

SCD is an **autosomal** recessively inherited condition, affecting the haemoglobin. SCD is a syndrome which encompasses

Table 10.3 Frequency of some haemoglobin variants

Sickle cell trait	Beta thalassaemia trait	Alpha thalassaemia trait
Afro-Caribbeans 1:10	Greek Cypriots 1:7	China/Far East 1:20
Nigerians 1:4	Turks 1:12	Mediterranean 1:30–100
Middle East/ Mediterranean/ Indian sub- continent 1:100	Gujaratis 1:10	
	Hindus 1:20	
	South Indians 1:20	
	Pakistanis 1:25	

Source: www.sickle-thal.nwlh.nhs.uk

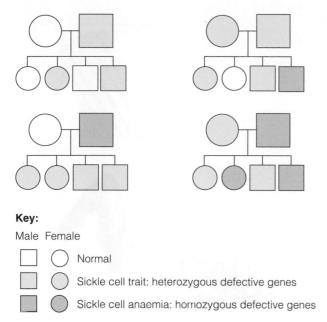

Key:

Male Female

☐ ○ Normal

☐ ○ Sickle cell trait: heterozygous defective genes

☐ ○ Sickle cell anaemia: homozygous defective genes

Figure 10.7 Inheritance pattern for sickle cell anaemia.

any abnormal haemoglobin genotype which combines with HbS. The most common combinations are: Hb SS–sickle cell anaemia (SCA), Hb SC disease (Hb SC) and sickle/beta thalassaemia (Hb S/Beta). The most common of all worldwide is SCA.

The terms sickle cell disease (SCD) and sickle cell anaemia (SCA) are sometimes used interchangeably, but should be seen as separate entities. Sickle cell trait is not included in SCD syndrome because it does not cause any illness. An example of inheritance of SCD is illustrated in Figure 10.7 related to SCA.

If both parents have sickle cell trait, there is a one in four chance (25%) the child will have HbAA (normal Hb genotype), 1 in 2 (50%) chance the child will have sickle cell trait (HbAS) and a 1 in 4 (25%) of having sickle cell anaemia. These risks remain the same for each and every pregnancy.

FAST FACTS

SCD

- There are approximately 12 500 people in the UK with SCD, making it one of the commonest genetic disorders found in the UK.

- SCD is diagnosed in 1 in 2400 births in the UK.

- It is important to note that symptoms of SCD do not occur before the age of three to six months because of foetal haemoglobin which has a high affinity for oxygen. However, during three to six months post-natally the percentage of foetal haemoglobin decreases and the haemoglobin genotype the infant has inherited increases, which then leads to the manifestations of the disease.

Source: www.sicklecellsociety.org.uk.

Pathophysiology

In SCD when the RBCs are oxygenated they retain the normal biconcave shape; however, when the haemoglobin gives up oxygen to tissues it is deoxygenated and valine, being a sticky protein, encourages the haemoglobin molecules to **polymerise**. This action leads to the distortion in the shape of the RBC, causing a sickle shape. Once these sickle-shaped RBCs are re-oxygenated they return to a biconcave shape. The continual changing of shape eventually leads to erythrocytes tiring and becoming irreversibly sickled, and they are destroyed by macrophages, leading to excessive haemolysis. The lifespan of sickle RBCs is approximately 10–20 days causing chronic haemolytic anaemia and haemoglobin is usually between 8 and 10 g/dL. The pathophysiology of sickle cell anaemia is illustrated in Figure 10.8.

The abnormal sickle-shaped erythrocyte has difficulty navigating through capillary blood vessels and periodically occludes blood flow to tissues and organs. As more sickle-shaped erythrocytes become trapped in a blood vessel, this leads to tissue hypoxaemia, tissue necrosis and the ultimate major significant problem known as painful vaso-occlusive crisis (VOC). The frequency and severity of these crises varies from person to person. Any organ can be affected which means any crisis can be life-threatening and potentially life-shortening.

There are some known precipitating factors which can cause a crisis, and these are:

- dehydration
- excessive exercise
- low oxygen levels
- infection
- smoking
- stress
- sudden change in temperature
- alcohol
- pregnancy.

VOC can lead to major life-threatening complications which are illustrated in Figure 10.9.

Hand foot syndrome is the first sign of SCD. Strokes are a major complication both in children and adults. Ten per cent of children will have a stroke before their 10th birthday. Sequestration (pooling of blood in an organ), particularly in the spleen in children and the liver in adults, can lead to hypovolaemic shock. Acute sequestration of the lungs can occur in both children and adults and is associated with significant mortality. Infections are a serious risk due to chronic anaemia and a dysfunctional spleen. Priapism (painful involuntary erection of the penis) can lead to erectile difficulties. In adults, multisystem organ failure is a major concern due to micro-sickling in organs causing their dysfunction.

Thalassaemia

Thalassaemia is an autosomal recessively inherited condition and relates to a defect in the synthesis of haemoglobin.

Haemoglobin S and Red Blood Cell Sickling

Sickle cell anaemia is caused by an inherited autosomal recessive defect in Hb synthesis. Sickle cell haemoglobin (HbS) differs from normal haemoglobin only in the substitution of the amino acid valine for glutamine in both beta chains of the haemoglobin molecule.

When HbS is oxygenated, it has the same globular shape as normal haemoglobin. However, when HbS off-loads oxygen, it becomes insoluble in intracellular fluid and crystallises into rod-like structures. Clusters of rods form polymers (long chains) that bend the erythrocyte into the characteristic crescent shape of the sickle cell.

The Sickle Cell Disease Process

Sickle cell disease is characterised by episodes of acute painful crises. Sickling crises are triggered by conditions causing high tissue oxygen demands or that affect cellular pH. As the crisis begins, sickled erythrocytes adhere to capillary walls and to each other, obstructing blood flow and causing cellular hypoxia. The crisis accelerates as tissue hypoxia and acidic metabolic waste products cause further sickling and cell damage.

Sickle cell crises cause microinfarcts in joints and organs, and repeated crises slowly destroy organs and tissues. The spleen and kidneys are especially prone to sickling damage.

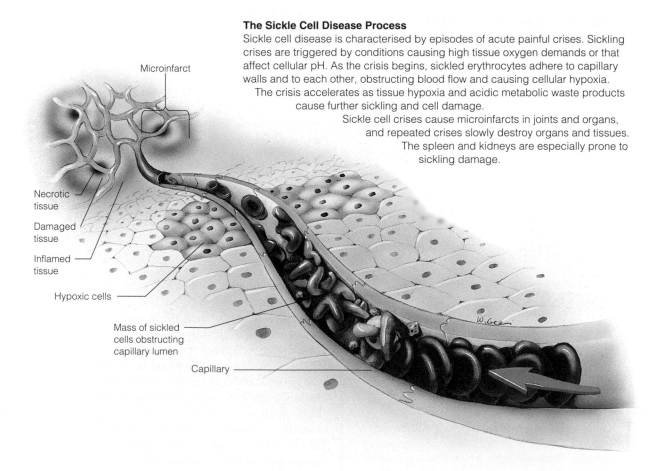

Figure 10.8 Pathophysiology illustrated: sickle cell anaemia.

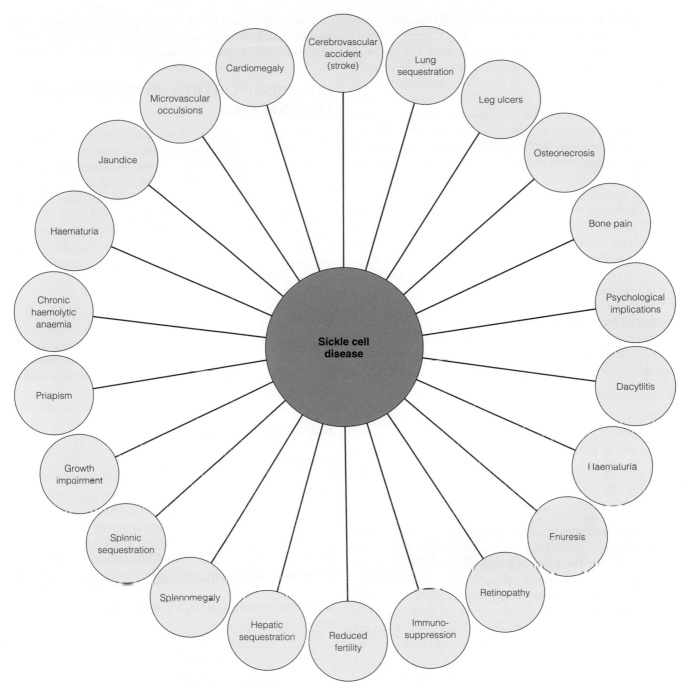

Figure 10.9 Complications of sickle cell disease.

Thalassaemia can affect either the alpha amino acids or the beta amino acids.

Alpha thalassaemia
Haemoglobin A comprises four alpha chains and deletion of one or two leads to alpha thalassaemia trait, which is asymptomatic. The deletion of three alpha chains leads to haemoglobin H disease, which causes chronic haemolytic anaemia. Deletion of all four alpha amino acid chains results in alpha thalassaemia major causing hydrops fetalis, leading to death *in utero* or stillbirth.

Beta thalassaemia trait
As with SCD, the individual with beta thalassaemia minor has inherited one defective beta-forming gene. If both beta genes are defective the person has beta thalassaemia major.

PRACTICE ALERT

Beta thalassaemia trait can mimic IDA and therefore haemoglobin electrophoresis should be undertaken to exclude it prior to iron administration.

In beta thalassaemia major, the individual is unable to synthesise haemoglobin and therefore the RBCs do not have any means to carry oxygen. This leads to anaemia and the body responds by increasing erythropoiesis. However, the erythropoiesis is ineffective because of the lack of haemoglobin synthesis, and this results in the erythrocytes being unable to function and being rapidly destroyed, leading to excessive haemolysis and chronic anaemia. The increase in erythrocytosis leads to hyperplasia (thinning of the bones), and potential fractures are possible as well as skeletal abnormalities, such as cranial bossing.

As in SCD, infants born with BTM do not present with any signs until after the age of three months, when they begin to fail to thrive, regress on milestones, become jaundiced, lethargic due to excessive haemolysis and present with splenomegaly. The prevalence of alpha and beta thalassaemia can be found in Table 10.3. Investigations to diagnose thalassaemia are the same for SCD.

Acquired haemolytic anaemia

Acquired haemolytic anaemia results from haemolysis due to factors outside of the RBC. Causes of acquired haemolytic anaemias include:

- autoimmune disorders;
- mechanical trauma to RBCs produced by prosthetic heart valves, severe burns, haemodialysis or radiation;
- bacterial or protozoal infection;
- immune-system-mediated responses, such as transfusion reactions;
- drugs, toxins, chemical agents or venoms.

The manifestations of acquired haemolytic anaemia depend on the extent of haemolysis and the body's ability to replace destroyed RBCs. The anaemia itself is often mild to moderate as erythropoiesis increases to replace the destroyed RBCs. The spleen enlarges as it removes damaged or destroyed RBCs. If the breakdown of haem units exceeds the liver's ability to conjugate and excrete bilirubin, jaundice develops. When the condition is severe, bone marrow expands, and bones may be deformed or may develop pathological fractures. The severity of generalised signs and symptoms of anaemia depends on the degree of anaemia and deficiency of tissue oxygenation.

Autoimmune disorders can be categorised as warm autoimmune haemolytic anaemia (AIHA) or cold autoimmune haemolytic anaemia, based on how the RBC reacts at a temperature of 37 °C or 4 °C. AIHA relates to patients producing antibodies against their own RBCs, 'coating' them, causing their haemolysis.

Ig (G) is the culprit antibody causing warm AIHA and Ig (M) causes cold AIHA. There are several options to manage warm AIHA, which include prednisolone in the first instance. If this is not effective, immunosuppressive drugs such as cyclophosphamide maybe prescribed. Other options are splenectomy or the monoclonal antibody, rituximab. In severe cases, blood transfusion and folic acid would be administered.

Treatment for cold AIHA is treating the underlying cause if identified and primarily advising the patient to keep warm. Chemotherapy or rituximab might be used in chronic cases.

INTERDISCIPLINARY AND NURSING CARE FOR ANAEMIAS

Anaemia causes weakness and shortness of breath on exertion. These symptoms are due to decreased circulating oxygen levels secondary to low haemoglobin levels. Weakness, fatigue and/or vertigo may occur during ALs, including those associated with self-care, home life, work and social roles. Care must be adapted to suit the individual's needs, with the aim being to alleviate symptoms, increase oxygen-carrying capacity of erythrocytes and prevent complications. Assessment and effective care planning are important in addressing and identifying the advice needed by patients.

Diagnosis

In addition to the blood values given in Table 10.1 on page 342, Table 10.4 lists investigations which may be undertaken to diagnose anaemia and thereby establish appropriate clinical treatment and nursing interventions.

Nutritional anaemias

Assessment

Assessment and effective care planning are important in identifying the advice needed by the individual and to address the impact of the anaemia on ALs. In Case Study 2, Kirsty was complaining of tiredness and difficulty with concentration. Nursing assessment should ascertain if she has shortness of breath with activity, fatigue, weakness, dizziness, fainting or palpitations. Identify any previous history of anaemia, chronic

Table 10.4 Investigations for anaemia

Test	Normal indices
Serum iron	10–30 μmol/L
Total iron binding capacity (TIBC)	40–75 μmol/L
Vitamin B_{12}	160–925 ng/L
Transferrin	1.7–3.4 g/L
Schillings test	Less than 11% ^{57}Co B_{12} excretion in urine.
Serum ferritin	40–300 μg/L
Haemoglobin electrophoresis	Determine haemoglobin genotype.
RDW–RBC distribution width	Change in width, size occurs in anaemias.
Bone marrow aspiration	If diagnosis is difficult this examination may be undertaken to directly examine the precursors to red cells.

diseases, bleeding episodes, menstrual history, and medications which may cause anaemia as a side-effect. Assess her usual diet and patterns of alcohol intake and/or cigarette smoking. In addition, her general appearance, skin colour, vital signs, abdominal tenderness and obvious bleeding or bruising should be recorded.

The majority of individuals with nutritional anaemia are cared for in the community. However, as nutritional anaemia can be secondary to major illnesses, it is important that nutritional assessments are undertaken regardless of whether the patient is in the community or in hospital.

Medication

IDA is primarily treated with oral iron medication and less commonly parenterally. The common oral ferrous compounds are ferrous gluconate (300 mg) three times a day or ferrous sulphate (200 mg) three times a day. Prior to the administration of oral iron, nurses should be aware of drugs that might adversely interact with iron. In syrup form, ferrous sulphate can stain the teeth and therefore it is best to use a straw.

Parenteral iron administration may be considered if:

- oral iron is not being absorbed from the gut;
- iron balance remains unresolved even with maximum oral dosage being prescribed; or
- malabsorption minimises iron absorption.

Iron Dextran or Venofer® (iron sucrose) are the parenteral iron sources used in the UK.

Anaphylaxis is a major concern with both drugs, but especially with Dextran, and therefore Venofer® is increasingly the drug of choice. Close monitoring of vital signs for early detection of anaphylactic shock is critical; these include erythema or flushing, oedema, wheezing, dyspnoea, nausea, vomiting, anxiety, metallic taste in the mouth, angioedema and urticaria. It is advisable to have an anaphylactic drug tray readily available.

Constipation, black stools and dysphagia are some side-effects of iron medication and laxatives may be required. Aim to encourage the individual to increase their fibre intake and fluids to help minimise the discomfort of constipation.

Nutrition

Individuals should be provided with advice on foods rich in iron to help with increasing iron intake. Iron is much more readily available as haem iron, which is found predominately in meat. Although green leafy vegetables contain iron it is not so easily absorbed because it is non-haem. People who are vegetarians or vegans need to be advised to increase their dietary intake of food which has a high iron content. Below is a list of foods rich in iron and folic acid.

- Food sources of haem:
  - beef
  - chicken
  - pork
  - clams
  - oysters

COMMUNITY-BASED CARE

PA is managed with an initial dose of 6 × of 1000 µg of hydroxocobalamin for two to three weeks to reverse the deficiency. Once established, the patient commences on a life long treatment of three-monthly intramuscular injections. This is usually administered in primary care in the general practitioner's surgery, as there is a risk of anaphylactic reactions. Generally, the individual is advised to stay in the surgery for 20–30 minutes to be monitored for such reactions.

Psychological support is very important for the individual as this is a change in lifestyle and they need to understand why it is important to have and maintain the treatment. Once started on their treatment, some symptoms, such as poor appetite, may resolve soon after commencement. However, neurological symptoms such as paraesthesia and numbness may take up to a year to resolve, and other complications such as degeneration of the optic nerve might be irreversible. Individuals who have neurological problems may require referral to a neurologist.

Encouraging attendance for out-patient appointments is important as PA is associated with gastric cancer and thyroid cancer. Periodic stool examination for occult blood and thyroid function tests are undertaken for early diagnosis of these cancers.

- egg yolk
- turkey
- veal
- Food sources of non-haem:
  - bran cereals
  - brown rice
  - whole grain breads
    dried fruits
  - greens (spring)
  - dried beans
- Food sources of folic acid (part of the B vitamin group):
  - oranges
  - broccoli
  - eggs
  - bananas
  - milk
  - brussels sprouts
  - liver
  - kidney beans
  - asparagus
- Food sources of vitamin B$_{12}$:
  - liver
  - kidney
  - cheese
  - beef
  - eggs
  - shrimps

Polyphenols found in tea and coffee can impair iron absorption and therefore patients should be advised to reduce their intake temporarily until the iron stores are increased.

Health promotion

It is important individuals are encouraged to continue their iron medication for the specified period of time, usually three to six months, since it can take three months for the body to replenish its stores. People can feel much better after a short period of taking iron and may discontinue before the body's stores have been replenished and IDA could return. As a teenager, this advice is very important for Kirsty (Case Study 2), especially as she will have blood loss from her menstrual cycle. Informing her mother of food sources of iron to help with meal preparation should also be considered.

PRACTICE ALERT

- Care should be taken not to give folic acid instead of B$_{12}$ to any patient who is B$_{12}$ deprived as this may result in fulminant neurological deficit.

- Oral iron therapy should be given before B$_{12}$ if iron deficiency is also present.

Nurses should be aware that the elderly are particularly at risk for developing folic acid deficiency due to a lack of interest in food, poverty, immobility and/or ill-fitting dentures. Therefore sensitive communication is needed to identify any of the above problems and make appropriate referral to other services, for example dentists or social services. Nurses should observe for signs of B$_{12}$ deficiency when elderly individuals are prescribed folate supplements and recommend folic acid supplements to women of child bearing age in order to prevent foetal neural tube defects.

FAST FACTS

Folate

- Folate is absorbed in the small intestine and a small reserve is stored in the liver.
- The daily intake of folic acid is 100–200 µg.

Eliminating the contributing causes of folic acid deficiency is important. Oral administration of folate preparations are 1–5 mg daily. If necessary the individual should be referred to a dietician to help them with planning meals. If individuals with IDA or folate deficiency smoke or drink regularly, they should be advised to stop or reduce these activities as both impair iron and folate absorption.

The oral cavity can be particularly affected in nutritional anaemia, and undertaking oral assessment using an oral assessment tool is important to reduce the risk of infection and haemorrhage. Glossitis can cause bleeding and increases the risk of fungal infections such as *Candida albicans*. The section on leukaemia addresses oral care (page 363).

Sickle cell anaemia

Diagnosis

To diagnose SCD, the following tests are undertaken:

- haemoglobin electrophoresis; or
- high-performance liquid chromatography; and
- FBC to determine haemoglobin and serum iron levels.

Treatment

Blood transfusion

Blood transfusion is not part of normal management in SCD crisis, but is used in certain circumstances – cerebrovascular accident, pre- and post-surgery, aplastic crisis, frequent sickling crisis causing organ damage, chest sequestration – and it might be an option in ante natal management.

Chemotherapy

An alternative to blood transfusion in recent years has been hydroxyurea (HU). This is a chemotherapy drug, prescribed to some children and adults with SCD who experience severe and/or frequent VOC. HU has been found to increase the percentage of foetal haemoglobin, thereby increasing the oxygen-carrying capacity of RBCs which could reduce the frequency of VOC.

Nursing diagnoses and interventions

The majority of hospital admissions in SCD are for acute painful VOC and therefore the main nursing care interventions are effective pain relief, monitoring for any deterioration and emotional support. Nurses should be familiar with local hospital guidelines and protocols in caring for patients experiencing a painful crisis.

Pain management

Effective pain assessment using a good pain assessment tool is important. Establish where the pain is and when it started and ascertain the last time the individual took any analgesia (this is essential to avoid the risk of overdose). Timely administration of analgesia is good practice and opioids, such as morphine or oxycodone, and NSAIDs, such as ibuprofen, are commonly prescribed in acute VOC. Patient-controlled analgesia (PCA) pumps are very effective in both administering and managing pain relief and are frequently used. Reassess the effectiveness of analgesia at least 30–40 minutes following administration. Keeping the person warm or use of distraction therapy, such as TV or massage, can help to manage the pain. For further information on pain management, see Chapter 2 on cancer.

Risk for health deterioration

The following issues should be considered as part of the nursing care plan for SCD:

✚ Regular monitoring of vital signs is essential to identify respiratory distress which could be caused by opioids or due to chest sequestration. Naloxone should be available to counteract the effects of morphine causing respiratory distress.

✚ Antiemetics and antihistamines may be prescribed to minimise the side-effects of morphine.

✚ Nurses should remember there are morphine receptors in the gut and that this can lead to constipation. Laxatives or stool softeners maybe prescribed and a high-fibre, high-protein diet should be encouraged. The fibre can help alleviate constipation and protein can aid in tissue repair.

✚ Hydration is very important and intravenous (IV) fluids of 2-4 L, over 24 hours is critical. Accurate fluid monitoring is essential to ensure fluid overload does not occur and to provide an early indication of kidney dysfunction.

✚ Infections are a common problem in SCD and prompt notification to the haematologist is important to instigate antimicrobial administration.

✚ Daily neurological assessment would be beneficial as part of the observation process as individuals can develop a stroke even if their primary admission was not for a neurological cause.

✚ Vitamin D deficiency may aggravate skeletal crisis, hence vitamin D medication may be prescribed.

Psychological support

Sickling crises are frightening because of their unpredictable nature and potential to cause death. This means that psychological support is essential. Educating the individual on the self-management practices outlined in the Community-based Care box is also important. Liaising with members of the MDT and specialist counsellors in sickle cell and thalassaemia centres is valuable in accessing support in the community.

Case Study 3 – Marcia
NURSING CARE PLAN Vaso-occlusive crisis

Marcia is admitted from the A&E Department having been assessed by the haematologist. She is having a VOC in her right hip.

Assessment

On admission to the ward, Marcia's vital signs are recorded. Her vital signs are temperature 38 °C, pulse 90 bpm, BP 125/80 mm/Hg and respirations 25 breaths per minute. Undertaking a pain assessment, using a numerical pain assessment tool, Marcia scores her pain as 8 out 10. She is anxious and fretful. She has physiological jaundice which is visible in conjunctival membranes over the sclera (whites of the eyes) and her skin is dry.

Marcia is prescribed intravenous fluids, 2–4 L/24 hours, and is prescribed morphine, 0.1 mg per kg intravenously. Once the pain has been controlled, PCA is to be set up. An antiemetic and antihistamine are also prescribed.

Diagnosis

✚ Pain – due to VOC causing tissue hypoxia and tissue damage.
✚ Deficient immune system – due to dysfunctional spleen and chronic haemolyticanaemia.
✚ Deficient fluid volume – due to reduced oral intake and pyrexia.
✚ Fear – due to pain not being relieved and of dying.

Expected outcomes

✚ Marcia to verbalise reduction in pain.
✚ Reduced dehydration.

✚ Marcia to feel reassured and fear reduced.
✚ Temperature to be returned to normal.

Planning and implementation

✚ Administer prescribed analgesia, antiemetic and antihistamine.
✚ Re-assess pain 30–40 minutes after administration.
✚ Consider with Marcia alternative therapies to manage the pain (distraction therapy).
✚ Monitor and record fluid input and urine output. As the pain reduces, encourage Marcia to drink orally.
✚ If receiving opiates, vital signs monitoring should be undertaken hourly and reduced to four-hourly once opiate management has been discontinued.
✚ Ensure Marcia has sufficient bedding to keep warm.
✚ Ensure the call bell is within easy reach.
✚ Reassure Marcia her pain is believed.
✚ Ensure Marcia has a high-protein, high-fibre diet.
✚ Provide emotional support.

Evaluation

The VOC is being controlled and her temperature is returning to normal. It was noted from Marcia's medical and nursing records that her last admission was a year ago. You ask Marcia whether she has any thoughts as to what triggered this VOC. She says it might have been due to being out all night with friends drinking alcohol.

Beta thalassaemia major

Treatment

Blood transfusion and iron chelation are the cornerstone of management for BTM. The haematologist will check the haemoglobin level to establish how many units of blood the individual will require. Individuals with BTM require lifelong monthly blood transfusion, and safe administration of blood to prevent ABO incompatibility occurring is vital in preventing life-threatening consequences from such an error.

Each 500 ml unit contains approximately 250 mg of iron. Humans do not have a normal excretory route for excess iron. Ultimately, due to the regularity of transfusions and iron being absorbed from the gut, iron overload will occur if chelation therapy is not administered. The main chelating drugs in the UK are deferoxaminemesylate (Desferal®), Deferiprone (Ferriprox®) and Deferasirox (Exjade®). Individuals may be prescribed one or a combination of these drugs.

PRACTICE ALERT

- Strict adherence to the 3Rs is crucial in blood administration – Right patient, Right blood, Right time.
- Are you familiar with your hospital protocol on blood transfusion management?

In addition to blood transfusion and chelation therapy, folic acid and vitamin C are prescribed. The role of the vitamin C is to enhance the efficacy of Desferal in taking up the iron.

Nursing diagnoses and interventions

Nurses should assess the individual for anaemia and its effects on ALs. In addition, nurses have a role in managing blood transfusion and iron chelation therapy and in offering psychological support.

Blood transfusion

Prior to the administration of a blood transfusion, the nurse should ensure that:

✚ indication of transfusion is written on the individual's notes;

✚ the individual is aware of the reason for transfusion;

✚ the individual has an identity bracelet;

✚ appropriate checks have been carried out (see In Practice box).

Iron chelation

Nurses play a key role in educating and supporting the individual with their iron chelation therapy. Individuals need to be supported in self-administration of Desferal. This is administered subcutaneously by the patient using an infusion pump. Dosage is initially 20–40 mg per kg per day. Nurses need to advise the individual on rotating the injection sites they use across the arms, abdomen and legs to avoid fibrotic tissue development and they need to monitor the individual for side-effects

IN PRACTICE

Pre-blood transfusion checks

- Check the individual's wristband details against the compatibility form. Involve the person in the process.
- Check the unit number details and record them on the prescription sheet.
- Record the date and time of commencement of transfusion.
- Ensure that a blood transfusion IV administration set is used.
- Record vital signs prior to commencement and 15 minutes after transfusion has started.
- Vital signs should again be recorded 30 minutes later and then hourly until transfusion has completed or as the person's condition dictates.
- On completion, vital signs are monitored and the time of completion is recorded.
- Ensure the call bell is within easy reach for the individual.

Consider this . . .

The Severe Hazards of Transfusion (SHOT) Committee over a number of years have reported the main cause of blood transfusion administration is ABO incompatibility, i.e. wrong patient, wrong blood and nurses are primarily the practitioners administering blood. There is a debate regarding whether two nurses should be checking and administering blood as it is currently, or whether this should change to a single registered practitioner. Some hospitals in the UK have changed towards a single checker. What are your thoughts? Would such a change make blood administration safer?

of Desferal, particularly auditory and visual disturbances and infections. Advising the individual on safe storage of Desferal in the fridge and safe disposal of needles and syringes must be addressed. Unsurprisingly, concordance is a major challenge.

Deferiprone was the first generation oral iron chelator. The amount of tablets a person has to take depends on weight and iron levels. This could mean having to take more than 10 tablets a day. Nurses must observe and advise the individual to report side-effects which include nausea, abdominal pain, diarrhoea and severe neutropenia or agranulocytosis.

Exjade is the second generation of oral chelation drugs. Exjade is one tablet per day which is dissolved in fruit juice and should be taken 30 minutes before having a meal. The initial dosage is usually 20 mg per kg. There are side-effects associated with Exjade such as renal and liver complications and gastric bleeding. Close monitoring of serum creatinine and serum transaminase is required and it is necessary to check these levels prior to commencement of Exjade, two weeks after initial dose and monthly thereafter.

Risk for excess iron

Iron is a 'double edge sword'. It is an essential requirement for RBC development; however, in excess iron is toxic, potentially a killer. Excess iron has a significant affinity for specific organs, particularly the heart, liver and endocrine glands. Endocrinological complications are very common and nurses will need to support individuals both emotionally and educationally. The liver is a major organ as it normally stores iron, but excess iron leads to liver failure. The beta cells in the islets of Langerhans in the pancreas which produces insulin become damaged by iron deposits, causing diabetes mellitus (see Chapter 6). Iron damages the pituitary gland, compromising its functions and leading to a reduction in testosterone and oestrogen, delayed sexual development and compromises fertility. The parathyroid and thyroid glands become damaged and osteoporosis is common in adults. The growth hormone can also be compromised because of excess iron, leading to short stature. Excess iron in the myocardium leads to cardiac dysfunction.

COMMUNITY-BASED CARE

SCD and BTM are chronic long-term conditions. Individuals with SCD have chronic pain and will require analgesia at home. They should be advised to drink at least 3 L a day and be reminded to take their prescribed medication of folic acid which aids in the maturation of red blood cells.

Due to chronic haemolytic anaemia and a dysfunctional spleen, some adult patients may also be prescribed prophylactic penicillin. The aim of the penicillin is to enhance the function of the immune system. For these reasons also, all children with SCD up to the age of 16 are prescribed prophylactic penicillin.

Extra fluids are important before, during and after any sports activity. Remind the individual of the importance of eating a high-protein, high-fibre diet and to keep warm to prevent vasoconstriction. Encourage attendance to their out-patient appointments.

For people with BTM nurses need to encourage continuation of iron chelation therapy and three monthly eye and ear examination should be arranged.

For both SCD and BTM, genetic counselling services should be advised. Provide individuals with information of support groups such as the Sickle Cell Society and the UK Thalassaemia Society.

Nurses need to be aware of how iron can cause major organ dysfunction and observe for signs of this. Understanding biochemistry and haematological results for prompt interventions is important.

Psychological support

Psychological support is necessary in helping individuals to live with BTM. Nurses play a pivotal role within the interdisciplinary team, particularly in timely referral for support. Referral to sickle cell and thalassaemia community services to support the patient at home is advisable.

The person with myelodysplastic syndrome (MDS)

MDS is a group of blood disorders characterised by an abnormal-appearing bone marrow and a reduction in the quantity and quality of circulating blood cells. MDS is not a single disease; at least five variations of the disorder have been identified. Anaemia that does not respond to treatment (refractory anaemia) is a characteristic of most forms of myelodysplasia.

Idiopathic MDS primarily affects older adults; men have a slightly higher incidence of the disorder than women. Risk factors for secondary MDS include exposure to environmental toxins such as cigarette smoke, benzene, radiation, radiation therapy or chemotherapy for cancer treatment, and other anaemias such as aplastic anaemia.

Pathophysiology of MDS

MDS is a stem cell disorder in which stem cells fail to reproduce and differentiate into the various types of blood cells. The genetic components of stem cells (nuclear DNA and/or mitochondrial DNA) are altered. The bone marrow loses its ability to produce normal blood cells, instead producing abnormal (dysplastic) cells. With significant alterations, malignant haematological conditions can occur.

Signs and symptoms of MDS

Signs and symptoms of MDS are varied but can include:

- anaemia;
- fatigue;
- weakness;
- dyspnoea;
- pallor;
- splenomegaly;
- abdominal discomfort;
- hepatomegaly;
- thrombocytopenia;
- neutropenia.

INTERDISCIPLINARY CARE FOR MDS

Diagnosis

Reduced haemoglobin and RBC count is common as is leuco-penia and thrombocytopenia. Abnormalities of size and shape of blood cells are also common. Bone marrow aspiration often appears normal, although precursor cells may have an abnor-mal appearance. Increased numbers of myeloblasts (granulo-cyte precursor cells) may be present in the bone marrow. In addition, serum erythropoietin, vitamin B_{12}, serum iron, total iron-binding capacity, ferritin levels and RBC folate levels are investigated to help guide supportive therapy.

Treatment

All individuals with MDS require monitoring, with regular visits to the clinic and laboratory investigations. Psychosocial support is vital in helping the individual and family manage a chronic, progressive and ultimately fatal disease.

Management of MDS is based on the severity of the disease. The International Prognostic Scoring System (IPSS) and the WHO system classify individuals into low-risk and high-risk on the basis of blood results, size and shape of blood cells and existence of genetic abnormalities. These systems are used to guide treatment options for MDS.

Individuals with MDS may require frequent RBC transfusions to treat the predominant anaemia. Like BTM, accumulation of excess iron may warrant iron chelation therapy. Please refer to the section on BTM for blood transfusion (p. 354) and iron chelation management (p. 354).

Platelet transfusions are given when bleeding occurs due to thrombocytopenia. Antibiotic therapy is initiated to treat bacterial infections. Chemotherapy regimens similar to those employed to treat leukaemia may be used. This is rare, but has been effective in treating MDS.

NURSING CARE FOR MDS

MDS is a chronic, usually progressive disorder, requiring active management to maintain functional status and quality of life.

Nursing diagnoses and interventions

Nursing diagnoses and interventions focus on monitoring for cardiac dysfunction and leukaemias, managing fatigue, and patient education and support.

Risk for cardiac dysfunction

Nurses need to assess the patient's vital signs to monitor and observe for increased cardiac workload which is due to anaemia and impaired oxygenation of tissues. Increased blood flow can lead to heart murmur or abnormal heart sounds. Furthermore, accumulated iron can lead to pericarditis and a pericardial friction rub.

Risk for leukaemias

Although neutropenia and thrombocytopenia may accompany the anaemia of MDS, these problems are less common. See the section on leukaemia (p. 362) for additional potential nursing diagnoses and interventions for the individual with MDS.

Managing fatigue

Identify with the individual, energy-conserving ways of performing activities. This might include alternative ways of performing tasks (for example, sitting while performing hygiene measures may reduce oxygen demands and fatigue). A balance between rest, activity and exercise is necessary and encourage 8–10 hours of sleep. Rest decreases oxygen demands and increases available energy for morning activities.

Suggest planning recreational activities following a trans-fusion and adjusting activity level between transfusions to match energy and minimise fatigue. The individual with MDS will have more energy and activity tolerance following a trans-fusion when RBC count, haemoglobin and haematocrit approach normal levels and oxygen transport is optimal.

Patient education and support

Assess the individual's knowledge about MDS as this will provide an opportunity to identify any gaps and provide additional information. As part of that process, the nurse can advise on the effects of MDS, prescribed medications and treatments. It is important the individual is advised to discontinue activities which are causing:

+ complaints of chest pain, breathlessness or vertigo;
+ palpitations or tachycardia that does not return to normal within four minutes of resting;
+ bradycardia;
+ tachypnoea or dyspnoea;
+ decreased systolic blood pressure.

These changes may signify cardiac decompensation due to insufficient oxygenation. The intensity, duration or frequency of the activity needs to be reduced. Advise the individual not to smoke as this causes vasoconstriction and increases carbon mono-xide levels in the blood, interfering with tissue oxygenation.

COMMUNITY-BASED CARE

The individual with MDS experiences fatigue, weakness and shortness of breath on exertion related to the lack of RBCs and ineffective oxygen transport. These symptoms may affect the person's ability to maintain self-care, home life, job performance and social roles.

Individuals with MDS require long-term supportive care and therapy to maintain their quality of life. Stem cell transplant offers the only real hope for cure in MDS. This high-risk therapy, however, is reserved for higher-risk individuals.

MDS is a challenging condition to live with. Therefore, emotional support and giving encouragement to enhance the ability of the individual and caregivers to manage the illness can be a real boost to their confidence.

The person with polycythaemia vera

Polycythaemia, or erythrocytosis, is an excessive production of RBCs, characterised by an increase in haematocrit and haemoglobin. Polycythaemia can be classified as primary polycythaemia (PV), secondary polycythaemia or relative polycythaemia.

Pathophysiology of polycythaemia

Primary polycythaemia (PV)

Polycythaemia vera (PV) is classified as a myeloproliferative disorder. It is a neoplastic stem cell disorder characterised by overproduction of RBCs and, to a lesser extent, WBCs and platelets. A single mutated stem cell produces a faulty precursor RBC that goes on to produce RBCs in excess. It is now recognised that this fault is associated with activation of the enzyme tyrosine kinase caused by a genetic fault of *JAK2*.

Signs and symptoms

Initially, PV is asymptomatic, and the diagnosis may be made during routine blood tests. Its manifestations are caused by increased blood volume and viscosity. Hypertension is common and may lead to headaches, dizziness and vision and hearing disruptions. Venous stasis causes plethora, a ruddy red colour of the face, hands, feet and mucous membranes. Splenomegaly, gastric bleeding and itching, particularly after a hot bath, are common. Excessive metabolic waste from RBC destruction increases the production of uric acid which can lead to gout (painful swelling of the joints). Retinal and cerebral vessels may be engorged. **Hypermetabolism** develops, causing weight loss and night sweats. Mental status may be altered, leading to drowsiness or delirium.

Thrombosis and haemorrhage are potential complications of PV. Thrombosis may cause transient ischaemic attacks, angina or manifestations of peripheral vascular disease.

FAST FACT

PV

PV commonly affects men of Jewish ancestry between 40 and 70 years of age.

Secondary polycythaemia

Secondary polycythaemia is the most common type of polycythaemia. It can occur due to abnormally high erythropoietin levels resulting from kidney disease or erythropoietin-secreting tumours (e.g. renal cell carcinoma). Chronic hypoxia that stimulates erythropoietin release is a more common cause of secondary polycythaemia. People living at high altitudes where the atmospheric oxygen pressure is lower develop a degree of polycythaemia, as do people with chronic heart or lung disease and smokers.

Signs and symptoms

The manifestations of secondary polycythaemia are similar to those of primary polycythaemia, although splenomegaly does not develop. Early symptoms are often overshadowed by the manifestations of the underlying disorder.

INTERDISCIPLINARY CARE FOR POLYCYTHAEMIA

Diagnosis

Blood investigations will show haemoglobin over 16.5 g/dL with a haematocrit over 0.48 for women and haemoglobin over 18.5 g/dL and a haematocrit over 0.51 for men. In PV, serum erythropoietin levels are low. Bone marrow studies show hyperplasia of all marrow cells. In secondary polycythaemia, serum erythropoietin levels are usually high and bone marrow studies show only red stem cell hyperplasia.

FAST FACTS

Relative polycythaemia

- Relative polycythaemia is also sometimes known as pseudo or apparent polycythaemia.
- This is because the RBC is normal, but plasma volume is reduced.
- The haematocrit is increased due to red blood cell concentration.
- This type of polycythaemia occurs in cases of burns, dehydration, stress and overweight middle-aged men. Corrected by hydration.

Treatment

For secondary polycythaemia, treatment focuses on the underlying cause of the disorder. If it is a physiological response in people living at high altitudes and the haematocrit is not too high or oxygen saturation levels are not low, no treatment is usually necessary. Smokers should be advised to stop. Measures to raise oxygen saturation levels and reduce tissue hypoxia will often relieve the polycythaemia.

In PV, phlebotomy is the mainstay of management. Approximately 300–500 ml of blood is removed. The aim of this is to reduce plasma viscosity, normalise blood volume and ameliorate symptoms. Individuals need to be advised that this is a long-term treatment.

PRACTICE ALERT

Regular venesection can cause IDA. Therefore it is essential to check the individual's iron levels prior to venesection.

If venesection is not effective in PV, chemotherapeutic drugs may be used to suppress marrow function but may increase the risk of developing leukaemia. Pruritus may be relieved by antihistamines, or may require more aggressive treatment with interferon alpha or other treatments. Low-dose aspirin may be prescribed to control thrombosis without increasing the risk of bleeding.

NURSING CARE FOR POLYCYTHAEMIA

Preventing polycythaemia begins with educating children and adults about the dangers of smoking. PV is a chronic condition and patients need to be educated as to why venesection is necessary. Advising on issues such as diet and exercise to reduce risk factors for cardiovascular disease may also be beneficial. Teaching the individual and family of the importance of maintaining adequate hydration and increasing fluid intake during hot weather and when exercising is important.

Discuss measures to prevent blood stasis such as: elevating legs and feet when sitting, using support stockings and continuing treatment measures. Advise the individual to report manifestations of thrombosis (leg or calf pain, chest pain, neurologic symptoms) or bleeding (black, tarry stools, vomiting of blood or coffee-ground emesis) immediately. Throughout treatment, nurses should monitor the haematocrit and marrow cell counts.

DISORDERS OF THE WHITE BLOOD CELLS AND LYMPHOID TISSUES

Disorders of the white blood cells include infectious mononucleosis, the leukaemias, multiple myeloma and malignant lymphomas. This section will provide an overview of the malignant pathologies and discuss treatment and key nursing interventions.

The person with a leukaemia

Leukaemic cells occur when at some stage during stem cell differentiation, the stem cell's development is arrested and

it fails to mature. At the stage at which it stops developing, there is a cloning of that immature, non-functioning cell, which proliferates in number. The increase in these abnormal cells leads to a reduction in erythrocytes, normal leucocytes and thrombocytes. As a consequence, individuals present with signs and symptoms of erythrocytopenia, leukopenia and thrombocytopenia.

Classification of leukaemias

There are four general classifications of leukaemia:

- acute myeloid leukaemia (AML);
- chronic myeloid leukaemia (CML);
- acute lymphoblastic leukaemia (ALL);
- chronic lymphoblastic leukaemia (CLL).

Myeloid leukaemias involve the myeloid stem cell lineage, interfering with granulocyte, erythrocyte and thrombocyte maturation. Lymphoblastic leukaemias affect the lymphoid stem cell lineage, interfering with lymphocytic maturation. The above classification is further subdivided as illustrated in Table 10.5.

Identifying the subtype of acute leukaemias is very important clinically for a number of reasons:

- enables appropriate treatment interventions;
- enables warning of potential side-effects;
- gives an indication of prognosis.

The FAB classification has been used for many years, but increasing knowledge of molecular abnormalities of haematological cancers and the significance of cytogenetics has led to a more detailed scientific classification system. In recent years,

FAST FACTS

Leukaemias

- Leukaemias as a whole account for 2.5% of all cancers and are the 11th greatest cause of death from cancer.
- There are approximately 7000 new cases per year in the UK.
- Leukaemia is more common in men than in women.
- ALL is more common in children whereas AML is more common in adults.
- CLL has a higher incidence in adults over 70 years whereas CML is more common in young adults.
- Leukaemias are more commonly found in Caucasians in western European and American populations and less commonly in Afro-Caribbean, South East and Far East Asians.

Source: Cancer Research UK 2011a.

Table 10.5 French American British (FAB) classification

Acute myeloid leukaemia	Predominate cell type	Prognosis
AML-0	Undifferentiated cells	Poor
AML-1	Immature myeloblasts	Good response in 65% of cases
AML-2	Mature myeloblasts	Good for two or more years of remission
AML-3	Promyelocytes	Good in adults
AML-4	Myeloblasts or monocytic maturation	Poorest in adults
AML-5	Monoblastic (M5a) or monocytic (M5b)	Poor
AML-6	Erythroblasts	Variable
AML-7	Megakaryoblastic	Poor
Acute lymphoblastic leukaemia	Predominate cell type	Prognosis
ALL-1	Immature lymphoblast blast cell	More than 90% remission rate in children
ALL-2	Mature lymphoblast blast cell	Relapse rate common after two years or more
ALL-3	Vacuolated* lymphoblast blast cell	Poor

* Vacuolated cells have holes which cause leakage of cellular materials.

the WHO classification system (Tefferi and Vardiman 2008) using cytogenetic data to provide more detailed information in classifying haematological malignancies is being used. Haematologists in the UK use both classification systems.

Aetiology of leukaemias

Although the cause of leukaemia is not always known, there are many risk factors associated with its development:

- Genetics – it is well known that some genetic and chromosomal aberrations are associated with leukaemia – e.g. there is a 30% increased risk of developing AML in Down's syndrome. Half of individuals with leukaemia have chromosomal abnormalities.
- Cigarette smoking is associated with AML.
- Ionising radiation – bone marrow cells are highly susceptible to radiation.
- Chemicals – in particular petroleum chemical benzene.
- Chemotherapy treatment for other cancers.
- Viruses, for example human T-cell lymphotropic/leukaemia virus – 1 (HTLV-1).
- Bone marrow diseases (myeloproliferative disorders, e.g. polycythaemia, essential thrombocytopenia, myelodysplastic

syndrome, e.g. myelofibrosis, aplastic anaemia) can transform into leukaemia.

Pathophysiology of leukaemias

Acute myeloid leukaemia (AML)
AML is characterised by uncontrollable proliferation of myeloblasts and hyperplasia of the bone marrow and spleen. AML is more common in adults than children.

Chronic myeloid leukaemia (CML)
CML, also known as chronic granulocytic leukaemia, is a clonal proliferation of myeloid cells (eosinophils, basophils, neutrophils). Approximately 85% of patients have the chromosomal abnormality, the Philadelphia chromosome (Ph). The Ph is a reciprocal translocation of protogenic material (Abl/Bcr), between chromosomes 9 and 22. This is usually denoted as t(9;22), (q34;q11). The Abl/Bcr triggers the production of protein p210, which causes the malignant myeloid cell development, known as Ph+ve cells. CML has three phases: chronic, accelerated and blast crisis. This last phase resembles AML with an extensive increase in blast cells in the marrow (greater than 5%). Keeping individuals in the chronic phase is the aim of treatment and to plan if appropriate for an allogeneic stem cell transplant.

Acute lymphocytic leukaemia (ALL)
Most cases of ALL result from malignant transformation of B cells and resemble immature lymphocytes (lymphoblasts), however, they do not mature or function effectively to maintain immunity. These lymphoblasts accumulate in the bone marrow lymph nodes and spleen as well as circulating in the blood.

ALL is the most common type of leukaemia in children. In adults ALL is rarely seen in adults until middle age.

Chronic lymphoblastic leukaemia (CLL)
CLL is a very slow progressive malignancy of lymphocytes. The majority of individuals have B-cell CLL. T-cell CLL tends to carry a poorer prognosis. In CLL lymphocytes appear normal but are not fully developed and are non-functioning. Humoral immunity and cellular mediated immunity tend to be compromised, increasing the risk of infections.

Often diagnosis is incidental and, if the individual is asymptomatic, a 'wait and watch' position is taken by the haematologist. Symptoms such as loss of weight, anaemia, night sweats, extensively high WCC and lymphadenopathy may indicate instigation of treatment.

Signs and symptoms of leukaemias

Acute leukaemias tend to be rapid in onset and are related to cytopenias of all the marrow cells. The symptoms are:

- anaemia;
- lethargy;
- tiredness;
- weakness;

- recurrent infections;
- petechiae, purpura, ecchymoses (bruising), epistaxis (nose-bleeds), haematomas, haematuria and gastrointestinal bleeding;
- bone infarctions of leukaemic cells which may cause bone pain.

In ALL, other symptoms such as

- headaches, lack of concentration;
- increased intracranial pressure;
- lymphadenopathy;
- testicular infiltrations

can also occur. In chronic leukaemias, symptoms are insidious and, in many cases, diagnosis is incidental. More constitutional problems such as priapism in men can occur.

INTERDISCIPLINARY CARE FOR LEUKAEMIAS

Diagnosis

Table 10.1 outlined the blood investigations which are commonly undertaken, but additional tests as listed below may be carried out to confirm and establish the severity/stage of the illness:

- bone marrow aspiration;
- bone marrow trephine;
- biochemistry tests – lactate dehydrogenase (LDH), uric acid;
- cytogenetic screening;
- clotting screening – prothrombin, fibrinogen;
- activated partial thromboplastin time (APTT);
- lumbar puncture;
- chest x-ray.

Table 10.6 outlines the diagnostic findings by type of leukaemia.

Treatment

Chemotherapy, radiotherapy, growth factors, steroids, mono-clonal antibodies and stem cell transplant form the basis of clinical management. Leukaemia and its treatment can cause significant problems which are illustrated in Figure 10.10.

Chemotherapy is the treatment of choice for most types of leukaemia. There are a number of chemotherapy drugs used, and the type of treatment, dosage, route of administration and length of treatment would depend on a number of factors. These include type of leukaemia, stage of the leukaemia, sub-type of the leukaemia presence/absence of genetic abnormalities, age of the individual and presence of any co-morbidities, such as liver, renal or cardiac dysfunction. The aims of treatment are to eradicate malignant cells, restore normal bone marrow functions and ameliorate the effects of the illness.

In the case of CML, chemotherapy is not first line. Instead, imatinib mesylate (Glivec®), a biological therapy which specifically targets Ph+ve cells, is prescribed.

In the case of acute leukaemias, because of their aggressive behaviour, patients are given combination chemotherapy. There are a number of benefits in using combination chemotherapy:

- The chemotherapy drugs can attack malignant cells at all stages of the cell cycle.
- It minimises the ability of the malignant cell to develop resistance.
- It helps to improve remission rates.
- It reduces the need (and danger) of giving very high dosage of a single drug.

Combination chemotherapy is usually given in 'cycles'. This is important as it allows for normal marrow to recover as well as attacking the malignant cells.

Table 10.6 Diagnostic findings by type of leukaemia

Test	AML	CML	ALL	CLL
RBC count	Low	Low	Low	Low
Haemoglobin	Low	Low	Low	Low
Haematocrit	Low	Low	Low	Low
Platelet count	Very low	High early, low late	Low	Low
WBC count	Varies	Increased	Varies	Increased
Myeloblasts	Present	–	–	–
Neutrophils	Decreased	Increased	Decreased	Normal
Lymphocytes	–	Normal	–	Increased
Monocytes	–	Normal/low	–	–
Blasts	Present	Present (crisis)	Present	–
Bone marrow	Hypercellular	–	Hypercellular	–
Myeloblasts	Present	–	–	–
Lymphoblasts	–	–	Present	–
Lymphocytes	–	–	–	Present

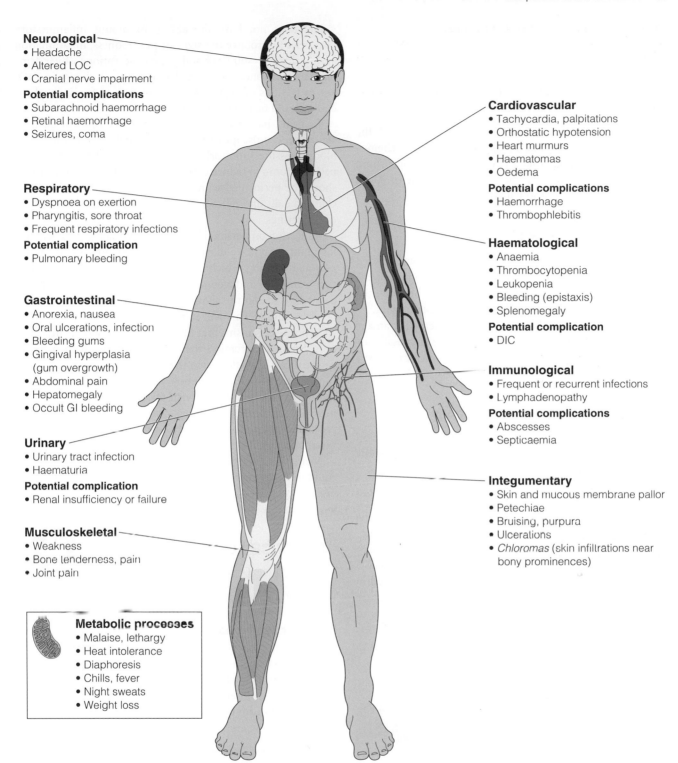

Neurological
- Headache
- Altered LOC
- Cranial nerve impairment

Potential complications
- Subarachnoid haemorrhage
- Retinal haemorrhage
- Seizures, coma

Respiratory
- Dyspnoea on exertion
- Pharyngitis, sore throat
- Frequent respiratory infections

Potential complication
- Pulmonary bleeding

Gastrointestinal
- Anorexia, nausea
- Oral ulcerations, infection
- Bleeding gums
- Gingival hyperplasia
  (gum overgrowth)
- Abdominal pain
- Hepatomegaly
- Occult GI bleeding

Urinary
- Urinary tract infection
- Haematuria

Potential complication
- Renal insufficiency or failure

Musculoskeletal
- Weakness
- Bone tenderness, pain
- Joint pain

Metabolic processes
- Malaise, lethargy
- Heat intolerance
- Diaphoresis
- Chills, fever
- Night sweats
- Weight loss

Cardiovascular
- Tachycardia, palpitations
- Orthostatic hypotension
- Heart murmurs
- Haematomas
- Oedema

Potential complications
- Haemorrhage
- Thrombophlebitis

Haematological
- Anaemia
- Thrombocytopenia
- Leukopenia
- Bleeding (epistaxis)
- Splenomegaly

Potential complication
- DIC

Immunological
- Frequent or recurrent infections
- Lymphadenopathy

Potential complications
- Abscesses
- Septicaemia

Integumentary
- Skin and mucous membrane pallor
- Petechiae
- Bruising, purpura
- Ulcerations
- *Chloromas* (skin infiltrations near
  bony prominences)

Figure 10.10 Multisystem effects of leukaemia.

In AML there are two phases of treatment.

- *Induction phase.* This is the first few cycles of treatment. This aims to kill the majority of the leukaemia cells. At the end of this phase there are usually no leukaemia cells detectable in a blood sample or in a bone marrow sample. This is called being 'in remission'. Remission does not mean

cure. It means that no abnormal cells can be detected by tests.

- *Consolidation (intensification) phase.* This is the remaining cycle of treatment and the type of drugs used may be different. This phase of treatment aims to kill any remaining leukaemia cells which may still be present.

In ALL, there are three phases of treatment:

● induction;

● consolidation;

● maintenance – this period of treatment can be up to two years.

Chemotherapy is the main treatment for ALL, but if the leukaemia has spread radiotherapy or intrathecal chemotherapy (injecting chemotherapy into the cerebrospinal fluid via a lumbar puncture) may be used. In the case of AML, radiotherapy is not commonly used.

NURSING CARE FOR LEUKAEMIAS

Leukaemia is a life-threatening illness which is compounded by the treatment necessary to manage or potentially cure the illness. Nurses must be skilled in managing the potential effects of both the illness and side-effects of the treatment.

Chemotherapy and radiotherapy cause systematic damage to cells, particularly fast dividing cells such as mucosal, hair follicles, gonads and gastrointestinal system, which can have a physical, emotional and psychological impact on the individual.

Nursing diagnoses and interventions

Key areas of nursing care are managing the risk of infection and haemorrhage, managing the side-effects of chemotherapy and radiation therapy, and psychological support.

Risk for infection

Infections are a major risk for leukaemic patients and the main cause of mortality due to the reduced normal production of WBCs and the damage caused by chemotherapy and radiotherapy to the marrow. Neutropenia is an inevitable consequence of treatment, and meticulous care is required in reducing the risk of cross-infection. Nurses should be aware of normal levels of neutrophils and monitor FBC results to determine the neutrophil count. Antimicrobial medication is usually prescribed to reduce the risk of infections as well as to treat any infection that may develop.

FAST FACT

Neutropenia

A neutrophil count of 0.1×10^9/L is neutropenia and below 0.5×10^9/L indicates a severe risk of infection.

The individual is usually nursed in protective isolation, in a single room, and some may have en suite facilities. Meticulous hand washing and hand drying procedures must be followed.

Temperature observation is critical in providing an early indication of infection. The absence of WBCs means the individual does not have the ability to mount inflammatory responses to produce the signs of pus, redness, inflammation and swelling. Respiratory and pulse observations which demonstrate tachypnoea, tachycardia, restlessness, change in PaO_2 are early signs of sepsis. Any complaints of fever, cough or chills should be investigated as a priority.

In some haematology units, clinical equipment such as stethoscope, otoscope (assess the ear canal for inflammation), blood pressure monitoring equipment may be kept in each patient's room to reduce cross-infection. Cleaning of the room should be performed with damp cloths, bed linen should be changed daily and pillows and mattresses should have protective coverings.

Education on personal hygiene is essential. Some haematology units may have disposable towelettes for patient use for personal washing, which is an efficient way of reducing infections caused by endogenous organisms. The individual should be advised to run the shower for approximately two minutes before washing. This will minimise contamination from any waterborne organisms that may reside in the shower head and hose. Sensitively, remind the individual to wash their hands before meals and after using the toilet.

Hospitals have their own policies on visitors, but all visitors should be advised not to visit if they have a cold or any infection themselves. Children who have received childhood vaccinations should not visit at least for several days post the vaccination until they have developed antibodies.

Meticulous management of intravenous devices which could include central venous catheter (CVC), peripherally inserted central catheter (PICC) or implantable ports is critical to prevent cross-infection.

PRACTICE ALERT

A temperature of 38 °C for more than one hour or one recording of 38.5 °C warrants immediate intervention.

Risk for haemorrhage

Bleeding is the second most common cause of death in leukaemia. As platelet counts decrease, the risk of bleeding increases. As part of the daily assessment, signs of bruising or easy bleeding should be observed. Individuals should be advised to ensure they inform nurses of any bleeding episodes. Common sites for bleeding are:

● skin and mucous membranes for petechiae, ecchymoses and purpura;

● gums, nasal membranes and conjunctiva;

● epistaxis;

● vaginal bleeding;

● occult blood;

● complaints of headaches, blurred vision, weakness, which could be an indication of intracranial bleeding;

● abdominal complaints of epigastric pain, diminished bowel sounds, increasing abdominal girth, rigidity or guarding.

Individuals should avoid using razor blades for shaving, and rectal or vaginal suppositories, vaginal tampons or enemas should be avoided.

Inadequate nutrition

Chemotherapy and radiotherapy take a significant toll on the body and nutritional support is essential in aiding recovery. Looking back at Malcolm in Case Study 1, he had lost weight and it would be important to address. Advising him of a high-energy, high-protein, high-fibre diet to aid in tissue repair, provide energy and aid normal bowel function is important. However, patients may have difficulty eating due to oral damage, nausea and vomiting (N&V), abdominal discomfort, diarrhoea, taste changes, dysphagia and pain. Individuals will have some restrictions on the type of food they are allowed to eat when they become neutropenic. These diets are sometimes called 'neutropenic' or 'clean' diets. There are no national guidelines on what constitutes a safe diet, but generally the food types listed below are considered prohibited whilst the individual is neutropenic.

- salads;
- cold meats;
- unpasteurised dairy products;
- soft cheese;
- bottled water;
- fruit which cannot be peeled.

Raw nuts and raw or rare-cooked meat, fish and eggs should be avoided.

Encouraging individuals to have drinks with their meals can aid in mastication of the food and help to keep the mouth moist. Pineapple can be very helpful in developing an appetite and keeping the mouth moist. Encourage small, frequent meals rather than large meals and advise the patient to avoid very sweet, rich or greasy foods. Nutritional supplements such as Ensure should be made available.

If relatives are providing meals, nurses must advise on safe hygiene in cooking and the storage of food in sealed containers in the fridge. When using a microwave to reheat meals, it is essential a temperature probe is used to ensure thorough heating of the meal.

Timely administration of antiemetics is important if the individual is experiencing N&V. Removing the covering lid off the plate prior to serving the meal to reduce the strong immediate aroma of the meal can be helpful in reducing nausea. Advising the individual to reduce intake of milk and milk products, which make mucus more tenacious, can be helpful.

If the individual has lost more than 5% of their admission weight or is still unable to eat well, referral to the dietician should be done. In some cases, parenteral or enteral feed may need to be instigated. Enteral feed is via an nasogastric tube or parenterally via a CVC.

Nausea and vomiting

N&V are other debilitating side-effects of chemotherapy and radiotherapy. It is embarrassing for the individual and requires sensitive management. Being aware of the treatment interventions should assist nurses in timely antiemetic management. It is important to recognise that N&V are separate phenomena, although related and controlling both is essential. Prompt administration of prescribed antiemetics is important.

In making the individual feel comfortable, ensure there are sufficient tissues at the bedside and have a vomit bowl at the bedside, which should be cleared away quickly if used, and assist the individual with oral care. Most of the interventions for nutrition apply to N&V, but in addition it could be suggested to the individual to eat dry biscuits such as crackers or ginger biscuits and eat prior to but not immediately before their chemotherapy treatment.

Stomatitis

Stomatitis is inflammation of the mucosal lining of the oral cavity. Damage to the mucosal lining of the oral cavity is a major complication of cytoreductive therapy. Mucosal cells are fast dividing cells and are directly and indirectly affected by chemotherapy. Direct effect is to the epithelial lining of the oral cavity, which naturally alters as it divides in the mouth to form the mucous lining. Chemotherapy damages the epithelial layer which prevents new mucosal cells being formed to replace the damaged ones, leading to stomatitis. Stomatitis is also further impacted indirectly by chemotherapy due to the myelosuppression which results in neutropenia creating an increased risk of infections or oral bleeds due to thrombocytopenia.

FAST FACTS

Opportunistic infections

- Herpes simplex virus and *Candida albicans* (yeast) are more common in patients with neutropenia.
- Herpes lesions are usually red, raised, fluid-filled blisters; candida causes a white coating and patches of white plaque.

Discussion in the section on nutrition is also relevant for stomatitis. Undertaking oral assessment is an essential part of nursing care. An oral assessment tool should be used and assessment should be done twice daily. Patient education on oral care is paramount in helping to reduce the risk of infection. Oral care should be done before and after every meal and prior to sleeping at night. A soft toothbrush is usually better tolerated by the individual, and they should be advised not to use commercial mouthwashes as they tend to contain alcohol which will cause pain. Chlorhexidine (CHX) is the usual mouthwash used, followed by an antifungal oral solution, usually nystatin. CHX is used undiluted but, if the individual is experiencing oral pain, it can be diluted with water.

Encourage the individual to drink fluids to help keep the mouth moist, and for comfort suggest using petroleum vaseline to keep the lips moist to prevent cracking and reduce the

PRACTICE ALERT

The individual must be advised to wait 30 minutes after using CHX before they administer the nystatin because the CHX needs to coat the mucosal lining. If the nystatin is taken immediately after the CHX it will not effectively coat the mucosal lining and will be less effective in its antimicrobial functions.

risk of an infection site. Cryotherapy, using ice cubes, can be soothing and aids in reducing pain and blood loss by causing vaso-constriction and reducing inflammation.

Oral pain can be a significant problem, and prompt administration of analgesia is important. Stomatitis not only has a physiological effect but a psychological and emotional impact which nurses must be aware of. Difficulty with speaking due to pain and lack of saliva or having halitosis (bad breath) can be embarrassing, and sensitive, empathetic care and reassurance is essential support.

Impaired skin integrity

This can be compromised for a number of reasons:

- the effects of radiation and chemotherapy on the skin can cause dryness, blisters and rashes;
- insertion of the CVC creates possible entry sites for infective organisms.

Nurses should assess the skin daily for any lesions and rashes and patients should be advised after showering to pat dry rather than rub the skin. Special care should be advised in drying the armpits, under the breasts, in the groin area to avoid leaving any moist areas which could encourage microorganism growth. Keeping the skin supple and reducing dryness, patients could use a non-perfumed moisturiser. Wearing cotton bed clothing is best as it allows the skin to 'breathe' and is more comfortable to wear.

Tumour lysis syndrome (TLS)

TLS is a risk with intensive chemotherapy. TLS develops when a large number of malignant cells are destroyed by chemotherapy or radiation. The resultant by-products of cell lysis can overwhelm the body's ability to effectively eliminate them, leading to significant alterations in electrolyte levels, and complications such as cardiac dysrhythmias, muscle weakness or tetany, paraesthesia and mental status changes can occur. Excess uric acid can compromise renal function and lead to metabolic acidosis and gout.

Monitoring and prompt reporting of abnormal blood levels of electrolytes, uric acid, urea nitrogen and creatinine is essential. Maintain adequate hydration and administer prescribed medications such as allopurinol and diuretics. Hydration is vital to maintain renal function and promote elimination of tumour lysis by-products. Allopurinol reduces the risk of uric acid crystallisation in the kidneys and other tissues.

Sexual dysfunction

Chemotherapy and radiotherapy can cause reduction in the sex hormones and, in women, loss of libido, vaginal dryness, amenorrhoea and dyspareunia are common symptoms. The ovaries can become fibrotic, leading to reduction in oocytes to enable menstruation. Pre-menopausal symptoms and permanent sterility can occur. In men loss of libido, difficulty with having an erection, premature ejaculation, azoospermia and gynaecomastia are significant problems.

Sexual dysfunction is an area warranting sensitive discussion and should not be ignored within the assessment and care of the patient. Nurses should not wait for the individual to instigate a conversation on this issue. For many individuals this is an important part of their life, but they may feel uncomfortable to ask any questions. Nurses should approach the issue by asking questions which can elicit information regarding the effect of the treatment on sexual dysfunction in a way that is comfortable for both the individual and nurse. Questions such as 'has the treatment affected how you feel about being a wife/husband/partner?' could be used.

Assess the individual's knowledge and understanding about the impact of the treatment on fertility and sexuality with the aim of providing accurate information and clarifying misconceptions. Discuss realistic measures for coping (for example, sperm banking prior to chemotherapy or radiation therapy). Remember in Case Study 1 that Malcolm mentioned during the assessment he and Sheila were planning to start a family. The option of sperm banking may still enable that to happen and this should be discussed with the patient. For women there are very limited fertility treatment options and all require hyperstimulation of a menstrual cycle which will take four weeks. This timing can be prohibitive, especially in acute leukaemias. Where appropriate refer for sexual counselling.

Contraception advice during treatment is important. Condoms should be used during sex within the first 48 hours after chemotherapy in order to protect the partner from any of the drug that may be present in semen or vaginal fluid. There is a possibility that treatment may harm the developing baby, and it is important to advise patients not try to conceive for at least one year after treatment.

Altered body image

The loss of weight, alopecia, N&V, loss of sexuality and the insertion of a CVC are some of the issues which can lead to individuals feeling quite negative about themselves.

Discuss the risks for and measures to cope with alopecia. Suggest wearing wigs, scarves, hats or caps. Teach proper scalp care using baby shampoo or mild soap, a soft brush, sunscreen and mineral oil to reduce itching. If eyelashes and eyebrows are lost, teach eye protection, such as wearing spectacles and caps with wide brims.

Interestingly, there tends to be more of a focus on the impact of alopecia in women, but men can be psychologically affected by alopecia, particularly young men. In addition, there can be religious importance to hair, particularly for Sikh men, and therefore nurses should be aware that alopecia can be just as devastating for men as it is for women.

Hair loss usually begins one to two weeks after initiation of chemotherapy, with maximum loss one to two months later. Alopecia may range from thinning to total hair loss. Regrowth depends on the treatment schedule and doses; however, it usually begins two to three months after treatment ends. New hair may be softer, curlier and slightly different in colour. Planning for hair loss can be helpful for the individual to prepare emotionally and identify self-care techniques to cope with hair loss.

Psychological support

Having a cancer diagnosis, individuals will have a sense of fear, anxiety and dread as Malcolm in Case Study 1 highlighted. Fear of an unknown future, issues regarding survivorship, how will loved ones be looked after are all major areas of concern for the individual. Supporting the individual and their family through the treatment is a fundamental part of holistic care. Good interpersonal skills are essential in creating an environment which encourages communication.

Reactions to the diagnosis may vary with many individuals going through Kübler-Ross 'five stages' of grief: denial, anger, bargaining, depression and acceptance.

If the individual does not have children but they were planned for in the future, it can be soul-destroying that this opportunity is no longer open to them.

Malcolm was highly anxious and very frightened, and his concerns are compounded by seeing his brother go through the treatment journey he is about to embark on. Ascertain from the individual what their perceptions are of the treatment and side-effects and identify their coping strategies to harness as sources of strength and support. Individuals may want to discuss changing roles within the family, resulting from leukaemia diagnosis, and its effect on spiritual, social and economic status and usual lifestyle. Culture, religion and ethnicity play a significant part in how patients respond to and cope with a cancer diagnosis.

Individuals are given a great deal of information at the time of diagnosis so it is important to establish the patient's understanding about their illness and the planned treatment. The provision of patient information from organisations such as Macmillan Cancer Relief, Leukaemia Care and Maggie's Centres could be provided.

As part of discharge planning, nurses should establish if assistance with physical care, finances and transportation may be required. Refer the individual and family to social services, support groups and home care services as needed.

The person with malignant lymphoma

Lymphomas are a heterogeneous group of diseases, related to malignant lymphoma, characterised by the proliferation of lymphocytes (T or B lymphocytes). Lymphomas are closely related to lymphocytic leukaemia. These cells accumulate in the lymph nodes but can infiltrate the bloodstream and other organs.

Pathophysiology of lymphoma

Although there are many types of malignant lymphoid cells, lymphomas are commonly identified as Hodgkin's lymphoma (HL) or non-Hodgkin's lymphoma (NHL).

Hodgkin's lymphoma (HL)

HL was first discovered by Thomas Hodgkin in 1832, identifying peculiar-shaped cells in post-mortem cases. These cells became known as Reed–Sternberg cells (RS); they have distinctive 'owl'-like appearance and are derived from B-lymphocytes.

FAST FACTS

HL

- HL is rarely seen in children but appears to have a bimodal age distribution, being seen in the 3rd decade of life, then seeming to decline in incidence before rising in the 6th decade.
- The incidence is slightly higher in men than women, at 3 per 100 000 and 2.4 per 100 000, respectively.

Source: Cancer Research UK 2011b.

Signs and symptoms

HL typically presents as painless lymphadenopathy (enlarged lymph nodes). This is a distinctive feature since normally swollen lymph glands are painful due to an infection. The cervical nodes are the most common sites, followed by axillary and inguinal nodes as other sites. Other symptoms include:

- splenomegaly
- hepatomegaly
- mediastinal involvement may occur
- constitutional symptoms – fever, pruritis, alcohol-induced pain at the site of enlarged nodes, weight loss, weakness, fatigue, night sweats.

Subtypes

Classification of HL is based on the REAL/WHO classification and there are four subtypes: nodular sclerosing, mixed cellularity, lymphocyte predominate and lymphocyte depleted. All the subtypes will contain RS cells in various degrees but, unlike NHL, the subtype does not affect prognosis.

Non-Hodgkin's lymphoma

This is much more complex than HL, with a greater diversity of malignant lymphoma and other immune cells involved. NHL is classified under B-cell and T-cell lymphomas.

Risk factors

There are a number of risk factors associated with the development of NHL, which include infective organisms such as HIV, Epstein–Barr virus, human T-cell lymphoma virus type 1.

FAST FACTS

NHL

- There were 10 917 new cases of NHL in 2007 in the UK.
- The ratio between men and women is roughly equal.
- NHL incidence rates in the UK have increased by more than a third since the late 1980s.
- The incidence increases with age, with a sharp rise in the 6th decade of life.
- Unlike HL, NHL can occur in both adults and children.
- NHL is the 5th most common cancer in the UK.

Source: Cancer Research UK 2011c.

Chromosomal abnormalities have been associated with NHL, and it has been recognised that if an individual has NHL, their siblings have a higher than average risk of developing NHL, compared to the general population.

Individuals who have had immunosuppressive drugs used in organ transplantation and those who have had previous chemotherapy have an increased risk of developing NHL as a secondary cancer. Certain environmental factors such as agricultural chemicals or working in carpentry have also been associated with NHL.

Signs and symptoms

These are quite similar to HL, although extranodal sites are more common and more extensive than in HL, with multinodal involvement. Systemic symptoms are common, including unexplained fevers, drenching night sweats and weight loss. These are known as 'B' symptoms.

In addition to disease at nodal sites, 15–20% of NHL occurs in lymphoid tissue elsewhere in the body. Extranodal lymphomas can occur at almost any anatomical site, which include:

- gastrointestinal system;
- respiratory;
- ocular;
- breast;
- lachrymal glands;
- thyroid;
- skin;
- testes;
- prostate;
- small intestine;
- central nervous system.

Subtypes

There are many subtypes of NHL, but they can all be put into one of two broad categories:

- *High-grade NHL*, where the cancer develops quickly, is aggressive, but potentially curable.
- *Low-grade or indolent NHL*, where the cancer is indolent, can be asymptomatic for many years, slow in progression, responds to chemotherapy but difficult to cure. This could possibly be because chemotherapy attacks fast-dividing cells, low-grade NHL malignant cells develop more slowly and therefore the impact of the treatment may not be as effective.

Table 10.7 illustrates the subtypes of NHL.

INTERDISCIPLINARY CARE FOR HL AND NHL

Diagnosis

Investigations to diagnose HL and NHL are outlined in Table 10.8.

Staging

Following investigations in diagnosing HL or NHL, staging of the disease is necessary to ascertain the most effective treatment interventions. The Ann Arbor Staging System is used and has four stages as outlined below. In addition to the staging, letters A or B will be used and are associated with the presence or absence of constitutional symptoms which are: weight loss, fever and night sweats.

- Stage I – involvement of a single lymph node area.
- Stage II – involvement of two or more lymph node regions on same side of the diaphragm.
- Stage III – involvement of lymph node regions on both sides of the diaphragm +/− spleen.
- Stage IV – disseminated extralymphatic spread.
- Category A = B symptoms absent.
- Category B = B symptoms present.
- Localised extralymphatic lesions with or without associated lymph node involvement are termed 'E' (extranodal) lesions.

The staging is based on chest x-rays to establish mediastinal, lung and hilar involvement, plus CT scan to detect intrathoracic, intra-abdominal or pelvic disease. More specialist investigations such as MRI or PET may be required for certain sites.

Treatment

Depending on the stage and severity of the disease, both HL and NHL will be treated by chemotherapy or radiotherapy or a combination of both.

Patients with stages I & IIa may receive radiotherapy only, and this can be highly effective. Usually approximately (40Gy) may be administered. The involved lymph node region is treated, with careful shielding to protect unaffected areas and minimise the extent of radiation burn and normal cell

Table 10.7 Subtypes of Non-Hodgkin's lymphoma

Subtype	Incidence	Course and prognosis
B-Cell Lymphomas		
Diffuse large B-cell lymphomas	Most common adult type (40%–50% of adult lymphomas) More common in males Incidence increases with ageing	Aggressive tumor 45%–50% cure rate
Follicular lymphoma	Accounts for 40% of adult lymphomas, rare in children Incidence increases with ageing	Bone marrow frequently involved Course slow, indolent; 72% 5-year survival
Extranodal marginal zone lymphoma (MALT lymphoma)	Accounts for about 5% of adult lymphomas, rare in children Incidence increases with ageing More common in Italy	Presents with tumors outside lymphatic system GI tract, lung, thyroid, urinary tract, skin, CNS Slow, indolent course; 74% 5-year survival
Mantle cell lymphoma	Accounts for 3% to 4% of adult lymphomas, rare in children Predominantly affects older men (74%)	Aggressive, difficult to cure 27% 5-year survival
Burkitt lymphoma	Rare in adults (<1% of lymphomas), more common in children (–30% NHL)	Rapidly progressive but responds well to therapy 45% 5-year survival
T-Cell Lymphomas		
Precursor T-cell lymphoblastic leukaemia/lymphoma	More common in children and young adults More common in males than females	Can present either as ALL or lymphoma Aggressive disease; 26% 5-year survival
Peripheral T-cell lymphoma	Most common T-cell lymphoma in adults	Often presents as disseminated disease 25% 5-year survival
Mycosis fungoides/cutaneous T-cell lymphoma	Onset typically during mid-50s; more common in African Americans	Cutaneous lymphoma Slow course, progressing from patchy skin lesions to plaque to cutaneous tumours

destruction. The 'mantle' and inverted 'Y' techniques of radiotherapy are used depending on the position(s) of the lymphadenopathy (Figure 10.11). These techniques aim to minimise radiation burns and limit damage to normal cells.

There are various combination chemotherapy regimens which are administered in a cyclic process and tend to be offered for stages III & IV as well as stages IB & IIB. Rituximab is a monoclonal antibody used as part of the treatment of some types of NHL. It may be used on its own or in combination with chemotherapy. Rituximab attaches to a protein called CD20 that is found on the surface of B lymphocytes and stimulates the body's natural defences to attack and destroy the lymphocytes.

In relapsed cases, alternative chemotherapy or possibly chemotherapy combined with radiation might be used. If lymphoma cells are chemosensitive, allogeneic stem cell transplant (SCT) might be offered as a curative option.

Stem cell transplantation (SCT)

SCT is the potential curative treatment for some haematological conditions. Preparation for SCT involves high-dose chemotherapy with or without total body irradiation (TBI).

Allogeneic SCT uses bone marrow cells from a donor (often from a sibling matched donor or closely matched unrelated donor). Prior to allogeneic SCT, high doses of chemotherapy and/or TBI are used to destroy the patient's marrow cells in the bone marrow. This is necessary to make space for the donor's marrow cells, which are collected either under general anaesthetic from the iliac crest or the marrow collected via apheresis. This involves the use of a cell separator machine.

Table 10.8 Investigations to diagnose HL and NHL

Investigation	Findings
Full blood count	Normocytic, normochromicanaemia Eosinophilia Leucocytosis
Erythrocyte sedimentation rate	Raised
C-reactive proteins	Increased
Serum lactate dehydrogenase (LDH)	Increased
Serum transaminase	Raised – may indicate liver involvement
Biopsy	Lymph node and of the bone marrow is done to establish the diagnosis for both Hodgkin's disease and NHL

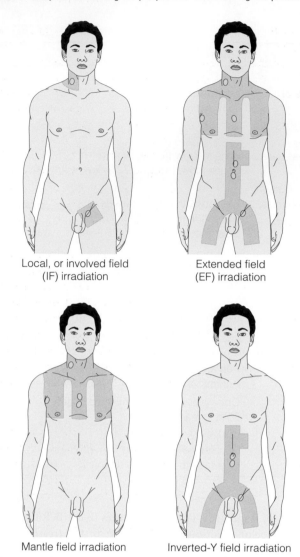

Local, or involved field
(IF) irradiation

Extended field
(EF) irradiation

Mantle field irradiation

Inverted-Y field irradiation

Figure 10.11 Patterns of radiation therapy.

Autologous SCT uses the individual's own bone marrow to restore bone marrow function after chemotherapy or radiation. In autologous SCT, about 1 L of bone marrow is aspirated (usually from the iliac crests) during a period of disease remission. Cryopreservation using liquid nitrogen is used to store the collected bone marrow cells. Autologous SCT is not a curative treatment but offered to increase longevity and ameliorate symptoms.

NURSING CARE FOR LYMPHOMA

Individuals undergoing chemotherapy and/or radiation will have significant side-effects, including bone marrow depression which can lead to immunosuppression, anaemia and bleeding. Secondary cancers and cardiac injury are the most serious late adverse effects of treatment. Some chemotherapy regimens carry a risk of acute leukaemia. Cancers such as breast or lung cancer may develop 10 or more years after thoracic radiation. Thoracic radiation also increases the risk for coronary heart disease and hypothyroidism.

Nursing diagnoses and interventions

Nursing interventions for the individual with leukaemia are similar to what is required for the individual with lymphoma, and the reader is guided to the nursing section (p. 362) in this chapter. What will be addressed here is fatigue which has a debilitating effect caused by both the treatment and the disease.

Assessment and management of fatigue

Fatigue can be extraordinarily overwhelming, with the individual having a sense of feeling drained, and the cumulative effect of treatment-associated fatigue can seem a never-ending road of tiredness.

General malaise and fatigue may accompany malignant lymphoma and are side-effects of chemotherapy. Malaise and fatigue are subjective experiences with physiological, situational and psychological components. In addition, the physical and psychological stress of coping with a chronic, debilitating disease and its treatment compounds the fatigue. Using a fatigue assessment tool to help establish the level of impact of the fatigue on ALs can be very helpful.

Provide an environment to encourage the individual to talk about what impact the disease is having on their lifestyle. This can help identify what interventions are required to help support the individual. These may include identifying and encouraging the individual to use energy-saving equipment. Keeping a diary to help with undertaking activities may help to highlight periods and activities which increase or decrease fatigue. It can also help in promoting concentration and aiding attention span.

Involve family members to delegate responsibilities of activities in the home to support the individual.

Encouraging a diet high in carbohydrates and fluids is important. A high-carbohydrate diet helps maintain muscle glycogen stores. A liberal fluid intake promotes excretion of metabolic by-products that may contribute to malaise and fatigue.

As an advocate, nurses can help to sensitively monitor the number of visitors in order to conserve the individual's energy.

As with leukaemia, discharge planning should identify any assistance with physical care, finances and transportation that may be required. Refer as appropriate to social services, support groups, home care services as needed, and other agencies that can provide needed support such as Lymphoma UK.

The person with multiple myeloma (MM)

Multiple myeloma (MM), also known as myelomatosis or Kahler's disease (named after the Austrian physician who first described MM), is a malignancy in which plasma cells multiply uncontrollably and infiltrate the bone marrow. Plasma cells are the functional mature cells of B-cell differentiation and they secrete antibodies (immunoglobulins).

FAST FACTS

MM

- MM is the second most common haematological malignancy in the UK.
- In 2007 4040 people in the UK were diagnosed with MM.
- IN 2008, 2660 deaths resulted from MM.
- MM affects men more frequently than women.
- MM predominately occurs after the 6th decade.
- There has been a rise in the number of younger people diagnosed for which reasons are not well understood.
- MM affects black persons twice as often as white persons.

Sources: Cancer Research UK 2010a, b.

Risk factors for MM

The cause of MM is unknown, but there are said to be possible risk factors, which include:

- Lower immunity – possibly caused by conditions such as HIV or drugs used for preventing organ rejection in transplant.
- Autoimmune diseases.
- Exposure to certain chemicals such as benzene.
- Genetic abnormalities, particularly of chromosome 13, which carries a poor prognosis.
- Monoclonal gammopathy of undetermined significance (MGUS) is linked to increased risk of developing myeloma. In MGUS there is an increase in antibodies, but there is no anaemia, no bone lesions and no renal dysfunction.

Pathophysiology of MM

The immunoglobulin (Ig) are 'Y'-shaped structures, composed of light chains which form the upper part of the Ig and are attached to the heavy chain which form the lower half of the immunoglobulin. The light chain of each immunoglobulin is known as either kappa or lambda, and the heavy chain determines the classification of the immunoglobulin. There are five classifications of immunoglobulins, namely:

- IgA – alpha;
- IgD – delta;
- IgE – epsilon;
- IgG – gamma;
- IgM – mu.

For further learning on antibodies, the reader is guided to Chapter 4 on immunology.

Myeloma cells produce a specific protein known as monoclonal protein (M-protein) in abundance, which is referred to as paraproteins. The increased production of antibodies leads to increased viscosity of the blood. This suppresses normal haemopoiesis and can lead to renal dysfunction.

In normal wear and tear of bones, there are complex interactions between osteoclasts and osteoblasts in bone remodelling to maintain a strong skeletal structure. The osteoclasts remove worn-out bone by resorption, creating lesions (holes). Osteoblasts are attracted to the lesions and repair the bone. See Chapter 12 on care of the patient with musculoskeletal problems for further details.

In MM there is an imbalance between the osteoclasts and osteoblasts, with osteoclasts overworking and creating more lesions which overwhelm the ability of the osteoblasts to repair the bone, ultimately leading to osteolytic lesions. These lesions allow calcium to 'leak' out leading to hypercalcaemia.

Cytokines play a significant role in the development and progression of MM. Osteoclast activating factors (OAFs), namely IL-1, stimulate the bone marrow to produce another growth factor RANKL (receptor activator for nuclear factor κ B ligand), also known as TNF-related activation-induced cytokine (TRANCE).

TRANCE encourages the development of osteoclasts, leading to an increase in their activity. This results in bone destruction and osteolytic lesions. Affected bones (primarily the vertebrae, ribs, skull, pelvis, femur, clavicle and scapula) are weakened and may break without trauma (pathological fracture).

Myeloma cells have an adhesive (sticky) structure on their surface, which allows them to bind onto VCAM-1 (vascular cell adhesion molecule-1). VCAM-1 is found on the stromal cells (the structural cells) of the bone marrow. Interleukin-6 (IL 6) plays a major role in the production of myeloma cells and prevents apoptosis (programmed cell death, i.e., cellular suicide). There are a number of other cytokines involved in MM, and their interactions ultimately disturb the bone marrow microenvironment, leading to increased tumour growth and bone expansion, inhibition of apoptosis and promotion of angiogenesis (development of new blood vessels) and bone resorption.

Signs and symptoms of MM

Bone pain is a common feature in MM, particularly of the spine, sternum and cranium, and compression of the vertebrae can cause spinal cord damage. Hypercalcaemia may present with polydipsia, polyuria, vomiting, lethargy, mental disturbances and constipation. Reduced normal immunoglobulins leads to an impaired humoral immune function and potential for frequent infections.

Impaired haemopoiesis will lead to anaemia, and platelet dysfunction leads to haemorrhagic manifestations. Hyperviscosity due to the large volume of antibodies can be characterised by neurological disturbance (dizziness, somnolence, coma).

Renal failure is commonly due to hypercalcaemia (see above) and tubular damage from excretion of light chains (known as Bence Jones proteins – BJPs). Other causes include glomerular deposition of amyloid, hyperuricaemia, recurrent infections (pyelonephritis) and local infiltration of tumour cells. Headaches, weakness, confusion and fatigue due to hypercalcaemia and hyperviscosity can occur. Retinopathy, carpel tunnel syndrome and loss of bowel and bladder control are other potential problems.

INTERDISCIPLINARY CARE FOR MM

Diagnosis

In addition to investigations listed in Table 10.1, additional investigations include:

- skeletal x-ray – to identify osteolytic lesions;
- CAT (computer-assisted tomography);
- MRI (magnetic resonance imaging);
- bone marrow aspiration – illustrates increases in plasma cells (pleomorphic plasma cells);
- eosinophils sedimentation rate (ESR) – increased;
- laboratory findings indicating impaired haemopoiesis, reduced Hb concentrations and rouleaux-shaped RBCs;
- protein electrophoresis to determine the abnormal paraprotein – most common are IgA & IgG;
- 24-hour urine collection to identify BJPs;
- renal function tests – blood urea greater than 14 mmol/L and serum creatinine, greater than 20%;
- serum calcium, uric acid are levels often elevated

Diagnosis of MM is usually based on three findings:

- Skeletal survey demonstrating osteolytic lesions. Fractures are a common presentation.
- Presence of plasma cells of greater than 4%, contains myeloma cells.
- M-proteins found in serum, urine or both. Presence of BJPs in urine.

Staging

This can be based on either the Durie–Salmon staging system (DSS) or the International Staging System (ISS). Neither has proven to be superior and different parameters are used in both systems and therefore, both tend to be commonly used.

The DSS has three categories (stages 1, 2 and 3) based on level of immunoglobulin, Hb and calcium concentrations, level of anaemia, platelet count and number of lesions. The stages 1, 2 and 3 can be divided into A or B depending on serum creatinine:

- A: serum creatinine less than 2 mg/dL (177 µmol/L);
- B: serum creatinine greater than 2 mg/dL (177 µmol/L).

The ISS is based on levels of serum β2 microglobulin and albumin. β$_2$-microglobulin is a protein which is shed by B lymphocytes and correlates with myeloma cell mass.

Plasma cell labelling index (PCLI) is also a useful prognostic indicator. PCLI indicates the percentage of plasma cells that are actively dividing and provides evidence of the level of plasma cell proliferation.

IN PRACTICE

The International Staging System (ISS)

- Stage I: β$_2$-microglobulin (β2M) less than 3.5 mg/L, albumin greater than 3.5 g/dL
- Stage II: β$_2$M less than 3.5 mg/L and albumin less than 3.5 g/dL; or β$_2$M 3.5–5.5 mg/L, irrespective of the serum albumin
- Stage III: β$_2$M greater than 5.5 mg/L

Source: adapted from the ISS for myeloma from the International Myeloma Working Group 2003.

Treatment

MM is incurable, but treatable. The aim of treatment is to extend the plateau phase of the disease, relieve any pain and anaemia and effectively manage other symptoms. Treatment may involve chemotherapy, radiation and surgery. If the individual is asymptomatic, chemotherapy and radiation will not be undertaken as this could lead to chemoresistance, particularly to alkylating drugs. When treatment is required it would depend on the symptoms, and there are various combined chemotherapy regimens.

Chemotherapy relieves pain through reducing tumour mass and reducing plasma cell proliferation, leading to a reduction in paraproteins, enabling improvement in marrow function and in quality of life.

Immunodulators and protease inhibitors are new developments in treatment for MM. In 2011 the National Institute for Health and Clinical Excellence (NICE) approved the use of thalidomide (an immunomodulator) and bortezomib (a proteaseome inhibitor) for newly diagnosed patients. These drugs are not chemotherapy but act against the activities of cytokines involved in myeloma, inhibiting their functions.

Radiotherapy is useful in reducing localised tumour mass and preventing pathological fractures, all of which can reduce pain. Surgical interventions include pinning of fractures or decompression laminectomy.

Supportive treatment would comprise bisphosphonates such as clodronate, pamidronate, zoledronic acid, calcium, vitamin D and fluoride supplements. These drugs strengthen bones, reduce pain and prevent destruction. Infections are treated promptly when they develop.

NURSING CARE FOR MM

The nurse has a pivotal role in ensuring interdisciplinary support for the person with MM. Nursing care priorities are to restore and preserve normal ALs and to provide and coordinate palliative care and physiotherapy with a view to enhancing the individual's quality of life. Emotional support is essential, particularly given that MM is an incurable condition.

Assessment should ascertain history of any pain, its duration and intensity. In addition, identify any signs of infection, fatigue and numbness. Discuss with the patient if there are any problems with mobility and if their gait is challenging.

Nursing diagnoses and interventions

Nursing diagnoses focus on infection, relieving pain, improving mobility, reducing the risk of injury, managing fatigue, monitoring kidney function and psychological support.

Risk for infection

Risk of infection is a major area for nursing care and prompt recognition is essential in managing the individual with MM; see the previous section on leukaemia (page 362) for specific interventions to reduce this risk.

Pain management

Individuals with MM typically experience chronic back pain and deep bone pain as myeloma cells saturate the bone marrow and invade the bone structure. Weakness caused by osteolytic lesions leads to pathological fractures being a common and reoccurring problem.

Effective pain assessment and management interventions are crucial in relieving pain and improving the patient's quality of life. The reader is guided to Chapter 2 on cancer, for detailed discussion on pain management.

Impaired physical mobility

Painful bony infiltrates and pathologic fractures may limit mobility. The spine usually is affected; the ribs and bones of the extremities also may be at risk of fracture. A brace or splint may be used to protect extremities or support the back.

Fatigue

It is also important to recognise that persistent weakness associated with MM and anaemia may limit the individual's ability to participate in usual activities. Therefore, encourage a balance between rest and activity. Resting conserves energy and gentle exercise such as walking can help with strengthening bones and muscles.

Risk for injury

Pathological fractures can occur with simple activities such as turning or reaching for an item. Ensure the individual has needed items within close reach, for example the call bell, drinks. Straining to reach objects increases the risk of falling or sustaining other injury. Support and advise the patient to change position regularly as this activity can improve comfort and also reduce risk of loss of skin and tissue integrity.

Consideration should be given to safety issues such as the height of the bed, lowering it to enable easy access and the use of side rails if necessary to prevent falls. Other safety issues to discuss with the individual are wearing shoes with non-skid soles, ensuring pathways are clear, particularly not having loose rugs on the floor, and not to lift or carry heavy items. Discuss, if appropriate, the use of walking aids. The damage to the vertebrae can lead to a reduction in height and it is not unusual for individuals to lose 2/3 inches off their height leading to the need for adjustment in clothes. Some individuals may be concerned about this and need to be reassured.

Risk for renal dysfunction

Careful monitoring of kidney function through accurate recording of fluid intake and urine output is critical to detect early signs of renal dysfunction. Individuals should be encouraged to drink at least 2L of fluid to help with minimising kidney dysfunction. Nurses should be familiar with normal levels of urea and creatinine levels, to recognise abnormal levels.

Psychological support

Provision of psychological support through listening to individuals' concerns, providing written patient information, informing individuals of support charities such as Myeloma UK is an important part of care.

COMMUNITY-BASED CARE

Interdisciplinary care involving the GP, district nurses and social services is essential to ensure the right facilities are available at home for the individual. An occupational therapist may need to do a home assessment to ascertain what facilities might be required to support the individual in their home.

Planning discharge, the individual should be advised of the following:

● Signs and symptoms of complications to be reported to the clinical nurse specialist or haematologist (e.g. symptoms of vertebral and extremity fractures).

● Signs and symptoms of infection to report: fever and chills; increased malaise, fatigue, or weakness; cough with or without sputum; sore throat; dysuria, nocturia, frequency or urgency.

● Fatigue is a significant debilitating feature of both MM and its treatment. Nursing issues of addressing fatigue are similar to those mentioned in the previous section (p. 368).

● Preventing and managing constipation should be discussed with the patient. A high-fibre diet, high in fluids should be encouraged. Stool softeners may be prescribed if constipation occurs.

HAEMOSTATIC DISORDERS

Platelet and coagulation disorders affect haemostasis and can either be acquired or inherited. Haemostasis maintains a relatively steady state of blood volume, blood pressure and blood flow through vessels. Bleeding disorders result from deficient, defective platelets or disruption of the clotting cascade.

PHYSIOLOGY REVIEW

Effective control of bleeding requires a series of complex interactions between the damaged tissue and blood vessel, platelets, clotting factors, and processes to dissolve clots once bleeding has been controlled. Platelets are formed in bone marrow under control of thrombopoietin, a protein produced by the liver, kidneys, smooth muscle and bone marrow. When a blood vessel wall becomes damaged, it changes in structure, becoming sticky. This enables platelets to aggregate at the site of injury, and they release many chemical mediators such as adenosine diphosphate (ADP), adenosine triphosphate (ATP) and thromboxane A_2 which leads to vasoconstriction, reducing blood loss and forms a platelet plug (Figure 10.12). Once the platelet plug is formed, it triggers the clotting factors into action in a sequential manner which ultimately leads to a fibrin clot being formed (Figure 10.13).

The person with thrombocytopenia

Thrombocytopenia is a platelet count of less than 100×10^9/L. A continuing decline in circulating platelets to less than 20×10^9/L can lead to spontaneous bleeding and haemorrhage from minor trauma. Thrombocytopenia can occur due to either failure of platelet production or increased platelet destruction. Failure of platelet production most often occurs from damage to megakaryocyte in the bone marrow.

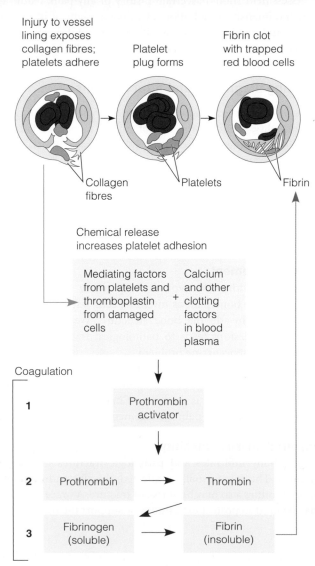

Figure 10.12 Platelet plug formation.

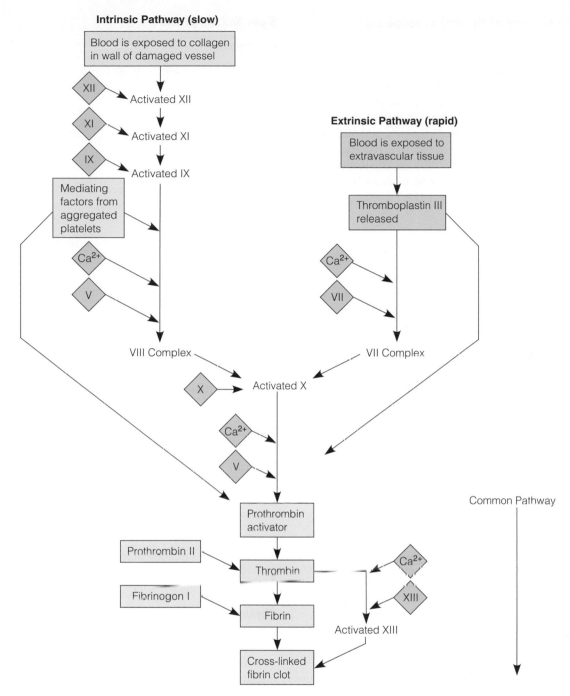

Figure 10.13 Clot formation.

Bleeding due to platelet deficiency usually occurs in small vessels, causing manifestations such as petechiae and purpura. The mucous membranes of the nose, mouth, gastrointestinal tract and vagina often bleed. Serious and potentially fatal bleeding occurs when the platelet count is less than 10×10^9/L.

Risk factors for thrombocytopenia

There are many causes of thrombocytopenia, which can be viral, drug-related or an effect of chemotherapy and radiotherapy.

A number of causes are related to increased destruction of platelets due to:

- autoimmune (idiopathic) thrombocytopenic purpura, which can either be acute or chronic (acute ITP or chronic ITP);
- post-transfusion purpura;
- drug-induced immune thrombocytopenia;
- thrombotic thrombocytopenic purpura (TTP);
- disseminated intravascular coagulation (DIC);
- splenic pooling.

Pathophysiology of thrombocytopenia

Acute ITP

Acute ITP is most commonly seen in children and tends to be preceded by a viral infection such as chicken pox or vaccination. Diagnosis is made by excluding all other causes of thrombocytopenia. If the platelet count is above 30×10^9/L, the majority of patients make a spontaneous recovery, and usually the patient is asymptomatic and no treatment is required.

If the platelet count is 20×10^9/L or where bleeding is severe, prednisolone may be prescribed. In about 10% of acute ITP this might transform to chronic ITP.

Chronic ITP

This is commonly seen in women in the 2nd–5th decade. Although known as idiopathic, it has been recognised that many individuals actually produce antibodies against their platelets, leading to their destruction. The culprit antibody is thought to be IgG which coats the platelets rendering them susceptible to destruction by splenic and liver macrophages. Chronic ITP is also associated with conditions such as systemic lupus erythematosis, HIV and CLL.

Being chronic, the symptoms are insidious. Easy bruising, prolonged bleeding, petechiae, haemorrhage and menorrhagia are common. Diagnosis is based on platelet count, usually, 10–50×10^9/L.

Drug-induced immune thrombocytopenia

It is generally believed that immune mechanisms are involved in drug-induced immune thrombocytopenia. Drugs associated with causing drug-induced thrombocytopenia include:

- thiazide diuretics;
- phenytoin;
- heparin;
- naproxen;
- diazepam;
- aspirin;
- digoxin.

Discontinuing the drug will generally enable the platelet count to recover.

Thrombotic thrombocytopenic purpura (TTP)

TTP or Moschcowitz syndrome causes extensive microscopic thromboses to form in small blood vessels throughout the body (thrombotic microangiopathy).

Most cases of TTP arise from inhibition of the enzyme ADAMTS13. When ADAMTS 13 is not present, this results in abnormally large von Willebrand factor multimers in plasma having a greater ability to react with platelets and causing the disseminated platelet thrombi characteristic of thrombotic thrombocytopenic purpura. As the platelets clump together in these clots, fewer platelets are available in the blood in other parts of the body to help with clotting.

Signs and symptoms

- Purpura.
- Malaise.
- Fever.
- Headache.
- Diarrhoea.
- Bruising.
- Kidney failure.
- Neurologic symptoms, such as hallucinations, bizarre behaviour, altered mental status, stroke or headaches.

Disseminated intravascular coagulation (DIC)

DIC is a pathological activation of coagulation mechanisms. DIC is never a primary illness but is always secondary to another illness. Below are some conditions which can lead to DIC:

- Adult Respiratory Distress Syndrome (ARDS);
- ABO incompatibility;
- obstetric complication – abruptio placentae, pre-eclampsia, amniotic fluid embolism;
- massive tissue injury – trauma, burns, extensive surgery;
- AML-M3;
- liver disease;
- heat stroke;
- vasculitis;
- aortic aneurysm;
- cancers of lung, pancreas, prostate and stomach;
- streptococcus pneumoniae;
- septicaemia.

Physiology

In DIC, widespread microthrombi occur throughout the body. This leads to consumption of platelets, clotting factors and calcium ions, disrupting normal coagulation processes. The utilisation of these components leads ultimately to bleeding. The sequence of DIC follows:

1. Endothelial damage, tissue factors or toxins stimulate the clotting cascade.
2. Excess thrombin within the circulation overwhelms naturally occurring anticoagulants.
3. Widespread clotting occurs within the microvasculature.
4. Thrombi and emboli impair tissue perfusion, leading to ischaemia, infarction and necrosis.
5. Clotting factors and platelets are consumed faster than they can be replaced.
6. Clotting activates fibrinolytic processes, which begin to break down clots.

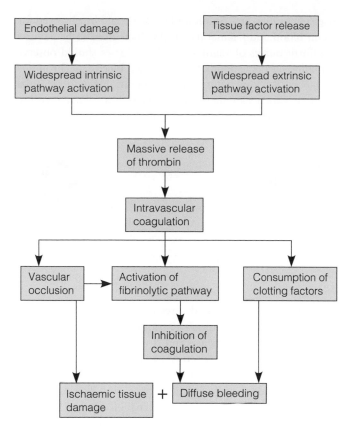

Figure 10.14 Disseminated intravascular coagulation (DIC).

7. Fibrin degradation products (FDPs, potent anticoagulants) are released, contributing to bleeding.

8. Clotting factors are depleted, the ability to form clots is lost and haemorrhage occurs (Figure 10.14).

Signs and symptoms

Generally, signs and symptoms are due to the reduction in platelets and clotting factors and are outlined below:

- haemorrhaging from wounds;
- oozing of blood from intravenous catheter sites;
- bruising, petechiae;
- hypotension;
- tachycardia;
- dyspnoea;
- gastrointestinal bleeding;
- signs of increased intracranial pressure, decreased level of consciousness, confusion;
- cyanosis of extremities;
- haematuria;
- oliguria;
- acute renal failure;
- septic shock may precipitate DIC;
- infections.

Diagnosis

Diagnosis is usually determined by the presence of:

- thrombocytopenia;
- prolongation of prothrombin time and activated partial thromboplastin time;
- a low fibrinogen concentration;
- increased levels of FDPs.

Heparin-induced thrombocytopenia (HIT)

HIT develops as a result of an abnormal response to heparin therapy. Unfractionated heparin carries a greater potential to precipitate HIT; however, it can develop in patients receiving low-molecular-weight heparin who have previously been treated with unfractionated heparin.

Heparin is a protein that occurs naturally in human tissues and inflammatory cells. It can react directly with platelets, causing them to agglutinate (clump) and be removed from circulation by phagocytosis. This form of HIT, called type I HIT, typically causes mild thrombocytopenia. The more severe form, type II HIT, results from an immune reaction to heparin. In type II HIT, heparin forms an immune complex with a platelet protein known as platelet factor 4 (PF4). This complex acts as a foreign antigen in some patients, stimulating antibody production. The antibody binds with the heparin–PF4 complex, and these antibody–heparin–PF4 complexes subsequently bind with circulating platelets, causing them to aggregate. As affected platelets aggregate, they are removed from circulation, leading to thrombocytopenia. In addition, small pieces of platelets can break loose, stimulating the clotting cascade and the development of thrombosis. The thrombocytopenia and the thrombosis can be reversed by prompt withdrawal of heparin therapy.

Signs and symptoms

Bleeding is usually a manifestation of HIT, probably because of the increased tendency to form clots that deplete clotting factors. The patient may develop manifestations of an arterial thrombosis (severe pain, paraesthesia, pallor and cool skin temperature, and pulselessness distal to the arterial occlusion) or of venous thrombosis (oedema, redness and warmth of the affected area). On rare occasions, an intravenous bolus of unfractionated heparin can precipitate an acute inflammatory response with manifestations that may mimic an acute pulmonary embolism which can manifest as: fever, chills, hypertension, tachycardia, dyspnoea, chest pain and cardiopulmonary arrest.

INTERDISCIPLINARY CARE FOR THROMBOCYTOPENIA

For acute and chronic ITP, corticosteroids tend to be quite effective in many cases. Dosage is usually prednisolone, 1 mg per kg daily and reduced after two weeks. If this fails, splenectomy may be considered, but it is usually successful in only

50% of cases. High-dose intravenous immunoglobulin may be used and gives a rapid response. Dosage of 400 mg per kg per day for five days or 1 g per kg per day for two days is common. Immunosuppressive drugs such as azathioprine may be the next option if splenectomy and steroid management are not successful. Other options may be anti-D, immunoglobulin and platelet transfusion given as a short-term measure in life-threatening situations.

TTP is usually treated with plasma exchange, using fresh frozen plasma or cryosupernatant. Platelet count and LDH are usually used as a means of monitoring the effectiveness of treatment. Individuals who do not respond to treatment may require high-dose steroids or chemotherapy. Unfortunately, relapses are very common and mortality is not uncommon.

PRACTICE ALERT

Individuals with TTP must NOT be given platelets as this will aggravate the thrombosis. Patients should be advised to wear a medi-alert.

DIC carries a high mortality rate and effective treatment is to stop the underlying cause, but this is clearly difficult if the cause is surgery or stopping chemotherapy treatment.

When bleeding is the major manifestation of DIC, fresh frozen plasma (FFP) and platelet concentrates are given to restore clotting factors and platelets. Heparin, although controversial, may be administered. Heparin interferes with the clotting cascade and may prevent further clotting factor consumption due to uncontrolled thrombosis. It is used when bleeding is not controlled by FFP and platelets, as well as when the patient has manifestations of thrombotic problems such as acrocyanosis and possible gangrene. Long-term heparin therapy (administered by injection or continuous infusion using a portable pump) may be necessary for patients with chronic DIC.

NURSING CARE FOR THROMBOCYTOPENIA

Patients with thrombocytopenia are at risk for bleeding. TTP causes extensive microscopic thrombosis. Patients with DIC are at risk of impaired tissue perfusion and gas exchange, pain and anxiety associated with their symptoms.

Nursing diagnoses and interventions

Risk for bleeding

Bleeding is a serious complication associated with thrombocytopenia and therefore four-hourly monitoring of vital signs and frequent assessment for signs of bleeding should be undertaken. The skin and mucous membranes should be assessed for petechiae, ecchymoses and haematoma formation. The nasal membranes and conjunctiva should also be assessed for bleeding. Stools and urine should be observed for occult blood and haematuria. Individuals need to be advised to inform nurses of vaginal bleeding. Nurses should observe puncture sites or wounds for prolonged bleeding. Thrombocytopenia can cause neurological problems due to intracranial bleeding which can manifest as headaches, blurred vision, confusion, seizures and decreasing level of consciousness.

PRACTICE ALERT

If possible avoid invasive procedures such as urinary catheterisation, intramuscular, intravenous injections as far as possible. Invasive procedures can cause tissue trauma and bleeding.

If venepuncture is required, pressure should be applied for three to five minutes and 15–20 minutes to arterial puncture sites to promote haemostasis and clot formation.

Patients should be advised to avoid forcefully blowing the nose or picking crusts from the nose, straining to have a bowel movement, and forceful coughing or sneezing. These activities increase the risk of external and internal bleeding.

Thrombocytopenia frequently leads to bleeding of the gums and oral mucosa. As a result, risk for infection and impaired nutrition increases. Oral care can be found in the earlier section on leukaemia (page 363).

TTP

TTP is a very challenging condition for individuals to live with. Lack of concentration can be a major problem and therefore giving patient information in small amounts with written information as an additional source is very important. Advising the individual to seek medical help early when they are experiencing symptoms is important.

DIC

Individuals with acute DIC are critically ill, with multiple nursing care needs. Priority nursing diagnoses discussed in this section focus on impaired tissue perfusion and gas exchange, pain and fear.

Nurses are instrumental in identifying early manifestations of DIC and facilitating timely intervention. Being aware of the individual's primary illness should heighten awareness of risks of developing DIC.

Assessment and observation

If the patient has had surgery, check the wound site for bleeding and IV sites. Vital sign monitoring to observe for abnormal cardiopulmonary functions is essential. Abdominal assessment should include girth measurements, bowel sounds, tenderness or guarding to palpation. Observations of skin colour, temperature, condition of hands, feet and digits, petechiae or purpura of skin, mucous membranes should all be undertaken.

Any complaints of chest pain, altered mental health status, respirations, gastro intestinal function and oliguria require prompt attention. Chest pain could be indicative of angina or pulmonary embolism. Reduced urine output could be indicative of renal dysfunction. Microclots in the pulmonary vasculature are likely to interfere with gaseous exchange. Monitor oxygen saturation continuously and administer oxygen as prescribed. Supplemental oxygen promotes gas exchange and reduces cardiac work, relieving dyspnoea. Maintaining bedrest reduces oxygen demands and cardiac work. Encouraging deep breathing and effective coughing aids in increasing respiratory depth and clearance of secretions from airways, improving alveolar ventilation and oxygenation.

Thrombi and emboli forming throughout the microcirculation affect the perfusion of multiple organs and tissues. Additionally, bleeding due to clotting factor consumption affects cardiac output and blood flow to these tissues. Therefore, assessment of extremity pulses, warmth and capillary refill are important.

PRACTICE ALERT

A painful, pale and cold extremity with no or diminished pulse indicates arterial occlusion. Prompt intervention is critical to save the extremity. Acute abdominal pain, decreased bowel sounds and GI bleeding may indicate mesenteric occlusion, which is a surgical emergency.

Tissue perfusion

Poor tissue perfusion warrants careful positioning and regular repositioning to prevent skin breakdown. Position changes facilitate circulation and tissue perfusion and also provide an opportunity to assess for purpura, pallor and bleeding. Minimise use of tape on the skin, using non-adhesive dressings, and other devices as needed. Preventing skin trauma reduces the risk for bleeding and potential infection.

Discourage crossing the legs, and do not elevate the knees on the bed or with a pillow. These positions may impair arterial and venous flow to the lower legs and feet, increasing vascular stasis and the risk for thrombosis.

PRACTICE ALERT

Cautious nasotracheal suctioning may be instituted if cough is ineffective or an endotracheal tube is in place. Removal of secretions facilitates ventilation and oxygenation. However, care must be used to minimise suction-induced hypoxia and airway trauma.

Pain management

Both the underlying cause of DIC and tissue ischaemia from microvascular clots can cause pain. Establishing the aetiology of pain is important to identify potential complications or harmful effect of DIC and to institute effective treatment.

Providing reassurance and comfort measures is extremely important. Individuals are highly anxious and frightened as they are very aware they are critically ill. Pain and anxiety increase the respiratory rate and decrease the depth of respirations, reducing effective ventilation and gas exchange. Please refer to Chapter 2 on cancer for more information on pain management.

Any sudden complaint or new complaints of pain should be reported urgently as it may be an indication of a worsening situation. It should also be remembered that ischaemic tissue can cause immense pain and therefore care and gentle handling to prevent/minimise any further injury is important.

If the individual is prescribed analgesia, it is critical that judicious, careful monitoring of vital signs and neurological observations are undertaken as analgesia can mask neurological impairment due to thromboembolism and depression of respiration.

Psychological support

Psychological support is important for both the individual and their family. The underlying serious illness and a complication such as DIC result in an uncertain prognosis, often accompanied by fear. Nurses should encourage the patient to verbalise their concerns in order to reduce anxiety. Being open and honest is critically important in developing a therapeutic nurse–patient relationship. Accurate responses allow the individual and family to set priorities as they plan for an uncertain future. Responding promptly to an individual's request for help can engender feelings of security and further enhances a trusting relationship. Providing an empathetic approach and calm environment can lessen anxiety, can instil confidence and provide a sense of control in the care being provided.

Identify and harness coping strategies the individual has used in the past to support them through this challenging time. It can be beneficial to teach relaxation techniques as these can reduce muscle tension and other signs of anxiety. Gaining control over physical responses can help the individual gain a sense of control over the situation.

The person with a hereditary coagulation disorder

Haemophilia is a group of hereditary disorders which are the most common causes of hereditary coagulation disorders. The main three hereditary coagulation disorders are haemophilia A (factor VIII deficiency), haemophilia B (Christmas disease, factor IX deficiency) and von Willebrand disease (vWD).

Pathophysiology of hereditary coagulation disorders

When tissue injury occurs, platelets collect at the site, adhering to the damaged vessel wall (the platelet plug). Activation of the clotting cascade, a sequential process of interactive reactions

Table 10.9 Blood coagulation factors

Factor	Name	Function or pathway
I	Fibrinogen	Converted to fibrin strands
II	Prothrombin	Converted to thrombin
III	Thromboplastin	Catalyees conversion of thrombin
IV	Calcium ions	Needed for all steps of coagulation
V	Proaccelerin	Extrinsic/intrinsic pathways
VII	Serum prothrombin conversion accelerator	Extrinsic pathway
VIII	Antihemophilic factor	Intrinsic pathway
IX	Plasma prothrombin component	Intrinsic pathway
X	Stuart factor	Extrinsic/intrinsic pathways
XI	Plasma prothrombin antecedent	Intrinsic pathway
XII	Hageman factor	Intrinsic pathway
XIII	Fibrin stabilising factor	Cross-links fibrin strands to form insoluble clot

of clotting factors, is vital to form a stable clot. Clotting factors are plasma proteins primarily produced by the liver. A number of these factors require the presence of vitamin K for synthesis and activation (Table 10.9). Once the clot has been formed and stabilised, it begins to retract, pulling together the edges of the damaged blood vessel to initiate the healing process.

Haemophilia A

Haemophilia A (or classic haemophilia) is the most common type of haemophilia, caused by deficiency or dysfunction of clotting factor VIII. The inheritance is X-linked and primarily it is carrier mothers who have a 50% chance of passing on their X chromosome with the factor VIII gene to their son (Figure 10.15). The factor VIII gene (known as F8) is on the long arm of the X chromosome. The genetic defect of haemophilia A on the X chromosome may cause deficient factor VIII production or a defective form of the protein.

When the concentration of clotting factor VIII is 5–35% of normal, the disease is mild. Bleeding is infrequent, and usually associated with trauma. Concentrations of 1–5% of normal result in moderate disease. Again, bleeding usually occurs secondary to trauma. Severe haemophilia occurs when concentrations are less than 1% of normal. Bleeding is frequent, often occurring without trauma.

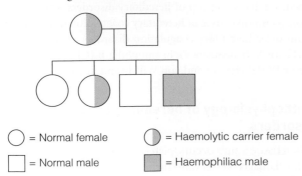

○ = Normal female   ◑ = Haemolytic carrier female
□ = Normal male   ■ = Haemophiliac male

Figure 10.15 The inheritance pattern of haemophilia A & B.

Haemophilia B

Haemophilia B (Christmas disease) accounts for about 15% of cases, and is caused by a deficiency in Factor IX. Despite the difference in clotting factor deficits, haemophilia A and haemophilia B are clinically identical.

Von Willebrand disease (vWD)

VWD is the most common hereditary bleeding disorder. It was discovered by von Willebrand in 1926 in families on islands in the Baltic (Åland Islands). VWD is caused by a deficit of or defective von Willebrand factor (vWF), a protein that mediates platelet adhesion. Reduced levels of factor VIII are also often present, because the vWF carries factor VIII. This clotting disorder affects men and women equally. Bleeding associated with vWD is rarely severe. It is often diagnosed when prolonged bleeding follows surgery or a dental extraction.

People with haemophilia form a platelet plug at the site of bleeding, but the clotting factor deficit impairs formation of a stable fibrin clot. The effect of vWF deficiency is somewhat different, in that platelet aggregation at the site of injury is impaired. In either case, prolonged or extensive bleeding may result. Often bleeding occurs in response to injury or as a result of surgery. However, a severe clotting factor deficit can lead to spontaneous bleeding into the joints (haemarthrosis), deep tissues and central nervous system. Haemarthrosis often causes joint deformity and disability, usually of the elbows, hips, knees and ankles.

Signs and symptoms of hereditary coagulation disorders

Signs and symptoms associated with haemophilia are:

- haemarthrosis;
- easy bruising and cutaneous haematoma formation with minor trauma (for example, an injection);

- bleeding from the gums and prolonged bleeding following minor injuries or cuts;
- gastrointestinal bleeding, with haematemesis (vomiting blood), occult blood in the stools, gastric pain or abdominal pain;
- spontaneous haematuria or epistaxis (nosebleed);
- pain or paralysis due to the pressure of haematomas on nerves;
- intracranial haemorrhage which is potentially life threatening.

FAST FACTS

Some hereditary disorders

- Haemophilia A is found in 1 in 5000–1 in 10 000 live male births and is five times more common than haemophilia B in the UK.
- VWD is thought to be clinically significant in 1 in 10 000 of the UK population.

INTERDISCIPLINARY CARE FOR HEREDITARY COAGULATION DISORDERS

Diagnosis

Diagnosis of haemophilia and vWD are based on findings from the following laboratory investigations. Serum platelet levels are measured and are usually normal. Coagulation studies such as activated partial thromboplastin time (APTT), bleeding time and prothrombin time are used to screen for haemophilia when abnormal bleeding occurs. APTT is increased in all types of haemophilia. Prothrombin time is unaffected in these disorders but may be measured to rule out other disorders. Bleeding time is prolonged in vWD but normal in haemophilia A and B. Factor assays are undertaken and factor VIII is decreased in haemophilia A and often in vWD. VWF is low in vWD and factor IX is decreased in haemophilia B. Amniocentesis or chorionic villus sampling is used to identify the genetic defect of haemophilia when there is a known family history of the disease.

Treatment

Managing individuals with haemophilia requires an interdisciplinary approach. Treatment of haemophilia focuses on preventing and/or treating bleeding, primarily by replacing deficient clotting factors. Specific treatment depends on the severity of the disorder and the specific factor deficiency. Haemophilia A is usually managed with factor VIII concentrate or cryoprecipitate. The factor VIII may be heat-treated as

this reduces the risk of transmitting disease, or recombinant factor VIII is used. The dose of factor VIII is determined by the severity of the deficit and the presence or prospect of active bleeding (for example, planned surgery). In milder cases of haemophilia A, DDAVP (desmopressin) might be used. This drug causes an increase in factor VIII and vWFs and will raise blood levels by two- or threefold for several hours, reducing the risk of bleeding and the need for clotting factor concentrate.

Haemophilia B is treated with factor IX (Christmas disease concentrate). Because factor IX concentrates also contain a number of other proteins, there is risk of thrombosis with recurrent use. Hence they are used judiciously. Products produced by recombinant technology or that are monoclonally purified carry a lower risk of stimulating thrombus formation.

VWD is managed with cryoprecipitate and DDAVP. Factor VIII concentrates contain functional vWF, and may also be used to treat vWD. Tranexamic acid, an antifibrinolytic agent, might be used in epistaxis or menorrhagia bleeding episodes in vWD.

In all cases, factor levels are frequently checked to ensure the treatment is adequate.

Deficient clotting factors are replaced regularly, as a prophylactic measure before surgery and dental procedures, and to control bleeding. Clotting factors may be given as fresh–frozen plasma, cryoprecipitate or concentrates. If the cause of bleeding is not yet determined, fresh–frozen plasma may be administered intravenously until a definitive diagnosis is made.

NURSING CARE FOR HEREDITARY COAGULATION DISORDERS

The inability to form stable clots and stem bleeding from injured blood vessels creates a significant risk for the individual with haemophilia. Nursing care measures focus on preventing injury and protecting the skin from damage.

Individuals should be advised to contact the clinical nurse specialist or consultant if any bleeding episodes occur. Early intervention with administration of clotting factor concentrate decreases the risk of haemorrhage and subsequent hypovolaemia.

If possible, avoid intramuscular injections, rectal temperatures and enemas. These can pose a risk of tissue and vascular trauma, which can precipitate bleeding.

If the individual is vomiting, the vomitus should be checked for blood. Similarly stools should be observed for occult blood. Bleeding may occur in cutaneous tissues as well as internal organs. Bleeding in the upper gastrointestinal tract may not be readily apparent in the stool.

If bleeding occurs, control blood loss using gentle pressure, ice or a topical haemostatic agent. Direct pressure occludes bleeding vessels. Ice, a vasoconstrictor, may facilitate bleeding control, as do topical haemostatic agents.

Advising on safety measures to minimise bleeding is important. For example, using an electric razor rather than a razor blade to shave minimises the development of superficial cuts that may result in bleeding. Contact sport is generally advised against, but activities such as swimming could be a useful substitute. Jobs which require excessive physical exertion should be avoided. Awareness of safety measures in the home should be considered. Aspirin is avoided in all types of haemophilia as it causes prolonged bleeding.

Health promotion

Haemophilia is a lifelong chronic disorder, requiring active management to prevent and control bleeding and complications. Frequent visits to the haematologist or clinic may be necessary. Education should involve ensuring the individual and their family have information about the disease and the rationale for treatment, and understand the importance of early interventions to reduce complications from bleeding. Nurses should teach the individual self-administration of clotting factors and measures to prevent complication. The adolescent period can be a difficult time in adjusting and accepting their condition and additional support may be required during this period. Impaired disease management may be due to lack of knowledge or a conscious decision not to follow the recommendations of the nurse or haematologist. Continuing emotional support and encouragement can enhance the confidence patients have in carrying out self-care activities.

Encourage individuals with a family history of haemophilia or bleeding disorders to seek genetic counselling during their family planning process.

COMMUNITY-BASED CARE

Discuss the following topics when preparing the individual with a bleeding disorder and the family for home care:

- Recognising the manifestations of internal bleeding: pallor, weakness, restlessness, headache, disorientation, pain and swelling. These manifestations require emergency medical care and should be reported immediately.
- Applying cold packs and immobilising the joint for 24–48 hours if haemarthrosis occurs.
- Using analgesics for pain; avoiding prescription and over-the-counter drugs containing aspirin.
- Ensuring a safe home environment (for example, padding sharp edges of furniture, using transition lighting or a night light; avoiding scatter rugs; and wearing protective gloves when working in the house or garden).
- Wearing a MedicAlert bracelet in case of accident.
- Practising good dental hygiene to decrease potential tooth decay and extractions. If dental procedures are necessary, discuss the need for prophylactic factor administration with the dentist and haematologist.
- Following safe sex practices.
- Preparing and administering intravenous medications.
- Refer the individual and family to a local haemophilia or bleeding disorders support group or to the UK Haemophilia Society.

CASE STUDY SUMMARIES

Haematology is a fascinating field of nursing and this chapter has illustrated the diversity of haematological conditions nurses might encounter. The challenges faced by individuals such as Malcolm with leukaemia highlight the need for nurses to have a wide breadth of skills in caring for a patient with a haemato-oncological diagnosis. Long-term conditions like SCD, illustrated by Marcia, underpin the need for nurses to have a wide repertoire of skills in pain management and a good understanding of genetics in haematology. Kirsty's case of IDA and anorexia nervosa demonstrate the importance of providing sound dietary advice to help with consequences of nutritional anaemias.

With the continual developments in treatments and interventions, haematology nursing continues to be dynamic, exciting, intriguing and highly rewarding.

CHAPTER HIGHLIGHTS

- This chapter has provided an overview of haemopoiesis and discussed the role growth factors play in the development of marrow cells.
- Anaemia is the most common disorder of red blood cells (RBCs); nutritional anaemias are the common causes of anaemia. The signs and symptoms of anaemia relate to the function of RBCs and haemoglobin-transporting O_2 and CO_2.
- Nursing care related to anaemia is primarily educational to prepare the patient for effective self-care, including diet and medication.
- Sickle cell disease (SCD) and beta thalassaemia major (BTM) are long-term conditions which can cause significant morbidities, impacting on quality of life. Continual education to support self-management is important. Effective pain management in SCD and

- safe administration of blood transfusion and iron chelation in BTM are essential.
- Polycythaemia vera (PV) is a myeloproliferative disorder which has the potential to transform into acute leukaemia. Skilled venepuncturing is necessary to manage these patients.
- Leukaemia and lymphoma are haematological disorders of white blood cells.
- Signs and symptoms of leukaemia reflect a poor immune surveillance system and reduced cytopenia.
- There are four major subtypes of acute leukaemia which impact on the different treatment options, potential side-effects and prognosis.
- Lymphocytic leukaemia and lymphomas are closely related.
- Nursing care of patients with leukaemia and lymphoma focuses on reducing the risk of bleeding and managing the side-effects of chemotherapy/radiotherapy.
- Multiple myeloma is a malignancy of plasma cells, resulting in the excessive production of abnormal antibodies. Myeloma cells cause excessive overactivity of osteoblasts leading to osteolytic lesion causing significant pain.
- Calcium leaks out from the osteolytic lesions causing hypercalcaemia which can cause acute renal failure in multiple myeloma (MM).

- Great care is required in managing mobility in patients with MM as pathological fractures can occur.
- Bleeding and clotting disorders can result from dysfunctional or inadequate platelets (thrombocytopenia) or disruption to clotting (haemophilia, disseminated intravascular coagulation (DIC)).
- DIC is a disorder of widespread microvascular coagulation, leading to consumption of platelets and clotting factors leading to haemorrhage. DIC is never a primary illness but is always secondary to another.
- Nursing care in DIC revolves around ensuring effective gaseous exchange, monitoring cardiac and renal function, managing pain and providing emotional and psychological support.
- Haemophilia A and B occur from a genetic fault on the X chromosomes, with women primarily being carries and males being affected. Von Willebrand disease (vWD), the most common bleeding disorder, is an autosomal dominant inherited condition and affects both sexes equally.
- Teaching self-care and safety to minimise bleeding episodes in haemophilia is very important. Advising against taking aspirin is important as this can cause prolonged bleeding.
- Referral to genetic counselling services is paramount in SCD, BTM and haemophilia.

TEST YOURSELF

1. What is haemopolesis?
   a. production of red blood cells
   b. production of neutrophils
   c. production of marrow cells
   d. production of aplastic cells

2. What does neutropenia mean?
   a. increase in white cells
   b. decrease in neutrophils
   c. increase in neutrophils
   d. decrease in insulin production

3. Why is the accuracy of height and weight important in patients receiving chemotherapy?
   a. it can affect the accuracy of chemotherapy/ radiotherapy the patient will require
   b. important for establishing when a referral to the dietician may be necessary
   c. it is relevant for deciding on iron medication
   d. it helps calculate the need for pressure-relieving aids

4. When a patient is neutropenic, what temperature recording is considered a medical emergency?
   a. 37.5°C
   b. 35.5°C
   c. 36.5°C
   d. 38.5°C

5. If both parents have sickle cell trait, what are the statistical chances of having a child with sickle cell disease?
   a. 2 in 4
   b. 3 in 4
   c. 1 in 4
   d. 1 in 10

6. In thalassaemia major what is the role of iron chelation?
   a. rid the body of excess potassium
   b. rid the body of proteins
   c. helps the body to store iron
   d. rid the body of excess iron

7. In multiple myeloma why is care required in mobilising a patient?

  a. they are very tired
  b. risk of pathological fractures
  c. patients tend to have ataxia
  d. risk of the patient becoming dependent

8. Why is hydration important in VOC?

  a. reduces the viscosity of the blood
  b. reduces splenic dysfunction
  c. unsickles red blood cells
  d. improves production of bile

9. What important advice should be given to patients prescribed thalidomide?

  a. avoid pregnancy and use contraception
  b. keep all hospital appointments
  c. enhance the uptake of iron
  d. do not drink fluids containing carotene

10. How is haemophilia inherited?

  a. autosomal recessive inheritance
  b. autosomal dominant inheritance
  c. sex linked inheritance
  d. through infected semen

Further resources

Myeloma UK
http://www.myeloma.org.uk
Myeloma UK provides information and support to those affected by myeloma and works to improve standards of treatment and care through research, education, campaigning and raising awareness.

Macmillan
http://www.macmillan.org.uk
Macmillan nurses provide information and support to individuals and their families affected by cancer, as well as educational materials, patient information and financial support.

The Haemophilia Society
http://www.haemophilia.org.uk
The Haemophilia Society provides information and support to individuals with haemophilia.

Leukaemia and Lymphoma Research
http://leukaemialymphomaresearch.org
A campaigning and fund-raising organisation for haematological cancers.

Sickle Cell Society
http://www.sicklecellsociety.org
The Sickle Cell Society provides support and information to individuals and their families and campaigns to raise awareness and improve care in SCD.

UK Thalassaemia Society
http://www.ukts.org
The UK Thalassaemia Society provides information and support for individuals and their families with thalassaemia and campaigns to raise awareness about the condition.

Bibliography

Allen L H (2009) How common is vitamin B-12 deficiency? *American Journal of Clinical Nutrition*, **89**, 693S–696S.

Allen S (2005) Understanding sickle cell anaemia. *The Pharmaceutical Journal*, **275**, 25–28.

Bain B J (2006) *Blood Cells – A practical guide*. Oxford, Blackwell.

Benner H, Rothenbacher D M and Arndt V (2009) Epidemiology of stomach cancer. In Verma M (ed.), *Methods of Molecular Biology, Cancer, Epidemiology*, Vol. 472. Totowa, NJ, Humana Press, 467–478.

Brown M (2010) Nursing care of patients undergoing allogeneic stem cell transplantation. *Nursing Standard*, **25** (11), 47–56.

Cancer Research UK (2010a) *Multiple Myeloma – UK incidence statistics*. London, available at: http://info.cancerresearchuk.org/cancerstats/

types/multiplemyeloma/incidence/#age (accessed September 2011).

Cancer Research UK (2010b) *Multiple Myeloma – UK mortality statistics*. London, available at: http://info.cancerresearchuk.org/cancerstats/types/multiplemyeloma/mortality/ (accessed September 2011).

Cancer Research UK (2011a) *Leukaemia – UK incidence statistics*. London, available at: http://info.cancerresearchuk.org/cancerstats/types/leukaemia/incidence/ (accessed September 2011).

Cancer Research UK (2011b) *Hodgkin Lymphoma – UK incidence statistics*. London, available at: http://info.cancerresearchuk.org/cancerstats/types/hodgkinslymphoma/incidence/ (accessed September 2011).

Cancer Research UK (2011c) *Non-Hodgkin Lymphoma – UK incidence statistics*. London, available at: http://info.cancerresearchuk.org/

cancerstats/types/nhl/incidence (accessed September 2011).

Cantril C A and Haylock P J (2004) Tumor lysis syndrome. *American Journal of Nursing*, **104** (4), 49–52.

Coleman R W, Marder V J, Clowes A W, George J N, and Goldhaber S Z (2005) *Hemostasis And Thrombosis; Basic priniciples and clinical practice* (5th edn). Hagerstown, MD, Lippincott.

Cook J D (2005) Diagnosis and management of iron deficiency anaemia. *Best Practice Research Clinical Haematology*, **18** (2), 319–332.

Demakos E P and Linebaugh J A (2005) Advances in myelodysplastic syndrome: Nursing implications of azacitidine. *Clinical Journal of Oncology Nursing*, **9** (4), 417–423.

Dougherty L and Lister S (2008) *The Royal Marsden Hospital Manual of Clinical Nursing Procedures* (7th edn). Oxford, Wiley-Blackwell.

Durie B G and Salmon S E (1975) A clinical staging system for multiple myeloma. Correlation of measured myeloma cell mass with presenting clinical features, response to treatment, and survival. *Cancer*, **36** (3), 842–854.

Goddard A F, James M W, McIntyre A S and Scott B (2005) *Guidelines for the Management of Iron Deficiency Anaemia*. London, British Society of Gastronenterology.

Grundy M (2006) *Nursing in Haematological Oncology* (2nd edn). Edinburgh, Elsevier.

Hoffbrand A V, and Moss P A H (2011) *Essential Haematology* (6th edn). Oxford, Blackwell Science.

Hughes-Jones N C, Wickramasinghe S N and Hatton C S R (2009) *Lecture Notes in Haematology* (8th edn). Oxford, Wiley-Blackwell.

International Myeloma Working Group (2003) Criteria for the classification of monoclonal gammopathies, multiple myeloma and related disorders: a report of the International Myeloma Working Group. *British Journal of Haematology*, **121** (5), 749–757.

Kübler-Ross E (2005) *On Grief and Grieving: Finding the meaning of grief through the five stages of loss*. New York, Simon & Schuster.

Lewis S M, Bain B J and Bates I (2006) *Practical Haematology* (10th edn). Philadelphia, PA, Churchill Livingston, Elsevier.

Raab M S, Podar K, Breitkreutz I, Richardson P G, and Anderson K C (2009) Multiple myeloma. *Lancet*, **374** (9686), 324–339.

Ress D C, Lujohungbe A D, Parker N E, *et al.* (2003) Guidelines for the management of acute painful crisis in sickle cell disease. *British Journal of Haematology*, **120**, 744–752.

Shelton B K (2003) Evidence-based care for the neutropenic patient with leukemia. *Seminars in Oncology Nursing*, **19** (2), 133–141.

UK Thalassaemia Society (2008) *Standards for the Clinical Care of Children and Adults with Thalassaemia in the UK*. London, UK Thalassaemia Society.

Sickle Cell Society (2008) *Standards for the Management of Adults with Sickle Cell Disease in the UK*. London, Sickle Cell Society.

Tefferi A and Vardiman J W (2008) Classification and diagnosis of myeloproliferative neoplasms: The 2008 World Health Organization criteria and point-of-care diagnostic algorithms. *Leukemia*, **22** (1), 14–22.

Toumba M, Sergis A, Kanaris C and Skordis N (2007) Endocrine complications in patients with Thalassemia major. *Pediatric Endocrinology Reviews*, **5** (2), 642–648.

Van Amsterdam J G V, Opperhuizen A and Jansen E M J M (2005) *Masking of Vitamin B12 Deficiency Associated Neuropathy by Folic Acid*. Bilthoven, RIVM.

Van Beers E J, van Tuiju C F J, MacGillavry M R, *et al.* (2008) Sickle cell disease-related organ damage occurs irrespective of pain rate; implications for clinical practice. *Haematologica*, **93** (5), 757–760.

WHO (2001) *Iron Deficiency Anemia. Assessment, Prevention, and Control. A Guide for Programme Managers*. Geneva, World Health Organization.

Caring for people with respiratory problems

Learning outcomes

- List the most common respiratory diseases seen in the UK and be aware of the epidemiology of respiratory problems.

- Relate the pathophysiological process – presenting signs and symptoms – of common respiratory problems to the physiology of breathing.

- Relate the signs and symptoms of respiratory disease to respiratory function.

- Relate the pathophysiology and signs and symptoms of lower respiratory infections and inflammation, chest wall problems and trauma to the ability to maintain effective ventilation and respiration (gas exchange).

- Compare and contrast the risk factors for lower respiratory infections and diseases affecting ventilation and gas exchange.

- Describe the nursing role in health promotion and caring for people with lower respiratory infections, chest wall problems and trauma.

Clinical competencies

- Assess functional health status and the effects of lower respiratory and chest wall problems on ventilation and gas exchange.

- Plan and implement individualised nursing care, including measures to promote ventilation and gas exchange, for people with lower respiratory problems.

- Plan and provide appropriate teaching for health promotion among vulnerable populations and to prepare people and families for community-based care.

- Assess functional health status of people with problems affecting ventilation and gas exchange.

CASE STUDIES

Below are three case studies that you may wish to consider before, during or after you have read this chapter. There are no right or wrong answers to these care studies, but you should think about the physical, psychological and social implications. For example, can you identify the major anatomical structures of the lower respiratory tract? You may also want to think about what nursing observations you are familiar with to assess people with respiratory problems.

Case Study 1 – Jim

Mr Jim Hunter, aged 58, was an emergency admission to the medical admissions unit (MAU) with a diagnosis of right lower lobe **pneumonia**. Jim is a cigarette smoker, with a history of acute chest infections (acute **bronchitis**)

Case Study 2 – Gemma

Ms Gemma Watson is a 24-year-old single woman who works as an office cleaner. She is admitted to the medical ward with an acute **asthma** attack.

Case Study 3 – Alan

Mr Alan Hoyle is 74. Living in the North West of Britain, all of his working life was spent in the textile industry and, like many of his peers, he smoked cigarettes from starting employment at the age of 15. Alan has a diagnosis of **chronic obstructive pulmonary disease** (COPD) and has been prescribed a variety of inhalers over the years by his GP. On most occasions he abandons them; in fact, at home he has a drawer full of part and unused medication. Alan is isolated because of his condition and relies on the support of his close neighbours for shopping. His daughter visits a couple of times a week to make sure that he is OK and to take care of his hygiene needs.

INTRODUCTION

It is of no surprise that the logo for the British Lung Foundation, a charitable organisation, is a balloon! Many people with lung problems could barely contemplate the simple task of blowing up a balloon; in fact, sadly, many people with long-term chronic lung disease would barely be able to take in a breath deep enough to make an impact on the first inflation. This chapter will explore acute and chronic conditions of the respiratory system and the effect that they have on the individual and those who care for them.

The impact of respiratory disease in acute and ongoing care in the UK is enormous. Often referred to as the 'poor relation' in medical care, respiratory diseases put a huge strain on resources within the NHS. According to the British Thoracic Society (BTS) (2006) respiratory diseases account for 20% of all mortality in the UK, that is more than deaths from cardio-vascular disease.

The future provision of care for people with respiratory disease is likely to be more readily focused within the primary healthcare setting, with a shifting emphasis towards prevention rather than treatment. National Health Service (NHS) Trusts have made headway in the provision of thoracic medical units with specialist respiratory nurses working in a clinical and advisory capacity. Despite not having a National

FAST FACTS

Respiratory disease

- Respiratory disease kills one in five people in the UK.

- Death rates from respiratory disease are higher in the UK than both the European and EU average. Only seven other European countries have a worse record than the UK – five of which are former Soviet Union countries with relatively under-funded, less sophisticated health services.

- In 2006, more women (59 105 deaths) than men (58 351) died from lung disease.

- Respiratory disease costs the NHS and society £6.6 billion: £3 billion in costs to the care system, £1.9 billion in mortality costs and £1.7 billion in illness costs per annum.

- Major respiratory diseases include tuberculosis, pneumonia, asthma, COPD, **cystic fibrosis**, lung cancer, occupational lung disease, sleep apnoea, scarring lung diseases and many others.

Source: BTS 2006.

Service Framework (NSF) for respiratory care, within the last 10 years, the NHS has seen the emergence of clinical guidance from the major influencers in respiratory medicine. The BTS and the National Institute for Health and Clinical Excellence (NICE) continue to promote evidence-based guidelines in relation to asthma care and COPD management. This chapter will provide the reader with an insight into these new developments.

The most common respiratory problems of the lower respiratory tract seen in the UK fall into two main categories:

- *problems of ventilation*, which include, for example, infections such as **tuberculosis (TB)**, pneumonia, acute bronchitis and people with pleural effusion
- *gas exchange problems*, for example asthma, COPD and those people who need artificial ventilation

ANATOMY, PHYSIOLOGY AND FUNCTIONS OF THE RESPIRATORY SYSTEM

Understanding the structures and workings of the respiratory system helps to inform our insight into the disease processes in people with respiratory problems. All human cells require oxygen, and it is the function of the respiratory system to carry oxygen throughout the body. As cells use oxygen, carbon dioxide (a waste gas) is produced and the transportation and elimination of carbon dioxide is a key feature of the respiratory system.

Breathing is a physical process by which living organisms take in oxygen from the surrounding air and emit carbon dioxide. The term *respiration* is used to refer to breathing. The physical process of respiration consists of several separately defined and linked steps:

- inspiration (breathing in), followed by
- gaseous exchange and the transportation of gaseous oxygen, which leads to
- cellular respiration which in turn produces adenosine triphosphate (ATP), the molecular unit of energy, then
- transportation of carbon dioxide and expiration (breathing out).

As a result of the above steps, the respiratory system provides the cells of the body with oxygen (O_2) and eliminates carbon dioxide (CO_2), formed as a waste product of cellular metabolism. The events in this process, called respiration, are:

- *Pulmonary ventilation:* Air is moved into and out of the lungs.
- *External respiration:* Exchange of oxygen and carbon dioxide occurs between the alveoli and the blood.
- *Gas transport:* Oxygen and carbon dioxide are transported to and from the lungs and the cells of the body via the blood.
- *Internal respiration:* Exchange of oxygen and carbon dioxide is made between the blood and the cells.

Pulmonary ventilation and external respiration are the sole task of respiratory function. Blood transportation of oxygen and carbon dioxide (gas transport and internal respiration) is also dependent on a healthy cardiovascular system. This is further discussed in Chapter 9.

RESPIRATORY STRUCTURES

The respiratory system functions as a whole, but is divided into the upper and the lower respiratory system. Because the air that we breathe can be polluted from a variety of sources, (e.g. smoke, industrial gases, car emissions, etc.), it is no surprise that respiratory diseases are so prevalent.

The upper respiratory system

The upper respiratory system (Figure 11.1) assists air moving into the lungs and carbon dioxide moving out to the external environment. As air moves through the structures of the nose, the pharynx and the oropharynx, it is filtered, humidified and warmed.

The nose

The nose is the external opening of the respiratory system. The external nose is given structure by the nasal, frontal and maxillary bones as well as plates of hyaline cartilage. The nostrils (also called the external nares) are two cavities within the nose, separated by the nasal septum. These cavities open into the nasal portion of the pharynx through the internal nares. The nasal cavities just behind the nasal openings are lined with skin that contains hair follicles, sweat glands and sebaceous glands. The nasal hairs filter the air as it enters the nares. The rest of the cavity is lined with mucous membranes that contain olfactory neurons and goblet cells that secrete thick mucus. The mucus not only traps dust and bacteria but also contains lysozyme, an enzyme that destroys bacteria as they enter the nose. As mucus and debris accumulate, mucosal ciliated cells move it toward the pharynx, where it is swallowed. The mucosa is highly vascular, warming air that moves across its surface.

Three structures project outward from the lateral wall of each nasal cavity: the superior, middle and inferior turbinates that cause air entering the nose to become turbulent and also increase the surface area of mucosa exposed to the air.

The sinuses

The nasal cavity is surrounded by paranasal sinuses (Figure 11.2), located in the frontal, sphenoid, ethmoid and maxillary bones.

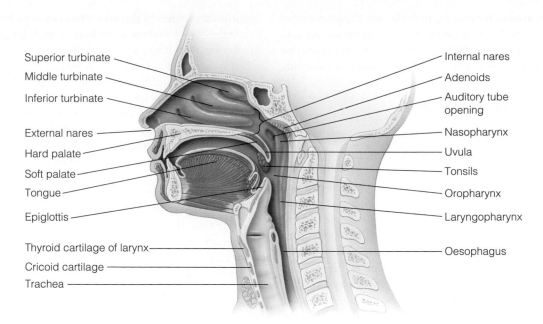

Figure 11.1 The upper respiratory system.

Sinuses lighten the skull, assist in speech, and produce mucus that drains into the nasal cavities to help trap debris.

The pharynx (throat)

This passage connects the nasal cavity with the larynx and the mouth with the oesophagus. It is anatomically divided into the oropharynx, nasopharynx and laryngopharynx.

The oropharynx lies behind the oral (mouth) cavity and extends from the soft palate to the level of the hyoid bone. It serves as a passageway for both air and food. An upward rise of the soft palate prevents food from entering the nasopharynx during swallowing. The oropharynx is lined with stratified squamous epithelium that protects it from the friction of food and damage from the chemicals found in food and fluids.

The laryngopharynx extends from the hyoid bone to the larynx. It is also lined with stratified squamous epithelium, and serves as a passageway for both food and air. Air does not move into the lungs while food is being swallowed and moved into the oesophagus.

The larynx (voice box)

The larynx is about 5 cm long. It opens at the laryngopharynx and is continuous with the trachea. The larynx provides an airway and routes air and food into the proper passageway. As long as air is moving through the larynx, its inlet is open; however, the inlet closes during swallowing. The larynx also contains the vocal cords, necessary for voice production.

The larynx is framed by cartilages, connected by ligaments and membranes. The thyroid cartilage is formed by the fusion of two cartilages; the fusion point can be visible as the Adam's apple. The cricoid cartilage lies below the thyroid cartilage; other pairs of cartilages form the walls of the larynx. The epiglottis, also a cartilage, normally projects upward to the base of the tongue; however, during swallowing, the larynx moves upward and the

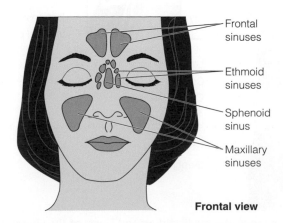

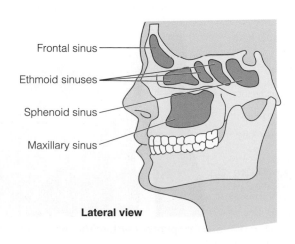

Figure 11.2 Frontal and lateral views of the sinuses.

epiglottis tips to cover the opening to the larynx. If anything other than air enters the larynx, a cough reflex expels the foreign substance before it can enter the lungs. It is important to note that this protective reflex does not work if the person is unconscious.

The lower respiratory system

Trachea (windpipe)

The structure of the trachea is made up of 16 to 20 'C'-shaped cartilage rings. These are joined by connective tissue and involuntary muscle enabling the trachea to be open and preventing it from collapse when breathing in. The mucosa lining the trachea consists of ciliated columnar epithelium containing seromucous glands that produce thick mucus. Dust and debris in the inspired air are trapped in this mucus, moved toward the throat by the cilia and then either swallowed or coughed out through the mouth. The powerful protective cough reflex is triggered by sensitive nerve endings lying within the trachea and extending into the bronchioles. Here, irritant receptors stimulate a cough which forces particles upwards. If an obstruction occurs above the larynx, for example a foreign object, trauma or inflammation, there may be a need for airway support in the form of tracheostomy.

The lungs

The centre of the thoracic cavity is filled by the mediastinum, which contains the heart, great blood vessels, bronchi, trachea and oesophagus. The mediastinum is flanked on either side by the lungs (see Figure 11.3). Each lung is suspended in its own pleural cavity, with the anterior, lateral and posterior lung surfaces lying close to the ribs. The hilus, on the mediastinal surface of each lung, is where blood vessels of the pulmonary and circulatory systems enter and exit the lungs. The primary

bronchus also enters in this area. The apex of each lung lies just below the clavicle, whereas the base of each lung rests on the diaphragm. The lungs are made of elastic connective tissue, called stroma, and are soft and spongy.

The two lungs differ in size and shape. The left lung is smaller and has two lobes, whereas the right lung has three lobes. Each of the lung lobes contains a different number of bronchopulmonary segments, separated by connective tissue. There are eight segments in the two lobes of the left lung and 10 segments in the three lobes of the right lung.

The vascular system of the lungs consists of the pulmonary arteries, which deliver blood to the lungs for oxygenation, and the pulmonary veins, which deliver oxygenated blood to the heart. Within the lungs, the pulmonary arteries branch into a pulmonary capillary network that surrounds the alveoli. Lung tissue receives its blood supply from the bronchial arteries and drains its blood supply via the bronchial and pulmonary veins.

The pleura

The pleura is a double-layered membrane that covers the lungs and the inside of the thoracic cavities (see Figure 11.3). The parietal pleura lines the thoracic wall and mediastinum. It is continuous with the visceral pleura, which covers the external lung surfaces. The pleura produces pleural fluid, a lubricating, serous fluid that allows the lungs to move easily over the thoracic wall during breathing. The pleura's two layers also cling tightly together and hold the lungs to the thoracic wall. The structure of the pleura creates a slightly negative pressure in the pleural space necessary for lung function.

The bronchi and alveoli

During inspiration, air enters the lungs through the primary bronchus and then moves through the increasingly smaller airways of the lungs to the alveoli (see Figure 11.4).

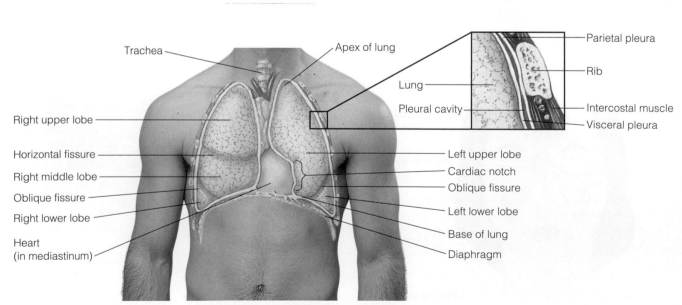

Figure 11.3 The lower respiratory system showing the location of the lungs, the mediastinum and layers of the visceral and parietal pleura.

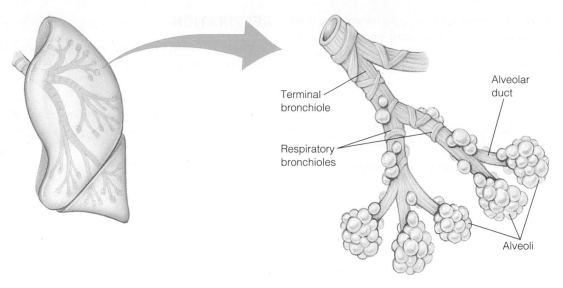

Figure 11.4 Respiratory bronchi, bronchioles, alveolar ducts and alveoli.

The trachea divides into right and left primary bronchi; in comparison to the left primary bronchus, the right primary bronchus is shorter, wider and situated more vertically (making aspiration of foreign bodies into the right primary bronchus more likely). The point where the trachea divides is innervated with sensory neurons; activities such as tracheal suctioning may cause coughing and bronchospasm from stimulation of these neurons. These main bronchi subdivide (or bifurcate) into the secondary (lobar) bronchi, with the right middle lobe bronchus being smaller in diameter and length, and sometimes it bends sharply near its bifurcation. The secondary bronchi then branch into the tertiary (segmental) bronchi, and then into smaller and smaller bronchioles, ending in the terminal bronchioles, which are extremely small. These branching airways collectively are called the bronchial or respiratory tree. From the terminal bronchioles, air moves into air sacs (called respiratory bronchioles), which further branch into alveolar ducts that lead to alveolar sacs and then to the tiny alveoli. During inspiration, air enters the lungs through the primary bronchus and then moves through the increasingly smaller airways of the lungs to the alveoli, where oxygen and carbon dioxide exchange occurs in the process of external respiration. During expiration, the carbon dioxide is expelled.

Alveoli cluster around the alveolar sacs, which open into a common chamber called the atrium. The adult lung has approximately 300 million alveoli, providing an enormous surface for gas exchange. Alveoli have extremely thin walls of a single layer of squamous epithelial cells over a very thin basement membrane. The external surfaces of the alveoli are covered with pulmonary capillaries. The alveolar and capillary walls form the respiratory membrane. Gas exchange across the respiratory membrane occurs by simple diffusion. The alveolar walls also contain cells that secrete surfactant, a substance necessary for maintaining a moist surface and reducing the surface tension of the alveolar fluid to help prevent collapse of the lungs.

The rib cage and intercostal muscles

The lungs are protected by the bones of the rib cage and the intercostal muscles. There are 12 pairs of ribs, which all articulate with the thoracic vertebrae. Anteriorly, the first seven ribs articulate with the body of the sternum. The eighth, ninth and tenth ribs articulate with the cartilage immediately above the ribs. The 11th and 12th ribs are called floating ribs, because they are unattached.

The sternum has three parts: the manubrium, the body and the xiphoid process. The junction between the manubrium and the body of the sternum is called the manubriosternal junction or the angle of Louis. The depression above the manubrium is called the suprasternal notch.

The spaces between the ribs are called the intercostal spaces (see Figure 11.5). Each intercostal space is named for the rib

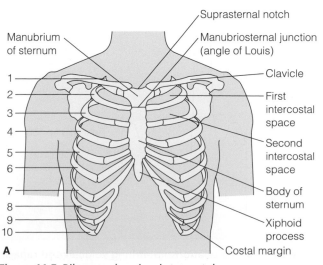

Figure 11.5 Rib cage showing intercostal spaces.

immediately above it (for example, the space between the third and fourth ribs is designated as the third intercostal space). The intercostal muscles between the ribs, along with the diaphragm, are called the inspiratory muscles.

RESPIRATION

Breathing is controlled both mechanically and chemically. Mechanical control occurs when the respiratory centre of the

---

IN PRACTICE

Pulmonary function tests – spirometry

Pulmonary function tests (PFTs) are performed in a pulmonary function laboratory. After preparing the person, a nose clip is applied and the unsedated person breathes into a spirometer, a device for measuring and recording lung volume in litres versus time in seconds. The person is instructed how to breathe for specific tests: for example, to inhale as deeply as possible and then exhale to the maximal extent possible. Using measured lung volumes, respiratory capacities are calculated to assess pulmonary status. The specific values determined by PFT and illustrated Figure 11.6 include the following.

- *Total lung capacity (TLC)* is the total volume of the lungs at their maximum inflation. Four values are used to calculate TLC:
  1. *total volume (TV)*, the volume inhaled and exhaled with normal quiet breathing (also called tidal volume);
  2. *inspiratory reserve volume (IRV)*, the maximum amount that can be inhaled over and above a normal inspiration;
  3. *expiratory reserve volume (ERV)*, the maximum amount that can be exhaled following a normal exhalation;
  4. *residual volume (RV)*, the amount of air remaining in the lungs after maximal exhalation.

- *Vital capacity (VC)* is the total amount of air that can be exhaled after a maximal inspiration. It is calculated by adding together the IRV, TV and the ERV.
- *Inspiratory capacity* is the total amount of air that can be inhaled following a normal quiet exhalation. It is calculated by adding the TV and IRV.
- *Functional residual capacity (FRC)* is the volume of air left in the lungs after a normal exhalation. The ERV and RV are added to determine the FRC.
- *Forced expiratory volume (FEV1)* is the amount of air that can be exhaled in 1 second.
- *Forced vital capacity (FVC)* is the amount of air that can be exhaled forcefully and rapidly after maximum air intake.
- *Minute volume (MV)* is the total amount or volume of air breathed in 1 minute.

In older people, residual capacity is increased, and vital capacity is decreased. These age-related changes result from the following:

- calcification of the costal cartilage and weakening of the intercostal muscles, which reduce movement of the chest wall;
- vertebral osteoporosis, which decreases spinal flexibility and increases the degree of kyphosis, further increasing the anterior–posterior diameter of the chest;
- diaphragmatic flattening and loss of elasticity.

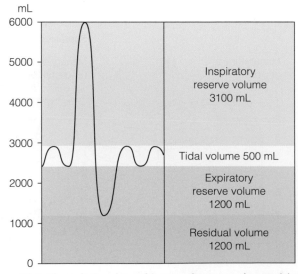
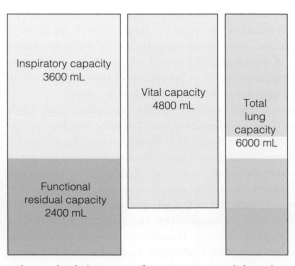

Figure 11.6 The relationship of lung volumes and capacities. Volumes (mL) shown are for an average adult male.

brain transmits regular nerve impulses to both the diaphragm and external intercostal muscles to cause inhalation. Nerve stretch receptors in the alveoli and bronchioles detect inhalation and send inhibitory signals to the respiratory centre to cause exhalation. This *negative feedback* system is continuous and prevents damage to the lungs.

When we begin to consider our own breathing pattern, we become aware that we are able to voluntarily alter our breathing, slow it down, take deep breaths or pant. External influences may play a part; outside temperature, the effect of exercise and excitement are examples of this. However, regulation of breathing occurs whilst we are not thinking about it, despite being able to make ourselves breathe faster or slower. This voluntary control sits in the higher centres of the brain, but the regulation of respiration (the respiratory centres) sit in the brainstem. So if we deliberately hold our breath, dangerously high levels of carbon dioxide and/or low levels of oxygen will activate chemoreceptor reflexes that will override this and make us breathe.

Factors affecting ventilation and respiration

Many factors affect ventilation and respiration. Those discussed here include changes in volume and capacity; air pressures; oxygen, carbon dioxide and hydrogen ion concentrations in the blood; airway resistance, lung compliance, elasticity; and alveolar surface tension.

Respiratory volume and capacity

Respiratory volume and capacity are affected by gender, age, weight and health status. Pulmonary function tests measure these and other respiratory volumes and capacities, and are described and illustrated in the In Practice box opposite.

Air pressures

Pulmonary ventilation depends on volume changes within the thoracic cavity. A change in the volume of air in the thoracic cavity leads to a change in the air pressure within the cavity. Because gases always flow along their pressure gradients, a change in pressure results in gases flowing into or out of the lungs to equalise the pressure.

The pressures normally present in the thoracic cavity are the intrapulmonary pressure and the intrapleural pressure. The intrapulmonary pressure, within the alveoli of the lungs, rises and falls constantly as a result of the acts of ventilation (inhalation and exhalation). The intrapleural pressure, within the pleural space, also rises and falls with the acts of ventilation, but it is always less than (or negative to) the intrapulmonary pressure. Intrapulmonary and intrapleural pressures are necessary not only to expand and contract the lungs, but also to prevent their collapse.

Pulmonary ventilation has two phases: inspiration (Figure 11.7), during which air flows into the lungs; and expiration (Figure 11.8), during which gases flow out of the lungs. The two phases make up a single breath, and normally occur from 12–20 times each minute. A single inspiration lasts for about 1–1.5 seconds, whereas expiration lasts for about 2–3 seconds.

During inspiration, the diaphragm contracts and flattens out to increase the vertical diameter of the thoracic cavity. The external intercostal muscles contract, elevating the rib cage and moving the sternum forward to expand the lateral and anteroposterior diameter of the thoracic cavity, decreasing intrapleural pressure. The lungs stretch and the intrapulmonary volume increases, decreasing intrapulmonary pressure slightly below atmospheric pressure. Air rushes into the lungs as a result of this pressure gradient until the intrapulmonary and atmospheric pressures equalise.

Expiration is primarily a passive process that occurs as a result of the elasticity of the lungs. The inspiratory muscles relax, the diaphragm rises, the ribs descend and the lungs recoil. Both the thoracic and intrapulmonary pressures increase, compressing the alveoli. The intrapulmonary pressure rises to a level greater than atmospheric pressure, and gases flow out of the lungs.

Oxygen, carbon dioxide and hydrogen ion concentrations

The rate and depth of respirations are controlled by respiratory centres in the medulla oblongata and pons of the brain and by chemoreceptors located in the medulla and in the carotid and aortic bodies. The centres and chemoreceptors respond to changes in the concentration of oxygen, carbon dioxide and hydrogen ions in arterial blood. For example, when carbon dioxide concentration increases or the pH decreases, the respiratory rate increases.

Airway resistance, lung compliance and elasticity

Respiratory airway resistance, lung compliance and lung elasticity also affect respiration.

- Respiratory airway resistance is created by the friction encountered as gases move along the respiratory airways, by constriction of the airways (especially the larger bronchioles), by accumulations of mucus or infectious material and by tumours. As resistance increases, gas flow decreases.

- Lung compliance depends on the elasticity of the lung tissue and the flexibility of the rib cage. Compliance is decreased by factors that decrease the elasticity of the lungs, block the respiratory airways or interfere with movement of the rib cage, for example the effects of age.

- Lung elasticity is essential for lung distention during inspiration and lung recoil during expiration. Decreased elasticity from diseases such as **emphysema** impairs respiration.

Alveolar surface tension

A liquid film of mostly water covers the alveolar walls. At any gas–liquid boundary, the molecules of liquid are more strongly attracted to each other than to gas molecules. This produces a state of tension, called surface tension, that draws the liquid molecules even more closely together. The water content of the alveolar film compacts the alveoli and aids in the lungs' recoil during expiration. In fact, if the alveolar

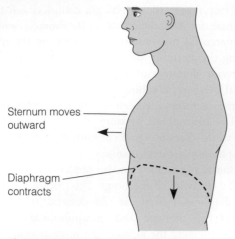

Sternum moves outward

Diaphragm contracts

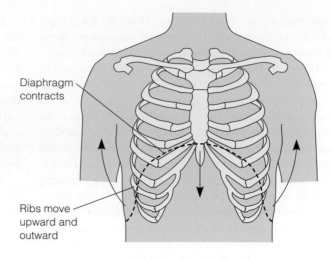

Diaphragm contracts

Ribs move upward and outward

Figure 11.7 Respiratory inspiration.

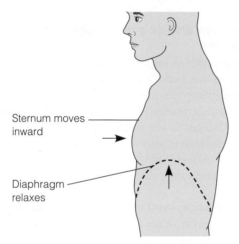

Sternum moves inward

Diaphragm relaxes

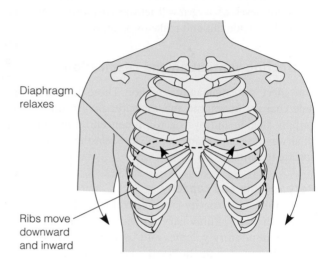

Diaphragm relaxes

Ribs move downward and inward

Figure 11.8 Respiratory expiration.

film were pure water, the alveoli would collapse between breaths.

Surfactant, a lipoprotein produced by the alveolar cells, interferes with this adhesiveness of the water molecules, reducing surface tension and helping expand the lungs. With insufficient surfactant, the surface tension forces can become great enough to collapse the alveoli between breaths, requiring tremendous energy to reinflate the lungs for inspiration.

Blood gases

Gases are transported by the blood to provide cells with oxygen and to remove carbon dioxide produced during cellular activities.

Oxygen transport and unloading

Oxygen is carried in the blood either bound to haemoglobin or dissolved in the plasma. Oxygen is not very soluble in water, so almost all oxygen that enters the blood from the respiratory system is carried to the cells of the body by haemoglobin. This combination of haemoglobin and oxygen is called oxyhaemoglobin.

IN PRACTICE

Normal values of blood gases

pH	7.35–7.45 (below 7.35 indicates acidosis, above 7.45 indicates alkalosis)
$PaCO_2$	4.7–6.0 kPa (25–45 mmHg)
PaO_2	12–15 kPa (90–110 mmHg)
Oxygen saturations	95% or greater
HCO_3	22–28 mmol
Base excess	–2/+2

Each haemoglobin molecule is made of four polypeptide chains, with each chain bound to an iron-containing haem group. The iron groups are the binding sites for oxygen; each haemoglobin molecule can bind with four molecules of oxygen.

Oxygen binding is rapid and reversible. It is affected by temperature, blood pH, partial pressure of oxygen (PaO_2), partial pressure of carbon dioxide ($PaCO_2$), and serum concentration of an organic chemical called 2,3-DPG. These factors interact to ensure adequate delivery of oxygen to the cells.

- Under normal conditions, the haemoglobin in arterial blood is 97.4% saturated with oxygen. Haemoglobin is almost fully saturated at a PaO_2 of 760 mmHg (atmospheric air – 760 mmHg at sea level).
- As arterial blood flows through the capillaries, oxygen is unloaded, so that the oxygen saturation of haemoglobin in venous blood is 75%.

Carbon dioxide transport

Active cells produce about 200 mL of carbon dioxide each minute; this amount is exactly the same as that excreted by the lungs each minute. Excretion of carbon dioxide from the body requires transport by the blood from the cells to the lungs. Carbon dioxide is transported in three forms: dissolved in plasma, bound to haemoglobin and as bicarbonate ions in the plasma (the largest amount is in this form).

Assessing respiratory function

Function of the respiratory system is assessed by findings from diagnostic tests; however, a health assessment interview to collect subjective data (i.e. the individual's experience and how they feel) and a physical assessment to collect objective data (from measuring the individual's health status). As a nurse, your observational and communication skills need to be used here. You will need to focus on factors that may influence the person's ability to breathe normally. These will include:

- pregnancy – due to fluid retention and enlargement of the uterus;
- obesity;
- circulatory problems – for example, pulmonary oedema and anaemia;
- environmental – exposure to cold;
- trauma – to the chest;
- allergies – in those with an allergic reaction;
- pathophysiological – for example, abdominal distension;
- psychological – fear can affect the ability to breathe correctly.

Respiratory assessment must be undertaken on all people as part of a routine clinical assessment and must include assessment of the airway. A structured approach to assessment incorporates the ABCDE method as shown in Table 11.1.

Assess all people with respiratory problems by looking, listening and feeling.

- *Looking* for obvious signs of airway obstruction; observe the pattern of breathing – see-saw breathing, where the chest and abdomen move in opposite directions, is abnormal.

Table 11.1 Respiratory assessment using a structured approach

A Airway	• Is the airway patent (unobstructed) and maintained? • Can the person speak? • Are there added noises? • Is there a see-sawing movement of the chest and abdomen?
B Breathing	• Observe rate and pattern. • Depth of respiration. • Symmetry of chest movement. • Use of accessory muscles. • Colour of the person. • Oxygen saturation.
C Circulation	• Manual pulse and BP. • Capillary refill time. • Urine output/fluid balance. • Temperature.
D Disability	• Conscious level. • Blood glucose level. • Pupil size and reaction. • Observe for seizures. • Pain assessment.
E Exposure	• Perform head to toe examination front and back.

Normal movement sees the chest and abdomen moving outwards as a breath is taken and moving inwards as a breath is expired.

- *Listening* to responses to a verbal command like 'how are you feeling today?' can give useful information with regard to an individual's ability to breathe effectively. Other sounds to listen for include snoring, which can indicate pharyngeal obstruction; gurgling, suggestive of fluids in the upper airway; stridor, a sign of obstruction in the upper airway.
- *Feeling* for air movement with the hand might help determine if the airway is obstructed.

The results of diagnostic tests of respiratory function (below) are used to support the diagnosis of a specific disease and to provide information to identify or modify the appropriate medications or therapy used to treat the disease.

FACTORS AFFECTING RESPIRATORY FUNCTION

Factors affecting respiratory function include:

- Lifestyle and occupation:
  - Regular physical exercise expands the lungs increasing the rate and depth of respiration.
  - Occupational exposure to irritants can cause respiratory disease. A classic example of this is asbestosis in those exposed to asbestos fibres and dust.

DIAGNOSTIC TESTS The respiratory system

Sputum studies (Culture and sensitivity, Acid-fast smear and sensitivity, Cytology)

To diagnose bacterial infection and identify the most effective antibiotic; to diagnose acid-fast bacillus, TB; to diagnose abnormal malignant cells.

RELATED NURSING CARE *If the person is unable to provide a specimen, this may be obtained during bronchoscopy; be aware that saliva is **not** a sputum specimen.*

Arterial blood gases (ABGs)

To assess acid–base balance caused by respiratory problems: pH of less than 7.35 indicates acidosis; pH of more than 7.45 indicates alkalosis.

RELATED NURSING CARE *Arterial blood is collected in a heparinised needle and syringe, and the sample is analysed immediately or sent to lab on ice. If the person is receiving oxygen, indicate this on lab form. Apply pressure to puncture site for 2–5 minutes.*

Pulse oximetry

Non-invasive test used to monitor oxygen saturation levels of the blood. Infrared light passes through the finger, toe, earlobe or nose. Normal value: 90–100%.

RELATED NURSING CARE *Factors such as skin tone, acrylic nails, faulty placement of equipment may alter findings.*

Chest x-ray

Identifies abnormalities in chest structure and lung tissue and diagnoses disease and lung injury. Used to monitor treatment.

RELATED NURSING CARE *No special preparation needed.*

Computed tomography (CT)

Shows cross-section of more complex structures of the thorax not clearly shown on x-ray, e.g. tumours and abscesses.

RELATED NURSING CARE No special preparation needed.

Magnetic resonance imaging (MRI)

To diagnose alterations in lung tissue more difficult to visualise by CT scan.

RELATED NURSING CARE *Assess person for metallic implants, e.g. pacemaker. The test will not be performed if present. The person needs to be aware of the claustrophobic nature of the MRI scanner and that it can cause anxiety.*

Positron emission tomography (PET)

The person is given radiographic substance and cross–sectional images appear on computer. Radiation from PET is only 25% of that from a CT scan.

RELATED NURSING CARE *Zero alcohol, coffee, tobacco for 24 hours prior to test. Increase fluid intake post test to help eliminate radioactive material.*

Pulmonary angiography

Identifies emboli, tumours, vascular changes, pulmonary circulation. A catheter is inserted into brachial or femoral artery which is then threaded into the pulmonary artery. Dye is injected and images are taken.

RELATED NURSING CARE *ECG monitoring during procedure. Monitor injection site and pulses distal to the site after the test.*

Pulmonary ventilation/perfusion scan (V/Q scan)

Scans the person inhaling radioactive gas. Useful for diagnosing airway obstruction and blood flow disruption.

RELATED NURSING CARE *No special preparation needed.*

- Age:
  - With increasing age, respiratory systems become less elastic and more rigid.
  - Osteoporosis can compromise lung expansion.
  - Air exchange is lessened.
  - Cilia action is decreased and mucous membranes become drier.
  - In older adults there is an associated risk of acute respiratory disease due to gradual decrease in immune responses.
- Environment: oxygenation can be affected by the following:
  - heat
  - cold
  - air pollution
  - altitude
- Stress: psychological and physiological responses affect oxygenation. Hyperventilation may cause dizziness. Adrenaline causes bronchioles to dilate, increasing blood flow and oxygen to active muscles.
- Medication: source medications decrease the rate and depth of respirations, for example sedatives and anti-anxiety drugs, barbiturates and narcotics.

THE LANGUAGE OF BREATHING

A variety of terms are used in the description of breathing. These include the rate, rhythm, volume and relative ease or effort of breathing:

- Tachypnoea (rapid respiratory rate) is seen in **atelectasis** (collapse of lung tissue following obstruction of the bronchus or bronchioles), pneumonia, asthma, pleural effusion, **pneumothorax**, congestive heart failure, anxiety and in response to pain.

- Damage to the brainstem from a stroke or head injury may result in either tachypnoea or bradypnoea (low respiratory rate).
- Bradypnoea is seen with some circulatory problems, lung problems and as a side-effect of some medications.
- Apnoea, cessation of breathing lasting from a few seconds to a few minutes, may occur following a stroke or head trauma, as a side-effect of some medications or following airway obstruction.
- Hyperventilation, increased movement of air into and out of the lungs, can be a response to stress.
- Orthopnoea – the inability to breathe except in the upright position.
- **Dyspnoea** is difficult or uncomfortable breathing.
- Stridor is the sound made on inspiration where there is obstruction of the trachea; tends to be harsh and high-pitched.

Consider this . . .

'Interpreting the language of breathlessness'

Research into dyspnoea and tools to measure its severity led the investigators to consider the language used by people to describe their breathlessness.

'Just like language developed to describe the sensation of pain, a common language for breathlessness quality has emerged', say the nurse researchers. People will often use terms such as 'air hunger', 'effort' or 'work' and 'chest tightness' to describe their quality of breathlessness.

'Important questions to ask people when assessing a change in their clinical condition should include an alteration in the work or effort of breathing, the urgency to breathe and the presence of any chest tightness.'

Source: Yorke and Russell 2008.

PROBLEMS OF VENTILATION

Respiratory problems can affect the way that air moves in and out of the lungs. In general, there are two ways in which these problems can affect the individual; first, in relation to the ability to maintain clear and patent airways to fully ventilate the lungs (considered in the next part of this chapter); and second, the inability to effectively maintain gas exchange for effective respiration (considered in the later part of the chapter). A person with respiratory and chest wall problems will have both local and systemic effects. Local effects include rhinitis, cough, excess mucous production, shortness of breath or dyspnoea (difficult or laboured breathing), **haemoptysis** (bloody sputum) and chest pain. Systemic effects may include fever, anorexia and malaise, **cyanosis** (grey to blue or purple skin colour caused by deoxygenated haemoglobin), and other signs and symptoms of impaired gas exchange.

INFECTIONS OF THE RESPIRATORY SYSTEM

Infections and inflammation of the respiratory system are common. The respiratory tract is constantly exposed to the environment as air moves into and out of the respiratory tract. In addition, the oropharynx is colonised by huge numbers of micro-organisms that may be aspirated into the bronchial tree. Both anatomical and physiological defences help maintain the sterility of the lower respiratory tract. When these defences are impaired, the risk for infection increases. For example, drugs, alcohol or neuromuscular disease may suppress the cough reflex, and the influenza virus can leave the respiratory epithelium vulnerable to bacterial infection.

FAST FACTS

Respiratory complaints

In 2004 in the UK community:

- An estimated 24 million consultations with GPs were for respiratory disease.
- Nearly one in five males and one in four females consulted a GP for a respiratory complaint.
- More than 62 million prescriptions were used in the prevention and treatment of respiratory disease.

Source: BTS 2006.

The person with sinusitis

Sinusitis is inflammation of the mucous membranes of one or more of the sinuses (see Figure 11.2). Sinusitis is a common condition that usually follows an upper respiratory infection such as acute viral upper respiratory infection or influenza. Common causative organisms include streptococci, *S. pneumoniae*, *Haemophilus influenzae* and staphylococci. The risk of sinusitis is higher when the immune system is suppressed by immunosuppressive drugs or HIV infection. Sinusitis is common and difficult to treat in people who have AIDS.

Pathophysiology of sinusitis

Sinusitis develops when nasal mucous membranes swell or other problems obstruct sinus openings, impairing drainage. Mucous secretions collect in the sinus cavity, serving as a medium for bacterial growth. The nasal and sinus mucous membranes are continuous; therefore, bacteria generally spread to the sinuses via the opening into the nasal turbinates. The inflammatory response provoked by bacterial invasion draws serum and leucocytes to the area to combat the infection, increasing swelling and pressure.

Any process that impairs drainage from the sinuses may precipitate sinusitis. These include nasal polyps, deviated septum, rhinitis, tooth abscess or swimming or diving trauma. In hospitalised people, sinusitis may develop following prolonged nasotracheal intubation. Usually more than one sinus is infected. The frontal and maxillary sinuses are usually involved in adults.

Sinusitis may be acute or chronic. Chronic sinusitis results when acute sinusitis is untreated or inadequately treated.

With continued infection, bacteria can become isolated, producing chronic inflammation. Over time, mucous membranes become thickened. Fungal infections may cause chronic infections, especially in immunosuppressed people. Other factors that may contribute to chronic sinusitis are smoking, a history of allergy and habitual use of nasal sprays or inhalants.

Signs and symptoms of sinusitis

The person with acute sinusitis often looks sick. Manifestations of sinusitis include pain and tenderness across the infected sinuses, headache, fever and malaise. The pain usually increases with leaning forward. When the maxillary sinuses are involved, pain and pressure are felt over the cheek. The pain may be referred to the upper teeth. Frontal sinusitis causes pain and tenderness across the lower forehead. Symptoms often worsen for three to four hours after awakening and then become less severe in the afternoon and evening as secretions drain. The intensity and location of headache pain may change as sinuses drain. In acute sinusitis, the pain is usually constant and severe. In chronic sinusitis, the pain is described as dull and may be constant or intermittent.

The person with obstructive sleep apnoea

Sleep apnoea, intermittent absence of airflow through the mouth and nose during sleep, is a serious and potentially life-threatening disorder. Sleep apnoea is a leading cause of excessive daytime sleepiness, and may contribute to other problems such as poor work performance and motor vehicle crashes. There is a link between sleep apnoea and an increased risk of hypertension, ischaemic heart disease and exacerbation of heart failure.

Risk factors for obstructive sleep apnoea

In addition to male gender, risk factors for obstructive sleep apnoea include:

- increasing age and obesity;
- large neck circumference (> 17 inches in men and > 16 inches in women) (Porth 2009);
- use of alcohol and other CNS depressants which may contribute to sleep apnoea.

Pathophysiology of obstructive sleep apnoea

During sleep, skeletal muscle tone decreases (except the diaphragm). The most significant decrease occurs during rapid eye movement (REM) sleep. Loss of normal pharyngeal muscle tone permits the pharynx to collapse during inspiration as pressure within the airways becomes negative in relation to atmospheric pressure. The tongue is also pulled against the posterior pharyngeal wall by gravity during sleep, causing further obstruction. Obesity or skeletal or soft-tissue changes that decrease inspiratory tone, such as a relatively large tongue in a relatively small oropharynx, contribute to the problem. Airflow obstruction causes the oxygen saturation, PaO_2, and pH to fall, and the $PaCO_2$ to rise. This progressive asphyxia causes brief arousal from sleep, which restores airway patency and airflow. Sleep can be severely fragmented because these episodes may occur hundreds of times each night.

The person with influenza

Influenza or 'flu' is a respiratory illness associated with infection by influenza virus. Symptoms frequently include headache, fever, cough, sore throat, aching muscles and joints.

FAST FACT

Influenza activity

Epidemic: outbreak of a disease in which more cases than expected appear suddenly.

Pandemic: an epidemic on a worldwide scale.

Overall, influenza activity in the UK in 2010/11 reached a level higher than that seen in the winter of the 2008/09 season and 2009/10 winter season of the pandemic, but lower than during the first wave of the pandemic in the summer of 2009.

Source: HPA 2011.

Influenza occurs most often in winter and usually peaks between December and March in the UK. Illnesses resembling influenza that occur in the summer are usually due to other viruses. There are two main types that cause infection: influenza A and influenza B. Influenza A usually causes a more severe illness than influenza B.

The influenza virus is unstable and new strains and variants are constantly emerging, which is one of the reasons why the flu vaccine should be given each year. Vaccine is available to protect against flu. Each year a new vaccine has to be produced to protect against the flu viruses expected to be in circulation that winter and to boost the immune response. The vaccine is very safe and side-effects are uncommon and usually mild. The vaccine is given in the autumn before the flu season begins. It is not recommended for everyone, but it is advisable for those likely to be more seriously affected by influenza. This includes:

- people of any age with chronic heart, lung, metabolic problems (including severe asthma and diabetes), kidney problems or a lowered immune system due to treatment or disease;
- pregnant women;
- everyone aged 65 years and over;
- those in long stay residential care accommodation where influenza, once introduced, may spread rapidly.

The most common complications of influenza are bronchitis and bacterial pneumonia, both of which will be considered next.

The person with acute bronchitis

Bronchitis refers to inflammation of the bronchi, and this can be an acute or long-term chronic condition. People will often be told that they have a chest infection; however, the medical term is *acute bronchitis*. Acute bronchitis is commonly seen in adults who may be more at risk because of smoking and immune deficiency. In otherwise healthy adults, it can often follow a viral upper respiratory tract infection (URTI). (**Chronic bronchitis** is a component of chronic obstructive pulmonary disease (COPD) and will be considered later in this chapter.)

Pathophysiology of acute bronchitis

Infectious bronchitis can be caused by either viruses or bacteria that damage the respiratory mucosa. The viruses (the most common cause of acute bronchitis) include those that might otherwise cause influenza. As viruses attack the bronchial lining they can become open to bacterial infection.

The inflammatory response to infection or tissue damage from inhaled substances causes capillary dilation and oedema of the mucosal lining of the bronchi. Inflammatory cells infiltrate the affected mucosa, leading to exudate formation and increased mucous production. Ciliated epithelium is damaged by the inflammatory response and ciliary function is impaired. The immune response of lymphocytes and tissue macrophages is inhibited by some viruses and mycobacteria, increasing the risk for bacterial infection. Mucosal irritation and increased mucous production initiate the cough reflex.

PRACTICE ALERT

People who have underlying lung problems, such as chronic bronchitis, are more likely to get acute bronchitis as their lung defence mechanism (immunity) against infection is lower than normal. Smoking is the commonest reason for this to happen.

Signs and symptoms of acute bronchitis

Signs and symptoms of acute bronchitis include:

- moderate pyrexia and general feeling of being unwell;
- chest pain when coughing;
- dry, irritable and painful cough which later becomes productive (i.e. producing mucus);
- increased production of mucus;
- may be associated wheezing as the airways narrow due to inflammation of the mucous membrane and increased mucous production.

COMMUNITY-BASED CARE

The majority of people with acute bronchitis will present at GP surgeries and walk-in centres within the community setting. At the first face-to-face contact in primary care, including walk-in centres and emergency departments, offer a clinical assessment, including: history (presenting symptoms), use of over-the-counter or self-medication, previous medical history, relevant risk factors, relevant co-morbidities (NICE 2008).

Nursing interventions for people with acute bronchitis are primarily educational and can include advice about the following health education topics.

What makes acute bronchitis worse?

- Cigarette smoking.
- Air pollution.
- Cold damp weather.

What can I do to help myself?

- Drink plenty of fluids to encourage mucous production.
- Cough naturally to remove mucus.
- Consider over-the-counter (OTC) products such as paracetamol to help relieve some of the symptoms.

Do I need antibiotics?

- Acute bronchitis is most commonly caused by a virus and it is not possible to treat these with antibiotics.
- Offer people reassurance that antibiotics are not normally needed immediately because they will make little difference to symptoms and may have side-effects, for example, diarrhoea, vomiting and rash.

The person with pneumonia

Pneumonia is an infection of the alveoli and bronchioles (small airways). Pneumonia may be either infectious or non-infectious. Bacteria, viruses, fungi, protozoa and other microbes can lead to infectious pneumonia. Non-infectious

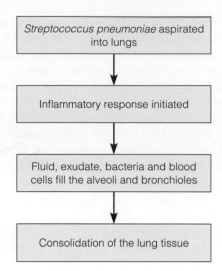

Figure 11.9 The pathogenesis of pneumococcal pneumonia.

causes include aspiration of gastric contents and inhalation of toxic or irritating gases.

Pathophysiology of pneumonia

When the invading micro-organisms colonise the alveoli, an inflammatory and immune response is initiated. Inflammation and subsequent oedema cause the alveoli to fill and to produce exudates. Infectious debris and exudate can fill alveoli, interfering with ventilation and gas exchange. The exudate quickly fills with neutrophils, erythrocytes and fibrin to form a solid mass called consolidation. Consolidation can manifest in a number of ways and affect the lobes and bronchi in patches of consolidated masses. The pathogenesis of pneumococcal pneumonia is illustrated in Figure 11.9.

Pneumonia can be either community or hospital acquired. In the community, many different bacteria, viruses and fungi cause pneumonia. One of the most common is *Streptococcus pneumoniae*. Other common causes include haemophilus and staphylococcus. Bacterial pneumonia is the most common form of pneumonia in adults and is usually more serious. It may be a secondary complication of a viral respiratory illness such as influenza, especially in people with immune deficiencies. Fungal pneumonia is almost always linked to an immunodeficiency.

Consider this . . .

- Reflect on your own lifestyle. What factors may put you at risk from pneumonia?
- In younger people, factors such as smoking, heavy drinking, chronic lung disease or underlying illness can sometimes increase their risk.

Older people are particularly at risk, as are people in hospital because of a combination of general illness, immobility and the presence of many more resistant bacteria within the hospital environment. In the care setting, inhalation pneumonia is due to inhalation of foreign material, such as food or vomit (for example, if someone falls unconscious or has a stroke and so loses the normal control that protects the airway). Chronic illness may also be a cause of inhalation pneumonia, for example in people with Parkinson's disease where the cough reflex may be restricted.

Some types of pneumonia are known as atypical. These are milder, with a more gradual onset and less severe symptoms and include infections caused by certain bacteria, such as *Legionella pneumophila*, *Mycoplasma pneumoniae* and *Chlamydia pneumoniae*.

Signs and symptoms of pneumonia

Symptoms vary depending on the cause. In older people, symptoms may be vague, for example their temperature may be only slightly raised or even normal. Confusion or disorientation may be the only clue something is wrong. Symptoms may include:

- pyrexia in response to bacterial infection;
- dehydration – pyrexia causes fluid loss;
- tachycardia;
- **hypoxaemia**;
- tachypnoea and dyspnoea;
- reduced lung expansion – consolidation makes it difficult to expand the lungs and to breathe normally;

- pain – pleuritic pain as inflammation spreads to the pleura, with people complaining of sharp localised pain that increases with breathing and coughing;
- productive cough – exudates present in the alveoli can produce rusty-coloured sputum;
- tiredness.

Some common investigations used in diagnosing pneumonia are given in Table 11.2.

Table 11.2 Common investigations in the diagnosis of people with pneumonia

Investigation	Rationale
Full blood count	High white cell count indicates inflammation, infection or immune response
Urea and electrolytes	Raised urea (≥ 7 mmol/L) is indicative of severe infection
Blood and sputum cultures	Identifies the cause and enables correct antibiotic therapy
Liver function tests	Acute pneumonia can affect liver function
X-ray	Shows the extent of lung tissue involvement

Case Study 1 – Jim
NURSING CARE PLAN Pneumonia

You will remember Jim Hunter from the introduction. Aged 58, he was an emergency admission to the medical admissions unit (MAU) with a diagnosis of right lower lobe pneumonia. Jim lives alone and is a smoker with a history of acute chest infections (acute bronchitis). He presented to his GP following 24 hours of fever-like symptoms and the development of a painful cough. He became alarmed when he began to cough up rust-coloured sputum.

On admission Jim was clean and well-nourished. He had obvious signs of respiratory distress with a respiratory rate of 32 breaths per minute. He describes his breathing as being 'hard work'. Other vital signs were pulse 120 beats per minute and a temperature of 38.7 °C. His blood pressure was recorded as 140/90 mmHg. His oxygen saturation levels were measured with a pulse oximeter (see Figure 11.10) and recorded as 88%.

Immediate nursing care

Immediate nursing care for Jim should include the following:

- Effective establishment of a therapeutic relationship between yourself and Jim will help him to stay calm and less anxious, and support his concordance to treatment and care.
- Position Jim in a comfortable upright position to promote diaphragm and intercostal muscle movement, this will help him to breathe more easily.

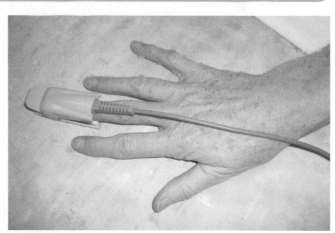

Figure 11.10 Pulse oxymeter applied to finger.

- Using an established pain assessment tool, assess Jim's pain levels. Effective pain management will help him to become more relaxed and to aid ventilation (see Chapter 2).
- Safely administer prescribed oxygen therapy to raise oxygen saturation levels above 90% and to correct hypoxia.
- Safely administer prescribed antipyretic and antibiotic therapy to reduce pyrexia and to combat bacterial infection.

NURSING CARE PLAN Pneumonia (continued)

✦ Jim's vital signs are recorded hourly to rule out deterioration of his condition which could be indicated by a fall in blood pressure and the onset of mental confusion. *A rising respiratory rate is a sensitive indicator of Jim's condition deteriorating.*

✦ Hydration is important to encourage Jim to expectorate sputum and combat the effects of a high temperature and

sweating. Intravenous fluids may be prescribed if Jim is severely dehydrated.

✦ Offer small light nourishment to Jim and encourage independent care as his symptoms subside.

✦ Allow Jim to rest. Cough suppressants can be considered at **night only** to support this.

The person with tuberculosis (TB)

FAST FACTS

Tuberculosis

● Figures released by the Health Protection Agency reveal a 30-year high in the incidence of TB in the UK in 2009.

● The figures were the highest since 1979 with 9266 cases in England and Wales (HPA 2010).

● One person dies from tuberculosis each day in the UK (BTS *et al.* 2009).

Incidence and prevalence of TB

The incidence of reported cases of TB has been rising in the UK since the 1980s, and in 2008 an incidence rate of 14.1 cases per 100 000 population was recorded (HPA 2010). The disease tends to have associated risk factors which include exposure to droplet infection in closed poorly ventilated environments.

Consider this . . .

Given the increasing incidence of TB in the UK, what do you think the risk factors are that might make an individual more susceptible to tuberculosis infection?

Risk factors for TB

Of course risk is associated with the extent of air contamination, the duration of exposure to the disease and the susceptibility of the individual. Risk factors might include pre-existing disease, for example diabetes, renal disease and anaemia. Chemotherapy and radiotherapy may weaken a person's immune system as can immunological problems such as HIV infection. Other risk factors might include age, nutritional status, stress and even pregnancy. In the UK, TB is associated with those in high-risk groups, and large proportions of cases occur in those people not born in the UK and

who have not had opportunity for immunisation, and in people aged between 15 and 44 years.

PRACTICE ALERT

● Communication to support infection control to minimise the spread of TB both in the hospital and the community setting is essential.

● Make sure that you consider communication in relation to any possible language barriers that might exist when supporting 'at risk' people.

Pathophysiology of TB

TB is a chronic, recurrent infectious disease that usually affects the lungs, although any organ can be affected. This disease is caused by *Mycobacterium tuberculosis*, an airborne slow-growing bacillus and as such is spread from one person to another. The well-chanted rhyme 'coughs and sneezes spread diseases' familiar to our grandparents in the UK came about to support the prevention and spread of common respiratory diseases (including TB). If minute droplets containing the tuberculosis bacilli are inhaled, they have the potential to infect the alveoli because of their small size. This initial infection is known as *primary TB* which can go on to develop *latent TB*.

Signs and symptoms of TB

The signs and symptoms of TB include:

● haemoptysis – this can present after initial dry cough that turns productive with purulent or blood-tinged sputum;

● localised chest pain;

● weight loss which is unexplained;

● pyrexia which is low grade and common in the afternoons;

● night sweats;

● fatigue.

Identifying the types of TB

Depending on the site of the disease, TB is defined as being either pulmonary (respiratory), where there is a high potential for infectious spread, or extra-pulmonary (non-respiratory), where there is a low potential for infectious spread of the disease. Those people with pulmonary TB are required to have their sputum screened to determine the potential for spread (NICE 2006). Bacteriological investigation of tuberculosis is the only certain way of confirming diagnosis. Sputum microscopy is critical in identifying infectious people and therefore nurses have a key role in managing the collection of samples and in the infection control of TB.

PRACTICE ALERT

- Sputum samples are referred to as *'smears'*.
- Sputum NOT saliva is required – clear advice is needed.
- Reports will show *'smear positive'* if acid-fast bacilli (indicative of *Mycobacterium*) are seen.
- *Smear positive* is not a conclusive diagnosis of TB and further culture of sputum is required.
- *'Smear negative'* is reported if acid-fast bacilli are not seen.
- People who produce three negative sputum samples on three consecutive days are usually regarded as non-infectious.

Tuberculin testing

Skin tests for evidence of immunological reaction to mycobacterial antigens are commonplace screening activities, in particular for those who are in the at-risk categories previously identified. Two types of tests are used, the Heaf or the Mantoux tests. Tuberculin protein is injected intradermally and an immune response develops on the surface of the skin to show reaction to mycobacterial antigens.

PRACTICE ALERT

- *Positive* reaction to skin tests are not in themselves an indication of TB (previous immunisation of the Bacille Calmette–Guerin (BCG) vaccine can cause some reactivity).
- *Negative* response to skin test cannot rule out active TB since people with severe immune-suppression may fail to react to the tuberculin protein.

TB is a notifiable disease in the UK. This is a legal requirement of the medical practitioner and supports the ongoing surveillance of outbreaks of TB in the community and the follow-up (contact tracing) of those at risk through prolonged exposure to infected people. Contact tracing endeavours to detect related cases that may be infected without disease

symptoms, to identify candidates for BCG vaccination and to screen local at-risk groups of individuals.

NURSING CARE FOR TB

The care of people with TB needs to be focused around helping them take their treatment consistently over the long period of time it takes to achieve a cure. This can often take months to achieve. Drug resistance is a key challenge to the treatment and control of TB with some strains of the disease resistant to one or more of the drugs commonly used to treat the infection. The term 'multi-drug resistance TB' (MDR-TB) refers to strains of the infection that are resistant to rifampicin and isoniazid, the two common anti-TB drugs.

NICE (2006) guidelines recommend that a key worker provide support in adherence to the treatment of TB. This support can include directly observed therapy (DOT) for those people who find compliance with the therapeutic regime difficult. DOT is a treatment control scheme where health workers directly observe and record people swallowing their drug therapy. Many people can become disillusioned and frustrated with the long-term nature of the treatment for TB. Nursing care should be mindful of the stigma associated with the disease. Closely associated with poverty, TB can leave people feeling ashamed and isolated. This means supporting each person throughout their treatment, if necessary arranging for the treatment to be taken under supervision, at a clinic or elsewhere; or helping with other aspects of their lives so that they can give their TB treatment the priority it needs.

Consider this . . .

Why might it be better to investigate tuberculosis in a clinic environment as opposed to hospital admission?

The British Thoracic Society (BTS 2000) and NICE (2006) recommend home treatment of TB whenever possible; this supports the reduction of infection to vulnerable people in hospital settings. Of those admitted to hospital care, the practice of isolating people who are known or suspected of TB infection varies within NHS Trusts in the UK. The Department of Health (DoH 2007) recommends that in high-incidence areas, people with suspected or confirmed TB are best managed in TB-specific out-patient clinics by specially designated multidisciplinary teams, and not alongside other general respiratory out-patients. Isolation facilities for hospitalised people with suspected or confirmed TB are recommended. Control of the spread of TB is encouraged through education, for example covering the mouth when coughing and sneezing, and the use of tissues.

DISORDERS OF THE PLEURA

The *pleura* is a thin membrane with two layers: the visceral pleura, which overlies the lung surface, and the parietal pleura, which lines the inner chest wall. Between the layers of pleura is the *pleural cavity*, which contains a thin layer of serous fluid. As the thoracic cavity expands during inspiration, the pressure in this space becomes negative in relation to atmospheric and alveolar pressure. The expansible lung is drawn out, and air rushes into the alveoli. When the pleura is inflamed or affected by disease or injury, air or fluid can collect in the pleural cavity, restricting lung expansion, air movement and ventilation.

The person with pleuritis (pleurisy)

Pleuritis (*pleurisy*), inflammation of the pleura, irritates sensory fibres of the parietal pleura, causing characteristic sharp or stabbing pain. Pleural inflammation usually occurs secondarily to another process, such as a viral respiratory illness, pneumonia or rib injury. The onset of pleuritis is typically acute.

Signs and symptoms of pleuritis

Some signs and symptoms of pleuritis are:

- The pain is usually one-sided and well-localised.
- Pain is usually sharp or stabbing in nature.
- Pain may be referred to the neck or the shoulder and can be aggravated by deep breathing, coughing and movement.
- Respirations are rapid and shallow, and chest wall movement is limited on the affected side.

INTERDISCIPLINARY CARE FOR PLEURITIS

Chest x-ray and ECG can rule out other causes of chest pain. Treatment for pleuritis is symptomatic. Analgesics and non-steroidal anti-inflammatory drugs (NSAIDs) in particular, help relieve the pain. Codeine may be prescribed, both to relieve pain and to suppress the cough.

NURSING CARE FOR PLEURITIS

Nursing care for the person with pleuritis is directed toward promoting comfort, including administration of NSAIDs and analgesics. Pleuritis isn't usually associated with long-term complications; however, nursing care should be focused on monitoring for increased pyrexia, productive cough, difficulty in breathing and shortness of breath.

The person with pleural effusion

The pleural space normally contains only about 10–20 ml of serous fluid. Pleural effusion is collection of excess fluid in the pleural space. Pleural effusions result from either systemic or local disease. Systemic problems that may lead to pleural effusion include heart failure, liver or renal disease, and connective tissue Problems, such as rheumatoid arthritis and systemic lupus erythematosus (SLE). Pneumonia, atelectasis, tuberculosis, lung cancer and trauma are local conditions that may cause pleural effusion.

> **Consider this . . .**
>
> With your understanding of the physiology of the lungs and surrounding tissues, what do you think might be the causes of pleural effusion?

> **PRACTICE ALERT**
>
> A large pleural effusion compresses adjacent lung tissue. This causes the characteristic manifestation of dyspnoea. Pain may develop, although with inflammatory processes pleuritic pain is often relieved by formation of an effusion, as the fluid reduces friction between inflamed visceral and parietal pleura. Breath sounds are diminished or absent, and chest wall movement may be limited.

Chest x-ray often provides the first evidence of a pleural effusion. Because fluid typically collects in dependent regions, it is seen at the base of the affected lung on an upright chest x-ray, and along the lateral wall when the person is positioned on the affected side. CT scans and ultrasound also are used to localise and differentiate pleural effusions.

The person with pneumothorax

Accumulation of air in the pleural space is called pneumothorax. Pneumothorax can occur spontaneously, without apparent cause, as a complication of pre-existing lung disease, as a result of blunt or penetrating trauma to the chest or from an iatrogenic cause, for example following chest drain insertion.

Pathophysiology of pneumothorax

Pressure in the pleural space is normally negative in relation to atmospheric pressure. This negative pressure is vital to the process of breathing. Contraction of the diaphragm and the intercostal muscles enlarges the thoracic space. Negative intra-pleural pressure draws the lung outward, increasing its volume so air rushes in to fill the expanded lung space.

When either the visceral or parietal pleura is breached, air enters the pleural space, equalising this pressure. Lung expansion is impaired, and the natural recoil tendency of the lung causes it to collapse to a greater or lesser extent, depending on the size and rapidity of air accumulation.

Spontaneous pneumothorax

Spontaneous pneumothorax (Figure 11.11) develops when an air-filled blister on the lung surface ruptures. Rupture allows air from the airways to enter the pleural space. Air accumulates until pressures are equalised or until collapse of the involved lung section seals the leak. Spontaneous pneumothorax may be either *primary* (*simple*) or *secondary* (*complicated*).

- *Primary pneumothorax* affects previously healthy people, and usually tall, slender men between ages 16 and 24 are more at risk. The cause of primary pneumothorax is unknown. Risk factors include smoking. Air-filled blisters tend to form in the apices of the lungs. This is considered to be a benign condition, although recurrences are common. Certain activities also increase the risk of spontaneous pneumothorax, such as high-altitude flying and rapid decompression during scuba diving.

- *Secondary pneumothorax*, generally caused by overdistension and rupture of an alveolus, is more serious and potentially life-threatening. It develops in people with underlying lung disease, usually COPD. Middle-aged and older adults are primarily affected. Secondary pneumothorax also may be associated with asthma, cystic fibrosis, pulmonary fibrosis, tuberculosis, **acute respiratory distress syndrome (ARDS)** and other lung diseases.

Signs and symptoms

The signs and symptoms of spontaneous pneumothorax depend on the size of pneumothorax, extent of lung collapse and any underlying lung disease. They include:

- Pleuritic chest pain and shortness of breath begin abruptly, often while at rest.

- The respiratory and heart rates increase as gas exchange is affected.

- Chest wall movement may be asymmetrical, with less movement on the affected side than the unaffected side.

- Breath sounds may be diminished or absent.

- Hypoxaemia may develop, although normal mechanisms that shunt blood flow to the unaffected lung often maintain normal oxygen saturation levels.

Traumatic pneumothorax

Traumatic pneumothorax (Figure 11.12) can be caused by blunt or penetrating trauma of the chest wall and pleura. Blunt trauma, for example due to a road traffic accident, falls or during cardiopulmonary resuscitation (CPR), can lead to a *closed pneumothorax*. Fractured ribs penetrating the pleura are the leading cause of pneumothorax due to blunt trauma. Fracture of the trachea and a ruptured bronchus or oesophagus also may result from blunt trauma, leading to closed pneumothorax.

Open pneumothorax (*sucking chest wound*) results from penetrating chest trauma such as a stab wound or impalement injury. With open pneumothorax, air moves freely between the pleural space and the atmosphere through the wound. Pressure on the affected side equalises with the atmosphere, and the lung collapses rapidly. The result is significant hypoventilation.

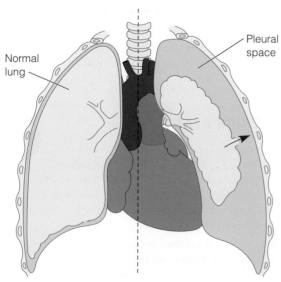

Figure 11.11 Spontaneous pneumothorax.

Normal lung

Pleural space

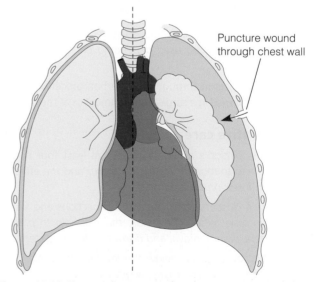

Figure 11.12 Traumatic pneumothorax.

Puncture wound through chest wall

Iatrogenic pneumothorax may result from puncture or laceration of the visceral pleura during central-line placement or lung biopsy. During bronchoscopy, bronchi or lung tissue can be disrupted. Alveoli can become overdistended and rupture during anaesthesia, resuscitation procedures, or mechanical ventilation.

Signs and symptoms

- With traumatic pneumothorax, symptoms of pain and dyspnoea may be masked or missed due to other injuries.

- Tachypnoea and tachycardia may be attributed to the primary injury. Focused assessment for evidence of pneumothorax is vital.

- Chest wall movement on the affected side is diminished, and breath sounds are absent. If a penetrating wound is present, air may be heard and felt moving through it with respiratory efforts.

- **Haemothorax** frequently accompanies traumatic pneumothorax.

- The signs and symptoms of iatrogenic pneumothorax are similar to those of spontaneous pneumothorax.

Tension pneumothorax

Tension pneumothorax (Figure 11.13) develops when injury to the chest wall or lungs allows air to enter the pleural space but

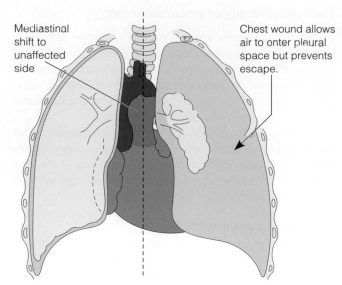

Mediastinal shift to unaffected side

Chest wound allows air to enter the pleural space but prevents escape.

Figure 11.13 Tension pneumothorax.

prevents it from escaping. Pressure within the pleural space becomes positive in relation to atmospheric pressure as air rapidly accumulates with each breath. The lung on the affected side collapses and pressure on the mediastinum shifts thoracic organs to the unaffected side of the chest, placing pressure on the

---

NURSING CARE PLAN The person having an intrapleural drain

Review Chapter 1 for routine pre- and post-operative care.

Pre-operative care

- This is an invasive procedure and will require informed consent.

- Explain that local anaesthesia will be used but that pressure may be felt by the person as the drain is inserted. *The person may be anxious and extremely dyspnoeic and may need reassurance that the procedure will provide relief.*

- The person needs to be positioned correctly. *Upright or side lying position may be used depending on the site of the pneumothorax.*

- Support the person through the insertion procedure which may be performed in a surgical environment or at the bedside.

Post-operative care

- Assess the person's respiratory status at least four hourly. *This will help to monitor respiratory status and the effect of the drain insertion on breathing.*

- Maintain a closed system. *Tape all connections and secure the drain tube to the chest wall, this will help to prevent inadvertent drain removal and disruption to the system.*

- Keep the collection jar below the level of the chest. *Fluid drains from the pleural cavity by gravity flow.*

- Check tube for kinks or loops.

- Check water seal frequently. The water level should fluctuate with breathing in and out. *Air bubbles can be seen in the chamber as air is being removed from the pleural cavity.*

- Measure drainage frequently. Report and record any changes that occur. *Red, free-flowing drainage indicates haemorrhage. Cloudiness may indicate infection.*

- Your person can be active with a drain *in situ*, and you can encourage gentle movement and change of position.

- When the drain is removed, immediately apply a sterile occlusive dressing to prevent air from re-entering the pleural space.

PRACTICE ALERT

- Provide emotional support to the person requiring intrapleural drainage, particularly in early stages and during intrapleural drain insertion. Dyspnoea and hypoxaemia can cause extreme anxiety and apprehension, impairing the ability to cooperate with procedures.

- Ensure intrapleural drain remains at a level below the chest at all times. This prevents backflow into the pleural space.

opposite lung as well. Ventilation is severely compromised, and venous return to the heart is impaired. Tension pneumothorax is a medical emergency requiring immediate intervention to preserve respiration and cardiac output.

Signs and symptoms

- In addition to signs and symptoms of pneumothorax, hypotension and distended neck veins are evident as venous return and cardiac output are affected.
- The trachea is displaced toward the unaffected side as a result of the mediastinal shift.
- Signs of shock may be present. (See Chapter 3 for the signs and symptoms and treatment of shock.)

Intrapleural drainage

The treatment of choice for significant pneumothorax is placement of an intrapleural drain to allow the lung to re-expand. When a tube is placed in the pleural cavity to remove air or fluid, it must be sealed to prevent air from also entering the tube and, in essence, creating an open pneumothorax. Chest tubes are sealed with a Heimlich (one-way) valve or connected to a closed drainage system with a 'water seal'. The valve or water seal prevents air from entering the chest cavity during inspiration and allows air to escape during expiration. Applying a low level of suction to the system helps to re-establish negative pressure in the pleural space, allowing the lung to re-expand.

The person with lung cancer

FAST FACTS

Lung cancer

- Lung cancer can be cured.
- One in eight people with lung cancer have never smoked; however, over 90% of lung cancers are caused by smoking.
- More women die from lung cancer than breast cancer.
- Half of all people in the UK know someone that has died or been affected by lung cancer.

Incidence and prevalence of lung cancer

Lung cancer is the most common cancer in the world, the vast majority of which are caused by cigarette smoking. Cancer Research UK (2011a) predicts that the lifetime risk of developing lung cancer is 1 in 14 for men and 1 in 19 for women in the UK. The picture in this country has seen the incidence of

lung cancer overtaken by breast cancer to make it the second most common UK cancer. Falls in the incidence of lung cancer have been attributed to smoking cessation, especially in younger men. Lung cancer is rare in younger people under the age of 40. Most commonly it occurs in the 60 and above age group, peaking between 75 and 85 years.

Risk factors for lung cancer

The causes in the main are attributed to cigarette smoking (which accounts for an estimated 85–90% of cases). Other causes include a number of pollutants (for example asbestos, diesel exhaust, silica, non-ferrous metals and nitrogen oxides). Exposure to environmental smoke, radon gas and industrial carcinogens is also linked to lung cancer.

Pathophysiology of lung cancer

Two types of lung cancer are seen (Figure 11.16). Around 20% are small-cell lung cancers (SCLC) and the rest are non-small-cell lung cancers (NSCLC). Of these, squamous cell carcinoma and adenocarcinoma are the most common forms.

Treatments for SCLC and NSCLC are very different and therefore accurate histological diagnosis is essential. In the UK about half of all people diagnosed with lung cancer are referred for investigation by their GP.
Bronchiogenic carcinoma is the most common type of lung cancer. Arising from the epithelial lining of the bronchi, it accounts for about 90% of all lung cancers.

Bronchoalveolar carcinoma originates in the lung parenchyma and spreads along the alveolar walls. All types of lung cancer can spread throughout the body in three ways: first by direct spread into surrounding tissue; second by the lymphatic system; and third by haematologic spread. The most common sites for lung cancer metastases are lung, brain, cervical nodes, liver, bone, adrenals and skin.

Signs and symptoms of lung cancer

People present with a variety of symptoms, usually relating to the primary tumour. The commonest symptoms include cough, dyspnoea (breathing difficulties), weight loss and chest pain. Haemoptysis (coughing up blood) and bone pain are also relatively common symptoms.

Multisystem effects of lung cancer are illustrated in Figure 11.14.

INTERDISCIPLINARY CARE FOR LUNG CANCER

Diagnosis

Investigations for lung cancer might include the following:

- X-ray;
- CT scan;
- bronchoscopy;

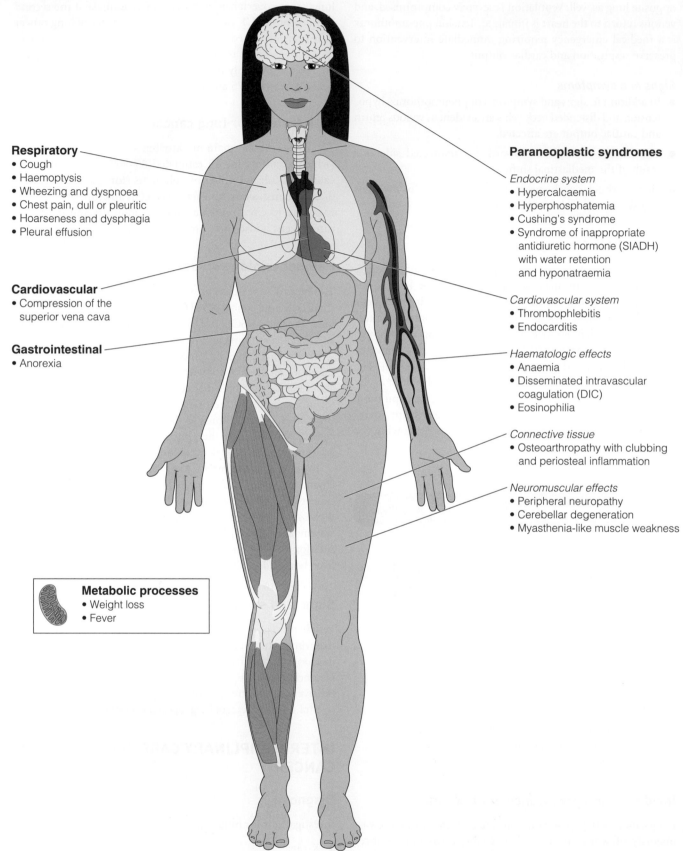

Respiratory
- Cough
- Haemoptysis
- Wheezing and dyspnoea
- Chest pain, dull or pleuritic
- Hoarseness and dysphagia
- Pleural effusion

Cardiovascular
- Compression of the superior vena cava

Gastrointestinal
- Anorexia

Metabolic processes
- Weight loss
- Fever

Paraneoplastic syndromes

Endocrine system
- Hypercalcaemia
- Hyperphosphatemia
- Cushing's syndrome
- Syndrome of inappropriate antidiuretic hormone (SIADH) with water retention and hyponatraemia

Cardiovascular system
- Thrombophlebitis
- Endocarditis

Haematologic effects
- Anaemia
- Disseminated intravascular coagulation (DIC)
- Eosinophilia

Connective tissue
- Osteoarthropathy with clubbing and periosteal inflammation

Neuromuscular effects
- Peripheral neuropathy
- Cerebellar degeneration
- Myasthenia-like muscle weakness

Figure 11.14 Multisystem effects of lung cancer.

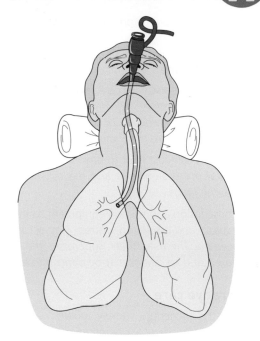

IN PRACTICE

Investigations for lung cancer

BRONCHOSCOPY
A bronchoscopy (Figure 11.15) is the direct visualisation of the larynx, trachea and bronchi through a bronchoscope to identify lesions, remove foreign bodies and secretions, obtain tissue for biopsy and improve tracheobronchial drainage. During the test, a catheter brush or biopsy forceps can be passed to obtain secretions or tissue for examination diagnostic purposes.

LUNG BIOPSY
A lung biopsy is carried out to obtain tissue to differentiate benign from malignant tumours of the lungs. It may be done during a bronchoscopy, or by surgical procedure. Nursing care is the same as for a bronchoscopy or a thoracotomy (incision through the chest wall) if a surgical biopsy is performed.

PNEUMOTHORAX
Done to obtain a specimen of pleural fluid for diagnosis (and used as a procedure to remove pleural fluid or instil medication). A large-bore needle is inserted through the chest wall and into the pleural space. Following the procedure, a chest x-ray is taken to check for a pneumothorax.

Figure 11.15 Fibre-optic bronchoscopy.

- image-guided lung biopsy;
- biopsy of lymph nodes;
- MRI scan;
- PET scan;
- ultrasound scan.

Staging

The size, position and extent of the disease is measured in stages and this helps in the decision of the best treatment options for the disease. Two types of staging are used: the number system (see Table 11.3) and the TNM (tumour, nodes, metastases) method. These are combined to show the extent and severity of the disease process, for example a very small cancer with no lymph and no spread is coded as T1 N0 M0.

The TNM staging system measures the tumour according to:

- the size of the tumour (T);
- cancer cell spread into lymph nodes (N);
- tumour spread anywhere else in the body – secondary cancer or metastases (M).

Outcome for people with lung cancer will depend on the severity and type of cancer at the first diagnosis. People with stage 1 cancer will have a five-year survival rate of between 43 and 73%. The five-year survival percentage rate decreases for stage 2, 3 and 4 with as few as 2–13% of people predicted to survive after five years in the most severe stages of lung cancer.

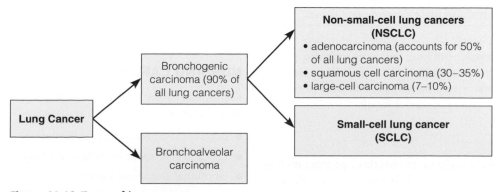

Figure 11.16 Types of lung cancer.

NURSING CARE PLAN The person undergoing a bronchoscopy

Review Chapter 1 for routine pre-operative and post-operative care.

Pre-operative care

✚ Provide routine pre-operative care as ordered. *Bronchoscopy is an invasive procedure requiring conscious sedation or anaesthesia. Care provided prior to the procedure is similar to that provided before many minor surgical procedures.*

✚ Provide mouth care just prior to bronchoscopy. *Mouth care reduces oral micro-organisms and the risk of introducing them into the lungs.*

✚ Bring resuscitation and suction equipment to the bedside. *Laryngospasm and respiratory distress may occur following the procedure. The anaesthetic suppresses the cough and gag reflexes, and secretions may be difficult to expectorate.*

Post-operative care

✚ Following the procedure, closely monitor vital signs and respiratory status. *Possible complications of bronchoscopy include laryngospasm, bronchospasm, bronchial perforation with possible pneumothorax or subcutaneous emphysema, haemorrhage, hypoxia, pneumonia or bacteraemia.*

✚ Instruct to avoid eating or drinking for approximately two hours or until fully awake with intact cough and gag reflexes. *Suppression of the cough and gag reflexes by systemic and local anaesthesia used during the procedure increases the risk for aspiration.*

✚ Provide a vomit bowl and tissues for expectorating sputum and saliva. *Until reflexes have returned, the person may be unable to swallow sputum and saliva safely.*

✚ Monitor colour and character of respiratory secretions. *Secretions normally are blood tinged for several hours following bronchoscopy, especially if biopsy has been obtained. Notify the physician if sputum is grossly bloody. Grossly bloody sputum may indicate a complication such as perforation.*

✚ Collect post-bronchoscopy sputum specimens for cytology examination as ordered. *Cells in the sputum may be examined if a tumour is suspected.*

Health education for the person and family

✚ Fibre-optic bronchoscopy requires 30–45 minutes to complete. It may be done at the bedside, in a special procedure room or in the surgical suite.

✚ The procedure usually causes little pain or discomfort, because an anaesthetic is given. The person is able to breathe during the bronchoscopy.

✚ Some voice hoarseness and a sore throat are common following the procedure. Throat lozenges or warm saline gargles may help relieve discomfort.

✚ A mild fever may develop within the first 24 hours following the procedure. This is a normal response.

✚ Persistent cough, bloody or purulent sputum, wheezing, shortness of breath, difficulty breathing or chest pain may indicate a complication. Notify the physician if they develop.

Table 11.3 The number staging system for lung cancer

Stage 1	Cancer is small and only in one area of the lung (localised).
Stage 2 and 3	Cancer is larger and may have grown into the surrounding tissues and there may be cancer cells in the lymph node (locally advanced).
Stage 4	The cancer has spread to another part of the body (secondary or metastatic spread).

Management of people with lung cancer by multidisciplinary teams is recommended in the 2005 NICE guidelines. Members of these teams work in accordance with standards of practice that aim to ensure quality of service for all.

Treatment

A variety of treatments exist to support those people with lung cancer. Surgery, radiotherapy and chemotherapy are the most common forms of treatment. New biological treatments aim to interfere with the way cancer cells interact and signal to each other. Treatments can be used in isolation or combined to create the best outcome for the individual with lung cancer.

PRACTICE ALERT

Strategies for supportive and palliative care should be considered by the interdisciplinary team from diagnosis onwards. Lung cancer significantly affects the physical, psychological and social health of individuals and their families.

NURSING CARE FOR LUNG CANCER

Key aspects of the nursing care for people with lung cancer should encompass the following:

● good communication and information;

● easy access to specialist help and advice;

● emotional and social support;

● expert symptom management and advice;

- coordinated care;
- continuity of care.

Nurses within the community setting are in a key position to ensure that people who are at risk from lung cancer are assessed and screened appropriately. This supports early diagnosis and potentially increases survival rates from initial diagnosis. Ongoing assessment of the care needs of people and their families helps to identify and initiate palliative care pathways for end-of-life care.

GAS EXCHANGE PROBLEMS

FAST FACTS

The relationship between social inequality and lung disease

According to the data, social inequality causes a higher proportion of deaths in respiratory disease than any other disease area:

- Almost a half of all deaths from lung disease (44%) are associated with social class inequalities compared with 28% of deaths from ischaemic heart disease.
- Furthermore, men aged 20–64 employed in unskilled manual occupations are around 14 times more likely to die from COPD and nine times more likely to die from TB than men employed in professional roles.

Burden of Lung Disease (BTS 2006) is the only publication that analyses the total death, disability and cost of respiratory disease in the UK. The report was compiled in 2006 for the British Thoracic Society by the Lung and Asthma Information Agency at St Georges, University of London.

PHYSIOLOGY REVIEW

Normal function of the lower respiratory system depends on several organ systems:

- the central nervous system, which stimulates and controls breathing;
- chemoreceptors in the brain, aortic arch and carotid bodies, which monitor the pH and oxygen content of blood;
- the heart and circulatory system, which provide for blood supply and gas exchange;
- the musculoskeletal system, which provides an intact thoracic cavity capable of expanding and contracting;
- the lungs and bronchial tree, which allow air movement and gas exchange.

Impaired function of any of these systems affects ventilation and respiration. As a result, tissues may become *hypoxic*, with inadequate oxygen to support metabolic activity. Signs of hypoxia are:

- rapid shallow breathing and dyspnoea;
- increased restlessness and dizziness;
- flaring of nostrils;
- cyanosis;
- rapid pulse;
- often a sitting position, leaning forward is adopted enabling more lung expansion;
- facial expression is one of anxiety and tiredness.

Although some of the problems discussed below can affect ventilation (air movement into and out of the airways and alveoli), all can have significant effects on gas exchange. The mechanisms by which they affect gas exchange differ:

- In reactive airway disease (asthma) and obstructive problems, air trapping reduces the amount of oxygen available to drive gas exchange.
- Interstitial lung problems affect the ability of the lungs to expand and the work of breathing, again reducing alveolar oxygenation and gas exchange.
- Pulmonary vascular problems affect blood flow to the lungs or a portion of the lungs, reducing gas exchange through their effects on perfusion of the lungs.
- Respiratory failure is the ultimate consequence of impaired gas exchange; the lungs cannot adequately oxygenate the blood or eliminate carbon dioxide.

With a few exceptions, the problems discussed in this chapter are relatively common, chronic lung diseases.

Problems of other body systems, such as neurologic problems (for example, head injury, spinal cord trauma or problems) can also affect gas exchange through their effects on the central or peripheral nervous systems. These problems and their effects on the respiratory system are discussed further in Chapter 13.

Ageing affects pulmonary ventilation and gas exchange as well. The number of alveoli decrease, and emphysematous changes (senile emphysema) reduce the surface area for gas exchange. Alveoli become less elastic, causing increased air trapping and dead space. For most older adults who remain active, these changes have minimal effect on exercise tolerance and activities of daily living (ADLs). When combined with lung disease, however, age-related pulmonary changes increase the person's risk for developing respiratory failure.

The person with asthma

Asthma is a chronic inflammatory disorder of the airways characterised by recurrent episodes of wheezing, breathlessness, chest tightness and coughing. Inflammation causes increased responsiveness of the airways to multiple stimuli such as pollutants which cause the individual to wheeze. The widespread airflow obstruction that occurs during acute episodes usually reverses, either spontaneously or with treatment. While most episodes or asthma 'attacks' are relatively brief, some people with asthma may experience longer episodes with some degree of airway impairment daily. In rare cases, an acute episode of asthma is so severe that respiratory failure and death result.

Risk factors for asthma

A number of risk factors can be identified for asthma, although many people develop the disease in the absence of known risk factors. Allergies play a strong role in childhood asthma, a lesser role in adults. There is a strong genetic component to the disease, although a specific pattern of inheritance has not been identified. Active and passive smoking as well as environmental factors, including air pollution and occupational exposure to industrial compounds, may contribute. Respiratory viruses such as rhinovirus and influenza can precipitate asthma attacks as can recurrent chest infections. Other contributory factors include socioeconomic status and maternal youth (having a young mother).

Pathophysiology of asthma

Airways within the lungs contain criss-crossing strips of smooth muscle that control their diameter. This muscle is innervated by the autonomic nervous system. Parasympathetic (cholinergic) stimulation leads to bronchoconstriction, or narrowing of the airways. Sympathetic stimulation through β_2-adrenergic receptors causes bronchodilation, or expansion of the airways. Slight bronchoconstriction normally predominates. However, when increased airflow is necessary (for example, during exercise), the parasympathetic system is inhibited, and stimulation of the sympathetic system causes bronchodilation. Inflammatory mediators (such as histamine) released during an antigen–antibody response act directly on bronchial smooth muscle to produce bronchoconstriction.

In asthma, the airways are in a persistent state of inflammation. During symptom-free periods, airway inflammation in asthma is subacute or quiet. Even during these periods, however, inflammatory cells such as eosinophils, neutrophils and lymphocytes may be found in airway tissues and oedema may be present.

Asthma attack triggers

Common triggers for an acute asthma attack (Figure 11.17) include exposure to allergens, respiratory tract infection, exercise, inhaled irritants and emotional upsets. This airway obstruction is partially or completely reversible, either spontaneously or in response to therapeutic interventions. Childhood asthma (which may continue into adulthood) is most often linked to inhalation of allergens such as pollen, animal dander or household dust. People with allergic asthma often have a history of other allergies. Environmental pollutants, such as tobacco smoke and irritant gases (for example, sulphur dioxide, nitrogen dioxide and ozone), can provoke asthma. Exposure to second-hand smoke as a child is associated with a higher risk for and increased severity of asthma. Agents found in the workplace, such as noxious fumes and gases, chemicals and dusts, may cause occupational asthma.

Respiratory infections, viral in particular, are a common internal stimulus for an asthmatic attack. Exercise-induced asthma attacks also are common; loss of heat or water from

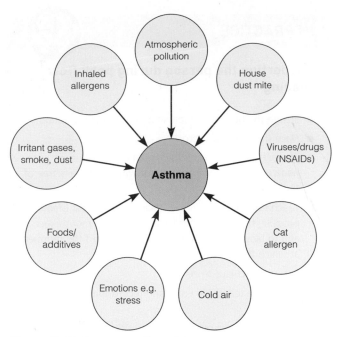

Figure 11.17 Common asthma triggers.

the bronchial surface may contribute to exercise-induced asthma. Exercising in cold, dry air increases the risk of an asthma attack in susceptible people.

Emotional stress is a significant aetiologic factor for attacks in as many as half of people with asthma. Common pharmacologic triggers include aspirin and other non-steroidal anti-inflammatory drugs, sulphites (which are used as preservatives in wine, beer, fresh fruits and salad) and beta-blockers.

Interactions between environmental and genetic factors contribute to hyper-responsiveness and airway inflammation. The resulting bronchiospasm develops in response to a number of triggers.

Responses to triggers

When a trigger such as inhalation of an allergen or irritant occurs, an *acute* or *early response* develops in the hyper-reactive airways predisposed to bronchospasm. Sensitised mast cells in the bronchial mucosa release inflammatory mediators such as histamine, prostaglandins and leukotrienes. Resident and infiltrating inflammatory cells also produce inflammatory mediators such as cytokines, bradykinin and growth factors. These mediators stimulate parasympathetic receptors and bronchial smooth muscle to produce bronchoconstriction. They also increase capillary permeability, which allows plasma to escape and leads to mucosal oedema. Mucous production is stimulated; excess mucus collects in the narrowed airways.

The attack is prolonged by the *late phase response*, which develops 4–12 hours after exposure to the trigger. Inflammatory cells such as basophils and eosinophils are activated, and they damage airway epithelium, produce mucosal oedema, impair mucociliary clearance and produce or prolong bronchoconstriction. The degree of hyper-reactivity depends on the extent of inflammation. Together, bronchoconstriction, oedema and inflammation, and mucous secretion narrow the airway. Airway resistance increases, limiting airflow and increasing the work of breathing.

To summarise, in an acute asthma attack, inflammatory mediators are released from sensitised airways followed by activation of inflammatory cells. These events lead to bronchoconstriction, airway oedema and impaired mucociliary clearance. Airway narrowing limits airflow and increases the work of breathing; trapped air mixes with inhaled air, impairing gas exchange.

Signs and symptoms of acute asthma

Signs and symptoms of acute asthma include:

- chest tightness;
- cough;
- dyspnoea;
- wheezing;
- tachypnoea and tachycardia;
- anxiety and apprehension.

The frequency of attacks and severity of symptoms vary greatly from person to person. Although some people have infrequent, mild episodes, others have nearly continuous signs and symptoms of cough, dyspnoea on exertion and wheezing with periodic severe exacerbations.

PRACTICE ALERT

Status asthmaticus is severe, prolonged asthma that does not respond to routine treatment. Without aggressive therapy, status asthmaticus can lead to respiratory failure with hypoxaemia, hypercapnia and acidosis. Endotracheal intubation, mechanical ventilation and aggressive drug treatment may be necessary to sustain life.

INTERDISCIPLINARY CARE FOR ASTHMA

Assessment of acute asthma

Assessment of the person experiencing an acute asthma attack must be very focused and timely. The structured ABCDE assessment discussed earlier can be applied.

The diagnosis of asthma is based on the recognition of the characteristic signs and symptoms that will eliminate any other problems. The key is to take a careful clinical history (BTS *et al.* 2009).

Presentation of the symptoms such as wheezing and shortness of breath is not specific to asthma alone. For this reason, diagnosis is made from a combination of a detailed history and the results of objective lung function tests.

Pulmonary function tests in asthma are known as objective lung measurements and will commonly include peak flow measurement and spirometry discussed below.

IN PRACTICE

Taking an individual's history to diagnose asthma

The following questions are important in establishing the diagnosis of asthma:

- What are the presenting symptoms?
- Past significant medical history, e.g. eczema, rhinitis, may indicate sensitivity to external irritants.
- Family history? Does anyone in the immediate family have any allergies?
- Occupation/hobbies/interests? May focus the cause of this attack.
- Current or ex-smoker? How many per day and for how many years?
- When do the symptoms occur, e.g. morning/evening?
- Any seasonal variation to symptoms? May indicate, for example, pollen or extreme temperature changes as an irritant.
- What is the severity of the symptoms? Have you been admitted to hospital/number of courses of oral steroids per year?
- Any known triggers, e.g. pets, exercise, pollen, etc.?
- Previous medication, prescription or over-the-counter?
- How effective is/was your medication?

Source: adapted from Scullion 2007.

IN PRACTICE

Supporting the person during peak flow reading

- Ensure the person is stable and in a standing position.
- Place the cursor on zero.
- The person should hold the peak flow meter in a horizontal position to the mouth with the fingers free of the cursor.
- Teach the person to inhale, taking the deepest breath possible, then to seal their lips around the mouthpiece and to blow out as hard as possible. Record the number at which the cursor rests.
- Return the cursor to zero.
- Repeat the test three times and record the highest reading.
- Teaching the person the correct technique and the interpretation of results can support self-management of the condition. Establishing 'best flow' can alert individuals to recognise deteriorating asthma and to either self-medicate or seek medical help.

Spirometry and FEV1

Spirometry (Figure 11.18) measures the levels and severity of obstruction in the airways. Large unobstructed airways will expel more air more quickly than obstructed ones. As discussed earlier in the chapter, a spirometer measures both the amount of *forced expiratory volume in one second* (FEV1) and the *forced vital capacity* (FVC) of the lungs. Measurements are made against the normal for age and gender. Like peak flow, a variation of between 15–20% before and after treatment with a bronchodilator is indicative of asthma.

PRACTICE ALERT

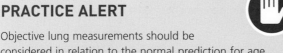

Objective lung measurements should be considered in relation to the normal prediction for age, gender and race. High levels of physical fitness, for example, may increase an individual's lung capacity.

Peak flow measurement

Recordings are taken morning and evening over a two-week period to assess the level of airway obstruction. The person maintains a diary and chart of the peak flow readings and any significant triggers encountered. The daily variation is monitored because persons with uncontrolled asthma may show morning dips in the peak flow due to natural reduction of ventilation that occurs overnight. Variation of about 20% is suggestive of asthma. The peak flow can also be used to measure the effectiveness of bronchodilators before and after treatment; here the variation indicative of asthma is about 15–20% variation (BTS/SIGN 2011).

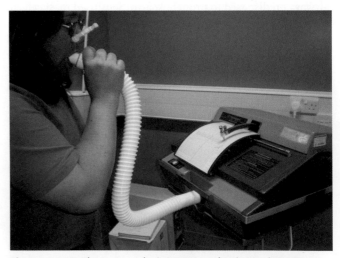

Figure 11.18 The person being assessed using spirometry.

Medication

Most asthma medications are administered by inhalation. In this way, treatments are in direct contact with the affected airways and this reduces the use of systemic medicines and the side-effects associated with them. The most common types are described below:

β_2 *agonists*:

- known as relievers or bronchodilators;
- stimulate β_2-adrenergic receptors in bronchial smooth muscle to create bronchodilation and relaxation;
- almost always given as a dry powder inhaler or metered dose inhaler;
- can be administered prior to activity to help ventilation;
- often prescribed as an 'as required' medication.

PRACTICE ALERT

- Use β_2 agonists with caution in people who have hypertension, a history of cardiovascular disease or diabetes.
- When given to a person who is hypoxic or acidotic, these drugs can potentially create cardiac stimulation.

Inhaled corticosteroids:

- are the core of asthma treatment;
- reduce inflammation (oedema) in the airways, reducing bronchial hyper-reactivity;
- are a long-term treatment that enables the reduced dosage of other drugs.

Long-acting β_2 agonists (LABA):

- part of the BTS 'stepwise' plan, step 3 (BTS *et al.* 2009);
- apart from relaxing smooth muscle for up to 12 hours, these drugs also aid in the effect of inhaled steroids.

Leukotriene receptor antagonists (LTRA):

- interfere with the inflammatory process in the airways by suppressing the effects of leukotrienes, a group of inflammatory mediators;
- are powerful bronchoconstrictors and vasodilators; blocking their synthesis or their receptors improves airflow, decreases symptoms, and reduces the need for short-acting bronchodilators;
- are used for maintenance therapy in adults and children over the age of 12 as an alternative to inhaled corticosteroid therapy. They are not used to treat an acute attack.

IN PRACTICE

Corticosteroids for asthma

- Administer inhaler doses after bronchodilators to facilitate transit of the medication to distal airways.
- Assess for common side-effects: sore throat, hoarseness and oropharyngeal or laryngeal *Candida albicans* infection.
- Administer antifungal medications or gargles as prescribed.
- Advise the person to rinse the mouth after using the inhaler and maintain good oral hygiene to reduce the risk of fungal infections.
- These medications should not be used to alleviate the symptoms of an acute attack.
- Several weeks of continued therapy may be required before a beneficial effect is noticed.
- Notify the doctor in the event of weight gain, fluid retention, muscle weakness, redistribution of fat or mood changes.

NURSING CARE FOR ASTHMA

Nurses encounter people with asthma in the acute care setting during an acute exacerbation, as out-patients or in homes. The priority nursing care needs differ with each setting.

An acute asthma attack causes fear as breathing becomes increasingly difficult and hypoxaemia develops. Anxiety in turn tends to increase the severity and signs and symptoms of the attack. Priority nursing care during an acute attack should focus on improving airway clearance and reducing fear and anxiety. Teaching about prevention of future attacks and home management must be postponed until adequate ventilation is restored.

The management and care pathway for asthma relates to the protocols highlighted by the British Thoracic Society and the Scottish Intercollegiate Guidelines Network (BTS/SIGN 2011) in the form of the 'stepwise' approach, ranging from step 1 (mild symptoms) to step 5 (most severe). Following assessment, people commence treatment at the step most appropriate to the initial severity of their asthma. In the example below, a person with severe symptoms is likely to be placed on step 4 of the protocol; as the symptoms subside, people step down the protocol of treatment options.

Case Study 2 – Gemma
NURSING CARE PLAN Asthma

Gemma Watson's case was presented briefly at the beginning of the chapter. Let us now return to Gemma.

Gemma has ineffective airway clearance

Bronchospasm and bronchoconstriction, increased mucous secretion and airway oedema narrow the airways and impair airflow during an acute attack of asthma. Both inspiratory and expiratory volume are affected, decreasing the oxygen available at the alveolus for the process of respiration. Narrowed air passages increase the work of breathing, increasing the metabolic rate and tissue demand for oxygen.

✚ Frequently assess Gemma's respiratory status (at least every one to two hours): respiratory rate and depth, chest movement or excursion, breath sounds and peak expiratory flow rate. Respiratory status can change rapidly during an acute asthma attack and its treatment. Decreasing peak flow rates indicate worsening airflow restriction. *Slowed, shallow respirations with significantly diminished breath sounds and decreased wheezing may indicate exhaustion and impending respiratory failure. Immediate intervention is necessary.*

✚ Monitor Gemma's skin colour and temperature and level of consciousness (LOC). *Cyanosis, cool clammy skin and changes in LOC (agitation, lethargy or confusion) indicate worsening hypoxia.*

✚ Assess Gemma's pulse oximetry readings; notify the doctor of abnormal values or changes in status. *These values provide information about gas exchange and the adequacy of alveolar ventilation. A fall in Gemma's oxygen saturation levels is an early indicator of impaired gas exchange.*

✚ Assess Gemma's cough effort and sputum for colour, consistency and amount. *Ineffective cough may also signal impending respiratory failure.*

✚ Place Gemma in orthopneic position (with her head and arms supported on her bed table) to facilitate breathing and lung expansion. *These positions reduce the work of breathing and increase lung expansion, especially of basilar areas.*

✚ Administer oxygen as ordered. If a mask is used, monitor closely for feelings that Gemma may have of claustrophobia or suffocation. *Supplemental oxygen reduces hypoxaemia. Although the mask is a very effective oxygen delivery system, it may increase Gemma's anxiety.*

✚ Administer prescribed nebuliser treatments to Gemma and provide humidification as ordered. *Nebuliser treatments are used to administer bronchodilators and other medications; humidity helps loosen secretions.*

✚ Initiate or assist with chest physiotherapy for Gemma, including percussion and postural drainage. *Percussion and postural drainage facilitate the movement of secretions and airway clearance.*

✚ Increase Gemma's fluid intake. *Increasing fluids helps keep secretions thin.*

✚ Provide endotracheal suctioning as needed. *Endotracheal suctioning may be necessary to remove secretions and improve ventilation if Gemma is unable to clear secretions by coughing.*

Gemma has an ineffective breathing pattern

The physiological changes in lung ventilation that occur during an acute asthma attack impair both lung expansion and emptying. Anxiety caused by hypoxia and dyspnoea compounds the problem by increasing the respiratory rate. Collaborative and nursing interventions can help restore a more normal breathing pattern and adequate lung ventilation.

✚ Frequently assess Gemma's respiratory rate, pattern and breath sounds. Note signs and symptoms of ineffective breathing, including rapid rate, shallow respirations, nasal flaring, use of accessory muscles, intercostal retractions and diminished or absent breath sounds. *Early identification of ineffective respirations allows timely initiation of interventions.*

✚ Monitor Gemma's vital signs and laboratory results. *Tachypnoea, tachycardia, an elevated blood pressure and increasing hypoxaemia and hypercapnia are signs of compromised respiratory status.*

✚ Assist with Gemma's ADLs as needed. *This acts to conserve Gemma's energy and reduce her fatigue.*

✚ Provide Gemma with rest periods between scheduled activities and treatments. *Scheduled rest is important to prevent fatigue and reduce oxygen demands.*

✚ Teach and assist Gemma to use techniques to control breathing pattern:
   a. pursed-lip breathing;
   b. abdominal breathing;
   c. relaxation techniques including visualisation and meditation.

Pursed-lip breathing helps keep Gemma's airways open by maintaining positive pressure, and abdominal breathing improves her lung expansion. Relaxation techniques can help to reduce Gemma's anxiety and its effect on the respiratory rate.

✚ Administer medications to Gemma, including bronchodilators and anti-inflammatory drugs, as prescribed. Tell her what is being given and how it will help to relieve her symptoms. Monitor Gemma for desired and possible adverse effects. *Medications are used to improve airway status and facilitate breathing.*

Gemma is anxious

Acute exacerbations of asthma can produce significant anxiety. Fear of being unable to breathe and feelings of suffocation associated with acute asthma are significant. Increasingly frequent and severe episodes may cause fear for the future. Hypoxia contributes to anxiety as well, stimulating the sympathetic nervous system and the fight-or-flight response.

+ Assess Gemma's level of anxiety. *Interventions for severe anxiety or panic differ from those for mild or moderate anxiety.*

+ Assist Gemma to identify coping skills that have been successful in the past. *Successful coping helps her to regain control of the situation, reducing anxiety.*

+ Provide physical and emotional support to Gemma. Remain with her during episodes of severe anxiety; schedule time every one to two hours to be with her and answer her call bell promptly. The severely anxious person may fear being alone or believe she will die if someone is not on hand. *Knowing that the nurse is readily available and will return regardless if help is needed reduces anxiety.*

+ Listen actively to Gemma's concerns; do not deny or negate the fear of dying or of being unable to breathe. *Active listening promotes trust and helps Gemma to express her concerns.*

+ Provide clear, concise directions and explanations about procedures to Gemma. Avoid presenting more information than she is able to deal with. Anxiety may interfere with her ability to understand what you are saying. *Explanations may need to be repeated frequently to Gemma.*

+ Include Gemma in care planning and decisions as appropriate, without making excessive demands. *Participating in decision-making increases Gemma's sense of control. Because high levels of anxiety interfere with the ability to make decisions, it is important to avoid placing demands on Gemma that may further increase her level of anxiety.*

+ Reduce excessive environmental stimuli, and remain calm. *This promotes rest.*

+ Allow supportive family members or friends to remain with Gemma. *Significant others provide additional support and can help reduce anxiety.*

+ Assist to use relaxation techniques, such as guided imagery, muscle relaxation and meditation. *These techniques help restore psychological balance and reduce sympathetic stimulation and responses.*

Gemma has neglected the treatment of her asthma

Once acute asthma is under control and effective respirations have been re-established, it is important to help the person identify contributing factors to the attack. This helps the person prevent future episodes.

+ Assess Gemma's level of understanding about her asthma and the prescribed treatment that she is on. Provide Gemma with additional information and teaching as indicated. *Assessment helps to identify and clarify misperceptions and difficulties with asthma management.*

+ Discuss Gemma's perception of her illness and its effect on her lifestyle. *Open discussion can help identify conflicts between Gemma's lifestyle and the treatment she is on.*

+ Assist to identify factors that contributed to the acute episode that Gemma suffered. *Identifying contributing factors increases will increase Gemma' awareness of the disease and strategies to prevent future exacerbations.*

+ Assist Gemma and significant friends and family to identify problems or difficulties integrating the treatment that she is on into her lifestyle *Asthma and its management may necessitate Gemma to modify her lifestyle to prevent acute exacerbations. This can significantly impact family members, for example eliminating cigarette smoking or pets from the household, removing carpets or daily damp-dusting to remove dust mites. Gemma needs to consider her working environment and the potential triggers around her.*

+ Assess Gemma's knowledge and understanding of prescribed medications and use of over-the-counter (OTC) preparations. *This is important to determine misperceptions or possible misuse of medications.*

+ Provide Gemma with verbal and written instructions. *Written instructions reinforce teaching and allow future reference.*

+ Refer Gemma to support groups or self-help organisations. *Support groups and self-help organisations can help Gemma adapt to living with asthma and the treatment that she is prescribed.*

COMMUNITY-BASED CARE

Asthma is a chronic disease that is best managed by the person with assistance from the specialist respiratory medical team. Teaching for home care focuses on promoting the highest level of wellness and preventing and managing acute episodes and exacerbations of the disease. Topics to include in teaching are as follows:

PREVENTIVE MEASURES
Asthma management aims to control the underlying disease process to support the management of persons' lives with least disruption.

Although specific measures to prevent asthma have not yet been identified, the link between parental smoking and childhood asthma is strong. Discuss this link with young people and families with children. Encourage all people to not start smoking and, if they do smoke, to quit. Provide referrals to smoking cessation clinics, help groups or a care provider for nicotine patches as needed to facilitate quitting.

ASTHMA MANAGEMENT
The most effective approach to asthma care is to work with the person towards common goals. Despite this, people continue to have poor asthma control and to accept unnecessary symptoms. There are two approaches to asthma treatment: *pharmacological* and *non-pharmacological.* When supporting people with asthma it is significant that they understand the combined importance of the two approaches, and support the notion of self-management of the disorder.

Pharmacological management of asthma in the UK follows the guidance of the British Thoracic Society and the Scottish Intercollegiate Guidelines Network (BTS/SIGN) (2011). Using 'Stepwise' people can be treated at the step most appropriate for the severity of their symptoms, stepping up

if the treatments are not effective, and stepping down as symptoms subside.

- Suggestions for lifestyle changes to avoid specific triggers for asthma attacks.
  - Warm up slowly before exercising in cold weather; wear a special mask or scarf to retain air warmth and humidity while exercising.
  - Substitute indoor exercises during cold, dry weather.
  - Reduce the risk for respiratory infections (e.g., adequate rest, good nutrition, and stress management to maintain immune function, yearly influenza vaccines and immunisation against pneumococcal pneumonia).
  - Use techniques to reduce or manage physical and psychological stress.
- Use of a PFR meter to monitor airway status; teach how to manage the disease based on results.
- Use of prescribed medications, including:
  - name, frequency, dose and desired effect;
  - potential adverse effects and their management, including effects to report to the physician;
  - potential interactions with other drugs (including OTC herbal preparations) or foods;
  - if tolerance is a potential risk, how to identify it and steps to take.
- Provide referrals to local or regional resources for further teaching and support as needed.
- Consider the need for home health services, home respiratory care services and others as needed.
- In primary care, people with asthma should be reviewed regularly by a nurse or doctor with appropriate training in asthma management. The review should incorporate a written action plan.

The person with chronic obstructive pulmonary disease (COPD)

People with chronic airflow obstruction due to chronic bronchitis and/or emphysema are said to have chronic obstructive pulmonary disease (COPD). An estimated three million people have COPD in the UK. Most people are not diagnosed until they are in their 50s.

Risk factors for COPD

Obstructive lung disease typically affects middle-aged and older adults. Cigarette smoking is clearly implicated as the primary cause of COPD. Even though COPD develops in a minority of smokers, smokers are 12–13 times more likely to die from COPD than non-smokers (NICE 2010). Cigarette

smoke and the irritants it contains impair ciliary movement, inhibit the function of alveolar macrophages and cause mucus-secreting glands to malfunction. It also produces emphysema or airway destruction and constricts smooth muscle, increasing airway resistance. Other contributing factors include air pollution, occupational exposure to noxious dusts and gases, airway infection and familial and genetic factors.

Pathophysiology of COPD

COPD is characterised by slowly progressive obstruction of the airways. The disease is one of periodic exacerbations, often related to respiratory infection, with increased symptoms of dyspnoea and sputum production. Unlike acute processes in which lung tissues recover, airways and lung tissue do not return to normal following an exacerbation; instead, they demonstrate progressive destructive changes.

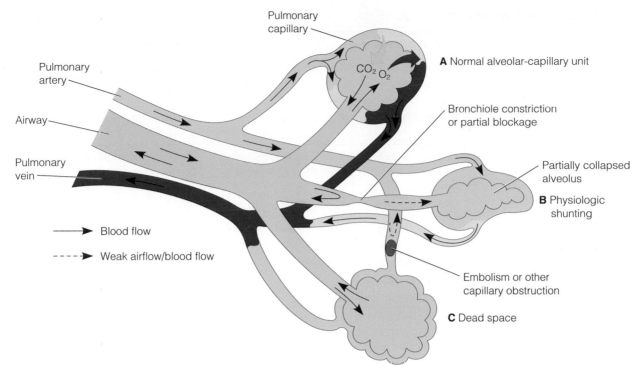

Figure 11.19 Ventilation–perfusion relationships.

Although one or the other may predominate, COPD typically includes components of both chronic bronchitis and emphysema, two distinctly different processes discussed below. Small airways disease, narrowing of small bronchioles, is also part of the COPD complex. Through different mechanisms, these processes cause airways to narrow, resistance to airflow to increase and expiration to become slow or difficult. The result is a mismatch between alveolar ventilation and blood flow or perfusion, leading to impaired gas exchange.

Chronic bronchitis

Chronic bronchitis is a disorder of excessive bronchial mucous secretion. It is characterised by a productive cough lasting three or more months in two consecutive years. Cigarette smoke is the major factor implicated in the development of chronic bronchitis. A smoking history of more than 20 pack years in people aged over 40 is significant (one pack year is the equivalent of smoking 20 cigarettes a day for one year).

Inhaled irritants lead to a chronic inflammatory process with vasodilatation, congestion and oedema of the bronchial mucosa. Goblet cells increase in size and number, and mucous glands enlarge. Thick, tenacious mucus is produced in increased amounts. Changes in bronchial squamous cells impair the ability to clear mucus. Narrowed airways and excess secretions obstruct airflow; expiration is affected first, then inspiration. Because ciliary function is impaired, normal defence mechanisms are unable to clear the mucus and any inhaled pathogens. Recurrent infection is common in people with chronic bronchitis (see Figure 11.19). An imbalance between ventilation and perfusion leads to hypoxaemia (low levels of oxygen in the blood), hypercapnia (high concent-

ration of carbon dioxide in the blood) and pulmonary hypertension. Pulmonary hypertension often leads to right sided heart failure.

Emphysema

Emphysema is characterised by destruction of the walls of the alveoli, with resulting enlargement of abnormal air spaces. As in chronic bronchitis, cigarette smoking is strongly implicated as a causative factor in most cases of emphysema. Deficiency of a_1-antitrypsin, an enzyme that normally inhibits the activity of proteolytic enzymes and tissue destruction in the lungs, contributes to the development of emphysema, especially when combined with exposure to cigarette smoke.

Inflammatory cells that collect in distal airway tissues appear to lead to destruction of elastic fibres in the respiratory bronchioles and alveolar ducts. Alveolar wall destruction causes alveoli and air spaces to enlarge with loss of corresponding portions of the pulmonary capillary bed. As a result, the surface area for alveolar-capillary diffusion is reduced, affecting gas exchange. Elastic recoil is lost, reducing the volume of air that is passively expired. The loss of support tissue also affects airways, increasing the risk of expiratory collapse and further air trapping. Anatomically, either respiratory bronchioles or alveoli may be the primary tissue involved.

To summarise, COPD is a progressive, non-reversible process of airway narrowing and loss of supporting tissue. Three separate processes typically are involved:

- Chronic bronchitis with persistent airway oedema, excessive mucous production and impaired airway clearance.

Table 11.4 Clinical features of COPD

	Feature	Chronic bronchitis	Emphysema
History	Onset	After age 35; recurrent respiratory infections.	After age 50; insidious progressive dyspnoea.
	Smoking	Usual.	Usual.
	Cough	Persistent, productive of copious mucus.	Absent or mild with scant clear sputum, if any.
Physical examination	Appearance	Often obese; oedematous and cyanotic; distended neck veins and other symptoms of right-sided heart failure.	Usually thin; barrel chest; prominent accessory muscles of respiration.
	Chest	Wheezing.	
Other features	Blood gases	Hypercapnia and hypoxaemia; respiratory acidosis.	Normal or mild hypoxaemia; normal pH.
	Pulmonary function studies	Normal or decreased total lung capacity; moderately increased residual volume.	Increased total lung capacity; markedly increased residual volume.
	Pulmonary hypertension	May be severe.	Only when advanced.

- Emphysema with loss of interstitial membranes and airway support tissue, resulting in airway collapse and loss of alveolar surface area for gas exchange.
- Small airways disease with bronchoconstriction.

The result of these processes and their combined effects is increased work of breathing, impaired expiration with air trapping and impaired gas exchange.

Signs and symptoms of COPD

The clinical presentation of COPD (see Table 11.4) varies from simple chronic bronchitis without disability to chronic respiratory failure and severe disability. Signs and symptoms are typically absent or minor early in the disease. When the person finally seeks care the following signs can be seen:

- Productive cough.
- Dyspnoea.
- Exercise intolerance which has often been present for as long as 10 years.
- The cough typically occurs in the mornings and is often attributed to 'smoker's cough.'
- Initially, dyspnoea occurs only on extreme exertion; as the disease progresses, dyspnoea becomes more severe and accompanies mild activity.
- Signs and symptoms characteristic of chronic bronchitis and emphysema develop.

INTERDISCIPLINARY CARE FOR COPD

NICE (2010) suggests that a diagnosis of COPD should be considered in people over the age of 35 who have a risk factor (commonly smoking), and who present with breathlessness on exertion, chronic cough, regular sputum production and winter bronchitis.

Although COPD can be prevented in most people, it cannot be cured. Smoking abstinence is the only certain way to prevent COPD and to slow its progression. To a certain extent, airway obstruction can be reversed and disability minimised early in the disease. Treatment generally focuses on relieving symptoms, minimising obstruction and slowing disability.

Assessment

Other assessment tools include the COPD Assessment Test (CAT). Current management guidelines – such as those produced by NICE (2010) and the Global Initiative for Chronic Obstructive Lung Disease (GOLD 2011) – emphasise the need for regular and effective person monitoring and assessment. The CAT has been developed in line with the goals of these guidelines, with the aim of making these tasks easier and less time-consuming.

IN PRACTICE

Medical Research Council Dyspnoea Scale

- Grade 1: 'I only get breathless with strenuous exercise'.
- Grade 2: 'I get short of breath when hurrying on the level or up a slight hill'.
- Grade 3: 'I walk slower than other people of the same age when walking at my own pace on the level, because of breathlessness'.
- Grade 4: 'I stop for breath after walking every 100 yards or after a few minutes on the level'.
- Grade 5: 'I am too breathless to leave the house, or I get breathless when I am dressing or undressing'.

Source: Fletcher *et al.* 1959.

The CAT measures the impact of COPD on a person's health status, in order to help address the fact that people with COPD tend to underestimate their condition and to improve the management of COPD. People are asked to score on a scale with opposing statements around an individual's limitation through breathlessness.

Management

Spirometry

Vital capacity of the lungs can be measured in two ways:

- slow vital capacity (SVC);
- forced vital capacity (FVC).

Another useful measurement is where the volume of air expired in the first second (FEV1) is measured. If a person has an obstructed airway, it will take them longer to exhale during the FVC manoeuvre. In affected people, the FEV1 will be reduced, and this defines the presence or absence of obstruction in the airways.

> **PRACTICE ALERT**
>
> Until recently, an FEV1 ratio of less that 70% was deemed to be indicative of obstructive lung disease. This practice has been challenged because normal values are affected by age, and the 70% cut off can over diagnose older and under-diagnose younger people.
>
> Source: NICE 2010.

Inhaled therapy

Inhaled therapy is the most common form of treatment in COPD. The most common delivery systems are inhalers, spacers and nebulisers. In all cases, person concordance is paramount and nurses are in a prime position to support correct inhaler technique. Most people can learn to use an inhaler unless they have a specific learning impairment (NICE 2010). If a person cannot use a particular device, another should be tried, and an opportunity for regular checking of technique is recommended.

Oxygen therapy

Long-term oxygen therapy is used for severe and progressive hypoxaemia. Oxygen therapy improves exercise tolerance, mental functioning and quality of life in advanced COPD. It also reduces the rate of hospitalisation and increases length of survival. Oxygen may be used intermittently, at night or continuously. For severely hypoxaemic people, the greatest benefit is seen with continuous oxygen. Home oxygen may be supplied as liquid oxygen, compressed gas cylinders or oxygen concentrators. An acute exacerbation of COPD may necessitate oxygenation and inspiratory positive-pressure assistance with a face mask or intubation and mechanical ventilation.

> **PRACTICE ALERT**
>
> Oxygen administered without intubation and mechanical ventilation requires caution: Administering oxygen to people with chronic elevated carbon dioxide levels in the blood can actually increase the $PaCO_2$, leading to increased fatigue and even respiratory failure.

The delivery of oxygen relies on individuals having a patent airway. A face mask is the most common way of delivering oxygen to an acutely breathless person. Masks vary and should be selected on the needs of the specific person. Simple face masks (used to deliver high concentrations of oxygen) fit over the mouth and nose and have open side ports that allow room air to mix with the oxygen inhaled and exhaled carbon dioxide to leave the contained space. Nasal cannula can be an effective means of delivering low-concentration oxygen (24–45%). The advantage of this method of oxygen therapy is the ease of speech and the ability to eat and drink (see Figure 11.20).

Partial rebreather masks have covered side ports with one-way discs to prevent room air from entering the mask, and can deliver 70–90% oxygen at a flow of 6–15 litres per minute. A soft plastic bag stores the first third of the person's exhaled air, and is designed to make use of carbon dioxide as a respiratory stimulant.

A non-rebreather oxygen mask is similar to a simple face mask but has one-way valves to prevent room air entering, but allow the flow of exhaled air. It too has a reservoir bag to store larger concentrations of oxygen and therefore deliver high concentrations of 90–100% oxygen at a flow of 15L per minute.

Venturi oxygen masks are similar to simple face masks but have an integrated valve that ensures specific mixes of oxygen and room air to deliver a fraction of inspired oxygen. In Table 11.5 you will see the number of litres of oxygen and the corresponding oxygen concentration delivered to the individual.

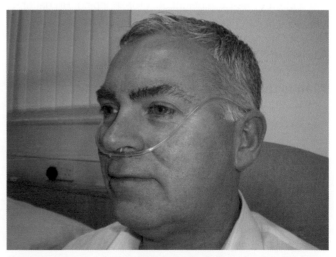

Figure 11.20 Person receiving oxygen via a nasal cannula.

Table 11.5 Flow rate and fraction of inspired oxygen (FiO₂) of different Venturi valves

Venturi valve colour	Flow rate (L min.)	FiO₂
Blue	2	24%
White	4	28%
Yellow	6	35%
Red	8	40%
Green	12	60%

Complementary therapies

Acupuncture may help the person with smoking cessation, and also has been used to treat asthma and other respiratory conditions. Hypnotherapy and guided imagery are used to assist with smoking cessation. These techniques can also help the person control anxiety and breathing patterns. Refer people to a trained professional. Breathing exercises are used to slow the respiratory rate and relieve accessory muscle fatigue. Pursed-lip breathing slows the respiratory rate and helps maintain open airways during exhalation by keeping positive pressure in the airways. Abdominal breathing relieves the work of accessory muscles of respiration.

Exercise

Unless disabling cardiac disease is present, a regular exercise programme is beneficial for:

- improving exercise tolerance;

- enhancing ability to perform ADLs;
- preventing deterioration of physical condition.

A programme of regular aerobic exercise (for example, walking for 20 minutes at least three times weekly) designed to gradually increase exercise tolerance is recommended. Activities that strengthen the muscles used for breathing and ADLs, such as swimming and walking, are also beneficial.

Education

As with any chronic disease, the person and family will have primary responsibility for disease management. Teaching is vital to promote optimal health and slow disease progression. Teaching for home care focuses on effective coughing and breathing techniques, preventing exacerbations and managing prescribed therapies.

Pulmonary rehabilitation

Pulmonary rehabilitation is an organised programme of exercise and education over a period of six to eight weeks. It is an evidence-based therapy of proven benefit for people with COPD in terms of increasing exercise tolerance and improving health-related quality of life. The success of pulmonary rehabilitation is attributed to the multidisciplinary approach to exercise and education, which aims to address both the physical and psychological limitations experienced by people with COPD. The BTS guidelines (BTS/SIGN 2011) state that pulmonary rehabilitation should be available to all people who consider themselves disabled by their lung disease.

Case Study 3 – Alan
NURSING CARE PLAN The person with COPD

Remember Alan Hoyle from the start of the chapter? He's a long-term cigarette smoker who's been diagnosed with COPD. He struggles to stick at his medication and has a drawer full of part-used inhalers. You will recall that he lives alone and relies on the support of his close neighbours for shopping. His daughter visits a couple of times a week to make sure that he is OK and to take care of his hygiene needs. Below is a care plan based on Alan's needs.

Alan is thin and appears malnourished

With advanced COPD, minimal activity, including eating, can cause fatigue and dyspnoea. Alan may be unable to consume a full meal without resting. At the same time, the increased work of breathing increases metabolic demands, and more calories are required. Alan may appear cachectic (thin and wasted). Poor nutritional status further impairs immune function and increases the risk of a complicating infection.

- Assess Alan's nutritional status, including diet history, weight for height (body mass index). *It is important to differentiate*

nutritional status from body type rather than assume a nutritional impairment.

- Observe and document Alan's food intake, including types, amounts and calorific intake. *This information can provide direction for supplementation of Alan's diet, if needed.*

- Monitor laboratory values, including serum albumin and electrolyte levels. *These values provide information about the adequacy of nutritional intake, including protein.*

- Consult with a dietitian to plan meals for Alan and nutritional supplements that meet calorific needs. *More concentrated sources of high-energy foods may be required to maintain calorific intake without excess fatigue. A diet high in proteins and fats without excess carbohydrates is recommended to minimise carbon dioxide production during metabolism (carbohydrates are metabolised to form CO₂ and water).*

- Encourage Alan to eat frequent, small snacks between meals to help maintain calorie intake and reduce fatigue associated with eating.

NURSING CARE PLAN The person with COPD (continued)

+ Advise Alan to eat whilst seated. *An upright position promotes lung expansion and reduces dyspnoea.*

+ Assist Alan to choose preferred foods. *Providing preferred foods encourages eating.*

Alan's family are finding it difficult to cope

Chronic illness affects the entire family structure. Roles and relationships change; additional demands are placed on the family. Family members may blame the person for causing the illness or have distorted perceptions about it, even denying its existence. They may refuse to assist or participate in care. The person may develop an attitude of helplessness or dependence or may demonstrate anger, hostility or aggression.

+ Assess interactions between Alan and his daughter. *To identify desired and potential destructive behaviours.*

+ Help Alan and his daughter identify strengths for coping with the situation. *To help the family regain a sense of control.*

+ Provide information to Alan and his daughter about COPD. *To help the family gain an understanding of the person's condition and needs.*

+ Encourage Alan to express his feelings. Avoid judging feelings expressed or family members as 'good' or 'bad', 'right' or 'wrong'. *The nurse must remain objective to maintain the therapeutic relationship.*

+ Help Alan's family members recognise behaviours and attitudes that may hinder effective treatment, such as continuing to smoke in the house. *Family members may be unaware of the effect of their behaviour on Alan's ability to change habits and cope with a disabling disease.*

+ Encourage Alan's family members to participate in care. *This helps develop skills for use at home.*

+ Discuss Alan's care with the wider healthcare team. Consider referral to the specialist respiratory nurse. *A wide range of perspectives and areas of expertise aids in problem-solving and facilitates communication.*

+ Refer Alan to support groups and pulmonary rehabilitation programmes, as available. *To enhance coping abilities.*

+ Arrange a social services assessment. *This can help Alan and his family identify care and support service needs. Agencies or community services can provide additional support beyond the family's means or capability.*

Alan is a smoker

Smoking is more than a habit; it is an addiction. The person who must quit is facing a significant loss, not only of nicotine but also of a lifestyle. Although the person may fully comprehend the consequences of continuing to smoke, the decision to give up a part of his or her life is not easy. This fear may be expressed in such concerns as 'I'll gain weight' or 'What will I do with my hands?' In addition to providing practical information, a plan and assistance with nicotine withdrawal, the nurse must support the person's decision-making process to comply with an order to stop smoking.

+ Assess Alan's knowledge and understanding of the choices involved and possible consequences of each. *The decision to quit smoking ultimately belongs to the person. Alan needs a full understanding of the consequences of quitting or continuing to smoke.*

+ Acknowledge concerns, values and beliefs; listen non-judgementally. *The nurse needs to avoid imposing his or her values and beliefs about smoking on Alan.*

+ Spend time with Alan, encouraging expression of feelings. *This demonstrates acceptance of him and his right to make the decision.*

+ Help Alan plan a course of action for quitting smoking and adapt it as necessary. *When the person develops the plan, he has more ownership in it and interest in making it work.*

+ Demonstrate respect for decisions that Alan makes and the right to choose. *Respect supports self-esteem and the ability to cope.*

+ Provide referral to a counsellor or other professional as needed. *Counsellors or other people trained to assist with smoking cessation can help with decision-making. (Smoking cessation is discussed in more detail in Chapter 9.)*

The person with pulmonary embolism

A **pulmonary embolism** (or *thromboembolism*) is obstruction of blood flow in part of the pulmonary vascular system by an embolus. Thromboemboli, or blood clots, that develop in the venous system (deep venous thrombosis or DVT) or right side of the heart are the most frequent cause of pulmonary embolism. Other sources of emboli include tumours that have invaded venous circulation, fat or bone marrow entering the circulation due to fracture or other trauma, amniotic fluid released into the circulation during childbirth and intravenous injection of air or other foreign substances.

Pulmonary embolism is a medical emergency. Fifty percent of deaths from pulmonary embolism occur within the first two hours following embolisation. In many cases, DVT has not been recognised or treated; often embolisation also goes undetected. Prevention is the most effective treatment strategy for pulmonary embolism.

Risk factors for pulmonary embolism

Although many substances can become emboli, thrombus arising from the deep veins of the legs is the leading cause of pulmonary embolism. The risk factors for pulmonary embolus are those for DVT: stasis of venous blood flow, vessel wall damage and altered blood coagulation. Risk factors for DVT are prolonged immobility; trauma, including hip and femur fractures; surgery (orthopaedic, pelvic and gynaecologic surgery in particular); myocardial infarction and heart failure; obesity; and advanced age. Women who use oral contraceptives or oestrogen therapy are at risk, as are women during pregnancy and childbirth.

Pathophysiology of pulmonary embolism

The impact of a pulmonary embolus depends on the extent to which pulmonary blood flow is obstructed, the size of the embolus, its nature and secondary effects of the obstruction. The effects can range widely:

- Occlusion of a large pulmonary artery with the result of sudden death. Gas exchange is significantly reduced or prevented, and cardiac output falls dramatically as blood fails to move through the pulmonary vascular system and return to the left heart.
- Lung tissue infarction due to occlusion of a significant portion of pulmonary blood flow. Fewer than 10% of pulmonary emboli result in pulmonary infarction.
- Obstruction of a small segment of the pulmonary circulation with no permanent lung injury.
- Chronic or recurrent, possibly multiple, small emboli with recurring symptoms.

Fat emboli are the most common non-thrombotic pulmonary emboli. A fat embolism usually occurs after fracture of long bone (typically the femur) releases bone marrow fat into the circulation. Adipose tissue or liver trauma may also lead to fat emboli.

Signs and symptoms of pulmonary embolism

Signs and symptoms of pulmonary embolism

- depend on size and location. Small emboli may be asymptomatic.
- Emboli usually develop abruptly, over a period of minutes.
- The most common symptoms are dyspnoea and pleuritic chest pain.
- Anxiety, a sense of impending doom and cough are also common.
- Diaphoresis and haemoptysis may develop.
- Massive pulmonary embolus can cause syncope and cyanosis.
- Tachycardia and tachypnoea are present.
- Crackles may be heard on auscultation of the chest.
- A low-grade pyrexia may develop.

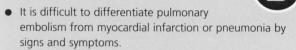

PRACTICE ALERT

- It is difficult to differentiate pulmonary embolism from myocardial infarction or pneumonia by signs and symptoms.
- Because DVT may not be identified until pulmonary embolism occurs, prevention is the primary goal in treating pulmonary embolism.

INTERDISCIPLINARY CARE FOR PULMONARY EMBOLISM

Early mobility of individuals is an effective way of preventing venous stasis and reducing the incidence of pulmonary embolism. External compression of the legs with anti-embolic stockings is also effective for people undergoing neurosurgery, urologic surgery or major surgery of the hip or knee, or when anticoagulant therapy is contraindicated. Other preventive measures include elevating the legs and active and passive leg exercises.

Medication

Anticoagulant therapy is the standard treatment to prevent pulmonary emboli. It is often instituted in high-risk individuals who have no evidence of pulmonary embolism, to prevent possible devastating effects. In the person with DVT or a pulmonary embolus, anticoagulants are administered to prevent further clotting and embolism. For pulmonary embolus, heparin therapy is typically continued for about five days or until oral anticoagulant therapy has become fully effective.

PRACTICE ALERT

Bleeding is a risk associated with anticoagulant therapy. Although major haemorrhage is uncommon, it occurs in approximately 5% of people receiving intravenous heparin. Cardiac, hepatic and renal disease increase the risk of significant bleeding, as does age over 60 years. Protamine, a protein that combines with heparin to inactivate it, is used to stop its anticoagulant effect if major bleeding occurs. Vitamin K is given to treat bleeding associated with anticoagulant therapy.

NURSING CARE FOR PULMONARY EMBOLISM

Health promotion

Nurses are key in preventing pulmonary embolism. Encouraging people to ambulate after surgery or illness, applying compression stockings or pneumatic compression devices, teaching and encouraging leg exercises, discouraging the use of pillows under the knees – all of these measures help prevent DVT and subsequent pulmonary emboli.

Teach individuals to reduce the risks associated with long periods of immobility, stopping every one to two hours during long automobile trips for a brief stretch and walk, getting up every hour or so and doing leg exercises while seated during long flights, and avoiding crossing the legs to prevent venous stasis and pooling. Regular exercise such as walking also reduces the risk of DVT. Instruct people who stand for long periods to use well-fitted elastic stockings, being careful to avoid hose that bind around the knee or thigh.

COMMUNITY-BASED CARE

Discuss the following topics when preparing the person with pulmonary embolism and family members for home care:

- Use of prescribed anticoagulant, including drug interactions, scheduled laboratory testing and manifestations of bleeding to report to the GP.
- Using a soft toothbrush and electric shaver to reduce the risk of bleeding.
- Avoiding aspirin (unless prescribed) and other OTC medications unless approved by the physician.
- Importance of wearing a MedicAlert tag for anticoagulant use.
- Health promotion measures to reduce the risk of recurrent pulmonary embolism.
- Symptoms of recurrent pulmonary embolism, such as sudden chest pain, shortness of breath and possibly bloody sputum need immediate attention.

The person with acute respiratory failure

Many of the conditions discussed in this chapter and in this book, from pneumonia to acute respiratory distress syndrome, can lead to respiratory failure. In respiratory failure, the lungs are unable to oxygenate the blood and remove carbon dioxide adequately to meet the body's needs, even at rest.

Respiratory failure is not a disease but a consequence of severe respiratory dysfunction. It is often defined by arterial blood gas (ABG) values. An arterial oxygen level (PaO_2) of less than 50–60 mmHg and an arterial carbon dioxide level ($PaCO_2$) of greater than 50 mmHg are generally accepted as indicators of respiratory failure. However, people with advanced COPD may be alert and functional with blood gas values that would indicate respiratory failure in someone whose respiratory function was previously normal. In people with COPD, respiratory failure is indicated by an acute drop in blood oxygen levels along with increased carbon dioxide levels.

Respiratory failure can result from inadequate alveolar ventilation (hypoventilation), impaired gas exchange, or a significant ventilation–perfusion mismatch. COPD is the most common cause of respiratory failure. Other lung diseases, chest injury, inhalation trauma, neuromuscular problems and cardiac conditions can also lead to respiratory failure.

Signs and symptoms of acute respiratory failure

Signs and symptoms of acute respiratory failure include:

- hypoxaemia and hypercapnia;
- hypoxaemia causes dyspnoea and neurologic symptoms such as restlessness, apprehension, impaired judgement and motor impairment;
- tachycardia and hypertension develop as the cardiac output increases in an effort to bring more oxygen to the tissues;
- cyanosis is present;
- as hypoxaemia progresses, dysrhythmias, hypotension and decreased cardiac output may develop.

Pathophysiology of acute respiratory failure

Increased carbon dioxide levels depress CNS function and cause vasodilation. Dyspnoea and headache are early signs. Other manifestations include peripheral and conjunctival vasodilation, papilloedema, neuromuscular irritability and decreased LOC. As hypercapnia worsens, the respiratory centre may be depressed, reducing dyspnoea and slowing respirations. Increased carbon dioxide and hydrogen ion concentrations no longer stimulate the respiratory centre; hypoxaemia provides the primary active breathing stimulus. Administering oxygen without ventilatory support may further reduce the drive to breathe, leading to respiratory arrest.

FAST FACTS

Ventilatory support

- Non-invasive ventilation (NIV) refers to the provision of ventilatory support through the upper airway using a mask or similar device.
- Invasive ventilation – the upper airway is bypassed by laryngeal mask, endo-tracheal tube or a tracheostomy is used (intubation).

Medication

Drugs used in treating respiratory failure depend on the underlying cause of the failure and the need for intubation and mechanical ventilation.

Sedation and analgesia are often required during mechanical ventilation to decrease pain and anxiety. Benzodiazepines such as diazepam (Valium) or lorazepam (Ativan) may be used for sedation and to inhibit the respiratory drive. Intravenous morphine or fentanyl provides analgesia and also inhibits the respiratory drive, allowing more effective mechanical ventilation.

Oxygen therapy

Oxygen is administered to reverse hypoxaemia in acute respiratory failure. In general, the goal is to achieve an oxygen saturation of 90% or greater without oxygen toxicity. A PaO_2 of about 60 mm Hg is usually adequate to meet the oxygen needs of body tissues. When respiratory failure is caused by hypoventilation or usual oxygen delivery systems do not correct hypoxaemia, a tight-fitting mask to maintain *continuous positive airway pressure* (CPAP) may be used. CPAP increases lung volume, opening previously closed alveoli, improving ventilation of underventilated alveoli and improving ventilation–perfusion relationships.

Airway management

If the upper airway is obstructed or positive-pressure mechanical ventilation is necessary to correct hypoxaemia and hypercapnia, an endotracheal tube that extends from the mouth or nose into the trachea is inserted. To maintain positive-pressure ventilation, the tube is cuffed with an air-filled or foam sac just above the end of the tube. When the cuff is inflated, it obstructs the upper airway, preventing air from escaping back into the nose or mouth. Excess pressure of the cuff can cause tissue ischaemia and necrosis of the trachea. To minimise this risk, high-volume, low-pressure ('floppy') cuffs are used. Tubes with low-pressure cuffs may be left in place for three to four weeks (Figure 11.21).

A tracheostomy may be performed if long-term ventilatory support is required. Although a tracheostomy is more comfortable and easier to secure in place, complications such as cuff necrosis and increased risk of infection are associated with tracheostomy as well as endotracheal intubation.

When the person is able to maintain effective respirations and ventilatory support is no longer required, the endotracheal tube is removed (*extubation*). Gag, cough and swallow reflexes must be intact to prevent aspiration. After oxygenation and suctioning, the cuff is deflated and the tube removed. Humidified oxygen is provided immediately following removal. Close observation for respiratory distress is vital following extubation. Sore throat and a hoarse voice are common after extubation. Oral intake is reinitiated slowly, with careful assessment of swallowing.

Non-invasive ventilation (NIV) provides ventilator support using a tight-fitting face mask, thus avoiding intubation. Its primary use is to support people with obstructive sleep apnoea, neuromuscular disease or impending respiratory failure (for example, advanced COPD). NIV may also be used for people in respiratory failure who refuse intubation. NIV tends to be more successful in people without significant underlying lung disease (for example, respiratory failure related to neuromuscular disease).

Acute respiratory failure resulting from an acute event such as pneumonia or near-drowning often resolves with few long-term complications. When respiratory failure results from an underlying disease such as COPD, the prognosis is less optimistic. People with end-stage COPD may have repeated episodes of respiratory failure, with a gradual loss of respiratory function and reserve.

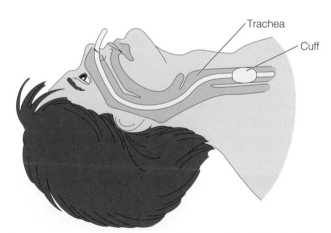

Figure 11.21 Nasal endotracheal (nasotracheal) intubation.

CASE STUDY SUMMARIES

Three case studies have been presented within this chapter to illustrate the care of people with respiratory problems. The first part of the chapter focused on nursing people with problems of ventilation. Jim, aged 58, was admitted to hospital with a diagnosis of right lower lobe pneumonia caused by a bacterial infection.

In the second part of the chapter, the focus shifted to the care of people with gas exchange problems and here you can gain an insight into the care of Gemma aged 24 who has an acute asthma attack. In addition, this part of the chapter gives a more detailed account of the care of Alan, a 74-year-old man who has neglected his medications for long-term COPD.

Case Study 1. Sputum cultures confirmed bacterial infection as the cause of Jim's pneumonia. He was discharged home three days following admission with information on the importance of completing the course of prescribed antibiotics. Jim was given advice on the link between his smoking and his increased risk of respiratory infection and on the importance of engaging in moderate exercise to promote lung expansion.

Case Study 2. Gemma was admitted to hospital suffering an acute asthma attack. With her acute asthma under control and effective respiration established, focus shifted to supporting Gemma in managing her asthma and its impact on her lifestyle. Discussions centred on identifying lifestyle elements which could contribute to exacerbating Gemma's asthma, ensuring that Gemma understands how to use her medications and referral to support or self-help groups.

Case Study 3. Alan has a diagnosis of COPD and lives alone and his chronic illness impacts on his family and neighbours. COPD is associated with poor nutritional status so input

from the dietician was instigated with a view to planning meals and nutritional supplements for Alan and advising him on strategies to improve his calorie intake. Alan and his family were offered support in coping with the emotional and practical demands placed upon them by his illness. A social services assessment identified needs and support services resources and referrals made to support groups and pulmonary rehabilitation programmes. Alan was given advice concerning the impact of smoking on his illness and support given in making and maintaining a decision to stop smoking.

CHAPTER HIGHLIGHTS

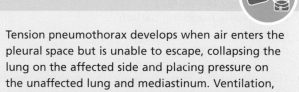

- All human cells require oxygen and it is the function of the respiratory system to carry oxygen throughout the body. As cells use oxygen, carbon dioxide (a waste gas) is produced and the transportation and elimination of carbon dioxide is a key feature of the respiratory system. Breathing is a physical process by which living organisms take in oxygen from the surrounding medium and emit carbon dioxide. The term *respiration* is used to refer to breathing.

- Respiration involves four distinct physiological processes. *Pulmonary ventilation* where air is moved into and out of the lungs. *External respiration*: where the exchange of oxygen and carbon dioxide occurs between the alveoli and the blood. *Gas transport*: Oxygen and carbon dioxide are transported to and from the lungs and the cells of the body via the blood. *Internal respiration*: the exchange of oxygen and carbon dioxide is made between the blood and the cells.

- Lower respiratory problems can affect the way that air moves in and out of the lungs. In general, there are two ways in which these problems can affect the individual. First, in relation to the ability to maintain clear and patent airways to fully ventilate the lungs, and second, the ability to effectively maintain gas exchange for effective respiration.

- Pneumonia, inflammation of the respiratory bronchioles and alveoli, usually is bacterial in origin. Different organisms are usually found in hospital-acquired pneumonia than in community-acquired pneumonia. Nursing care focuses on promoting airway clearance, supporting effective gas exchange and promoting rest.

- Infection control measures, including standard, airborne and contact precautions, are vital to prevent the spread of infection.

- Effective tuberculosis treatment is a public health concern, requiring therapy and compliance monitoring, contact follow-up, and assessment for adverse treatment effects.

- Tension pneumothorax develops when air enters the pleural space but is unable to escape, collapsing the lung on the affected side and placing pressure on the unaffected lung and mediastinum. Ventilation, gas exchange, venous return and cardiac output can be significantly affected.

- In an acute asthma attack, inflammatory mediators are released from sensitised airways followed by activation of inflammatory cells. These events lead to bronchoconstriction, airway oedema and impaired mucociliary clearance. Airway narrowing limits airflow and increases the work of breathing; trapped air mixes with inhaled air, impairing gas exchange.

- COPD is a progressive, non-reversible process of airway narrowing and loss of supporting tissue. Three separate processes typically are involved:
  - Chronic bronchitis with persistent airway oedema, excessive mucous production and impaired airway clearance
  - Emphysema with loss of interstitial membranes and airway support tissue, resulting in airway collapse and loss of alveolar surface area for gas exchange
  - Small airways disease with bronchoconstriction.

  The result of these processes and their combined effects is increased work of breathing, impaired expiration with air trapping and impaired gas exchange.

- Pulmonary embolism is a medical emergency. Fifty per cent of deaths from pulmonary embolism occur within the first 2 hours following embolisation. In many cases, DVT has not been recognised or treated; often embolisation also goes undetected. Prevention is the most effective treatment strategy for pulmonary embolism.

- Trauma may affect the chest wall (rib fracture, **flail chest**), the surface of the lungs (pulmonary contusion), or the airways and alveoli (smoke inhalation and near-drowning). Chest trauma (chest wall or airways) can endanger effective ventilation and gas exchange.

TEST YOURSELF

1. Where is the apex of each lung located?
   a. in the mediastinum
   b. resting on the diaphragm
   c. within the parietal pleura
   d. just below the clavicle

2. Which of the following does the nurse identify as of highest priority for a person with tension pneumothorax?
   a. decreased cardiac output
   b. ineffective breathing pattern
   c. acute pain
   d. risk for aspiration

3. The older adult is prone to respiratory problems due to which age-related changes in the respiratory system? (Select all that apply.)
   a. loss of skeletal muscle strength in the thorax
   b. increased elastic recoil of lungs during expiration
   c. alveoli that are less elastic and more fibrotic
   d. decreased residual volume of lung
   e. decreased effectiveness of coughing

4. Which of the following is true in relation to pneumonia:
   a. community- and hospital-acquired pneumonia are the same thing
   b. the most common cause is *Streptococcus pneumoniae* bacteria
   c. smoking is not a risk factor for pneumonia
   d. pneumonia is never associated with pleuritic pain

5. Which are early signs and symptoms of pulmonary tuberculosis?
   a. tachypnoea, tachycardia, activity intolerance
   b. bradypnoea, foul-smelling sputum, weight gain
   c. blood-tinged sputum, high-grade fever, fatigue
   d. low-grade fever, night sweats, dry cough

6. What colour sputum would most likely indicate acute bronchitis?
   a. clear
   b. rust
   c. white
   d. pink and frothy

7. The presence of air in the pleural space is known as:
   a. haemothorax
   b. pneumothorax
   c. pleuritis
   d. pleural effusion

8. Which of the following statements regarding COPD is false?
   a. COPD is an umbrella term for emphysema and chronic bronchitis
   b. the main cause of COPD is smoking
   c. a person with COPD will have an FEV1 of 80% or higher
   d. wherever possible COPD people should be cared for at home

9. Tracheal deviation may indicate that a person has
   a. asthma
   b. a pneumothorax
   c. anaphylaxis
   d. emphysema

10. What does the abbreviation FEV1 mean?
    a. fixed expiratory volume in one second
    b. forced expiratory volume in one second
    c. forced expiratory value
    d. failed expiratory value

Further resources

British Thoracic Society (BTS)
www.brit-thoracic.org.uk
Aims to improve the care offered to those people suffering from respiratory disease. It provides up-to-date resources for people, carers and professionals.

Global Initiative for Obstructive Lung Disease (GOLD)
www.goldcopd.com
Works with people and healthcare professionals to raise the profile of COPD worldwide.

Education for Health
www.nrtc-usa.org
Founded in the UK in 1986, offers training and development to professionals working in respiratory care.

National Institute for Health and Clinical Excellence (NICE)
www.nice.org.uk
Provides guidance, sets quality standards and manages a national database to improve people's health and prevent and treat ill health. There are many excellent resources on this website that can help guide and inform practice.

British Lung Foundation (BLF)
www.lunguk.org
UK charity offering support for people with lung disease.

Cancer Research UK
www.cancerresearchuk.org
Cancer information for everyone. Up-to-date research and support for people, carers and healthcare professionals.

Bibliography

Asthma UK (2004) *Where do we Stand? Asthma in the UK Today*, London, Asthma UK.

BTS (2000) *Control and Prevention of Tuberculosis in the United Kingdom: Code of Practice 2000*. London, British Thoracic Society.

BTS (2006) *Burden of Lung Disease* (2nd edn). London, British Thoracic Society.

BTS/SIGN (2011) *British Guideline on the Management of Asthma. A National Clinical Guideline*, revised edition. Edinburgh, Scottish Intercollegiate Guidelines Network, available at: http://www.sign.ac.uk/pdf/sign101.pdf (accessed September 2011).

BTS, Royal College of Nursing TB Forum, All Party Parliamentary group on Global TB (2009) *Turning UK TB Policy into Action: The view from the frontline*. London, British Thoracic Society, available at: http://www.appg-tb.org.uk/documents/RCN_APPG_BTS_report_final.pdf (accessed September 2011).

Cancer Research UK (2010) *Mesothelioma Statistics – Key Facts*. London, available at: http://info.cancerresearchuk.org/cancerstats/types/Mesothelioma/ (accessed September 2011).

Cancer Research UK (2011a) *Mortality UK: UK Lung Cancer Incidence Statistics*. London, available at: http://info.cancerresearchuk.org/cancerstats/types/lung/incidence (accessed September 2011).

Cancer Research UK (2011b) *Lung Cancer Stages*. London, available at: http://cancerhelp.cancerresearchuk.org/type/lung-cancer/treatment/lung-cancer-staging (accessed September 2011).

Doll (2007) *Tuberculosis Prevention and Treatment: A toolkit for planning, commissioning and delivering high quality services in England*. London, Department of Health.

European Respiratory Society and European Lung Foundation (2003) *European Lung White Book. The First Comprehensive Survey on Respiratory Health in Europe*. Huddersfield, The Charlesworth Group.

Fletcher C M, Elmes P C, Fairbairn M B *et al.* (1959) The significance of respiratory symptoms and the diagnosis of chronic bronchitis in a working population. *British Medical Journal*, 2, 257–266.

Francis C (2006) *Respiratory Care*. Oxford, Blackwell.

GOLD (2011) *Teaching Slide Kit*. Global Initiative for Chronic Obstructive Lung Disease. Available at: http://www.goldcopd.org/other-resources-gold-teaching-slide-set.html (accessed September 2011).

Healthcare Commission (2006) *Clearing the Air: A national study of chronic obstructive pulmonary disease*. London, Healthcare Commission.

Hoare Z and Lim W S (2006) Pneumonia: Update on diagnosis and management. *British Medical Journal*, **332**, 1077–1079.

HPA (2010) *Enhanced Surveillance of Tuberculosis*. London, Health Protection Agency, available at: http://www.hpa.org.uk/web/HPAweb&Page&HPAwebAutoListName/Page/1294739536811 (accessed September 2011).

HPA (2011) *Surveillance of Influenza and Other Respiratory Viruses in the UK: 2010–2011 Report*. London, Health Protection Agency.

ICS (2008) *Standards for the Care of Adult Patients with Temporary Tracheostomy*. London, Intensive Care Society.

Kennedy S (2007) Detecting changes in the respiratory status of ward people. *Nursing Standard*, **21**(49), 42–46.

Laws D, Neville E and Duffy J (2003) British Thoracic Society Guidelines for the insertion of an intrapleural drain. *Thorax*, **58**, 53–59.

Lawson L and Henneter D L (2010) *Medicines Management in Adult Nursing*. Exeter, Learning Matters Ltd.

Moore S (2004a) Guidelines on the role of the specialist nurse in supporting people with lung cancer. *European Journal of Cancer Care*, **13**(4), 344–348.

Moore T (2004b) Respiratory assessment. In Moore T and Woodrow P (eds), *High Dependency Nursing Care: Observation, intervention and support*. London, Routledge, 135–145.

NAC (2001) *National Asthma Audit*. London, National Asthma Campaign.

Nair M and Peate I (2009) *Fundamentals of Applied Physiology. An essential guide for nursing students*. Chichester, Wiley-Blackwell.

NHS QIS (2008) *Management of Lung Cancer Services*. Edinburgh, NHS Quality Improvement Scotland.

NICE (2005) *Lung Cancer: Diagnosis and treatment*, CG24. London, National Institute for Health and Clinical Excellence.

NICE (2006) *Tuberculosis: Clinical diagnosis and management of tuberculosis, and measures for its prevention and control*, CG33. London, National Institute for Health and Clinical Excellence.

NICE (2008) *Respiratory Tract Infections – Antibiotic prescribing: Prescribing of antibiotics for self-limiting respiratory tract infections in adults and children in primary care*, CG69. London, National Institute for Health and Clinical Excellence.

NICE (2010) *Chronic Obstructive Pulmonary Disease. Management of chronic obstructive pulmonary disease in adults in primary and secondary care*, update of CG12. London, National Institute for Health and Clinical Excellence.

NICE (2011) *Chronic Obstructive Pulmonary Disease Quality Standard*. London, National Institute for Health and Clinical Excellence.

Porth C (2009) *Pathophysiology: Concepts of altered health states*. Philadelphia, PA, Lippincott.

Pratt R J, Grange J M and Williams V G (2005) *Tuberculosis: A Foundation for nursing and health care practice*. London, Hodder Arnold.

Price D, Foster J, Scullion J and Freeman D (2004) *Asthma and COPD*. London, Churchill Livingstone.

Reis A L, Carlin B W, Carrieri-Kohlman V *et al.* (1997) Pulmonary rehabilitation: joint ACCP/AACVPR evidence-based guidelines. *Chest*, **112**, 1363–1396.

Scullion J (2005) A proactive approach to asthma. *Nursing Standard*, **20**(9), 57–65.

Scullion J (2007) *Fundamental Aspects of Nursing Adults with Respiratory Problems*. London, Quay Books.

Yorke J and Russell A-M (2008) Interpreting the language of breathlessness. *Nursing Times*, **104**(23), 36–39.

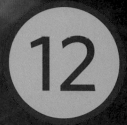

12

Caring for people with musculoskeletal problems

Learning objectives

- Describe the anatomy, physiology and functions of the musculoskeletal system.

- Examine how trauma and damage through normal wear and tear to this system affects mobility and function, restricting and disrupting life.

- Examine the effects of genetic and autoimmune diseases, metabolic diseases and infections have on the musculoskeletal system.

- Explain the principles of management and care of people affected by altered function to this system.

Clinical competencies

- Assess the nursing needs of people who have sustained traumatic injury or who have developed problems related to mobility and function disorders arising from disease in the musculoskeletal system.

- Use evidence-based research to plan and implement nursing care for people with skeletal injuries and disorders.

- Provide teaching appropriate for prevention of further injury and self-care of traumatic injuries of the musculoskeletal system.

- Evaluate and monitor the person's needs, providing advice on rehabilitation or adaption of lifestyle to manage their situation.

CASE STUDIES

Below are three case studies that you may wish to consider before, during or after you have read the chapter. There are no right or wrong answers to these case studies, but you should think about the physical, psychological and social implications.

Case Study 1 – Stephen

Mr Stephen Jones is 18 years old and has recently acquired a motorbike. He has been involved in a road traffic accident involving no other vehicles; however, the road was wet following a heavy burst of rain and he has sustained a fractured femur and dislocated his shoulder. He was just about to sit his school exams and planned a gap year before starting university. He is extremely popular, with a large circle of friends and has been captain of the school soccer team.

Case Study 2 – Joy

Mrs Joy Dennis is 58 years old, divorced with two adult children and has already gone through the menopause; she has worked in a solicitor's office for a number of years and does not exercise regularly. Her pastimes are sedentary: reading, sewing and doing crosswords. She enjoys dining out and usually has a glass or two of wine with her meals and maybe another when she returns home. She slips on wet pavement and fractures her wrist. X-rays suggest that there is thinning of the bone density.

Case Study 3 – Ben

Mr Ben Brown, aged 70 years, moved to England from the Caribbean as a young man. He now lives alone in an upstairs flat and does not venture out much. He worked shifts, including night shifts, on the London Underground network and, as a consequence, his type 2 diabetes was poorly controlled as his daily routines and mealtimes were constantly changing. He also had a tendency to snack between meals. He has suffered with leg ulcers in the past and now presents with gangrenous toes. The only course of treatment is a below knee **amputation**.

INTRODUCTION

Orthopaedic nursing was one of the first specialist nursing roles developed in the UK. The first specialist certificates were awarded in 1918 by Dame Agnes Hunt, the first nurse to specialise in and develop this field of care, opening a home for crippled children in 1907 in Shropshire. Development in this area has been driven following treatment of injuries received by people involved in the trauma of war, Dame Agnes Hunt being given a Red Cross Insignia for her contribution, and this continues through to this day. Although we have not experienced another world war since the 1940s, there are wars throughout the world involving many people who are subsequently repatriated to the UK for treatment. Traumatic injury can occur at any time and trauma may result from a fairly innocuous event, like slipping over on wet grass, or from a major one, as in a motorcycle accident or car crash. Many people engage in sport to maintain their health; unfortunately, this can lead to injury and A&E departments deal with many persons presenting with injuries which may be just **sprains** and **strains**, but may also involve **fractures** of the bone. Injuries may heal over time, and normal function may be resumed; however, some injuries may result in major surgery such as amputation which can lead to alterations in lifestyle.

FAST FACTS

Motorcycle accidents

- Motorcycle accidents:
  - occur in young inexperienced riders; or
  - older experienced riders on more powerful bikes.
- The main causes of accidents are:
  - car drivers who do not look properly at junctions (these are referred to as 'right of way' accidents);
  - motorcyclists losing control on bends;
  - motorcyclists taking more risks when overtaking and passing other vehicles.
- The number of motorcyclists killed or seriously injured in accidents is double that of pedal cyclists and 16 times more than car drivers.
- Motorcyclists represent less than 1% of road traffic, but account for 14% of road traffic accidents.
- Men are seven times more likely to ride a motorbike than women.

Source: Clarke *et al.* (2004).

Various metabolic, degenerative, autoimmune, Inflammatory, infectious, neoplastic (tumours), connective tissue and structural disorders may also affect the musculoskeletal system. Many of these diseases have significant physical, psychosocial and financial consequences. When these problems occur, people experience a variety of individualised responses to their altered health status.

Consider this . . .

Look at the case studies at the start of the chapter. Which of these will experience permanent changes to their lifestyle? Which individuals will recover from their experiences and resume the life they had before or a similar life?

● Joy may well resume the life she had before once the fractured wrist heals. The changes she may need to make to her lifestyle could be minor; she may alter her diet and take care to prevent falls. She should attend a follow-up clinic to determine whether she is suffering from **osteoporosis** and whether she needs to make further adaptations in light of the results.

● Stephen's accident, however, has come at a pivotal time in his life. The disruption to his school exams may impact on his results and determine his future life. Any plans he had may change permanently and he may lose contact with his peer group. However, he may adapt well to his situation and resume his studies and career choices at a later date, thus making the impact transient.

● Ben, on the other hand, has permanent changes to adapt to which may include structural changes to his home or even moving from his home or losing his independence completely. The impact of his altered body image may affect his mental health status; he may become depressed, moody and withdrawn.

This chapter will examine the anatomy and physiology of the musculoskeletal system as this enables better understanding of the rationale for treatments used to manage the problems that arise from trauma or disease to this system. It will also examine degenerative, metabolic and autoimmune diseases and the manner in which these also affect structure and function.

ANATOMY, PHYSIOLOGY AND FUNCTIONS OF THE MUSCULOSKELETAL SYSTEM

The musculoskeletal system consists of

● the bones of the skeletal system;
● the muscles;
● the ligaments, tendons and joints.

THE SKELETON

Bones form the body's structure and provide support for soft tissues. They protect vital organs from injury and serve to move body parts by providing points of attachment for muscles. Bones also store minerals and serve as a site for **haematopoiesis** (blood cell formation).

The human skeleton (Figure 12.1) is made up of 206 bones, divided into the axial skeleton and the appendicular skeleton. The *axial* skeleton includes the bones of the skull, the ribs and sternum and the vertebral column. The *appendicular* skeleton consists of all the bones of the limbs, the shoulder girdles and the pelvic girdle.

Bone structure

Bone cells include:

● osteoblasts (cells that form bone);
● osteocytes (cells that maintain bone matrix);
● osteoclasts (cells that resorb bone).

The bone matrix between the cells consists of collagen fibres, minerals (primarily calcium and phosphate), proteins, carbohydrates and ground substance. Ground substance is a gelatinous material that facilitates diffusion of nutrients, wastes and gases between the blood vessels and bone tissue. Bones are covered with periosteum, a double layer of connective tissue. The outer layer of the periosteum contains blood vessels and nerves; the inner layer is anchored to the bone.

Bones consist of a rigid connective tissue called osseous tissue, of which there are two types: compact bone is smooth and dense; spongy bone contains spaces, forming a meshwork of bone (trabecular bone). Both types contain the same elements and are found in almost all bones of the body.

The basic structural unit of compact bone is the Haversian system (also called an osteon) (Figure 12.2 on p. 432). The Haversian system consists of a central canal, called the Haversian canal; concentric layers of bone matrix, called lamellae; spaces between the lamellae, called lacunae; osteocytes within the lacunae; and small channels, called canaliculi.

Spongy bone has no Haversian systems. Instead, the lamellae are arranged in concentric layers called trabeculae that branch and join to form a mesh. The spongy sections of long bones (humerus and head of femur) and flat bones (sternum) contain tissue for haematopoiesis (development of blood cells); these sections are called red marrow cavities.

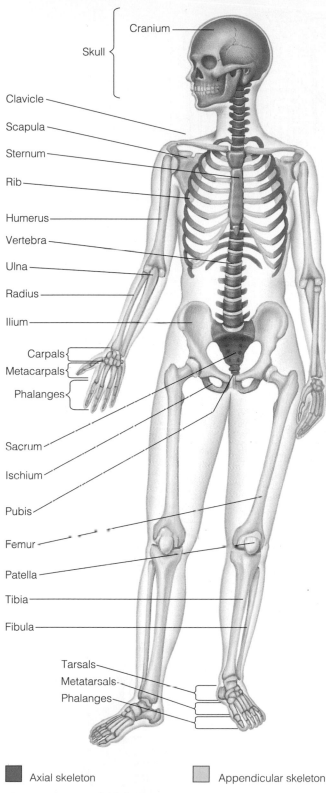

Cranium
Skull
Clavicle
Scapula
Sternum
Rib
Humerus
Vertebra
Ulna
Radius
Ilium
Carpals
Metacarpals
Phalanges
Sacrum
Ischium
Pubis
Femur
Patella
Tibia
Fibula
Tarsals
Metatarsals
Phalanges

Axial skeleton   Appendicular skeleton

Figure 12.1 Bones of the human skeleton.

Bone shapes

Bones are classified by shape (Figure 12.3):

- *Long bones*, which have a mid-portion called a diaphysis and two broad ends, called epiphyses. The diaphysis is compact bone and contains the marrow cavity, which is lined with endosteum, a thin layer of connective tissue. Each epiphysis is spongy bone covered by a thin layer of compact bone. Long bones are the bones of the arms, legs, fingers and toes.

- *Short bones* are cuboid, spongy bone covered by compact bone. They are the bones of the wrist and ankle.

- *Flat bones* are thin and flat and most are curved. Their disc-like structure consists of a layer of spongy bone between two thin layers of compact bone. Flat bones are mostly bones of the skull, the sternum and the ribs.

- *Irregular bones* are of various shapes and sizes and, like flat bones, are plates of compact bone with spongy bone between. Irregular bones include the vertebrae, the scapulae and the bones of the pelvic girdle.

Bone remodelling in adults

Although the bones of adults do not normally increase in length and size, constant remodelling of bones, as well as repair of damaged bone tissue, occurs throughout life. In the bone remodelling process, bone reabsorption and bone deposition occur at all periosteal and endosteal surfaces. Hormones and forces that put stress on the bones regulate this process, which involves a combined action of the osteocytes, osteoclasts and osteoblasts. Bones that are in use and are therefore subjected to stress, increase their osteoblastic activity to increase **ossification** (the development of bone). Bones that are inactive undergo increased osteoclast activity and bone reabsorption.

The hormonal stimulus for bone remodelling is controlled by a negative feedback mechanism that regulates blood calcium levels through the interaction of parathyroid hormone (PTH) from the parathyroid glands and calcitonin from the thyroid gland. When blood levels of calcium decrease, PTH is released; PTH then stimulates osteoclast activity and bone reabsorption, which releases calcium from the bone matrix. As a result, blood levels of calcium rise and the stimulus for PTH release ends. Rising blood calcium levels stimulate the secretion of calcitonin, which inhibits bone reabsorption and calcium salts are deposited in the bone matrix. Thus, bones regulate blood calcium levels. Calcium ions are necessary for the transmission of nerve impulses, the release of neurotransmitters, muscle contraction, blood clotting, glandular secretion and cell division. Of the body's 1200–1400 g of calcium, over 99% is present as bone minerals.

Bone remodelling is also regulated by the response of bones to gravitational pull and to mechanical stress from the pull of muscles. Although the exact mechanism is not fully understood, it is known that bones that undergo increased stress are heavier and larger. This finding supports Wolff's law, which states that bone develops and remodels itself to resist the stresses placed on it.

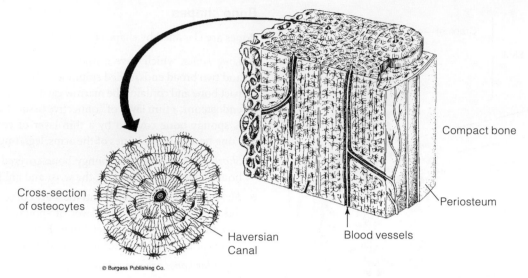

Figure 12.2 The microscopic structure (Haversian system) of compact bone.

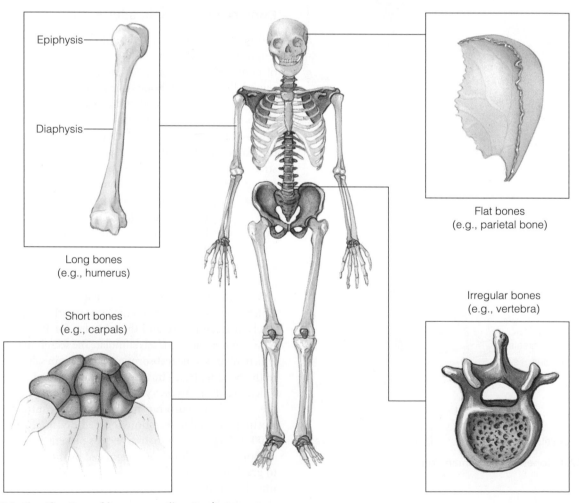

Figure 12.3 Classification of bone according to shape.

THE MUSCLES

The three types of muscle tissue in the body are:

- *skeletal muscle*, which is striated (striped in appearance), voluntary muscle as in the biceps, triceps, deltoid and gluteus maximus muscles;
- *smooth muscle*, which is non-striated, involuntary muscle as found in the walls of the stomach, bladder and bronchi;
- *cardiac muscle*, which is striated, involuntary and only found in the heart, (see Chapter 9).

Skeletal muscles attach to and cover the bones of the skeleton. They promote body movement, help maintain posture, produce body heat and may be moved by conscious, voluntary control or by reflex activity. The body has approximately 600 skeletal muscles (Figure 12.4).

Skeletal muscles are thick bundles of cell fibres. Each single muscle fibre is a bundle of smaller structures called myofibrils. The myofibrils have alternating light and dark bands conferring a striated (striped) appearance when seen under an electron microscope. Myofibrils are strands of smaller repeating units called sarcomeres, which consist of thick filaments of myosin and thin filaments of actin, proteins that contribute to muscle contraction. Bundles of muscle are encased in connective tissue, called fascia, which tapers at each end to form a tendon forming a compartment of muscle. The fascia is not elastic and does not stretch.

Skeletal muscle cells have typical functional properties:

- *Excitability:* they are able to receive and respond to a stimulus, usually a neurotransmitter which is released by a neuron.
- *Contractibility:* they respond to a stimulus by forcibly shortening.
- *Extensibility:* they respond to a stimulus by extending and relaxing; muscle fibres shorten when they contract and lengthen when they relax.
- *Elasticity:* this is the ability to resume its resting size after it has shortened or lengthened.

Prolonged strenuous activity causes continuous nerve impulses and eventually results in a buildup of lactic acid and reduced energy in the muscle or muscle fatigue. However, continuous nerve impulses are also responsible for maintaining muscle tone; lack of use results in muscle atrophy, whereas regular exercise increases the size and strength of muscles.

THE JOINTS, LIGAMENTS AND TENDONS

Joints are regions where two or more bones meet. Joints hold the bones of the skeleton together while allowing the body to move. Joints may be classified by function as:

- *synarthroses*, an immovable joint as found in the skull;
- *amphiarthroses*, the joints that move slightly as in the vertebrae;
- *diarthroses*, joints that move freely as in the limbs and at the shoulders and hips.

Joints are also classified by structure as:

- *fibrous*, permitting little movement – the binding connective tissue fibres are short as in the skull;
- *cartilaginous*, that is made of hyaline (shiny pink) cartilage that fuse articulating bone ends together as in the ribs, or fuse with a plate of flexible fibrocartilage (disc) as in the spine;
- *synovial*.

Synovial joints

Synovial joints (Figure 12.5) are freely movable, allowing many kinds of movements (see Table 12.1), and are found at all limb joints. They have several characteristics:

- The articular surfaces are covered with articular cartilage.
- The joint cavity is enclosed by a tough, fibrous, double-layered articular capsule; internally, the cavity is lined with a synovial membrane that covers all surfaces not covered by the articular cartilage.
- Synovial fluid fills the free spaces of the joint capsule, enhancing the smooth movement of the articulating bones.

Inflammation of the synovial membrane is referred to as **synovitis**.

Bursae are small sacs of synovial fluid that cushion and protect bony areas that are at high risk for friction, such as the knee and the shoulder. Inflammation of these is called **bursitis** (see section on repetitive strain injury on page 447). Tendon sheaths are a form of bursae, but they are wrapped around tendons in high-friction areas.

Table 12.1 Movements allowed by synovial joints

Movement	Description
Abduction	Move limb away from body midline
Adduction	Move limb toward body midline
Extension	Straighten limbs at joint
Flexion	Bend limbs at joint
Dorsiflexion	Bend ankle to bring top of foot toward shin
Plantar flexion	Straighten ankle to point toes down
Pronation	Turn forearm to place palm down
Supination	Turn forearm to place palm up
Eversion	Turn out
Inversion	Turn in
Circumduction	Move in circle
Internal rotation	Move inward on a central axis
External rotation	Move outward on a central axis
Protraction	Move forward and parallel to ground
Retraction	Move backward and parallel to ground

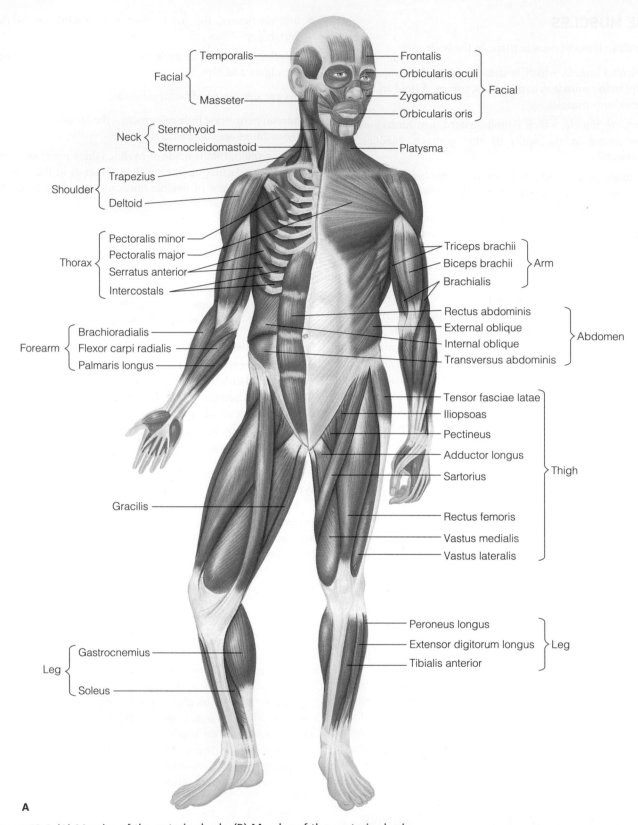

A

Figure 12.4 (A) Muscles of the anterior body. (B) Muscles of the posterior body.

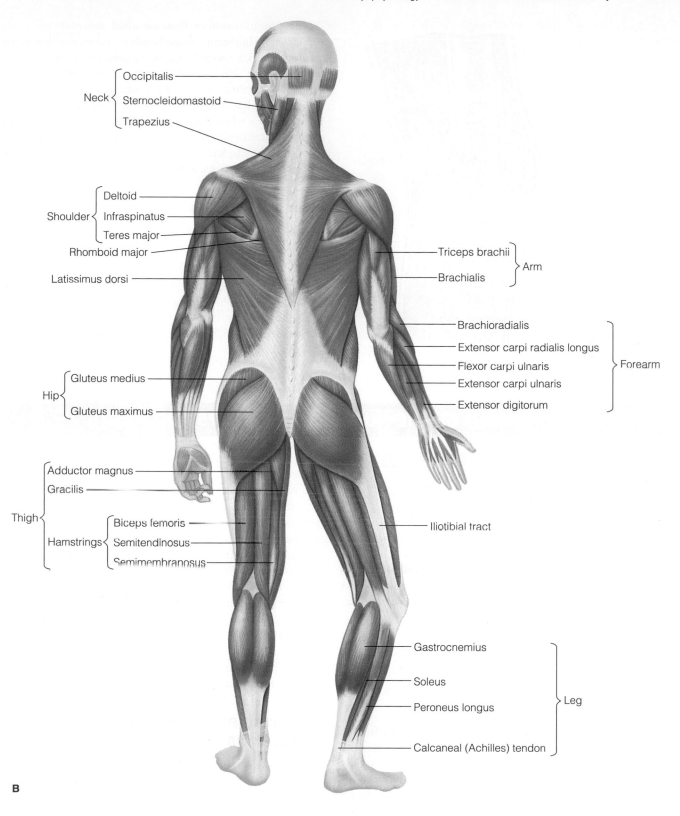

Neck
- Occipitalis
- Sternocleidomastoid
- Trapezius

Shoulder
- Deltoid
- Infraspinatus
- Teres major

Rhomboid major

Latissimus dorsi

Triceps brachii } Arm
Brachialis

Brachioradialis
Extensor carpi radialis longus
Flexor carpi ulnaris } Forearm
Extensor carpi ulnaris
Extensor digitorum

Hip
- Gluteus medius
- Gluteus maximus

Thigh
- Adductor magnus
- Gracilis

Hamstrings
- Biceps femoris
- Semitendinosus
- Semimembranosus

Iliotibial tract

Gastrocnemius
Soleus } Leg
Peroneus longus
Calcaneal (Achilles) tendon

B

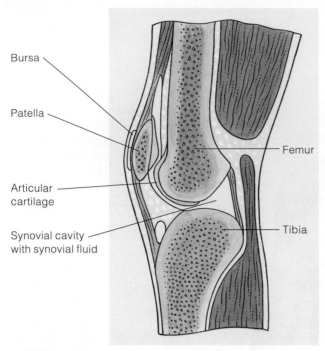

Figure 12.5 Structure of a synovial joint (knee).

The fibrous capsules that surround synovial joints are supported by ligaments, dense bands of connective tissue that connect bones to bones. Ligaments limit or enhance movement, provide joint stability and enhance joint strength. Tendons are fibrous, non-elastic, connective tissue bands that connect muscles to the periosteum of bones and enable the bones to move when skeletal muscles contract. When muscles contract, increased pressure causes the tendon to pull, push or rotate the bone to which it is connected. It is the muscle that shortens and lengthens, not the tendons.

Other types of joints

- *Fibrous joints* have little or no movement as between the bones forming the skull. The joints are made up of very short fibres of connective tissue.
- *Cartilaginous joints* are found in the rib cage and spinal column where hyaline cartilage joins the two bone ends. In the spine, in between the vertebral bones, the hyaline cartilage sandwiches flexible fibrocartilage which is disc-shaped.

TRAUMATIC INJURIES OF THE MUSCLES, LIGAMENTS AND JOINTS

The person with a contusion, strain or sprain

Contusions, strains and sprains are among the most commonly reported injuries. They account for about 50% of work-related injuries, with lower back injuries being the most commonly reported occupational injury. However, many sprains and strains are not work-related and often are not reported. The lower back and cervical region of the spine are the most common sites for muscle strains; the ankle is the most commonly sprained joint, usually caused by twisting it suddenly.

Pathophysiology and signs and symptoms of contusions, strains or sprains

A contusion is bleeding into soft tissue that results from a blunt force, such as a kick or striking a body part against a hard object. The skin remains intact, but small blood vessels underneath rupture and bleed into the tissues, resulting in swelling and discoloration. The blood in the soft tissue initially results in a purple and blue colour, commonly referred to as a bruise; as it begins to be reabsorbed, the area involved becomes brown and then yellow until it disappears. A large bleed is called a haematoma.

A strain is a stretching injury to muscle or muscle and tendons by mechanical overloading. A muscle that is forced to extend past its elasticity will become strained. Lifting heavy objects without bending the knees or a sudden acceleration–deceleration, as in a motor vehicle crash, can cause strains. The most common sites for a muscle strain are the lower back and cervical regions of the spine. Strains result in pain, limited motion, muscle spasms swelling and possible muscle weakness.

A sprain is a stretch and/or tear of one or more ligaments surrounding a joint. Forces going in opposite directions cause the ligament to overstretch and possibly tear either partially or completely. Although any joint may be involved, sprains of the ankle and knee are most common. Sprains result in a loss of the ability to move or use the joint, a feeling of a 'pop' or tear, discoloration, pain and rapid swelling. Motion increases the joint pain. The intensity of the symptoms depends on the severity of the sprain.

INTERDISCIPLINARY CARE FOR CONTUSIONS, STRAINS OR SPRAINS

The initial goal is to reduce swelling and pain. A useful way to remember the care that is needed is the mnemonic RICE, which stands for:

- *Rest*, that is not putting any weight or strain on the affected area, using slings or crutches and splints to immobilse the joint if necessary.
- *Ice*, that is applying ice packs three or four times a day for 20 minutes, and warning patients that applying it for longer may lead to frostbite-type injuries.

- *Compression*, that is using special bandages, splints or support hosiery which will help reduce swelling.
- *Elevation*, that is keeping the injured limb raised on a pillow to help reduce swelling.

Physiotherapy is usually recommended once the initial swelling has gone down so that the patient regains muscle tone and proper use of the joint affected. Time required for healing depends on the severity of the injury; for example, a mild ankle sprain may require up to three to six weeks of rehabilitation, whereas a severe sprain may require up to 8–12 months to return to full activities.

When soft tissue trauma is suspected, x-rays are taken to rule out soft tissue injury, and magnetic resonance imaging (MRI) may be done if further assessment is necessary.

IN PRACTICE

Managing analgesic preparations

Pain and the inflammatory responses to injury are managed by taking non-steroidal anti-inflammatory drugs (NSAIDs) and analgesics such as paracetamol. The two drugs can be alternated for maximum benefit, providing the person is not allergic to either.

The person with a joint dislocation

A dislocation of a joint means the ends of bones are forced from their normal position; usually as a result of trauma such as a fall or blow, with the bone ends displaced or separated from their normal position in the joint capsule. They are commonly seen in people who take part in contact sports such as football or from falls during activities such as skiing. Although dislocations may occur in any joint, they occur most frequently in the shoulder and acromioclavicular joints. Dislocations may also result from a disease such as **rheumatoid**

arthritis. A sub-luxation is a partial dislocation in which the bone ends are still partially in contact with each other.

Pathophysiology of joint dislocation

Dislocations may also be congenital, or pathological (resulting from disease). Congenital dislocations are present at birth and are seen in the hip and shoulder. Pathological dislocations result from disease of the joint, including infection, rheumatoid arthritis, paralysis and neuromuscular diseases. Dislocations cause pain, deformity and limit movement.

INTERDISCIPLINARY CARE FOR JOINT DISLOCATION

The dislocation is usually reduced (bone ends realigned) by means of manual traction (pulling the bone into position by hand). Treatment of a shoulder joint dislocation depends on the severity of the dislocation. Immobilisation is no longer recommended unless it is a recurring injury and only the most severe dislocations are surgically reduced. A dislocated hip requires immediate reduction in the emergency room to prevent necrosis of the femoral head and injury to the nerves. After reduction, the person is placed on bedrest. In some cases, mechanical traction is needed for several weeks. The application of traction is illustrated in Figure 12.6.

If a hip dislocation is accompanied by a fracture, then surgery is required to increase mobility, decrease complications and rapidly stabilise the joint.

NURSING CARE FOR JOINT DISLOCATION

Once seen in the emergency department, most people are usually allowed home with the following advice:

- Rest the joint initially. Engaging in exercises before the joint has had time to recover may cause more damage.
- Introduce exercise gradually as this will strengthen the muscles surrounding the joint.
- Take analgesics regularly initially to control the pain and wean off gradually as the joint heals.

TRAUMATIC INJURIES OF THE BONES

The person with a fracture

A fracture is any break in the continuity of a bone. They vary in severity according to the location and type. Fractures occur in all age groups. They are more common in people who have sustained trauma, but can occur spontaneously because of bone disease such as cancer. Any of the 206 bones in the body

can be fractured. Fractures may result from a direct blow, a crushing force (compression), a sudden twisting motion (torsion), a severe muscle contraction or disease that has weakened the bone (called a stress or pathological fracture).

Pathophysiology of fractures

Fractures are either:

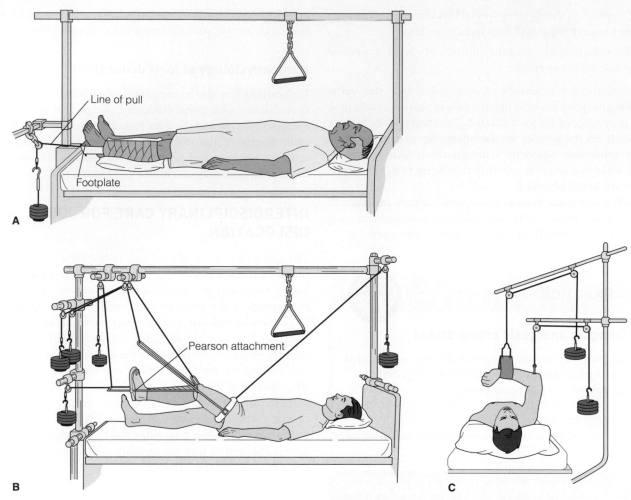

Figure 12.6 Traction is the application of a pulling force to maintain bone alignment. **(A)** Skin traction. **(B)** Balanced traction. **(C)** Skeletal traction.

- *closed (simple) fracture*, where the skin is intact over the site; or
- *open (compound) fracture*, where the skin is broken.

They are also described as being:

- *oblique*, at an angle to the bone;
- *spiral*, curving around the bone;
- *avulsed*, where the fracture pulls bone and other tissues away from the point of attachment;
- *comminuted*, broken in many pieces;
- *compressed*, crushed;
- *impacted*, where the broken bone ends are forced into each other;
- *depressed*, where the broken bone is forced inward.

Different types of fractures are illustrated in Figures 12.7 and 12.8.

Fractures can be complete, involving the whole width of the bone, or incomplete, where only part of the width of the

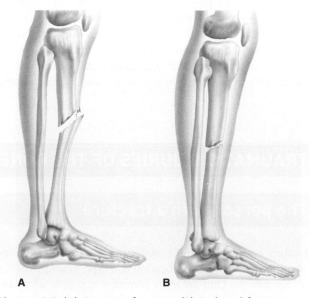

Figure 12.7 (A) An open fracture. (B) A closed fracture.

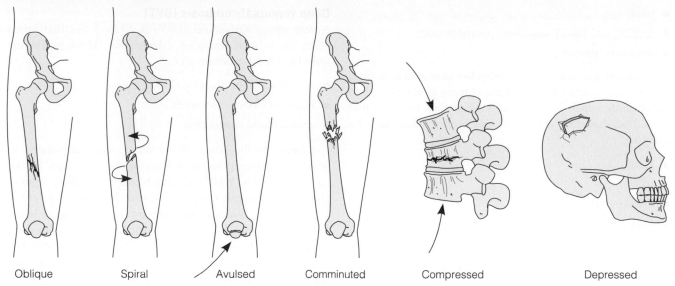

| Oblique | Spiral | Avulsed | Comminuted | Compressed | Depressed |

Figure 12.8 Types of fracture.

bone is damaged. They can also be stable (or non-displaced), meaning they maintain their anatomic alignment, or unstable (displaced), where they are no longer aligned as expected. Displaced fractures require immediate attention to minimise damage to the surrounding tissues.

Fracture healing

Regardless of classification or type, fracture healing progresses over three phases:

- *The inflammatory phase,* where a haematoma forms between the bone ends, resulting in a lack of oxygen and necrosis at the site, which in turn stimulates the body's inflammatory response. Lymphocytes and macrophages migrate to the site to deal with the inflammatory response, and then fibroblasts build up a network of capillaries which bring in nutrients and collagen, into which calcium is deposited.
- *The reparative phase,* where osteoblasts form new bone and osteoclasts remove the dead tissue.
- *The remodelling phase,* where a callus forms over the fracture site and new bone is formed along the fracture line.

The age and physical condition of the patient and the type of fracture sustained influence the healing of fractures. Healing time varies with the individual. An uncomplicated fracture of the arm or foot can heal in six to eight weeks. A fractured vertebra will take at least 12 weeks to heal. Healing of a fractured hip may take from 12–16 weeks.

Signs and symptoms of fractures

Fractures are often accompanied by soft tissue injuries that involve muscles, arteries, veins, nerves or skin. The degree of soft tissue involvement depends on the amount of energy or force transmitted to the area. Usual signs and symptoms are:

- deformity from the position of the broken bone;
- swelling and oedema around the site of the break;
- pain and tenderness at the site of the break;
- numbness because of nerve involvement;
- crepitus, which is the grating sound of the bone ends rubbing against each other;
- shock;
- muscle spasm;
- **ecchymosis** (bleeding from surrounding tissue at the site of the break).

Complications that may arise following a fracture

Complications of fractures are associated with pressure from oedema and haemorrhage, development of fat emboli, deep venous thrombosis, infection, loss of skeletal integrity or involvement of nerve fibres.

Compartment syndrome

Muscles are bound by a covering of non-elastic fibrous membrane or fascia (see page 433) which forms a 'compartment'. When bleeding and swelling occur within this compartment, as there is no stretch, pressure builds up on cells in the encased tissue; these cells are also deprived of oxygen and nutrients which results in cell death. **Compartment syndrome** may occur because of haemorrhage and oedema following an accident or if a plaster cast is too tight which also reduces circulation to the muscles and nerves. Compartment syndrome usually develops within the first 48 hours of injury, when oedema is at its peak.

Signs and symptoms of compartment syndrome are:

- pain;
- tingling and loss of sensation (paraesthesias);
- weakness (paresis).

It is important to note that arterial pulses may remain normal, even when pressure within the compartment is high enough to significantly impair tissue perfusion. There are five signs that should be checked every one to two hours, called the 5 Ps. They are:

- pain;
- pallor;
- distal pulses;
- paraesthesias – tingling sensations;
- paresis or paralysis.

If compartment syndrome develops, interventions to alleviate pressure will be implemented; these may include removal of a tightly fitting cast. If the pressure is internal, a *fasciotomy*,

PRACTICE ALERT

Checking whether circulation is impaired is relatively easy. When pressure is lightly applied to the nail bed, it blanches then returns to its normal colour. If it does not return to its normal colour spontaneously, it implies that circulation is not at its optimum level and immediate action needs to be taken.

a surgical intervention in which muscle fascia is cut to relieve pressure within the compartment, may be necessary. After a fasciotomy, the incision is left open and passive ranges of movement (ROM) exercises are performed on the extremity.

Volkmann's contracture, a common complication of elbow fractures, can result from unresolved compartment syndrome. Arterial blood flow decreases, leading to ischaemia, degeneration and contracture of the muscle. Arm mobility is impaired and the person is unable to completely extend the arm.

Fat embolism syndrome (FES)

Fat embolism syndrome can occur when long bones fracture or following hip surgery. There is a risk of fat globules being released from the site of injury, entering the circulation and causing an emboli (blockage) in the capillaries. Symptoms usually develop within a few hours to a week after injury. Altered cerebral blood flow causes confusion and changes in level of consciousness. The blockage can occur in the lungs and cause oedema and, if untreated, respiratory arrest. FSE is suspected if the person becomes confused, or suddenly breathless. Petechial rashes (small red pinprick dots) appear on the chest, axilla and upper arms. Stabilising long bone fractures early may prevent this complication. In severe cases, the person may require intubation and mechanical ventilation to prevent hypoxaemia, therefore, it is important to identify and treat the syndrome quickly.

Deep venous thrombosis (DVT)

A *deep venous thrombosis (DVT)* is a blood clot that forms along the intimal lining of a large vein. Three precursors linked to DVT formation are:

- venous stasis, or decreased blood flow;
- injury to blood vessel walls;
- altered blood coagulation.

Damage to the lining of the vein causes the platelets to aggregate or clump together, forming the thrombus. Fibrin, white blood cells (WBCs) and red blood cells (RBCs) begin to cling to the thrombus and a tail forms. This tail or the entire thrombus may dislodge and move to the brain, lungs or heart. Five per cent of DVTs dislodge and enter the pulmonary circulation to form a pulmonary embolus. If the thrombus remains in the vein, venous insufficiency may result from scarring and valve damage.

The symptoms are usually swelling, leg pain, tenderness or cramping. A Doppler ultrasound of lower leg confirms the diagnosis; it is non-invasive investigation which can be performed at the bedside.

Early immobilisation of the fracture and early ambulation of the person is imperative to prevent this complication occurring. Antiembolism stockings and compression boots increase venous return and prevent stasis of blood. If the person is diagnosed as having a DVT, they are usually given anticoagulant therapy as described in Chapter 9, p. 332.

Infection

Infection is more likely to occur in an open fracture than a closed fracture, but any complication that decreases blood supply (like compartment syndrome described above) increases the risk of infection. Surgical treatment to reduce fractures is another potential for contamination and increases the risk of infection. *Pseudomonas*, *Staphylococcus* or *Clostridium* organisms may invade the wound or bone. *Clostridium* infection is particularly serious because it may lead to severe gas gangrene and cellulitis, but any infection may delay healing and result in **osteomyelitis**, infection within the bone that can lead to tissue death and necrosis (see Chapter 4).

Wounds and pin sites need to be cared for using strict aseptic techniques. Any indication of infection (e.g. redness, increase in temperature) should be reported immediately so that antibiotic treatment can be commenced.

Delayed union and non-union

Occasionally, fractures do not heal in the expected time. This is called delayed union and there are many reasons for this:

- poor nutritional status;
- the broken ends of the bone have not been immobilised properly so continue to move;
- infection is present;
- too many bone fragments at the site of injury;

Pin sites

There is a great deal of debate in orthopaedic nursing as to the most appropriate method of managing pin sites; whether they are skeletal traction pins or pins and wires from external fixation.

Grant *et al.* (2005) found that when pin sites were treated daily with an application of povidone–iodine solution as opposed to the application of soft white paraffin ointment there were fewer cases of infection. They state that many nurses are reluctant to use povidone–iodine solution in the belief that this corrodes the stainless steel pins, yet there is no research-based evidence to support this view.

Santy and Newton-Triggs (2006) found that nursing practice in the UK was varied, with some advising showering daily and drying the pin sites with a clean towel. They cite research that indicates cleansing with normal saline solution to be less effective at keeping infection at bay than using clean tap water.

Pin sites remain an open wound until they are removed, and infection can track in and lead to osteomyelitis, which is extremely difficult to treat and requires hospitalisation and parenteral antibiotic treatment. According to Santy and Newton-Triggs, infection rates have been recorded as occurring in 86% of pin sites. Further research is needed to standardise care.

- the person's immune response is compromised (may be taking drugs for another condition that affects the immune response);
- age, older people take longer to heal.

Delayed union is diagnosed by means of serial x-ray studies. It is important to note that x-ray findings may lag one to two weeks behind the healing process; for example, a patient may be completely healed by week 13, but this fact may not be apparent on the x-ray until week 14.

Non-union may require surgical interventions, such as internal fixation and bone grafting. If infection is present, the bones are surgically debrided (cleaned).

INTERDISCIPLINARY CARE FOR FRACTURES

A fracture requires to be stabilised and the fractured bone(s) need to be immobilised to prevent pain and the development of further complications, and to restore function. This may involve a closed reduction and the application of a plaster cast or may require traction, which will be discussed below. The diagnosis of a fracture is primarily based on physical assessments and x-rays. Preliminary treatment of fractures may be undertaken by someone with first aid knowledge as most fractures are the result of an accident.

Case Study 1 – Stephen
NURSING CARE PLAN Fracture

Stephen, as you will recall, was involved in a motorcycle accident and requires initial care at the roadside and then further care in the hospital A & E department.

Emergency care

Stephen receives emergency care from paramedics at the site of the road traffic accident. They assess Stephen for his injuries and make sure he did not receive a head injury and his airway is patent. Gas (Entonox) and air may be used to give pain relief, but he may be numbed from shock.

With regard to his injuries, it is important to immobilise the fractured femur which may be done by using an air splint. If he has any open wounds, these will be covered with a sterile dressing. The extremities are assessed for the presence of pulses, movement and sensation. The joint above and below the deformity is immobilised. Pulses, movement and sensation are re-evaluated after splinting.

The fracture is splinted to maintain normal anatomic alignment and prevent the fracture from dislocating. Splinting relieves pain and prevents further damage to the arteries, nerves and

bones. If equipment is not available, the limb may be secured to the body. For example, an arm may be secured to the torso with a sling or the broken leg may be strapped to the other leg.

Diagnosis

Once in the A & E department, diagnosis of a fracture begins with the history taking, followed by further assessment and is usually confirmed by radiographic tests. X-rays and bone scans are used to identify fractures (see Figure 12.8 on pages 438 and 439). Blood chemistry studies, complete blood count and coagulation studies may be used to assess blood loss, renal function, muscle breakdown and the risk of excessive bleeding or clotting.

Pain relief

Most people with a fracture require pharmacological interventions for the management of pain. In the case of multiple fractures or fractures of large bones, opioids are administered initially. As healing progresses, the person begins to take oral medication for pain.

Stephen may experience pain from:

+ the fracture site;

+ muscle spasm;

+ swelling of the tissues around the injury or inside the cast or splint;

+ infection if there was an open wound.

The pain is often severe and may be described as sharp, aching or burning.

Besides giving pain medication regularly, Stephen can be taught to relax by using distraction therapies and visualisation. Wriggling his toes and fingers increases circulation and helps to reduce oedema. Giving pain medication regularly at this point prevents the development of pain syndromes which occur when pain is poorly managed.

Consider this . . .

Stephen will probably need skeletal traction and the pin will be inserted under general anaesthesia.

● What might be Stephen's main concerns at this point in his care?

● How will Stephen's accident impact on his family, friends and peers?

● What nursing care will be required to support him as he adjusts to his situation?

Traction

The muscles surrounding a fractured bone can go into spasm and pull the bones out of alignment, requiring a great deal of force to counteract this. The force is usually applied by traction. For smaller bones or where the muscle spasm is not too great, traction can be performed manually with two people pulling in opposite directions above and below the fracture and the bones held in alignment until a plaster cast is applied. However, manual traction is not suitable in many situations and traction is applied mechanically with weights providing the counterbalance. Types of traction are as follows:

● *Skin traction* (also called straight traction), which is used to control muscle spasms and immobilise a part of the body before surgery. This is usually undertaken for fractures of the neck of the femur, where the leg is bandaged and a weight suspended from this (see Figure 12.6 on page 438). The advantage is that it is easy to apply and quickly provides comfort. The disadvantage is that the weight required to keep normal body alignment or fracture alignment cannot exceed the tolerance of the skin, about 6 lb per extremity.

● *Balanced suspension traction* involves more than one force of pull. Several forces work together to raise and support the person's injured limb off the bed and pull it in a straight line away from the body (see Figure 12.6). The advantage of this type of traction is that it enables the person a greater range of movement. The disadvantage is that the use of multiple weights makes the person more likely to slide down in the bed.

● *Skeletal traction* is the application of a pulling force through placement of pins into the bone (see Figure 12.6). The patient may receive a local, spinal or general anaesthetic, and the pins are inserted into the bone. This type of traction must be applied under sterile conditions because of the increased risk of infection. One or more pulling forces may be applied with skeletal traction. The advantage of this type of traction is that more weight can be used to maintain the proper anatomic alignment if necessary. The disadvantages include increased anxiety, increased risk of infection and increased discomfort.

For traction to be successful, the weights must not be removed, with the person's weight providing the countertraction. Therefore, the person's foot should not be wedged or placed flush with the bottom of the bed. The weights must hang freely and nothing should impede their movement, so care is required to ensure knots do not get caught up in the pulleys.

Plaster casts

Plaster casts are bandages impregnated with Plaster of Paris that are immersed in water before being applied over a thin cushion of padding and moulded gently to the contour of the body. As the plaster dries and sets, it warms up and the person needs to be aware that this normally occurs. An alternative to plaster is fibreglass, which is much lighter, and is not affected by water (allowing the wearer to wash more easily), unlike Plaster of Paris which softens when wet. The plaster cast should be applied to ensure that the injured bones are maintained in alignment and are immobile. If the cast is too short, it will not maintain immobility and the alignment may be lost as the oedema around the fracture subsides.

Surgery

Surgery is indicated for a fracture that:

● requires direct visualisation and repair;

● has common long-term complications;

● is severely comminuted and threatens vascular supply.

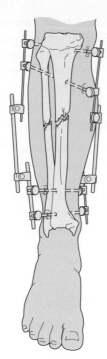

Figure 12.9 External fixation of a bone above and below the fracture site.

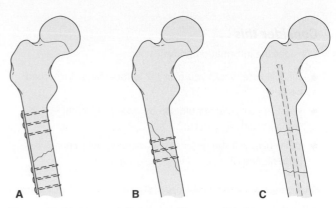

Figure 12.10 Internal fixation of bones. **(A)** Plate and screws. **(B)** With screws. **(C)** With medullary nail.

The simplest form of surgery is done by external fixation (Figure 12.9) with an external fixator device which consists of a frame connected to pins that are inserted perpendicular to the long axis of the bone. The number of pins inserted varies with the type and site of the fracture, but in all cases the same number of pins is inserted above and below the fracture line. The pins require care similar to that of skeletal traction pins and are monitored for signs of infection. The fixator increases independence while maintaining immobilisation.

Internal fixation is referred to as an *open reduction and internal fixation (ORIF)* and is used for open fractures of the arms or legs, and hips in older people. In this procedure, the fracture is reduced and nails, screws, plates or pins are inserted to hold the bones in place (see Figure 12.10). Barry Sheene, the former British World Champion Grand Prix Motorcycle road racer, published x-rays of his legs which were pinned and plated following a crash at Silverstone to gain publicity for his return to the sport (the pictures are still available on the Internet).

NURSING CARE FOR FRACTURES

There are various nursing interventions which are appropriate, directed at patient education, pain relief, infection prevention and prevention of neurovascular dysfunction. Here, we will focus on care for the person having a plaster cast and on the person having an internal fixation.

Nursing care of the person with a plaster cast entails checking that the cast is not too tight and that the fingers or toes protruding from the cast maintain a healthy colour and the person still has sensation there. Advise the person not to get the cast wet if it is made of Plaster of Paris. If the cast encases

an open wound, it should be checked for warmth which may indicate an area of infection under the cast.

Plaster casts may cause itching and irritation, particularly in warm weather and the advice is not to poke sticks or other objects down inside the cast to scratch the area, but blowing cold air from a hair dryer may offer some relief. If oedema is suspected, the cast may be split to relieve pressure and prevent compartment syndrome.

Following an internal fixation, the nurse should:

+ assess the wound for drainage or bleeding;
+ administer analgesics as prescribed;
+ ensure the patient is comfortable, the affected areas are well supported and assist with moving;
+ check that the circulation is good to the extremities of the injured limb;
+ if it is an injured limb, ensure it is raised to assist venous return of blood thus minimising the development of oedema.

Case Study 2 – Joy

NURSING CARE PLAN Fracture

Joy has slipped on the wet pavement outside her home when getting out of her car. Her neighbours come to her rescue and they remove her jewellery, especially her rings, before making a short journey to their local emergency centre.

Joy is taken into the treatment area and her arm is supported in a sling. She is given analgesics before being seen by a doctor and going to the x-ray department. The x-rays confirm that she has broken the ulna. Morphine is injected into the area of the break and two doctors reduce the fracture, applying manual traction, and a plaster cast is applied. Joy then returns for another x-ray to ensure that the bone is aligned properly.

Consider this . . .

Consider the information above:

● What advice would you give Joy before she is discharged home?

● What in particular should she be aware of? What complications may occur?

● What help will she require with meeting her general hygiene needs?

The person having an amputation

An amputation is the partial or total removal of an extremity. It may be required following a traumatic event like stepping on a landmine or because of a chronic condition, such as peripheral vascular disease (PVD) or diabetes mellitus, where the circulation is compromised or because of an infection that is unresponsive to antibiotics. Regardless of the cause, an amputation is devastating. The loss of all or part of an extremity has a significant physical and psychosocial effect on the person and their family. Adaptation may take a long time and require much effort. Interdisciplinary healthcare is always important, but is especially necessary to meet the person's physical, spiritual, cultural and emotional needs after an unexpected or planned amputation.

Causes of amputation

Peripheral vascular disease (PVD) developing secondary to hypertension, diabetes or hyperlidaemia is the major cause of amputation of the lower extremities. Peripheral neuropathy also places the person with diabetes at risk for amputation as loss of sensation frequently leads to unrecognised injury and infection which may lead to gangrene, osteomyelitis (infection in the bone) and the need for amputation. The risk of needing an amputation is 15–46 times higher in diabetics than the general population.

The incidence of traumatic amputations is highest among young men. Most amputations in this group result from accidents; either motor vehicle or involving machinery at work. These people present with an injury that may be life-threatening; significant loss of blood and tissue may have already occurred, and shock may develop. Other traumatic events that may necessitate an amputation are frostbite, burns or electrocution, and war injuries.

In acute trauma situations, the limb is partially or completely severed, and tissue death ensues. However, replantation of fingers, finger tips and entire limbs has been successful. In some chronic diseases, circulation is impaired, venous pooling begins, proteins leak into the tissues and oedema develops. This increases the risk of injury and further decreases circulation.

Stasis ulcers develop and readily become infected because impaired healing and altered immune processes allow bacteria to proliferate. Circulation is further compromised by progressive infection which can lead to gangrene and, ultimately, amputation is the only solution.

Levels of amputation

The level of amputation is determined by local and systemic factors. Local factors include ischaemia and gangrene; systemic factors include cardiovascular status, renal function and severity of diabetes mellitus. The goals are to alleviate symptoms, to maintain healthy tissue and to increase functional outcome. When possible, the joints are preserved because they allow greater function of the extremity. Figure 12.11 illustrates common sites of amputation.

Types of amputation

Amputations may be open (*guillotine*) or closed (*flap*). Open amputations are performed when infection is present. The wound is not closed but remains open to drain. When infection is no longer present, surgery is performed to close the wound. In closed amputations, the wound is closed with a flap of skin that is sutured in place over the stump. For the prosthesis (artificial limb) to fit well, the amputation site must heal properly. To promote healing, a rigid or compression dressing is applied to prevent infection and minimise oedema. A rigid dressing is made by placing a cast on the stump and moulding the stump to fit the prosthesis. A soft compression dressing is applied when frequent wound checks are necessary. When this type of dressing is used, a splint is sometimes applied to help mould the extremity to fit the prosthesis. After the wound is dressed, the person is encouraged to toughen the stump skin by pushing it into first soft and then harder surfaces. The stump is wrapped in a self-adhering (ACE) bandage to allow a conical shape to form and to prevent oedema developing.

Stump care includes:

● daily washing of the stump and inspecting it for redness or soreness;

● massaging the stump to prevent the formation of scar tissue, to keep the skin healthy and to help desensitise the area;

● keeping stump socks/bandages clean.

Complications associated with amputation

Complications that may occur after an amputation include infection, delayed healing, contractures forming, chronic stump pain and phantom limb pain.

Infection

The person who suffers a traumatic rather than planned amputation has a greater risk of infection. However, planned amputations carry a risk of infection if the patient is older, has diabetes mellitus or suffers peripheral neurovascular problems.

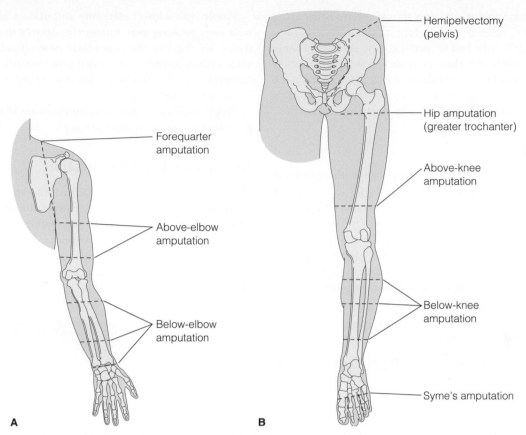

Figure 12.11 Common sites of amputation. **(A)** The arm. **(B)** The leg.

Local signs of infection include drainage, odour, redness and increased discomfort at the suture line. Systemic symptoms include fever, an increased heart rate, a decrease in blood pressure, chills and positive wound or blood cultures.

Delayed healing
Factors which lead to delayed healing are:

- presence of infection;
- poor circulation;
- electrolyte imbalances;
- compromised nutritional status;
- smoking;
- decreased cardiac output.

Chronic stump pain and phantom limb pain
Phantom limb pain is not the same as phantom limb sensation. A majority of amputees experience phantom limb sensation (sensations such as tingling, numbness, cramping or itching in the phantom foot or hand) early in the post-operative period. It is often self-limited, but may last for decades in some people. When phantom limb sensation is painful, it is referred to as phantom limb pain. The condition was first described by a French military surgeon in the sixteenth century. Although various theories have been proposed, the exact cause of this experience is unknown.

Ronald Melzack, a Canadian doctor who has researched extensively into pain, has proposed the neuromatrix theory to explain the phenomena. Pain messages are transmitted by neurons to the thalamus in the brain and are then relayed to the cognitive and sensory cortex of the brain through the neuromatrix, establishing a neurosignature or pain memory. Melzack hypothesises that in prolonged episodes or severe pain, these neurosignatures become sensitised and keep transmitting pain messages, so that even when the pain stimulus stops, the neurons keep firing the pain message. To break the cycle, cognitive behaviour therapy helps the person revise their memories and cognitions about pain. Other treatments to manage pain include using a TENS (transcutaneous electrical nerve stimulation) machine and massage. People with phantom limb pain often benefit from referral to a pain clinic for a comprehensive pain management programme.

Contractures
Contracture of the joint above the amputation is a common complication; it is an abnormal flexion and fixation of a joint caused by muscle atrophy and shortening. The person with an above-the-knee amputation needs to extend the joint by lying prone for short periods throughout the day and should not sit for long periods of time as this can lead to hip contractures. The person with a below-the-knee amputation should elevate the stump, keeping the knee extended. The same principles apply

to the upper extremities. All joints should receive either active or passive exercises every two to four hours. A trapeze frame should be added to the bed to encourage the person to change position every two hours. The person who has an upper extremity amputation should exercise both shoulders. Physiotherapy and occupational retraining are necessary for patients following amputation and the rehabilitative phase may be lengthy.

Prosthesis

The type of prosthesis selected for the person with an amputation depends on the level of the amputation as well as the person's occupation and lifestyle. The prosthesis is based on a detailed prescription and is custom-made for each person, based on the specific characteristics of the stump. Most are made of plastic and foam materials. Many factors influence the person's use of the prosthesis, including the status of the remaining limb and the motivation to use the prosthesis.

People with a lower extremity amputation are often fitted with early walking aids. Pneumatic devices that fit over the stump are used in the immediate post-operative period to allow early ambulation, decreased post-operative swelling and improved morale. Weight bearing may be encouraged as soon as two weeks after surgery.

People with upper extremity amputations may be fitted for prosthesis immediately after surgery.

Nursing care for amputation

The goals of nursing care for a person with an amputation are to relieve pain, promote healing, prevent complications developing, support the patient and family during the process of grieving and adaptation to alterations in body image and restore mobility. Care is individualised and the circumstances that led to the amputation (e.g., traumatic injury or disease) may also need to be addressed.

Case Study 3 – Ben
NURSING CARE PLAN Post–amputation

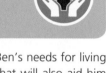

Ben lives in an inner city suburb; he is retired now but worked for London Transport on the underground. Years of working shifts has meant his diabetes was often out of control and he eventually developed peripheral neuropathies, which means he is not always aware that he has damaged his toes. He did not notice the damage until the toes were painful and infected and they became gangrenous when he failed to respond *to* courses of antibiotic treatment. Reluctantly, he agreed to a below-the-knee amputation.

Post-operative care includes:

✚ learning to adapt to the loss of a limb;
✚ learning to care for the stump;
✚ learning to prevent contractures from occurring;
✚ learning to use a wheelchair.

Ben will require physiotherapy and occupational therapy. The physiotherapist will teach Ben exercises that prevent contractures of the knee joint, strengthen his upper body limbs, enable him to move from his bed to the wheelchair safely and become independent.

The occupational therapist will assess Ben's needs for living and instigate modifications to his home that will also aid him to become independent. He may need safety rails and ramps fitted to allow easy access to his home and modifications to his kitchen and bathroom to accommodate his wheelchair.

Social services need to be contacted to ensure that Ben receives all the appropriate support that he needs. He may need rehousing if his present accommodation cannot be adapted for someone who is now wheelchair dependent. He may also require help with shopping and preparing meals.

Consider this . . .
Not all amputees become wheelchair dependent following a lower limb amputation. Younger people adapt well with prosthetic limbs and they are not totally reliant on a wheelchair for mobility.

● How will Ben's amputation affect his diabetes?
● What else in Ben's life will be affected by this surgery?

Psychosocial issues

Although amputation is reconstructive surgery, it affects the person's sense of self, their body image. Young people, for whom body image is a particularly important component of self-image, are at greater risk of not adapting well and may grieve the loss of their 'old' self. This is termed as non-finite grief. The intensity of the grief reaction

depends on the meaning that the loss has for the person, their personality and the support network that is available to them. Grief is an individual response; some people are resilient in the face of adversity and cope extremely well. They probably have a good support network and strong sense of who they are and their role in society, but at times may still be overcome with feelings of sadness, which could result in depression.

COMMUNITY-BASED CARE

Preparing the amputee for home care includes a careful assessment of the patient's family and support services, and the home for possible barriers to the patient's safety and independence. In Case Study 3, Ben lives in rented accommodation that is owned by the local council so the adaptations are organised by social services and it may be possible to exchange his accommodation for one that is more suitable to meet his changed needs. However, if Ben owned his own property, he will have to organise adaptations himself and at his own expense, although he may be entitled to some government support.

The person with repetitive strain injury (RSI)

Repeatedly twisting and turning the wrist, pronating and supinating the forearm, kneeling or raising arms over the head can result in repetitive use injuries. Often people appear puzzled as they relate a history of symptoms that have worsened over time.

Pathophysiology of RSI

Common repetitive use injuries include carpal tunnel syndrome, bursitis and epicondylitis.

Carpal tunnel syndrome

Carpal tunnel syndrome is one of the three most common work-related injuries. The incidence is related to long-term use of computer keyboards, repetitive tasks and using tools that vibrate. It is higher in women, especially post-menopausal women, as it has a link to hormonal levels. There does appear to be a genetic predisposition and people with small wrists are inclined to suffer more.

The carpal tunnel is a canal through which flexor tendons and the median nerve pass from the wrist to the hand. The syndrome develops when the tunnel narrows because of inflammation or swelling of the joint, and irritation of the median nerve ensues. The person complains of numbness and tingling of the thumb, index finger and lateral ventral surface of the middle finger. They may also complain of pain in this area that interferes with sleep and is alleviated by shaking or massaging the hand and fingers. The affected hand may become weak and the person may be unable to hold utensils or perform activities that require precision. People who complain of a hot burning sensation probably have nerve damage from lack of oxygen and other nutrients.

Bursitis

Bursitis is an inflammation of a bursa which is an enclosed sac found between muscles, tendons and bony prominences. The bursae that commonly become inflamed are in the shoulder, hip, knee and elbow. Constant friction between the bursa and the musculoskeletal tissue around it causes irritation, oedema and inflammation. Symptoms develop as the sac becomes engorged, the area becomes tender and extension and flexion of the joint near the bursa produce pain. The inflamed bursa is hot, red and oedematous. The person guards the joint to decrease pain and may point to the area of the bursa when identifying joint tenderness.

Epicondylitis

Epicondylitis is the inflammation of the tendon at its point of origin into the bone and is also referred to as *tennis elbow* or *golfer's elbow*. Tears, bleeding and oedema are thought to cause avascularisation and calcification of the tendon.

NURSING CARE FOR RSI

The nursing care of a patient with a repetitive strain injury focuses on relieving pain. Using splints can relieve pain because it prevents movement of the inflamed area and application of either hot or cold packs can reduce swelling and inflammation. A referral may be made to a physiotherapist who will show the person exercises that will prevent joint stiffness. It may be that they need educating about their posture when working with computers and how to avoid repetitive use of certain joints.

PRACTICE ALERT

The patient with a repetitive strain injury usually receives NSAIDs. Opioids also may be administered for acute flare-ups and severe pain. For the person who has epicondylitis or carpal tunnel syndrome, corticosteroids may be injected into the joint.

METABOLIC BONE DISORDERS

Metabolic bone disorders originate in the bone remodelling process, which normally involves a sequence of events of bone reabsorption and formation. In adults, this process is primarily internal remodelling involving replacement of trabecular (spongy) bone. Adults replace about 25% of trabecular bone every four months through reabsorption of old bone by osteoclasts and formation of new bone by osteoblasts. Metabolic bone disorders may result from a variety of factors, including ageing, calcium and phosphate imbalances, genetics and changes in levels of hormones.

The person with osteoporosis

From the age of 35 years onwards, more bone cells are lost than replaced in the body (referred to as bone thinning). Women are affected by this more than men, probably because men's bones are denser than those of women. It is thought that by the time women reach the age of 60, 15% have osteoporosis. It is referred to as a silent disease, that is, people do not know they have it until they have had a fracture following a fall, as in Case Study 2.

Risk factors for osteoporosis

It is known that the following hormone-related problems contribute to osteoporosis:

- hyperthyroidism;
- Cushing's syndrome;
- diabetes;
- coeliac disease.

Other factors include:

- low levels of calcium and vitamin D in the diet;
- drinking alcohol;
- smoking;

FAST FACTS

Osteoporosis

- 230 000 fractures occur each year because of osteoporosis, costing health and social services in the UK over £1.8 billion a year.
- 50% of people with fractures from osteoporosis lose their mobility and independence.
- People over the age of 60 years with these fractures utilise two million hospital bed days!
- 14 000 people die each year from hip fractures.
- Hip fractures cost the NHS and government more than £2.3 billion a year – that's £6 million a day.

Source: National Osteoporosis Society 2005.

- iatrogenic (treatment-induced) causes due to long-term use of steroid medication.

Content *et al.* (2003) found that when osteoporosis nurse practitioners informed patients and their GPs that their wrist fracture could have been due to osteoporosis, more patients availed themselves of screening programmes and took precautions such as modifying their diet.

Case Study 2 – Joy
NURSING CARE PLAN Osteoporosis screening

It is six weeks since Joy has had the plaster removed from her fractured wrist. She has had physiotherapy as an out-patient and has regained full use of her hand and wrist. Joy is contacted by the fracture liaison service, who would like Joy to undertake some bone density measurements which are taken from the hip, using a dual energy x-ray absorptiometry (DEXA) scanner. A family history is taken from Joy, as evidence suggests that there is a genetic link and, as Joy's mother and aunt have had fragility fractures, it would suggest that she is at increased risk.

The fact that Joy has had a sedentary lifestyle is another contributing factor and, as seen from her case history at the beginning of the chapter, she regularly consumes alcohol. Kanis *et al.* (2005) state that four units of alcohol a day can double the risk of hip fractures in women over retirement age.

Joy is given nutritional advice to ensure that her diet includes calcium and vitamin D. These can be taken as dietary supplements. Joy may wish to consider reducing her alcohol and caffeine intake.

Another way in which Joy can reduce her risk of further osteoporosis is by engaging in regular exercise, walking for at least 30 minutes a day at least four times a week is very beneficial. Exercise has to be weight bearing, which is why walking is advocated over, say, swimming.

INTERDISCIPLINARY CARE FOR OSTEOPOROSIS

NICE (2011) recommend the following:

- oral bisphosphonates – alendronate, etidronate and risedronate;
- the oestrogen receptor modulator Raloxifene;
- strontium ranelate.

The person with Paget's disease

Paget's disease is an age-related, progressive skeletal disorder that results from metabolic activity in bone, where reabsorption and formation of new bone is excessive. This chronic remodelling leaves the affected bones larger and softer than normal, resulting in bone pain, **arthritis**, obvious skeletal deformities, fractures and nerve compression syndromes. The disorder affects the femur, pelvis, vertebrae and skull; it may affect one bone or several. There are several theories as to why people develop Paget's disease, and recent research would suggest that it is genetic with 15–40% of people having a family history of the disease. More people in the UK present with Paget's disease than anywhere else in the world, and it affects men more than women (www.paget.org.uk). Although people have the disease in certain parts of Europe and in New Zealand, it is very rare in Scandinavia and Asia, which suggests that as well as being genetic there may be some environmental reasons for it developing. Most cases are asymptomatic, but for about 15% of sufferers, the condition can be treated successfully with medication.

Signs and symptoms of Paget's disease

The most common symptom is localised pain which is described as mild to moderate, a deep ache that is aggravated by pressure and weight bearing or persistent and nagging. It is more noticeable at night or when the person is resting. There is flushing and warmth in the overlying skin because of the increased blood flow to pagetic bone. People may present with deformities, fractures and muscle weakness, hearing loss, hypercalcaemia and spinal cord injuries.

Complications of Paget's disease

Complications of Paget's disease are:

- **osteoarthritis;**
- cardiac failure;
- loss of hearing – if the skull is affected;
- hypercalcaemia;
- **gout;**
- nerve compression.

INTERDISCIPLINARY CARE FOR PAGET'S DISEASE

Diagnosis

The condition can be seen in x-rays and bone scans, which illustrate localised areas of demineralisation in the early stages, seen as 'punched-out' areas that lend a coarse, irregular appearance to the bone. In the later phase, x-rays show enlargement of the bones, tiny cracks in the long bones and bowing of the weight-bearing bones. CT scans and MRIs help identify possible causes of pain, including degenerative problems, spinal stenosis or nerve root impingement.

Medication

People with mild symptoms often find relief using aspirin or NSAIDs, such as ibuprofen and indomethacin.

Bisphosphonates and calcium supplements are the primary treatments used for severe Paget's disease. Pamidronate and zoledonic acid are given as injections; one injection of zoledonic acid can instigate a two-year remission. After bisphosphonate treatment, patients often experience remission of symptoms for a year or more.

Calcitonin inhibits osteoclastic reabsorption of bone. It also works as an analgesic for bone pain. The two derivatives of this medication are salmon and human. Salmon calcitonin is generally preferred because it is inexpensive and widely available. Human calcitonin is derived from human thyroid glands, which makes it more expensive and difficult to obtain.

NURSING CARE FOR PAGET'S DISEASE

A diagnosis of Paget's disease can be frightening for the individual and their family. It is important that they understand that this is a treatable disease and that many manifestations of the disease will be relieved with treatment. The Paget Association, UK should be suggested as a useful resource for up-to-date information and support.

The person with gout

Gout has been a recognised disorder for centuries; it is believed that Charles V of Habsburg abdicated in the 1500s after a particularly bad episode of gout. It was known as a rich man's illness because only the rich could afford a diet that led to the disorder, but is increasing in incidence now because of changes in lifestyle and diet.

Pathophysiology of gout

Gout is an arthritis that arises from inflammation that is caused following a buildup of serum uric acid (hyperuricaemia) which precipitates as sodium monourate crystals in the joints causing erosion of cartilage and bone; and it is a metabolic disease because it results from by-products of metabolism of alcohol, particularly beer, and purine-rich foods, for example meat, full-fat dairy products and seafood. The liver produces uric acid in response to high levels of metabolites from the digestion of red meats and alcohol, and suppresses insulin production. The kidneys are unable to excrete all the uric acid, resulting in higher levels of serum uric acid. The sodium monourate crystals can lead to the development of renal stones.

The joint most affected is the big toe, but it can occur elsewhere, and the buildup of crystals results in nodules called tophi. Men over the age of 50 are more susceptible than women.

Signs and symptoms of gout

The person usually presents with a large, swollen, reddened big toe that is extremely painful. The onset is usually sudden.

Diagnosis is confirmed following a blood test where the serum uric acid and ESR (eosinophils sedimentation rate) is raised. Approximately 50% of initial attacks of acute gouty arthritis occur in the metatarsophalangeal joint of the big toe.

INTERDISCIPLINARY CARE FOR GOUT

Medication

In an acute attack, pain management is the main objective and usually the person is prescribed NSAIDs, such as diclofenac, indomethacin or ibuprofen. Colchicine can be given to those who cannot tolerate NSAIDs; however, its use is limited because of the side-effects, which are principally nausea and vomiting and abdominal pain.

If the person has several bouts of gout, the condition can be controlled with allopurinol, and this is started after an acute attack has subsided.

Nutrition

Shulten *et al.* (2009), in a study conducted in Australia, found that dietary modifications were as effective at controlling episodes of gout as prophylactic treatment with drugs such as allopurinol, but that people were not always compliant. However, those people who reduced their intake of beer and exchanged full-fat dairy products for low-fat products and reduced their intake of red meat and seafood did see benefits. Choi *et al.* (2007) provide evidence that consumption of coffee (five to six cups a day) also reduces the risk of gout.

The problem with the dietary advice as seen by Shulten *et al.* (2009) is that the population considers fish as a healthy food because the omega-3 oils are beneficial in reducing heart disease and a large increase in coffee raises the blood pressure. It would seem sensible to advocate moderation and variation in diet for a healthy lifestyle.

A liberal fluid intake to maintain a daily urinary output of 2000 mL or more is recommended to increase urate excretion and reduce the risk of urinary stone formation.

NURSING CARE FOR GOUT

Nursing care primarily focuses on management of the acute phase, which involves managing the person's pain. Medical management can be augmented by encouraging the person to rest, elevate the foot and apply hot or cold compresses for comfort. The affected joints are so painful that even the weight of a sheet can be unbearable so using a bed cradle to keep the weight off the toe is beneficial.

Degenerative disorders, of which arthritis is one, are the most common form of arthritis and develop over time, thus affecting older people more than younger. However, athletes who put more pressure on the musculoskeletal system may experience problems much earlier.

We have now finished our discussion of metabolic bone disorders and will proceed to look at degenerative disorders.

Degenerative disorders, of which arthritis is one, develop over time.

The person with osteoarthritis (OA)

Risk factors for OA

There is some debate over the aetiology of osteoarthritis. There is evidence that there is a genetic tendency affecting more females in a family than males. However, age, weight and mechanical loading are implicated in most instances. Repetitive tasks and movements aggravate the situation.

The causes of secondary OA include trauma, mechanical stress, inflammation of joint structures, joint instability, neurological disorders, endocrine disorders and selected medications.

Other risk factors that are linked to OA are hormonal factors such as decreased oestrogen in menopausal women, excessive growth hormone and increased parathyroid hormone.

Pathophysiology of OA

OA is the most commonly occurring of all forms of arthritis. This disease is characterised by loss of articular cartilage in articulating joints and hypertrophy of the bones at the articular margins. It may be idiopathic (without known cause) or secondary (associated with known risk factors). Men are affected more than women at an earlier age, but the rate of OA in women exceeds that in men by the middle adult years. The joints most affected are in the hand, wrist, neck, lower back, hip, knee, ankle and feet. Men are more likely than women to have OA in the hips, whereas post-menopausal women more often have OA in their hands.

Localised OA affects only one or two joints whereas generalised OA affects three or more joints. Idiopathic OA most commonly affects the terminal interphalangeal joints (*Heberden's nodes*). Secondary OA may occur in any joint from an articular injury.

Signs and symptoms of OA

OA usually develops gradually and insidiously. Pain and stiffness in one or more joints are the first signals, with pain being localised and described as a deep ache. It is aggravated by use or movement of the joint and relieved by rest; some people feel the change in weather aggravates the area. Pain at night may be accompanied by paraesthesias (numbness, tingling); patients wake up feeling stiff and sore and, following periods of immobility, like in a long car ride, joints may stiffen. Usually only a few minutes of activity are necessary to relieve the stiffness. The range of movement of the joint decreases as the disease progresses and crepitus (grating sound of bones rubbing together) may be noted during movement. Disc degeneration and joint space narrowing alter the mechanics of the spinal column, promoting osteoarthritic changes in the articular processes (the facet joints) of the vertebrae. The cartilage covering the inferior and superior articular processes degenerates, causing localised pain, stiffness, muscle spasm and limited range of movement. Osteophytes may form on articular processes, further contributing to pain and muscle spasm.

The presentation of OA in older people is similar to that in younger adults. However, in this population, the risk of debilitation because of OA is greater and the disease may progress faster.

INTERDISCIPLINARY AND NURSING CARE FOR OA

Medication

There are no treatments available to arrest the process of joint degeneration. OA is initially treated conservatively, the initial focus of care being to manage pain through the use of analgesics such as aspirin or acetaminophen. NSAIDs such as ibuprofen or naproxen may also be prescribed.

Potent anti-inflammatory medications, such as systemic corticosteroids, are seldom prescribed for people with OA, although intra-articular corticosteroid injections may be used. With intra-articular injections, a long-acting corticosteroid medication, often mixed with a local anaesthetic such as lidocaine, is injected directly into the joint space of the affected joints. Although this procedure may provide marked pain relief, it can hasten the rate of cartilage breakdown if performed more frequently than every four to six months.

The nursing assessment should include finding out what the person has done in the past to relieve pain and how successful the measures were. Given that the medication can cause gastric bleeding and constipation, the assessment should include questions about their tolerance of the drugs used, their bowel movements and whether there has been any rectal bleeding noticed.

Surgery

Arthroscopy

An arthroscopy may be done to diagnose the type of arthritis or to perform debridement (cleaning) by smoothing rough cartilage and flushing out the joint to remove debris.

Osteotomy

An osteotomy is an incision into the bone, which may be performed to realign an affected joint, particularly when significant bony overgrowth or osteophyte formation has occurred. This procedure may also be used to shift the joint load toward areas of less severely damaged cartilage, improving function and reducing pain.

Joint arthroplasty

A joint arthroplasty is the reconstruction or replacement of a joint. Arthroplasty is usually indicated when the person has severely restricted joint mobility and pain at rest. Pain is

virtually eliminated and the function of the joint is generally improved. Arthroplasty may involve partial joint replacement or reshaping of the bones of a joint. For most people with OA, both surfaces of the affected joint are replaced with prosthetic parts in a procedure known as a *total joint replacement*. Joints that may be replaced include the hip, knee, shoulder, elbow, ankle, wrist and joints of the fingers and toes.

FAST FACTS

Joint replacements

- 160 000 hip and knee replacements are performed each year in the UK.
- 23% of hip operations are on people younger than 60 years of age (a rising trend because of obesity)
- between a third and a half of the operations are carried out in the independent sector – figures for 2010 show that 48 093 operations were carried out in the independent sector and 115 398 operations were carried out in the NHS.
- 85% of people are satisfied with their post-operative outcomes.

Source: National Joint Registry, www.njrcentre.org.uk (accessed September 2011).

In a total joint replacement, some or all of the synovium, cartilage and bone on both sides of the joint are removed. A metallic prosthesis is inserted to replace one joint surface (generally the load-end or distal portion of a weight-bearing joint). The other joint surface is replaced by a silicone-lined ceramic or plastic prosthesis.

In a *total hip replacement* (Figure 12.12), the articular surfaces of the acetabulum and femoral head are replaced with a prosthesis of high-molecular-weight polyethylene.

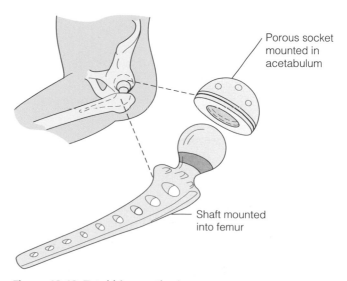

Porous socket mounted in acetabulum

Shaft mounted into femur

Figure 12.12 Total hip prosthesis.

Most hip replacements last 10–15 years, after which a second joint replacement, called a revision, can be performed. Potential problems associated with a total hip replacement include blood clots in leg veins, dislocation within the prosthesis, loosening of joint components from surrounding bone and infection. Infection is a major problem as there is a 20% risk of acquiring infection. If infections are recurrent or ineffectively treated, it may necessitate removal of the prosthesis, resulting in severe shortening of the extremity and an unstable joint. The other joints that frequently require surgical intervention are the knees (see Figure 12.13 for an example of joint replacement).

NURSING CARE PLAN The person undergoing a joint replacement

Nursing care should start as soon as the decision is made to perform a joint replacement. People make a better recovery following surgery if they have been well prepared physically and mentally beforehand.

Review Chapter 1 for routine pre- and post-operative care.

Pre-operative care

Pre-operative preparation should include:

+ a range of exercises that they will have to do post-operatively to be practised now

+ introduction to crutches so that they can use them and build up confidence before surgery

+ a home assessment to ascertain that they will not be using low chairs, beds or toilet seats. Modifications may need to be made by the occupational therapists to raise toilet seats and chair levels.

+ Assessment of infection risk which should include a dental checkup.

Prior to the date of the planned surgery, the person will be screened for MRSA and checked that they are suitable for anaesthesia. At this point, the nurse should discuss the post-operative pain management protocols as this allays anxiety.

Post-operative care

Post-operatively, the key to good care is pain management as this enables the person to mobilise much more quickly. Initially, the person may receive opioids via a patient controlled analgesia (PCA) pump intravenously or given epidural opiates. A step-down approach is used, that is opioids are reduced gradually and oral analgesics and NSAIDs are increased.

The person returns from surgery with a wound that is closed with either sutures or staples, covered with a semi-permeable dressing which should not be removed unless there is a significant amount of seepage to prevent infection. When it is hip replacement surgery, a drain is usually inserted to prevent a haematoma forming at the site of the operation.

As the person is at risk of developing thromboembolisms (blood clots in the veins – DVTs), antiembolism stockings are applied. For the person over 60 years of age, a prophylactic dose of heparin (an anticoagulant) may also be given.

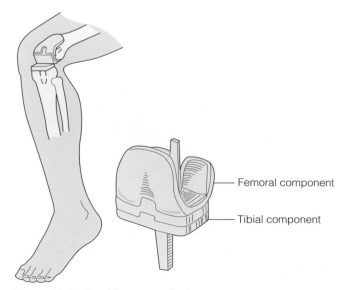

— Femoral component

— Tibial component

Figure 12.13 Total knee prosthesis.

Physical therapy and rehabilitation

Recovery from all types of joint replacement requires post-operative physical therapy, focusing on building strength and regaining joint flexibility. Following a total knee replacement, people have to use crutches or walking sticks for four to six weeks. Following a hip replacement, people have to do their exercises three times a day to improve muscle strength. They will usually be up and walking on crutches from the first day after surgery without putting any weight on the leg which has been operated on, and they may have to be partially non-weight-bearing for six weeks, depending on the surgical procedure and whether cement was used to fix the prostheses. Recovery takes between three and six months and people often report pain in their buttocks up to 12 weeks following surgery.

AUTOIMMUNE AND INFLAMMATORY DISORDERS

Autoimmune and inflammatory disorders of the musculo-skeletal system are chronic systemic disorders, characterised by diffuse inflammatory lesions and degenerative changes in connective tissues. The disorders have similar clinical features and may affect many of the same structures and organs.

The person with rheumatoid arthritis (RA)

Rheumatoid arthritis (RA) is the most common form of inflammatory arthritis, of which there are approximately 200 variations, affecting 580 000 people in England with 26 000 new cases being reported each year (Finney and Thwaites 2010). RA affects all people irrespective of where they live and what climate they live in; however, Martin (2004) states it is less prevalent in Asian communities and absent in certain parts of Africa. RA is considered a systemic disease because it affects the whole body, producing flu-like symptoms, anaemia and general malaise. Unlike osteoarthritis where only one joint may be affected, RA is a symmetrical, i.e. affecting both sides of the body, disease affecting the synovial membranes covering the joints in the hands, wrists, feet, ankles, knees and shoulders.

Risk factors for RA

Whilst siblings can develop the disease, it is not classified as hereditary. Rankin (2005) questions whether it is autoimmune in origin and believes that the autoimmune response develops after the person has had either a bacterial or viral infection. This is based on evidence gleaned from molecular biology, where it would appear that proteins from micro-organisms can mimic proteins in host cells and lead to an immunological response that then becomes autoimmune because it can no longer differentiate between itself and the non-self proteins. Because patients with RA respond in different ways, it would suggest that there are variants of the disease and, as yet, no definitive cause has been established.

INTERDISCIPLINARY CARE FOR RA

The main aims of care are:

- diagnosis;
- relief of symptoms;
- preserving function;
- preventing deformity.

Diagnosis

There is no single blood test that can categorically lead to a diagnosis so a range of tests are undertaken before the disease is confirmed and these include:

- Full blood count as patients often prove to be anaemic.
- Liver function tests; alkaline phosphatase and gamma glutamyl transferase levels are raised when inflammation is present in the body.
- ESR, CRP and plasma viscosity levels are other indicators of inflammation.
- Immunological tests measuring rheumatoid factor, nuclear antibody and anti-cyclic citrullinated peptide levels. Eighty per cent of people with RA have raised levels of rheumatoid factor, and 5% of the population may have the factor but not the disease. Anti-cyclic citrullinated peptide is raised with inflammation of the synovial membrane.

Other diagnostic tests include x-rays which show joint deterioration and the bones have small puncture-like holes and ultrasound which is useful at delineating early disease.

Medication

Pain is managed with regular analgesia, e.g. paracetamol and NSAIDs; however, this requires close monitoring because of the gastrointestinal and other side-effects. Newer medication includes disease modifying antirheumatic drugs (DMARDs) and slow-acting antirheumatic drugs (SAARDs). Corticosteroids can be injected into a joint if there is a flare-up of disease or given orally as a low maintenance dose.

Thwaites and Finney (2010) state that immunotherapy in the form of monoclonal antibodies such as Infliximab, Etanercept and Adulimumab are now being used but these drugs are expensive and a year's treatment can cost £10,000.

NURSING CARE FOR RA

When patients are experiencing acute phases of illness they will require nursing care. The main emphasis of care is to control pain using hot or cold compresses, provide support for painful joints and provide psychological support and education to help sufferers and their families cope with the effects of RA on their lives.

The impact of RA

As a disease, RA fluctuates with periods when people are asymptomatic. However, when suffering pain and fatigue people have real problems, especially when there are no other visible signs and symptoms of illness, and this can cause tension in families and at work. The National Rheumatoid Arthritis

Society (NRAS 2007) reports that many RA sufferers cannot continue in paid employment within six years of their diagnosis. People report that:

- Home life is disrupted because of their physical limitations.
- They cannot engage in hobbies to distract themselves.
- They lose control and independence.
- Although they are fatigued, they are unable to sleep and rest (50% of those with RA report having persistent fatigue that is not associated with any other symptoms).

The illness results in body changes and altered body image. The loss of life as they knew it can precipitate grieving reactions and depression with 21–34% of cases being unrecognised and untreated.

Nursing diagnoses and interventions

Nursing diagnoses and interventions for RA focus on the management of fatigue and on psychological issues.

Fatigue

Fatigue is a notoriously difficult symptom to manage and, whilst the obvious advice is to rest, it is evident from research undertaken with cancer patients and other chronic conditions that exercise is the best way to combat this. In a systematic review conducted by Neill *et al.* (2006), it is evident aerobic exercise such as walking for 15–20 minutes at least three times a week leads to significant levels of improvement. An alternative form of exercise is Tai Chi which brings additional benefit by being a group activity. Neill *et al.* (2006) also found that cognitive behavioural therapy was beneficial in altering perceptions of fatigue. It may be that patients need advice as to timing their periods of activity to coincide with the time of day that they feel more enabled to do this, given that joint stiffness tends to be experienced in the mornings.

Psychological issues

People with RA have expressed feelings of frustration, fear and anger. People have different coping styles so it is important that these are recognised and that the resilient person is allowed to be self-caring and that nursing actions do not undermine this resilience. The person who is demonstrating a fatalistic coping style should be offered support and strategies that may enable them to cope better. Coping strategies can be summarised as:

+ *Accepting the challenge* where they take charge of their situation and deal with it proactively.
+ *Palliative coping* where they distract themselves by watching TV or talking to a friend.
+ *Fatalistic coping* where they just put up with the situation.
+ *Supportant coping* where they discuss their problems and issues with a friend.
+ *Self-reliant coping* where they strive to do as much for themselves as best they can without obtaining support elsewhere.

The person with systemic lupus erythematosus (SLE)

Systemic lupus erythematosus (SLE) is a chronic inflammatory connective tissue disease affecting mainly women of childbearing age. It frequently affects the musculoskeletal system but also affects kidneys, lungs, heart, skin and central nervous system. In the UK, about 12.5–26 people per 100 000 are affected. Relatively few people experience the disease in the same way (www.lupusuk.org.uk). For some it may lead to repeated miscarriages, and those who are pregnant require close medical monitoring. The disease can be triggered at any point; at puberty, following childbirth, after trauma, through sunlight and by some drugs. Although the exact aetiology of SLE is unknown, genetic, environmental and hormonal factors play a role in its development.

The course of SLE is mild in most people, with periods of remission and exacerbation. The number and severity of exacerbations tend to decrease with time. In some people, however, SLE is a virulent disease with significant organ system involvement.

Signs and symptoms of SLE

In the early stages, the symptoms are similar to those of RA, with joint and muscle pain, fatigue, skin rashes or flu-like symptoms. The skin rashes tend to be across both cheeks, evocative of butterfly wings. Some people develop photosensitivity and are advised not to sunbathe as this may precipitate a flare-up of the disease. Between 20 and 40% of people may develop renal disease. Some may develop depression (www.edren.org) as a result of the disease.

Diagnosis may take years depending on the severity of the symptoms. A full haematological screen, liver function tests and antinuclear antibody screening is undertaken.

INTERDISCIPLINARY CARE FOR SLE

Eighty per cent of patients do not need any treatment. However, if internal organs are affected, people may be treated with immunosuppressant drugs such as azathioprine and cyclophosphamide. The antimalarial drugs chloroquine and hydroxychloroquine are sometimes used to treat skin eruptions.

Because of the photosensitivity associated with SLE, the person should be cautioned to avoid sun exposure. They should use sunscreens with a sun protection factor (SPF) rating of 15 or higher when out of doors. Topical corticosteroids may be used to treat skin lesions.

NURSING CARE FOR SLE

Teaching is a critical factor in preparing patients with SLE for self-care at home. There are several websites which offer help and advice, such as Lupus UK, which is considered the best by professionals. Patients need to be aware that the disease can flare up and should seek medical advice when this occurs.

PRACTICE ALERT

The following are warning signs that SLE may flare up:

● increased fatigue;
● pain, abdominal discomfort;
● rash;
● headache;
● fever;
● dizziness.

The person with osteomyelitis

Osteomyelitis is an infection of the bone, caused by a pathogen. It can be acute, sub acute or chronic. Acute osteomyelitis occurs more in children; however, it is a rare condition. Adults usually develop sub-acute or chronic osteomyelitis following trauma or surgery; this is called contiguous osteomyelitis. It can also occur as a complication in diabetes and sickle cell anaemia (NHS Choices accessed 29.6.2010). The infection can be either bacterial or viral.

Signs and symptoms of osteomyelitis

Patients developing osteomyelitis will present with:

● pyrexia (elevated temperature);
● pain;
● nausea;
● anorexia.

In addition, the area over the site of infection will be warm and reddened.

Blood tests measuring ESR and WBC counts will be raised, and examination using MRI and CT scans will identify abscesses, sinus tracts and bone changes.

INTERDISCIPLINARY CARE FOR OSTEOMYELITIS

The care of the person with osteomyelitis focuses on relieving pain, eliminating the infection and preventing or minimising complications. Early diagnosis is important to prevent bone necrosis and to enable administration of the appropriate antibiotic. Most patients require both debridement of bone and a long period of antibiotic administration.

Medication

Antibiotic therapy is the first line of treatment, given over four to six weeks. Parenteral (intravenous) antibiotic therapy begins as soon as cultures (blood and/or wound) are obtained. A penicillinase-resistant semi-synthetic penicillin (for example, methicillin, oxacillin) may be given until the culture and sensitivity results are known. These antibiotics are used initially because many cases of osteomyelitis are caused by *Staphylococcus aureus*. When the detailed sensitivity report is obtained from the cultures, more definitive antibiotics are prescribed.

Surgery

Surgical debridement is the primary treatment for the patient with chronic osteomyelitis. The periosteum (outer bone casing) is excised and the cortex (middle) is drilled to release the pressure from accumulated pus. During this procedure, cultures will be obtained and sent to the laboratory for analysis. The wound holes are irrigated and the wound is then closed. The cavity may be kept clean by inserting drainage tubes that are connected to an irrigation and suction system. Post-operatively, the nurse is responsible for instilling and removing dilute antibiotic solutions through the drainage tubes.

A musculocutaneous (myocutaneous) flap is another approach used for the treatment of the dead space caused by extensive debridement of the infected site. The procedure involves moving or rotating a muscle and the section of skin fed by the arteries from that muscle into the cavity created by the surgery. A skin graft is performed later.

NURSING CARE FOR OSTEOMYELITIS

The person with chronic osteomyelitis faces frequent and lengthy hospitalisations and/or treatment. The prognosis is uncertain; they face a future of possible disability and perhaps an amputation if the infection does not clear.

Compromised immune status places the patient with osteomyelitis at risk for 'super' infection, which may be resistant to antibiotic therapies. To minimise the risk of infection for people who have undergone surgery for orthopaedic procedures, nurses must be vigilant and observe strict hand washing practices to maintain a safe environment for their patients.

Antibiotic therapy needs to be given at the exact time it is prescribed to ensure blood concentrations of the drugs remain constant and are not subject to peaks and troughs. It is when there are peaks and troughs that bacteria can develop resistance to the drugs.

Nurses must ensure that analgesia is given as prescribed and regularly to prevent the development of chronic pain syndromes occurring which are notoriously difficult to manage.

The nurse should ensure that the person with osteomyelitis receives a balanced diet containing plenty of protein and vitamins to aid recovery.

NEOPLASTIC DISORDERS

The person with a bone tumour

Pathophysiology of bone tumours

Bone tumours may be either primary (arising in the bone itself) or metastatic (seeded from a tumour elsewhere in the body), secondary to prostatic, breast, kidney, thyroid and lung cancers. Five to ten per cent of people with advanced cancer develop bone metastases. Like other tumours, bone tumours can be either benign or malignant.

Primary bone tumours can be of the:

- cartilage (chondrogenic); as in osteochondroma, which is a benign tumour or chondrosarcoma which is malignant;
- bone (osteogenic) as in osteosarcoma;
- collagen (collagenic) as in fibrosarcoma;
- bone marrow cells (myelogenic).

Osteosarcomas are the most common form; however, even they are rare. They are bimodal; that is 75% of these tumours occur in people under the age of 20 and represent 5% of cancers occurring in children. The second peak occurs in people over the age of 75, associated with other conditions such as Paget's disease. The cancer usually presents in the metaphysis of long bones (Figure 12.14).

Signs and symptoms of bone tumours

The three main manifestations of bone tumours are pain, a mass and impaired function. Bone pain usually comes on slowly and lasts for as long as a week, is constant or intermittent, and may be worse at night. The mass is described as a swelling or lump on the bones that is firm, slightly tender to touch and may be felt through the skin. The mass may interfere with normal movement and/or cause the bone to break.

INTERDISCIPLINARY CARE FOR BONE TUMOURS

The extent of the disease or staging is established following MRI and isotope bone scans. CT scans of the lungs are performed to establish whether the cancer has metastasised.

As with other malignant tumours, bone tumours are treated with chemotherapy, radiotherapy and surgery as described in Chapter 2.

NURSING CARE FOR BONE TUMOURS

The person with a bone tumour requires nursing care to meet many health problems, including prevention of injury, relief of pain, assistance with mobility and teaching about the disease process and treatment. The threat that is associated with cancer requires the nurse to provide psychological and emotional support as well as physical care. Survival rates have improved now that treatment includes combination of chemotherapy, radiotherapy with surgery. Chemotherapy is usually administered pre- and post-surgery. Once surgery

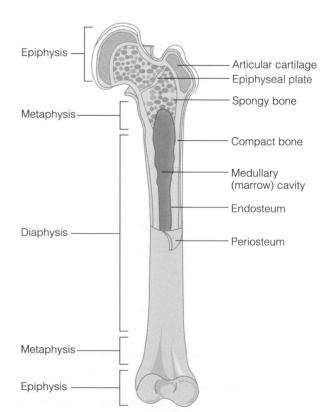

Figure 12.14 Anatomy of a long bone.

has been undertaken, the person may be discharged home and have chemotherapy and radiotherapy on an out-patients' basis.

The person with spinal cord compression

In cancer, spinal cord compression is an oncological emergency requiring immediate attention. The vertebral column is the most common site for bone metastases with:

- 70% of cancer deposits in the thoracic vertebrae;
- 20% in the lumbar vertebrae;
- 10% in the cervical region.

Signs and symptoms of spinal cord compression

The first indication that a person has developed spinal metastases may be a sensation of muscle weakness, or they may experience constipation. As the disease progresses, they may experience loss of feeling, or pins and needles and a tingling sensation in the legs. Ninety-five per cent of people report pain, which is worse at night when they are resting. The pain is described as burning and shooting which indicates that it is neuropathic (because of damage to the nerves).

INTERDISCIPLINARY CARE FOR SPINAL CORD COMPRESSION

Anyone suspected of having spinal cord compression needs to be immobilised to prevent pathological fractures and further damage to the spinal cord.

Diagnosis

People with suspected spinal cord involvement require an MRI scan. Scans can take up to an hour to perform; the machines are noisy and may prove very uncomfortable particularly if the person suffers from claustrophobia. If they cannot tolerate an MRI scan, a CT scan can be performed.

Medication

The main goal is to reduce the pain. NSAIDs are usually given, but this depends on the person's current pain medication. Stronger analgesics may be advocated in line with the World Health Organization guidelines as discussed in Chapter 2. As the person requires regular analgesia, which is constipating, they will need to take a laxative regularly to prevent straining and incurring further damage to the spinal cord.

The person with spinal cord compression secondary to cancer is usually treated with steroids; dexamethasone 8 mg twice a day initially.

Radiotherapy

Radiotherapy is the preferred treatment and is very effective at achieving pain control. The disadvantage of radiotherapy is that it does leave the person feeling fatigued and they may question its value, given that it signifies a deterioration in the condition.

CONNECTIVE TISSUE AND STRUCTURAL DISORDERS

Connective tissue is the most abundant and widely distributed body tissue. It not only connects body parts but also provides support; forms bones, cartilage and the walls of blood vessels; and attaches muscles to bones. Connective tissue consists of three elements:

- long fibres embedded in a
- non-cellular ground substance, and
- cells specific to the class of connective tissue.

Fibres made up primarily of collagen, a protein, are the most abundant in connective tissue. Connective tissue disorders, also known as collagen diseases, are a group of immune-mediated disorders and are often managed by rheumatologists.

The person with scleroderma

Scleroderma is an umbrella term that incorporates a group of rare conditions that may be either localised, affecting the skin only, or generalised (systemic sclerosis), with both skin and visceral organ involvement. Localised involvement may occur as irregularly shaped patches of skin (morphea) or a line of disease on the arm, leg or side of the face (linear scleroderma) and is usually seen in children only.

Systemic sclerosis literally translates as hardening of the skin; it is a chronic disease characterised by the formation of excess fibrous connective tissue and diffuse fibrosis of the skin and internal organs. Women are five times more likely to develop the condition than men.

Raynaud's phenomenon is also classified as scleroderma. In Raynaud's phenomenon, people report pain, numbness, tingling and blanching in the fingers when exposed to cold. The cause of the condition is unclear, and it involves blood vessels and neural function. For most people, it is a condition that is treated conservatively; however, a few develop symptoms of systemic sclerosis, hence its inclusion in this chapter although not strictly a condition of connective tissue *per se*.

Ninety per cent of scleroderma cases are systemic sclerosis and these tend to be in two subgroups: limited scleroderma, with long-standing Raynaud's phenomenon, skin and gastrointestinal involvement and some lung fibrosis, or diffuse scleroderma, with skin changes occurring within a year of developing Raynaud's phenomenon and significant involvement of lungs, kidneys, heart and gastrointestinal tract.

It is a difficult disease to diagnose as patients present with different disease profiles. There is evidence to support that there is a genetic component to the disease, but something is required to trigger disease activity. Antinuclear antibodies are present in the blood, which classifies this disease as being an autoimmune rheumatic disorder. Whilst there is as yet no treatment for systemic scleroderma, disease progression can be slowed down with the use on immunosuppressant drugs such as methotrexate, cyclophosphamide and azathioprine; however, some rheumatology centres are interested in exploring biological therapies such as infliximab.

As the disease is rare, it is important that patients are seen and treated in specialist centres so that they get the most effective treatment and care.

NURSING CARE FOR SCLERODERMA

Nursing care needs of patients with systemic sclerosis are individualised to the effects and the signs and symptoms of the disease. Nurses have a role in providing advice and guidance on physical care and in providing psychological support. The disease can have a poor prognosis similar to cancer.

Patients need referring to the various self-help groups and websites that offer valuable information and guidance such as www.scleroderma.royalfree.org.uk.

Skin care is very important, and the person should be taught to moisturise the skin and particularly the affected joints with oil-based moisturisers. Paraffin wax baths and massage are useful in bringing calcitonin lumps that develop in the skin to the fore.

The person with fibromyalgia

Fibromyalgia can be literally translated from the Greek to mean pain in the muscle fibres; however, it is not a muscular disorder as such but an idiopathic condition, that is, the cause is unknown and the condition comes on suddenly. It has been noted that people with fibromyalgia have low levels of

serotonin and high levels of substance P, a chemical present in the spinal cord that triggers pain receptors. It can be associated with rheumatoid arthritis and may be a bacterial or viral illness or trauma. It is a chronic condition affecting 1.7 million people in the England and Wales (NHS Choices accessed 29.6.2010). As with other chronic conditions outlined in this chapter, it is subject to flare-ups which can occur suddenly and disrupt life to such an extent that it makes work, socialising and other activities of living difficult.

Signs and symptoms of fibromyalgia

People with fibromyalgia present with a history of:

● sudden onset of pain;
● pain in four quadrants of the body, shoulders, arms, back and hips and legs – when these pain points are palpated they are tender and swollen;
● pain on waking associated with stiffness all over;
● insomnia;
● fatigue;
● headaches;
● irritable bowel syndrome;
● dizziness;
● sensitivity to light or noise or smoke or changes in the weather.

INTERDISCIPLINARY CARE FOR FIBROMYALGIA

Fibromyalgia is difficult to manage, and symptoms are treated as they arise. Pain can be treated with analgesics and non-steroidal anti-inflammatory drugs; however, there is no inflammation so NSAIDs are not very effective. Antidepressants such as amitriptyline are used as an adjuvant drug (see pain management in Chapter 2) because they stimulate the production of serotonin in the body. Non-pharmacological interventions offer the best relief. Henderson (2002) advocates cognitive behavioural therapy, autogenic training and exercise. Guided imagery, meditation and relaxation techniques have all been reported as helpful. Acupuncture offers some relief as does TENS.

NURSING CARE FOR FIBROMYALGIA

As there is no specific treatment for this chronic and debilitating condition, the nurse is pivotal in supporting people with fibromyalgia. The key supportive measures are:

✚ Demonstrate belief in the person; pain is what the person says it is and occurs when they say it does, at the intensity they describe.
✚ Listen to the person in a non-judgemental fashion.
✚ Explain the condition's idiosyncrasies so the person knows what to expect and can take charge of their condition.

+ Provide advice on supportive strategies, such as exercising, meditating, etc., that can be used to promote wellbeing and manage flare-ups of the condition.
+ Provide advice on sleep management.
+ Provide information on websites to access and support groups that are available.

The person with low back pain

Back pain is the largest single cause of absence from work in the UK (NHS Choices 2009). Acute or chronic low back pain involves the lumbar, lumbosacral or sacroiliac areas of the back. In most cases, low back pain is due to strains in the muscles and tendons of the back caused by abnormal stress or overuse.

In general, the five causes and types of back pain are as follows:

- Local pain is caused by compression or irritation of sensory nerves. Fractures, strains and sprains are common causes of local pain; tumours also may press on pain-sensitive structures.
- Referred pain may originate from abdominal or pelvic viscera.
- Pain of spinal origin, that is, pain associated with pathology of the spine such as disc disease or arthritis, may be referred to other structures such as the buttocks, groin or legs.
- Radicular back pain is sharp, radiating from the back to the leg along a nerve root. This pain may be aggravated by movements such as coughing, sneezing or sitting.
- Muscle spasm pain is associated with many spine disorders, although its origin may be unclear. This type of back pain is dull and may be accompanied by abnormal posture and taut spinal muscles.

Signs and symptoms of low back pain

People with low back pain report pain ranging from mild discomfort lasting a few hours to chronic debilitating pain. Acute pain is usually caused when the person participates in an activity that is not usually pursued, such as unusual lifting or bending, playing an active sport or shovelling snow. However, it may come on suddenly from a small movement and the person may find that they are unable to move.

INTERDISCIPLINARY CARE FOR LOW BACK PAIN

Care of the patient with low back pain focuses on relieving pain, correcting the condition if possible, preventing complications and educating the patient.

Medication

The medications of choice for low back pain include NSAIDs and analgesics. NSAIDs block prostaglandin production and reduce inflammation, thus relieving the pain. Epidural steroid injections may be used to help reduce intense, intractable pain. A steroid solution is injected into the epidural space, which helps decrease the swelling and inflammation of the spinal nerves.

Conservative treatment

The majority of people with acute low back pain need only a short-term treatment. Limited rest, combined with appropriate exercise and education, is often the primary method of treatment. There is no evidence that activity is harmful or aggravating to the source of pain. In fact, activity promotes bone and muscle strength and may increase endorphin levels. Therefore, active rehabilitation helps to restore function and reduce pain. Pain may be relieved by an ice bag or hot water bottle (or heating pad) applied to the back for short periods of time and, for optimum treatment, it is best to alternate the applications of heat and cold.

NURSING CARE FOR LOW BACK PAIN

Nursing care of the patient with low back pain focuses on relieving the pain. In addition, most people have very little understanding of the anatomy of the spine, the reasons for the pain, the choices for treatment and the importance of self-management. Therefore, education is another essential aspect of treating low back pain.

Health promotion

Recommendations for preventing back pain include the following:

+ Have a regular exercise programme.
+ Stretch before working in the garden, jogging and playing sports.
+ Lose weight, if needed.
+ Maintain a correct posture.
+ Use supportive seats when driving.
+ Lift by bending at the knees rather than at the waist.
+ Reduce emotional stress that causes muscle tension.

In industrial and work settings, nurses should be alert for situations that increase the risk of back pain and injury. Office workers should have chairs with appropriate seat height and length and back support. Modifications of workspace or machinery may be necessary for industrial workers to avoid excess stresses on back muscles. Finally, it is important to remember that back pain is a leading cause of lost work time for nurses themselves. Remind co-workers to use good body mechanics and to seek help when lifting or moving patients.

CASE STUDY SUMMARIES

Orthopaedic nursing has changed since Dame Agnes Hunt first set up and awarded certificates to nurses specialising in this field of care in the early 1900s. Whether having emergency or elective procedures, people remain in hospital for much shorter periods of time. The bones may heal over six to eight weeks, but the recovery period can be as long as six months to a year and much of this is spent in the community, managing on one's own for the most part.

Case Study 1. Stephen is typical of many new users of motorcycles and his accident is typical for his age group. Once emergency care has been given and the fractured femur is realigned and maintained in position through traction, Stephen has to wait until the bone heals, which means he is in hospital for a long time. This does have implications for him. His friends may get bored of hospital visiting, and they may initially arrive in a group and not know how to behave, which may cause embarrassment and offence. If friends do not maintain contact, Stephen may feel isolated which could lead to depression.

The timing of his accident will cause disruption to his school examinations, but arrangements can be made for these to be completed in hospital. Whatever the outcome, Stephen may have to revise his life plans at this moment in time, which may cause him a great deal of concern. His nursing care needs may well diminish; he will be able to attend to his hygiene needs. Initially, he may have problems with constipation as he is not eating or exercising as he used to. However, he will establish a new routine and this may only be a transient problem.

Case Study 2. Joy will recover fully following her wrist fracture. She will need physiotherapy once the plaster cast has been removed to regain strength and mobility. She may change her diet to reduce the risk of osteoporosis. As it is unlikely that Joy will be admitted to a ward following the setting of her fracture, she will need advice regarding pain management. Pain will be a problem until the bone starts to heal and Joy will need to take analgesics regularly. The type of analgesic taken depends on whether Joy is taking any other medication for other existing conditions such as hypertension.

Joy needs to be advised not to get her plaster cast wet; her arm can be encased in a plastic bag whilst she showers. She will require assistance with washing and dressing. The nurse needs to enquire whether this will pose a problem for Joy as she may need social care for the first few weeks until she can manage herself. It is usual to recommend a diet high in calcium to enhance bone healing and, whilst there is calcium and vitamin D in dairy products, rich sources of calcium are available in nuts and seeds, particularly sesame seeds, and green vegetables such as broccoli.

Case Study 3. Ben will need a great deal of ongoing care following his amputation. His losses may not just be limited to altered body image. If Ben has difficulty in adapting to being wheelchair dependent, he may well lose his home. Being transferred into residential care will entail many losses, such as loss of independence and friends and acquaintances from his neighbourhood. Ben faces many challenges that will affect him psychologically and socially, and he will require support in dealing with these issues.

CHAPTER HIGHLIGHTS

- Metabolic bone disorders are varied, and many of these diseases can have significant physical, psychosocial and financial consequences. When these problems occur, people experience a variety of individualised responses to their altered health status.

- Degenerative and autoimmunine disorders of the musculoskeletal system are chronic systemic disorders, characterised by diffuse inflammatory lesions and degenerative changes in connective tissues. These disorders have similar clinical features and may affect many of the same structures and organs.

- Osteomyelitis, an infection of the bone, can be acute, sub-acute or chronic. The condition typically develops sub-acutely or as chronic osteomyelitis after trauma or surgery; this is called contiguous osteomyelitis. The infection may be either bacterial or viral.

- Neoplastic disorders, bone tumours, may be either primary (arising in the bone itself) or metastatic (seeded from a tumour elsewhere in the body), secondary to prostatic, breast, kidney, thyroid and lung cancers. Between 5 and 10% of people with advanced cancer develop bone metastases. As is the case with other tumours, bone tumours can be either benign or malignant.

- Connective tissue disorders include scleroderma and fibromyalgia. Connective tissue is the most abundant and widely distributed body tissue. It not only connects body parts but also offers support, forms bones, cartilage and the walls of blood vessels, and attaches muscles to bones.

- Structural disorders include back pain, and this is the largest single cause of absence from work in the UK. Acute or chronic low back pain involves the lumbar, lumbosacral or sacroiliac areas of the back. In the majority of cases, low back pain is due to strains in the muscles and tendons of the back caused by abnormal stress or overuse.

TEST YOURSELF

1. With ageing, bone mass and calcium absorption decrease. What risk is increased as a result?

   a. obesity
   b. weakness
   c. fractures
   d. deformity

2. What term is used to describe a grating sound when a joint is moved?

   a. crackles
   b. arthritis
   c. synovitis
   d. crepitus

3. What are the most common signs and symptoms of musculoskeletal disorders?

   a. pain and limited mobility
   b. swelling and exaggerated reflex responses
   c. cyanosis and decreased pulses
   d. pallor and decreased range of movement

4. A woman has a cast applied to her left lower arm (from below the elbow down to her fingers). Which of the following assessments indicates a possible complication?

   a. slightly oedematous fingers
   b. warm pink skin above the cast
   c. pale cold fingers
   d. throbbing pain

5. The day after a below-the-knee amputation, the person describes pain in his amputated foot. What is this experience called?

   a. chronic stump pain
   b. contracture pain
   c. attention seeking
   d. phantom limb pain

6. A post-operative nursing care plan for someone who has had a total knee replacement includes monitoring vital signs because:

   a. it ensures regular contact with the person
   b. it ensures that there is adequate circulation to the affected limb
   c. it monitors whether the person has developed an infection
   d. it ascertains whether the person has altered mood

7. When a bone is broken into many pieces it is said to be:

   a. a comminuted fracture
   b. a compacted fracture
   c. a compressed fracture
   d. an avulsed fracture

8. Which of the following is not a complication of Paget's disease?

   a. osteoarthritis
   b. deafness
   c. respiratory depression
   d. cardiac failure

9. Muscles that are overstretched result in a:

   a. sprain
   b. contusion
   c. strain
   d. tear

10. Which of the following minerals is essential to bone healing?

   a. sodium
   b. calcium
   c. potassium
   d. magnesium

Further resources

WHO Fracture Risk Assessment Tool
www.shef.ac.uk/FRAX
This website provides links to other sites providing information about osteoporosis. The site has a tool for self-assessing the potential of developing fractures which is internationally recognised and helps standardise care.

International Osteoporosis Association
http://www.iofbonehealth.org/
This website has a special section for healthcare professionals. The focus is on osteoporosis, and there is access provided to professional journals which contain articles on the latest research being undertaken.

Arthritis Care
http://www.arthritiscare.org.uk/
This website offers a wealth of information which is useful to professionals. The society responds to government strategies and comments are available. There is a discussion forum which makes it a useful site for people who have recently received a diagnosis of arthritis.

Arthritis Research UK
http://www.arc.org.uk/
This website features a section for healthcare professionals; the charity provides bursaries and grants for healthcare professionals wishing to extend their expertise in this field of medicine. It advertises professional conferences and provides information on current research.

UK Fibromyalgia
http://www.ukfibromyalgia.com
This website is very useful for people with this disease as it specifies all the help they can access including financial benefits they may be entitled to. It is a useful resource that nurses can recommend to people with this debilitating disease.

Scleroderma Society
http://www.sclerodermasociety.co.uk/newsite/links.php
This UK-based charity website has links to the Royal Free Hospital which is a specialist centre treating people with this disease. It provides useful information about the disease but also about support groups and annual events where people can meet others who have problems or issues similar to their own.

Bibliography

Brown S (2003) Systemic lupus erythematosus. *Nursing Times.Net*, available at: http://www.nursingtimes.net/nursing-practice-clinical-research/systemic-lupus-erythematosus/205276.article (accessed August 2011).

Choi H K, Wilett W and Curham G (2007) Coffee consumption and risk of incident gout in men. *Arthritis and Rheumatism*, **56**(6), 2049–2055.

Clarke D D, Ward P, Bartle C and Truman W (2004) In depth study of motorcycle accidents, *Road Safety Research Report No 54*, London, Department for Transport.

Content G, Hajela V and Lucas B (2003) Osteoporosis screening and education following distal radial fracture: an expanding role for fracture clinic nurses. *Journal of Orthopaedic Nursing*, **7**, 137–140.

Finney A and Thwaites C (2010) Rheumatoid Arthritis 1: background, symptoms and ensuring prompt diagnosis and treatment, *Nursing Times*, **9**(106), 22–24.

Grant S, Kerr D and Wallis M (2005) Comparison of povidone–iodine solution and soft white paraffin ointment in the management of skeletal pin-sites: a pilot study. *Journal of Orthopaedic Nursing*, **9**, 218–225.

Hannon C and Murphy K (2007) A survey of nurses' and midwives' knowledge of risks and lifestyle factors associated with osteoporosis. *Journal of Orthopaedic Nursing*, **11**, 30–37.

Henderson H (2002) The causes, symptoms and management of fibromyalgia, *Nursing Times.Net*, available at: http://www.nursingtimes.net/nursing-practice/clinical-specialisms/pain-management/the-causes-symptoms-and-management-of-fibromyalgia/199405.article (accessed September 2011).

Kanis J A, Johansson H, Johnell O et al. (2005) Alcohol intake as a risk factor for fracture. *Osteoporosis International*, **16**, 737–742.

Love C (2003) Carpal tunnel syndrome. *Journal of Orthopaedic Nursing*, **7**, 33–42.

Lucas B (2008a) Total hip and total knee replacement: preoperative management, *British Journal of Nursing*, **17**(21), 1346–1350.

Lucas B (2008b) Total hip and total knee replacement: postoperative nursing management. *British Journal of Nursing*, **17**(22), 1410–1414.

Martin L (2004) Rheumatoid arthritis: symptoms, diagnosis and management. *Nursing Times.Net*, available at: http://www.nursingtimes.net/nursing-practice-clinical-research/rheumatoid-arthritis-symptoms-diagnosis-and-management/204381.article (accessed September 2011).

Melanson PM and Downe-Womboldt B (2003) Confronting life with rheumatoid arthritis. *Journal of Advanced Nursing*, **42**(2), 125–133.

National Osteoporosis Society (2005) *New Horizons in Bone Health. Research Executive Summary 2006–2009*. Bath, National Osteoporosis Society.

Nazarko L (2007) Care of the feet: common problems and how to treat them. *British Journal of Health Care Assistants*, **10**(1), 27–30.

Neill J, Belan I and Reid K (2006) Effectiveness of non-pharmacological interventions for fatigue in adults with multiple sclerosis, rheumatoid arthritis, or systemic lupus erythematosus: a systematic review. *Journal of Advanced Nursing*, **56**(6), 617–635.

NHS Choices (2009) Back pain, *Nursing Times.Net*, available at: http://www.nursingtimes.net/nursing-practice/clinical-specialisms/pain-management/back-pain/1984671.article (accessed August 2011).

NICE (2011) Alendronate, etidronate, risedronate, raloxifene, and strontium ranelate for the primary prevention of osteoporotic fragility fractures in post menopausal women (amended), available at http://publications.nice.org.uk/alendronate-etidronate-risedronate-raloxifene-and-strontium-ranelate-for-the-primary-prevention-ta160 (accessed 21 December 2011).

NRAS (2007) *NRAS Survey. I want to work. Employment and rheumatoid arthritis. A national picture*. Maidenhead, National Rheumatoid Arthritis Society.

Pellatt G C (2008) Nontraumatic spinal cord injury part 3: care for spinal cord compression. *British Journal of Neuroscience Nursing*, **4**(11), 549–553.

Ralston S H, Langston A L and Reid I R (2008) Pathogenesis and management of Paget's bone disease. *The Lancet*, **372**(9633), 155–163.

Ramjeet J, Smith J and Adams M (2008) The relationship between coping and psychological and physical adjustment in rheumatoid arthritis: a literature review. *Journal of Clinical Nursing*, **17**(11), 418–428.

Rankin J A (2005) Immunogenetics and rheumatoid arthritis: a review for orthopaedic nurses. *Journal of Orthopaedic Nursing*, **9**(2), 64–76.

Repping-Wuts H, Fransen J, van Achterberg G and van Riel P (2007) Persistent fatigue in patients with rheumatoid arthritis. *Journal of Clinical Nursing*, **16**(11), 377–383.

Richardson C (2008) Nursing aspects of phantom limb pain following amputation. *British Journal of Nursing*, **17**(7), 422–426.

Santy J and Newton-Triggs L (2006) A survey of current practice in skeletal pin site management. *Journal of Orthopaedic Nursing*, **10**, 198–205.

Shulten P, Thomas J, Miller M, Smith M and Ahern M (2009) The role of diet in the management of gout: a comparison of knowledge and attitudes to current evidence. *Journal of Human Nutrition and Dietetics*, **22**, 3–11.

Swinson D, Snaith J, Buckberry J and Brickley M (2010) High performance liquid chromatography (HPLC) in the investigation of gout in palaeopathology. *International Journal of Osteoarchaeology*, **20**, 135–143.

Sutcliffe A (2009) Paget's disease 1: epidemiology, causes and clinical features, *Nursing Times.Net*, available at: http://www.nursingtimes.net/nursing-practice-clinical-research/guided-learning-archive/pagets-disease-1-epidemiology-causes-and-clinical-features/1992719.article (accessed August 2011).

Tanna N (2009) Osteoporosis and fragility fractures: identifying those at risk and raising public awareness. *Nursing Times*, **105**(38), 28–31.

Thwaites C and Finney A (2010) Rheumatoid Arthritis 2: exploring treatment options to achieve early control and remission. *Nursing Times*, **106**(10), 18–20.

Weiss E and Jurmain R (2007) Osteoarthritis revisited: a contemporary review of aetiology. *International Journal of Osteoarchaeology*, **17**, 437–450.

Whigham J (2009) Managing malignant spinal cord compression in a patient with advanced progressive disease. *British Journal of Neuroscience Nursing*, **5**(2), 73–78.

Wilson D J (2005) Amputation and the diabetic foot: learning from a case study. *British Journal of Community Nursing*, **10**(12), S18–S24.

Wilson H and Vincent R (2006) Autoimmune connective tissue disease: scleroderma, *British Journal of Nursing*, **15**(15), 805–809.

Wilson M (2009) Preparing a patient for an X-Ray: a student nurse's perspective of radiographic imaging, *Journal of Orthopaedic Nursing*, **13**, 115–118.

Wright K (2009) A practical guide to foot care for older adults. *Nursing and Residential Care*, October, **11**(10), 496–501.

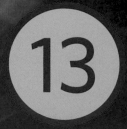

13

Caring for people with neurological problems

Learning outcomes

- Describe the anatomy, physiology and functions of the nervous system.

- Explain techniques for assessment of neurological function.

- Identify signs and symptoms of impairment of neurological function.

- Identify prevalence, incidence and risk factors responsible for problems of the nervous system.

- Explain the pathophysiology, signs and symptoms, complications, interdisciplinary care and nursing care of common neurological conditions.

- Discuss the purposes, nursing implications and health education for the person and family.

Clinical competencies

- Conduct and document a health history and assessment of neurological function.

- Monitor people with neurological problems for expected and unexpected signs and symptoms, reporting and recording findings and results from diagnostic tests.

- Determine priority nursing diagnoses, based on assessed data, to select and implement individualised nursing interventions for persons with neurological disorders.

- Provide skilled care to people with neurological conditions.

CASE STUDIES

Below are three case studies that you may wish to consider before, during or after you have read the chapter. There are no right or wrong answers to these case studies, but you should think about the physical, psychological and social implications. Consider the immediate care and management as well as the longer-term consequences for the person and their family.

Case Study 1 – Ali

Mr Ali Everett is a 21-year-old student studying at the local technical college. Whilst out drinking with his friends he falls and bangs his head. He is taken to the local A&E where he is nauseous and headachy with a Glasgow Coma Score of 14.

Case Study 2 – Bob

Mr Bob Andrews is a 78-year-old retired factory worker who bangs his head on the car door whilst getting out. His wife calls an ambulance because he becomes increasingly confused and unsteady on his feet. On admission to A&E he is confused, localising to painful stimuli and rousable to speech with a Glasgow Coma Score of 12. On examination he is found to have a mild left-sided arm and leg weakness. Bob's wife informs the A&E nurses that he has been suffering from headaches for the last four to five weeks. Bob's CAT scan revealed a right subdural haematoma.

Case Study 3 – Jane

Mrs Jane Kennedy is a 67-year-old retired schoolteacher who has been suffering dizziness and blurred vision the week before her stroke. However, these symptoms lasted only a few minutes and she believed them to be due to 'old age'. On the morning of admission, Jane woke up with a right-sided facial weakness and could not move her right arm. Jane also could not speak sensibly.

INTRODUCTION

This chapter first introduces the anatomy and physiology of the nervous system, then discusses altered consciousness and increased intracranial pressure followed by intracranial disorders that might manifest these and other signs. Degenerative neurological disorders are introduced to the reader in the final section. Nursing care considerations are discussed including both short- and long-term healthcare needs.

ANATOMY, PHYSIOLOGY AND FUNCTIONS OF THE NERVOUS SYSTEM

The nervous system is the most complex of the body's systems and regulates and integrates all body functions, muscle movements, senses, mental abilities and emotions. The nervous system is divided into two parts: the central nervous system (CNS), which consists of the brain and spinal cord, and the peripheral nervous system (PNS), which consists of the cranial and spinal nerves that are outside the CNS. The CNS controls and integrates the whole nervous system, receiving information (input) about the changes in the internal and external environment, processing and interpreting this information and providing signals that are manifested in sensory or motor outputs. The PNS provides input and output information to the CNS.

CELLS OF THE NERVOUS SYSTEM

The basis anatomical and functional unit of the nervous system is the *neurone* which receives impulses and sends them on to other cells. The supporting cells in the CNS are called *neuroglia* (also called glia). These provide protection, support and nourishment to the neurones, and far outnumber them.

Neurones

Each neurone consists of a cell body, an axon and dentrites (Figure 13.1).

Cell bodies vary in size and in the PNS are found in clusters known as ganglia. In the CNS these clusters are called a centre, and a centre with a discrete boundary is called a nucleus. The thin tubes (projections) that radiate from the cell body are neuritis, and there are two types: dendrites and axons. The dendrites are short processes arising from the cell body that conduct impulses toward (afferent) the cell body. The cell bodies and dendrites comprise what is often called the grey matter of the CNS. The axon, a single long process usually arising from the cell body, conducts impulses away (efferent) from the cell body. Axons may be insulated by a white lipid sheath known as myelin (myelinated) or not (unmyelinated).

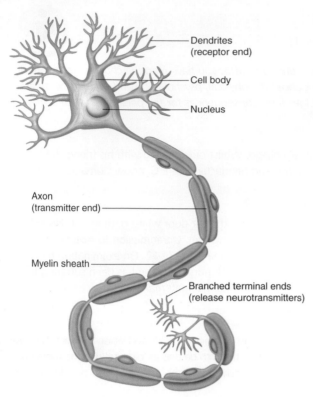

Dendrites
(receptor end)

Cell body

Nucleus

Axon
(transmitter end)

Myelin sheath

Branched terminal ends
(release neurotransmitters)

Figure 13.1 A typical neurone.

The myelin sheath is formed by Schwann cells in the PNS and oligodendrocytes in the CNS (see Table 13.1). The myelin sheath insulates the axon and contains gaps (bare segments) called *Nodes of Ranvier*, which allow movement of ions between the axon and the extracellular fluid and serve to increase the speed of nerve impulse conduction in axons.

Table 13.1 Summary of common neurotransmitter and receptor sites within the nervous system

Neurotransmitters	Receptor sites
Excitatory neurotransmitter	
Acetylcholine (ACh) released by cholinergic synapses in motor neurones in spine and brainstem.	Cholinergic; can be mucarinic or nicotinic receptors.
Norepinephrine (NE) (noradrenaline) released by adrenergic synapses (amine).	Adrenergic receptors found in CNS and PNS.
Glutamate (amino acid) at most CNS synapses.	Throughout the CNS.
Inhibitory neurotransmitters	
Gamma aminobutyric acid (GABA) (amino acid).	Throughout the CNS.
Dopamine (amine) (is also excitatory at other synapses).	CNS (5 types D_1–D_5).
Serotonin (5-hydroxtryptamine; 5-HT) (is excitatory at other synapses).	7 subtypes in CNS and PNS.

Action potentials

Neurones communicate with each other and other cells via the electrical changes (impulses) that occur in their membranes referred to as *action potentials*. An action potential is a transient (< 1 millisecond) reversal in the polarity of this transmembrane potential, initiated by a stimulus propagated by the rapid movement of charged ions through the cell membrane, which then moves down the axon to the axon terminals. At rest the neurone is polarised, that is the semi-permeable membrane separates excess positive charge on the outside from the excess negative charge on the inside. This separation is referred to as *potential difference*. In addition, the extracellular fluid (outside) contains relatively higher concentrations of sodium (Na+) ions than intracellular (inside the cells), and relatively higher concentrations of potassium ions (K+) exist intracellular compared to extracellular. Any stimulus alters this membrane permeability to Na+ and K+ resulting in the movement of these ions across the membrane, and the neurone is said to depolarise. When a neurone reaches a certain level of stimulation (threshold potential), an electrical impulse is generated (the action potential) only at the point of the stimulus; but, once generated, it is propagated along the entire length of the axon regardless of whether the stimulus continues. The conduction of the impulse is rapid in myelinated fibres, with the action potential 'jumping' from one node of Ranvier to the next (saltatory propagation), and slower in unmyelinated fibres. After the impulse the membrane potential moves back to its resting state, referred to as repolarisation.

The movement of impulses to and from the CNS is made possible by afferent and efferent neurones. Afferent, or sensory, neurones have receptors in skin, muscles and other organs and relay impulses to the CNS. Efferent, or motor, neurones transmit impulses from the CNS to cause some type of action.

Neurotransmitters

Neurotransmitters are the chemical messengers of the nervous system. When the action potential reaches the end of the axon at the presynaptic terminal, a neurotransmitter is released from the neurone and travels across the gap between one neurone and another, called the synaptic cleft, binding (like a key) with specific receptors in the post-synaptic neurone dendrite or cell body. At least 50 known neurotransmitters exist, which may be either inhibitory or excitatory, and different neurones in the brain release different neurotransmitters (see Table 13.1).

Neuroglia

There are a number of different neuroglia cells to be found in the CNS and PNS. Table 13.2 summarises the main types and functions.

THE CENTRAL NERVOUS SYSTEM (CNS)

The CNS consists of the brain and spinal cord, highly evolved clusters of neurones that act to accept, interconnect, interpret

Table 13.2 Types of neuroglia cells and their functions

Type of neuroglia	Located in the central nervous system (CNS)	Located in the peripheral nervous system (PNS)
Macroglia	Astrocytes – largest and most numerous, star-shaped cells. Fill the space between the neurones. Regulate the chemical content of this extracellular space, form part of the blood–brain barrier, and are involved in repair of damaged neural tissue.	Capsular cells – surround the neuroneal cell bodies in sensory and autonomic ganglia.
	Oligodendroglia – small cells. Form the myelin sheath of several neurones and are involved in growth of damaged CNS axons.	Schwann cells – form part of the myelin shealth on one neurone.
Microglia	Smallest, rarest glia cells; are phagocytic engulfing debris resulting from injury, infection or diseases and release cytokines (for further information see Chapter 4).	
Ependymal cells	Line the central canal of the spinal cord and ventricles in the brain. Involved in the formation and flow of cerebral spinal fluid (CSF).	

and generate a response to nerve impulses originating throughout the body.

The brain

The brain is the control centre of the nervous system and also generates thoughts, emotions and speech. Averaging 3–4 lb in weight, the brain is protected from the external environment by three barriers: the skull, a bony structure, the meninges, a three-layer membrane, and the CSF. The brain has four major regions: the cerebrum, the diencephalon, the brainstem and the cerebellum (Figure 13.2). The general functions of these regions are summarised in Table 13.3.

The two hemispheres of the cerebrum account for almost 60% of brain weight. The surface of the cerebrum is folded into elevated ridges of tissue called gyri, which are separated by shallow grooves called sulci. Deep grooves called fissures further divide the surface of the cerebrum. The longitudinal fissure separates the hemispheres, and the transverse fissure separates the cerebrum from the cerebellum. In addition, each cerebral hemisphere is divided into frontal, parietal, temporal and occipital lobes (Figure 13.3).

The cerebral hemispheres are connected by a thick band of axons of the corpus callosum, which allows communication between the two hemispheres. Each hemisphere receives sensory and motor impulses from the opposite side of the body. One of the cerebral hemispheres tends to develop more than the other. Approximately 95% of people have a more highly

Table 13.3 General functions of the four regions of the brain

Region	Functions
Cerebrum	• Interprets sensory input. • Controls skeletal muscle activity. • Processes intellect and emotions. • Contains skills memory.
Diencephalon	• Conducts sensory and motor impulses. • Regulates autonomic nervous system. • Regulates and produces hormones. • Mediates emotional responses.
Brainstem	• Serves as conduction pathway. • Serves as site of crossing of nerve tracts (decussation). • Contains respiratory nuclei. • Helps regulate skeletal muscles.
Cerebellum	• Processes information. • Provides information necessary for balance, posture and coordinated muscle movement.

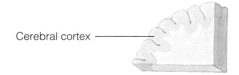

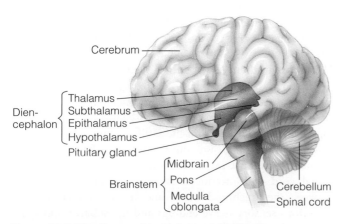

Cerebral cortex

Cerebrum

Dien-cephalon
Thalamus
Subthalamus
Epithalamus
Hypothalamus
Pituitary gland

Brainstem
Midbrain
Pons
Medulla oblongata

Cerebellum
Spinal cord

Figure 13.2 The four major regions of the brain.

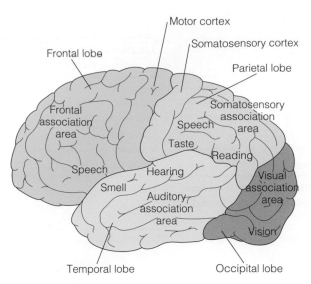

Figure 13.3 Lobes of the cerebrum and the functional areas of the cerebral cortex.

Table 13.4 General functions of the lobes of the cerebrum and areas of the cerebral cortex

Area	Functions
Parietal lobe (somatic sensory area of cerebral cortex)	• Processing of the somatic sensory system – recognition of pain, temperature, touch and proprioceptive sensation, e.g. position, vibration and two-point discrimination. • Perception and awareness of body image; drawing ability. • Identification of objects by contact.
Occipital lobe	• Receives and interprets visual stimuli.
Temporal lobe	• Receives and interprets sensory information (smell and hearing). • Recognition of face and shapes. • Wernicke's area – understanding the spoken word.
Frontal lobe	• Primary motor control area – facilitates voluntary movement of skeletal muscles, coordinates voluntary eye movement. • Broca's area – motor expression of speech and receives inputs from Wernicke's area via long connecting fibres (arcuate fasciculus). • Regulation of emotion, behaviour and cognition processes, e.g. reasoning, insight, personality, social behaviour, working (short-term) memory.
Insula or 'Island of Reil'	• Pyramid-shaped area that receives and interprets taste (gustatory) stimuli.

developed, dominant left hemisphere, which is responsible for the control of language. The right hemisphere has greater control over non-verbal perceptual functions, such as facial recognition.

The cerebral cortex is the outer surface of the cerebrum. It consists of neurone cell bodies, unmyelinated fibres, neuroglia and blood vessels. The functions of the different lobes of the cerebrum and the specific areas of the cerebral cortex are listed in Table 13.4.

Diencephalon

The diencephalon is embedded in the cerebrum superior to the brainstem. It consists of four main divisions: the thalamus, hypothalamus, epithalamus and the subthalamus (see Figure 13.2). The thalamus, the largest component, integrates and processes sensory impulses before they ascend to the cerebral cortex, and plays a role in motor control. It serves as a sorting, processing and relay station for input into the cortical region. The hypothalamus, located inferior to the thalamus, regulates temperature, water metabolism, appetite and emotional expressions, is part of the sleep–wake cycle (circadian rhythm) and synthesises various releasing hormones that target the anterior pituitary, for example vasopressin and oxytocin. The epithalamus forms the dorsal part of the diencephalon and is concerned with emotions and behaviours. The subthalamus is mostly situated in the posterior third of the diencephalon and is involved in motor function associated with the basal ganglia.

Brainstem

The brainstem consists of the midbrain, pons and medulla oblongata (see Figure 13.2). The midbrain is a centre for auditory and visual reflexes. In addition, it functions as a nerve pathway between the cerebral hemispheres and lower brain. The pons is located just below the midbrain. It consists mostly of fibre tracts, but it also contains nuclei that control respiration. The medulla oblongata, located at the base of the brainstem,

is continuous with the superior portion of the spinal cord. Nuclei of the medulla oblongata play an important role in controlling cardiac rate, blood pressure, respiration and swallowing.

Cerebellum

The cerebellum is connected to the midbrain, pons and medulla. Its functions include coordinating skeletal muscle activity, maintaining balance and controlling fine movements.

Meninges and cerebral spinal fluid

The brain and spinal cord are covered and protected by three connective tissue membranes called meninges; dura mater, arachnoid mater and pia mater (see Figure 13.4). The meninges form divisions within the skull, enclose venous sinuses and contain CSF. The outer dura mater, a tough fibrous double membrane, and the inner pia mater are continuous with the spinal cord and provide a structural support. The layer between the arachnoid mater and the pia mater contains numerous sensory nerve endings and the subarachnoid space filled with CSF and cerebral blood vessels. The innermost

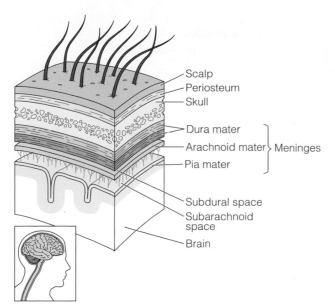

Figure 13.4 Anatomy of the meninges.

layer, the pia, is the thin translucent membrane adherent to the brain, spinal cord and segmental nerves and is filled with small blood vessels.

CSF is a clear and colourless liquid, produced largely by the choroid plexus, a group of ependymal specialised cells located in the brain ventricles. Derived from blood plasma, normal CSF chemical content varies according to location and contains few cells if any.

CSF serves three main functions:

- supporting the weight of the brain and spine acting as a buoyancy aid;
- providing a cushion/buffer for the brain tissue, protecting the brain and spinal cord from trauma and providing nourishment for the brain;
- removal of waste products of cerebrospinal cellular metabolism.

CSF circulates within and around the CNS and is often referred to as *the third circulation* (the first and second circulatory systems being the cardiovascular and lymphatic systems). Daily production of CSF is approximately 15–20 ml/hr (500 ml/day) with a total circulating volume of 90–140 ml. Of this, approximately 30 ml is located in the chambers in the brain known as ventricles with the remainder in the subarachnoid space. CSF is normally produced and absorbed in equal amounts, with the entire volume being replaced roughly every eight hours. The brain contains four ependymal lined chambers or ventricles forming the ventricular system. There are two lateral ventricles (one in each hemisphere) and a third and fourth ventricle. They are linked by ducts that allow the CSF to circulate. CSF circulates from the lateral ventricle which connects with the third ventricle through two channels called the foramen of Monro. The third ventricle communicates with the fourth ventricle through a short channel called the aqueduct of Sylvius. Finally, the fourth ventricle communicates

with the central canal of the spinal cord and over the cerebral hemispheres in the subarachnoid space where it is reabsorbed through the arachnoid granulations (large collections of arachnoid villi) into the venous system.

FAST FACTS

CNS

- The brain does not contain pain receptors (nociceptors).
- The CNS cannot store nutrients.
- By 80 years of age, the brain will have lost 15% of its weight due to shrinkage of neurones.

Source: Young *et al.* 2008.

Blood supply of the CNS

The brain receives about 700–750 ml/min of blood and consumes 20% (50 ml/min) of cardiac output. The total intracranial blood volume at any one time is 100–150 ml. The large amount of oxygen is necessary for metabolism of glucose, the brain's sole source of energy. Blood flow to the brain is maintained at a constant via cerebral autoregulation which is closely related to the brain's metabolic needs: carbon dioxide (major stimulus for vasodilation), hydrogen ion and oxygen concentrations.

The brain receives blood from four arteries: two internal carotid arteries (anterior or carotid system) and two vertebral arteries (posterior or vertebral–basilar system). The internal carotid artery branches into further arteries: the ophthalmic, posterior communicating, anterior choroidal, anterior cerebral and middle cerebral. The brainstem and cerebellum receive their blood supply from the basilar artery. These major arteries are connected by small anterior and posterior communicating arteries, which form a circle of connected blood vessels called the circle of Willis (see Figure 13.5). The cerebral blood drains via two systems, superficial and deep veins, and drains into the dural sinuses which then empty into the right and left internal jugular veins.

Blood–brain barrier (BBB)

The blood–brain barrier is an exclusive barrier between capillary walls and brain tissue, preventing the movement of large molecules into the brain tissue. This protects the brain from many harmful substances in the blood. This barrier is made up of brain endothelial cells forming a physical barrier and certain chemicals forming a chemical barrier. There are certain areas within the CNS, known as '*circumventricular organs*' that lack a BBB, for example the posterior pituitary gland. This barrier also presents difficulties in delivering drugs to the CNS, with only a few small fat-soluble molecules being able to cross the BBB, for example morphine, alcohol, caffeine and nicotine. BBB breakdown is found in a number of CNS diseases, for example brain tumours, multiple sclerosis and Alzheimer's disease.

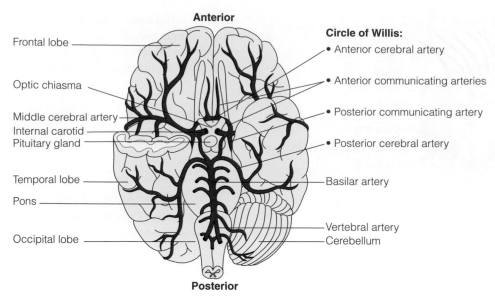

Figure 13.5 Major arteries serving the brain and the circle of Willis.

The limbic system and reticular formation

The limbic system and the reticular formation are functional brain systems. The limbic system consists of structures that form a ring of interconnections in each hemisphere, surrounding the upper portion of the brainstem and corpus callosum. The limbic system integrates and modulates input to make up the affective part of the brain, providing emotional and behavioural responses to environmental stimuli.

The reticular formation is located through the central core of the medulla oblongata, pons and midbrain. This system has widespread connections throughout the brain and relays sensory input from all body systems to all levels of the brain. The reticular formation includes the reticular activating system (RAS), a stimulating system for the cerebral cortex, keeping it alert (awake) and responsive to incoming sensory stimuli while filtering out repetitive or unwanted stimuli, motor nuclei that help maintain muscle tone and coordinated movements through interconnections with spinal nerves, and the vasomotor and cardiovascular regulatory centres, which are part of autonomic regulation of the cardiovascular system.

The spinal cord

The spinal cord extends from the medulla to the level of the first lumbar vertebra (Figure 13.6). It serves as a centre for conducting messages to and from the brain and as a reflex centre. The spinal cord is about 17 inches (42 cm) long and 0.75 inch (1.8 cm) thick. It is protected within the spinal canal by a bony arch formed by each vertebra and by the meninges and CSF. The grey matter of the cord is on the inside, and the white matter is on the outside (the reverse of the arrangement in the brain). There are 33 vertebrae: seven cervical, 12 thoracic, five lumbar, five sacral and four fused, which form the coccyx. Intervertebral discs, a thick capsule surrounding a gelatinous core called the nucleus pulposus, are located between each of the movable vertebrae. On either side of each vertebra, nerves

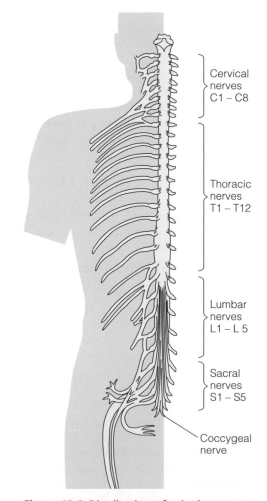

Figure 13.6 Distribution of spinal nerves.

exit the spinal canal allowing them to collect and transmit sensory messages to and from the brain. Messages to and from the brain are conducted via ascending (sensory) pathways and descending (motor) pathways (see Figure 13.7).

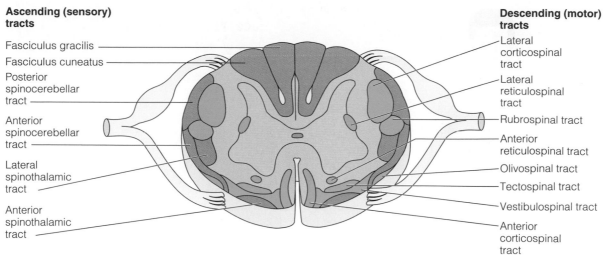

Figure 13.7 Ascending and descending tracts in the spinal cord.

Upper and lower motor neurones

Upper motor neurones, such as those of the corticospinal and extrapyramidal tract, carry impulses from the cerebral cortex to the anterior grey column of the spinal cord. Damage to upper motor neurones results in increased muscle tone, decreased muscle strength, decreased coordination and hyperactive reflexes. Lower motor neurones begin in the anterior grey column of the spinal cord and end in the muscle. Damage to these results in decreased muscle tone, muscle atrophy, **fasciculations** and loss of reflexes.

THE PERIPHERAL NERVOUS SYSTEM (PNS)

The PNS links the CNS with the rest of the body. It is responsible for receiving and transmitting information from and about the external environment. The PNS consists of nerves, ganglia (groups of neurone cell bodies) and sensory receptors located outside or peripheral to the brain and spinal cord. The PNS is divided into a sensory (afferent) division and a motor (efferent) division. Most nerves of the PNS contain fibres for both divisions and all are classified regionally as either spinal nerves or cranial nerves.

Spinal nerves

The 31 pairs of spinal nerves are grouped according to the region of the vertebral column from which they originate (see Figure 13.6). Spinal nerves exit the vertebral column through intervertebral foramina to travel to the body regions they serve, called a dermatome. Each spinal nerve contains both sensory and motor fibers (see Figure 13.8). The sensory fibres are located in the dorsal root, and their cell bodies are located within the dorsal root ganglion. The motor fibres are located in the ventral root, and their cell bodies are located within the spinal cord. The dorsal and ventral roots merge outside the vertebral canal just past the dorsal root ganglion, forming a spinal nerve. Each spinal nerve further divides into branches called rami. The ventral rami of the cervical, brachial, lumbar and sacral regions form complex clusters of nerves called plexuses of which there are four.

The spinal cord does not reach the end of the vertebral column; as a result, the lumbar and sacral nerve roots travel inferiorly through the vertebral canal for some distance before exiting the vertebral column through their associated intervertebral foramina. This collection of descending nerve roots is called the cauda equina.

Cranial nerves

Twelve pairs of cranial nerves originate from brain tissue; the forebrain and brainstem (Figure 13.9). All emerge from the brain except the IX accessory which emerges from the spinal cord. To reach their targets, they exit the cranium through various openings in the skull. Although most are mixed nerves, with a motor and sensory component, three pairs (olfactory, optic and acoustic) are solely sensory. The motor components of the cranial nerves are derived from cells that are located in the brain. These cells send their nerve out of the cranium where they will ultimately control muscle (for example, eye movements), glandular tissue (for example, salivary glands) or specialised muscle (for example, heart or stomach). The sensory components of cranial nerves originate from collections of cells that are located outside the brain (for example taste receptors on the tongue), and send sensory information back to the brain. The vagus nerve extends into the ventral body cavity, but the 11 other pairs innervate only head and neck regions. The cranial nerves and their related functions are summarised in Table 13.5.

Reflexes

A reflex is a rapid, involuntary, predictable motor response to a stimulus. Reflexes are categorised as either somatic or autonomic. Somatic reflexes result in skeletal muscle contraction.

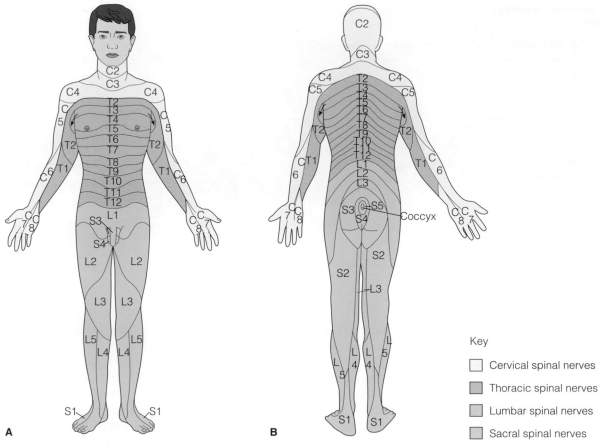

Key

☐ Cervical spinal nerves

▨ Thoracic spinal nerves

▨ Lumbar spinal nerves

▨ Sacral spinal nerves

Figure 13.8 Dermatomes of the body. (A) Anterior. **(B)** Posterior.

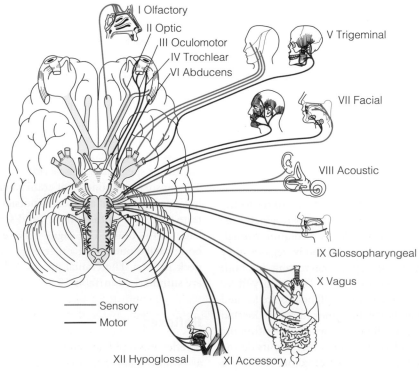

Figure 13.9 Cranial nerves.

Table 13.5 Cranial nerves summary and testing for function

Cranial nerve	Classification	Major function
I Olfactory	Sensory	**Chemoreceptors** – receptors in the nasal mucosa send smell signals to the olfactory cortex in the temporal lobe.
II Optic	Sensory	Vision (acuity and field of vision) – messages are relayed via pathways to the occipital cortex.
III Oculomotor	Motor	• Eye movement – inferior, medial and superior rectus, and inferior oblique muscles. • Eyelid elevation – levator palpebrae superioris muscle. • Efferent parasympathetic fibres innervate the cillary muscle and the constrictor pupillae muscle – control constriction of pupils.
IV Trochlear	Motor	Eyeball movement – supplies one muscle, the superior oblique muscle (turns eye downward and laterally).
V Trigeminal	Sensory and motor	• Sensory (has three large branches) – sensation of head/neck (corneal reflex), sinuses, meninges and external surface of tympanic membrane. • Motor function (mandibular branch) – muscles of mastication (biting and chewing).
VI Abducens	Motor	Eye movement – supplies one muscle, the lateral rectus muscle (lateral movement of the eyeball).
VII Facial	Motor and sensory	• Motor – movement of facial muscles – facial expression, corneal reflex (motor), eyelid and lip closure. • Parasympathetic to all glands of head except the parotid. • Sensory – anterior two-thirds of the tongue (taste) and the external auditory meatus and tympanic membrane of the ear.
VIII Acoustic	Sensory	Two special senses: hearing (audition) and balance (vestibular).
IX Glossopharyngeal	Motor and sensory	• Motor – input to the muscles involved in swallowing and gag reflex • Parasympathetic input to the parotids (salivary glands) to release saliva. • Sensory – posterior third of the tongue (taste) and external ear, inner surface of the tympanic membrane and pharynx. • Chemoreceptors in the carotid body regulate blood pressure.
X Vagus	Sensory and motor	• Longest cranial nerve with branches of the nerve distributed from the ear to the rectum. • Motor – muscles of pharynx and larynx (swallowing), thorax and abdomen. • Sensory – regulation of cardiac rate and respirations, sensation pharynx, thoracic and abdominal organs.
XI Accessory	Motor	Innervates the muscles in the head and neck (shoulder movement and head rotation), palate and the pharynx.
XII Hypoglossal	Motor	Movement of tongue for speech (articulation) and swallowing.

Autonomic reflexes activate cardiac muscle, smooth muscle and glands. A reflex occurs over a pathway called a reflex arc.

The essential components of a reflex arc are a receptor, a sensory neurone to carry afferent impulses to the CNS, an integration centre in the spinal cord or brain, a motor neurone to carry efferent impulses and an effector (the tissue that responds by contracting or secreting) (Figure 13.10).

Somatic reflexes mediated by the spinal cord are called spinal reflexes. Many spinal reflexes occur without impulses travelling to and from the brain, with the cord serving as the integration centre, whereas others require brain activity and modulation. Deep tendon reflexes (DTRs) occur in response to muscle contraction and cause muscle relaxation and lengthening.

THE AUTONOMIC NERVOUS SYSTEM (ANS)

The ANS is a division of the PNS that regulates the internal environment of the body. It is also called the general visceral motor system, because it consists of motor neurones that innervate the body's viscera. Whereas skeletal muscle activity and reflexes are regulated by a division of the PNS called the somatic nervous system, the ANS regulates the activity of cardiac muscle, smooth muscle and glands.

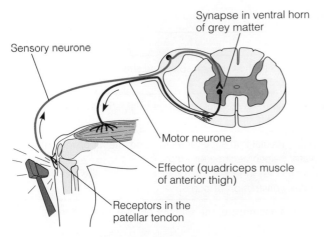

Figure 13.10 A typical reflex arc of a spinal nerve.

The ANS is primarily controlled by the reticular formation in the brainstem. Stimulation of centres in the medulla initiates reflexes that regulate cardiac rate, blood vessel diameter and gastrointestinal function.

The ANS has sympathetic and parasympathetic divisions. Although fibres from both divisions affect the same structures, the actions of the two divisions are opposite in effect, and they serve to counterbalance each other. The effects of these two divisions are summarised in Table 13.6.

Table 13.6 Summary of the effects of the autonomic nervous system on target organs or tissues

Sympathetic division – stress response (fright, fight and flight)	Parasympathetic division – rest and digest
• Main neurotransmitter – acetylcholine	• Main neurotransmitter – noradrenaline
• Dilated pupils	• Constricted pupils
• Circulation – increased rate and force of heartbeat and increased blood pressure. Vasodilation of the coronary arteries, vasoconstriction of arteries and abdominal and skin blood vessels.	• Circulation – decreased rate and force of heartbeat, vasoconstriction of the coronary arteries
• Respiratory system – dilation of the bronchioles and increased rate of respiration.	• Respiratory system – constricted bronchioles and decreased rate of respiration
• Digestive system – increased metabolic rate, decreased digestion, increased release of glucose by the liver.	• Digestive system – increased peristalsis and secretion of gastrointestinal fluids
• Decreased urine output	• Constriction of the bronchioles
• Increased mental alertness	
• Increased sweat (*diaphoresis*)	

Sympathetic division

The sympathetic division of the ANS prepares the body to handle situations that are perceived as harmful or stressful and to participate in strenuous activity, often referred to as the 'fight or flight' response, i.e. increased heart and respiratory rate, dilated pupils and increased blood supply to the voluntary muscles. Cell bodies for this division arise in the lateral horns of the spinal cord in the area from T1 through L2. The fibres separate after leaving the cord and form a chain of ganglia that extends from the neck to the pelvis. Long fibres then extend to the organs that are supplied by the sympathetic division.

Parasympathetic division

The parasympathetic division of the ANS operates during non-stressful situations, for example rest and recuperation of the body. In contrast to the widespread influence of the sympathetic division, the parasympathetic division has a very localising influence. Cell bodies for this division are located in the brainstem (for the cranial nerves) or in the spinal cord (S2 through S4).

Assessing the person with neurological problems

A comprehensive assessment of the structures and functions of the neurological system is extremely important in the care of the person with neurological conditions. Neurological assessment begins when the nurse first meets the person, assessing appearance, including dress, hygiene, grooming, gait and posture. Assessment involves a number of processes: a person interview, physical assessment to collect objective data and findings from diagnostic testing. An interview with the person aims to collect subjective data, such as the person's history of seizures, fainting, dizziness, headaches, and any trauma, tumours, or surgery of the brain, spinal cord or nerves and any family history of neurological health problems, diabetes mellitus, hypertension, seizures or mental health problems. A thorough neurological examination is discussed in this chapter but, in most instances, the nurse will conduct a focused assessment specific to the person's health status. In addition to the assessment processes, nurses should also be alert to other signs and symptoms discussed later in this chapter. Whilst assessing a person's mental status and cognition, be aware that fatigue or illness may alter findings and, when interpreting findings, consider the person's age, educational background and cultural orientation.

ALTERED CONSCIOUSNESS

Neurological observations are a set of parameters which help to describe the neurological status of a person and determine

IN PRACTICE

The Glasgow Coma Scale

In practice, it is important to document how the GCS score is made up as well as the sum score, e.g. (best eye response) E = 2 + (best verbal response) V = 3 + (best motor response) M = 5 = Total GCS score of 10 (see Table 13.7). The lowest score that a person can achieve is 3, indicating total unresponsiveness and the maximum score is 15, indicating that the person is alert and oriented and fully responsive.

Table 13.7 Assessment of consciousness – Glasgow Coma Scale

Feature	Response	Score
Best eye response (record C if unable to open eyes, e.g. from orbital swelling or facial fractures)	Opens spontaneously	4
	Opens to verbal commands	3
	Opens to pain	2
	No eye opening	1
Best verbal response (record 'T' if the person has a endotracheal or tracheostomy tube in place and record 'D' if the person is dysphasic)	Orientated to questions	5
	Disorientated /confused	4
	Inappropriate words	3
	Incomprehensible sounds	2
	No verbal response	1
Best motor response (record best upper arm response)	To verbal commands obeys	6
	To painful stimuli localises pain	5
	Withdrawal from pain	4
	Flexion to pain	3
	Extension to pain	2
	No response to pain	1

problems with neurological structure and/or function. The main reason for performing a neurological examination is to determine if a person's neurological condition is improving, remaining static or deteriorating and to establish a baseline assessment of the patient's neurological function against which to determine any further changes. Assessment includes level of consciousness (orientation and cognition) with responses to sound and pain, pupil size and response to light and motor function.

Consciousness is a condition in which the person is aware of self and environment and is able to respond appropriately to stimuli. It has two major components:

- *Arousal or alertness* – level of consciousness, depends on the integrity of the reticular activating system extending from the brainstem to the thalamic nuclei in the cerebral hemispheres.
- *Awareness* – content of the consciousness, largely a function of the cerebral hemispheres (cortex); includes all mental activities controlled by the cerebral hemispheres and reflects cognition.

A person's level of consciousness may be assessed by using the Glasgow Coma Scale (GCS) (Teasdale and Jennett 1974). Developed as an objective measure of neurological status in head-injured patients, the tool is used universally to assess the

level of consciousness in a patient. Its graphic format enables the assessment of the three modes of behaviour, each assessed separately – eye opening (arousal), verbal response (cognition), motor response (activity) – and arranges them in a scale of increasing dysfunction. The three parameters are then added together to give an overall Glasgow Coma Score.

Altered consciousness consists of abnormal behaviour in one or more of these three functional areas. Level of consciousness is the most important aspect of the neurological assessment as it is the earliest and most sensitive indicator of neurological deterioration (Hickey 2009). If not experienced in using the GCS, the AVPU scale (see Table 13.8) can give information easily and quickly about the patient's level of consciousness. It is often incorporated into the early-warning scores systems and is ideal in the initial rapid ABCDE assessment (see Chapter 1). However, in patients with neurological conditions the AVPU is not an adequate assessment tool and not a replacement for the GCS.

Patients may present in practice with varying levels of consciousness, and these are presented in Table 13.9.

As well as assessment of consciousness, other higher cortical functioning is also assessed. This includes thought processes (both content and perceptions) by noting responses to questions, ability to understand what is said and to express thoughts, for example language, and the ability to make

Table 13.8 The AVPU scale

A = alert	• Are you alert?
V = responds to voice	• Do you response to verbal stimulation?
P = responds to pain	• Do you respond to pain?
U = unresponsive	• Do they respond at all?

logical and safe judgements. In addition, note attention span and recent and remote memory. This may be assessed by asking the person to:

1. Repeat five to seven numbers.
2. Recall three items after five minutes.
3. Recall his or her address, breakfast or birthday.

The person should be oriented to time, place and person; demonstrate attention and ability to remember recent and past events; respond appropriately to questions; and be able to

Table 13.9 Terms used to describe varying levels of consciousness

Term	Characteristics of person
Full consciousness	Alert; oriented to time, place and person; comprehends spoken and written words.
Confusion	Unable to think rapidly and clearly; easily bewildered, with poor memory and short attention span; misinterprets stimuli; judgement is impaired.
Disorientation	Not aware of or not oriented to time, place or person.
Obtundation	Lethargic, somnolent; responsive to verbal or tactile stimuli but quickly drifts back to sleep.
Stupor	Generally unresponsive; may be briefly aroused by vigorous, repeated or painful (**nociceptive**) stimuli; may shrink away from or grab at the source of stimuli.
Semi-comatose	Does not move spontaneously; unresponsive to stimuli, although vigorous or painful stimuli may result in stirring, moaning or withdrawal from the stimuli, without actual arousal.
Coma	Unrousable; will not stir or moan in response to any stimulus; may exhibit non-purposeful response (slight movement) of area stimulated but makes no attempt to withdraw.
Deep coma	Completely unrousable and unresponsive to any kind of stimulus, including pain; absence of reflexes.

make judgements. More specific tests of cognition ability include the Mini-Mental Status Examination (MMSE). In addition, elicit information about memory, feeling state (such as anxiety or depression), recent changes in sleep patterns, ability to perform self-care and activities of daily living, sexual activity and weight. If the person is taking prescribed medications, over-the-counter medications or herbal supplements, ask about the type and purpose, frequency and duration of use. If the patient's level of consciousness is altered, the nurse may need to rely on family members/carers for information.

Pupil size and response to light

Testing the eyes' reaction to light and assessing the character of the pupils is not part of the scoring system of the GCS, but is a vital component of neurological assessment. It can assist in identifying the location of an expanding space-occupying lesion and is a later sign of increased intracranial pressure. Any changes in pupil reaction, shape or size should be reported and documented immediately. The light reflex tests two cranial nerves:

• optic nerve (II) – the sensory nerve of visual acuity;
• oculomotor nerve (III) – the motor nerve that controls pupillary reaction.

IN PRACTICE

Assessing pupillary reaction

This is performed by shining a light (pen torch) from the temple into each eye in turn and observing and recording the pupillary reaction.

A normal pupillary reaction to light should provide a brisk constricting of the pupil immediately when the light is shone into the eye. This is recorded as '+'; unreactive pupils are recorded as '−' and sluggish pupils as 'S'.

Withdrawal of the light should produce an immediate and brisk dilatation of the pupil. This is called the *direct light reflex*. Introducing the light into one pupil should cause similar constriction to occur simultaneously in the other pupil, and when the light is withdrawn from one eye, the opposite pupil should also dilate simultaneously. This response is called the *consensual light reaction*.

Record the size of the pupil by using the millimetre scale (as indicated on the neurological observation chart or pen torch) to estimate the size of each pupil.

It is important to make a baseline assessment of pupillary size and compare subsequent assessments with the baseline.

The shape of the pupil should be round; abnormal pupil shapes may be described as ovoid, keyhole or irregular. Sluggish or suddenly dilated unequal pupils are an indication that the oculomotor cranial nerve is being compressed. If this is left unrelieved, the pupil will become fixed and dilated ('blown pupil') and the oculomotor nerve on the opposite side will also become compressed, resulting in bilateral and dilated and fixed pupils. The person should also be observed for spontaneous eye movements as this may indicate in the case of the otherwise unresponsive person conditions such as locked-in syndrome, catatonia or complex partial seizure status (pp. 490–493).

PRACTICE ALERT

- 17% of the normal population have inequality in size between the pupils known as *anisocoria*.
- Certain medication may influence the size of the pupil, e.g. very small pupils (1–2 mm) may suggest the use of opiates, fentanyl or barbiturates, and the use of eye drops, such as atropine, can dilate the pupils.
- Pre-existing ophthalmic conditions can produce a unilaterally dilated pupil, e.g. cataract or localised injury or misshapen pupils, e.g. 'keyhole' pupils in people who have undergone cataract surgery.

MOTOR FUNCTION ASSESSMENTS

The motor function assessment can be divided into the following:

- muscle tone and bulk;
- muscle strength;
- involuntary movements, for example **tremors** (rhythmic movements) and fasciculations (irregular movements);
- gait and posture and body positioning – resting position and during spontaneous movement.

Motor function assessment proceeds from the upper limbs down to the lower limbs with each limb assessed separately, and includes assessment for bilateral symmetry, size of the muscle, muscle tone and muscle strength. In addition, the patient's movements at rest (not making a purposeful movement) and during activity (making a purposeful movement, such as reaching for a glass of water) are observed.

Assessment of muscle size includes assessing for muscle wasting atrophy and hypertrophy.

Assessment of muscle tone includes a decrease in tone with the muscle being weak, soft flabby and fatigues easily. This is referred to as *flaccidity*. An increase in tone, evident by an increased resistance to passive movement, is referred to as *spasticity*. The muscles may be in a state of increased resistance or rigidity. This may result in muscles moving in small, regular jerky movements caused by alternating episodes of resistance and relaxation to passive movement known as 'cogwheel rigidity', or there may be a persistent resistance to passive movement throughout the entire range of movement known as 'lead pipe rigidity'.

Assessment of muscle strength and movement in the conscious cooperative person is performed by active, passive and

Table 13.10 Grading of muscle strength

Grade	Strength
5	Full range of motion against gravity and resistance, normal muscle strength (normal power).
4	Full range of motion against gravity and a moderate amount of resistance, slight weakness (mild weakness).
3	Full range of motion against gravity and only moderate muscle weakness (moderate weakness).
2	Full range of motion when gravity is eliminated, severe weakness (the patient is unable to move against gravity – severe weakness).
1	A weak muscle contraction felt, but no movement is noted (very severe weakness).
0	Complete paralysis.

active resistive movements. With the person in bed, assess motor strength bilaterally. Have the person flex and extend the arm against your hand, squeeze your fingers, lift the leg while you press down on the thigh, hold the leg straight and lift it against gravity, and flex and extend the foot against your hand. Grade each extremity using a motor scale (see Table 13.10). Muscle strength and movement should be bilaterally equal and strong.

In the unconscious person, muscle strength assessment begins with observation of spontaneous movements progressing to the application of a noxious stimulus with the purpose of eliciting a motor response. There are two ways of applying noxious stimuli: a peripheral or a central painful stimulus. The choice of stimulus depends on the reaction that the practitioner needs to generate. For upper limbs, apply central stimuli (e.g. pinching the pectoralis major muscle); for lower limbs this is applied peripherally.

In the unconscious person, motor function and tone can exhibit specific abnormal motor responses and postural patterns depending upon the underlying site of injury and motor tract interruption. These can be divided into two main patterns of posturing:

- *Decorticate posturing*. Upper arms are close to the sides; elbows, wrists and fingers are flexed; legs are extended with internal rotation; and feet are plantar flexed. Occurs with lesions of the corticospinal tracts (Figure 13.11).
- *Decerebrate posturing*. Neck is extended, jaw clenched; arms are pronated, extended and close to the sides; legs are extended straight out; and feet are plantar flexed. Decerebrate posturing occurs with lesions of the midbrain, pons or diencephalon (Figure 13.12).

Involuntary movements, posture and gait

These include a number of abnormal movements such as tremors, tics, spasms and ballism. Assessment of gait and

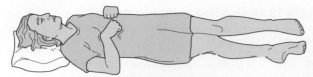

Figure 13.11 Decorticate posturing.

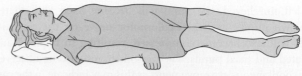

Figure 13.12 Decerebrate posturing.

posture includes a variety of simple tests. Ask the person to walk normally, then in a heel-to-toe fashion (tandem walking), then on toes and finally on heels. A person with appropriate gait can walk heel-to-toe, on toes and on heels. **Ataxia** is a lack of coordination and a clumsiness of movements, with staggering, wide-based and unbalanced gait due to a lack of coordination in voluntary muscle movements.

The Romberg test assesses balance. Ask the person to stand with the feet together and eyes closed. Stand close to the person to prevent falling. There should be minimal swaying for up to 20 seconds. A positive Romberg sign is indicated when the person sways and falls. Assessment of coordination may include checking the cooperative conscious person for the following:

● Observe ability to pat knees, alternating front and back of hands and increasing speed.

● Observe ability to touch their nose, then one of the assessor's fingers, then their nose again.

● Observe ability to run each heel down each shin, while in a supine position.

SENSORY FUNCTION ASSESSMENTS

Sensory function is an important component of the neurological assessment in people with spinal cord disease or a condition that affects the spinal cord or spinal nerves. Assess ability to perceive various sensations. Touch both sides of various parts of the body (chest, abdomen, arms and legs) with one or more of the following: cotton wisp, Neurotip ™ (single-use neurological examination pins) and a vibrating tuning fork placed on bony prominences. Patients should be able to differentiate between soft and sharp, and feel vibrations appropriately.

Assess the person's sense of position (kinesthesia). There are a number of tests that can be performed. For example, with the person's eyes shut, move a finger or the big toe up or down. The person should be able to accurately describe the position of the finger or toe.

A number of age-related changes also need to be considered during neurological assessment and these are listed in Table 13.11.

DIAGNOSTIC TESTS

The results of diagnostic tests of neurological structures and functions are used to support the diagnosis of a specific injury or disease, to provide information to identify or modify the appropriate medications or therapy used to treat the disease,

Table 13.11 Age-related changes in the neurological system

Age-related change	Significance
Decreased number of brain cells, cerebral blood flow and metabolism. Slower nerve conduction velocity.	Delayed response to multiple stimuli and slower reflexes; may need additional time to process and respond to verbal stimuli.
Slower retrieval of information from long-term memory.	There is some age-related forgetfulness, which can be improved by using memory aids such as making lists.
Slower response to changes in balance.	May contribute to increased risk for falls.
May exhibit less readiness to learn and depend on prior experiences to solve problems. Is more easily distracted and has a decrease in the ability to maintain attention.	Learning new skills or knowledge is improved when they are related to previously learned information and when limits are set on times for learning (e.g. no more than 30 minutes at one time).

and to help nurses monitor the patient's responses to treatment and nursing care interventions. Diagnostic tests to assess the structures and functions of the neurological system are described on pages 479–480.

REFLEX ASSESSMENT

Reflex testing provides an important indication of the status of the nervous system. Reflexes are classified into deep reflexes and superficial reflexes. Testing deep reflexes involves the use of a patellar hammer to strike the tendon of various reflex sites. These include the patellar, biceps, brachioradialis, triceps and achilles deep tendon. These reflexes test the integrity of specific nerve roots. Normally there is a stretching of the tendon followed by a contraction of the attached muscle and movement of the part of the body innervated by the muscle. For this reason, deep reflexes are also referred to as stretch reflexes. Abnormal findings include:

● *Hyperactive reflexes* are present with lesions of upper motor neurones, for example brain injury.

● *Decreased reflexes* are present with lower motor neurone involvement, for example spinal cord injury.

● *Absent reflexes* are a result of lower motor neurone lesions.

DIAGNOSTIC TESTS AND PROCEDURES Neuroscience

RADIOLOGICAL EXAMINATIONS
Skull and spine x-rays

Standard x-rays of the skull/face and spine are done to identify fractures, displacement of vertebrae, spinal curves and tissue displacement.

Computed tomography (CT) scan

CT scans take a series of x-rays of an area of the body from different angles and give a series of cross-sections or 'slices' through the part of the body being scanned. The computer builds a three-dimensional (3D) picture in grey tones which correlate with tissue density (the denser the structure the whiter it appears, e.g. bone appears white, brain grey and air and CSF appear black). Contrast medium may be given prior to scan to provide anatomical clarity. Useful for identifying intracerebral haemorrhage, tumours, cysts, aneurysms, oedema, ischaemia, atrophy and tissue necrosis and may also be used to evaluate a shift in intracranial contents and to differentiate types of stroke.

Magnetic resonance imaging (MRI), functional MRI (fMRI)

A MRI scan uses a powerful magnetic field to create a computerised map or image of radio signals emitted by the human body. Three types of images dependent upon the type of radio frequency (RF) waves patterns are available. Tesla (T) is the unit of measurement quantifying the strength of a magnetic field – the stronger the magnetic field, the better the image of the MRI. Available MRI scanners are termed T1-weighted images, T2-weighted images and T3-weighted images. Gadolinium contrast medium may be used to enhance visualisation. An MRI is done to identify and monitor conditions of the brain and spinal cord, including stroke, tumours, trauma, seizures and multiple sclerosis. A fMRI is done to evaluate metabolic or blood flow responses of the brain to specific tasks, such as activity and rest.

Positron emission tomography (PET) and single-photon emission computed tomography (SPECT)

PET can assess normal brain function and cerebral blood flow and volume; can differentiate different types of dementia; and can identify stages of brain tumours, strokes and seizure disorders. A small amount of radioactive drug (tracer), to show differences between healthy tissue and diseased tissue is given, which is then detected and displayed by the computer.

CEREBRAL BLOOD FLOW TESTS
Cerebral angiogram

The definitive diagnostic procedure for aneurysms, arteriovenous malformations, blood vessel patency and stenosis, thrombosis, vasospasm, aneurysm and space-occupying lesions (e.g. tumours or haematomas). This technique allows for accurate imaging of the blood supply of the brain and involves injecting a contrast medium and taking films at various time intervals.

CT angiography (CTA)

CT scanning may allow very detailed imaging of the blood vessels supplying blood to the brain and within the brain itself. This technique involves an intravenous injection of contrast medium.

Magnetic resonance angiography (MRA)

MRA can provide information about the blood vessels of the brain and identify vascular lesions. Uses the signals from blood vessels to reconstruct only those vessels with blood flow. Can also be performed using contrast medium.

NEUROPHYSIOLOGY TESTS

This includes tests such as nerve conduction studies and EMG (electromyogram) and EEG (electroencephalogram). These tests are performed by a medical specialist trained in this technique – a consultant clinical neurophysiologist.

EMG and nerve conduction studies

This technique allows the integrity and functioning of nerves in the arms and legs to be tested. It is used to diagnose and identify nerve trapping or compression, as well as to identify damage to peripheral nerves or muscle disorders. This test involves using small electrical pulses to stimulate the nerves and record their activity and function. EMG involves inserting a very fine needle into muscles to record and analyse the electrical activity of the muscle. The test takes approximately 30–40 minutes.

Evoked potentials

Evoked responses measure the electrophysiological responses of the nervous system to a variety of stimuli. These may include: visual evoked responses (VER) which measure the visual pathway from the retina to the occipital cortex, somatosensory evoked responses (SSER) which measures the brain and spinal cord response to nerves in an arm or leg being stimulated, and auditory evoked responses (AER) or brainstem AER in which hearing is stimulated by listening to a test tone. Used to diagnose and evaluate neuromuscular diseases and identify nerve damage.

Electromyogram (EMG)

An EMG measures the electrical activity of skeletal muscles at rest and during contraction; useful in diagnosing neuromuscular diseases. Needle electrodes are inserted into skeletal muscle (as on the legs) and electrical activity can be heard, viewed on an oscilloscope, and recorded on graph paper. Normally, there is no electrical activity at rest.

Electroencephalogram (EEG)

An EEG is used to measure the electrical activity of the brain in order to analyse patterns of brain wave rhythms and diagnose brain disease and brain death. Electrodes are applied to the scalp with skin clips and a graphic picture is obtained (similar to an ECG of the heart). It is particularly useful in the diagnosis and management of epilepsy, differentiating different types of epilepsy and helping to identify the part of the brain that is producing the abnormal electrical activity. EEG involves placing several small electrical contacts on the scalp. Recordings may be carried out over a specified period of time.

- *24-hour EEG* involves wearing EEG recording electrodes attached to a recording device at home for a day and night.
- *Video EEG telemetry* involves admission to a specialist hospital unit for 24–72 hours. During this time, the EEG is constantly monitored and continuous video recording allows seizures or attacks that occur to be analysed and correlated with the simultaneous EEG recording.

OTHER NEUROLOGICAL DIAGNOSTIC TESTS AND PROCEDURES
Lumbar puncture (LP)

Used to measure CSF pressure and to obtain a sample of CSF to use in diagnosis of various conditions such as multiple sclerosis. After local anaesthetic is injected into the skin over the area of the needle insertion, a needle is inserted in L_3–L_4 or L_4–L_5 and CSF is withdrawn (see Figure 13.13).

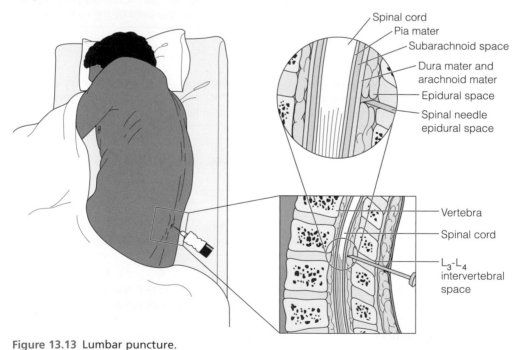

Figure 13.13 Lumbar puncture.

Muscle biopsy

A muscle biopsy is a minor operation in which a small sample of muscle is removed, normally the muscles in the leg or arm, for viewing under the microscope to provide information about muscles and the severity of musculoskeletal system problems. Various diseases can cause muscle weakness or pain. These conditions may be related to problems with the nervous system, connective tissue, vascular system or musculoskeletal system.

Superficial reflexes are assessed by lightly stroking the area with the end of a tongue depressor. These include abdominal and cremasteric reflexes and the plantar reflex (Babinski). The plantar reflex is an important spinal withdrawal reflex that is normally suppressed by the cerebral cortex. A normal response (negative) plantar reflex produces flexion of all toes, whilst an abnormal response called a Babinski sign produces a dorsiflexion of the big toe and fanning of all other toes. This is commonly seen with upper motor neurone disease affecting the pyramidal tract (for example, brain tumour or head injury).

INTRACRANIAL DISORDERS

Patients with intracranial disorders present a unique nursing challenge. Problems that patients experience in the acute stage are often a prelude to long-term problems requiring ongoing management which may affect both the patient's quality of life and that of their family. Accurate assessment helps determine the extent of the cerebral dysfunction and improvement or deterioration of cerebral function. Except in the case of direct damage to the brainstem and RAS, brain function deterioration usually follows a predictable progression, from impaired higher levels of function progressing to impairment of more primitive functions. Signs and symptoms of progressive deterioration of cerebral function are outlined in Table 13.12.

Table 13.12 Progression of deteriorating brain function

Level of consciousness	Pupillary response	Oculomotor responses	Motor responses	Breathing
Alert; oriented to time, place and person	Brisk and equal; pupils regular.	Eyes move as head turns; caloric testing (ear irrigation) produces **nystagmus**.	Purposeful movement; responds to commands.	Regular pattern with normal rate and depth.
Responds to verbal stimuli; decreased concentration; agitation, confusion, lethargy; disoriented	Small and reactive.	Roving eye movements; doll's eyes positive, with gaze fixed straight ahead; eye deviation away from cold caloric stimulus and toward warm stimulus.	Purposeful movement in response to pain stimulus.	Yawning, sighing respirations.
Requires continuous stimulation to rouse			Decorticate posturing with upper extremity flexion.	Cheyne–Stokes respirations (crescendo–decrescendo pattern in rate and depth followed by period of apnoea).
Reflexive positioning to pain stimulus	Pupils fixed (non-reactive) in midposition.	Caloric testing produces nystagmus.	Decerebrate posturing with adduction and rigid extension of upper and lower extremities.	Central neurogenic hyperventilation with rapid, regular and deep respirations; apneustic breathing with prolonged inspiration and pauses at full inspiration and following expiration.
No response to stimuli	Pupils fixed in midposition.	No spontaneous eye movement or nystagmus.	Extension of upper extremities with flexion of lower extremities; flaccidity.	Irregular pattern and depth of respirations; gasping respirations or apnoea.

The person with altered level of consciousness (LOC)

The function of the brain, especially the cerebral hemispheres, depends on continuous blood flow with unimpeded supplies of oxygen and glucose. Processes that disrupt this flow of blood and nutrients may cause widespread damage to the cerebral hemispheres, impairing arousal and cognition.

Pathophysiology of LOC

LOC may be altered by processes that affect the arousal functions of the brainstem, the cognitive functions of the cerebral hemispheres or both. The major causes are:

1. Lesions or injuries that affect the cerebral hemispheres directly and widely or that compress or destroy the neurones of the RAS. Intracranial causes which may directly destroy or compress neurological structures include the following:
   - cerebral oedema (brain swelling) and increased intracranial pressure (ICP);
   - hydrocephalus (dilation of the ventricular system);
   - stroke;
   - haematomas and intracranial haemorrhage;
   - infections–meningitis, encephalitis and brain abscess;
   - injury from excitatory amino acids;
   - demyelinating disorders (for example, multiple sclerosis).

2. Extracranial causes including metabolic disorders (such as hypoglycaemia), fluid and electrolyte imbalances (such as hyponatraemia or hyperosmolality) (see Chapter 3) and acid–base alterations, such as hypercapnia (an elevated arterial CO_2 level) (see Chapter 11).

> ### Consider this . . .
>
> What other contributing factors may lead to altered consciousness? Consider the ageing process, seizures and drugs that may depress the CNS.

Coma states and brain death

Possible outcomes of altered level of consciousness (LOC) and coma include full recovery with no long-term residual effects, recovery with residual damage (such as learning deficits, emotional difficulties or impaired judgement) or more severe consequences such as persistent vegetative state (cerebral death) or brain death. These are described below in more detail.

- *Persistent vegetative state* (also called irreversible coma) is a permanent condition of complete unawareness of self and the environment and loss of all cognitive functions. The brain continues its homeostatic regulatory functions but the person cannot interact with the environment. Usually results from severe brain trauma or global ischaemia.

- *Minimally conscious state* refers to the person being aware of the environment and able to follow simple commands, manipulate objects, gesture or verbalise to indicate 'yes/no' responses and make meaningful movements (such as blinking or smiling) in response to a stimulus. With appropriate supportive care, the person may remain in this state for years.

- *Locked-in syndrome* is distinctly different from persistent vegetative state in that the person is alert and fully aware of the environment and has intact cognitive abilities, but is unable to communicate through speech or movement because of blocked efferent pathways from the brain. Motor paralysis affects all voluntary muscles, although the upper cranial nerves (I through IV) may remain intact, allowing the person to communicate through eye movements and blinking. In essence, the person is 'locked' inside a paralysed body while remaining fully conscious of self and environment.

- *Brain death* is the cessation and irreversibility of all brain functions, including the brainstem. It is generally agreed that this occurs when there is no evidence of cerebral or brainstem function for an extended period.

INTERDISCIPLINARY CARE FOR LOC

Management of the person with an altered LOC or coma must begin immediately. The focus of management is to identify the underlying cause, preserve function and prevent deterioration if possible. Airway and breathing must be maintained. Intravenous fluids are used to support circulation and to correct fluid, electrolyte and acid–base imbalances. Treatment protocols to reduce increased intracranial pressure or control seizure activity (discussed later in this chapter) may be initiated. Appropriate antibiotics are administered intravenously to the person with suspected or confirmed meningitis (see pp. 498–500 for more information).

Diagnosis

Although the person history and physical examination findings often indicate the cause of alterations in LOC, several diagnostic tests may be useful in establishing the diagnosis. The tests used to identify and evaluate for possible metabolic, toxic or drug-induced disorders include both radiologic (CT and MRI scans) and laboratory tests such as blood glucose, serum electrolytes, serum osmolality, arterial blood gases (ABGs), liver function tests and toxicology screening. For further information on specific neurological diagnostic tests see pages 479–480 .

Surgery

Changes in LOC associated with intracerebral tumours, trauma or haematomas often require immediate surgical intervention. When there is a risk of increased intracranial pressure, the person is monitored continuously. This is discussed later (see p. 486).

Case Study 1 – Ali
NURSING CARE PLAN Mild head injury

You will remember Ali who, whilst out drinking with his friends, sustained a mild head injury (MTBI). He is admitted to the medical assessment unit for assessment and further observations. On examination his GCS is 14 (E4, V4, M6), he is complaining of a headache, has vomited twice and is nauseous and his breath smells strongly of alcohol. Skull x-ray revealed a fractured skull. CT scan was normal. On questioning, Ali can't recall events immediately after his fall (amnesia).

Immediate nursing care

Immediate nursing care for Ali includes:

+ Assessment and reassessment of neurological function using the GCS according to his clinical condition at least four hourly.

+ Assess and reassess vital signs, blood pressure, pulse and respirations.

+ Using a validated pain assessment tool, assess Ali's level of pain and safely administer analgesia as prescribed, reassessing for effectiveness, for example paracetamol and/or codeine phosphate.

+ Assess Ali's nausea and safely administer prescribed antiemetics, ensuring that a vomit bowl is close at hand.

+ Encourage fluid and food as tolerated. Ali may require a intravenous infusion to ensure hydration. Record intake and output on a fluid balance chart.

Discharge

Ali was discharged home to his flat where he lives with friends after 48 hours of observations with information that a post-concussion syndrome (PCS) (headache, dizziness, fatigue, lack of concentration, impaired memory, irritability and mood changes) sometimes occurs post-MTBI and rehabilitation including neuropsychology may help the person compensate for memory impairment and attention deficits. Ali was informed that the majority of people with MTBI are likely to be symptom-free at six months.

NURSING CARE FOR LOC

Nursing care for an unconscious person is both general and specific. For general care issues, the reader will need to consult other chapters in this book, for example respiration (Chapter 11), nutrition (Chapter 7) and mobility (Chapter 12).

Nursing diagnoses and interventions

More specific aspects of nursing care considerations discussed in this section include problems with airway maintenance, nutrition, mobility and specific hygiene requirements.

Risk for ineffective airway clearance and risk of aspiration

Support of the airway and respirations is vital in the person with an altered LOC. The person who is drowsy but rousable may need little more than an oral pharyngeal airway such as a Guedel airway or a nasopharyngeal tube. With more severe alterations in consciousness, the person may need endotracheal intubation or a tracheostomy to maintain airway patency, particularly if the cough and gag reflexes are absent. Mechanical ventilation is indicated when hypoventilation or apnoea is present. Ineffective airway clearance related to loss or impaired cough reflex and the inability to remove secretion to discharge matter from the throat or lungs by coughing and spitting (expectoration) is a major problem for the unconscious patient. This occurs when conditions that produce coma depress the function of the medullary centres. A depressed or absent gag and swallowing reflex also presents a high risk for aspiration. Drainage, mucus or blood may obstruct the airway and interfere with oxygenation. Pooling of aspiration secretions in the lungs also increases the risk of pneumonia.

+ Monitor breath sounds, rate and depth of respirations.

+ Report signs and symptoms of aspiration: crackles and wheezes, dyspnoea, tachypnoea and cyanosis.

+ Ensure airway patency. This may require the insertion of a Guedel airway or a nasopharyngeal tube or a tracheostomy tube.

+ Maintain an open airway by suctioning as required to clear the oropharyngeal/tracheostomy of secretion that might otherwise be aspirated.

+ Position the person to allow secretions to drain from the mouth rather than into the pharynx, for example lateral position.

+ Maintain oxygen saturation levels via prescribed oxygen therapy, monitoring results of arterial blood gas analysis and pulse oximetry.

+ Assess swallowing and gag reflexes.

Risk for imbalanced nutrition

The unconscious person is at risk of imbalance in nutrition due to reduced or complete inability to eat and the potential increase in metabolic requirements as result of trauma and/or infection. In the person with long-term alterations in consciousness, such as vegetative state or locked-in syndrome, or if the person is unable to take enough food by mouth without aspirating then alterative measures to maintain nutritional status are required. This may include enteral feeding, for example nasogastric, gastrostomy or jejunostomy tube feeding. For further information on nutrition see Chapter 7.

Risk for impaired physical mobility

Patients who are unconscious are unable to maintain normal musculoskeletal movement and are at high risk for contractures related to decreased movement. Because the flexor and adductor muscles are stronger than the extensors and abductors, flexor and adductor contractures develop quickly without preventive measures. Passive range-of-motion exercises must be performed routinely to maintain muscle tone and function, to prevent additional disability and to help restore impaired motor function. Measures to maintain muscle tone and function include:

+ The use of proper support devices, for example splints in preventing plantar flexion.

+ Collaborate with a physical therapist to develop and implement passive range-of-motion (ROM) exercises (unless contraindicated).

Risk to integrity of skin and related structures

The unconscious person may clench their fists, making their hands sweaty, and long or broken fingernails may cause injury. File, clip nails and maintain hand hygiene to prevent injury and infection. The unconscious person often presents with diminished or absent corneal reflex, preventing the normal protective mechanisms, which may result in an increased risk of drying and damage to the cornea. In addition, tear production may be reduced and the person's eyelids often do not close completely. Following regular assessments of the eyes, care may include the following:

+ Regular eye cleansing and monitoring for redness, oedema, exudate and ulceration.

+ The regular instillation of methylcellulose drops or artificial tear ointment, for example Lacri-lube, to prevent drying.

+ Eye closure with the use of polyethylene films/polyacrylamide gel placed over closed eyelids.

+ Application of an eye shield or patch for patients with incomplete lid closure.

For further information on skin and eye care see Chapters 5 and 14 respectively.

PRACTICE ALERT

- Both active and passive exercises increase venous return, decreasing the risk of thrombophlebitis and maintaining joint mobility.

- Correct poistioning reduces the risk of spasticity and contractures.

- Do not position the unconscious person on their back as their tongue may slide back and occlude their airway, and any vomit cannot drain out.

- Assess the patient's swallow reflex before starting any feeding programme.

The person with increased intracranial pressure

Increased intracranial pressure (IICP) is sustained elevated pressure (10 mmHg or higher) within the cranial cavity. Transient increases in ICP occur with normal activities such as coughing, sneezing, straining or bending forward. These transient increases are not harmful; however, sustained IICP alters cerebral perfusion and oxygenation of brain cells and can result in significant tissue ischaemia and damage to delicate neural tissue. A significant number of neurological patients are at risk of developing IICP. Regular neurological assessments to identify trends and changes in LOC and specific signs and neurological function are vital for early detection; even subtle changes may be clinically significant. Sign and symptoms may differ according to the speed and cause of the IICP.

Pathophysiology of increased intracranial pressure

Essential to understanding the pathophysiology of IICP is the *Monro–Kellie hypothesis*. In the adult, the rigid cranial cavity created by the skull is normally filled to capacity (1400–1700 ml) with three non-compressible interchangeable components. Of these, the brain makes up approximately 85% (comprising 5% extracellular fluid, 45% glial tissue and 35% neuroneal tissue); the remaining approximately 15% comprises 7% blood and 8% CSF (Littlejohns and Bader 2001). The hypothesis states that these components are in a state of dynamic equilibrium. If any one of these components increases, then the others will need to decrease to compensate (maintain normal pressures within the cranial cavity).

Displacement of some CSF to the spinal subarachnoid space and increased CSF absorption are early compensatory mechanisms. The low-pressure venous system is also compressed, and cerebral arteries constrict to reduce blood flow. However, brain tissue's ability to accommodate change is relatively restricted. Once the compensatory mechanisms are exhausted then ICP rises, cerebral perfusion falls, cerebral tissue becomes ischaemic and signs and symptoms of cellular hypoxia appear. If significant ICP elevations are not aggressively treated then severe, permanent neurological deficits or death will occur.

Cerebral haemodynamics

Changes in the cerebral haemodynamics can have an effect on the ICP, and several parameters are measured and calculated when caring for a person at risk of or with raised ICP:

- Cerebral perfusion pressure (CPP) is the pressure it takes for the heart to provide the brain with blood, calculated by the following equation:

    MAP (mean arterial blood pressure) − ICP (intracranial pressure) = CPP (normal CPP is 70–95 mmHg).

For example, MAP (systolic 145 − diastolic 60 = 85) 85 − ICP 25 = CPP 60

- Cerebral blood flow (CBF) – cerebral blood volume is the amount of blood in the brain at a given time. Adequate blood flow, 750 mL/min, and oxygen are required for normal neural function. CBF is influenced by changes in blood pressure and cardiac function. Cerebral blood flow is represented by the following equation:

$$\text{CBF} = \text{mean arterial pressure (MAP)} - \text{central venous pressure (CVP)}$$

FAST FACTS

CNS

- Normal ICP ranges from 0–10 mmHg.
- ICP persistently above 20 mmHg is termed intracranial hypertension.
- An increase in body temperature of 1 °C increases cerebral metabolism by up to 10%.

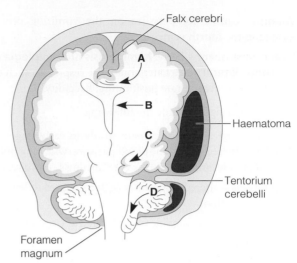

Figure 13.14 Forms of brain herniation due to intracranial hypertension. (A) Cingulate herniation occurs when the cingulate gyrus is compressed under the falx cerebri. **(B)** Central herniation occurs when a centrally located lesion compresses central and mid-brain structures. **(C)** Lateral herniation occurs when a lesion at the side of the brain compresses the uncus or hippocampal gyrus. **(D)** Infratentorial herniation occurs when the cerebellar tonsils are forced downward, compressing the medulla and top of the spinal cord.

Brain herniation

If IICP is not treated, cerebral tissue is displaced from its normal compartment through the tentorium cerebelli (double fold of dural mater) which separate the cerebrum from the cerebellum. If the ICP continues to rise then a proportion of the cerebrum will exert pressure on the brainstem and eventually cerebellar herniation and death will ensue as a result of compression of the respiratory centre in the medulla. See Figure 13.14 for various forms of brain herniation.

Cerebral oedema

Cerebral oedema is an increase in the volume of brain tissue due to abnormal accumulation of fluid. Cerebral oedema is the most frequent cause of sustained increases in ICP and can also result from the following mechanisms:

- Increase in intracranial contents (often referred to as 'mass effect') due to oedema and/or space-occupying lesions (for example, tumour, haemorrhage or abscess).
- Obstruction in the flow or absorption of CSF – hydrocephalus.
- Increased venous failure (for example, venous thrombosis, heart failure, depressed fracture over major venous sinus).

Brain function becomes disrupted when cerebral oedema causes an increase in ICP. This can result in decreased cerebral blood flow, and brain tissue becomes hypoxic and ischaemic. Autoregulatory mechanisms cause vasodilation and increase cerebral blood flow, further increasing cerebral oedema and intracranial pressure. Without effective intervention, condition can deteriorate rapidly with intracranial pressure increasing to the point where brain structures herniate.

Hydrocephalus

Hydrocephalus refers to a progressive dilatation of the ventricular system, which becomes dilated as the production of CSF exceeds its absorption (Hickey 2009). It is generally classified as either non-communicating, occurring when CSF drainage from the ventricular system is obstructed, or communicating hydrocephalus in which CSF is not effectively reabsorbed through the arachnoid villi.

Sign and symptoms of increased intracranial pressure

Signs and symptoms of increased intracranial pressure:

- Decreased level of consciousness – Early: confusion; restlessness, lethargy; disorientation, first to time, then to place and person. Late: comatose with no response to painful stimuli.
- Pupillary dysfunction – sluggish response to light progressing to fixed pupils (pupillary dysfunction is first noted on the same (**ipsilateral**) side).
- Oculomotor dysfunction – inability to move eye(s) upward; **ptosis** (drooping) of eyelid due to compression of the occulomotor nerve.
- **Papilloedema** which will eventually lead to visual abnormalities such as decreased visual acuity, blurred vision and even blindness.
- Double vision (**diplopia**).
- Generalised headache worse on rising in the morning, position changes and coughing.

- Vomiting caused by pressure on the vomiting centre located in the fourth ventricle.
- Motor impairment – Early: **hemiparesis** or **hemiplegia** of the **contralateral** side. Late: abnormal responses such as decorticate or decerebrate positioning; flaccidity.

Changes in vital signs include the following.

- Blood pressure and pulse remain steady in early stages of raised ICP. Increased systolic blood pressure, widening pulse pressure, bradycardia known as the Cushing's response.
- Respirations – altered respiratory pattern related to level of brain dysfunction.
- Temperature may be significantly elevated as compensatory mechanisms fail.

Consider this . . .

Ali has sustained a mild TBI and is complaining of a headache. What pain relief might you consider and why? What alternative measures could you consider to reduce Ali's pain?

PRACTICE ALERT

- Often, the earliest signs of raised intracranial pressure are altered respiration pattern and conscious level.
- A sluggishly reactive pupil may be one of the first signs of herniation.
- A lumbar puncture is not performed when raised ICP is suspected because the sudden release of the pressure in the skull may cause cerebral herniation.

INTERDISCIPLINARY CARE FOR INCREASED INTRACRANIAL PRESSURE

Diagnosis

The diagnosis is made on the basis of observation and neurological assessment. Diagnostic tests focus on identifying the presence of raised ICP and its underlying cause. A CT or MRI scan is generally the initial test used to identify the possible causes and to evaluate therapeutic options.

Medication

Medications play an important role in the management of raised ICP and include:

- Diuretics, particularly osmotic diuretics such as Mannitol, are commonly used to reduce ICP. These hyperosmotic agents draw fluid out of extracellular space by increasing the osmolality of the blood. Loop diuretics, for example frusemide, are also commonly used.

- Sedation – proprofol is the sedation of choice in the neuroscience patient. It is used when patients are receiving mechanical ventilation to control restlessness and agitation, because these movements increase blood pressure, ICP and cerebral metabolism.
- Antipyretics to reduce hyperthermia, decreasing the high cerebral metabolism that contributes to ICP.
- Anticonvulsants may be prescribed to manage seizure activity associated with brain injury.

Monitoring

Assessing patients who are receiving sedatives, analgesics or neuromuscular blocking agents is not optimal for detecting IICP. For this reason, ICP monitoring is essential in the patient's management; preserving brain function and preventing secondary brain damage from raised ICP. Monitoring provides continual assessment of ICP and quickly detects ICP elevations and diminished compliance. It also facilitates the monitoring of the effects of medical therapy and nursing interventions on ICP. Several ICP monitoring methods are available, including intraventricular catheter, subarachnoid bolt or screw (Figure 13.15).

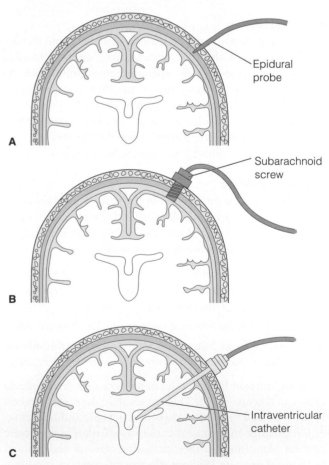

Figure 13.15 Types of intracranial pressure monitoring. (A) Epidural probe. (B) Subarachnoid screw. (C) Intraventricular catheter.

Surgery

Patients with raised ICP may undergo various intracranial surgical techniques to treat the underlying cause, for example infarcted or necrotic tissue may be resected to reduce brain mass. A drainage catheter or shunt may be inserted laterally via a burr hole into a ventricle to drain excess cerebrospinal fluid and reduce hydrocephalus. This is known as an external ventricular drain.

NURSING CARE FOR INCREASED INTRACRANIAL PRESSURE

Nurses caring for patients at risk for or having IICP need to perform and document regular neurological assessments in order to detect any subtle neurological changes which require timely interventions and management. Management of the person is directed toward identifying and treating the underlying cause of the disorder, and controlling ICP to prevent herniation syndrome. This includes the following:

+ Maintain adequate oxygenation and control of respiratory gases. This may involve respiratory support, thus preventing hypoxaemia and hypercapnia, both of which can increase intracranial pressure.

+ Regularly monitor consciousness level using the GCS and neurological function.

+ Continuously monitor and recording of ICP readings.

+ Maintain CPP at around 70 mmHg.

+ Monitor for signs and symptoms of IICP.

+ Maintain a head-up position at 30° which facilitates intracranial blood outflow to the jugular veins, decreasing venous blood volume in the brain.

+ Maintain the head in a neutral position with the head in line with the thorax, to avoid hyperextension or exaggerated neck flexion, as obstruction of jugular veins can impede venous drainage from the brain causing localised changes in cerebral blood flow and IICP.

+ As clinically appropriate, interventions should be spaced over time, avoiding clustering activities in order to limit a cumulative effect on increasing ICP.

+ Monitor intracranial compliance. In those patients with a compromised intracranial compliance, measures to reduce stimuli need considering, for example suctioning, turning, bathing, coughing, sneezing and straining to have a bowel movement all initiate Valsalva's manoeuvre, which constricts the jugular veins and impairs venous return from the brain.

+ Maintain accurate fluid balance and management to ensure normovolemia.

+ If an external ventricular drainage system is in place, avoid kinks in tubing and maintain the drainage collecting device and the person's head at the prescribed levels.

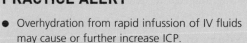

PRACTICE ALERT

● Overhydration from rapid infussion of IV fluids may cause or further increase ICP.

● IV glucose and dextrose solutions should be avoided as they worsen cerebral oedema.

● Analgesics which have a depressant effect on the CNS (e.g. opiates) and which can depress respiration rates should be avoided to prevent masking early signs and symptoms of deteriorating LOC.

● Constipation and bladder distention increase intrathoracic or intra-abdominal pressure and increase the risk of reducing venous drainage from the brain.

● Suctioning for more than 15 seconds in the person with increased ICP may cause hypercapnia.

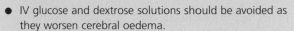

The person with a headache

Headache refers to pain within the cranial vault and is one of the most frequent signs and symptoms of a health problem people experience. The International Headache Society (2004) classifies headaches into 14 groups and lists 150 headaches, which can be categorised broadly into either primary or secondary (see Table 13.13 for common causes of headache). Signs and symptoms of headache vary according to the cause,

Table 13.13 Common causes of headaches

Primary – those that exist independent of any other medical condition	Secondary – headaches caused by some underlying condition
Migraine Tension-type headache (TTH) Cluster headache (CH) and other trigeminal autonomic cephalalgias Other primary headaches, e.g. thunderclap headache, exertion headache	Vascular: ● Subarachnoid haemorrhage (SAH) ● Strokes Non-vascular: ● Tumours and other space–occupying lesions causing raised ICP ● Benign intracanial hypertension (BIH) ● Infections in the nasal or sinus passages and CNS infections (meningitis, encephalitis) ● Neck and head injuries ● Post-lumbar puncture headache ● Substance abuse ● Headaches related to psychiatric disorders

type and precipitating symptoms. The most common types of headaches are migraine, cluster and tension headaches.

Pathophysiology of headache

The bones and brain tissue itself lack pain-sensitive nerve fibres. Pain-sensitive structures include supporting structures, such as the skin, muscles and periosteum; the nasal cavities and sinuses; portions of the meninges, cranial nerves II, III, IV, V, VI, IX and X; and cerebral vessels, including extracranial arteries and the venous sinuses. Most facial and scalp structures are sensitive to pain. Headache is experienced when there is traction, pressure, displacement, inflammation or dilation of nociceptors (nerve endings that are receptors of noxious stimuli) in areas sensitive to pain (Hickey 2009).

Tension headache

Tension headache is characterised by bilateral pain, with a sensation of a band of tightness or pressure in the head, neck or scalp. Sharply localised painful spots (trigger points) may be present. The onset is gradual, and the intensity, frequency and duration of the attack vary greatly. It is typically caused by sustained contraction of the muscles of the head and neck and often precipitated by stressful situations and anxiety. Secondary causes include prolonged computer use and disorders of the eyes, ears, sinuses or cervical vertebrae; slouching while reading or watching television can lead to muscle contraction. Most primary headaches are tension-type headaches.

Migraine headache

Migraine headache is a complex, common disorder which affects 1:6 women and 1:12 men and is more common between the ages of 15 and 55 years (Lipton and Scher 2001). Typically, attacks are characterised by sensory symptoms of pulsating headaches usually on one side of the cranium associated with other symptoms such as nausea, vomiting and sensitivity to light. Most (80%) migraineurs will have a family member who suffers from migraines. Migraine affects eight million people in the UK and is the most common long-term neurological condition. The World Health Organization (WHO 2001) ranks it 19th among all causes of 'years lived with disability'. Most sufferers commonly have approximately one attack per month. Migraine can be divided into episodic (occurs on fewer days than 15 in a month) and chronic (occurs on more than 15 days in a month). Migraines can be broadly classified as with or without **auras** (symptoms immediately before the headache, for example visual disturbances). Migraines with aura typically occur in three phases: **prodromal** (symptoms that occur hours or days before the headache), aura and headache. The underlying mechanism for migraine was originally thought to be vascular, but it is now understood to be a disorder of the cerebral nerve and blood vessel dysfunction (Durham and Garrett 2009). Migraine attacks may be triggered by certain internal or external factors. These include low blood glucose levels, stress, emotional excitement, fatigue, hormonal changes due to menstruation, stimuli such as bright lights, food high in tyramine, low level of magnesium and dehydration.

Signs and symptoms

- Prodromal phases include abdominal migraines in children.
- Aura phase – the person often experiences a visual disturbance prior to the pain, such as bright spots or flashing lights zigzagging across the visual fields lasting from 5–60 minutes or, less commonly, sensory symptoms, for example numbness or tingling of the face or hand, weakness of an arm or leg, mild **aphasia**, confusion, drowsiness and lack of coordination.
- Headache phase is characterised by vasodilation, a decline in serotonin levels in the brain and the onset of throbbing headache.

FAST FACTS

Headaches

- Headaches are the commonest neurological symptom.
- Headache disorders are under-recognised and under-treated.
- 1:7 people suffer from migraines.
- Cluster headaches or 'suicide headache' are one of the most painful conditions known to man.

Cluster headache

A cluster headache, also known as histamine headache, is a form of neurovascular headache. Men are affected more commonly than women in a proportion of 6:1 and between the ages of 20 and 50 years. About 75% of attacks occur between 9 pm and 10 am, typically occurring two to three hours after falling asleep. The headache awakens the person and then lasts from 15–180 minutes. The headaches occur without auras in groups or 'clusters' of one to eight each day for several weeks or months, followed by remission lasting months to years. The underlying physiological mechanism is not well understood, but it is believed to involve a vascular disorder, a disturbance of serotonergic mechanisms, a sympathetic defect or dysregulation of the hypothalamus.

Signs and symptoms

- Extremely severe, unilateral, burning intense stabbing, icepick-like pains located behind or around the eyes.
- Autonomic symptoms, including reddening and lacrimation (tearing) of the affected eye, flushing, sweating and pallor on the forehead.
- Ipsilateral nasal congestion.
- Transitory partial Horner's syndrome (constricted pupil and ptosis) occurs in two-thirds of patients.
- Restlessness, rocking and walking about during pain.

INTERDISCIPLINARY CARE FOR HEADACHE

Diagnosis

Diagnosis and treatment are based on history, identifying triggering or precipitating events and the type of headache. A thorough history and physical examination are integral parts of the assessment. Neurodiagnostic testing may be done to rule out other causes for the headache, such as structural disease process. Tests may include CT scan, MRI, x-ray studies of the skull and cervical spine, EEG or lumbar puncture for CSF if inflammation is suspected.

Medications

Pharmacological management depends on the type of headache and includes prevention (prophylactic therapy), reducing the frequency and medication to limit or relieve a headache that is beginning or in progress. Using a stepwise approach to treatment, initially simple analgesia and an antiemetic may be prescribed to control nausea and vomiting, progressing to combined treatment options.

IN PRACTICE

Headache medication

Medication for the treatment of tension headaches includes:

● analgesics – simple analgesic, e.g. asprin, ibuprofen and paracetamol.

Medication for the treatment of cluster headaches may include:

● antriptan drugs such as sumatriptan;

● 100% oxygen inhalation.

Drugs used to reduce the frequency and severity of migraine may include:

● analgesics – simple analgesic, e.g. asprin, ibuprofen and paracetamol;

● antimigraine drugs, e.g. triptans (5-HT agonists) – drugs that act directly on the 5-HT receptors to correct the 5-HT imbalance.

● migraine prophylaxis:
  – beta-blockers such as propanolol hydrochloride; atenolol prevents dilation of vessels in the pia mater and inhibits serotonin uptake;
  – Botox (botulinum toxin) injections into multiple head and neck muscle sites in chronic migraineurs.

Alternative and complementary therapies

Alternative and complementary therapies are used to relieve the pain of headaches. These include vitamin D, riboflavin (vitamin B), magnesium, acupuncture, relaxation, guided imagery, massage, melatonin, magnetic field therapy, herbal therapy and osteopathic manipulation.

Surgery

Deep-brain stimulation (DBS) or neurostimulation to the hypothalamus may be offered to patients with chronic cluster headaches.

NURSING CARE FOR HEADACHE

Assessment includes a detailed history and description of headache characteristics; family history; triggering factors; usual diet; effects of recurring headaches on lifestyle. In addition to implementing comfort measures, nurses can play an important role in education, focused on limiting attacks and providing relevant information to help people to manage their headaches. This may include:

+ Teach the person how to limit attacks, for example by avoiding precipitating factors and using stress management techniques and relaxation techniques.

+ Provide help and advice on how to keep a headaches diary: identify triggers, time of onset, frequency and site of pain.

+ For tension headaches, intervention is directed toward reducing the person's level of stress and relieving pain. The application of heat can help to reduce muscle tension and improve circulation.

+ Information about current medications, dietary advice, for example foods to avoid and sources of magnesium, and available resources and support groups (Migraine Action, http://www.migraine.org.uk/, and The Migraine Trust, www.migrainetrust.org.uk/).

+ Referrals to specialist clinics for management options may be necessary for people with chronic headaches.

The person with epilepsy

Epilepsy (also called *seizure disorder*) is a chronic disorder of abnormal recurring, excessive and self-terminating electrical discharge from neurones. This abnormal neuroneal activity, which may involve all or part of the brain, disturbs skeletal motor function, sensation, autonomic function of the viscera, behaviour and/or consciousness.

Incidence and prevalence of epilepsy

Epilepsy is one of the most common neurological conditions, affecting up to 50 million people worldwide. The incidence of epilepsy is increasing due to several contributing factors: technologic advances in obstetric and paediatric care that allow extremely high-risk neonates to survive; other technologic advances that have improved survival rates after traumatic brain injury; and the ageing population.

Epilepsy may be *idiopathic* (no identifiable cause) with multiple episodes diagnosed as a seizure disorder or it may be secondary to conditions affecting the brain or other organs such as:

- birth injury and toxaemia of pregnancy;
- drug and alcohol overdose and withdrawal;
- systemic metabolic conditions (e.g. hypoglycaemia, hypoxia, uraemia and electrolyte imbalances);
- brain pathologies, for example meningitis, cerebral bleeding, cerebral oedema, infection, vascular abnormalities, trauma or tumours.

Seizures may also be provoked or unprovoked. The clinical signs or symptoms of seizures depend on the brain location of the epileptic discharges and the extent and pattern of the epileptic discharge in the brain. Typical symptoms include:

- temporary changes in mental status and LOC;
- abnormal sensory changes;
- abnormal movements.

FAST FACTS

Epilepsy

- Epilepsy affects people of all ages, races and ethnic backgrounds.
- Epilepsy is the most common chronic disabling neurological condition in the UK.
- Epilepsy is estimated to occur in 15% of people with mild learning disabilities and 30% of those with severe learning disabilities.
- Misdiagnosis for epilepsy is estimated at an annual cost in the UK of up to £189 million.

Source: Stokes *et al.* 2004.

Pathophysiology of epilepsy

A seizure results when a sudden imbalance occurs between the excitatory and inhibitory forces within the network of cortical neurones. During a seizure, these neurones produce a rhythmic and repetitive hypersynchronous discharge. It is believed that most seizures arise from a few unstable, hypersensitive and hyper-reactive neurones in the brain. Although the exact initiating factor for seizure activity has not been identified, several theories have been proposed (Porth 2009). All people have a seizure threshold; when this threshold is exceeded, a seizure may result. The neurones that initiate seizure activity are called the *epileptogenic focus*.

The metabolic needs of the brain increase dramatically during seizure activity. Consequently, the demand for glucose and oxygen increases, and oxygen consumption increases by about 60%. To supply this increased oxygen need and remove carbon dioxide and other metabolic by-products, cerebral blood flow increases to about 2.5 times the normal rate. If cerebral blood flow cannot meet these needs, cellular exhaustion and cellular destruction may result.

Classification of epilepsy

Focal or partial seizures

Abnormal neuronal activity may remain localised, causing partial or focal seizures, usually involving a restricted part of one cerebral hemisphere at the onset. Partial seizures can be further subdivided:

- simple partial seizure, without impaired consciousness;
- complex partial seizure, with impaired consciousness;
- partial seizures evolving into secondary generalised seizures.

Both types of partial seizures can spread, resulting in secondary generalised tonic–clonic seizures, the signs and symptoms of which will depend on the area of brain involved. Typically, a portion of the motor cortex is affected, causing recurrent muscle contractions. This motor activity may stay confined to one area or spread sequentially to adjacent areas, a phenomenon known as *Jacksonian march* or *Jacksonian seizure*. In complex partial seizures, consciousness is impaired and the person may engage in repetitive, non-purposeful activity, such as lip smacking, aimless walking or picking at clothing. These behaviours are known as *automatisms*. Complex partial seizures usually originate in the temporal lobe and may be preceded by an aura, such as an unusual smell, a sense of déjà vu or a sudden intense emotion.

Generalised seizures

Generalised seizures affect both hemispheres of the brain as well as deeper brain structures. Consciousness is always impaired, and these can be further subdivided into six major categories: (1) generalised tonic–clonic seizures; (2) tonic seizures; (3) clonic seizures; (4) myoclonic seizures; (5) atonic seizures; and (6) absence seizures. Tonic–clonic and absence seizures are the common forms of generalised seizure activity; they occur more frequently (especially in children) than partial seizures.

Tonic–clonic seizures

Tonic–clonic seizures, also known as the '*grand mal*' seizures, are the most common type of seizure activity in adults. This type of seizure activity follows a typical pattern.

- *Aura.* A warning may precede generalised seizure activity. This may a vague sense of uneasiness or an abnormal gustatory, visual, auditory or visceral sensation (e.g. metallic taste in the mouth, a smell of burning rubber or seeing a bright light). Often, however, the seizure occurs without warning.

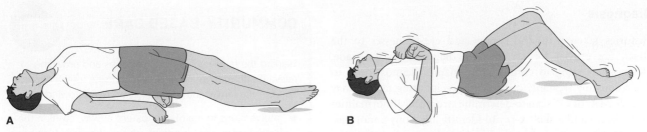

Figure 13.16 Tonic–clonic seizures in grand mal seizures. **(A)** Tonic phase. **(B)** Clonic phase.

- *Tonic phase.* Sudden loss of consciousness and sharp tonic muscle contractions. The person may cry out as air is forced out of the lungs. Postural control is lost, and the person falls to the floor in the opisthotonic posture (Figure 13.16A). Muscles are rigid, with the arms and legs extended and the jaw clenched. Urinary incontinence is common; bowel incontinence may also occur. Breathing ceases and cyanosis develops during the tonic phase of a seizure. The pupils are fixed and dilated. The tonic phase lasts an average of 15 seconds, although it may persist for up to a minute.

- *Clonic phase.* Follows the tonic phase and is characterised by alternating contraction and relaxation of the muscles in all the extremities along with hyperventilation (Figure 13.16B). The eyes roll back, and the person may froth at the mouth. The clonic phase varies in duration and subsides gradually.

- *Post-ictal period or phase.* Following the clonic phase, the person remains unconscious and unresponsive to stimuli. The person then regains consciousness gradually, and may be confused and disoriented on waking. Headache, muscle aches and fatigue often follow the seizure, and the person may sleep for several hours. Amnesia of the seizure is usual and amnesia of the events just prior to the seizure activity may occur.

Tonic seizures

These seizures involve a sudden onset of stiffening of the muscles resulting in increased muscle tone, usually leading to falling.

Clonic seizures

These are rapidly alternating contraction and relaxation of a muscle (repeated jerking) of the arms and legs. This type of seizure is uncommon.

Myoclonic seizures

These are brief, arrhythmic, jerking, motor movements that last less than a second and often occur in clusters.

Atonic seizures (drop attacks)

These seizures consist of brief loss of postural tone, often resulting in falls and injuries.

Absence seizures

Absence seizures, often called '*petit mal*' seizures, are characterised by a sudden brief cessation of all motor activity accompanied by a blank stare and unresponsiveness. Absence seizures are more common in children than in adults. The seizure typically lasts only 5–10 seconds, although some may last for 30 seconds or more. Movements such as eyelid fluttering or automatisms such as lip smacking may occur during an absence seizure. Seizure activity may vary from occasional episodes to several hundred per day.

Status epilepticus

Status epilepticus can develop during seizure activity. In this case, the seizure activity becomes continuous, with only very short periods of calm between intense and persistent seizures. The person is in great danger of developing hypoxia, acidosis, hypoglycaemia, hyperthermia and exhaustion if the seizure activity is not halted. Status epilepticus is considered a life-threatening medical emergency that requires immediate treatment to preserve life.

Non-epileptic seizures (NESs)

These are events that resemble epileptic seizures and are relatively common. There are two major types of NESs:

- *Psychogenic NES (PNES)* are episodes of altered movement, sensation or experience, caused by a psychological process and not associated with abnormal electrical discharges in the brain.

- *Physiological NESs* are caused by physiological dysfunction, for example cardiac arrhythmias, hypotensive episodes or cerebrovascular disease. Such conditions may result in loss of consciousness with or without associated motor signs.

NESs are often difficult to differentiate from events due to epilepsy, and misdiagnosis leads to inappropriate treatment with antiepileptic drugs (AEDs) (also called anticonvulsant drugs). They can be life-threatening, for example cardiac causes. A correct diagnosis is important to ensure appropriate interventions and improvement in quality of life.

INTERDISCIPLINARY CARE FOR EPILEPSY

Initial treatment focuses on controlling the seizure; the long-term goal is to determine the cause and prevent future seizures. Interdisciplinary care includes diagnostic testing, medications and, in some cases, surgery.

Diagnosis

Histories taken from the person and eye-witnesses to the attack are crucial for an accurate diagnosis to be made. Diagnostic testing to confirm the seizure diagnosis and to determine any treatable causes and precipitating factors may include MRI or CT scan to determine structural abnormalities in the brain and a skull x-ray to identify any bony abnormalities. An EEG helps localise any brain lesions and confirm the diagnosis. Other tests may include LP to assess spinal fluid for CNS infections (increased white blood cells), blood studies (plasma electrolytes, glucose and calcium). Confirmed diagnosis should be carried out by a specialist in the field of epilepsy. Other causes of LOC may need to be explored, including cardiac **syncope** and vasovagal syncope (uncomplicated faint) (NICE, 2010).

Medication

The goals of medications for epilepsy are to protect the person from harm and to reduce or prevent seizure activity without impairing cognitive function or producing undesirable side-effects. Ideally, the lowest possible dose of a single medication that will control the seizures is prescribed on an individual basis. AEDs can reduce or control most seizure activity in one of two ways: by acting on the motor cortex in the brain to raise the seizure threshold or by limiting the spread of rapidly firing epileptic foci in the brain. Several factors are considered when determining the most appropriate AED, including type of seizure and/or epilepsy syndrome, age and the presence of other diseases; individual and/or carer preferences, potential interactions with other drugs, potential adverse effects and the licensed indication of the drug. There are numerous AEDs available, and people may be prescribed one AED or a combination of AEDs.

Surgery

People may be suitable for surgery which involves the removal of the epileptogenic focus. This may involve stereotactic radiotherapy (Gamma Knife), neurostimulation therapy, such as deep brain stimulation and, more commonly and most effective for partial complex seizures, temporal lobectomies which involves resection of the temporal lobe.

Vagus nerve stimulation (VNS) is designed to prevent seizures by sending regular small pulses of electrical energy to the brain via the vagus nerve. These pulses are supplied by a device something like a pacemaker.

NURSING CARE FOR EPILEPSY

Nursing care of patients with a seizure disorder focuses on providing care during and immediately after the seizure and person/family teaching to promote safety and reduce the incidence of seizure activity.

COMMUNITY-BASED CARE

Helping the family adjust to a diagnosis and providing relevant information are important nursing interventions. Educate the family and the person on the following:

- Interventions to maintain a patent airway; cushion the head, loosen anything tight around the neck, turn on the side, do not force anything into the mouth and, if prescribed and available, administer oxygen by mask.

- When to call for medical assistance: if the seizure lasts for more than five minutes, there is slow recovery, a second seizure, or difficulty breathing after the seizure and if there are signs of injury (such as bleeding from the mouth).

- The importance of follow-up care, of keeping medical appointments and of continuing to take AEDs as prescribed even when no seizures are experienced.

- Relevant legislation that applies to people with seizure disorders, for example driving a motor vehicle.

- Awareness of drug interactions with other prescribed drugs, over-the-counter drugs, street drugs and alcohol.

- Identifying factors that may trigger a seizure, such as abrupt withdrawal from medication, constipation, fatigue, excessive stress, fever, menstruation, sights and sounds such as television, flashing video and computer screens.

- Taking showers versus tub baths, because of safety issues during a generalised seizure.

- Information about resources and support groups, for example the Epilepsy Society www.epilepsysociety.org.uk.

PRACTICE ALERT

- Syncope maybe misdiagnosed as epilepsy as sometimes during a syncopal 'attack' the person may exhibit limb twitching, jerking and even urinary incontinence.

- Other causes of transient loss of consciousness need to be excluded as some of these can be fatal if misdiagnosed.

Nursing assessment before, during and after a seizure is shown in Table 13.14.

Consider this . . .

Epilepsy is misdiagnosed in more than 90 000 people in England and Wales each year. What could the impact of a misdiagnosis be for the person and their family? You may want to consider the consequences of inappropiate treatment on their health and the impact on their lifestyle as well as social and financial issues.

Table 13.14 Nursing assessments before, during and after a seizure

Assessment	Rationale
Past medical history – past seizures, age when the first seizure occurred, most recent seizure, factors precipitating a seizure, any warning signs (aura), prophylactic AEDs	Indicates type of seizure and area of the brain involved.
What was the person's level of consciousness? If consciousness was lost, at what point?	Indicates area of brain involved and type of seizure.
What was the person doing just before the attack?	May suggest precipitating factors.
In what part of the body did the seizure start?	May indicate the site of seizure activity in the brain tissue; for example, if jerking movements were first observed in right hand, the seizure focus may be in left motor cortex.
Was there an epileptic cry?	Usually indicates the tonic stage of a generalised tonic–clonic seizure.
Were any automatisms such as eyelid fluttering, chewing, lip smacking or swallowing observed?	Often seen in complex, partial and absence seizures.
How long did movements last? Did the location or character change (tonic to clonic)? Did movements involve both sides of the body or just one?	Indicates areas in which focal activity originated.
Did the head and/or eyes turn to one side and, if so, which side?	Helps localise the focus of the seizure. During the seizure, the head and eyes typically will turn away from the side of the epileptogenic focus.
Were there changes in pupillary reactions?	Indicates involvement of the ANS.
If the person fell, was the head hit?	Skull x-ray and CT scan may be needed to exclude head trauma or skull fracture.
Was there foaming or frothing from the mouth?	Usually indicates a tonic–clonic seizure.

This section has discussed disorders related to cerebral function. We will now go on to look at traumatic injuries to the brain.

The person with a traumatic brain injury (TBI)

Traumatic brain injury (TBI) refers to any injury of the scalp, skull (cranium or facial bones) or brain. TBI is a leading cause of death and disability in the UK. The National Head Injury Foundation defines TBI as a traumatic insult to the brain capable of causing physical, cognitive, emotional and behavioural changes. A TBI may be classified as a penetrating (open) head injury (for example, resulting from a knife, bullet or baseball bat) or a closed head injury (a blunt injury to the brain that does not result in an open skull fracture).

Pathophysiology of TBI

Traumatic head injuries are commonly categorised according to their severity, i.e. mild to severe. Mild brain injuries, if repeated over an extended period of time, can result in cumu-

FAST FACTS

Traumatic brain injury (TBI)

● TBI is the leading cause of morbidity and mortality for young people throughout the world.
● Leading causes of TBI are falls, followed by road traffic accidents and assaults.
● Approximately one million people will sustain a head injury in the UK each year.
● Highest incidences occur between 16 and 25 years of age and the ratio of male to female ranges from 2:1–3:1.

lative neurological and cognitive deficits. Specific damage following craniocerebral injuries is related to the mechanism of the injury (how it occurs), the nature of the injury (type) and the location of the injury (where it occurs). TBIs can occur through several mechanisms:

● Acceleration injury is sustained when the head is struck by a moving object, for example sports injuries.

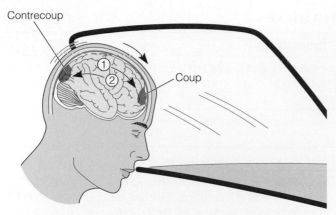

Figure 13.17 Coup-contrecoup head injury. Following an initial injury (coup) the brain rebounds within the skull and sustains additional injury (contrecoup) in the opposite part of the brain.

- Deceleration injury occurs when the head hits a stationary object, for example falls.
- Acceleration–deceleration injury (also called a *coup-contrecoup* phenomenon) occurs when the head hits an object and the brain 'rebounds' within the skull (Figure 13.17). The brain is injured at the point of impact (the *coup*) and on the opposite side of the impact (the *contrecoup*).
- Penetrating brain injury (PBI) is caused by high-velocity objects such as bullets, missiles and shrapnel and low-velocity objects such as knives.

Further classification includes the types of craniocerebral trauma, including injuries to the skull (including fractures), injuries to the brain (including concussion and contusion) and intracranial haemorrhage (including haematomas).

Types of skull fractures

A *skull fracture* is a break in the continuity of the skull. It may occur with or without damage to the brain; however, intracranial trauma often results from skull fractures. Skull fractures

Table 13.15 Types of skull fractures

Type	Description
Linear (simple) 80% of all skull fractures	• Simple, clean break in skull. • Occurs with low-velocity injuries.
Comminuted	• Bone is crushed into small, fragmented pieces. • Usually seen with high-impact injuries.
Depressed	• Inward depression of bone fragments. • Usually due to a powerful blow to the skull. • The dura may or may not be intact. • Bone fragments may penetrate into the brain tissue or tear blood vessels.
Basal skull (basilar) 20% of all skull fractures	• Occurs at the base of the skull. • May be linear, comminuted or depressed.

are classified as open (the dura is torn) or closed (dura is not torn). Skull fractures are further classified into one of four categories: linear, comminuted, depressed or basilar (see Table 13.15). If the fracture results in a tear in the dura, CSF leakage may occur and the person is at increased risk for infection or air may enter the intracranial compartment.

Even when the skull and other structures overlying the brain remain intact, a blow to the head can cause significant brain injury. Closed head injuries may result in either focal or diffuse damage to the brain. Brain injury results from both primary and secondary mechanisms. Primary injury results from the direct impact of the trauma on the brain, and may be focal (contusions, haematomas) or diffuse (contusions, diffuse axonal injury). Secondary injury is the progression of the initial injury, resulting from events that affect perfusion and oxygenation of brain cells which can result in intracranial oedema, haematoma, infection, hypoxia or ischaemia.

Focal brain injuries

Focal brain injuries are specific, grossly observable brain lesions confined to one area of the brain. They include contusions, lacerations and intracranial haemorrhages.

Contusions

Contusions refers to bruises of the surface of the brain (cerebral paraenchyma), typically accompanied by small, diffuse venous haemorrhages. Both white and grey matter may have a bruised, discoloured appearance. Contusions occur most frequently near bony prominences of the skull and as a result of penetrating wounds, acceleration and deceleration and closed head injuries. Signs and symptoms of the contusion depend on the size and location of the brain injury, but cerebral oedema can follow contusion, resulting in IICP.

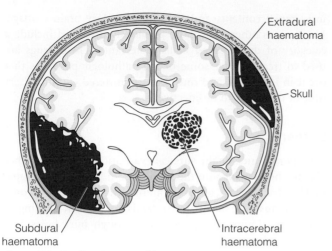

Figure 13.18 Three types of haematoma: extradural, subdural and intracerebral.

Intracranial haemorrhage

This can result directly from the trauma (for example, beneath a fracture) or from shearing forces on cerebral arteries and veins that occur with acceleration–deceleration. Depending on the site and rate of bleeding, signs and symptoms may appear immediately or may not become evident for hours or even weeks. Intracranial haemorrhages and the haematomas they cause place pressure on surrounding structures, causing signs and symptoms of an expanding space-occupying lesion. They also cause IICP, leading to altered levels of consciousness and potential herniation syndromes. Intracranial haematomas are classified by their location as extradural, subdural or intracerebral. Figure 13.18 illustrates their locations.

Extradural haematoma (EDH) refers to the collection of blood in the potential space between the dura and the skull, which normally adhere to one another. As the blood collects, the expanding haematoma strips the dura away from the skull, commonly occurring over the temporal bone (over the middle meningeal artery). EDH tends to develop rapidly, requiring immediate surgical evacuation to prevent significant increases in ICP and herniation.

Subdural haematoma (SDH) refers to bleeding between the dura mater and the arachnoid mater. Approximately 30% of post-traumatic intracranial lesions are SDH, generally caused by tearing of the bridging veins located over the convexity of the brain but also by tearing of small arteries. SDHs are further subdivided into acute SDH (within 48 hours), subacute SHD (within 48 hours–two weeks) and chronic SDH (about three weeks–several months). SDH can result from direct or indirect trauma; as the blood collects it places direct pressure on underlying brain tissue.

Intracerebral haematoma (ICH) refers to bleeding into the cerebral parenchyma. These may be single or multiple, associated with contusions and tend to occur in the frontal or temporal lobes. They behave as expanding space-occupying lesions and may result from closed head trauma or occur without trauma, for example spontaneously due to hypertension or excessive coagulation or a bleeding or vasculitic disorder.

Intraventricular and subarachnoid haemorrhage (SAH) refers to bleeding into the ventricular system (ventricles) or the subarachnoid space (see p. 505 for care of the person with cerebrovascular disorders). Traumatic SAH is common in severe head injuries.

Diffuse injury

Diffuse brain injury, referred to as *diffuse axonal injury* (DAI) is a common feature of any type of brain. It affects the entire brain and is caused by a shaking motion, with twisting movement (rotational acceleration) as the primary mechanism of injury. The shearing stresses on brain tissue cause axonal damage from shearing, tearing or stretching of nerve fibres.

Concussion or mild traumatic brain injury (MTBI) involves temporary axonal disturbances and is defined as a momentary interruption of brain function. A concussion is associated with an immediate, brief loss of consciousness on impact.

Table 13.16 Systemic effects of acute brain injury

Cause	Effect
Stimulation of the sympathetic nervous system, which stimulates the adrenal cortex and medulla to increase glucocorticoid and mineralocorticoid levels	• Increased metabolism of carbohydrates, fats and proteins • Retention of sodium and water
Stimulation of the sympathetic nervous system, increasing the serum catecholamine levels	• Hypertension • EEG changes • Dysrhythmias (bradycardia, sinus tachycardia)
Altered release of ADH from the posterior pituitary	• Retention of water or diuresis and diabetes insipidus
Neurogenic pulmonary dysfunction	• Abnormal respiratory patterns • Reduced residual capacity with retention of CO_2, vasodilation and increased ICP • Pulmonary oedema
Stress response to trauma	• Hyperglycaemia
Increased platelet, plasma fibrinogen and thromboplastin levels	• Decreased clotting and prothrombin times • Vascular occlusion • Disseminated intravascular coagulation • Anaemia
Immunosuppression	• Infection
Decreased gastric motility and increased gastric acidity	• Gastritis • Gastric ulcers

Altered consciousness may last only seconds or persist for several hours. Amnesia for events immediately preceding (antegrade amnesia) and following (retrograde amnesia) the injury is common. Other signs and symptoms of concussion include headache, drowsiness, confusion, dizziness and visual disturbances such as double vision (diplopia) or blurred vision. Following concussion (MTBI), post-concussion syndrome may last for several weeks or up to a year with symptoms including persistent headache, dizziness, irritability, insomnia, impaired memory and concentration and learning problems.

Acute brain injury affects all body systems as well as the CNS. Systemic effects of acute brain injury are listed in Table 13.16.

INTERDISCIPLINARY CARE FOR TBI

Diagnosis

Diagnostic testing may be done to monitor haemodynamic status and detect conditions that may contribute to cerebral oedema. Radiological examinations include skull x-rays (to identify skull fractures and assess penetrating objects) and CT scan or MRI to detect contusions and lacerations associated with diffuse axonal injury. ABGs are analyed, with particular attention to oxygen and carbon dioxide levels.

Medication

The person with a TBI has or is at high risk for IICP. IICP is managed (see page 484) to re-establish equilibrium of the intracranial contents and prevent secondary brain damage. Medications other than those previously discussed include a category of drugs called neuroprotectants. These drugs are used to treat or alter some of the pathologic pathways that occur in ischaemia, and must be administered within a short time of the injury to be effective.

Surgery

Surgery may include the surgical evacuation of the clot either via burr holes made into the skull (Figure 13.19), for example EDH and acute SDH, or via a craniotomy, for example chronic SDH because the haematoma tends to solidify, making it difficult or impossible to remove through burr holes (see Figure 13.20).

A decompressive craniectomy may also be considered, allowing the brain to expand and thus reducing ICP (for further information on common neurosurgical procedures see p. 502).

NURSING CARE FOR TBI

The person who has intracranial surgery does not have normal human defences against changes in intracranial pressure and is also at risk from cerebral oedema and a shift of intracerebral contents. Surgery may cause cerebral oedema, bleeding or haematoma formation. Accurate and repeated neurological assessments including GCS is important in order to monitor for signs and symptoms of increased intracranial pressure and provide early recognition and treatment of problems and complications so that treatment can be instigated.

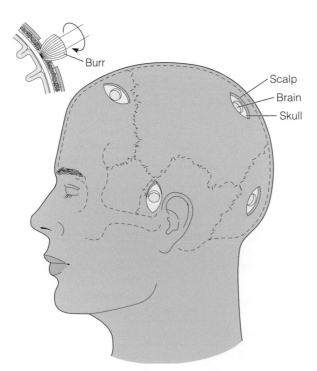

Figure 13.19 Possible locations of burr holes.

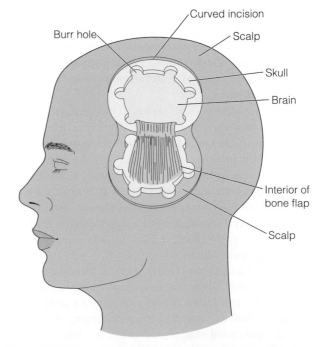

Figure 13.20 In a craniotomy a portion of the skull and overlying scalp is removed to allow access to the brain.

Case Study 2 – Bob
NURSING CARE PLAN Haematoma

Bob is 78 years old and lives with his wife. He has developed a right-sided subacute haematoma. Bob was taken to theatre and via two burr holes his haematoma is evacuated. A subdural drain is inserted and he is returned to the ward for post-operative care. Bob remains confused and agitated with a mild right-sided weakness and a GCS score of 14. Vital signs are BP 180/90 mm/Hg, pulse 78 per minute, temperature of 36.5 °C and oxygen saturations are 97% on 4 L of oxygen via a face mask.

Immediate nursing care

Immediate nursing care should include:

+ Establish an effective therapeutic relationship with Bob and his wife to facilitate compliance and cooperation with treatment and care.

+ Initially assess and repeatedly reassess Bob's neurological function to detect neurological deterioration and increases in ICP using the GCS (see sections in this chapter on neurological assessment and care of the person with increased ICP).

+ Initially assess and repeatedly assess Bob's vital signs, including blood pressure, pulse and temperature.

+ Initially assess and repeatedly assess Bob's respiratory function, including respiratory rate and pattern and oxygen saturation in order to maintain normocapnia.

+ Assess level of discomfort/pain (headache) related to stretching and cutting of the brain tissues and increase in intracranial pressure using a recognised pain assessment tool and administer analgesics as prescribed.

+ Nurse Bob flat in bed, usually for the first 24–48 hours post-operative and then gently mobilise to facilitate brain re-expansion by increasing the intracranial venous pressure, and optimise drainage of fluid into the wound drain.

+ Ensure Bob is hydrated. Administer IV fluids to maintain fluid intake as ordered and record intake and output on a fluid balance chart. Adequate patient hydration is needed to help re-expand the brain.

+ Empty and record outputs from the closed drainage system often inserted post-operatively into the subdural space for 24–72 hours. Maintain asepsis and remove the drain as instructed, usually when drainage is minimal. Monitor wound site for signs of infection and CSF leakage.

+ Post-operative coagulation studies (for example, prothrombin time) and platelet counts should be observed closely and adjustments made, when possible, to reduce the risk of additional bleeding.

Nursing diagnoses and interventions

Many nursing interventions associated with traumatic brain injury correspond with those outlined previously in the sections on caring for a person with altered LOC and monitoring for signs and symptoms of IICP. Specific nursing care discussed in this section focuses on potential problems associated with intracranial surgery. Assessment includes history of injury, for example nature of the craniocerebral trauma, period of loss of consciousness.

Risk for impaired airway management

The primary objective in the care of any trauma person is maintaining a patent airway to prevent hypoxia. However, in the initial acute care phase, the risk of cervical vertebral fractures and spinal cord injury may complicate the process of establishing a patent airway. In addition, other multisystem injuries may complicate the interpretation of vital signs. In general, all unconscious people with a TBI should be intubated with an endotracheal tube to prevent aspiration. Patients with head trauma may also require a tracheostomy to provide an airway and be placed on a ventilator. If the person is self-ventilating then continuously monitor respiratory pattern for rate, depth and rhythm.

PRACTICE ALERT

● Never suction a person nasally if they have a basilar skull fracture, or have CSF draining from the ears or nose as catheters could be inadvertently advanced into the cranial cavity.

● People who have had a large bone flap removed are at risk of venous congestion. Position the person on the unoperated side to decrease venous congestion in the operative area.

● People with a traumatic head injury may develop neuroendocrine disorders, i.e. diabetes insipidus (DI).

● **Anosmia** (loss of smell) commonly occurs following frontal head injuries.

Risk for infection

The person who has had intracranial surgery is at risk for infection from multiple invasive lines, the scalp wound and introduction of bacteria into the operative area. Surgical trauma, for example during transsphenoidal pituitary surgery or other neurosurgical procedures, also increases the risk of

CSF leakage, and this exposes the CNS to the external environment, predisposing the person to infection. Nursing care includes providing interventions to monitor for and prevent infection, including:

- Monitor for signs and symptoms of CSF leakage:
  a. presence of glucose in clear watery drainage from ears, nose or wound;
  b. complaints of 'something dripping down the back of the throat;'
  c. constant swallowing and salty taste;
  d. staining on the patient's pillow – '*halo or ring sign*'.
- Provide interventions to prevent contamination of area leaking CSF, which may include:
  a. if leaking from the nose: keep head of bed elevated 20 degrees unless contraindicated; do not suction nasally; do not clean nose; tell person not to put finger in nose; do not insert packing;
  b. if leaking from the ear: position person on side of leakage unless contraindicated; do not clean ear; tell person not to put finger in ear;
  c. if leaking from wound site: place a sterile dressing over the area of drainage and change as soon as it becomes damp.
- Monitor for and report signs and symptoms of infection as intracranial surgery increases the risk of meningitis (see below on CNS infections and Chapter 5 for further information on wound care).

Consider this . . .

Bob is agitated, pulling at his intravenous infusion line and his wound drain. You know that restlessness increases ICP. How might this be managed? You might want to consider the following management options: one-to-one nursing, behavioural programmes, pharmacological management and restraint.

The person with a CNS infection

CNS infections are serious illnesses, with potentially life-threatening effects and complications. The CNS, including the meninges, neural tissues and blood vessels, can be affected.

Infection may be caused by a number of organisms, including bacteria, viruses, fungi, protozoans, prions and rickettsiae. In general, organisms enter the brain in two ways: through the bloodstream by crossing the BBB or by direct invasion, for example through a skull fracture.

Pathophysiology of CNS infection

The major CNS infections include meningitis, encephalitis and brain abscesses.

Meningitis

Meningitis is an inflammation of the pia mater, the arachnoid and the subarachnoid space and may be bacterial, viral, fungal or parasitic in origin. The organism responsible for meningitis must overcome the host's defence mechanisms to invade and replicate in the CSF. These include: skin barrier, the BBB the non-specific inflammatory response and the immune response. Once penetrated, the CNS inflammation spreads rapidly throughout the CNS because of the circulation of CSF around the brain and spinal cord. In the case of bacterial meningitis, purulent exudate infiltrates the CSF and cranial nerve sheaths and blocks the choroid plexus and subarachnoid villi. IICP occurs as brain tissue responds to the pathogen and cerebral perfusion decreases and cerebral perfusion autoregulation is lost.

There are two major types of meningitis: *bacterial meningitis* and *viral meningitis*.

Bacterial meningitis

Causative organisms are varied, the most common including: *Neisseria meningitis* (Meningococcus), *Streptococcus pneumoniae* and *Mycobacterium tuberculosis*. Mortality rates for adults are approximately 25%, although vaccination programmes have reduced the incidence of disease.

The person with bacterial meningitis typically presents with the following symptoms:

- restlessness, agitation and irritability;
- signs of meningeal irritation: stiff neck (**nuchal rigidity**), positive **Brudzinski's sign** (flexion of the neck that causes the hip and knee to flex) (see Figure 13.21) and positive **Kernig's sign** (inability to extend the knee while the hip is flexed at a 90-degree angle) (see Figure 13.22);

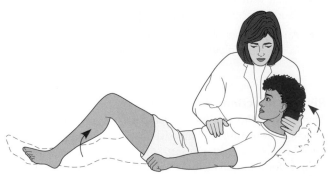

Figure 13.21 Assessing for Brudzinski's sign.

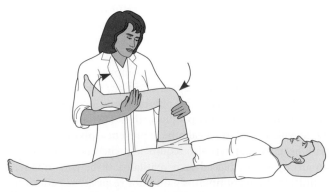

Figure 13.22 Assessing for Kernig's sign.

- chills and high fever;
- raised ICP (see page 484);
- **photophobia** (aversion to light);
- joint stiffness and muscle pains;
- petechial rash (small spots) (in meningococcal meningitis);
- Seizures.

Complications include cranial nerve damage; cranial nerve VIII, the auditory nerve, is frequently affected, with resulting nerve deafness. Hydrocephalus can develop as a result of pus clogging the arachnoid villi, reducing CSF absorption and causing adhesion which may obstruct CSF flow. Thrombophlebitis may develop in cerebral vessels, with infarction of surrounding tissues and septicaemia.

Viral meningitis

Viral meningitisis is more common than the bacterial form and many cases go unreported because the disease is often mild and recovery is uneventful. Causative organisms are numerous viruses, such as herpes simplex, herpes zoster, Epstein–Barr virus or cytomegalovirus (CMV). Although viral infection also triggers the inflammatory response, the course of the disease is benign and of short duration.

The signs and symptoms of viral meningitis are similar to those of bacterial meningitis, although usually milder.

Encephalitis

Encephalitis is an acute inflammation of the parenchyma of the brain or spinal cord. Few studies provide accurate data on the prevalence rates in the UK; however, data from the USA provide some indication with reported prevalence rates 7.3 per 100 000 people (Khetsuriani et al. 2002). It is almost always caused by a virus, but it may also be caused by bacteria, fungi and other organisms. Viral encephalitis is commonly caused by herpes simplex virus (cold sore virus), and the mortality rate is high, 40% even with treatment. Viruses depend on living tissue for reproduction and become highly destructive when they invade brain tissue. The virus gains access to the CNS via the bloodstream or along peripheral or cranial nerves or it may already be present in the meninges in the person with meningitis. The inflammatory response extends over the cerebral cortex, the white matter and the meninges, with degeneration of the neurones. The pathology of encephalitis includes local necrotising haemorrhage, which ultimately becomes generalised, with prominent oedema.

Signs and symptoms

The signs and symptoms of encephalitis vary, depending on the organism and area of the brain affected. Encephalitis frequently starts with flu-like symptoms. Patients often present with meningeal irritation, fever, headache, seizures, stiff neck and altered LOC. Other clinical symptoms include behavioural and speech disturbances and focal or diffuse neurological symptoms. These symptoms distinguish the encephalitic person from those with meningitis. As the disease progresses, the LOC deteriorates, and the person may become comatose. People are often left with cognitive, psychological and physical deficits.

Brain abscess

A brain abscess is a focal collection of (pus) purulent material within the brain tissue. They are extremely rare; approximately 80% are found in the cerebrum and 20% are cerebellar. Causes include open trauma and neurosurgery and the spread of infection from other nearby areas, for example teeth, middle ear, nasal cavity or nasal sinuses. If the abscess is encapsulated, it has the ability to enlarge and, therefore, behaves as a space-occupying lesion within the cranium. This can result in raised intracranial pressure. Occasionally, the abscess does not become encapsulated; instead, it spreads through the brain tissue to the subarachnoid space and ventricular system. The most common causative pathogens include streptococci staphylococci and bacteroids. Yeast and fungi may also cause brain abscess.

Signs and symptoms

Initially, the person exhibits the general symptoms associated with an acute infectious process, such as chills, fever, malaise and anorexia. Because brain abscess generally forms after infection, the person may consider these signs to be an exacerbation of that illness. The person may experience seizures, focal neurological deficits, altered LOC and signs and symptoms of raised ICP. As the abscess enlarges, specific symptoms are related to location of the mass in the brain. Cerebral abscesses are associated with significant mortality and morbidity rates.

FAST FACTS

CNS infections

- Meningitis is inflammation of the meninges and is a life-threatening disease affecting all ages.
- Encephalitis is inflammation of the brain tissue and can damage nerve cells resulting in 'acquired brain injury'.
- Brain abscesses are rare but behave as space-occuping lesions and can cause raised ICP.

INTERDISCIPLINARY CARE FOR CNS INFECTION

Diagnosis

The diagnosis of meningitis is based on signs and symptoms and diagnostic tests results. Tests include LP with Gram stain and culture of the CSF to determine the presence of bacterial infection and the specific infectious agent (unless contraindicated i.e. signs of raised ICP). The CSF may be turbid (cloudy) with markedly increased white blood cell and protein content and decreased glucose content.

Diagnosis in those patients with encephalitis is often difficult due to the broad symptoms. CSF protein and lymphocytes may be slightly raised. Diagnosis may be confirmed by a specific CSF test [polymerase chain reaction (PCR) test]. CAT and MRI scanning may show the extent of the inflammation, and an EEG may reveal abnormal brain activity.

CT scans with contrast medium in persons with suspected abscess will reveal a ring of enhancement surrounding the abscess.

Medication

Bacterial meningitis is a medical emergency and can be fatal. Successful management depends on rapid diagnosis and aggressive treatment with intravenous antibiotics that cross the BBB into the subarachnoid space to eradicate the infecting organism and support vital functions. Corticosteroids such as dexamethasone may be prescribed to suppress inflammation in bacterial meningitis.

Treatment for viral meningitis focuses on managing patient symptoms and is supportive. Antipyretic and analgesic medications may provide symptomatic relief.

Treatment for encephalitis consists of administering specific medications, such as intravenous acyclovir for viral encephalitis, and preventing complications.

Treatment of the person with a brain abscess focuses on aggressive and early initiation of antibiotic therapy. A combination of broad-spectrum antibiotics is used if the infecting organism is unknown. Other symptoms are treated symptomatically, as with the person diagnosed with meningitis or encephalitis. If pharmacological management is not effective, the abscess may be surgically drained or, if it is encapsulated, removed (see section on neurosurgical procedures p. 502). Anticonvulsant medications may be prescribed to control seizure activity, and antiemetics to control nausea and vomiting.

NURSING CARE FOR CNS INFECTION

The person who presents with a CNS infection is often very ill, and the combination of fever, dehydration and cerebral oedema may predispose the person to seizures. Neurological deterioration, airway obstruction, respiratory arrest or cardiac dysrhythmias may occur. Nursing care associated with altered LOC, IICP and seizures is also appropriate for the person with a CNS infection. Other interventions include:

- Liaison with the infection control team for precautionary measures.

- Health promotion information should be provided, for example vaccinations and mosquito control with repellants, insecticides and protective clothing.
- Advise people about signs and symptoms of meningitis, and the importance of early recognition and urgent medical treatment.

The person with an intracranial tumour

Intracranial tumours are growths within the cranium, including tumours in brain tissue, meninges, the pituitary gland or blood vessels. Brain tumours may also be classified as primary intracranial lesions or metastatic tumours, can be further subdivided according to their origin in the brain and are classified according to the WHO classification of tumours (see Table 13.17). Regardless of type or location, brain tumours are potentially lethal as they grow within a closed cranial vault and displace or impinge on CNS structures. In general CNS tumours have a poor prognosis.

Incidence and prevalence of intracranial tumour

CNS tumours are rare, accounting for less than 2% of all cancers. There are many types of primary tumours (nearly 100 types), with differing incidence rates, clinical behaviour and response to treatment and prognosis. The most numerous primary CNS tumours are brain tumours. The incidence of CNS tumours rises throughout adulthood and peaks in the late 70s. The cause of many brain tumours is unknown.

Pathophysiology of intracranial tumour

Primary intracranial tumours can arise from the cells and structures that are found within the brain, for example neurones and neuroglia, or from supporting structures such as the meninges, pituitary gland and pineal gland. Primary brain tumours rarely metastasise outside the CNS. Focal disturbances take place when there is compression of brain tissue and infiltration or direct invasion of brain parenchyma with destruction of neural tissue. As the tumour grows, oedema develops in adjacent tissues, and some tumours may cause haemorrhage.

Brain metastases are more common than primary intracranial tumours and originate from structures outside the brain. An estimated 25% of people with cancer develop brain metastasis, and presentation is the same as for primary brain tumours, with IICP and focal and/or diffuse cerebral dysfunction. Common sources of intracranial metastasis are cancers of the lung, breasts, melanoma, prostate gland, kidney and gastrointestinal tract. The metastasis reaches the brain through the circulation and, in most cases, the tumours are multiple.

Table 13.17 Summary of CNS tumours

Tumour type	Tumour name and characteristics
Tumours originating from neuroglia and invading brain tissue. Account for around 50% of all brain tumours.	*Gliomas*: • Astrocytoma develop from the astrocytes • Oligodendroglioma arising form the oligdentrocytes • Ependymoma uncommon but prevalent in 5–15 years, arising from the linings of the ventricles (considered malignant) • Glioblastoma multiforme (most common glioma, 45–50% of all gliomas) • Mixed gliomas or oligoastrocytomas containing a mixture of astrocytic and oligodendrocytic cells
Tumours of the sellar regions arising from the pituitary gland. Originate from embryonal cells found in pituitary gland known as Rathke's pouch	*Pituitary adenoma*: • Hypersecretory (functioning), e.g. prolactinoma, 10–15% of all intracranial tumours • Non-functioning macroadenomas *Craniopharyngioma*: rare and about 50% occur in children
Extracerebral tumours	*Medulloblastoma*: fast growing, may be encapsulated and malignant; occurs primarily in children; common in the cerebellum.
Cranial nerve tumours (originate from Schwann cells)	*Schwannoma*: accounts for 6–7% of all intracranial tumours *Acoustic neuroma*: slow growing but may also affect cranial nerves V, VII, IX and X
Meningioma (arise from the meninges)	*Meningioma*: arise from the meningeal cells and account for around 20% all brain tumours, affecting women 2–3 times more often than men
Ependymal tumours	*Ependymomas*: develop from lining of ventricles
Congenital tumours (developmental)	*Hemangioblastoma*: a vascular tumour associated with von Hippel–Lindau syndrome account for 1–2% of all brain tumours
Familial	*Neurofibromatosis*: type 1 and type 2 (autosomal dominant)

Signs and symptoms of intracranial tumour

The signs and symptoms of intracranial tumours are determined by location and size. Some of the more common signs and symptoms include:

- headache that is usually worse in the morning;
- seizures;
- limb weakness, difficulty walking, abnormal gait, deficits;
- changes in cognition, personality, confusion and loss of memory;
- visual disturbances, for example double vision, visual loss;
- altered consciousness;
- focal deficits including speech disturbances.

Compression of brain tissue and the invasion of the brain tumour into the cerebral tissue may lead to changes typically seen with cerebral oedema and IICP. Cerebral blood supply may diminish as the tumour compresses blood vessels. Shifts in brain tissue can occur, leading to brain herniation syndromes and, if untreated, death.

INTERDISCIPLINARY CARE FOR INTRACRANIAL TUMOUR

Advances in technologies and techniques have improved diagnostic modalities and treatment options which may involve chemotherapy, radiation therapy, surgery or any combination of these. This is dependent upon the type of tumour, its size and location and related symptoms (such as neurological deficits), and the person's overall condition.

Diagnosis

The following diagnostic tests may be ordered.

- A CT scan or an MRI with contrast can locate the brain tumour and define its size, shape, extent to which normal anatomy is distorted and the degree of any associated cerebral oedema.
- CT angiogram may show stretching or displacement of cerebral vessels as well as the presence of tumour vascularity, for example meningioma.
- EEG provides information about cerebral function, may demonstrate focal or diffuse changes and is useful if seizures are present.
- Endocrine studies are conducted if a pituitary tumour is suspected.
- Visual field studies to chart the patient's visual fields (often affected due to compression from expanding pituitary tumours). (See Figure 13.24 on p. 504 and Figure 14.14 on p. 525 for further information on visual fields.)
- Once a brain tumour has been found, a biopsy is normally performed which involves taking a small sample of the tumour tissue via a burr hole for examination (see section on common cranial surgical procedures p. 502).

Medication

The choice of chemotherapy is based on the type of tumour, its location and the person's response to therapy. Other medications that may be prescribed include corticosteroids and anticonvulsants.

Surgery

For intracranial tumours, surgery is used to obtain a diagnosis, to remove or reduce the size of the tumour or for symptom relief (palliation). The type of procedure, the surgical approach and the timing of surgery (emergency versus planned procedure) influence the overall nursing management of the person having intracranial surgery. For pituitary tumours, transsphenoidal surgery (either microscopically or endoscopically) involves approaching the tumour at the skull base via the nostril and the sphenoid bone at the base of the brain. This approach makes surgery easier and safer. Some of the more common intracranial neurosurgical procedures follow:

- *Burr hole* – a hole made in the skull with a special drill. The hole may facilitate the evacuation of an extracerebral clot/biopsy, or a series of holes may be made in preparation for craniotomy (see Figure 13.19).
- *Craniotomy* – surgical opening into the cranial cavity (see Figure 13.20).
- *Craniectomy* – excision of a portion of the skull and complete removal of the bone flap. This procedure may be done to provide space for expansion after cerebral oedema.
- *Cranioplasty* – repair to the skull in which synthetic material is inserted to replace the cranial bone that was removede.g. titanium.

Radiation therapy

Patients may be offered radiation therapy alone or as adjunctive therapy with surgery. Radiation is often the treatment of choice for surgically inaccessible tumours; it may also be used to decrease the size of a tumour prior to surgery or after incomplete surgical removal. Chemotherapy may also be offered as an adjunctive therapy to surgery. For further information see Chapter 2.

Specialist treatment

- Stereotaxic techniques to precisely locate a specific area of the brain that controls specific functions and exact locations of deep brain lesions.
- Advances in radiotherapy, for example external beam radiation, intense-modulating radiation and Gamma Knife (linear accelerator) which delivers a focused beam of radiation capable of destroying deep and otherwise inaccessible lesions in a single treatment session.
- Chemotherapy in the form of biodegradable anhydrous wafers, which are impregnated with the chemotherapy drug and implanted into the tumour bed after surgical resection, releasing the drug over a period of time.

NURSING CARE FOR INTRACRANIAL TUMOUR

Nursing care for a person following intracranial surgery is both general and specific. For general care issues, the reader will need to consult other chapters in this book, for example pain relief is covered in Chapter 1, respiration in Chapter 11, nutrition in Chapter 7 and mobility in Chapter 12.

Nursing diagnoses and interventions

More specific aspects of nursing care considerations discussed in this section include the risk of diabetes insipidus, disturbed self-esteem and anxiety.

Risk for diabetes insipidus

Observe for signs of DI caused by decreased secretion of anti-diuretic hormone (ADH), as a result of surgical manipulation of the pituitary gland, for example production of large quantity of urine with low specific gravity. Maintain an accurate fluid balance and assess the person for serum electrolyte levels, urine osmolality, urine specific gravity and urine sodium levels.

Risk for disturbed self-esteem

Encourage the person to verbalise feelings about the surgery and potential disturbed body image and self-esteem related to loss of hair on the scalp, cranial incision and facial swelling and bruising and perhaps indentation of the skull. Suggest measures that may help minimise this effect, for example hats and wigs.

Risk for anxiety

The diagnosis of an intracranial tumour brings anxiety and feelings of uncertainty about the future. Both the person and family members are likely to be apprehensive and require education and emotional support. Clear, relevant and timely information is important and may include overall treatment plan, procedures and investigations along with management of deficits and/or disabilities. Refer to the neuro-oncology specialist nurse for additional support and guidance.

PRACTICE ALERT

- Post-operative headache may be an indication of either compression or displacement of brain tissue or from raised ICP and may be a sign of meningitis.
- Fluid and electrolyte imbalance may occur post-transsphenoidal surgery due to the major potential transient complication of DI.
- The main post-operative complication post-transsphenoidal surgery is rhinorrhoea (CSF leakage).

The person with a cerebrovascular disorder

A stroke is a 'brain attack' caused by a sudden decrease in blood flow to a localised area of the brain. It is characterised by a gradual or rapid onset of neurological deficits due to compromised cerebral blood flow. Stroke is a major medical emergency requiring rapid treatment in order to prevent avoidable death and long-term disability. There are two main types of stroke:

- *Ischaemic.* This is the most common form of stroke (approximately 80%), caused when the blood supply to a part of the brain is suddenly interrupted by a *thrombus* (blood clot), *embolus* (foreign matter travelling through the circulation), or *stenosis* (narrowing), which leads to the death of brain cells due to lack of oxygen.

- *Haemorrhagic.* There are two types of haemorrhagic strokes (approximately 20%): intracerebral haemorrhage and sub-arachnoid haemorrhage, both caused by a bursting of blood vessels producing bleeding into the brain. Subarachnoid haemorrhages (SAH) are a type of haemorrhagic stroke where bleeding occurs in the subarachnoid space. Ruptured cerebral aneurysms are the cause for the majority of SAHs and are associated with high morbidity and mortality rates. A small number are caused by arteriovenous malformations (AVMs) (a complex conglomerate of abnormal arteries and veins which displace rather than encompass normal brain tissue).

Transient ischaemic attacks (TIA), also known as minor strokes, occur when stroke symptoms resolve themselves within 24 hours. TIAs are clear warning signs that a further stroke may occur.

Incidence and prevalence of cerebrovascular disorder

Stroke is the third largest cause of death in the UK, responsible for 11% of deaths in England. Every year in England, approximately 110 000 will have a stroke and there are over 900 000 people living in England who have had a stroke (DoH 2007). Strokes carry a high mortality rate, and an estimated 20–30% of people who have had a stroke will die within one month.

Aneurysmal SAH occurs in 15 per 100 000 of the population per annum, is most common in adults aged 30–60 and is more prevalent in women than men (Hickey 2009). The exact aetiology is unknown, but hypertension and cigarette smoking may be contributing factors.

Risk factors for cerebrovascular disorder

Certain diseases, lifestyle habits and ethnic backgrounds increase the risk of a stroke. Recognised causative factors are as follows:

FAST FACTS

Cerebrovascular disorders – stroke

- Strokes cost the NHS and the economy approximately £7 billion/year.
- Stroke is the largest single cause of severe disability; a third of people who have a stroke are left with long-term disability.
- The risk of stroke doubles every decade after the age of 55.
- 50% of persons with subarachnoid haemorrhages die at onset and for those that survive there is an increased risk of rebleeding.
- Of the 110 100 new strokes per annum in the UK, one-third will go on to to have a further stroke.

Sources: DoH 2007, Intercollegiate Stroke Working Party 2008.

- *Hypertension.* This prevents the greatest risk. People with hypertension have a four to six times greater risk for stroke than do those without hypertension.
- *Cardiac arrhythmias.* Atrial fibrillation is the second greatest risk factor for stroke.
- *Diabetes mellitus.* People with diabetes are three times more likely to have a stroke compared to those without diabetes.
- *Smoking.* Cigarette smoking doubles a person's risk for ischaemic stroke and increases the risk for cerebral haemorrhage by up to 3.5%.
- *Blood cholesterol levels.* Increased blood cholesterol levels contribute to the risk of atherosclerosis, including arteries in the cerebral circulation.

Other risk factors include heart disease, sickle cell disease, substance abuse, family history of stroke, obesity, dietary factors such as saturated fats, alcohol consumption, a sedentary lifestyle, recent viral and bacterial infections and previous TIAs. Risk factors specific to women include oral contraceptive use, pregnancy, childbirth, menopause, migraine headaches with aura, autoimmune disorders (such as diabetes and lupus) and clotting disorders. In addition, having a stroke is a major risk factor for having another stroke (called recurrent stroke). Race (higher incidences are found in Asian and Africa Caribbean) and gender, with strokes more common in men than women, are relevant, and the incidence of stroke increases dramatically with age.

Pathophysiology of cerebrovascular disorder

When blood flow to and oxygenation of cerebral neurones are decreased or interrupted, pathophysiological changes at the cellular level take place in four to five minutes. Cellular metabolism ceases as glucose and other vital substances are depleted

504   Chapter 13 Caring for people with neurological problems

and the cells swell as sodium draws water into the cell. Cerebral blood vessels also swell, further decreasing blood flow. Severe or prolonged ischaemia leads to cellular death. The neurological deficits caused by ischaemia and the resultant necrosis of cells in the brain vary according to the area of the brain involved, the size of the affected area and the length of time blood flow is decreased or stopped. Because the motor pathways cross at the junction of the medulla and spinal cord (decussation), strokes lead to loss or impairment of sensorimotor functions on the side of the body opposite the side of the brain that is damaged. This effect, known as a *contralateral deficit*, causes a stroke in the right hemisphere of the brain to be manifested by deficits in the left side of the body (and vice versa). A thrombotic stroke usually affects only one region of the brain that is supplied by a single cerebral artery. Embolic strokes result when parts of the thrombus break off from either the cerebral circulation or from outside the brain and are carried through the arterial system to the brain.

A haemorrhagic stroke, or intracranial haemorrhage, occurs when a cerebral blood vessel ruptures. Although hypertension is the most common cause, a variety of factors may contribute to a haemorrhagic stroke, including rupture of a brittle plaque-encrusted artery wall, ruptured intracranial aneurysms, trauma, and erosion of blood vessels by tumours, arteriovenous malformations, anticoagulant therapy and blood disorders. As a result of the blood vessel rupture, blood enters the brain tissue, the cerebral ventricles or the subarachnoid space, compressing adjacent tissues and causing blood vessel spasm and cerebral oedema. Blood in the ventricles or subarachnoid space irritates the meninges and brain tissue, causing an inflammatory reaction and impairing absorption and circulation of CSF. Intracranial aneurysms tend to occur at the bifurcations and branches of the carotid arteries and the vertebrobasilar arteries at the circle of Willis, with most aneurysms (85%) located anteriorly.

Signs and symptoms of cerebrovascular disorder

Signs and symptoms vary according to the cerebral artery involved and the area of the brain affected and are always sudden in onset, focal and usually one-sided. Signs and symptoms are dependent on the location of the haemorrhage, but may include loss of consciousness and raised intracranial pressure (see sections earlier in this chapter). In the case of a SAH, the person typically complains of the following:

- severe, sudden explosive headache ('like being hit with a sledge hammer');
- nausea and vomiting;
- loss of consciousness;
- neck stiffness (nuchal rigidity) and photophobia;
- raised temperature (pyrexia);
- seizure activity.

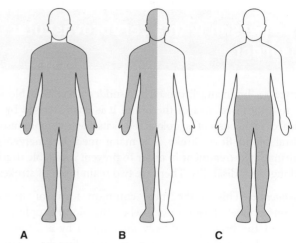

Figure 13.23 Types of paralysis. **(A)** Quadriplegia is complete or partial paralysis of the upper extremities and complete paralysis of the lower part of the body. **(B)** Hemiplegia is paralysis of one half of the body when it is divided along the median sagittal plane. **(C)** Paraplegia is paralysis of the lower part of the body.

Other signs and symptoms following a stroke are listed below:

- Motor deficits depending on the area of the brain involved causing hemiplegia or paralysis of the left or right half of the body (see Figure 13.23), hemiparesis (weakness) of the left or right half of the body and flaccidity and spasticity.
- Communication disorders are usually the result of a stroke affecting the dominant hemisphere, for example aphasia, expressive and receptive dysaphasia and **dysarthria**.
- Visual disturbances, for example **hemianopia** (loss of half of the visual field of one or both eyes) (see Figure 13.24).
- Behavioural changes, for example emotional lability, depression, loss of social inhibitions, loss of self-control and decreased tolerance for stress.

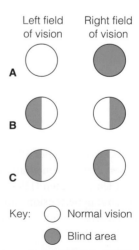

Figure 13.24 Abnormal visual fields. **(A)** Normal left field of vision with loss of vision in right field. **(B)** Loss of vision in temporal half of both fields (bitemporal hemianopia). **(C)** Loss of vision in nasal field of right eye and temporal field of left eye (homonymous hemianopia).

- Cognitive changes, for example memory loss, short attention span, poor problem-solving ability.
- Difficulties with balance and swallowing (**dysphagia**).
- Disorders of bladder and bowel elimination are common.

As a result of the neurological deficits, the person with a stroke has complications that involve many different body systems. The disabilities resulting from a stroke often cause serious alterations in functional health status. Those people who survive the initial insult of the subarachnoid haemorrhage are faced with the high possibility of developing one or more life-threatening complications. These include delayed cerebral vasospasm, which often results in delayed ischaemic deficits, and cerebral infarction, rebleeding and hydrocephalus. Vasospasm is caused by narrowing of the vessels sustained by smooth muscle contraction.

INTERDISCIPLINARY CARE FOR CEREBROVASCULAR DISORDER

Diagnosis

Rapid diagnosis and treatment of stroke is essential to minimise the possibility of a resultant disability. Diagnosis begins with a complete history and careful physical assessment, including a thorough neurological examination. The FAST tool is a validated tool for quick assessment of patients outside the hospital to screen for a diagnosis of stroke or TIA. The score is based on three specific symptoms of stroke. If any one of the three symptoms is positive then the person should seek urgent medical attention (see the In Practice box below).

IN PRACTICE

FAST assessment

- **F**acial weakness: Can the person smile? Has their mouth or eye drooped?
- **A**rm weakness: Can the person raise both arms?
- **S**peech problems: Can the person speak clearly and understand what you say?
- **T**ime to call 999 if you see any single one of these signs.

Source: DoH 2009.

CT scans are used to identify pathophysiological changes after a stroke has occurred, in order to demonstrate the presence of blood, oedema, tissue necrosis. Other imaging tests that may be used for diagnosis include a cerebral arteriogram, a transcranial ultrasound Doppler, an MRI, an MRA, a PET and a SPECT (see p. 479 for further information). A LP may be performed to obtain CSF for examination in patients with suspected SAH revealing blood-tinged CSF or xanthochromia (yellowish discoloration of CSF resulting from lysis of red blood cells).

The person may receive medical and/or surgical treatment depending on the type and severity of the stroke. In addition to the medical and surgical management of a stroke, management includes secondary prevention, the prevention of further complications and promoting recovery.

Medication

The type of medication used varies according to the type of stroke. Medications are administered to prevent a stroke in patients with TIAs or a previous stroke, and to treat the person during the acute phase of a stroke. Prevention drugs include antiplatelet agents used to prevent clot formation and blood vessel occlusion, for example aspirin and dipyridamole. Medications used during the acute phase of an ischaemic stroke include those to prevent further thrombosis formation, increase cerebral blood flow and protect cerebral neurones; these include anticoagulant drug therapy, thrombolysis, fibrinolytic therapy and antithrombotic drugs. Anticonvulsants may be prescribed if IICP causes seizures (increased intracranial pressure is discussed on pp. 484–487).

The prevention of vasospasm following SAH includes the administration of nimodipine, a calcium channel antagonist which blocks the influx of calcium in the arteries, resulting in an increase in vascular smooth muscle relaxation. In addition, continuous infusion of intravenous magnesium sulphate to raise the serum magnesium to above normal range may be administered. Triple-H therapy (hypertension, hypervolaemia and haemodilution) is aimed at augmenting cerebral blood flow by increasing the blood pressure, expanding the blood volume and reducing blood viscosity.

Surgery

Surgery may be performed to prevent the occurrence of a stroke, to restore blood flow when a stroke has already occurred or to repair vascular damage or malformations. This may include carotid endarterectomy at the carotid artery bifurcation to remove atherosclerotic plaque (Figure 13.25) and stenting to treat cerebral stenosis.

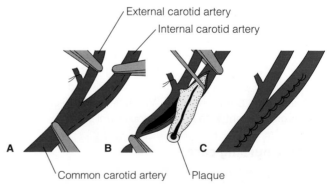

Figure 13.25 Carotid endarterectomy. (A) The occluded area is clamped off and an incision is made in the artery. **(B)** Plaque is removed from the inner layer of the artery. **(C)** To restore blood flow through the artery, the artery is sutured or a graft is completed.

Treatment for ruptured aneurysms is to secure the aneurysm to prevent rebleeding by prompt neurosurgery or radiologically guided interventions. Neurosurgery includes a craniotomy and fixing a clip around the ruptured aneurysm neck to prevent the entry of blood into the aneurysm and further bleeding, known as '*clipping*'. Alternative endovascular non-invasive occlusion of brain aneurysms are also performed intravascularly by inserting Guglielmi detachable coils (GDCs) into the aneurysm in the angiography suite. Other procedures include stenting (coil or mesh tubes) which may be used to cover the neck of an aneurysm and balloon occlusion.

PRACTICE ALERT

- Maintaining a positive fluid balance and avoiding hypovolaemia reduces the risk of vasospasm.

- Avoid constipation, straining to pass stools and the administration of emenas as the increase in intra-abdominal pressure can increase ICP and precipitate rebleeding.

- When lying on the affected side, patients may be restless because they do not have normal sensation and feel as if they may fall.

- After eating, check the person's mouth for 'pocketing' of food, especially in the affected cheek.

- Voiding small amounts of urine frequently may be a manifestation of a bladder dysfunction. Assess for a distended bladder.

- Coughing may be indicative of dysphagia.

AVM treatments include: surgical excision; embolisation, where substances are introduced to cause emboli to form and obstruct blood flow in the malformation; and stereotactic radiation therapy or laser therapy, intended to coagulate blood in the malformation and thicken its vascular elements, eventually obstructing it.

NURSING CARE FOR CEREBROVASCULAR DISORDER

Nursing assessment may include a health history, identifying risk factors and when signs and symptoms began. Even though many people who have a stroke have full recovery, a substantial number are left with disabilities that affect their physical, emotional, interpersonal and family status. The required nursing care is often complex and multidimensional, requiring consideration of continuity of care for patients in acute care settings, long-term care settings, rehabilitation centres and the home. The priority intervention in the acute stages of the person with aneurysmal SAH is cerebral perfusion. The reader is directed to the earlier sections in this chapter on IICP and the prevention of secondary brain damage. Care for the unconscious person and the person following intracranial surgery are also relevant. More specific interventions are directed at precautions to prevent rebleeding. These include:

✚ Nurse in a quiet environment (reducing noxious stimuli that could result in a rise in blood pressure) avoiding overhead bright lights as the person may be photophobic.

✚ Management of the acute severe headache with analgesia (see Chapter 2 for further information on pain management).

Case Study 3 – Jane
NURSING CARE PLAN Stroke

Remember Jane who was admitted to hospital having suffered a stroke. Following a brain CT scan, Jane is diagnosed with left-sided ischaemic stroke due to a thrombosis in the right middle cerebral artery. Following her immediate care, she is now on the stroke unit for further management and rehabilitation. For the past year, she has been taking medication for hypertension and smokes 30 cigarettes per day. Physical assessment findings include the following: alert, responsive to verbal stimuli but with muddled speech. Right facial weakness and hemiplegic right arm (Jane is right-handed). Visual fields are decreased in a pattern consistent with homonymous hemianopia.

Specific nursing care

Specific nursing care includes:

✚ Monitor and document Jane's neurological status to detect changes.

✚ Monitor Jane's mental status. *Early recognition and treatment of depression may improve the outcome of the stroke.*

✚ Assess Jane for types of communication difficulty. Refer to the speech and language therapist for speech therapy. Support attempts to communicate verbally and provide alternative methods of communication, for example pen and paper, using props, recapping, using simple language, checking for comprehension.

✚ Refer Jane for a swallowing assessment. *Impaired gag reflex presents a high risk of aspiration.*

✚ Discuss Jane with the interdisciplinary team with referrals to the physiotherapist and occupational therapist. Develop individualised safe-handling techniques and limb and body positioning schedule. *Incorrect handling and positioning can result in shoulder pain and subluxation of the glenohumeral joint and other potential complications, for example skin breakdown. Educate the family about the correct handling of Jane's arm.*

✚ Provide passive ROM exercises for her left arm *to prevent venous thromboembolism or deep vein thrombosis.* Encourage Jane to carry out bed exercises.

Case Study 3 – Jane   **NURSING CARE PLAN Stroke**

+ Provide adaptive devices (cutlery with thick handles and non-slip plates).
+ Place objects (for example, call bell, tissues) on unaffected side and approach Jane from that side. Remind Jane to turn her head to compensate for the loss of visual field.
+ Encourage Jane to do as much for herself as possible, teaching activities of daily living such as dressing techniques. *This will help to foster a sense of independence and increase Jane's sense of control.*
+ In collaboration with the interdisciplinary team, set realistic expectations and goals. *This may help Jane to manage her symptoms.*
+ Spend time with Jane encouraging her to express her feelings and concerns. Recognise emotional deficits such as emotional lability, reduced tolerance to stress, fear, anger and depression. Explain that behaviours are a manifestation of brain injury.
+ Arrange a social services assessment.

Health promotion

● Provide Jane with information, education and interventions to instigate and support lifestyle modifications, for example smoking cessation, physical exercise, to reduce the risk of secondary stroke.
● Provide information to facilitate adherence to prescribed medication.
● Provide Jane and her family with information about support groups to encourage coping capability.

Consider this . . .

Jane writes down on her writing pad, 'Why are you bothering to teach me how to dress when I can't do it anyway?'

The person with a spinal cord tumour (SCT)

Spinal cord tumours (SCTs) may be benign or malignant, primary or metastatic, and affect men and women equally, commonly between the ages of 20 and 60 years. They may arise at any level of the spinal column. They constitute about 0.5–1% of all tumours (Hickey 2009). Spinal cord tumours are classified by anatomic location as either intramedullary or extramedullary tumours. Intramedullary tumours (around 30% of SCT) arise from within the neural tissues of the spinal cord; for example, astrocytomas, ependymomas, glioblastomas and medulloblastomas. Extramedullary tumours arise from tissues outside the spinal cord and account for 60% of all SCTs, for example neurofibromas, meningiomas, sarcomas, chordomas and vascular tumours. Primary tumours, arising from the epidural vessels, spinal meninges or glial cells, have an unknown cause. Secondary tumours are metastatic in origin, most commonly the result of malignancies of the lung, breast, prostate, bowel and kidney.

Pathophysiology of SCT

Depending on their anatomic location, SCTs result in pathological changes as a result of compression, invasion or ischaemia secondary to arterial or venous obstruction. Extramedullary tumours alter normal function through compression of the spinal cord, with destruction of white matter and eventual filling of the space around the spinal cord. Spinal cord compression

(SCC) interferes with normal blood flow and membrane potentials, altering afferent and efferent motor, sensory and reflex impulses and resulting in a variety of neurological disturbance related to mobility, sensation, bladder, bowel and sexual function. SCC also causes oedema, ischaemia and ultimately cell death. Intramedullary tumours both compress and invade. As the tumour grows within the cord, the cord also enlarges and distorts the white matter. Common sources of spinal cord metastatic tumours are lung, breast or prostate, gastrointestinal tract cancer and bone metastases.

Signs and symptoms of SCT

The signs and symptoms of a spinal cord tumour depend on the anatomic location, level of occurrence, type of tumour and spinal nerves involved. People with SCT often present with the following:

● Dull ache or radicular pain (often the first sign and made worse by any activity that causes intraspinal pressure, such as sneezing or coughing).
● Motor and sensory deficits, including paresis and paralysis below the level of the tumour, spasticity and hyperactive reflexes. The Babinski reflex may be positive.
● Changes in bowel and/or bladder elimination, and changes in sexual function, especially in lower cord tumours.
● Syringomyelia is a disorder in which a cyst forms (syrinx) within the spinal cord which expands and elongates over time, destroying the centre of the cord. Syringomyelia is a complication of a SCT causing pain, motor weakness and spasticity.

INTERDISCIPLINARY CARE FOR SCT

Diagnosis

MR scan with or without contrasts is the preferred radiographic assessment for SCT.

Radiation therapy

Radiation therapy is used to treat metastatic SCTs for several different reasons. It is often used to treat the person with rapidly progressing neurological deficits, to reduce pain and following surgical excision of the tumour.

Surgery

Surgery for intramedullary and extramedullary tumours involves surgical resection of the tumour and decompression of the spinal cord to avert progression of neurological compromise whenever possible. Metastatic tumours may be partially excised to reduce cord compression; rapidly growing metastatic lesions may require surgical decompression to preserve motor, bowel or bladder function.

Medication

The person with a spinal cord tumour is given medications to relieve pain and control oedema. Pain management for persons with a SCT is provided by narcotic analgesics (see Chapter 2). Steroids, such as dexamethasone, are administered to control oedema of the cord.

NURSING CARE FOR SCT

Nursing care is individualised in accordance with the type of tumour and the type of treatment. The person with a benign tumour that is removed by surgery has different healthcare needs than the person with a metastatic tumour, even though they may have similar neurological deficits. The person with a SCT (regardless of type) requires nursing care to monitor for neurological changes, provide pain management and manage motor and sensory deficits in order to preserve quality of life.

DEGENERATIVE NEUROLOGICAL DISORDERS

Degenerative neurological disorders are diverse, chronic and challenging to treat, and presentations are varied depending on the part of the nervous system affected. They are often disabling and progressively disrupt cognitive processes or motor functions, affecting the core of an individual's sense of personal autonomy and wellbeing. They can be psychologically and emotionally devastating to family members and caregivers, and most of them have no cure. The goal of treatment is usually to improve symptoms, relieve pain and increase mobility. In this section three common disorders are discussed: multiple sclerosis, Parkinson's disease and Alzheimer's disease.

The person with multiple sclerosis (MS)

Multiple sclerosis (MS) is a complex, chronic demyelinating neurological disease of the CNS. It is incurable and associated with increasing disability. The signs and symptoms vary according to the area of the nervous system affected. The initial onset may be followed by a total remission, making diagnosis difficult. In about 60% of persons, MS is characterised by periods of exacerbation, when signs and symptoms are highly pronounced, followed by periods of remission, when signs and symptoms are not obvious. The end result, however, is progression of the disease with increasing loss of function.

Incidence and prevalence of MS

MS is the most common neurological disease in young adults, onset usually occurring between 20 and 40 years of age. Prevalence rates increase with distance from the equator in both northern and southern hemispheres, occurring mostly in white women of European descent. The reasons for these variations are unclear, but it is known that certain environmental and genetic factors contribute to the individual developing MS, for example exposure to UVB light enabling vitamin D3 synthesis (Rog *et al.* 2009).

FAST FACTS

Multiple sclerosis

- Approximately 100 000 people in the UK have MS (Multiple Sclerosis Society).
- Females are affected two times more often than males, and the incidence is highest in young adults.
- 40–70% of MS patients will suffer cognitive deficits.

Sources: Rao *et al.* 1991, Chiaravalloti and DeLuca 2008.

Pathophysiology of MS

MS is an autoimmune response to a prior viral infection or environmental exposure in childhood in a genetically susceptible

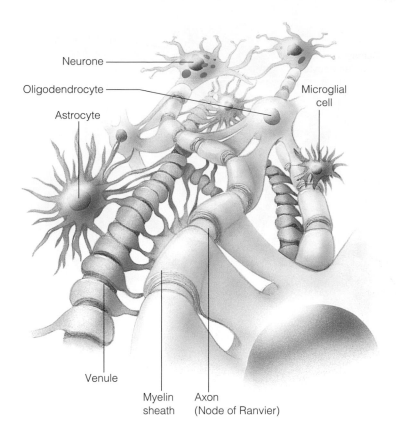

Normal anatomy of the central nervous system

The central nervous system (CNS) is composed of several cell types arranged in a dense, interconnected lattice. The basic functional cell of the CNS is the *neurone*, which transmits electrochemical impulses. Dendrites, thin projections extending from the neurone body, receive impulses that are passed down the neuroneal axon for transmission to other cells. Myelin, a lipid–protein substance, surrounds the axons, insulating them and speeding nerve impulse transmission.

Neurones are surrounded by a network of cells:

- *Astrocytes* support neurones and connect them to surrounding capillaries and venules.
- *Microglia* are motile phagocytic cells.
- *Oligodendrocytes* wrap concentric layers of myelin around nearby axons.

Acute attack

Multiple sclerosis (MS) is a demyelinating disease in which axonal myelin in the central nervous system is eroded, destroyed, and replaced by scar tissue.

An autoimmune process apparently triggered by genetic and environmental factors is believed to cause inflammation of venules in the CNS. This disrupts the blood–brain barrier, allowing lymphocytes to enter CNS tissue. These lymphocytes proliferate and produce IgG, an antibody that attacks and damages myelin and causes the release of inflammatory chemicals and oedema. As the inflammation subsides, the myelin regenerates and manifestations of the disease subside.

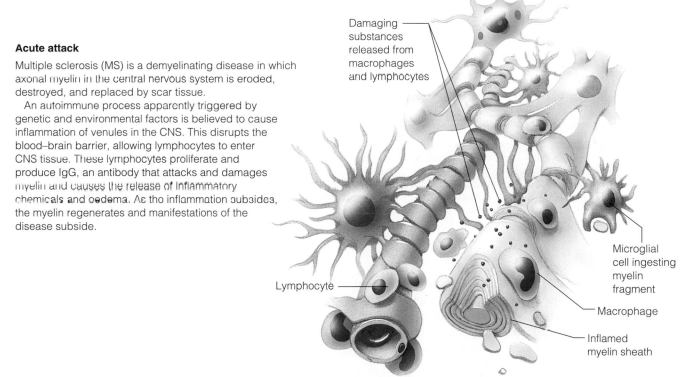

Figure 13.26 Pathophysiology illustrated: multiple sclerosis.

person. However, the aetiology is not fully understood. The infection or trigger activates T-cells, facilitating infiltration by other leucocytes, and an inflammatory process follows. Inflammation destroys myelin and oligodendrocytes (myelin-producing cells), in patches known as plaques along the axon, leading to axon dysfunction. The demyelination and plaque formation result in scarring of glia (gliosis) and degeneration of axons (see Figure 13.26).

Chronic lesion

After repeated inflammatory attacks, myelin is irreparably damaged. Segments of axons become totally demyelinated and may degenerate. Astrocytes proliferate in damaged regions of the CNS (a process called *gliosis*), forming plaques. The plaques are scattered throughout the CNS, appearing as grey or pinkish lesions. The relapsing–remitting character of MS and the scattered areas of damage within the CNS account for the variable nature of MS manifestations.

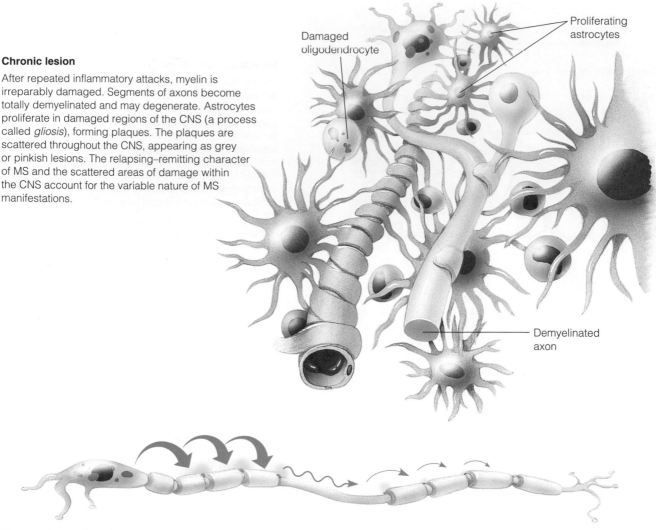

Abnormal nerve impulse transmission

In an undamaged neurone, nerve impulses travel down the axon by 'leaping' from one node of Ranvier to the next, thus greatly increasing the speed of impulse transmission. When nerve impulses travel down an axon damaged by MS, they are significantly slowed and weakened as they pass across the surface of demyelinated areas. Impulses may be blocked entirely when axons degenerate. The weakening or interruption of the transmission of nerve impulses and plaque formation within the CNS cause the manifestations of MS, including extremity weakness, paraesthesias, visual disturbances, bladder dysfunction and vertigo.

Figure 13.26 Continued

Neurones usually affected by MS are located in the spinal cord, brainstem, cerebral and cerebellar areas, and the optic nerve. Various stressors have been suggested as triggers for MS. These stressors include febrile states, pregnancy, extreme physical exertion and fatigue. There are four main types of MS:

● *Relapsing–remitting.* Most common type of MS (85%), characterised by exacerbations (acute attacks) with either full recovery or partial recovery with disability. 40% of relapses will leave permanent axonal damage and disability.

● *Primary progressive.* Steady worsening of disease from the onset. The person is left with residual disability from the onset. Diagnosed in about 10–15% of MS cases.

● *Secondary progressive.* Begins as with relapsing–remitting, but the disease steadily becomes worse between exacerbations.

● *Progressive–relapsing.* This rare form continues to progress from the onset but also has exacerbations.

Signs and symptoms of MS

The symptoms of MS vary widely in location and severity according to the areas destroyed by demyelination and the affected body system. Common symptoms include fatigue (most disabling symptoms), focal weakness, visual changes (diplopia and visual loss), numbness, spasticity, urinary problems, cognitive dysfunction and depression (see Figure 13.27).

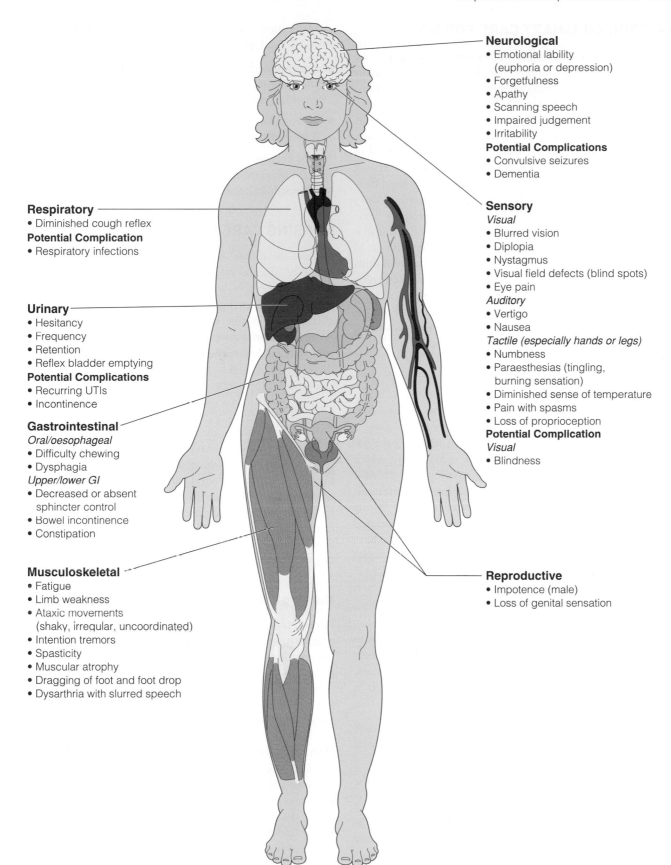

Neurological
- Emotional lability
  (euphoria or depression)
- Forgetfulness
- Apathy
- Scanning speech
- Impaired judgement
- Irritability
Potential Complications
- Convulsive seizures
- Dementia

Sensory
Visual
- Blurred vision
- Diplopia
- Nystagmus
- Visual field defects (blind spots)
- Eye pain
Auditory
- Vertigo
- Nausea
Tactile (especially hands or legs)
- Numbness
- Paraesthesias (tingling,
  burning sensation)
- Diminished sense of temperature
- Pain with spasms
- Loss of proprioception
Potential Complication
Visual
- Blindness

Respiratory
- Diminished cough reflex
Potential Complication
- Respiratory infections

Urinary
- Hesitancy
- Frequency
- Retention
- Reflex bladder emptying
Potential Complications
- Recurring UTIs
- Incontinence

Gastrointestinal
Oral/oesophageal
- Difficulty chewing
- Dysphagia
Upper/lower GI
- Decreased or absent
  sphincter control
- Bowel incontinence
- Constipation

Musculoskeletal
- Fatigue
- Limb weakness
- Ataxic movements
  (shaky, irregular, uncoordinated)
- Intention tremors
- Spasticity
- Muscular atrophy
- Dragging of foot and foot drop
- Dysarthria with slurred speech

Reproductive
- Impotence (male)
- Loss of genital sensation

Figure 13.27 Multisystem effects of multiple sclerosis.

INTERDISCIPLINARY CARE FOR MS

Management of the person with MS varies according to the severity of the manifestations. The focus is on retaining the optimal level of functioning possible, given the degree of disability. There is no cure for MS, but many of the symptoms can be controlled, leading to a better quality of life for the person and their families and a reduction in complications. Rehabilitation therapies are tailored to the person's level of functioning, providing supportive services such as speech therapy for problems with phonation and occupational therapy to maintain strength in the upper extremities and carry out activities of daily living (ADLs). It may also require referrals to a urologist for urinary problems. The long-term goal is to enable the person to retain as much independence as possible. During exacerbations, the focus of intervention shifts to controlling signs and symptoms and quickly returning to remission. MS management involves treatment of acute relapses, disease modification and symptom management. All three aspects of care require an individualised approach based on illness course and tolerability of treatments.

Diagnosis

Diagnosis of MS is challenging because the disease does not present uniformly and there is no single test to make a definitive diagnosis. Diagnosis is based on history, neurological assessment and various tests such as MRI scans which may reveal brain lesion where there is scarring of the myelin sheath, CSF analysis [80% have elevated levels of immunoglobulin G (IgG) in the CSF] and evoked response testing (visual, auditory and somatosensory) which may show delayed conduction. Generally, a diagnosis requires the person to have at least two or more episodes of neurological symptoms separated in time.

Medication

Medications are used for a variety of reasons, including to modify the course of the disease, treat the signs and symptoms (relapse) or to interrupt the progression of the disease. Disease-modifying therapies used to reduce exacerbations in patients with relapsing–remitting MS include:

- *Interferon beta-1a and interferon beta-1b*, which intervene in the inflammatory process by reducing the passage of inflammatory cells into the brain.
- *Glatiramer acetate (Copaxone)*, thought to prevent the T-cells attacking the myelin and reduce inflammation.

The medications used during a relapse are aimed at decreasing inflammation to inhibit signs and symptoms and induce remission. These include:

- Adrenal corticosteroid therapies such as Methylprednisolone, administered to decrease inflammation and suppress the immune system as soon as possible after relapse.

Medications used in the treatment of signs and symptoms are varied and may include:

- Anticholinergics, administered for bladder spasticity and cholinergics, given if the person has a problem with urinary retention related to flaccid bladder.
- Muscle relaxants such as baclofen are prescribed to relieve muscle spasms and antidepressant drugs for depression.

New therapies include monoclonal antibodies which prevent the migration of immune cells across the BBB, which would result in inflammation and myelin destruction.

NURSING CARE FOR MS

Because the disease most often affects young adults in the prime of life, the psychosocial and economic effect can be devastating. People with MS have to make adjustments to the body image changes while simultaneously adapting to the altered relationships usually encountered with the disease. A once-healthy spouse becomes wheelchair bound; a person once independent may eventually become dependent for even the most basic ADLs. The unpredictable course of MS is a challenge for long-term planning.

Assessment

Collect the following data through the health history and physical examination (see neurological assessment on p. 474): history of childhood viral illnesses; geographical residence when a child; exposure to physical or emotional stressors (pregnancy/delivery, extremes of heat), medications; symptom onset; severity of symptoms. Physical assessment includes: affect, mood, speech, eye movements, gait, tremors, vision and hearing, reflexes, muscle strength and movement, sensation.

Nursing diagnoses and interventions

Interventions for the person with MS vary with the acuity of exacerbations and the presenting problems. Many nursing interventions relate to the inability to perform ADLs. Others reflect problems with musculoskeletal changes or altered nerve conduction together with measures to reduce the risk of respiratory and urinary tract infections. The specific nursing intervention discussed in this section is fatigue.

Management of fatigue

MS is characterised by fatigue with and without exertion, worsening of symptoms with exertion and the limited ability to sustain physical activity. Fatigue affects every aspect of the life of the person with MS. Nurses can help the person and family understand how to prevent fatigue and exacerbations. This may include the following:

+ Assess degree of fatigue and identify contributing factors.
+ Arrange daily activities to include rest periods and psychological relaxation.

+ Suggest performing tasks in the morning hours and consider whether they are necessary.

+ Advise to avoid temperature extremes, such as hot showers or exposure to cold, as heat can delay impulse transmission across demyelinated nerves, which contributes to fatigue.

+ Refer to the appropriate healthcare professional for help managing fatigue: stress management groups, support groups, occupational or physical therapist, as indicated.

+ Also, address preventive measures to avoid secondary fatigue (as a result of non-MS-related factors) such as bladder problems and respiratory and urinary tract infections.

PRACTICE ALERT

● It may be difficult to differentiate fatigue from depression.

● It is important to remember that fatigue from chronic illnesses such as MS is very different from being 'tired', and that rest and sleep may not result in improvement.

The person with Parkinson's disease (PD)

Parkinson's disease (PD) is a progressive, degenerative neurologic disease characterised by tremor (shaking), muscle rigidity and bradykinesia (slowness of movement) (Porth 2009).

Incidence and prevalence of PD

PD is one of the most common neurological disorders affecting older adults. The disorder usually develops after the age of 60 years, but 15% of those diagnosed are under 40 years of age. PD is more common in men than in women. Recent discovery of inherited forms of PD suggests a genetic role in the development of this disease.

Parkinson's-like manifestations, called secondary parkinsonism, may result from other disorders such as trauma, encephalitis, tumours, toxins and drugs. Drug-induced parkinsonism, which is usually reversible, may occur in people taking neuroleptics, antiemetics, antihypertensives and illegal designer drug MPPP containing MPTP, a toxic chemical (Porth 2009). Carbon monoxide or cyanide poisoning can also cause secondary parkinsonism.

Pathophysiology of PD

PD involves the loss of dopamine-producing cells in the substantia nigra and in the connections in the basal ganglia region in the brain. The consequential depletion of dopamine results in motor dysfunction.

FAST FACTS

Parkinson's disease

● There are approximately 120 000 people in the UK with Parkinson's disease (PDS 2008).

● In the majority of cases, the cause is not known.

● Mainstay treatment is medication aimed at controlling symptoms, maintaining function and minimising side-effects.

Signs and symptoms of PD

PD begins with subtle symptoms: complaining of feeling tired and moving about more slowly; a slight tremor may accompany the fatigue. Over time, the signs and symptoms progressively increase in severity. The common signs and symptoms are listed below:

● Tremor at rest 'pill-rolling' motion of the thumb and fingers. The tremor may be controlled with purposeful, voluntary movement, and is worsened by stress and anxiety.

● Rigidity and bradykinesia – Rigidity (resulting from involuntary contraction of all skeletal muscles) makes both active and passive movement difficult with increased resistance to passive ROM. Although the extremity moves, it does so in a jerky motion, called *cogwheel rigidity*. Bradykinesia is experienced as difficulty in starting, continuing or coordinating movements. Patients have a staring gaze with minimal change in expression.

● Cognitive and psychological dysfunction is common. These may include dementia (50%), apathy (up to 70%), depression (30%), memory loss and lack of insight and problem-solving ability.

● Loss of normal postural reflexes results in postural abnormalities, including disorders of postural fixation, equilibrium and righting.

● Sleep disturbances: poor sleep onset, poor sleep maintenance and nightmares (up to 90%).

INTERDISCIPLINARY CARE FOR PD

Prognosis is poor, owing to the progressive degeneration that ultimately affects multiple physiologic systems and their function. Total disability is usually seen 10–20 years after diagnosis. Interventions vary with the clinical stage of the disorder and include medication, surgery and rehabilitation to retain the optimal level of functioning possible.

Diagnosis

No test clearly differentiates PD from other neurologic disorders (Hickey 2009). Diagnosis is based primarily on a thorough history and physical examination, and is made based on having two of the following signs and symptoms: tremor at rest, bradykinesia, rigidity and postural instability.

Medication

The goal of drug therapy is to control manifestations to the extent possible. Generally, medications vary with the stage of the disease; however, response is individualised and guides the selection of medications. Types of drugs used include monoamine oxidase (MAO) inhibitors, dopaminergics, dopamine agonists and anticholinergics. Other medications may be used to treat problems related to PD. Antidepressants may be prescribed. Propranolol (Inderal) may be used to treat tremors; it should be used cautiously when patients have orthostatic hypotension. Botulism toxin injections may be given to treat eyelid spasms and abnormal posturing (dystonia) involving the extremities.

> ## PRACTICE ALERT
>
> - People with suspected PD should be referred to a specialist in PD for accurate diagnosis and treatment.
> - People with PD are at risk of falls resulting from orthostatic hypotension, osteoporosis, poor vision and other problems causing disorientation and confusion.
> - Adherence to medication times is vital as uneven release of dopamine may suddenly render a person unable to move, get out of bed or walk, known as 'off period'.

Surgery

Various neurosurgical techniques may be used, for example pallidotomy and stereotaxic thalamotomy.

Deep brain stimulation (DBS) is an effective treatment option for some PD patients who generally have had the condition for some time and whose symptoms are not controlled effectively by medications.

NURSING CARE FOR PD

Patients with PD have complex and, ultimately, multisystem needs. People with PD are faced with multiple problems: deficits in mobility and self-care are common and emotional wellbeing, financial security and relationships with caregivers. Psychosocial needs may include problems related to ineffective coping, powerlessness and disturbed body image. Refer to the nursing care sections throughout this chapter for discussions of fatigue, self-care deficit, ineffective airway clearance and other pertinent nursing care.

Health promotion

Teaching preventive measures is extremely important when caring for patients who have PD. Preventing malnutrition, falls and other environmental accidents, constipation, skin breakdown from incontinence or immobility and joint contracture requires teaching and reinforcement. In addition, provide the following information about safety:

- The importance of taking medication as directed, especially dose and time of administration. Not to alter the dosages or suddenly stop medications.
- Watch for the '*on–off*' phenomenon, in which periods of symptom control alternate with periods when the drug fails to control symptoms.
- Observe and report any new signs and symptoms.
- Inform their practitioner when starting any new medications or if any new symptoms are noticed, for example difficulty making voluntary movements or cardiac or psychological symptoms develop.
- Advise on how to manage potential complications of postural hypotension.

The person with dementia

Dementia is a generic term that describes a progressive and irreversible disease, affecting multiple cortical functions, calculation, learning capacity, language and judgement. The progressive nature results in a variety of issues which can be devastating for the individual and their family and carers. All forms of dementia result from death of neurones and/or the loss of communication among the cells. Although the exact cause is not always known, many forms of dementia are characterised by abnormal structures in the brain called inclusions, and there is clearly a genetic component in the development of some kinds of dementia. Table 13.18 provides an overview of the most common causes of dementia.

Incidence and prevalence of dementia

The incidence of dementia rises with age, and 1 in 20 over the age of 65 years will have dementia. The incidences are not greater in men than women, however, as women live longer than men the number of women living with dementia is greater. Alzheimer's disease (AD) is the most common degenerative neurologic disorder and the most common cause of cognitive impairment in older adults (Porth 2009).

> ## FAST FACTS
>
>
>
> ### Dementia
>
> - About 822 000 people in the UK have dementia (Luengo-Fernandez *et al.* 2010).
> - By 2050, it is estimated that there will be 15 million people with dementia (European Commission 2009).
> - Dementia has a major impact on the person, their family and carers.
> - Dementia costs the UK economy £23 billion per year (Luengo-Fernandez *et al.* 2010)

Table 13.18 Common causes of dementia

Name	Cause and primary pathophysiology
Alzheimer's disease (AD) (the most common cause of dementia in people age 65 and older)	Unknown cause. Characterised by two abnormalities in the brain: plaques and neurofibrillary tangles and acetylcholine depletion.
Vascular dementia (the second most common cause of dementia), accounting for approximately 20% of dementias	Caused by brain damage from cerebrovascular and cardiovascular problems (usually strokes). May also be caused by small cerebral blood vessel damage, e.g. endocarditis, vasculitis and profound hypotension.
Lewy body dementia	Cause usually unknown, although familial cases have been reported. Characterised by small spherical protein deposits found in neurones in the subcortical and cortical brain called Lewy bodies. Parkinsonian motor symptoms commonly occur due to the dopamine receptor deficiency.
Fronto-temporal dementia (including Pick's disease), relatively uncommon	Nerve cells, especially in the frontal and temporal lobes, degenerate. In many people, abnormal tau protein accumulates in neurofibrillary tangles.

Risk factors for dementia

For the majority of dementias, the cause is unknown. However, a number of factors are known to increase the risk of dementia. These include the following:

- genetic – although no clear genetic cause has been identified, small numbers of gene mutations have been linked with familial forms of AD;
- diabetes hypertension (most predictive risk for vascular dementia) and atherosclerosis;
- high cholesterol and vitamin deficiencies;
- ageing;
- unhealthy lifestyle – smoking, drinking excessive alcohol and reduced physical activity;
- menopause;
- familial Creutzfeldt–Jakob disease (CJD);
- depression.

Pathophysiology of dementia

Characteristic findings in the brains of AD patients are loss of nerve cells far greater than would normally happen, and the presence of *neurofibrillary tangles* and *amyloid plaques* (see Figure 13.28). Neurofibrillary tangles result when an abnormal form of the tau protein found in neurones becomes distorted and twisted. Tau normally holds together the microtubules, forming a kind of scaffold which guides nutrients and molecules to the end of the axon. Because tau no longer maintains the transport system, communication is lost between neurones. Death of neurones may follow, contributing to the development of dementia.

Amyloid plaques are deposits of insoluble beta-amyloid, a protein fragment from a larger protein called amyloid precursor protein, mixed with other neurones and non-nerve cells. It is not yet known if plaque formation causes AD or if plaques are a by-product of the AD process. Groups of nerve cells (and

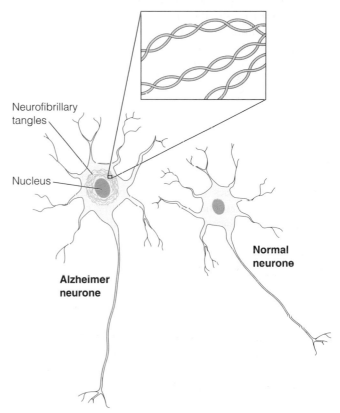

Figure 13.28 Neurone with neurofibrillary tangles in Alzheimer's disease.

especially the terminal axons) degenerate and clump around an amyloid core as plaques, found in the spaces between the neurones of the brain. These plaques, which develop first in areas used for memory and cognition, disrupt transmission of nerve impulses.

Signs and symptoms of dementia

These vary according to the type of dementia and the individual, but common symptoms include the following:

- chronic confusion, agitation and wandering related to deterioration of brain function and dementia;
- cognitive deficits accompanied by a deterioration in emotional control, social behaviour and motivation;
- self-care deficits related to forgetfulness and declining physical abilities, for example sensorimotor skills;
- risk for injury related to decreased orientation;
- disturbed sleep pattern related to time disorientation.

In addition people with AD have a high prevalence rate of depression, estimated between 30 and 50%.

INTERDISCIPLINARY CARE FOR DEMENTIA

The care and management of people with dementia is complex and requires nurses, doctors, physical therapists and social workers collaborating with the person's family to provide the least restrictive environment in which the person can safely function. There is no cure for Alzheimer's dementia. The main objective of care is to provide an environment that matches the person's functional abilities.

Diagnosis

NICE (2006) recommend that when people are being assessed for a possible diagnosis of dementia they are asked if they wish to be informed of the diagnosis along with other family members. Diagnosis involves a process of exclusion, to eliminate rare reversible causes of dementia, for example hypothyroidism. The process should include history, cognitive, functional and physical assessment. A definite diagnosis for AD can only be made on post-mortem examination; however, doctors often make a highly probable diagnosis based on both clinical examination and investigations. For example, the significant impairment of at least two brain functions without loss of consciousness, for example, language skills, perception, reasoning or judgement. Investigations may include cognitive and neuropsychological testing, CT or MRI imaging and EEG. Other investigations should focus on looking for risk factors for underlying contributing diseases. These may include blood glucose and calcium levels, thyroid function tests and full blood count.

Often it is difficult to distinguish dementia from depression and delirium as they share similar features. Thus, it is important that accurate assessments are made to ensure appropriate treatment options can be offered.

Medication

There is no cure for AD, and no way of preventing the disease; however, reducing some of the known risk factors may have some benefit, for example treating high blood pressure and high cholesterol levels. There are a number of medications that may have a beneficial effect on treating the symptoms of the disease, for example acetylcholinesterase (AChE) inhibitors

(Donepezil and Mementine), although the scientific evidence as to their effectiveness is limited (NICE 2011).

Behavioural and environmental factors

A number of strategies can be deployed to support people with dementia and their carers. Techniques to help with memory loss should be included in the teaching for both the person and the caregiver.

- Suggest using a calendar, keeping lists of reminders or asking someone else to remind them of appointments and events. Written or verbal reminders are helpful if memory is impaired.
- Recommend using a dosette box (e.g. pill organisers, calender blister packs) with medications organised into compartments by day and time. A medication box is a good way to remember to take medications.
- If safety is a concern, such as turning on the oven and forgetting it, suggest using alternatives such as a microwave. Programme emergency numbers into the telephone. Door alarms help reduce the risk of wandering. These measures can increase safety.
- Suggest using cues, such as an alarm on a watch or a pocket computer, to trigger actions at designated times. Cues are often helpful when memory loss is a problem.

Alternative and complementary therapy

The following types of alternative and complementary therapies may be used in treating the manifestations of dementia:

- Aromatherapy, acupuncture and massage
- Multisensory therapy – Snoezelen
- Dietary supplements, such as zinc, selenium and evening primrose oil
- Therapies involving art, music, sound and dance
- Herbs such as Ginkgo biloba and vitamin E.

NURSING CARE FOR DEMENTIA

Persons with dementia often require intensive, supportive nursing interventions directed at the physical and psychosocial responses to illness. Equally important, the nurse can facilitate the long-term support of these people by providing teaching and referrals to follow-up care in the community.

If the person is being cared for at home, then nurses need to address safety considerations as well as the caregivers' abilities to meet the person's needs, such as maintaining hygiene and other ADLs. In addition, it is important that the nurse provides support and education for the caregivers on coping with their family member. This may include addressing the following topics for home care of the person with dementia and for the caregiver:

✚ Plan care that matches the person's level of coping, using a consistent routine.

✚ Support groups and peer counselling are helpful in handling caregiver stress.

✚ A person with AD who is confused or agitated is not comfortable and is usually frightened.

✚ Provide regular rest periods to decrease the person's stress and fatigue (these do not increase night-time wandering).

✚ Plan care for the caregiver. Periodic adult day care or respite care during the initial stages, with plans for increasing assistance to meet the person with dementia daily needs as the disease progresses, may be sufficient. Referrals to the appropriate agency for long-term care, including skilled nursing facilities, may be indicated.

✚ Provide information on available resources, for example Alzheimer's Society and Admiral nurses (specialist community mental health nurses working to support those affected by dementia).

PRACTICE ALERT

● A person-centred apporach to care may reduce the need for physical and pharmacological restraint.

● Nurses should provide support and education to caregivers of people with dementia as they are at risk of role strain, distress, burden and stress.

● Avoid antihistamines and tricylic antidepressants that have high anticholinergic activity because they can increase AD manifestations such as cognitive impairment and precipitate delirium.

CASE STUDY SUMMARIES

Three case studies have been presented within this chapter to illustrate the care of people with neurological problems. In the first part of this chapter, you were introduced to Ali who sustained a mild TBI and required admission to hospital for close observation and monitoring. Second, you were introduced to Bob a 78-year-old with a cerebral haematoma who presented with signs of raised intracranial pressure and required an evacuation of his haematoma. The later sections of this chapter focused on the more long-term neurological conditions and introduced you to Jane, a 65-year-old lady who suffers an ischaemic stroke.

People who survive ABI often require rehabilitation and life long care, and neurological recovery can take many months or years. This impacts on the whole family, potentially disrupting equilibrium within the family unit. Whilst some may regain consciousness, others remain in a coma or vegetative state. Although physical disabilities post-ABI are well recognised, it is the psychological condition – the cognitive, behavioural and emotional changes – that account for the greatest share in long-term disability. These changes are complex and variable and often cause dramatic alterations in identity and structure of self of the person with the ABI, with devastating consequences for the family. Family and carer support is crucial in these circumstances.

● Ensure that family and carers appreciate the seriousness of the situation and evaluate their readiness to receive explanations regarding treatment and care.

● Include family members in caring for the person as much as they wish to be involved.

● Reinforce information provided by the interdisciplinary team, and encourage family and carers to talk to the person as though he or she were able to understand.

● Understand that family members of a person with an altered level of consciousness are often very anxious due to the uncertain prognosis. They may experience various conflicting emotions, such as guilt and anger.

● Provide timely and appropriate information to family and carers. This may include the following:

   – the real possibility of residual deficits in self-care, emotional responses, cognition, communication and movement;

   – information to enhance recovery, such as help in understanding the cognitive, emotional and behavioural responses that they will experience in their injured family member;

   – information on community resources including support groups such as the Brain and Spinal Injury Charity, www.BASIC.org.uk.

● Help families and carers to adapt to their changed role and to develop coping strategies that will support their wellbeing and reduce their stress and distress.

● Help families and carers to cope with the grief associated with the loss of the person that once was.

CHAPTER HIGHLIGHTS

- Altered level of consciousness (LOC) is a common response to intracranial disorders, and is an early manifestation of deterioration of the function of the cerebral hemispheres.

- Increased intracranial pressure (IICP) is a sustained elevated pressure (≥ 10 mmHg) within the cranial cavity. IICP may result from a number of causes intracranial and extracranial and, if untreated, can be fatal.

- A neurological assessment is conducted to assess the function and integrity of the nervous system and should be conducted in a systematic way. Initial assessment provides a baseline against which subsequent assessment can be compared.

- Headaches, a common type of intracranial pain, are categorised as tension, migraine and cluster. Headaches are a sign and symptom of increased intracranial pressure.

- Epilepsy is a chronic disorder of abnormal, recurring, excessive and self-terminating electrical discharges from neurones.

- Traumatic brain injury (TBI) refers to any injury of the scalp, skull or brain, and is a leading cause of death and disability. TBI affects all body systems, and carries the risk of secondary injury to the brain from hypoxia and ischaemia.

- Central nervous system infections may be caused by a variety of organisms. The major CNS infections are meningitis, encephalitis and brain abscess.

- Brain tumours are growths within the cranium, including on or in brain tissue, the meninges, the pituitary gland or blood vessels, and are potentially lethal because they displace or impinge on CNS structures within a closed bony system.

- A stroke is a condition in which neurological deficits result from a sudden decrease in blood flow to a localised area of the brain. Strokes may be ischaemic or haemorrhagic.

- Multiple sclerosis (MS) is a complex, chronic demyelinating neurological disease of the CNS occurring in the young to middle-aged adults.

- Parkinson's disease (PD) is a progressive degenerative neurologic disease characterised by tremor, muscle rigidity and bradykinesia.

- Alzheimer's disease (AD) is a form of dementia (a disease of the brain) of older adults with progressive irreversible deterioration of general intellectual functioning. The disease is characterised by atrophy of brain tissue, loss of neurones, neurofibrillary tangles and amyloid plaques. AD finally leaves the person unable to communicate, maintain continence and recognise self or others.

TEST YOURSELF

1. What component of the brain protects it from harmful substances?

   a. the circulation of cerebrospinal fluid
   b. the large oxygen demand
   c. the structure of neurones
   d. the blood–brain barrier

2. What pathophysiology results from damage to the lower motor neurones?

   a. loss of cognitive ability
   b. inability to communicate verbally
   c. loss of reflexes
   d. decreasing levels of consciousness

3. Which of the following statements about cerebrospinal fluid (CSF) is true?

   a. if CSF contains glucose, the person has a metabolic disorder.
   b. CSF circulates through the brain via the meninges.
   c. CSF protects the brain and spinal cord from trauma.
   d. A lumbar puncture is done to withdraw CSF from the brain.

4. Your body responses to stress are caused by which division of the autonomic nervous system?

   a. sympathetic
   b. parasympathetic
   c. cholinergic
   d. adrenergic

5. Which position best describes decorticate posturing?

   a. neck extended, arms extended and pronated, feet plantar flexed
   b. arms close to sides, elbows and wrists flexed, legs extended
   c. in prone position with arms and knees sharply flexed
   d. in supine position, spine extended, legs extended

6. Which of the following pathophysiological events results in irregular respiratory patterns as LOC decreases?

   a. pressure on the meninges
   b. reflexive motor responses
   c. loss of the oculocephalic reflex
   d. brainstem responses to changes in $PaCO_2$

7. What is the rationale for the use of osmotic diuretics to treat IICP?

   a. Hyperthermia increases the cerebral metabolic rate and exacerbates IICP.

   b. Increased blood osmolality draws oedematous fluid into the vascular system.

   c. Patients with ICP are at increased risk for gastrointestinal haemorrhage.

   d. Brain injury and IICP often cause seizures.

8. What signs and symptoms are consistently assessed in patients with generalised seizures?

   a. loss of consciousness

   b. repetitive non-purposeful activity

   c. tonic movements

   d. clonic movements

9. Although all of the following are risk factors for a stroke, which one is the greatest risk?

   a. hypertension

   b. heart disease

   c. diabetes

   d. high cholesterol level

10. You are preparing information to teach a person about medications for MS. What drugs would you expect to be used?

    a. antibiotics

    b. antihistamines

    c. interferon

    d. levedopa

Further resources

Brain Tumour UK
http://www.braintumouruk.org.uk
Brain Tumour UK is the leading, caring charity providing support, funding research and raising awareness for everyone affected by a brain tumour.

British Association of Neuroscience Nurses (BANN)
http://www.bann.org.uk
The mission of BANN is to support and enhance the development of competence in neuroscience nursing by improving the exchange of information between neuroscience nurses in the UK.

Epilepsy Society
http://www.epilepsysociety.org.uk
The epilepsy society is the leading national epilepsy medical charity working for everyone affected by epilepsy, through cutting-edge research, awareness campaigns and expert care.

Migraine Action
http://www.migraine.org.uk
Provides information and support to migraineurs and their families throughout the UK and overseas. Migraine Action strives to provide an excellent patient-led, compassionate and empathetic support community for individuals affected by migraine.

Multiple Sclerosis Society
http://www.mssociety.org.uk
The MS Society is the UK's largest charity for people affected by multiple sclerosis (MS).

Parkinson's Disease Society
http://www.parkinsons.org.uk
Offers education and training and develops resources for health and social care professionals to help improve services for people affected by Parkinson's.

The Stroke Association
http://www.stroke.org.uk
Funds research into prevention, treatment and better methods of rehabilitation, and helps stroke patients and their families directly through its Life After Stroke Services.

Spinal Injuries Association
http://www.spinal.co.uk
The Spinal Injuries Association (SIA) is the leading national charity for spinal cord injured people.

Bibliography

Afifi A K and Bergman R A (2005) *Functional Neuroanatomy: Text and Atlas* (2nd edn). New York, McGraw-Hill Professional.

Aird T and McIntosh M (2004) Nursing assessment. Nursing tools and strategies to assess cognition and confusion. *British Journal of Nursing*, **13**(10), 621–625.

Arbour R (2004) Intracranial hypertension: Monitoring and nursing assessment. *Critical Care Nurse*, **24**(5), 19–20, 22–26, 28–34.

Bear M F, Connors B W and Paradiso M A (2007) *Neuroscience: Exploring the brain* (3rd edn). Philadelphia, PA, Lippincott.

Bickley L and Szilagyi P (2008) *Bates' Guide to Physical Examination and History Taking* (10th edn). Philadelphia, PA, Lippincott.

Braine M E (2005) The management of challenging behaviour and cognitive impairment. *British Journal of Neuroscience Nursing*, **1**(2), 67–74.

Braine M E (2011) The experience of living with a family member with challenging behavior post acquired brain injury. *Journal of Neuroscience Nursing*, **43**(3), 156–164.

Breen K and Heisters D (2007) A guide to deep brain stimulation surgery: A treatment for Parkinson's disease. *British Journal of Neuroscience Nursing*, **3**(12), 554–559.

Burgess M (2002) *Multiple Sclerosis: Theory and practice for nurses*. Oxford, Wiley-Blackwell.

Calne S M and Kumar A (2003). Nursing care of patients with late stage Parkinson's disease. *Journal of Neuroscience Nursing*, **35**(5), 242–251.

Chiaravalloti N D and DeLuca J (2008) Cognitive impairment in multiple sclerosis. *Lancet Neurology*, **7**(12), 1139–1151.

Cook N F (2005) Fundamentals of fluids and hydration in the nursing of the neuroscience patient. *British Journal of Neuroscience Nursing*, **1**(2), 61–66.

DoH (2007) *National Stroke Strategy*. London, Department of Health.

DoH (2009) *Stroke: Act; F.A.S.T. Awareness Campaign*. London, Department of Health.

Durham P L and Garrett F G (2009) Neurological mechanisms of migraine: potential of the gap-junction modulator tonabersat in prevention of migraine, *Cephalalgia*, **29**(s2), 1–6.

European Commission (2009) *Communication on an European Initiative on Alzheimer's Disease and other Dementias* (COM (2009) 380/4). Brussels, European Commission.

Fan J (2004) Effect of backrest position on intracranial pressure and cerebral perfusion on pressure in individuals with brain injury: A systematic review. *Journal of Neuroscience Nursing*, **36**(5), 278–288.

Finlayson M. Van Denend T and Hudson E (2004) Aging with multiple sclerosis. *Journal of Neuroscience Nursing*, **36**(5), 245–251, 259.

Garner A and Amin Y (2007) The management of raised intracranial pressure: A Multidisciplinary approach. *British Journal of Neuroscience Nursing*, **3**(11), 516–521.

Giacino J and Whyte J (2005) The vegetative and minimally conscious states: Current knowledge and remaining questions. *Journal of Head Trauma Rehabilitation*, **20**(1), 30–50.

Hickey J V (2009) *Clinical Practice of Neurological & Neurosurgical Nursing* (6th edn). Philadelphia, PA, Lippincott.

Intercollegiate Stroke Working Party (2008) *National Clinical Guideline for Stroke* (3rd edn). London, Royal College of Physicians.

International Headache Society (2004) The International Classification of Headache Disorders (2nd edn). *Cephalalgia*, **24**(suppl 1), 1–160.

Kao H and Stuifbergen A (2004) Love and load: The lived experience of the mother–child relationship among young adult traumatic brain-injured survivors. *Journal of Neuroscience Nursing*, **36**(2), 73–81.

Khetsuriani N, Holman R C and Anderson L J (2002) Burden of encephalitis-associated hospitalizations in the United States, 1988–1997. *Clinical Infectious Disease*, **35**(2), 175–182.

Lipton R B and Scher A I (2001) Epidemiology and economic impact of migraine. C*urrent Medical Research and Opinion*, **17** (supplement1), s4–12.

Littlejohns L R and Bader M K (2001) Guidelines for the management of severe head injury: Clinical application and changes in practice. *Critical Care Nurse*, **21**(6), 48–65.

Luengo-Fernandez R, Leal J, Gray A (2010) *Dementia 2010: The Prevalence, Economic Cost and Research Funding Compared With Other Major Diseases*. Oxford, Alzheimer's Research Trust.

Mantri P (2007) Distinguishing between seizure types in adult epilepsy: A key role for nursing observation. *British Journal of Neuroscience Nursing*, **3**(12), 560–567.

Mini-mental state exam (1975) *Journal of Psychiatric Research*, **12**, 189–198.

NICE (2006) *Dementia the NICE-SCIE Guideline on Supporting People with Dementia and Their Carers in Health and Social Care*, CG 42. London. National Collaborating Centre for Mental Health; Leicester, The British Psychological Society; London, Gaskell.

NICE (2010) *Transient Loss of Consciousness ('Blackouts') Management in Adults and Young People*, Clinical guidelines CG109. London, National Institute for Health and Clinical Excellence available at: http://guidance.nice.org.uk/CG109, last accessed August 2011.

NICE (2011) *Donepezil, Galantamine, Rivastigmine and Memantine for the Treatment of Alzheimer's disease. Review of NICE technology appraisal guidance 111*, Technology appraisal TA s217. London, National Institute for Health and Clinical Excellence.

PDS (2008) *Life with Parkinson's Today – Room for Improvement*. London, Parkinson's Disease Society.

Porth C M (2009) *Pathophysiology: Concepts of altered health states* (9th edn). Philadelphia, PA, Lippincott.

Rao S M, Leo G J, Bernardin L *et al.* (1991) Cognitive dysfunction in multiple sclerosis: Frequency, patterns, and predictions. Neurology, **41**, 685–691.

RCP (2008) *STROKE: National clinical guideline for diagnosis and initial management of acute stroke and transient ischaemic attack (TIA)*, The National Collaborating Centre for Chronic Conditions. London, Royal College of Physicians.

RCP, National Council for Palliative Care, British Society of Rehabilitation Medicine (2008) *Long-term Neurological Conditions: Management at the interface between neurology, rehabilitation and palliative care*, Concise Guidance to Good Practice series, No 10. London, Royal College of Physicians.

Roberts I, Schierhout G and Wakai A (2005) Mannitol for acute traumatic injury. *The Cochrane Library (Oxford)* (2) (ID#CD001049).

Rog D, Burgess M, Mottershead J and Tolbort, P (2009) *Multiple Sclerosis: Answers at your fingertips* (2nd edn). London, Class Publishing.

Rubin R (2005) Communication about sexual problems in male patients with multiple sclerosis. *Nursing Standard*, **19**(24), 33–37.

Russell C and Matta B (2004). (eds) *Tracheostomy: A multiprofessional handbook*. London, Greenwich Medical Media Limited.

Spratt P, Cook N F and Gillespie M (2007) The care of patients with subarachnoid haemorrhage in the emergency department. *British Journal of Neuroscience Nursing*, **3**(5), 210–216.

Stokes T, Shaw E J, Juarez-Garcia A, Camosso-Stefinovic J and Baker R (2004) *Clinical Guidelines and Evidence Review for the Epilepsies: Diagnosis and management in adults and children in primary and secondary care*. London, Royal College of General Practitioners.

Teasdale G and Jennett B (1974) Assessment of the coma and impaired consciousness. A practical scale. *Lancet*, **2**, 81–84.

Warner R (2006) Understanding fatigue in multiple sclerosis: A case study inquiry. *British Journal of Neuroscience Nursing*, **2**(9), 462–469.

Waterhouse C (2005) The Glasgow Coma Scale and other neurological observations. *Nursing Standard*, **19**, 56–64.

Waterhouse C (2009) The use of painful stimulus in relation to Glasgow Coma Scale observations. *British Journal of Neuroscience Nursing*. 5(5), 209–215.

Whitehurst E (2009) The importance of nutrition support in the head-injured patient. *British Journal of Neuroscience Nursing*, **5**(1), 8–12.

WHO (2001) *World Health Report – Mental Health: New understanding, new hope*. Geneva, World Health Organization.

Woodward S and Mestecky A (eds) (2011) *Neuroscience Nursing Evidence-Based Practice*. Oxford, Wiley-Blackwell.

Young P A, Young P H and Tolbert D L (2008) *Basic Clinical Neuroscience* (2nd edn). Philadelphia, PA, Lippincott.

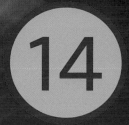

14

Caring for people with eye and ear problems

Learning outcomes

- Describe, identify and relate the anatomy, physiology and functions of the eye and the ear.
- Explain change processes related to vision and hearing.
- Identify specific topics for consideration during a health history.
- Describe normal variations in assessment findings for the older adult and discuss some of the diagnostic tests.
- Identify abnormal findings indicating impairment of the eye and the ear.
- Describe surgical and other invasive procedures.

Clinical competencies

- Assess vision, hearing and functional health of persons with eye and ear disorders.
- Conduct and document a health history.
- Monitor the results of diagnostic tests reporting abnormal findings.
- Conduct and document physical assessment.
- Implement individualised nursing interventions.

CASE STUDIES

Below are two case studies that you may wish to consider before, during or after you have read the chapter. There are no right or wrong answers to these case studies, but you should think about the physical, psychological and social implications.

Case Study 1 – Reggie

Mr Reggie Madison is a 65-year-old Afro-Caribbean seen in the eye clinic for a routine examination. He states he has not had any recent eye infections or eye injuries. He denies pain in the eyes. Vital signs are temperature 37.1 °C, pulse rate 84 beats per minute, respiratory rate 16 breaths per minute, BP 168/88 mmHg. His height is 1.72 m and his weight is 90.7 kg. His medical history indicates that he has hypertension and type 2 diabetes. He is taking hydrochlorothiazide, captopril and glibenclamide. He states that he is on a 2000-calorie diabetic diet, but he does not often stick to the diet. He sees the practice nurse about once a year but has not had an eye examination in about 10 years. He is married with five grown children and six grandchildren. Mr Madison states that he does not know if there is any family history of **glaucoma** because his father died of a heart attack at age 50 years and his mother died of cancer at 60 years of age.

An examination of his eyes is performed revealing an increase in intraocular pressure, pallor and an increase in the size and depth of the optic cup on the optic disc. Visual field testing shows significant peripheral vision loss. The results of these tests indicate a diagnosis of glaucoma.

Case Study 2 – Georgia

Ms Georgia Stanley, a 45-year-old is admitted with complaints of feeling like she is spinning or falling and has ringing and a feeling of fullness in her left ear. Vital signs are temperature 37.0 °C, pulse rate 78 beats per minute, respiratory rate 16 breaths per minute, BP 102/68 mmHg. She is sweating and complains of nausea. She has no other nursing or medical history to note but informs staff nurse Megan Howell that she is allergic to penicillin. She is scheduled for x-rays and a CT scan of her head at 1600h. An intramuscular injection of a prescribed antiemetic has been given and her father has been informed of her admission to the ward. Ms Stanley is self-employed and works as a telephone interpreter. She is very anxious and is concerned about the care of her 79-year-old diabetic father who is at home alone as well as the impact hospitalisation may have on her work. A diagnosis will not be made until the results of the various examinations are concluded, but a provisional diagnosis of **Ménière's disease** is made. Ms Stanley is nil by mouth and has an intravenous infusion *in situ*.

INTRODUCTION

Vision and hearing allow us to experience the world in which we live, providing the primary means of input for much of what we know about the world. Loss of sight or a disturbance of vision may have a damaging effect on health and wellbeing. The eyes and ears provide pathways for visual and auditory stimuli to reach the brain. Specialised structures within the ear help maintain position sense and equilibrium. Deficits may limit self-care, mobility, safety, independence, communication and relationships with others. The ability to receive and organise information orientates us to our surroundings. These senses allow us to communicate easily, gain access to information and derive pleasure from sights and sounds, and to maintain a safe environment.

Hearing and sight are two of the five special senses. The role and function of the nurse is to ensure that those people who are at risk of injury as result of a hearing or visual defect are kept safe. To offer care effectively, safely and with confidence, an understanding of the anatomy and physiology of the eyes and ears is required.

This chapter discusses conditions affecting vision and hearing as the result of eye and ear disorders. Care focuses on persons with vision and hearing deficits resulting from the disorders presented. The anatomy, physiology and functions of the eyes will be discussed first and then the ears. There are a number of complex-looking words and conditions used when discussing vision. Take your time to learn them and you will become more confident when using these terms and conditions.

ANATOMY, PHYSIOLOGY AND FUNCTIONS OF THE EYES

The eyes are complex structures, containing 70% of the sensory receptors of the body. Each eye is a sphere measuring about 2.5 cm in diameter, surrounded and protected by a bony orbit and cushions of fat. The primary functions are to encode the patterns of light from the environment through photo-receptors and to carry the coded information to the brain. The brain gives meaning to the coded information, so we can make sense of what we see.

EXTRAOCULAR STRUCTURES

These structures are outside the eyeball and they are vital to its protection. They are the eyebrows, eyelids, eyelashes, conjunctiva, lacrimal apparatus and extrinsic eye muscles (Figure 14.1).

The eyebrows shade the eyes and keep perspiration away from them. The eyelids are thin, loose folds of skin covering the anterior (front) eye, protecting the eye from foreign bodies, regulating the entry of light into the eye and distributing tears by blinking. Eyelashes are short hairs projecting from the top and bottom borders of the eyelids. An unexpected touch to the eyelashes initiates the blinking reflex.

The conjunctiva is a thin, transparent membrane lining the inner surfaces of the eyelids and also folds over the front of the eyeball. The palpebral conjunctiva lines the upper and lower eyelids, whereas the bulbar conjunctiva loosely covers the anterior sclera (the white part of the eye). The lacrimal apparatus is composed of the lacrimal gland, the puncta, the lacrimal sac and the nasolacrimal duct. These structures secrete, distribute and drain tears to cleanse and moisten the eye's surface.

The six extrinsic eye muscles control movement of the eye, allowing it to follow a moving object and move precisely. The muscles also help maintain the shape of the eyeball. The cranial nerves control the extrinsic muscles (Figure 14.2).

INTRAOCULAR STRUCTURES

These structures transmit visual images and maintain physiological consistency of the inner eye. These include the sclera and the cornea (forming the outermost coat of the eye, called the fibrous tunic), the iris and the pupil (Figure 14.3).

Sclera and cornea

The white sclera lines the outside of the eyeball, protecting and giving shape to it. The sclera gives way to the cornea over the iris and pupil. This is transparent, avascular (without blood vessels) and sensitive to touch. It forms a window allowing light to enter the eye and is a part of its light-bending apparatus.

Iris

This is a disc of muscle surrounding the pupil, lying between the cornea and the lens; it gives the eye its colour and regulates light entry by controlling pupil size. The pupil is the dark centre of the eye through which light enters: it constricts when bright light enters the eye and when used for near vision; it dilates when light conditions are dim and when the eye is used for far vision. In response to intense light, the pupil constricts rapidly.

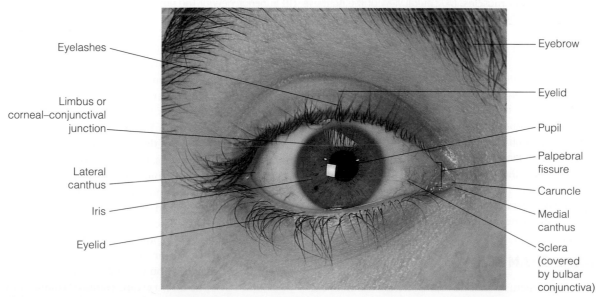

Figure 14.1 Accessory and external structures of the eye.

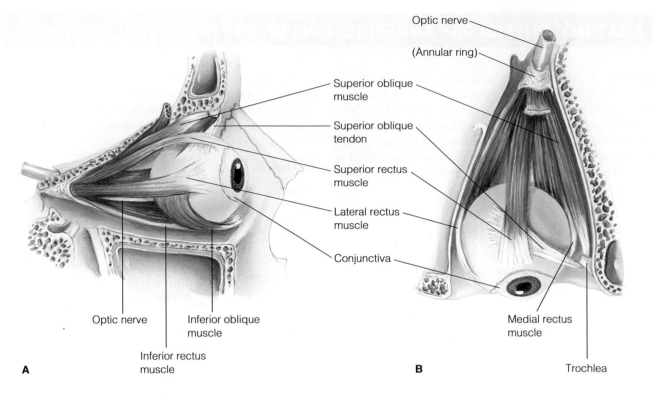

Figure 14.2 Extraocular muscles. (A) Lateral view of the right eye. (B) Superior view of the right eye. (C) Innervation of the extraocular muscles by the cranial nerves.

AQUEOUS FLUID

The anterior cavity is made of the anterior chamber (the space between the cornea and the iris) and the posterior chamber (the space between the iris and the lens). The anterior cavity is filled with aqueous humour, a clear fluid, constantly formed and drained to maintain a relatively constant pressure in the eye. The canal of Schlemm, a network of channels that circles the eye in the angle at the junction of the sclera and the cornea, is the drainage system for fluid moving between the anterior and posterior chambers. Aqueous humour provides nutrients and oxygen to the cornea and the lens.

INTERNAL CHAMBER

The intraocular structures that lie in the internal chamber are the lens, the posterior cavity and vitreous humour, the ciliary body, the uvea and the retina.

The lens is an avascular, transparent structure located directly behind the pupil which changes shape to focus and refract light onto the retina. The posterior cavity lies behind the lens, filled with a clear gelatinous substance, the vitreous humour, which supports the posterior surface of the lens, maintains the position of the retina and transmits light. The uvea is the middle layer of the eyeball. This pigmented layer has three components: the iris, the ciliary body and the choroid.

The retina is the innermost lining of the eyeball and has an outer pigmented layer and an inner neural layer. The outer layer, next to the choroid, serves as the link between visual stimuli and the brain. The transparent inner layer is made up of millions of light receptors in structures called rods and cones. Rods enable vision in dim light as well as peripheral vision. Cones enable vision in bright light and the perception of colour. The optic disc, a cream-coloured round or oval area within the retina, is the point at which the optic nerve enters the eye. The slight depression in the centre of the optic disc is

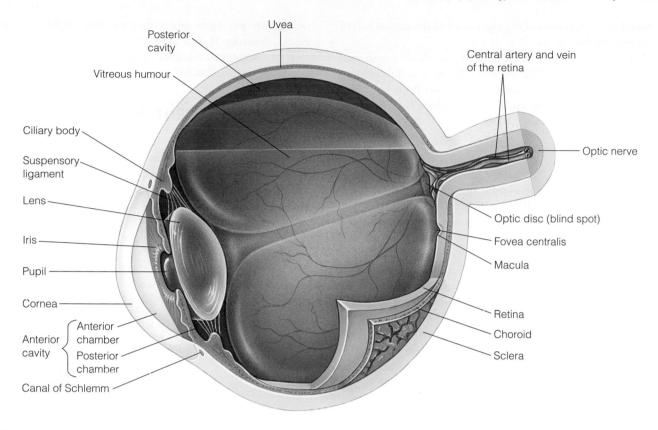

Figure 14.3 Internal structures of the eye.

called the physiologic cup. Located laterally to the optic disc is the macula, a darker area with no visible blood vessels, containing primarily cones.

THE VISUAL PATHWAY

The optic nerves are cranial nerves and meet at the optic chiasma, anterior to the pituitary gland in the brain. At the optic chiasma, axons from the medial half of each retina cross to the opposite side to form pairs of axons from each eye; these continue as the left and right optic tracts (Figure 14.4). The crossing of the axons results in each optic tract carrying information from both eyes; the left carries visual information from the lateral (towards the side) half of the retina of the left eye and the medial (towards the centre) half of the retina of the right eye, whereas the right one carries visual information from the

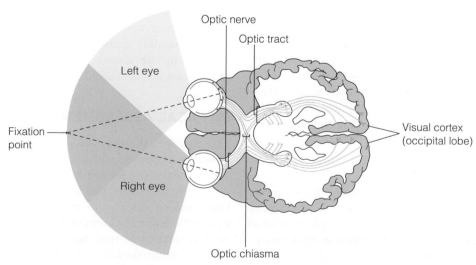

Figure 14.4 The visual fields of the eye and the visual pathways to the brain.

lateral half of the retina of the right eye and the medial half of the retina of the left eye.

The visual fields of each eye overlap considerably, with each eye seeing a slightly different view. Because of this overlap and the crossing of the axons, information from both eyes reaches each side of the visual cortex, which then fuses the information into one image.

REFRACTION

Refraction is the bending of light rays as they pass from one medium to another medium of different optical density. As light rays pass through the eye, they are refracted at several points: as they enter the cornea, as they leave the cornea and enter the aqueous humour, as they enter the lens and as they leave the lens and enter the vitreous humour. At the lens, the light is bent so that it converges at a single point on the retina. This is called **accommodation** (accommodation is to change the focal length of the lens by changing the curvature of the lens). Because the lens is convex, the image projected onto the retina (the real image) is upside down and reversed from left to right. This real image is coded as electric signals sent to the brain. The brain decodes the image so that the person perceives it as it occurs in space.

Now that you have some understanding of how the eyes function and how we see, you can now move on to the important aspect of assessment. Remember to go back to the anatomy and physiology described above at any time should you need clarification.

Assessing the eyes

Structures and functions of the eyes are assessed by findings from diagnostic tests, a health assessment interview to collect subjective data and a physical assessment to collect objective data.

DIAGNOSTIC TESTS

Diagnostic tests are used to support the diagnosis of a specific injury, disease or vision problem; to provide information to identify or modify the appropriate medications or assistive devices used to treat the disease or problem; and to help monitor responses to treatment and care interventions.

GENETIC CONSIDERATIONS

It is important to consider genetic influences on a person's health when conducting a health assessment. Several diseases of the eyes have a genetic component (for example, strabismus and glaucoma). Ask about a family history of glaucoma or blindness during the interview.

Assess for any signs and symptoms that might indicate a genetic disorder. If data are found to indicate genetic risk factors or alterations, ask about genetic testing and refer for appropriate genetic counselling.

HEALTH ASSESSMENT INTERVIEW

This can be conducted during a health screening. It may focus on a chief complaint (such as blurred vision or an eye infection), or it may be part of a total health assessment. If the person has a health problem involving one or both eyes, analyse its onset, characteristics and course, severity, precipitating and relieving factors and any associated symptoms, noting the timing and circumstances, you may ask the person:

● Describe the type of pain you experience in your eyes. When did it begin? How long does it last?

● Have you noticed rings of colour around streetlights at night?

● When did you first notice having difficulty reading the paper?

Be alert to non-verbal behaviours (such as squinting or abnormal eye movements) that suggest problems with eye function. Explore problems such as watery, irritated eyes or changes in vision. Assess the person's use of corrective eyewear or contact lenses. If the person uses eye medications, ask about the type and purpose as well as the frequency and duration of use. Find out about eye trauma, surgery or infections, as well as the date and results of the last eye examination. Ask the person about a medical history of diabetes, hypertension, thyroid disorders, glaucoma, **cataracts** and eye infections. Include questions about a family history of nearsightedness or farsightedness, colour blindness and any other eye or vision disorders.

Interview questions are listed in the Functional Health Pattern Interview box on page 527. Collect information about environmental or work exposure to irritating chemicals, participation in sports or hobbies that pose the risk of eye injury and the use of protective eyewear.

Understanding these important issues associated with anatomy and physiology and assessment will help you to provide care that is safe and effective.

PHYSICAL ASSESSMENT AND VISION

This may be performed as part of a total assessment or separately for persons with known or suspected eye problems. The eyes and vision are primarily assessed through inspection of external structures and assessment of visual fields and visual acuity, extraocular muscle function and internal structures. Before the examination, explain the techniques to decrease anxiety. Normal age-related findings for the older adult are summarised in Table 14.1.

FUNCTIONAL HEALTH PATTERN INTERVIEW The eye

Functional health pattern	Interview questions and leading statements
Health perception–health management	• Describe your vision. Rate it on a scale of 1 to 10, with 10 being excellent vision. Is it the same in both eyes? If not, which eye is better? • Describe your current vision problems. • What eye medications do you use and how often? • Have you ever had eye surgery? • Describe the type of corrective lens that you use. • Describe how you care for your eyes each day. • Do you wear sunglasses when you are outside? • When was your last eye examination? Have you been tested for glaucoma?
Nutritional–metabolic	• Do you have any redness, swelling, watering or dryness of your eyes?
Activity–exercise	• Does your vision problem interfere with your usual activities of living? • Do you wear protective goggles when you take part in activities that increase the risk of injury to your eyes (such as at work or when operating machinery at home)?
Sleep–rest	• Does your eye problem interfere with your ability to rest or sleep (for example, from pain)?
Cognitive–perceptual	• Do you have any difficulty focusing on objects? If so, do you have more difficulty with near objects or far objects? • Is your vision blurry? Do you see halos around lights? Do you see flashes of light or 'floaters'? Do you see double? • Do you have pain in or around your eyes?
Self-perception–self-concept	• Has this problem with your eyes affected how you feel about yourself?
Role–relationships	• How has having this condition affected your relationships with others? • Has having this condition interfered with your ability to work? • Has anyone in your family had problems with eye disease?
Sexuality–reproductive	• Has this condition interfered with your usual sexual activity?
Coping–stress-tolerance	• Has having this condition created stress for you? If so, does your health problem seem to be more difficult when you are stressed? • Have you experienced any kind of stress that makes the condition worse? • Describe what you do when you feel stressed.
Value–belief	• Describe how specific relationships or activities help you cope with this problem. • Describe specific cultural beliefs or practices that affect how you care for and feel about this problem. • Are there any specific treatments that you would not use to treat this problem?

Assessing visual fields

Visual fields are tested to assess the functioning of the macula and peripheral vision. The visual fields of the examiner (which must be intact to perform this assessment) are used as the standard. Sit directly opposite the person at a distance of 45–30 cm. Ask the client to cover one eye with the occluding cover while you cover your own eye opposite to the person (for example, if the person covers the right eye, you cover your left eye). Ask the person to look directly at you. Move the

Table 14.1 Age-related changes in the eye

Age-related change	Significance
The lens: • ↓ Elasticity, decreasing focus and accommodation for near vision (**presbyopia**) • ↑ Density and size, making lens more stiff and opaque • Yellowing of the lens and changes in the retina affect colour perception	Most older adults require corrective lenses to accommodate close and detailed work. Increased opacity leads to the development of cataracts; they increase sensitivity to glare and interfere with night vision.
The cornea: • Fat may be deposited around the periphery and throughout the cornea • ↓ Corneal sensitivity	A partial or complete white circle may form around the cornea (*arcus senilis*). Lipid deposited in the cornea can cause vision to be blurred. Decreased sensitivity increases the risk of injury to the eye.
The pupil: • ↓ Size and responsiveness to light sphincter hardens	Increased light perception threshold and difficulty seeing in dim light or at night means increased light is needed to see adequately.
The retina and visual pathways: • Visual fields narrow • Photoreceptor cells are lost • Rods work less effectively • Macular degeneration is a risk • Depth perception is distorted • Adaptation to dark and light takes longer	Peripheral vision is decreased and central vision may be lost from macular degeneration. Increased risk of falls as a result of changes in depth perception and adaptation to changes in light. Vision progressively declines with age.
The lacrimal apparatus: • ↓ Reabsorption of intraocular fluid • ↓ Production of tears	Increased risk of developing glaucoma; eyes feel and look dry.
The posterior cavity: • Debris and condensation become visible • Vitreous body may pull away from the retina	Vision is blurred and distorted and 'floaters' are often seen by the older person.

penlight from the periphery toward the centre from right to left, above and below, and from the middle of each of these directions. Both you and the person should see the penlight enter the field of vision at the same time. This is done for both eyes.

Eye and vision assessments

VISION ASSESSMENT

This is assessed with an eye chart such as the Snellen chart or the E chart for testing distance vision and the Rosenbaum chart for testing near vision. The Snellen chart contains rows of letters in various sizes, with standardised numbers at the end of each row. If the person is unable to read or does not read English, you can use the E chart (a set of random tumbling Es). The Snellen chart provides a standardised test of visual acuity and is placed 6 m from the subject. The chart consists of a series of symbols.

Cover one eye with an opaque cover. Then ask the person to read each row of letters, moving from the largest letters to the smallest that the person can see. Measure visual acuity in the other eye in the same way, and then assess visual acuity while the person has both eyes uncovered. Test the person who wears corrective lenses with and without the lenses.

EYE MOVEMENT ASSESSMENT

Assess the cardinal fields (there are six cardinal fields testing each muscle of the eye) of vision to gain information about extraocular eye movements. Ask the person to follow a pen or your finger while keeping the head stationary. Move the pen or your finger through the six fields, one at a time, returning to the central starting point before proceeding to the next field (Figure 14.5). *The eyes should move through each field without involuntary movements.*

● Failure of one or both eyes to follow the object in any direction may indicate extraocular muscle weakness or cranial nerve dysfunction.

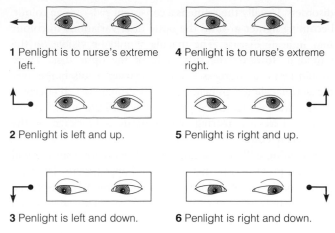

1 Penlight is to nurse's extreme left.

2 Penlight is left and up.

3 Penlight is left and down.

4 Penlight is to nurse's extreme right.

5 Penlight is right and up.

6 Penlight is right and down.

Figure 14.5 The six cardinal fields of vision.

- An involuntary rhythmic movement of the eyes, **nystagmus**, is associated with neurological disorders and some medications.

The cover–uncover test tests for strabismus, a weakening of a muscle that causes one eye to deviate from the other when focusing on an object. Hold a pen or your finger about 30 cm from the eyes and ask the person to focus on that object. Cover one eye and note any movement in the uncovered eye; as you remove the cover, assess for movement in the eye that was just uncovered. Repeat with the other eye.

Assess **convergence**. Ask the person to follow an object as you move it toward the person's eyes. Normally both eyes converge toward the centre.

- Failure to converge equally on an approaching object may indicate a neuromuscular disorder or improper eye alignment.

Assess the corneal light reflex. Direct a light source onto the bridge of the nose from 30 cm–35 cm. Observe for equal reflection of the light from each eye.

- Reflections of the light from different sites on the eyes reveal improper alignment.

PUPILLARY ASSESSMENT

Observe pupil size and equality: these should be of equal size, 3–5 mm.

- Unequal pupils may indicate a severe neurological problem, such as increased intracranial pressure.

Assess direct and consensual pupil response. Ask the person to look straight ahead. Shine a light obliquely into one eye at a time. Observe for constriction of the pupil in the illuminated eye. Test both eyes. To test consensual pupil response, again shine a light obliquely into one eye at a time as the person looks straight ahead. Observe constriction of the pupil in the opposite eye. The normal direct and consensual pupillary response is constriction.

- Failure to respond to light may indicate degeneration of the retina or destruction of the optic nerve.
- A person who has one dilated and unresponsive pupil may have paralysis of the oculomotor nerve.
- Some eye medications may cause unequal dilation, constriction or inequality of pupil size. Morphine and narcotic drugs may cause small, unresponsive pupils, and anticholinergic drugs such as atropine may cause dilated, unresponsive pupils.

Test for accommodation. Hold an object at a distance of about 60 cm from the person. The pupils should dilate. Ask the person to follow the object as you bring it to within a few centimetres of the person's nose. The pupils should constrict and converge as they change focus to follow the object.

- Failure of accommodation along with lack of pupil response to light may signal a neurological problem.
- Lack of response to light with appropriate response to accommodation is often seen in persons with diabetes.

EXTERNAL EYE ASSESSMENT

Inspect the eyelids; these should be the colour of the person's facial skin, without redness, discharge or drooping. The sclera should not be visible. Unusual redness or discharge may indicate an inflammatory state due to trauma, allergies or infection. Drooping of one eyelid, called **ptosis**, may be the result of a stroke, indicate a neuromuscular disorder or be congenital. Unusual widening of the lids may be due to exophthalmos (protrusion of the eyeball). This is associated with hyperthyroid conditions.

Inspect the puncta; this should be free of redness or discharge. Unusual redness or discharge may indicate an inflammation due to trauma, infection or allergies.

Inspect the conjunctiva; this should be clear, moist and smooth, without redness or swelling. Increased redness or discharge may indicate acute **conjunctivitis**. A fold in the conjunctiva, called a *pterygium*, may be seen as a clouded area that extends over the cornea and may interfere with vision if it covers the pupil. Inspect the sclera: this is white in Caucasians; people with darker skin normally have yellow sclera. Unusual redness may indicate an inflammatory state as a result of trauma, allergies or infection. Yellow discoloration of the sclera in persons with fair skin may be seen in liver conditions, such as hepatitis. Bright red areas in the sclera are often subconjunctival haemorrhages, indicating trauma or bleeding disorders. The cornea is normally transparent; dullness, opacities or irregularities may be abnormal. Assess corneal sensitivity. Lightly touch a wisp of cotton to the person's cornea; this should cause a **corneal reflex** (blinking the eye). Failure of the corneal reflex may indicate a neurological disorder.

INTERNAL EYE ASSESSMENT

This is undertaken by a skilled practitioner using the ophthalmoscope, an instrument which allows visualisation of the lens, the vitreous humour and the retina. Inspection can reveal opacity of the pupil by a cataract or a haemorrhage into the vitreous humour. The lens should be clear. A cataract is an opacity of the lens due to ageing, trauma, diabetes or congenital defect. When inspecting the retina there should be no visible haemorrhages, discharge or white patches. If present, these may be the result of diabetes or long-standing hypertension. The optic disc should be round to oval with clear, well-defined borders; loss of shape and increase in the size is seen in papilloedema (optic disc swelling) caused by increased intracranial pressure. Inspection of the blood vessels of the retina can reveal glaucoma as a result of increased intraocular pressure. Hypertension may cause a narrowing of the vein. Engorged veins may occur with diabetes, atherosclerosis and blood

disorders. Usually the retina is a consistent red–orange colour, becoming lighter around the optic disc. Variations in colour may indicate disease. The macula should be visible on the temporal (towards the side) side of the optic disc. There should be no tenderness, excessive tearing or discharge over the lacrimal glands, puncta and nasolacrimal duct. Tenderness or any drainage from the puncta may indicate an infectious process. Excessive tearing may indicate a blockage of the nasolacrimal duct.

Becoming skilled in assessing people with eye disorders will help you provide care that is safe and appropriate. The next section of the chapter considers some common eye disorders. These are only a selection of eye disorders; you are encouraged to consult other sources should you need to.

DISORDERS OF THE EYE

The eye and protective structures may be affected by an acute or chronic condition. Many disorders of the eye are minor and have little or no effect on vision. However, some can result in permanent vision impairment, cause discomfort and may have cosmetic effects. Damage to the cornea can present the greatest risk to vision. Eye surgery or minor trauma can have either temporary or permanent visual impairment.

FAST FACTS

Vision impairment

- In England at 31 March 2008, 153 000 people were registered blind.
- 64% of blind and 66% partially sighted people were aged 75 or over.
- About 2.5% of the UK population have some degree of visual impairment that is not correctable.
- In the UK every day another 100 people begin to lose their sight.

Sources: Denniston and Murray 2008, Centre for Health and Social Care 2008.

Although disorders that affect vision often cannot be prevented or cured, some can be controlled and vision corrected. Regardless of the real threat a disorder poses to vision, there may be anxiety related to a perceived threat.

Consider this . . .

Working with people who have visual impairment means devising ways of communicating effectively with that person, or using tried and tested methods. When providing a meal

for the person, use the plate as a clock face, for example, at 12 o'clock there are peas, at 3 o'clock there is fish. Think about alternative modes of communication needed to be used when assisting a person who is visually impaired.

The person with conjunctivitis

The conjunctiva is vulnerable to inflammation and infection due to its constant exposure to the environment. *Conjunctivitis*, inflammation of the conjunctiva, is the most common eye disease. Its usual cause is infection. These can be transmitted to the eye by direct contact (e.g., hands, towels). Allergens, chemical irritants and exposure to radiant energy such as ultraviolet light from the sun or tanning devices can also lead to this condition. Severity can range from mild irritation with redness and tearing to conjunctival oedema, haemorrhage or a tissue destruction.

Pathophysiology of conjunctivitis

Infectious conjunctivitis may be bacterial, viral or fungal. Bacterial conjunctivitis is highly contagious, and often is caused by the organisms *Staphylococcus* and *Haemophilus*. Systemic infections affecting the eyes include herpes simplex and other viral infections. Contact with genital secretions infected with *Gonococcus* (the organism responsible for gonorrhoea) can cause gonococcal conjunctivitis that can lead to corneal perforation.

Consider this . . .

How can the process of bereavement (losing a loved one) and losing a significant amount of sight be compared? You may have considered:

- disbelief;
- bargaining;
- anger, sadness, despair and pain;
- acceptance;
- feeling guiltily or experiencing shame for being envious of others;
- social stigma when some people may be nasty, unkind, patronising, over-protective, unhelpful and thoughtless.

Signs and symptoms of conjunctivitis

Signs and symptoms of conjunctivitis include:

- redness and itching;
- feelings of scratching or burning;
- photophobia may occur;
- tearing and discharge – this may be watery, purulent (pus) or mucoid (mucus), depending on the cause;
- associated signs and symptoms such as sore throat, fever, malaise and swollen lymph nodes near the ears.

Pain is uncommon.

Scarring of the conjunctival lining of the lid causes entropion (eyelid turns inwards). The lashes abrade the cornea, causing ulceration and scarring. The scarred cornea is opaque, causing loss of vision.

INTERDISCIPLINARY CARE FOR CONJUNCTIVITIS

Care focuses on establishing an accurate diagnosis and prompt treatment.

Diagnosis

Accurate diagnosis is especially important, because other potentially vision-threatening conditions, such as acute uveitis

or acute angle-closure glaucoma, can also cause a red eye (Table 14.2). Diagnostic procedures may include:

- *Culture and sensitivity* of exudates to determine presence of infection and identifing infecting organism.
- *Fluorescein stain* with slit-lamp examination to identify corneal ulcerations or abrasions.
- *Conjunctival scrapings* are examined microscopically or cultured to identify the organisms.

Additional laboratory testing such as blood counts or antibody titres may be used to identify underlying infectious or auto-immune processes.

Medication

Conjunctivitis is treated with antibiotic, antiviral or anti-inflammatory drugs as appropriate. Topical anti-infectives applied as eyedrops or ointment may include erythromycin, gentamicin, penicillin, bacitracin, amphotericin B or idoxuridine. For severe infections or cellulitis, anti-infectives may be administered by subconjunctival injection or systemic intravenous infusion. Antihistamines are used to minimise symptoms of conjunctivitis when there is an allergic response.

Complementary therapies

Frequent eye irrigations may be ordered to remove the copious purulent discharge. Soaking the lids with warm saline compresses prior to cleansing promotes comfort and facilitates the removal of crusts and exudate.

NURSING CARE FOR CONJUNCTIVITIS

The nursing role is primarily one of education to prevent the disorder and prevent its spread when it does occur.

Health promotion

Education is a vital strategy for preventing conjunctivitis. Teach all persons about proper eye care, including the importance of

Table 14.2 Possible causes of acute red eye

	Acute conjunctivitis	Corneal trauma or infection	Acute uveitis	Acute angle-closure glaucoma
Incidence	Very common	Common	Common	Rare
Pain	Mild	Moderate to severe	Moderate	Severe
Vision	Normal	Blurred	Blurred	Markedly blurred
Discharge	May be copious	Watery, may be purulent	None	None
Conjunctival erythema	Diffuse	Primarily around cornea	Primarily around cornea	Primarily around cornea
Cornea	Clear	Depends on cause	Usually clear	Cloudy
Pupils	Normal size, response to light	Normal size, response to light	Small, minimal response to light	Moderately dilated, fixed

not sharing towels, makeup or contact lenses, and avoiding rubbing or scratching the eyes. Instruct to avoid using old eye makeup, which can cause eye infections. Teach contact lens users appropriate care.

Assessment

+ *Health history:* presence of redness, discomfort, tearing, photophobia and drainage; symptom onset; care measures; use of contact lenses; recent travel; allergies; previous history of conjunctivitis; presence of any chronic diseases.
+ *Physical assessment:* visual acuity; inspect eyelids, conjunctiva, sclera and cornea; vital signs including temperature.

Nursing diagnoses and interventions

Care focuses on preventing complications from the disorder. The priority nursing diagnoses include risk for infection and risk of altered vision.

Risk for infection

Acute conjunctivitis is highly contagious. Most persons experience no more than discomfort, but the infection carries a risk for scarring and damage to the cornea. Preventing spread of infection is a vital nursing role.

+ Teach to wash hands thoroughly before instilling eye medications. Instruct to avoid touching or rubbing eyes. Advise to use a new, clean cotton-tipped swab or cotton ball for cleaning each eye.
+ Teach to instil prescribed eyedrops as ordered.
+ Discuss the importance of avoiding contact lens use until the infectious process has cleared and treatment completed.

IN PRACTICE

Contact lens care

● Wash hands before handling contact lenses.
● Keep storage case clean.
● Remove lenses before sleep, cleaning and storing as recommended by manufacturer.
● Use cleaning and wetting solutions recommended by eye care professional or lens manufacturer. Do not use water or home-made solutions for wetting or cleaning lenses.
● If eye redness, tearing, vision loss or pain occurs, remove lenses, contact eye care professional as soon as possible.
● Do not share contact lenses.

Risk for disturbed sensory perception

Conjunctivitis can disrupt the integrity or clarity of the cornea. Corneal damage can impair visual acuity.

+ Assess vision with and without corrective lenses, providing a baseline to evaluate possible changes in vision resulting from infection.
+ Advise the person to avoid activities requiring high visual acuity until the infection has cleared.
+ Suggest that the person use dark sunglasses with appropriate UV protection when out of doors, even on cloudy days.

COMMUNITY-BASED CARE

People with conjunctivitis are usually cared for in the community, reinforcing the need for effective teaching for home care. Emphasise ways to prevent transmission of infection. If unable to administer eye medications, involve the family in teaching. Include:

● Safety and medical asepsis when cleansing the eye
● Instillation of prescribed eyedrops and ointments
● Comfort measures such as reducing lighting intensity and wearing sunglasses
● Avoidance of activities such as excessive reading while eye is inflamed.

The person with a corneal disorder

The clear cornea allows light rays to enter the eye and transmits images onto the retina, helping to focus light on the retina and protect the internal structures. The cornea can be affected by a variety of disorders, including infection and trauma. The cornea heals quickly after minor injuries or abrasions; injury to its deeper layers can delay healing or result in scarring.

Refractive errors

Refractive errors, resulting from an abnormal curvature of the cornea or an altered shape of the eyeball, are the most common problem affecting visual acuity. Those with normal

FAST FACTS

Myopia

● Around five million people in the UK have myopia.
● 200 000 will have high degree myopia.
● Myopia can be associated with cataract formation, retinal detachment and glaucoma.
● Myopia can run in families (there is a genetic component).

Source: RNIB 2008.

vision see near and far objects clearly because light rays focus directly on the retina. In **myopia** (nearsightedness) the curvature of the cornea is excessive or the eyeball is elongated, causing the image to focus in front of the retina instead of on it. Objects in close range are seen clearly and those at a distance are blurred. The eyeball is too short in **hyperopia** (farsightedness), causing the image to focus behind the retina, objects clearer at a distance than those close to them.

Astigmatism develops due to an irregular or abnormal curvature of the cornea. Instead of the round, even curvature of the normal cornea, the cornea curves more in one direction than the other in astigmatism, resembling the back of a spoon. As a result, light rays focus on more than one area of the retina, distorting both near and distance vision.

Corneal ulcer

This may be caused by infection, exposure trauma or the misuse of contact lenses and bacterial infection following trauma or contact lens overuse. Herpes viruses are a leading cause of ulcerative corneal disease. Persons who are immunosuppressed are at particular risk for developing corneal ulcers due to infection.

In corneal ulceration, a portion of the epithelium and/or stroma is destroyed. This may be superficial or deep, penetrating underlying layers, posing a risk of perforation. Fibrous tissue may form during healing, causing scarring and opacity of the cornea. Perforation can lead to infection of deeper eye structures or extrusion of eye contents and loss of vision.

INTERDISCIPLINARY CARE FOR CORNEAL DISORDERS

Focus is on establishing an accurate diagnosis and ensuring prompt treatment. History and physical assessment are key in diagnosing.

Eye disorders can be treated in the community, but the person with a severe corneal infection or ulcer may require hospitalisation. Corneal ulcers are medical emergencies, requiring prompt referral to an ophthalmologist. Pressure dressings may be applied to both eyes for comfort and to reduce the risk of perforation and loss of eye contents.

Diagnosis

Visual acuity is tested. The following tests may be needed:

- *Fluorescein stain* with slit-lamp examination allows visualisation of any corneal ulcerations or abrasions.
- *Conjunctival* or *ulcer scrapings* are examined microscopically or cultured to identify the organisms.

Additional laboratory testing such as blood counts or antibody titres may be used to identify any underlying infectious or autoimmune processes.

Medication

Infectious processes are treated with antibiotic or antiviral therapy as appropriate. Topical anti-infectives may include erythromycin, gentamicin, penicillin, bacitracin, amphotericin B or idoxuridine. For severe infections, central ulcers or cellulitis, anti-infectives may be administered by subconjunctival injection and/or systemic intravenous infusion.

Corrective lenses

Corrective lenses, eyeglasses or contact lenses, are generally prescribed to restore visual acuity for persons with refractive errors such as myopia, hyperopia and astigmatism. Specially fitted contact lenses to reduce vision distortion are ordered for persons with keratoconus. Contact lenses are a risk factor for corneal infection and ulcers, and teaching appropriate care is vital.

Laser eye surgery

This is performed to correct refractive errors such as myopia, hyperopia and astigmatism. A laser is used to permanently change the shape of the cornea, so that the need to use corrective lenses is reduced or eliminated. Several surgical procedures are available. These reshape the cornea using laser technology to remove a thin layer of epithelial cells or to shrink and reshape the cornea. Candidates for laser surgery should be in good health and have adequate corneal thickness such that perforation is not a risk.

Following surgery, persons may experience a temporary loss of contrast sharpness (images do not appear as crisp), over- or undercorrection of visual acuity, dry eyes or temporarily decreased night vision with halos, glare and starbursts.

Phototherapeutic keratectomy (PTK) provides an alternative to corneal transplant in treating corneal dystrophies, scars and some infections. Diseased corneal tissue is vaporised and surface irregularities corrected with little trauma to surrounding tissue. Healing occurs rapidly. See page 534 for nursing care of the person undergoing eye surgery.

NURSING CARE FOR CORNEAL DISORDERS

Caring for persons with corneal disorders may involve direct care, but more often focuses on prevention and education.

Health promotion

Education is a vital strategy for preventing many corneal disorders. Teach all persons about proper eye care, including the importance of not sharing towels and makeup and avoiding rubbing or scratching the eyes as well as preventing trauma and infection. Teach contact lens users appropriate care and cleaning techniques and periodic removal of lenses. Lenses should be removed at night, despite manufacturers claiming it is safe to wear them while sleeping. Emphasise the need to follow cleaning instructions precisely, avoiding bacterial contamination of lenses and possible corneal infection.

Assessment

Collect the following data through history and physical examination. Additional focused assessments are described with the interventions below.

✦ *Health history*: risk factors; presence of redness, discomfort, tearing, photophobia, oedema and drainage; symptom onset; presence of pain; effect on vision.

✦ *Physical assessment*: visual acuity; inspect external eye, including conjunctiva, sclera and cornea; extraocular movements.

Nursing diagnoses and interventions

Care focuses primarily on preventing complications and promoting healing. The priority nursing diagnoses include risk of altered vision, pain and risk for injury.

Risk for disturbed sensory perception: visual

Disorders affecting the cornea may disrupt its integrity or clarity; the cornea plays a vital role in focusing light on the retina, and corneal damage can affect vision. Mitigating against risk will be similar to those issues discussed earlier concerning conjunctivitis and include:

✦ Assess vision with and without corrective lenses.

✦ Advise concerning handwashing and eye care.

✦ Proper care of contact lenses specific to the type of lens used.

✦ Teach the importance of using eye protection when engaging in potentially dangerous activities.

✦ If corneal perforation is suspected, place in the supine position, close the eye and cover it with a dry, sterile dressing. Notify the doctor immediately. Corneal perforation may occur without warning in persons with corneal ulcers with a high risk for loss of eye contents. Emergency measures are taken to reduce intraocular pressure and maintain eye integrity to preserve vision.

NURSING CARE PLAN The person having eye surgery

Review Chapter 1 for routine pre- and post-operative care.

Pre-operative care

✦ Assess visual acuity of the non-operative eye prior to surgery. The person with limited vision in the non-operative eye may need additional attention and assistance post-operatively to ensure safety.

✦ Assess the person's support systems.

✦ Teach measures to prevent eye injury post-operatively: avoid vomiting, straining at stool, coughing, sneezing, lifting more than 2.5 kg and bending over at the waist as this can temporarily increase intraocular pressure.

✦ Remove all eye makeup and contact lenses or glasses prior to surgery. Store safely and make them readily available to the person on return from surgery.

✦ Administer pre-operative medications as prescribed. Mydriatic (pupil-dilating) or cycloplegic (ciliary-paralytic) drops. Prescribed drops to lower intraocular pressure may be required pre-operatively.

Post-operative care

✦ Assess eye dressing for bleeding or drainage.

✦ Maintain the eye patch or shield in place; this helps prevent inadvertent injury to the operative site.

✦ Nurse in the recovery position on the unaffected side. Elevating the head of the bed and lying on the unaffected side reduces intraocular pressure in the affected eye.

✦ Remind the person to avoid coughing, sneezing or straining as needed.

✦ Assess and medicate as necessary for complaints of pain, aching or a scratchy sensation in affected eye. Immediately report complaints of sudden, sharp eye pain as this may indicate haemorrhage or another ocular emergency.

✦ Assess for potential complications:
   a. Haemorrhage with blood in the anterior chamber
   b. Flashes of light, floaters or the sensation of a curtain being drawn over the eye
   c. Cloudy appearance to the cornea

Evidence of complications or unusual complaints should be reported at once to prevent loss of sight.

✦ Approach the person on the unaffected side, facilitating eye contact and communication.

✦ Place personal articles and the call bell within easy reach.

✦ Administer all medications as prescribed.

✦ Prevent vomiting to maintain normal intraocular pressures; administer antiemetic medication as needed.

Health education for the person and family

✦ Teach about home care:
   a. How to instil eyedrops correctly and to follow the prescription
   b. How and when to use the eyepatch and eyeshield
   c. The importance of avoiding scratching, rubbing, touching or squeezing the affected eye

d. Measures to avoid constipation and straining
e. Activity limitations, if needed
f. Symptoms to report, including eye pain or pressure, redness or cloudiness, drainage, decreased vision, floaters or flashes of light, or halos around bright objects
g. The need to wear sunglasses with side shields when outdoors.

+ Remind the person that vision may not stabilise for several weeks following surgery. New corrective lenses, if necessary, are not prescribed until vision has stabilised.
+ Emphasise the importance of keeping recommended follow-up appointments. Provide referral to the community nursing services for assistance with home care after discharge.

Risk for acute pain

The cornea is extremely sensitive; corneal disorders frequently cause significant pain, and this increases the stress response, interfering with rest and potentially impairing healing.

+ Assess pain, using verbal and non-verbal cues.
+ Administer prescribed analgesia.
+ Patch both eyes if necessary, reducing eye movement and irritation of the affected eye.
+ Teach to apply warm compresses, reducing inflammation and pain, promoting comfort.
+ Advise to use dark sunglasses with appropriate UV protection when out of doors, even on cloudy days.
+ Teach to instil prescribed eyedrops as ordered.

Risk for injury

Corneal transplantation has an increased risk for injury for several reasons. The eye on which surgery was performed is patched for 24 hours after surgery, changing depth perception and increasing the risk for falls. Increased intraocular pressure or trauma to the eye may damage the graft, resulting in graft rejection.

PRACTICE ALERT

Administer prescribed antiemetics and stool softeners post-operatively to prevent vomiting and straining at stool, activities that increase intraocular pressure, damaging suture lines.

The person with eye trauma

Millions of eye injuries occur each year. Many are minor, but without timely and appropriate intervention, even a minor injury can threaten vision. All eye injuries should be considered medical emergencies requiring immediate evaluation and intervention.

Pathophysiology and signs and symptoms of eye trauma

Any part of the eye, especially the exposed parts, may be affected by trauma. Foreign bodies, abrasions and lacerations are common types of eye injury. Traumatic injury may also be due to burns, penetrating objects or blunt force.

Hyphema, bleeding into the anterior chamber, is a potential result of blunt eye trauma. When the highly vascular uveal tract is disrupted by blunt force, haemorrhage may result, filling the anterior chamber. The person complains of eye pain, decreased visual acuity and seeing a reddish tint. Blood is visible in the anterior chamber.

An orbital blowout fracture is another result of blunt eye trauma. Any part of the orbit may be fractured, but the ethmoid bone on the orbital floor is the most likely site. Orbital contents, including fat, muscles and the eye itself, may herniate through the fracture into the underlying maxillary sinus. The person complains of *diplopia* (double vision), pain with upward movement of the affected eye and decreased sensation on the affected cheek. The eye appears sunken and has limited movement on examination.

INTERDISCIPLINARY CARE FOR EYE TRAUMA

A thorough examination is conducted to determine the type and extent of the injury. Unless immediate treatment is indicated, as with a chemical burn, vision is evaluated initially. If the person normally wears corrective lenses, vision assessment is performed while glasses are worn. Eye movement is evaluated unless a penetrating object is present, and the lid and eye are inspected for lacerations. Inspection is performed using strong light and magnification with a headband loupe or slit lamp. Topical anaesthesia may be used prior to inspection if eye pain and photophobia make eye opening difficult. Fluorescein staining can help identify foreign bodies and abrasions. Any conjunctival or anterior chamber haemorrhage is noted, and ophthalmoscopic examination is used to detect haemorrhage or trauma to the interior chamber.

Facial x-rays and CT scans are used to identify orbital fractures or foreign bodies within the globe. Ultrasonography may be employed to detect a detached retina or vitreous haemorrhage.

Foreign bodies are removed using irrigation, a sterile cotton-tipped applicator or other instrument. Antibiotic ointment, such as erythromycin, is applied after their removal. In corneal abrasions and large foreign bodies in the eye, an eyepatch is applied firmly after the antibiotic application to keep the eye closed for approximately 24 hours.

The immediate priority of care with chemical burns is flushing the affected eye with copious amounts of fluid. Normal saline is preferred; however, water may be used if saline is not available. A special contact lens irrigating unit or a bottle of irrigant with intravenous tubing held to flush all eye surfaces may be useful. The eyelid is everted to identify and remove material from the conjunctival sac. A topical anaesthetic drops helps relieve pain, making inspection and irrigation easier. During irrigation, fluid is directed from the inner canthus to the outer. Tipping the head slightly to the affected side prevents contamination of the unaffected eye. Irrigation is continued until the pH of the eye is normal (in the range 7.2–7.4). Following irrigation, a topical antibiotic ointment is applied.

Penetrating wounds generally require surgical intervention by an ophthalmic surgeon. Immediate care focuses on relieving pain and protecting the eye from further injury. To prevent loss of intraocular contents, do not place pressure on the eye itself, but gently cover with sterile gauze or an eye pad. If a foreign body is embedded in or sticking out of the eye, do not attempt to remove it; it should be immobilised and the eye protected with a metal eyeshield until an ophthalmologist can see the person. Patching the unaffected eye decreases ocular movement. Pain is managed using narcotic analgesics; sedation may also be required as well as antiemetic medications to prevent vomiting. Intravenous antibiotics are prescribed to prevent infection.

Interventions for the person with blunt trauma to the eye include placing the person on bedrest and protecting the eye from further injury with an eyeshield. The unaffected eye is also patched minimising eye movement. A carbonic anhydrase inhibitor such as acetazolamide may be prescribed to reduce intraocular pressure.

NURSING CARE FOR EYE TRAUMA

The nursing role involves educating people about the prevention of injuries and providing direct care to the person. People with eye injury will be cared for and treated in the A&E department, the minor injuries clinic or other primary care facilities. Ocular injuries require immediate interventions simultaneously with assessment and accurate history collection.

The person with cataracts

A cataract is an opacification (clouding) of the lens. This opacification can significantly interfere with light transmission to the retina and the ability to perceive images clearly.

Incidence and risk factors for cataracts

Cataracts are a common and significant cause of visual deficits. By age 80, nearly half of the population is affected. In many cases, cataract does not significantly impair vision. Cataract affects slightly more women than men, and more white people than people of colour.

FAST FACTS

Cataracts

- 16 million people globally have cataracts; it is the most common cause of reversible loss of useful vision.
- Over 200 000 cataracts are removed in the UK per year.
- 492 cases per 100 000 occur in those who are aged over 80 years.

Source: Desai *et al*. 1999.

Age is the greatest single risk factor; genetics may contribute to the risk, although the link is unclear. Environmental and lifestyle factors play a role: long-term exposure to sunlight (UV-B rays) contributes; cigarette smoking and heavy alcohol consumption are associated with earlier cataract development. Senile cataracts are the most common, but cataracts may also be congenital or acquired in origin. Eye trauma, including injury to the lens capsule by a foreign body, blunt trauma or exposure to heat or radiation, can precipitate cataract formation. Diabetes mellitus is associated with earlier development of cataracts, especially when blood glucose level is not controlled at or near normal levels. Systemic or inhaled corticosteroids, chlorpromazine and busulfan also prompt the formation of cataracts.

Pathophysiology of cataracts

As the lens ages, its fibres and proteins change and degenerate; proteins clump, clouding the lens and reducing light transmission to the retina. This generally begins at the periphery of the lens, gradually spreading to involve the central portion. As the cataract continues to develop, the entire lens may become opaque. When only a portion of the lens is affected, the cataract is called immature. A mature cataract is opacity of the entire lens. In addition to clouding, the lens may discolour over time, affecting the ability to accurately discriminate colours.

Signs and symptoms of cataracts

Cataracts tend to occur bilaterally unless related to eye trauma. Fortunately, they tend to develop at different rates, one cataract generally maturing more rapidly than the other. As a cataract interferes with light transmission through the lens, visual acuity decreases, affecting both close and distance vision. Light rays are scattered as they pass through the lens, causing complaints of glare and affecting the ability to adjust between light and dark environments. Colour discrimination is impaired, particularly in the blue to purple range. When the cataract is mature, the pupil may appear cloudy grey or white rather than black.

INTERDISCIPLINARY CARE FOR CATARACTS

The diagnosis is made based on the history and eye examination. Ophthalmoscopic examination confirms diagnosis by identifying the location and extent of a cataract.

Surgery

Surgical removal is the only treatment used at this time for cataracts; no medical treatment is available to prevent or treat them. Surgery is only performed on one eye at a time. If an intraocular lens (an artificial lens to replace the diseased lens) is to be implanted during surgery, measurements are needed. Surgery is indicated when the cataract has developed to the point that vision and activities of living are affected. A mature cataract may also be removed when it causes a secondary condition such as glaucoma or uveitis.

Surgery is usually performed as an out-patient case, using local anaesthesia. If general anaesthesia is needed, hospitalisation may be required.

Using an operating microscope, a small incision is made at the edge of the cornea and extracts the lens intact or via emulsification and aspiration. Ultrasound vibrations break the lens material into fragments (phacoemulsification), which are then suctioned out of the eye.

After removal of the lens, the eye can no longer focus light on the retina and vision is seriously affected. Usually an intraocular lens is implanted at the time of surgery, rapidly restoring binocular vision and depth perception. Following extracapsular lens removal, the intraocular lens is positioned in the posterior capsule behind the iris (see Figure 14.6).

If an intraocular lens cannot be implanted, convex corrective glasses or contact lenses may be used to correct vision. Although contact lenses can provide excellent vision correction following cataract surgery, they may be difficult for some persons to adapt to or manipulate. The person with a pre-existing refractive error may continue to require corrective lenses and often needs a prescriptive change after surgery.

Complications are unusual and occur in less than 1% of the surgeries. Loss of vitreous humour, corneal oedema, increased intraocular pressure, haemorrhage, inflammation or infection, retinal detachment and displacement of the implanted lens are potential complications.

NURSING CARE FOR CATARACTS

Health promotion

Advise all persons about the importance of protecting the eyes from UVB rays by wearing eye protection during activities such as welding and sunglasses with UVB protection when out of doors. Discuss the link between heavy smoking and cataract development.

Assessment

+ *Health history:* effect of vision changes on lifestyle and activities (e.g., ability to read, watch television, participate in work and recreational activities); history of smoking, diabetes, use of prescription drugs associated with increased risk of cataract.
+ *Physical examination:* general health; visual acuity in each eye; presence of red reflex.

Nursing diagnoses and interventions

The person with cataracts has few physical care nursing needs. Patient advocacy, psychological and emotional support and

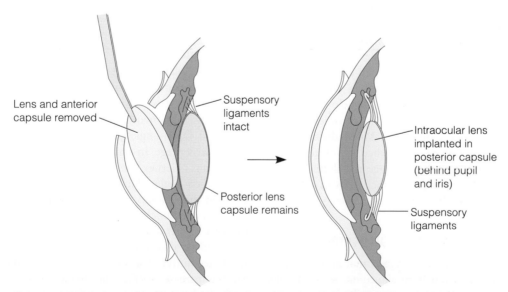

Figure 14.6 Extracapsular cataract extraction with removal of the lens and anterior capsule, leaving the posterior capsule intact. The intraocular lens is implanted within the posterior capsule.

teaching/learning needs are typically of higher priority for these persons.

Risk for decisional conflict: cataract removal

With the initial diagnosis of cataract, the nurse becomes an important information resource for the person.

+ Explain the non-emergent nature of the condition and help the person determine the extent to which the cataract is affecting daily life, helping the person decide when to proceed with surgery.

+ Attend to verbalised concerns about surgery and its outcome. Address questions factually and completely. Fear of blindness is second only to fear of cancer for many; therefore, a caring, understanding attitude can help the person deal with this fear.

Risk for ineffective therapeutic regimen management

+ Assess for factors that may interfere with the ability to provide self-care post-operatively; for example, arthritis affecting the ability to administer eyedrops which may indicate the need to include a family member in teaching.

+ Assess for other care needs that may be impacted by vision changes in the early post-operative period.

The person with glaucoma

Glaucoma is usually a primary condition without an identified cause. Primary glaucoma is most common in those over 60 years, but may also be congenital. Secondary glaucoma can develop as a result of infection or inflammation of the eye, cataract, tumour, haemorrhage or eye trauma.

The condition is characterised by *optic neuropathy* (complications associated with the optic nerve) with gradual loss of peripheral vision and increased intraocular pressure. Usually there are no signs and symptoms other than narrowing of the visual field, occurring so gradually that it often goes unnoticed until late in the disease process. It might be helpful if you go back to the beginning of the chapter and consider the case study related to glaucoma. Think about Mr Madison's health history and his medication regimen when trying to understand the issues associated with glaucoma. You should also be considering the psychosocial aspects associated with glaucoma and how Mr Madison may be feeling.

Incidence and risk factors for glaucoma

The World Health Organization suggests that approximately 12.5 million people are blind from glaucoma, with the total number affected being in the region of 66 million. Nearly 10% of UK blindness registrations are attributed to glaucoma and about 2% of people older than 40 years have *chronic open angle*

glaucoma (damage to the optic nerve caused by increased pressure in the eye). This figure rises to almost 10% in those who are older than 75 years. With changes in population demographics, the number of individuals who are affected by glaucoma will rise (NICE 2009a).

When an individual is diagnosed, they will require lifelong monitoring so that their condition can be controlled and potential complications detected early. When vision has been lost it cannot be re-established; therefore, disease control with prevention of complications is essential.

Pathophysiology of glaucoma

Aqueous humour, a thick fluid, occupies both the anterior and posterior chambers. The normal intraocular pressure of approximately 12–15 mmHg is maintained by a balance between the production of aqueous humour in the ciliary body, its flow through the pupil from the posterior to the anterior chamber and its outflow or absorption through the trabecular meshwork and canal of Schlemm. When this balance is disrupted, the intraocular pressure increases. Although the exact relationship is unclear, it appears that increased intraocular pressure injures the optic nerve. Axons in the periphery of the optic disc are damaged first. As optic fibres are destroyed, the rim of the optic disc shrinks, and the normal depression in its centre (the *optic cup*) becomes larger and deeper. These changes to the optic disc are visible before visual field changes can be detected (Porth 2009). As the disease progresses, there is a painless, progressive narrowing of the visual field and eventual blindness. Vision loss is often significant before the person seeks treatment and glaucoma is diagnosed.

Primary glaucoma has two major forms: open-angle glaucoma and angle-closure glaucoma. Both terms refer to the angle formed at the point where the iris meets the cornea in the eye's anterior chamber. Forms of primary glaucoma are compared in Table 14.3.

Open-angle glaucoma

Open-angle glaucoma, often called chronic simple glaucoma, is the most common, accounting for approximately 90% of all glaucoma. Its cause is unknown; it is thought to have a hereditary component, but no clear inheritance pattern can be identified. Open-angle glaucoma occurs more frequently and at an earlier age in those with African ancestry than in Caucasians (Tierney *et al.* 2005, RNIB 2009).

In open-angle glaucoma, the anterior chamber angle between the iris and cornea is normal (Figure 14.7), hence the term *open angle*. However, the flow of aqueous humour through the trabecular meshwork and into the canal of Schlemm is relatively obstructed; the cause is unknown. Restricted outflow leads to an increased amount of fluid in the eye and increased intraocular pressure. Open-angle glaucoma tends to be a chronic, gradually progressive disease. The trabecular meshwork increasingly inhibits the outflow of aqueous humour, and the intraocular pressure gradually

Table 14.3 A comparison of open-angle and angle-closure glaucoma

	Open-angle glaucoma	Angle-closure glaucoma
Incidence	• Common • Accounts for 90% of all cases of glaucoma	• Uncommon
Risk factors	• Over age 35 • Genetic link • African ancestry	• Narrow anterior chamber angle • Ageing • Asian ancestry
Pathophysiology	• Impaired aqueous outflow through the canal of Schlemm • Cause unknown • Gradual, consistent increase in intraocular pressure • Usually bilateral	• Pupil dilation or lens accommodation causes already narrowed angle to close, blocking aqueous outflow • Rapid rise in intraocular pressure • Usually unilateral
Signs and symptoms	• No initial signs and symptoms • Frequent lens changes in glasses • Impaired dark adaptation • Halos around lights • Gradual reduction of visual fields with preservation of central vision until late in the disease • Mild to severe increased intraocular pressure	• Abrupt onset of eye pain, headache • Decreased visual acuity • Nausea and vomiting • Reddened conjunctiva • Cloudy cornea • Fixed pupil • Rapid, significant increase in intraocular pressure
Management	• Topical medications such as miotics, beta-blockers, prostaglandin analogues • Carbonic anhydrase inhibitors • Laser trabeculoplasty, trabeculectomy	• Topical miotics or beta-blockers • Systemic osmotic agents, carbonic anhydrase inhibitors • Laser iridotomy or peripheral iridectomy

increases. The result is optic nerve degeneration, leading to gradual loss of vision.

Open-angle glaucoma typically affects both eyes, although the pressures and progression may not be symmetric. It is painless, with gradual loss of visual fields (Kasper *et al.* 2005).

Angle-closure glaucoma

Acute angle-closure (also called narrow-angle or closed-angle) glaucoma is a less common form of primary glaucoma, accounting for approximately 5–10% of all cases of glaucoma (Porth 2009). Approximately 1% of people over the age of 35 have narrowed anterior chamber angles; the incidence is higher in older adults and in people of Far Eastern, Asian ancestry (Porth 2009).

Narrowing of the anterior chamber angle occurs because of corneal flattening or bulging of the iris into the anterior chamber. When the lens thickens during accommodation or the iris thickens during pupil dilation, this angle can close completely. Closure of the angle blocks the outflow of aqueous humour through the trabecular meshwork and canal of Schlemm, and the intraocular pressure rises abruptly. This increase in intraocular pressure damages the neurones of the retina and the optic nerve, leading to a rapid and permanent loss of vision if not treated promptly.

Episodes of angle-closure glaucoma are typically unilateral. However, a history of angle-closure glaucoma of one eye increases the risk that it will occur in the other eye.

Because of the effect of pupil dilation on aqueous outflow in angle-closure glaucoma, episodes often occur in association with darkness, emotional upset or other factors that cause the pupil to dilate. Intermittent episodes can last several hours before having a more typical prolonged attack of angle-closure glaucoma. For persons with a history of the condition, it is vital to avoid medications such as atropine and other anti-cholinergics, which have a mydriatic or pupil-dilating effect.

INTERDISCIPLINARY CARE FOR GLAUCOMA

Glaucoma cannot be predicted, prevented or cured, but in most cases it can be controlled and vision preserved if diagnosed early. The most prevalent type of glaucoma, open-angle glaucoma, has few symptoms, and routine eye examinations are recommended for early detection. Measurement of intraocular pressure, fundoscopy to assess the optic disc and visual field testing are used for diagnosis and monitoring of treatment effectiveness.

Diagnosis

The following diagnostic studies are used to detect and evaluate for the presence, severity, type and effects of glaucoma.

● *Tonometry* indirectly measures intraocular pressure. Routine tonometry screening is recommended for those over the age of 60. A single elevated pressure reading does not warrant a diagnosis of glaucoma; variations occur throughout the day.

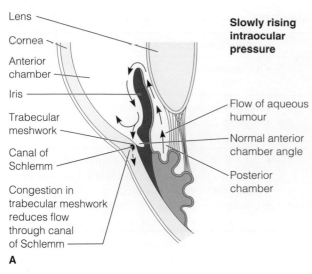

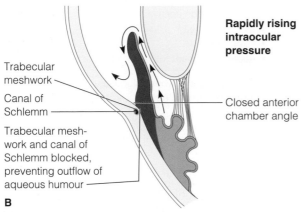

Figure 14.7 Forms of primary adult glaucoma. **(A)** In chronic open-angle glaucoma, the anterior chamber angle remains open, but drainage of the aqueous humour through the canal of Schlemm is impaired. **(B)** In acute angle-closure glaucoma, the angle of the iris and anterior chamber narrows, obstructing the outflow of aqueous humour.

- *Fundoscopy* (visual inspection of the optic fundus using an ophthalmoscope) identifies pallor and an increase in the size and depth of the optic cup on the optic disc.
- *Gonioscopy* uses a gonioscope to measure the depth of the anterior chamber. This test differentiates open-angle from angle-closure glaucoma.
- *Visual field testing* identifies the degree of central visual field narrowing and peripheral vision loss.

Medication

Although medications cannot cure glaucoma, many people with open-angle glaucoma can control intraocular pressure and preserve vision indefinitely with medications. Medications are used alone or in combination with the timing and dosage individually determined by pressure measurements. The primary pharmacological agents used to treat glaucoma are topical beta-adrenergic blocking agents, adrenergics (mydriatics),

prostaglandin analogues or carbonic anhydrase inhibitors. Oral carbonic anhydrase inhibitor may also be used.

Topical beta-adrenergic blocking agents decrease the production of aqueous humour in the ciliary body and can be used once or twice a day, depending on the drug and dosage form. When administering beta-blockers or teaching about their use, it is important to remember that ophthalmic preparations can produce systemic effects, including bronchospasm, bradycardia and heart failure.

Prostaglandin analogues such as latanoprost are a newer class of medications prescribed to increase aqueous outflow. They are similar to beta-blockers in their longer duration of action, requiring only a daily dose. Although they have fewer systemic effects, these drugs may cause conjunctival hyperaemia and permanent changes in the colour of the iris and eyebrows.

The adrenergic agonist brimonidine may be prescribed with a beta-blocker or if beta-blockers are contraindicated (e.g., in those with heart failure, asthma or COPD). Another adrenergic agonist, apraclonidine, may be prescribed when other drugs do not sufficiently reduce intraocular pressure, but adverse effects make it inappropriate for long-term use (Tierney *et al.* 2005).

Dorzolamide, a carbonic anhydrase inhibitor, decreases the production of aqueous humour and reduces intraocular pressure. It is used with other drugs to control pressures and in persons for whom beta-blockers are contraindicated because of heart failure or reactive airway disease. Acetazolamide, a systemic carbonic anhydrase inhibitor, may also be used. The nurse must ensure that any medication prescribed for the person is administered in line with local policy and procedure.

In acute angle-closure glaucoma, diuretics may be administered intravenously, achieving a rapid decrease in intraocular pressure prior to surgery. Both the carbonic anhydrase inhibitor acetazolamide and osmotic diuretics, such as mannitol, are used. Fast-acting miotic drops, such as acetylcholine, are also administered to constrict the pupil and draw the iris away from the angle and from the canal of Schlemm.

Surgery

Surgical intervention is indicated for persons with acute angle-closure glaucoma and for those with chronic open-angle glaucoma that is not effectively controlled by medication. Surgical management of chronic open-angle glaucoma involves improving the drainage of aqueous humour from the anterior chamber. Trabeculoplasty and trabeculectomy filtration surgery are the most common procedures.

In a *laser trabeculoplasty*, a laser is aimed to create multiple laser burns spaced evenly around the trabecular meshwork. As the burns heal, the scars they create cause tension, stretching and opening the meshwork. This non-invasive technique is the treatment of choice because it requires no incision and can be performed as an out-patient procedure.

Trabeculectomy is a type of filtration surgery in which a permanent fistula is created to drain aqueous humour from the anterior chamber. A portion of trabecular meshwork is removed, and a flap of sclera is left unsutured to create a channel or fistula between the anterior chamber and the subconjunctival space. Aqueous humour is able to drain into the space under the conjunctiva, where it can be absorbed into the systemic circulation. A trabeculectomy is usually performed under general anaesthesia and requires hospitalisation.

If these procedures are not fully effective, either photocoagulation using a laser (heat) or cyclocryotherapy using a probe to freeze tissue may be employed to destroy portions of the ciliary body. This tissue destruction reduces the production of aqueous humour, reducing intraocular pressure. Another surgical procedure involves insertion of a glaucoma drainage device that regulates the outflow of aqueous humour.

Surgical procedures used in the treatment of acute angle-closure glaucoma include gonioplasty, laser iridotomy and peripheral iridectomy. Because of the high risk for a future attack of angle-closure glaucoma in the unaffected eye, these procedures are often performed prophylactically.

NURSING CARE FOR GLAUCOMA

When planning and providing care for the person with glaucoma, the specific form of the disease and its actual or potential effects on the person's vision, lifestyle, safety and psychosocial wellbeing must be considered. In the hospitalised person, glaucoma is typically a concurrent diagnosis rather than the primary reason for seeking care, unless the diagnosis is acute angle-closure glaucoma.

Health promotion

Although glaucoma cannot be prevented, its severity and potentially permanent effects can be limited with early visual screening. The nurse assumes an important role in educating the public about the risk factors for glaucoma, such as increased age, and the higher incidence in those with African and Asian ancestry. All people over the age of 40 are encouraged to receive an eye examination every two to four years, including tonometry screening. Those with a predominant family history should be evaluated more frequently, every one to two years. After the age of 65, yearly ophthalmologic examinations are recommended.

Assessment

Collect the following data through a health history and physical examination.

✚ *Health history:* family history; presence of altered vision, halos and excessive tearing; sudden, severe eye pain; use of corrective lenses; most recent eye examination.

✚ *Physical examination:* distant and near vision, peripheral fields, retina for optic nerve cupping.

Nursing diagnoses and interventions

Nursing care focuses on problems associated with the temporary or permanent visual impairment, the resultant increased risk for injury and the psychosocial problems of anxiety and coping.

Risk for disturbed sensory perception: visual

Whether glaucoma and resulting impaired vision is the person's primary problem or a pre-existing condition in a person with another disorder, it must be a primary consideration in nursing care planning.

✚ Address by name and identify yourself with each interaction. Orient to time, place, person and situation as indicated. State the purpose of your visit.

✚ Provide any visual aids that are routinely used. Keep them close, making sure that the person knows where they are and can reach them easily.

✚ Orient to the environment. Explain the location of the call bell, personal items and the furniture in the room. If able, tour person's room, including the bathroom and sink.

Provide other tools or items that can help compensate for diminished vision, for example, bright, non-glare lighting, books, magazines and instructions in large print, books on tape, telephones with oversize pushbuttons, a clock with numbers and hands that can be felt. Help and assist the person with meals by reading menu selections and marking choices. Describing the position of foods on a meal tray according to the clock system, placing the utensils in a readily accessible position, removing lids from containers, buttering the bread and cutting meat, as needed. If the visual impairment is new or temporary, the person may need feeding or continued assistance during the meal. Assist with mobility and ambulation as needed. If the vision loss is unilateral and recent, provide instructions related to unilateral vision loss and change in depth perception, for example caution about the loss of depth perception and teach safety precautions, such as reaching slowly for objects and using visual cues as to distance.

Risk for injury

Whether the person is experiencing a sudden loss of vision due to acute angle-closure glaucoma or significant visual impairment due to inadequately managed chronic glaucoma, both are at an increased risk for injury. Persons who have had surgical interventions for glaucoma are at even greater risk.

✚ Assess ability to perform the activities of living.

✚ Notify housekeeping/domestic services and place a sign on the person's door to alert all personnel not to change the arrangement of the person's room.

✚ Discuss possible adaptations in the home to help the person remain as independent as possible and prevent falls or other injuries.

Risk for anxiety

The actual or potential loss of sight threatens self-concept (an individual's perception of self), role functioning and patterns of interaction. The person with impaired vision who functions well in a familiar environment will feel anxious in the unfamiliar setting of a hospital or care facility.

+ Assess for verbal and non-verbal indications of level of anxiety and for normal coping mechanisms. Repeated expressions of concern or denial that the vision change will affect the person's life indicate anxiety. Non-verbal indicators include tension, difficulty concentrating or thinking, restlessness, poor eye contact and changes in vocalisation (rapid speech, voice quivering). Physical indicators include tachycardia, dilated pupils, cool and clammy skin and tremors.

+ Encourage to verbalise fears, anger and feelings of anxiety.

+ Discuss perception of the eye condition and its effects on lifestyle and roles.

+ Introduce yourself when entering the room, explain all procedures fully before and as they are being performed and use touch to convey proximity and caring.

+ Identify coping strategies that have been useful in the past and adapt these strategies to the present situation.

COMMUNITY-BASED CARE

Persons with glaucoma require teaching about lifetime strategies for managing the disease at home. They need to understand the importance of lifetime therapy to control the disease and prevent blindness. If a permanent visual impairment has resulted, the person needs information on achieving the maximum possible independence while maintaining safety. Discuss the following:

● Prescribed medications including proper way to instil eye drops.

● Importance of not taking certain prescription and over-the-counter medications without consulting a pharmacist, general practitioner or practice nurse.

● Periodic eye examinations with intraocular pressure measurement.

● Risks, warning signs and management of acute angle-closure glaucoma.

● Possible surgical options.

The person with diabetic retinopathy

Diabetic retinopathy is a vascular disorder affecting the capillaries of the retina. The capillaries become sclerotic and lose their ability to transport sufficient oxygen and nutrients to the retina. The risk of developing diabetic retinopathy is related to the duration of the diabetes and the degree of glycaemic control. Hypertension is also a risk factor (Kasper

et al. 2005). Retinopathy is seen in both type 1 and type 2 diabetes. Nursing care of the person with diabetes is discussed in Chapter 6.

Pathophysiology and signs and symptoms of diabetic retinopathy

Diabetic retinopathy progresses through four stages (NHS 2010):

1. mild *non-proliferative* or background retinopathy;

2. moderate non-proliferative retinopathy;

3. severe non-proliferative retinopathy;

4. *proliferative* retinopathy.

Non-proliferative retinopathy is typically the initial form seen. Venous capillaries dilate and develop microaneurysms that may then leak, causing retinal oedema, or they may rupture, causing small haemorrhages into the retina. On ophthalmoscopic examination, yellow exudates, cotton-wool patches indicative of retinal ischaemia and red-dot haemorrhages are observed. When the peripheral retina is involved, few symptoms other than light glare are apparent. Oedema of the macula or a large haemorrhage may cause vision loss.

Diabetic retinopathy may progress to the proliferative form, marked by large areas of retinal ischaemia and the formation of new blood vessels (neovascularisation) spreading over the inner surface of the retina and into the vitreous body. These vessels are fine and fragile, making them permeable and easily ruptured. Blood and blood protein leakage contribute to retinal oedema, and haemorrhage into the vitreous body may occur. The vessels gradually become fibrous and firmly attached to the vitreous body, increasing the risk of retinal detachment.

INTERDISCIPLINARY CARE FOR DIABETIC RETINOPATHY

Diabetics should have eye examinations annually. The development of any new visual signs is an additional indication for ophthalmological examination and possibly retinal angiography.

Laser photocoagulation is used to treat the non-proliferative and proliferative forms of diabetic retinopathy. Leaking microaneurysms are sealed and proliferating vessels destroyed, reducing the risk of haemorrhage, retinal oedema and retinal detachment. This also slows the progress of aneurysms and new vessel formation; it does not cure the disorder. Severe proliferative retinopathy may require vitrectomy (removal of the vitreous humour) to remove vitreous haemorrhage or treat associated retinal detachments (Tierney *et al.* 2005).

NURSING CARE FOR DIABETIC RETINOPATHY

The nursing care focus for diabetic retinopathy is primarily educational. The newly diagnosed diabetic person needs to understand the importance of regular eye examinations. Changes of diabetic retinopathy may already be present when type 2 diabetes is diagnosed.

Teach the person to report any new visual manifestation, including blurred vision; black spots (floaters), cobwebs or flashing lights in the visual field; or a sudden loss of vision in one or both eyes. Emphasise that careful blood glucose control may help prevent diabetic retinopathy from developing; it may also slow its progress. Blood pressure should also be maintained within normal limits to prevent further damage to retinal vessels. Although diabetic retinopathy cannot be halted or cured, its progress can be slowed with aggressive management.

The next feature of the chapter concentrates on issues associated with the ears. In order to understand and help the people you care for you must understand the anatomy, physiology and function of this important sense, the sense of hearing.

ANATOMY, PHYSIOLOGY AND FUNCTIONS OF THE EARS

The ears have two primary functions, hearing and maintaining equilibrium. Each ear is divided into three areas: the external ear, the middle ear and the inner ear (Figure 14.8), each with a unique function. All three are involved in hearing, but only the inner ear is involved in equilibrium.

THE EXTERNAL EAR

The external ear consists of the auricle (or pinna), the external auditory canal and the tympanic membrane (ear drum).

The auricles are elastic cartilage covered with thin skin, containing sebaceous and sweat glands and sometimes hair. Each auricle has a rim (the helix) and a lobe. The auricle serves to direct sound waves into the ear.

The external auditory canal, about 2.5 cm long, extends from the auricle to the tympanic membrane and is lined with skin that contains hair, sebaceous and ceruminous glands. It serves as a resonator for the range of sound waves typical of human speech and increases the pressure that sound waves in this frequency range place on the tympanic membrane. The canal's ceruminous glands secrete a yellow to brown waxy substance called **cerumen** (earwax). This traps foreign bodies and has bacteriostatic properties, protecting the tympanic membrane and the middle ear from infections.

The tympanic membrane lies between the external ear and the middle ear. It is a thin, semi-transparent, fibrous structure covered with skin on the external side and mucosa on the inner side. The membrane vibrates as sound waves strike it; these are transferred as sound waves to the middle ear.

THE MIDDLE EAR

This is an air-filled cavity in the temporal bone, containing three auditory ossicles: the malleus, the incus and the stapes. These bones extend across the middle ear. The medial side of the middle ear is a bony wall containing two membrane-covered openings, the oval and the round windows. The posterior wall of the middle ear contains the *mastoid* (a bony prominence in the ear). This cavity communicates with the mastoid sinuses, helping the middle ear adjust to changes in pressure. It also opens into the eustachian tube, connecting with the nasopharynx. The eustachian tube helps to equalise the air pressure in the middle ear by opening briefly in response to differences between middle ear pressure and atmospheric pressure. This action ensures that vibrations of the tympanic membrane remain adequate. The mucous membrane lining the middle ear is continuous with the mucous membranes lining the throat.

The malleus attaches to the tympanic membrane and articulates with the incus, which in turn articulates with the stapes. The stapes fits into the oval window. When the tympanic membrane vibrates, vibrations are conducted across the middle ear to the oval window by the ossicles. The vibrations then set in motion the fluids of the inner ear, which stimulate hearing receptors. Two small muscles attached to the ossicles contract reflexively in response to sudden loud noises, decreasing vibrations and protecting the inner ear.

THE INNER EAR

Also called the labyrinth, the inner ear is a maze of bony chambers located deep within the temporal bone, behind the eye socket. The labyrinth is further divided into two parts: the bony labyrinth, a system of open channels that houses the second part, the membranous labyrinth. The bony labyrinth is filled with a fluid (similar to cerebrospinal fluid) called perilymph, bathing the membranous labyrinth. Within the chambers of the membranous labyrinth is a fluid called endolymph.

The bony labyrinth has three regions: the vestibule, the semi-circular canals and the cochlea. The vestibule is the central portion of the inner ear, one side of which is a bony wall containing the oval window. Two sacs within the vestibule (the saccule and the utricle) join the vestibule with the cochlea and the semi-circular canals. The saccule and the utricle contain receptors for equilibrium that respond to changes in gravity and changes in position of the head. The three semi-circular canals each project into a different plane (anterior, posterior and lateral). Each contains a semi-circular duct communicating with the utricle of the vestibule, with an enlarged area at one end containing an equilibrium receptor responding to angular movements of the head.

The cochlea is a tiny bony chamber housing the organ of Corti, the receptor organ for hearing. The organ of Corti is a series of sensory hair cells, arranged in a single row of inner

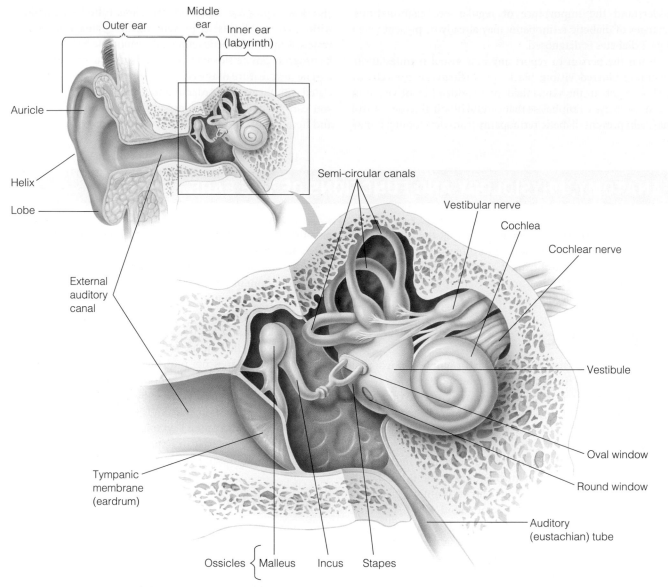

Figure 14.8 Structures of the external ear, middle ear and inner ear.

hair cells and three rows of outer hair cells. The hair cells are innervated by sensory fibres from cranial nerve VIII. The organ of Corti is supported in the cochlea by the flexible basilar membrane, which has fibres of varying lengths responding to different sound wave frequencies.

SOUND CONDUCTION

Hearing is the perception and interpretation of sound. Sound is produced when the molecules of a medium are compressed, resulting in a pressure disturbance evidenced as a sound wave. The intensity or loudness of sound is determined by the amplitude (height) of the sound wave, greater amplitudes causing louder sounds. The frequency of the sound wave determines the pitch or tone; higher frequencies result in higher sounds.

Sound waves enter the external auditory canal causing the tympanic membrane to vibrate at the same frequency. The

ossicles transmit the motion of the tympanic membrane to the oval window and amplify the energy of the sound wave. As the stapes moves against the oval window, the perilymph in the vestibule is set in motion. The increased pressure of the perilymph is transmitted to fibres of the basilar membrane and then to the organ of Corti. The up-and-down movements of the fibres of the basilar membrane pull the hair cells in the organ of Corti, which generate action potentials that are transmitted to cranial nerve VIII and then to the brain for interpretation.

EQUILIBRIUM

The inner ear also provides information about the position of the head, helping to coordinate body movements so that equilibrium and balance are maintained. The types of equilibrium are *static balance* (affected by changes in the position of the head) and *dynamic balance* (affected by the movement of the head).

Receptors called maculae detect changes in the position of the head. Maculae are groups of hair cells that have protrusions covered with a gelatinous substance. Embedded in this gelatinous substance are tiny particles of calcium carbonate called *otoliths* (ear stones), which make the gelatin heavier than the endolymph that fills the membranous labyrinth.

The receptor for dynamic equilibrium is in the crista, a crest in the membrane lining the ampulla of each semicircular canal. The cristae are stimulated by rotatory head movement (acceleration and deceleration) as a result of changes in the flow of endolymph and of movement of hair cells in the maculae. The direction of endolymph and hair cell movement is always opposite to the motion of the body.

To assess the ears effectively you have to understand the anatomy and physiology in order to provide you with a framework for the implementation, planning and evaluatory stages of nursing care. This next section provides information required to undertake an assessment of the ear and hearing.

Assessing the ears

The structure and functions of the ears are assessed by findings from diagnostic tests, a health assessment interview to collect subjective data and a physical assessment to collect objective data.

DIAGNOSTIC TESTS

The results of diagnostic tests support the diagnosis of a specific injury, disease or hearing problem; to provide information to identify or modify the appropriate medications or assistive devices used to treat the disease or problem; and to help monitor responses to treatment and care interventions.

Regardless of the type of diagnostic test, the nurse is responsible for explaining the procedure and any special preparation needed, for assessing for any medication use that might affect the outcome of the tests, for supporting the person during the examination as necessary, for documenting the procedures as appropriate and for monitoring the results of the tests. Diagnostic tests are described below.

GENETIC CONSIDERATIONS

When conducting a health assessment interview and a physical assessment, it is important to consider genetic influences on the person's health. Several diseases of the ears have a genetic component. Ask about a family history of congenital deafness, deafness associated with a thyroid goitre or tumours of the auditory nerve.

If data are found to indicate genetic risk factors or alterations, ask about genetic testing and refer for appropriate genetic counselling.

HEALTH ASSESSMENT INTERVIEW

The aim is to collect subjective data about the ears and hearing and may be part of a health screening. It may focus on a chief complaint (such as hearing problems or pain in the ear), or it may be part of a total health assessment. If the person has a problem involving one or both ears, analyse onset, characteristics and course, severity, precipitating and relieving factors and any associated symptoms, noting the timing and circumstances. You might ask the following:

- Have you noticed any difficulty hearing high-pitched sounds, low-pitched sounds, or both?
- When did you first notice the ringing in your ears?
- Is your workplace noisy? If so, do you wear protective ear equipment at work?

DIAGNOSTIC TESTS Ear disorders

Audiometry

Evaluates and diagnoses conductive and sensorineural hearing loss. Person sits in soundproof room and responds by raising a hand when sounds are heard.

RELATED NURSING CARE *No special preparation is needed.*

Auditory evoked potential (AEP)

Identifies electrical activity of the auditory nerve. Electrodes are placed on various areas of the ear and on the forehead, a graphic recording is made.

RELATED NURSING CARE *No special preparation is needed.*

Auditory brainstem response (ABR)

Measures electrical activity of the auditory pathway from inner ear to brain, diagnoses brainstem pathology, stroke and acoustic neuroma.

RELATED NURSING CARE *No special preparation is needed.*

DIAGNOSTIC TESTS Ear disorders (continued)

Caloric test

Used to assess vestibular system function. Cold or warm water is used to irrigate the ear canals one at a time and the person is observed for *nystagmus* (repeated abnormal movements of the eyes). Normally, the nystagmus occurs opposite to the ear being irrigated. If no nystagmus occurs, the person needs further testing for brain lesions.

RELATED NURSING CARE *Assess person for use of alcohol, central nervous system depressants and barbiturates. These may alter the test results.*

Throughout the examination, be alert to non-verbal behaviours (such as inappropriate answers or requests to repeat statements) that suggest problems with ear function. Explore changes in hearing, ringing in the ears (**tinnitus**), ear pain, drainage from the ears or the use of hearing aids. Ask about trauma, surgery or infections of the ear as well as the date of the last ear examination; ask about a medical history of infectious diseases, such as meningitis or mumps, as well as the use of medications that may affect hearing. Ear problems tend to run in families. Ask about a family history of hearing loss, ear problems or diseases that could result in such problems. If the person has a hearing aid, ascertain the type and assess measures for its care. Interview questions are listed in the Functional Health Pattern Interview box below.

FUNCTIONAL HEALTH PATTERN INTERVIEW The ear

Functional health pattern	Interview questions and leading statements
Health perception–health management	• Describe your hearing. Rate it on a scale of 1 to 10, with 10 being excellent hearing. Is it the same in both ears? If not, which ear is better? • Describe current hearing problems. • Do you use ear medications? What type? How often? • Have you ever had ear surgery? • Do you use a hearing aid? What type is it? How do you care for it? • Have you ever had your hearing tested? When?
Nutritional–metabolic	• Do you have any swelling or tenderness in the ears or drainage from the ears?
Activity–exercise	• Does your hearing problem interfere with your usual activities of living? • Do you wear protective earplugs when taking part in activities that increase the risk of injury to your ears (such as at work or when operating machinery)?
Sleep–rest	• Does your ear problem interfere with your ability to rest or sleep? If so, what do you do?
Cognitive–perceptual	• Do you have pain in or around your ears? Have you ever had ringing in your ears? If so, describe its location, intensity, what makes it worse and how long it lasts. How do you treat it? • Do you have difficulty hearing conversations, in person or on the telephone? Do you have trouble hearing the television? Do you have difficulty hearing when you are in crowds or there is background noise? • Have you noticed your hearing is different in each ear? • Do you have buzzing, ringing or crackling noises in one or both ears? • Do you ever feel dizzy?
Self-perception–self-concept	• Has this problem with your ears affected how you feel about yourself?

FUNCTIONAL HEALTH PATTERN INTERVIEW The ear (continued)

Functional health pattern	Interview questions and leading statements
Role–relationships	• How has having this condition affected your relationships? • Has having this condition interfered with your ability to work? • Has anyone in your family had problems with ear disease?
Sexuality–reproductive	• Has this condition interfered with your usual sexual activity?
Coping–stress-tolerance	• Has having this condition created stress for you? Have you experienced any kind of stress that makes the condition worse? • Describe what you do when you feel stressed.
Value–belief	• Describe how specific relationships or activities help you cope with this problem. • Describe specific cultural beliefs or practices that affect how you care for and feel about this problem. • Are there any specific treatments that you would not use to treat this problem?

PHYSICAL ASSESSMENT OF THE EARS AND HEARING

This may be performed as part of a total health assessment or separately for those with known or suspected problems. Assessment is primarily through inspection of external structures, the external auditory canal and the tympanic membrane. Disorders of the middle ear may be identified with tympanometry. Hearing acuity is assessed by voice tests and tuning fork tests. The external structures may be palpated. Normal age-related findings for the older adult are summarised in Table 14.4.

Ear and hearing assessments

HEARING ASSESSMENT

Tuning forks are used to determine the type of hearing loss. Hold the tuning fork at the base and make it ring softly by stroking the prongs or by lightly tapping them on the heel of the opposite hand. The vibrating tuning fork emits sound waves of a particular frequency, measured in hertz (Hz).

Table 14.4 Age-related changes in the ear

Age-related change	Significance
The inner ear: • Loss of hair cells, ↓ blood supply, less flexible basilar membrane, degeneration of spiral ganglion cells, and ↓ production of endolymph result in progressive hearing loss with age (presbycusis). • High-frequency sounds are lost; middle and low-frequency sounds may also be lost or decreased. • Vestibular structures degenerate, organ of Corti and cochlea atrophy.	Older adults may require hearing aids. With loss of high-frequency sounds, speech may be distorted, contributing to problems with communication. Degeneration and atrophy of inner ear structures concerned with balance and equilibrium increase the risk for falls.
The middle ear: • Muscles and ligaments weaken and stiffen, decreasing the acoustic reflex.	Sounds made from one's own body and speech are louder and may interfere with hearing, speech and communication.
The external ear: • Cerumen has a higher keratin content, contributing to increased cerumen in the ear canal.	Accumulated cerumen may impair hearing.

EXTERNAL EAR ASSESSMENT

Inspect the auricle.

- Unusual redness or drainage may indicate an inflammatory response.
- Scales or skin lesions around the rim of the auricle may indicate skin cancer.
- Small, raised lesions on the rim of the ear are known as *tophi* and indicate gout.

Inspect the external auditory canal with the otoscope.

- Unusual redness, lesions or purulent drainage may indicate an infection.
- Cerumen varies in colour and texture. Hardened, dry or foul-smelling cerumen may indicate an infection or an impaction of cerumen that requires removal. People with darker skin tend to have darker cerumen.

Inspect the tympanic membrane.

- White, opaque areas on the tympanic membrane are often scars from previous perforations.
- Inconsistent texture and colour may be due to scarring from previous perforations caused by infection, allergies or trauma.
- Bulging membranes, indicated by a loss of bony landmarks and a distorted light reflex, may be the result of **otitis media** or malfunctioning auditory tubes.
- Retracted tympanic membranes are indicated by accentuated bony landmarks and a distorted light reflex, often due to an obstructed auditory tube.

Palpate the auricles and over each mastoid process.

- Tenderness, swelling or nodules may indicate inflammation of the external auditory canal or mastoiditis.

You will be able to offer a better, safer service to the people you care for and their families now that you have read and understood the issues associated with assessment of hearing. In the next section some ear disorders are discussed.

DISORDERS OF THE EAR

Trauma or disease involving any portion of the hearing pathway can affect hearing. Tinnitus, the perception of sound such as ringing, buzzing or roaring in the ears, is another potential result of problems affecting the auditory system.

Disorders of the external ear can affect the conduction of sound waves and hearing. Obstruction of the external auditory canal or damage to the tympanic membrane, which separates the outer from the middle ear, may lead to conductive hearing loss. Infection or inflammation, trauma and obstruction of the ear canal with cerumen or a foreign body are the most common conditions affecting the external ear.

Middle ear disorders may be acute or chronic. Unless treated promptly and effectively, damage and scarring of middle ear structures can result in a permanent conductive hearing loss. Infectious or inflammatory disorders are the most common conditions affecting the middle ear. Otosclerosis, a genetic condition, can affect the middle ear structures.

The person with otitis externa

Otitis externa is inflammation of the ear canal. Swimmers, divers and surfers are particularly prone to otitis externa. Wearing a hearing aid or ear plugs, which hold moisture in the ear canal, is an additional risk factor. Although *Pseudomonas aeruginosa* or other bacterial infections are the most common cause, external otitis can be due to fungal infection, mechanical trauma (such as cleaning the ear with a toothpick) or an allergic reaction.

Pathophysiology and signs and symptoms of otitis externa

Disruption of the normal environment within the external auditory canal precedes the inflammatory process. Retained moisture, cleaning or drying of the ear canal can remove the protective layer of cerumen, leaving the skin of the ear canal vulnerable to invasion and infection.

The person with otitis externa often complains of a feeling of fullness in the ear. Ear pain is present and may be severe. The pain of otitis externa can be differentiated from that associated with otitis media by manipulation of the auricle. In external otitis, this manoeuvre increases pain; in otitis media there is no change in pain perception. Odourless watery or purulent drainage may be present. The ear canal appears inflamed and oedematous.

INTERDISCIPLINARY CARE FOR OTITIS EXTERNA

The aim is to restore the normal balance of the external ear and canal and to teach how to prevent future problems. For otitis externa, the following are recommended:

- Thorough cleansing of the ear canal, particularly if drainage or debris is present.
- Treatment of the infection with local antibiotics; if cellulitis is present, systemic antibiotics may be necessary.
- Medication to relieve the pain and itching.
- Teaching on the prevention of future episodes.

Topical antibiotics are often prescribed to treat otitis externa. Topical corticosteroid may be ordered in combination with antibiotics to provide immediate relief from pain, swelling and itching. Polymyxin B-neomycin-hydrocortisone is a combination preparation used to treat external otitis. Identify any known sensitivity to any of the drugs in this preparation prior to administration. Other preparations may be prescribed for a fungal infection of the ear canal.

NURSING CARE FOR OTITIS EXTERNA

External otitis can cause severe pain and discomfort. The disorder is rarely serious enough to require hospitalisation. The nurse teaches the person about the disorder, comfort measures and prevention of future episodes.

Nursing diagnoses and interventions

Risk for impaired tissue integrity

External otitis may result from attempts to clean the ear canal with a toothpick, cotton-tipped applicator or other implement that damages the skin, allowing an infectious organism to invade the tissue. Even if the canal is not damaged by attempts to clean it, the cleaning process often interrupts normal mechanisms, causing cerumen and debris to collect. This traps water within the canal, causing *maceration* (skin that is constantly wet) of the skin.

+ Inform that ear canals rarely need cleansing beyond washing of the external meatus with soap and water. Teach persons of all ages not to clean ear canals with any implement.

+ Teach person (and, if necessary, a family member) how to instil prescribed eardrops:

   a. Wash hands.
   b. Warm medication briefly by holding the container in the hand or placing it in a pocket for approximately five minutes before instilling drops.
   c. Lie on the unaffected side; if sitting, tilt the head toward the unaffected side.
   d. Partially fill the ear dropper with medication.
   e. Using the non-dominant hand, straighten the ear canal by pulling the pinna of the ear up and back.
   f. Administer the prescribed number of drops into the ear canal.
   g. Remain in the side-lying position for approximately five minutes after instillation.

+ Loosely place a small piece of cotton wool in the auditory meatus for 15–20 minutes.

+ Teach to avoid getting water in the affected ear until it is fully healed. Cotton balls may be used while showering, preventing water from entering the ear canal. Refrain from water sports and activities until approved by the practice nurse.

The person with impacted cerumen or a foreign body

The external auditory canal can be obstructed by cerumen or foreign bodies. The shape and narrow lumen make it vulnerable to obstruction.

Pathophysiology and signs and symptoms of impacted cerumen or a foreign body

As cerumen dries, it moves down and out of the ear canal. In some individuals it tends to accumulate, narrowing the canal. Ageing is a risk factor for impaction; less cerumen is produced and it is harder and drier. Accumulated cerumen can be aggravated by attempting to remove it using cotton-tipped swabs or hairpins, packing it more deeply into the ear canal.

A variety of foreign bodies may be lodged in the ear canal. Implements used to clean the ear canal may break and become lodged. Insects can enter the ear canal and be unable to exit.

When the ear canal becomes occluded with either cerumen or a foreign body, a conductive hearing loss in the affected ear occurs. Symptoms include a sensation of fullness, along with tinnitus and coughing due to stimulation of the vagal nerve. The foreign body or impacted cerumen may be visualised on otoscopy.

INTERDISCIPLINARY CARE FOR IMPACTED CERUMEN OR A FOREIGN BODY

Treatment focuses on clearing the canal. If there is no evidence of tympanic membrane perforation, irrigation is often the initial therapy.

Impacted wax or objects may require physical removal using an ear curette, forceps or right-angle hook inserted via an otoscope and ear speculum. Mineral oil or topical lignocaine (Lidocaine) drops are used to immobilise or kill insects prior to their removal from the ear. When an organic foreign body such as a bean or an insect is suspected, water should not be instilled into the ear canal. This may cause the object to swell, making removal more difficult. Smooth, round objects present the biggest challenge. Suction applied using a piece of soft intravenous tubing may be effective.

NURSING CARE FOR IMPACTED CERUMEN OR A FOREIGN BODY

Nurses often identify and relieve obstructions of the ear canal in out-patient and community settings. Any person with evidence of a new conductive hearing loss or complaints of discomfort and fullness in one ear should be evaluated for possible obstruction. Inability to visualise the tympanic membrane or observation of a dark, shiny mass obstructing the canal may indicate a need for irrigation or other procedure to clear the canal. It is important to ensure the tympanic membrane is intact before irrigating; assessment by an advanced practitioner, practice nurse or general practitioner may be necessary if a ruptured membrane is suspected.

Obstruction of the ear canal with cerumen or a foreign body is generally preventable; teaching is a key component of care. People need to know appropriate care measures for the external ear. The ear canal rarely needs cleaning. The person prone to cerumen impaction needs teaching about the use of commercial products to soften wax and, if irrigation to remove it is needed, a pharmacist or practice nurse would be ideally suited to do this. All persons should understand the importance of not inserting anything smaller than a finger wrapped with a flannel into the ear canal. Stress the risk of impacting cerumen against the tympanic membrane when using cotton-tipped swabs to clean the ear canal; the swab may break and lodge in the canal. If eardrops have been prescribed, teach how to instil them.

It is essential that the nurse applies a sound evidence base to care. This will include communicating with persons and providing safe and effective practical ear care. Fox and Bartlett (2001) discuss the importance of professional requirements in ear care provision from an ethical, legal and professional perspective. They consider the contradictions to ear syringing and the problems associated with water in the ears. The use of aural toilet is described as an alternative to the potentially dangerous activity of ear syringing. Aural toilet is the term used for manually cleaning the external auditory meatus of wax, debris or water. Contraindications to ear syringing include any history of ear surgery, profound hearing loss in one ear, history of perforated tympanic membrane, recent or current middle ear infection and recent or current otitis externa.

The person with otitis media

Otitis media, inflammation or infection of the middle ear, primarily affects infants and young children, but it can occur in adults. The tympanic membrane separates the middle ear from the external auditory canal, protecting the middle ear. The eustachian (auditory) tube connects the middle ear with the nasopharynx, helping equalise the pressure in the middle ear with atmospheric pressure. This connecting tube also provides a route by which infectious organisms enter the middle ear from the nose and throat, causing otitis media, the most common disease of the middle ear.

Pathophysiology of otitis media

There are two primary forms of otitis media: (1) serous and (2) acute or suppurative (discharging pus). Both are associated with upper respiratory infection and eustachian tube dysfunction. The eustachian tube is narrow and flat, normally opening only during yawning and swallowing. Allergies or upper respiratory tract infections can cause oedema of the tube lining,

impairing function. Air within the middle ear is trapped and gradually absorbed, creating negative pressure in this space.

Serous otitis media

This occurs when the eustachian tube is obstructed for a prolonged time, impairing equalisation of air pressure in the middle ear. Air within the middle ear space is gradually absorbed; the tube obstruction prevents more air from entering the middle ear. The resulting negative pressure in the middle ear causes sterile serous fluid to move from the capillaries into the space, forming a sterile effusion of the middle ear.

Upper respiratory infection or allergies predispose the person to serous otitis media. Those with narrowed or oedematous eustachian tubes may also be subject to *barotrauma* or *barotitis media*. The middle ear cannot adapt to rapid changes in barometric pressure, for example during air travel or underwater diving. Barotrauma tends to occur during descent in an airplane, as negative pressure within the middle ear causes the eustachian tube to collapse and lock. However, underwater diving places even greater stress on the eustachian tube and middle ear (Tierney *et al.* 2005).

Signs and symptoms

- Decreased hearing in the affected ear.
- Sensation of 'snapping' or 'popping' in the ear.
- On examination, the tympanic membrane demonstrates decreased mobility, retraction or bulging.
- Fluid or air bubbles are visible behind the eardrum.
- Acute pain.
- Haemorrhage into the middle ear.
- Rupture of the tympanic membrane or even rupture of the round window.
- Sensory hearing loss.
- Severe **vertigo**.
- *Haemo-tympanum*, bleeding into or behind the tympanic membrane, may be observed on otoscopic examination.

Acute otitis media

The eustachian tube also provides a route for the entry of pathogens into the normally sterile middle ear, resulting in acute or suppurative otitis media. This follows an upper respiratory infection. Oedema of the eustachian tube impairs drainage of the middle ear, causing mucus and serous fluid to accumulate, and this is an excellent environment for the growth of bacteria, which may enter from the oronasopharynx via the eustachian tube. Although a viral upper respiratory infection may predispose the person to a middle ear infection, the bacteria *Streptococcus pneumoniae*, *Haemophilus influenzae* and *Streptococcus pyogenes* account for most cases of otitis media in adults. Pus formation occurs and middle ear pressure increases sufficiently to rupture the tympanic membrane. Bacterial infection may migrate internally, causing mastoiditis, brain abscess or bacterial meningitis. A common complication of otitis media is a persistent conductive hearing loss, which resolves when the middle ear effusion clears.

Signs and symptoms

- Mild to severe pain in the affected ear.
- Pyrexia.
- Diminished hearing, dizziness, vertigo and tinnitus.
- Pus within the mastoid air cells causing mastoid tenderness.
- Otoscopic examination reveals a red and inflamed or dull and bulging tympanic membrane.
- Tympanometry or air insufflation demonstrates decreased movement of the membrane.

Spontaneous rupture of the tympanic membrane releases a purulent discharge. *Myringotomy* (an incision of the tympanic membrane) may be performed to relieve the pressure.

INTERDISCIPLINARY CARE FOR OTITIS MEDIA

Diagnosis of otitis media is usually based on history and physical examination. The tympanic membrane can be visualised and its mobility evaluated using a pneumatic otoscope that allows a puff of air to be instilled into the ear canal. Generally, the tympanic membrane moves slightly when air is instilled or the person performs the Valsalva manoeuvre. Less movement is seen in those with eustachian tube dysfunction and acute otitis media with effusion.

Diagnosis

- *Impedance audiometry*, also known as tympanometry, is a diagnostic test for otitis media with effusion. A continuous tone is delivered to the tympanic membrane by an audiometer with a sealed probe tip.
- A *full blood count (FBC)* may be undertaken to assess for an elevated white blood count and increased numbers of immature cells indicative of acute bacterial infection.
- If the tympanic membrane has ruptured or a *tympanocentesis* (drainage of fluid from the middle ear) or **myringotomy** (a surgical incision into the eardrum) is performed, drainage is cultured to determine the infecting organism.

Medication

When eustachian tube dysfunction and serous otitis media do not spontaneously resolve or lead to hearing loss, a short course of an anti-inflammatory drug (e.g., oral prednisone) is prescribed to reduce mucosal oedema and improve patency. A decongestant or antihistamine may be used, but there is little evidence of their effectiveness in treating serous otitis media.

The person with eustachian tube dysfunction may be taught to autoinflate the middle ear by performing the Valsalva manoeuvre or by forcefully exhaling against closed nostrils. The person is advised to avoid air travel and underwater diving.

Acute otitis media is usually treated with antibiotic therapy for 5–10 days. This course of treatment is long enough to ensure eradication of the infective organism, yet short enough to reduce the incidence of bacterial resistance. Symptomatic relief may be provided by analgesics, antipyretics, antihistamines and local application of heat.

Surgery

A myringotomy or tympanocentesis may be performed to relieve excess pressure in the middle ear and prevent spontaneous rupture of the eardrum. A special needle is inserted through the inferior portion of the tympanic membrane, allowing aspiration of fluid and pus from the middle ear to relieve pressure and, if necessary, obtain a specimen for culture. Myringotomy may be performed to relieve severe pain or when complications of acute otitis media, such as mastoiditis, are present. As soon as the pressure is released, pain subsides and hearing improves.

Those who do not respond to antibiotic therapy may require myringotomy with insertion of ventilation (tympanostomy) tubes. Small tubes are inserted into the inferior portion of the tympanic membrane, providing for ventilation and drainage of the middle ear during healing. The tube is eventually extruded from the ear, and the tympanic membrane heals. While the tube is in place, it is important to avoid getting any water in the ear canal because it may then enter the middle ear space.

NURSING CARE FOR OTITIS MEDIA

Persons with otitis media are commonly treated in out-patient and community settings. The nursing role is primarily one of support and education.

Health promotion

Health promotion for otitis media focuses on the importance of seeking medical care for prolonged, severe ear pain with or without drainage, combined with an upper respiratory tract infection. Untreated or repeated attacks can progress to a chronic form of otitis media, acute mastoiditis or eardrum perforation.

Assessment

Collect assessment data through a health history and physical examination.

- *Health history*: recent upper respiratory infection; presence, intensity and nature of pain in affected ear; sense of fullness or pressure in the ear; change in hearing; snapping or popping sensation in the affected ear; presence of vertigo.
- *Physical examination*: temperature; hearing test; inspect tympanic membrane.

Nursing diagnoses and interventions

Pain can be a significant problem for those with otitis media, as can the risk of damage to delicate tissues of the middle ear by the infectious and inflammatory processes.

Risk for pain

Tissue oedema, effusion of the middle ear and the inflammatory response can affect the pain-sensitive tissues of the middle ear in otitis media, causing acute discomfort. This is increased by pressure changes, such as those that occur during air travel or underwater diving.

✦ Assess pain for severity, quality and location.

✦ Encourage the use of mild analgesics such as aspirin or paracetamol every four hours as needed to relieve pain and fever.

✦ Advise to apply heat to the affected side unless contraindicated.

✦ Instruct to avoid air travel, rapid changes in elevation or diving.

✦ Instruct to report promptly an abrupt relief of pain to the GP or practice nurse (this may indicate spontaneous perforation of the tympanic membrane).

The person with chronic otitis media

Chronic otitis media involves permanent perforation of the tympanic membrane, with or without recurrent pus formation. Changes in mucosa and bony structures (ossicles) of the middle ear often accompany chronic otitis media. It is usually the result of recurrent acute otitis media and eustachian tube dysfunction, but may also result from trauma or other diseases.

Marginal perforations, occurring in the posterior–superior portion of the tympanic membrane, are associated with more complications than central perforations. With marginal perforations, squamous epithelium may migrate from the canal into the middle ear, where it begins to *desquamate* (shed) and accumulate, forming a *cholesteatoma* (a cyst or mass filled with epithelial cell debris). This continues to accumulate and remains infected, producing enzymes that destroy adjacent bone. The inflammatory process impairs blood supply to the stapes, causing its destruction and conductive hearing loss.

Cholesteatomas are benign and slow-growing tumours, which enlarge to fill the entire middle ear. The cholesteatoma can progressively destroy the ossicles and erode into the inner ear, causing profound hearing loss.

Systemic antibiotics are prescribed for exacerbations of purulent otitis media. Perforation is repaired with a **tympanoplasty**, restoring sound conduction and integrity of the middle ear. A cholesteatoma may require surgery for its removal. If possible, radical mastoidectomy with removal of the tympanic membrane, ossicles and tumour is avoided.

A priority of care is prevention of chronic otitis media and cholesteatoma. Persons with chronic otitis media need to understand treatment options, their risks and benefits and the long-term risk of not treating a perforated tympanic membrane. They are also taught how to instil eardrops, to clean the external auditory meatus and not to irrigate the ear when the tympanic membrane is or may be perforated.

If surgery will affect the person's hearing, include this information in pre-operative teaching. Teach the person and family how to use alternative means of communication if this will be necessary post-operatively. When an assistive device is ordered explain its use.

NURSING CARE PLAN The person having ear surgery

Review Chapter 1 for routine pre- and post-operative care.

Pre-operative care

✦ Assess hearing or verify documentation of pre-operative hearing assessment.

✦ Establish a means of communication to be used post-operatively.

✦ Explain that blowing the nose, coughing and sneezing are restricted post-operatively to prevent pressure changes in the middle ear and potential disruption of the surgical site. Keeping the mouth open during a cough or sneeze minimises pressure changes in the middle ear.

Post-operative care

✦ Assess for bleeding or drainage from the affected ear.

✦ Administer antiemetics as ordered. Vomiting may disrupt the surgical site.

✦ Elevate the head of the bed and position the person on the unaffected side.

✦ Assess for vertigo or dizziness, especially with ambulation or movement in bed. Avoid unnecessary movements such as turning.

✦ Assess hearing post-operatively. Stand on the unaffected side to communicate and use other measures such as written messages as needed for effective communication. Reassure the person that decreased hearing acuity immediately after surgery is expected.

✦ Remind to avoid coughing, sneezing or blowing the nose.

The person with an inner ear disorder

These disorders are much less common than disorders of the outer or middle ear. Inner ear disorders affect equilibrium and may also affect sensorineural hearing, the perception of sound. Labyrinthitis and Ménière's disease are the most common. Vertigo may be a disorder of the inner ear itself or a manifestation of other disorders.

Pathophysiology and signs and symptoms of inner ear disorders

The inner ear (also called the labyrinth) contains the cochlea and the semi-circular canals. The hair cells and neurones allowing sound perception and transmission to the auditory centre of the brain are in the cochlea. The semi-circular canals filled with endolymph are the primary organs involved in maintaining equilibrium. Disruption of this portion of the ear by an inflammatory process or excess endolymph affects balance and may also result in permanent hearing loss.

Vertigo

The integration of input from the labyrinths, eyes, muscles, joints and neural centres maintains balance and posture, and this can be affected by disorders of the labyrinth, vestibular nerve or nuclei, eyes, cerebellum, brainstem or cerebral cortex, causing vertigo. Vertigo, the sensation of movement when there is none, is a disorder of equilibrium. The sensation of whirling, rotation or movement is described as either subjective or objective.

Persons with subjective vertigo report the sensation of being in motion in a stable environment. There is not always a sense of spinning; there may be a sense of tumbling or falling forward or backward. The sensation is reversed in objective vertigo; persons report a sensation of stability in a moving environment. This motion may be perceived as the room spinning around or the ground rocking beneath the feet. Dizziness, which can be mistaken for vertigo, is a sensation of unsteadiness, lack of balance, light-headedness or movement within the head. The person who is dizzy does not have the rotational sensation felt with vertigo.

Vertigo may be disabling, resulting in falls, injury and difficulty walking. Attacks of vertigo are often accompanied by nausea and vomiting, nystagmus and autonomic symptoms such as pallor, sweating, hypotension and salivation.

Ménière's disease

Ménière's disease, also known as *endolymphatic hydrops*, is a chronic disorder characterised by recurrent attacks of vertigo with tinnitus and a progressive unilateral hearing loss. The cause is unclear, although the most common form of the disease is thought to result from viral injury to the fluid transport system of the inner ear. Other factors that may increase risk include trauma, bacterial infections such as syphilis, autoimmune processes and vascular disorders (Porth 2009, Copstead and Banasik 2010). A family history increases risk, suggesting a possible genetic link.

Ménière's disease results from an excess of endolymph. The precise pathophysiological mechanism leading to accumulation of endolymph is unclear, but it is thought to result from impaired filtration and excretion of the fluid by the endolymphatic sac (Tierney *et al.* 2005, Porth 2009). Excessive pressure causes neural organs of the cochlea to degenerate.

Signs and symptoms

Onset of Ménière's disease may be gradual or sudden.

- Recurrent attacks of vertigo.
- Gradual loss of hearing and tinnitus.
- A feeling of fullness in the ears and a roaring or ringing sensation (unilateral or bilateral).
- Attacks occur abruptly and often unpredictably, lasting from minutes to hours.

Attacks may be linked to increased sodium intake, stress, allergies, vasoconstriction or premenstrual fluid retention. Hearing loss progresses and vertigo can be severe enough to cause immobility, nausea and vomiting. Attacks are often accompanied by hypotension, sweating and *nystagmus*.

INTERDISCIPLINARY CARE FOR AN INNER EAR DISORDER

The signs and symptoms associated with inner ear disorders are similar, making testing necessary to establish a diagnosis. When diagnosis is determined, collaborative care is directed toward managing symptoms and preventing permanent hearing loss. Hospitalisation to manage the vertigo and its effects may be required.

Diagnosis

The following diagnostic studies may be ordered:

- *Caloric testing* evaluates the vestibulo-ocular reflex by identifying eye movements (nystagmus) in response to caloric testing. In people with impaired vestibular function, the normal nystagmus response is blunted or absent. This portion of the test is contraindicated in people who have a perforated tympanic membrane.
- *Rinne* and *Weber tests* of hearing show decreased air and bone conduction on the affected side if a sensorineural hearing loss is present. In Ménière's disease, audiology shows sensorineural hearing loss involving the low tones.
- *X-rays* and *CT scans* of the petrous bones are used to evaluate the internal auditory canal. In Ménière's disease, the vestibular aqueducts may be shorter and straighter than normal.
- *Glycerol test* is conducted by giving the person oral glycerol to decrease fluid pressure in the inner ear. An acute temporary hearing improvement is considered diagnostic for Ménière's disease.

Medication

In Ménière's disease, a diuretic may be prescribed to reduce endolymphatic pressure. A central nervous system depressant such as diazepam may halt an attack of vertigo. Droperidol (intramuscularly or intravenously) provides a sedative and antiemetic effect, making it a useful drug for acute attacks. Antivertigo/antiemetic medications such as prochlorperazine or hydroxyzine hydrochloride are prescribed to reduce the whirling sensation and nausea. If the nausea and vomiting are severe, intravenous fluids may be necessary to maintain fluid and electrolyte balance.

Treatment

Bedrest in a quiet, darkened room with minimal sensory stimuli and minimal movement provides the most comfort for the person experiencing an acute attack of vertigo.

Between acute attacks, management of the person with Ménière's disease is directed at preventing future attacks and preserving hearing. A low-sodium diet helps reduce labyrinthine pressure. Persons should avoid tobacco, which causes vasoconstriction and can precipitate an attack, as well as alcohol and caffeine.

Surgery

When episodes of vertigo are not controlled through medical interventions, surgery may be necessary. Surgical *endolymphatic decompression* relieves the excess pressure in the labyrinth; a shunt is inserted between the membranous labyrinth and the subarachnoid space to drain excess fluid away from the labyrinths and maintain lower pressure. This procedure preserves hearing for most people. Vertigo is relieved in approximately 70% of persons, but about half undergoing this procedure continue to experience sensations of fullness and tinnitus.

After surgery on the inner ear, the person is positioned to minimise ear pressure and vertigo. Movement is restricted, and assistance is provided when getting up. Antiemetics and antivertigo medications are used to manage symptoms resulting from disruption of the inner ear. Complications include infection and leakage of cerebrospinal fluid.

Go back and revisit the case study presented at the beginning of the chapter concerning Georgia Stanley. Compare some the issues Ms Stanley is experiencing and the topics discussed in this section concerning Ménière's disease. It is important when caring for people to care for them holistically. How might you help Ms Stanley alleviate the anxiety she is experiencing? Here are some issues you might want to think about:

● The impact of hospitalisation on a person's ability to work and earn a living.

● The role of society in assisting those who are unable to work.

● The care of Ms Stanley's father.

● How might you offer Ms Stanley support during bouts of nausea and vomiting?

● What comforting actions might you offer?

● What activities of living might be affected in the case of Georgia Stanley?

NURSING CARE FOR AN INNER EAR DISORDER

The person with an inner ear disorder has multiple nursing care needs related to the signs and symptoms of the disorder.

Health promotion

Health promotion focuses on identifying persons with potential inner ear disorders. Persistent episodes of dizziness, ringing in the ears, balance problems or loss of hearing should be reported to a healthcare provider. Persons diagnosed early may have a lower risk for injury and can be taught strategies for maintaining as near normal as possible their work and social life.

Assessment

In addition to the following, assess the older person for other medical causes of imbalance and dizziness, such as neurological dysfunction, musculoskeletal and cardiovascular disorders and endocrine problems.

✚ *Health history:* medication use; presence of vertigo, tinnitus, nausea and vomiting and hearing loss; balance problems; frequency and duration of symptoms, precipitating factors for an attack.

✚ *Physical examination:* vital signs, general health; hearing, nystagmus, balance.

Nursing diagnoses and interventions

The risk for trauma in persons with inner ear disorders is great. Attacks of vertigo may occur without warning and can be so severe that the person is unable to remain upright. If frequent attacks are accompanied by nausea, nutrition may be compromised. Constant or intermittent tinnitus can interfere with sleep and rest. Nearly all inner ear disorders are associated with some degree of hearing loss, which may be progressive. The person has significant psychosocial needs.

The person with hearing loss

Hearing loss impairs the ability to communicate effectively. Hearing deficits can be partial or total, congenital or acquired. One or both ears may be affected. In some types of hearing loss, the ability to perceive sound at specific frequencies is lost. In others, hearing is diminished across all frequencies.

People with a hearing loss often display signs that caregivers can recognise. Voice volume frequently increases, and the person positions the head with the better ear toward the speaker. The person may frequently ask people to repeat what they have said or respond inappropriately to questions or statements. A question may elicit a blank look if has not been heard or understood.

Pathophysiology and signs and symptoms of hearing loss

Lesions in the outer ear, middle ear, inner ear or central auditory pathways can result in hearing loss. The process of ageing can also affect the structures of the ear and hearing. Hearing loss is classified as conductive, sensorineural or mixed, depending on what portion of the auditory system is affected. Profound deafness is often a congenital condition.

Conductive hearing loss
Disruption of the transmission of sound from the external auditory meatus to the inner ear results in a conductive hearing loss. The most common cause is obstruction of the external ear canal. Impacted cerumen, oedema of the canal lining, stenosis and neoplasms all may lead to canal obstruction. Other causes include a perforated tympanic membrane, disruption or fixation of the ossicles of the middle ear, fluid, scarring or tumours of the middle ear.

With conductive hearing loss, there is an equal loss of hearing at all sound frequencies. If the level of sound is greater than the threshold for hearing, speech discrimination is good, and the person with conductive hearing loss benefits from amplification by a hearing aid.

Sensorineural hearing loss
Disorders that affect the inner ear, the auditory nerve or the auditory pathways of the brain may lead to a sensorineural hearing loss. Here, sound waves are effectively transmitted to the inner ear. In the inner ear, lost or damaged receptor cells, changes in the cochlear apparatus or auditory nerve abnormalities decrease or distort the ability to receive and interpret stimuli.

A significant cause of sensorineural hearing deficit is damage to the hair cells of the organ of Corti. Noise exposure is the major cause. Damage may result from either loud impulse noise (e.g., an explosion) or loud continuous noise (e.g., machinery). Exposure to a high level of noise (e.g., standing close to the stage or speakers at a concert) on an intermittent or continuing basis damages the hair and supporting cells of the organ of Corti. Ototoxic drugs also damage the hair cells; when combined with high noise levels, the damage is greater and resultant hearing loss more profound. Ototoxic drugs include aspirin, furosemide, aminoglycosides, streptomycin, vancomycin, antimalarial drugs and chemotherapy such as cisplatin. Other causes of sensory hearing loss include prenatal exposure to rubella, viral infections, meningitis, trauma, Ménière's disease and ageing.

Tumours such as acoustic neuromas, vascular disorders, demyelinating or degenerative diseases, infections (bacterial meningitis in particular) or trauma may affect the central auditory pathways and produce a neural hearing loss.

Sensorineural hearing losses typically affect the ability to hear high-frequency tones more than low-frequency tones. This makes speech discrimination difficult, especially in a noisy environment. Hearing aids are often not useful; they amplify both speech and background noise. The increased sound intensity may actually cause discomfort.

INTERDISCIPLINARY CARE FOR HEARING LOSS

The best treatment for hearing loss is prevention. Knowing the risk for hearing damage can help prevent it. Awareness of the effects of noise exposure, especially when combined with the ototoxic effects of drugs, is important to prevent sensorineural hearing loss.

Diagnosis

Hearing evaluation includes gross tests of hearing – the Rinne and Weber tests – and audiometry.

- *Rinne* and *Weber tests* compare air and bone sound conduction. When bone conduction of sound is better than air conduction, the hearing deficit is a conductive loss. The Rinne test involves placing a vibrating tuning fork on the base of the mastoid and the Weber test uses a vibrating tuning fork placed on the forehead equidistant from the person's ears.
- *Audiometry* identifies the type and pattern of hearing loss.
- *Speech audiometry* identifies the intensity at which speech can be recognised and interpreted. *Speech discrimination* evaluates the ability to discriminate among various speech sounds.
- *Tympanometry* is an indirect measurement of the compliance and impedance of the middle ear to sound transmission.
- *Acoustic reflex testing* uses a tone presented at various intensities to evaluate movement of the structures of the middle ear.

Amplification

A hearing aid or other amplification device can help with hearing deficits. These devices do nothing to prevent, minimise or treat hearing; they amplify the sound presented to the hearing apparatus of the ear, which may bring the level of sound above the hearing threshold, allowing more accurate perception and interpretation of its meaning. When sound perception is distorted, a hearing aid may be less helpful, because it simply amplifies the distorted sound.

For the person who does not have a hearing aid, an *assistive listening device*, or 'pocket talker', with a microphone and 'Walkman' – type earpieces, is useful. Pocket talkers are available over the counter or through an audiologist. The earpiece requires no special fitting, and the external microphone allows the person to focus on the desired sound rather than simply amplifying all sounds. Assistive listening devices may also be used in conjunction with a hearing aid.

Consider this . . .

If you wear glasses there is often no stigma associated with this. They are put on and people usually say, 'Great, now I can see.' This is not always the case with hearing aids. The stigma attached to wearing one can have a profound effect on a person's health and wellbeing. Hearing aids are often seen as undesirable items, whereas glasses may be seen as fashion accessories.

Consider why there is stigma attached to wearing hearing aids. The notions of deaf and dumb (often used interchangeably) are used incorrectly: some people assume deaf means dumb – with dumb in this instance meaning stupid. Some think that because a person has hearing loss their ability to function effectively is questioned.

Surgery

Reconstructive surgeries of the middle ear, such as a stapedectomy or tympanoplasty, may help restore hearing with a conductive hearing loss. *Stapedectomy* is used to treat hearing loss related to otosclerosis. In a *tympanoplasty*, the structures of the middle ear are reconstructed to improve conductive hearing deficits.

A *cochlear implant* may be the only option for restoring sound perception in sensorineural hearing loss. The implant consists of a microphone, speech processor, transmitter and receiver/stimulator and electrodes (Figure 14.9). Its function is similar to the way the ear normally receives and processes sounds. The microphone picks up sounds, sending them to the speech processor, which selects and processes useful sounds.

Cochlear implants provide sound perception but not normal hearing. The person is able to recognise warning sounds such as cars, sirens, telephones and doors opening or closing. They also receive stimuli to alert them to incoming communication so they can focus on the person speaking.

NURSING CARE FOR HEARING LOSS

In planning and implementing nursing care, the type and extent of hearing loss, the person's adaptation to the loss and the availability of assistive hearing devices are considered, together with the person's ability and willingness to use assistive devices.

Health promotion

Healthcare staff can be instrumental in preventing hearing loss through education. It is important to promote environmental noise control and the use of ear protection. Teaching for primary prevention focuses on:

+ Care of the ears and ear canals, including cleaning and treatment of infection
+ Not placing hard objects into the ear canal
+ Use of plugs to protect the ears during swimming or diving
+ Avoiding intermittent or frequent exposure to loud noise
+ Monitoring for side-effects with ototoxic medications
+ Hearing evaluation when hearing difficulty is present.

Assessment

+ *Health history:* perceived ability to hear; effect of hearing loss on function and lifestyle; risk factors such as use of ototoxic medications; upper respiratory tract or frequent ear infection; noise exposure; presence of vertigo, tinnitus, unsteadiness or imbalance.

+ *Physical examination:* apparent perception of normal speech; inspection of external ear, tympanic membrane; Rinne, and Weber tests; tests of balance and cranial nerve function.

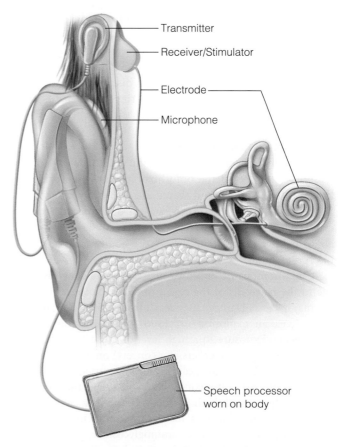

Figure 14.9 A cochlear implant for sensorineural hearing loss.

Nursing diagnoses and interventions

This section focuses on the problems of having a hearing deficit, impaired communication, and social isolation for the person who is hearing impaired.

Risk for disturbed sensory perception: auditory

Whether the hearing deficit is partial or total, impaired sound perception is the primary problem. The person needs to understand what causes the deficit and what to expect for the future. Nursing interventions focus on maximising available hearing and preventing further deterioration to the extent possible.

✚ Encourage to talk about the hearing loss and its effect on activities of living.

✚ Provide information about the type of hearing loss. Refer to an audiologist for evaluation of the hearing loss and possible exploration of amplification devices.

✚ Replace batteries in hearing aids regularly and as needed.

✚ If the hearing aid has a toggle switch for microphone/telephone, be sure it is in the appropriate position.

PRACTICE ALERT

Check hearing aids for patency, ensure batteries are working, cleaning out cerumen as necessary. Regular hearing tests are advocated.

Risk for impaired verbal communication

A hearing deficit impairs the ability to receive and interpret verbal communication. Hearing loss affects the ability to follow conversations, use the telephone and enjoy television or other forms of entertainment.

✚ Use the following techniques to improve communication:
   a. Wave the hand or tap the shoulder before beginning to speak.
   b. If the person wears corrective lenses, ensure that they are clean, and encourage the person to wear them.
   c. When speaking, face your patient and keep your hands away from your face.
   d. Keep your face in full light.
   e. Reduce the noise in the environment before speaking.
   f. Use a low voice pitch with normal loudness.
   g. Use short sentences and pause at the end of each sentence.
   h. Speak at a normal rate, do not overarticulate.
   i. Use facial expressions or gestures.

✚ Be sure hearing aid is properly placed, is turned on and has fresh batteries.

✚ Do not place intravenous catheters in the dominant hand.

✚ Rephrase sentences when there is difficulty understanding.

✚ Repeat important information.

✚ Inform other staff about the client's hearing deficit and effective strategies for communication.

Risk for social isolation

The person with impaired hearing often becomes socially isolated. This may be self-imposed because of difficulty communicating, especially in a group, and isolation comes about gradually and without intention. Social settings and events become increasingly difficult. Friends and family become frustrated trying to communicate with someone who has a hearing impairment, and invitations to participate in social activities dwindle.

✚ Identify the extent and cause of the social isolation. Help to differentiate the reality of the isolation and its cause from the person's perception of isolation.

✚ Encourage to interact with friends and family on a one-to-one basis in quiet settings.

✚ Treat with dignity and remind friends and family that a hearing deficit does not indicate loss of mental faculties.

✚ Involve in activities that do not require acute hearing, such as board games.

✚ Refer to an audiologist for evaluation and possible hearing-aid fitting.

✚ Refer to resources such as support groups.

COMMUNITY-BASED CARE

Teaching for home and community-based care for the person with hearing loss focuses on managing the deficit and developing coping strategies. Referral to an audiologist for evaluation of the deficit and to see whether a hearing aid may be appropriate. In addition, discuss the following:

● use, care and maintenance of a hearing aid;

● strategies for coping with the hearing deficit;

● voicing a preference for individual visits and small group interactions rather than large social functions.

CASE STUDY SUMMARIES

Return to the two people discussed at the beginning of the chapter – Mr Reggie Madison and Ms Georgia Stanley. Both people underwent surgery to help with their conditions.

Case Study 1. Mr Madison needed more intensive postoperative care than Ms Stanley as his diabetes needed careful monitoring and control. His eye became infected and he needed to have intravenous antibiotics. After four days he was discharged home and went to stay with his eldest son and his family. Referral to his endocrinologist was required so that he could be reassessed in relation to his diabetes; this was also the case for his hypertension. He returned to see the ophthalmologist two weeks post-operatively and was deemed fit and in good health, but a referral to the optician was required for an eye test and a new lens prescription.

Case Study 2. Ms Stanley struggled after her operation with pain, nausea and vomiting. She was given analgesia and an antiemetic and comforted to help with this and remained nil by mouth for six hours post-operatively. She was discharged the next day with an out-patient appointment. Her diabetic father was looked after by a kindly neighbour during Ms Stanley's hospitalisation. She gradually returned to her work and by the sixth day was undertaking full-time duties.

CHAPTER HIGHLIGHTS

- Structures of the external eye are vulnerable to trauma and infection. These problems can cause significant pain, scarring and clouding of the cornea and loss or impairment of vision.

- Cataracts, glaucoma and diabetic retinopathy are leading causes of visual impairment in the UK.

- Age, smoking, diabetes and long-term use of certain drugs are risk factors for cataract development. Removal of the clouded lens with insertion of an intraocular lens is the treatment of choice.

- Glaucoma is progressive loss of visual fields associated with increased intraocular pressure and impaired aqueous humour drainage. Open-angle glaucoma, the predominant form of the disorder, can be controlled using medications and, as needed, laser surgery to promote drainage.

- Angle-closure glaucoma is a medical emergency requiring immediate treatment to lower intraocular pressure to preserve vision.

- Diabetic retinopathy eventually affects nearly all people with diabetes. It is a disease of the small blood

vessels of the retina, leading to formation of aneurysms, retinal ischaemia and growth of fragile new vessels that easily rupture leading to haemorrhage.

- Otitis media is related to eustachian tube dysfunction, with impaired pressure equalisation of the middle ear. Otitis media may be either serous (sterile) or infectious (suppurative). Both cause acute discomfort with diminished hearing. There is a risk of complications, including rupture of the tympanic membrane, damage to structures of the middle ear and spread of infection to surrounding tissues.

- Potential complications of acute otitis media include mastoiditis, chronic otitis media with tympanic membrane perforation and cholesteatoma formation. Hearing loss in the affected ear is a possibility.

- The primary symptoms of disorders of the inner ear are vertigo and possible hearing loss. Severe vertigo can interfere with safety, nutrition and the person's ability to maintain activities of living and life roles.

TEST YOURSELF

1. What occurs when light enters the lens?
   a. accommodation
   b. convergence
   c. pupillary reflex
   d. hyperopia

2. During an eye assessment, you touch the part of the eye covering the iris and pupil. What normal response would you expect from the person?
   a. excess tearing
   b. blinking of eyelids
   c. bilateral nystagmus
   d. pupil dilates

3. What equipment would be necessary to test sound conduction during an assessment of the ear?
   a. ophthalmoscope
   b. tuning fork
   c. otoscope
   d. penlight

4. Why is the Snellen eye chart used during vision assessment?
   a. to test distant vision
   b. to test near vision
   c. to determine visual fields
   d. to examine convergence

5. What is another name for cerumen?

   a. blood
   b. lymph
   c. ear wax
   d. pus

6. What function, in addition to hearing, is provided by the inner ear?

   a. coordinates visual pathways
   b. integrates efferent neurone messages
   c. provides information about head position
   d. maintains middle ear structure and function

7. What is a high-priority risk for the older adult with age-related changes in the vestibular structures of the ear?

   a. infection
   b. falls
   c. medication errors
   d. constipation

8. Which of the following is not one of the three smallest bones in the ear?

   a. anvil
   b. hammer
   c. bridle
   d. stirrup

9. The semi-circular canals can help:

   a. breathe
   b. maintain balance
   c. see
   d. feel

10. Another name for the tympanic membrane is:

   a. the iris
   b. the palate
   c. the conjunctiva
   d. the eardrum

Further resources

Royal National Institute of Blind People (RNIB)
www.rnib.org.uk
The UK's leading charity offering information, support and advice to over two million people with sight loss.

Royal National Institute for Deaf People (RNID)
www.rnid.org.uk
The RNID helps people identify whether they have a hearing loss. They campaign for change and provide services and training.

National Institute for Health and Clinical Excellence (NICE)
www.nice.org.uk
Provides guidance, sets quality standards and manages a national database to improve people's health and prevent and treat ill health.

Bibliography

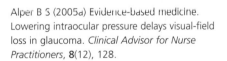

Alper B S (2005a) Evidence-based medicine. Lowering intraocular pressure delays visual-field loss in glaucoma. *Clinical Advisor for Nurse Practitioners*, **8**(12), 128.

Bickley L and Szilagyi P (2009) *Bates' Guide to Physical Examination and History Taking* (10th edn). Philadelphia, PA, Lippincott.

Bremridge T (2005) Caring for those with age-related impaired sight. *Nursing & Residential Care*, **7**(11), 507–509.

Centre for Health and Social Care (2008) *Registered Blind and Partially Sighted People Year ending 31 March 2008 England*. Leeds, Centre for Health and Social Care.

Cohen A S and Ayello E A (2005) Diabetes has taken a toll on your patient's vision: How can you help? *Nursing*, **35**(5), 44–47.

Conley Y P and Gorin M B (2003) The genetics of age-related macular degeneration. *Medsurg Nursing*, **12**(4), 238–241, 259.

Copstead L E and Banasik J L (2010) *Pathophysiology* (4th edn). Philadelphia, PA, W. B. Saunders.

Cox C, Boswell G, McGrath A, Reynolds T and Cole E (2004) Cranial nerve damage. *Emergency Nurse*, **12**(2), 14–21.

Davies S and de Guzman A (2004) Ear drops containing steroids were better than acetic acid for otitis externa. *Evidence-Based Nursing*, **7**(2), 43.

Denniston A K O and Murray P I (2008) *Oxford Handbook of Ophthalmology*. Oxford, Oxford University Press.

Desai P, Minassian D C and Reidy A (1999) National cataract surgery survey 1997–8: A report of the results of the clinical outcomes. *British Journal of Ophthalmology*, **83**(12), 1336–1340.

Dougherty L and Lister S (2008) *The Royal Marsden Hospital Manual of Clinical Nursing Procedures* (7th edn). Oxford, Wiley-Blackwell.

Eliopoulos E (2010) *Gerontological Nursing* (7th edn). Philadelphia, PA, Lippincott.

Ervin S (2004) Ménière's disease. Identifying classic symptoms and current treatments. *AAOHN Journal*, **52**(4), 156–158.

Fontaine K L (2010) *Healing Practices: Alternative therapies for nursing* (3rd edn). Upper Saddle River, NJ, Prentice Hall Health.

Fox A and Bartlett P (2001) Nurse-led ear care: training needs and the latest techniques. *Professional Nurse*, **17**(4), 256–258.

Gallacher R (2004). Understanding the nursing role in patients who have cataract. *Nursing Times*, **100**(21), 31.

Greenlee E C (2005) Laser and surgical treatments for glaucoma: an overview. *Insight: The Journal of the American Society of Ophthalmic Registered Nurses*, **30**(4), 32–37.

Hudspeth A (2002) How hearing happens. *Hearing Loss*, **23**(1), 25–27.

IGA (2010) *What is Glaucoma?* Ashford, International Glaucoma Association, available at: http://www.glaucoma-association.com/the-eye-and-glaucoma/what-is-glaucoma.html (accessed September 2011).

Jarvis C (2007) *Physical Examination & Health Assessment* (5th edn). St Louis, MO, Mosby.

Heimink A L and Sego S (2005) Advisor forum. Chronic tinnitus treatment. *Clinical Advisor for Nurse Practitioners*, **8**(4), 56.

Holcomb S S (2004) This just in. New guidelines improve treatment of otitis media. *Nurse Practitioner: American Journal of Primary Health Care*, **29**(10), 6, 8, 13.

Holman C, Roberts S and Nicol M (2005) Promoting good care for people with hearing impairment. *Nursing Older People*, **17**(2), 31–32.

Houde S C and Huff M A (2003) Age-related vision loss in older adults: A challenge for gerontological nurses. *Journal of Gerontological Nursing*, **29**(4), 25–33, 51–52.

Kahari K, Zachau G, Eklof M, Sandsjo L and Moller C (2003) Assessment of hearing and hearing disorders in rock/jazz musicians. *International Journal of Audiology*, **42**(5), 179–288.

Kasper D L, Braunwald E, Fauci A S, *et al.* (eds) (2005) *Harrison's Principles of Internal Medicine* (16th edn). New York, McGraw-Hill.

Kee J (2010) *Prentice Hall Handbook of Laboratory & Diagnostic Tests with Nursing Implications* (8th edn). Upper Saddle River, NJ, Prentice Hall.

Kertes P J and Johnson T K (2007) *Evidence Based Eye Care*. Philadelphia, PA, Lippincott.

Kleinbeck C and Williams A S (2004) Disabilities, diabetes, and devices. *Home Healthcare Nurse*, **22**(7), 469–475.

Levinson D (2003) Many elderly patients with chronic eye disease don't get recommended exams. *Report on Medical Guidelines & Outcomes Research*, **14**(20), 1, 5–6.

Lusk S L, Ronis D L, Kazanis A S, *et al.* (2003) Effectiveness of a tailored intervention to increase factory workers' use of hearing. *Nursing Research*, **52**(5), 289–295.

Marsden J (2004a) Clinical. Cataract: The role of nurses in diagnosis, surgery and aftercare. *Nursing Times*, **100**(7), 36–40.

Marsden J (2004b) Clinical. Implications of and treatment options for retinal detachment. *Nursing Times*, **100**(37), 44–47.

McGrory A and Remington R (2004) Optimizing the functionality of clients with age-related macular degeneration. *Journal of Rehabilitation Nursing*, **29**(3), 90–94.

Meadows M (2002) Saving your sight. Early detection is critical. *FDA Consumer*, **36**(2), 22–28.

Moore L W and Miller M (2003) Older men's experience of living with severe visual impairment. *Journal of Advanced Nursing*, **43**(1), 10–18.

Moore L W and Miller M (2005) Driving strategies used by older adults with macular degeneration: Assessing the risks. *Applied Nursing Research*, **18**(2), 110–116.

National Health Service (2010) *Diabetic Retinopathy the Facts*. Available at: http://www.retinalscreening.nhs.uk/userFiles/File/diabeticRetinopathyFacts.pdf, last accessed August 2011.

NICE (2009a) *Glaucoma: Diagnosis and Management and Chronic Open Angle Glaucoma and Ocular Hypertension*, CG85. London, National Institute for Health and Clinical Excellence.

NICE (2009b) *Cochlear Implants for Children and Adults with Severe to Profound Deafness*, TAG 166. London, National Institute for Health and Clinical Excellence.

Neault G (2005) Self-care needs of cataract patients following ambulatory surgery. *Insight: The Journal of the American Society of Ophthalmic Registered Nurses*, **30**(4), 7–11.

Porth, C M (2009) *Pathophysiology: Concepts of altered health states* (9th edn). Philadelphia, PA, Lippincott.

Quinlan K (2003) The importance of discharge instructions. *Journal of Emergency Nursing*, **29**(4), 308.

Rask E M (2004) Recognize cholesteatomas early. *The Nurse Practitioner*, **29**(2), 24–27.

Rassin M, Gorlansky N, Shahin E, *et al.* (2005) NT research. Importance of early referral in sudden loss of hearing. *Nursing Times*, **101**(49), 34–36.

RCN (2009) *The Nature and Scope of Ophthalmic Nursing*. London, Royal College of Nursing.

RNIB (2008) *High Degree Myopia*. London, Royal National Institute of Blind People, available at: http://www.rnib.org.uk/eyehealth/eyeconditions/eyeconditionsdn/Pages/high_degree_myopia.aspx (accessed September 2011).

RNIB (2009) *Could Your Family Hold a Clue to a Risk of Sight Loss?* Press release. London, Royal National Institute for Blind People, available at: http://www.rnib.org.uk/aboutus/mediacentre/mediareleases/media2009/Pages/Mediarelease16Oct2009.aspx (accessed September 2011).

RNIB (2011) *Clear Print Guidelines*. London, Royal National Institute of Blind People, available at: http://www.rnib.org.uk/professionals/accessibleinformation/text/Pages/clear_print.aspx, last accessed August 2011.

Rothrock J C (2007) *Alexander's Care of the Patient in Surgery* (13th edn). St Louis, MO, Mosby.

Smeeth L and Iliffe S (2005) Community screening for visual impairment in the elderly. *The Cochrane Library (Oxford)*, **1**, ID#CD001054.

Smith S C, Lamb P and Liu J (2005) Age-related macular degeneration: answers to some common questions. *Insight: The Journal of the American Society of Ophthalmic Registered Nurses*, **30**(3), 17–23.

Stuen C and Faye E (2003) Vision loss: Normal and not normal changes among older adults. *Generations*, **27**(1), 8–14.

Tierney L M, McPhee S J and Papadakis M A (eds) (2005) *Current Medical Diagnosis & Treatment* (44th edn). Stamford, CT, Appleton & Lange.

Wallhagen M, Pettengill E and Whiteside M (2006) Sensory impairment in older adults: Part 1: Hearing loss. *American Journal of Nursing*, **106**(10), 40–48.

Wandell B and Wade A (2003) Functional imaging of the visual pathways. *Neurologic Clinics*, **21**(2), 417–443.

Watkinson S (2005) Visual impairment in older people: The nurse's role. *Nursing Standard*, **19**(17), 45–52, 54–55.

Watkinson S and Seewoodhary R (2007) Common eye conditions and practical considerations in eye care. *Nursing Standard*, **21**(44), 42–47.

Way L W and Doherty G M (2003) *Current Surgical Diagnosis & Treatment* (11th edn). New York, McGraw-Hill.

Weber J and Kelley J (2009) *Health Assessment in Nursing* (4th edn). Philadelphia, PA, Lippincott.

Whiteside M, Wallhagen M and Pettengill E (2006) Sensory impairment in older adults: Part 2: Vision loss. *American Journal of Nursing*, **106**(11), 52–61.

Wilkinson J M (2005) *Nursing Diagnosis Handbook* (8th edn). Upper Saddle River, NJ, Prentice Hall.

Williams D (2005) Does irrigation of the ear to remove impacted wax improve hearing? *British Journal of Community Nursing*, **10**(5), 228–232.

Wright J (2005) Common ear problems in the primary care setting. *Journal of Community Nursing*, **19**(9), 43–44, 46.

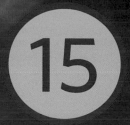

15

Caring for women with reproductive problems

Learning outcomes

- Describe the anatomy, physiology and functions of the female reproductive system.
- Identify specific topics for consideration during a health history.
- Identify signs and symptoms of impairment in the female reproductive system.
- Explain pathophysiological changes and nursing care.
- Discuss nursing implications and health education required.
- Describe various surgical procedures associated with the female reproductive system.

Clinical competencies

- Conduct and document a health history and physical assessment.
- Monitor the results of diagnostic tests and report abnormal findings.
- Assess the functional status of women and monitor, document and report abnormal signs and symptoms.
- Provide care to women using an evidence-base.
- Implement individualised nursing interventions.

CASE STUDIES

Below are three case studies that you may wish to consider before, during or after you have read the chapter. There are no right or wrong answers to these case studies, but you should consider the physical, psychological and social implications.

Case Study 1 – Megan

Mrs Megan Jones is 46 years old, married with two children. Ebrill is 22 years old and Dfydd is 8 years old. She presents to the general practice nurse with symptoms of premenopause. The practice nurse assesses Mrs Jones and she tells the nurse that she has not had a period in three months and her last four periods were irregular and short. Mrs Jones has been experiencing hot flushes and mood changes. She also reports a change in libido – her sex drive has fallen and she says that this it is affecting her relationship with her husband. She is on 'birth control pills' and has not had a cervical smear in three years. She does not perform breast self-examination as she tells the nurse 'she never knows what she is supposed to feeling or looking for'. Ebrill, her daughter, is expecting a baby in two months and she is worried that she will be unable to care for the new baby because of her frequent episodes of depression and mood swings.

Case Study 2 – Rohinee

Ms Rohinee Jenson is a 32 year-old. This is her first visit to the general practitioner for problems associated with her reproductive system. She complains of 'burning and pain in my crotch area' and notes that 'it really hurts to pee.' She adds that she had unprotected sex about two weeks ago. Oral temperature is 38.3 °C. Vaginal examination reveals findings of vesicles and red ulcerations on the labia majora and vaginal mucosa. Inguinal lymph nodes are enlarged and tender. A culture of ulcerations is taken and the specimen is sent to the laboratory for analysis.

Case Study 3 – Rachel

Mrs Rachel Clemments is a 42-year-old mother of two, Sarah, age 12, and Jennifer, age 18. Because of a family history of breast cancer, she has been closely monitored (annual mammograms and clinical breast examination, monthly breast self-examination (BSE), a needle aspiration biopsy with negative findings) for four years prior to her diagnosis. Mrs Clemments discovers a lump in her left breast during her monthly BSE. An incisional biopsy reveals invasive lobular carcinoma in the left breast. Mrs Clemments is debating whether to have reconstructive breast surgery. One of her greatest concerns is how her illness will affect her ability to support and care for her daughters. The breast cancer diagnosis seems part of the family legacy. She wonders, 'When will it happen to Jennifer? To Sarah?'

INTRODUCTION

Caring for women with gynaecological problems provides the nurse with the opportunity to offer physical, emotional and practical help. The nurse must be aware that some people are embarrassed about issues related to their reproductive health. When the nurse takes time to explain things in a language the person understands as well as to listen they can help relieve the embarrassment or at least make it more tolerable.

The pink ribbon

Encouraging women to speak openly can help to save lives, enhance quality of life and improve health and wellbeing. For many years the international symbol of awareness of breast cancer has been wearing of a pink ribbon or pink ribbon emblem. Breast cancer, the most common form of cancer diagnosed among women, is still killing today.

Whenever you see a pink ribbon you instinctively know what the symbol stands for. There are no words or pictures needed; automatically people connect it with breast cancer. In the early 1990s people were urged to wear the ribbons to raise awareness. The number of women coming forward for screening has increased since the campaign was introduced, demonstrating an increase in awareness amongst the population.

To care effectively and safely for women with problems associated with their reproductive system the nurse must have an understanding of this system. This next section provides an understanding of the associated anatomy and physiology.

The female reproductive system

The female reproductive organs, along with the neuroendocrine system, produce hormones important in biological development and sexual behaviour. Parts of the female reproductive organs are integral to the function of the urinary system. Assessment of the reproductive and urinary systems requires sensitivity when asking questions about topics that the person may be hesitant to talk about. Skill is also required in conducting physical examinations. The more experience and practice you acquire, the more skilled you will become.

Disorders range from a minor discomfort of menstrual cramps to life-threatening diseases. These disorders can occur at any point in a woman's adult life and can affect her ability to bear children, her sexuality and her sense of wellbeing.

A holistic approach is required to meet physical, emotional and educational needs along with sensitivity and understanding. When planning and implementing care, consideration is needed within the context of culture, socioeconomic, educational level and lifestyle.

This chapter summarises disorders of female sexual function. Sexually transmitted infections are discussed in Chapter 17. Treatment of cancer with chemotherapy and radiation is discussed in Chapter 2. Understanding the important issues discussed in this chapter helps you appreciate the care and treatment a woman needs for it to be safe and effective.

ANATOMY, PHYSIOLOGY AND FUNCTIONS OF THE FEMALE REPRODUCTIVE SYSTEM

The female reproductive system consists of the external genitalia and internal organs. The breasts are a part of women's reproductive organs. In women, the urethra and urinary meatus (the passage where urine passes) are separated from the reproductive organs, but they are so close to each other that a health problem with one often affects the other.

THE BREASTS

The breasts (or mammary glands) are located between the third and seventh ribs on the anterior (towards the front) chest wall supported by the pectoral muscles and supplied with nerves, blood and lymph (Figure 15.1). A pigmented area – the areola – is located below the centre of each breast, containing sebaceous glands and a nipple. The nipple usually protrudes and becomes erect in response to cold and stimulation.

The breasts are made of adipose (fat) tissue, fibrous connective tissue and glandular tissue. Bands of fibrous tissue support the breast, extending from the outer breast tissue to the nipple, dividing the breast into 15–25 lobes. Lobes are made of alveolar glands connected by ducts that open to the nipple.

THE EXTERNAL GENITALIA

Collectively, these are called the vulva, including the mons pubis, the labia, the clitoris, the vaginal and urethral openings and glands (Figure 15.2).

The mons pubis is a pad of adipose tissue covered with skin. The labia are divided into two structures. The labia majora, folds of skin and adipose tissue covered with hair, are outermost; they begin at the base of the mons pubis and end at the anus. The labia minora, located between the clitoris and the base of the vagina, are enclosed by the labia majora, made of skin, adipose tissue and some erectile tissues.

Between the labia is the vestibule, containing the openings for the vagina and the urethra and the Bartholin's glands. Skene's glands open onto the vestibule. These glands secrete

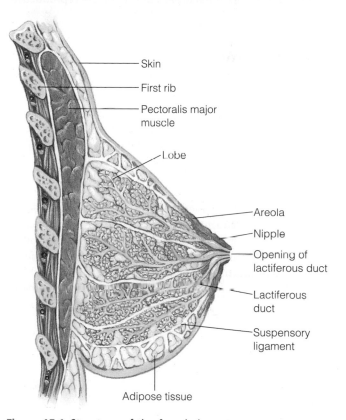

Figure 15.1 Structure of the female breast.

lubricating fluid during the sexual response and before **menopause**.

The clitoris is an erectile organ (akin to the penis), formed by the joining of the labia minora. It is highly sensitive, distending during sexual arousal.

The vaginal opening (the introitus) opens between the internal and the external genitals. Prior to intercourse or trauma, this is surrounded by the hymen.

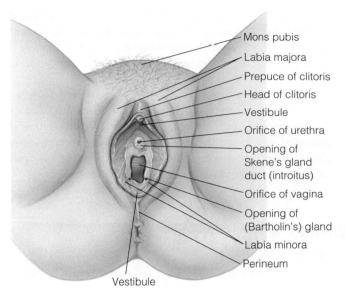

Figure 15.2 The external organs of the female reproductive system.

THE INTERNAL ORGANS

The vagina and cervix, uterus, fallopian tubes and ovaries are the internal organs of the female reproductive system (Figure 15.3). The ovaries are the primary reproductive organs, also producing female sex hormones. The vagina, uterus and fallopian tubes are accessory ducts for the ovaries and developing foetus.

The vagina and cervix

The vagina is a fibromuscular tube 8–10 cm in length located posterior to the bladder and urethra and anterior to the rectum. The upper end contains the uterine cervix in the fornix. The walls are membranes that form folds, called rugae, and are composed of mucous-secreting stratified squamous epithelial cells. The vagina excretes secretions, including menstrual fluid; it is an organ of sexual response and a passageway for the birth of an infant.

The walls are usually moist maintaining a pH ranging from 3.8–4.2. This is bacteriostatic (inhibits the growth of bacteria) and is maintained by the action of **oestrogen** and normal vaginal flora (healthy micro-organisms). Oestrogen stimulates the growth of vaginal mucosal cells so that they thicken and have increased glycogen content. Glycogen is fermented to lactic acid by lactobacilli (organisms that produce lactic acid) normally inhabiting the vagina.

The cervix projects into the vagina forming a pathway between the uterus and the vagina. The uterine opening of the cervix is the internal os, the vaginal opening the external os. The space between, the endocervical canal, is a route for discharge of menstrual fluid, entrance for sperm and expulsion of the infant during birth. The cervix is a firm structure, protected by mucus changing consistency and quantity during the **menstrual cycle** and pregnancy.

The uterus

This is a hollow pear-shaped muscular organ with thick walls located between the bladder and the rectum. It has three parts: the fundus, the body and the cervix. It is supported in the abdominal cavity by the broad ligaments, the round ligaments, the uterosacral ligaments and the transverse (lying across) cervical ligaments. The uterus receives the fertilised ovum providing a site for growth and development of the foetus. There are three layers:

- *The perimetrium* – outer serous layer merging with the peritoneum.

- *The myometrium* – middle layer making up most of the uterine wall; it has muscle fibres running in various directions, allowing contractions during menstruation or childbirth, and expansion as the foetus grows.

- *The endometrium* lines the uterus; its outermost layer is shed during menstruation.

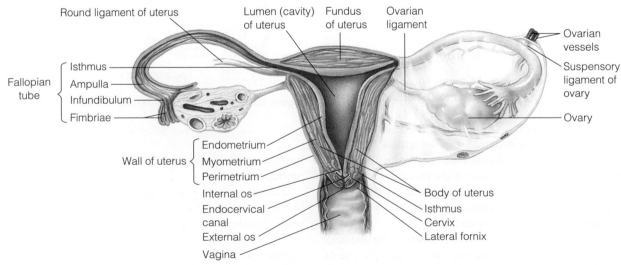

Figure 15.3 The internal organs of the female reproductive system.

The fallopian tubes

These are thin cylindrical structures 10 cm long and 1 cm in diameter, attached to the uterus on one end and supported by the broad ligaments. The lateral ends are open and made of projections called fimbriae draping over the ovary; these pick up the ovum after discharge from the ovary.

These tubes are made of smooth muscle and lined with ciliated, mucous-producing epithelial cells. The movement of the cilia and contractions of the smooth muscle move the ovum through the tubes toward the uterus. Fertilisation of the ovum by the sperm usually occurs in the outer portion of a fallopian tube.

The ovaries

In the adult woman these are flat, almond-shaped structures located on either side of the uterus below the ends of the fallopian tubes, attached to the uterus by ligaments. Ovaries store the germ cells and produce the oestrogen and progesterone. The total number of ova is present at birth.

Ovaries contain ovarian follicles. Each contains an immature ovum, an oocyte. Monthly, several follicles are stimulated by follicle-stimulating hormone (FSH) and luteinising hormone (LH) to mature. The developing follicles are surrounded by graafian follicles, which produce oestrogen, stimulating the development of endometrium. Ovulation occurs each month. The ruptured follicle then becomes a structure called the corpus luteum. This produces both oestrogen and progesterone, supporting the endometrium until conception occurs or the cycle begins again. The corpus luteum degenerates, leaving a scar on the surface of the ovary.

FEMALE SEX HORMONES

The ovaries produce oestrogens, **progesterone** and androgens in a cyclic pattern. Oestrogens are steroid hormones occuring naturally in three forms: estrone (E_1), estradiol (E_2) and estriol (E_3). Estradiol is the most potent and secreted in the greatest amount. Oestrogens are secreted throughout the menstrual cycle, and they are at a higher level during certain phases of the cycle, as discussed shortly.

Oestrogens are essential for the development and maintenance of secondary sex characteristics; with other hormones, they stimulate the female reproductive organs to prepare for growth of a foetus. Oestrogens are responsible for the normal structure of skin and blood vessels, decreasing the rate of bone resorption (bone breakdown), promoting increased high-density lipoproteins (chemicals containing proteins and lipids), reducing cholesterol levels and enhancing the clotting of blood. Oestrogens also promote the retention of sodium and water.

Menopause, a normal physiological process, occurs as a result of the gradual decrease and final cessation of oestrogen. As menstruation ceases tissues that had been supported by oestrogen change. Oestrogen deprivation increases the risk of osteoporosis (a bone disease) and cardiovascular disease.

Progesterone primarily affects the development of breast glandular tissue and the endometrium. During pregnancy, progesterone relaxes smooth muscle decreasing uterine contractions and increasing body temperature.

OOGENESIS AND THE OVARIAN CYCLE

All of a woman's ova are present at birth as primary oocytes in ovarian follicles. Each month, from puberty until menopause, the remaining events of oogenesis (the production of ova) occur. Collectively, this is known as the **ovarian cycle**.

The ovarian cycle has three consecutive phases occurring cyclically each 28 days (the cycle may be longer or shorter):

- *The follicular phase*, lasting from the 1st to 10th day of the cycle.
- *The ovulatory phase*, lasting from the 11th to 14th day of the cycle ending with ovulation.
- *The luteal phase*, lasting from the 14th to 28th day.

During the follicular phase, the follicle develops, the oocyte matures, controlled by the interaction of FSH and LH. On day 1 of the cycle, gonadotropin-releasing hormone (GnRH) increases and stimulates increased production of FSH and LH; they stimulate follicular growth and the oocyte grows. The structure, now called the primary follicle, becomes a multicellular mass surrounded by a fibrous capsule, the theca folliculi. As the follicle continues to increase in size, oestrogen is produced and a fluid-filled space forms within the follicle. The oocyte is enclosed by a membrane, the zona pellucida. By about day 10, the follicle is a mature graafian follicle bulging out from the surface of the ovary. Only one follicle becomes dominant and matures to ovulation, while the others degenerate.

The ovulatory phase begins when oestrogen levels are high enough to stimulate the anterior pituitary gland, and a surge of LH is produced. The LH stimulates meiosis (cell division) in the developing oocyte, and its first meiotic division occurs. The LH also stimulates enzymes that act on the bulging ovarian wall, leading to rupture and discharge. The oocyte is expelled from the mature ovarian follicle during ovulation.

During the luteal phase, the surge in LH stimulates the ruptured follicle to change into a corpus luteum and then stimulates the corpus luteum to begin immediately producing progesterone and oestrogen. The increase of progesterone and oestrogen in the blood has a negative feedback effect on the production of LH, inhibiting the further growth and development of other follicles.

If pregnancy does not occur, the corpus luteum degenerates and hormone production ceases. The declining production of progesterone and oestrogen at the end of the cycle allows the secretion of LH and FSH to increase, and a new cycle begins. The ovarian cycle is compared to the menstrual cycle in Figure 15.4.

THE MENSTRUAL CYCLE

The endometrium responds to changes in oestrogen and progesterone during the ovarian cycle, preparing for implantation

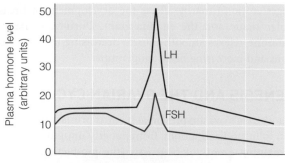

A Fluctuation of gonadotropin levels

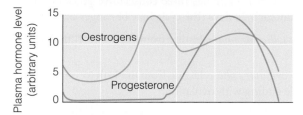

B Fluctuation of ovarian hormone levels

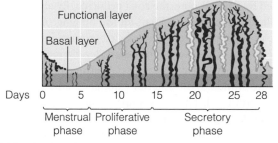

C Ovarian cycle

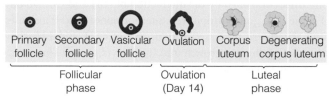

D Menstrual cycle

Figure 15.4 Comparison of the ovarian and menstrual cycles.

of the fertilised embryo. The endometrium is receptive to implantation of the embryo for a brief period each month, coinciding with the time when the embryo would normally reach the uterus from the uterine tube (usually seven days).

The menstrual cycle begins with the menstrual phase, lasting from days 1 to 5. The inner endometrial (functionalis) layer detaches and is expelled as menstrual fluid for three to five days. As the maturing follicle begins to produce oestrogen (days 6 to 14), the proliferative phase begins. In response, the functionalis layer is repaired and thickens. Cervical mucus changes to a thin substance helping sperm move up into the uterus.

The final phase, lasting from days 14 to 28, is the secretory phase. As the corpus luteum produces progesterone, rising

levels act on the endometrium, causing increased vascularity, changing the inner layer to secretory mucosa, stimulating the secretion of glycogen into the uterine cavity, causing the cervical mucus again to thicken and block the internal os (an os is mouth or mouth-like opening). If fertilisation does not occur, hormone levels fall. The endometrial cells begin to degenerate and slough off. The process begins again with the sloughing of the functionalis layer.

Understanding the anatomy and physiology can instil confidence in those you care for. Now the anatomy and physiology has been explained, the chapter will now move on and introduce to you assessment.

Assessing the female reproductive system

Assessment requires understanding, care and compassion. As you become an experienced practitioner your ability to use higher-level assessment skills will follow. Assessment occurs through diagnostic tests, health assessment interview to collect subjective data and physical assessment to collect objective data. Information is used to individualise the questions asked; for example, the post-menopausal woman would not be asked specific questions about her menstrual cycle, but it would be important to ask about vaginal dryness.

DIAGNOSTIC TESTS

The results of diagnostic tests are used to:

● monitor the health of reproductive structures;

● support the diagnosis of a specific sexual problem, injury or disease;

● provide information to identify or modify medications or treatments;

● help nurses monitor the responses to treatment and nursing care interventions.

Diagnostic tests to assess the female reproductive system are described on pages 568–569 and summarised below.

A number of tests are needed to ensure full assessment. The following may be required:

● Blood tests to diagnose hormonal changes and sexually transmitted infections.

● Cultures (types of tests that may include a swabbed specimen or blood specimen) and smears of discharge or mucous membranes.

● A mammogram (a radiographic examination of the breast) is used to detect breast tumours, followed by a breast biopsy (a small sample of breast tissue is removed and taken for analysis) for a definitive diagnosis.

- The Papanicolaou smear (often called cervical smear or smear).

- Space-occupying lesions (abnormal tissue occupying a space) and abnormalities of the vagina, cervix or uterus may be evaluated with ultrasound (a test used to produce a visual graphic of tissue being examined), a hysterosalpingogram (a test used to outline the uterus and fallopian tubes), a colposcopy (visualisation of the cervix), a cervical biopsy, a

laparoscopy (a procedure using a laparoscope to examine the fallopian tubes, ovaries and uterus) and/or an endometrial biopsy.

The nurse assists the woman before, during and after the examination and is responsible for explaining the procedure and any special preparation needed as well as for documenting the procedures as appropriate, and for monitoring the results of the tests.

IN PRACTICE

Cervical smear

Most cervical smears are undertaken by the practice nurse. This test does not diagnose cancer, it determines the health of the cervix (Higgins 2007). The intention is to collect squamous epithelial cells and endocervical cells from the transformation zone and squamo-columnar junction of the cervix (World Health Organization (WHO) 2006). A number of devices can be used to collect the specimens:

- wooden spatula;
- plastic spatula;
- plastic brush;
- plastic broom;
- endocervical brush.

It is vital that the cells collected are transferred immediately to a glass slide and preserved (fixed) immediately. Slides are then placed in a refrigerator prior to transportation to the laboratory. The best time to collect a slide is when the women is in mid-cycle (pre-menopausal), ensuring that the specimen is not contaminated with menstrual flow and debris (WHO 2006).

The equipment required for collecting a smear is taken from www.cancerscreening.nhs.uk/cervical, www.ic.nhs.uk

and Dougherty and Lister (2009). At all times local policy and procedure must be adhered to.

1. Alcohol hand rub, clean disposable gloves, plastic apron.
2. A variety of different sized speculae (instruments that are used to help view the cervix).
3. A variety of spatulae and brushes (as described opposite).
4. Glass slide with frosted edge.
5. Pencil for labelling the specimen.
6. Fixative solution.
7. Plastic slide container.
8. Specimen form and bag.
9. Box of tissues.
10. Clinical waste container.

Ensure there is a good light source available; the woman should be positioned on an appropriate examining couch. Make sure all of the equipment is available in the room prior to the examination. The room should be warm. Ensure that during the examination privacy and dignity will be maintained.

GENETIC CONSIDERATIONS

When conducting a health assessment interview and a physical assessment, consider genetic influences on health of the woman – some diseases of the reproductive system have a genetic component. During the health assessment interview, ask about a family history of ovarian or breast cancer. During physical assessment, assess for signs and symptoms that might indicate a genetic disorder (see below). If data are found to indicate genetic risk factors or alterations, refer for genetic counselling.

A number of genetic considerations are associated with the female reproductive system:

- There is a genetic link for some of the cases of breast and ovarian cancer. Two breast cancer susceptibility genes have been identified: BRCA1 and BRCA2. Having either of these genes increases risk for having breast or ovarian cancer.

- A family history of endometrial, colon or breast cancer increases risk for endometrial cancer.

- Turner syndrome is caused by complete or partial absence of one of the two X chromosomes and is characterised by short stature and the lack of sexual development at puberty.

Understanding of the various tests will help you deliver high-quality, informed care.

DIAGNOSTIC TESTS The female reproductive system

SCREENING TESTS, SMEARS AND CULTURES

Papanicolaou smear

Helps to diagnose malignant and premalignant lesions of the cervix; assesses the effects of hormone replacement; identifies viral, bacterial, fungal and parasitic conditions; evaluates response to chemotherapy or radiation therapy. Cells are obtained during a pelvic examination. Sample collected is smeared on a glass slide or put into a special liquid preservative. Cells are then stained and examined.

RELATED NURSING CARE *Explain that the test should be done during a time when the woman is not menstruating, she should not have intercourse, douche, or use vaginal medications for 36 hours before the examination. The woman should void urine prior to the examination.*

BREAST EXAMINATIONS

Mammogram

Detects tumours in the breast. Breasts are flattened in the mammography machine and low-dose x-rays taken.

RELATED NURSING CARE *The woman should not apply body powder or underarm deodorant before mammogram.*

Breast ultrasound

Uses high-frequency sound waves passing through tissues to detect masses in the breast. Performed if lesions are identified in mammogram.

RELATED NURSING CARE *No special preparation is needed.*

Breast biopsy and fine-needle aspiration

Core needle biopsy

Vacuum-assisted mammotome

Large core surgical biopsy

Open surgical biopsy

- Fine-needle aspiration withdraws fluid from cysts. It may be used to sample cells from masses in the breast. A needle is used to collect five to six samples of fluid or cells.
- Core needle biopsy obtains a sample of tissue from a solid mass or calcium deposits in the breast. A needle is used to collect five to six tissue samples.
- Vacuum-assisted mammotome evaluates calcifications. A needle is inserted through a small half centimetre incision and 8 to 10 samples are removed.
- Large core surgical biopsy evaluates breast masses or calcification identified with a mammogram but non-palpable. An incision is made and a 5–20 mm cylinder of breast tissue removed.
- Open surgical biopsy evaluate breasts masses, hard-to-reach lesions, multiple lesions and masses with calcifications. A 4–5 cm incision is made and a golf ball size (or larger) area of tissue is removed.

RELATED NURSING CARE *For all types, wearing a bra, applying ice packs and mild analgesics decrease discomfort post-procedure.*

✛ *Explain that some procedures may be performed with or without a local anaesthetic.*

✛ *Explain that if a local anaesthetic is used, no stitches are required for a core needle biopsy or mammatome.*

✛ *Explain that a local anaesthetic is used and stitches will be used to close the incision for a large-core biopsy.*

✛ *Explain that a general anaesthetic is usually used and that the incision requires stitches and that, for an open surgical biopsy, there will be scarring.*

DIAGNOSTIC TESTS The female reproductive system (continued)

TESTS OF THE INTERNAL REPRODUCTIVE SYSTEM

Ultrasound (abdominal, vaginal)

Detects the presence of space-occupying lesions. The abdomen is coated with transducing gel and a graphic visualisation is made. For vaginal ultrasound, a transducer is covered with a condom or vinyl glove coated with transducer gel, then introduced into the vagina.

RELATED NURSING CARE *Explain the need to increase intake of fluids, not to void until the test is completed to ensure a full bladder.*

Hysterosalpingogram

Diagnoses causes of infertility and abnormalities of the uterus or fallopian tubes. Contrast medium is instilled through the cervix, through the uterus and out of the fallopian tubes while x-rays are taken.

RELATED NURSING CARE *Assess for allergy to seafood (iodine) or previous contrast media. Explain that this procedure is briefly painful.*

Colposcopy

Conducted to further study abnormal smear tests; a microscope is used to directly visualise the cervix.

RELATED NURSING CARE *No special preparation required.*

Conisation

Loop electrosurgical excision of transformation zone (LEETZ)
Loop electrosurgical excision procedure (LEEP)
A conisation LEETZ or LEEP is performed to remove cervical tissue for evaluation. A cone-shaped area of tissue surrounding the cervical os is removed.

RELATED NURSING CARE *Explain that the procedure requires general anaesthesia. Post-operative self-care includes rest for two to three days. Minor vaginal bleeding and discharge are expected for several days post-procedure; perineal pads (not tampons) should be used. Avoid sexual intercourse until discharge stops. Notify nurse or doctor if increased bleeding or signs of infection (pain, foul-smelling discharge, fever) occur.*

Cervical biopsy

Performed when smear test results indicate possible cervical cancer or cervical intraepithelial neoplasia (CIN) and for screening for women at high risk for vaginal and cervical cancers from intrauterine exposure to diethylstilbestrol (DES). Cervix is cleaned and a sample of tissue taken for analysis.

RELATED NURSING CARE *Explain that minor vaginal bleeding and discharge are expected for several days post-procedure; perineal pads (not tampons) should be used. Avoid sexual intercourse until discharge stops. Notify nurse or doctor if increased bleeding or signs of infection (pain, foul-smelling discharge, fever) occur.*

Laparoscopy

Visualises the organs in the peritoneal cavity: in order to withdraw fluid for analysis and to perform a tubal ligation (tying off). A fibre-optic scope is inserted through small abdominal incisions and carbon dioxide is inserted into the peritoneal cavity for better visualisation.

RELATED NURSING CARE *Ask the woman to void prior to the examination. A general anaesthetic will be used. Shoulder pain is common after the procedure (referred pain from the retained carbon dioxide); some vaginal bleeding may occur and the woman should use a perineal pad. Excess bleeding, pain or signs of infection should be reported to the nurse or doctor.*

Now that you know more about the various tests and investigations, this can help to broaden your understanding of assessment.

HEALTH ASSESSMENT INTERVIEW

This may be conducted during health screening, and it may focus on a chief complaint or be part of a total health assessment. Questions should be asked in a non-threatening, matter-of-fact manner. Consider the psychological, social and cultural factors that affect sexuality and sexual activity. Use words that the woman can understand. Begin the interview with more general questions and then progress to specific questions; asking questions this way gives the woman permission to describe behaviours and signs and symptoms. At all times observe the women's body language and also be aware of your own.

Assessing sexual function

Questions asked may be tailored to the specific health problem of the woman. The nurse should analyse and document the onset of the problem, duration, frequency, precipitating and relieving factors, any associated symptoms, treatment, self-care and outcome.

With respect to Case Study 2 you could ask Rohinee:

- Have you noticed vaginal bleeding after intercourse?
- Does over-the-counter medication relieve the vaginal itching and discharge?
- Have you had any fever or abdominal pain with this vaginal infection?

To help you structure the assessment process a number of interview questions categorised by functional health patterns are listed in the Functional Health Pattern Interview below. You should observe other healthcare professionals you work with, noting how they conduct a health interview with women.

The health pattern interview questions are presented in list format. Use this only as a guide and tailor the questions you ask.

FUNCTIONAL HEALTH PATTERN INTERVIEW The female reproductive system

Functional health pattern	Interview questions and leading statements
Health perception–health management	• Have you ever had problems with your reproductive organs (ovaries, tubes, uterus, vagina) or with menstruation or menopause? Explain. If so, how was this problem treated? • Do you routinely take any prescribed or herbal medications for symptoms of menopause? If so, what and when do you take it? • Did you ever take hormone replacement therapy for menopausal symptoms? • Do you practise breast self-examination? When and how often do you do this? • Have you noticed any lumps in your breasts or discharge from your nipples? If so, describe. • Have you ever had a breast examination or mammogram? When was your last one? How often do you have these? • When was your last gynaecological examination? Cervical smear? How often do you have these done? • Do you use birth control? If so, what do you use? • What do you do to provide self-care if you have mood swings or menstrual cramps? • Have you ever had a sexually transmitted infection or an infection of the reproductive organs? What was it? How was it treated? • Do you use douches or vaginal sprays? If so, what type and how often? • Do you smoke? If so, how much and for how long?
Nutritional–metabolic	• Do you notice a change in your appetite right before your menstrual period? • Have you gained weight recently? If so, why do think this happened? • Describe your usual food intake for a 24-hour period.
Elimination	• When was your last menstrual period? • At what age did you start/end having menstrual periods? • Describe the length, amount of flow and clotting with your menstrual periods. Do you ever have bleeding between your menstrual periods? If so, describe the type and amount. • Describe any unusual vaginal discharge you have had (colour, consistency, odour, itching or rash). • Have you noticed any changes in urination (frequency, urgency, burning)? • Have you noticed changes in bowel elimination during your menstrual periods?

FUNCTIONAL HEALTH PATTERN INTERVIEW The female reproductive system (continued)

Functional health pattern	Interview questions and leading statements
Activity–exercise	• Describe your usual activities of daily living. • Have you noticed any change in activity or energy during your menstrual period? • Have you noticed any change in activity or energy since menopause (if applicable)? If so, how?
Sleep–rest	• How long do you sleep at night? • Do night sweats wake you? • Do menstrual cramps ever wake you at night?
Cognitive–perceptual	• Do you have pain or other symptoms (such as headache, mood swings, irritability, bloating, constipation, diarrhoea and/or breast tenderness) before your menstrual period? Describe. What do you do about this? • Do you have cramping before or during your menstrual period? Describe the type of cramping, how long it lasts and what you do to be more comfortable. • Do you ever have vaginal itching, pain, burning or dryness? If so, is it affected by sexual intercourse? Does dryness interfere with intercourse?
Self-perception–Self-concept	• Has this problem affected how you feel about yourself as a woman? • Do you believe your needs for intimacy and affection are being met?
Role–relationships	• How has having this condition affected your relationships with others? • Has having this condition interfered with your ability to work? Explain. • Has anyone in your family had problems with breast or ovarian cancer? Explain.
Sexuality–reproductive	• Are you currently in a sexual relationship? If so, has this condition interfered with your usual sexual activity? How long have you been with your current partner? Have you had any other partners during this time? • What is your sexual preference? • Has having this problem affected your relationship with your spouse or sexual partner? • Have you ever been pregnant? How many times? Have you ever had a miscarriage? • Do you practise birth control? If so, what do you use? • Do you ensure that your partner of the opposite gender uses a condom every time you have intercourse? • Do you use a vaginal condom?
Coping–stress tolerance	• Has having this condition created stress for you? If so, does your health problem seem to be more difficult when you are stressed? • Have you experienced any kind of stress that makes the condition worse? Explain. • Describe what you do when you feel stressed.
Value–belief	• Describe how specific relationships or activities help you cope with this problem. • Describe specific cultural beliefs or practices that affect how you care for and feel about this problem. • Are there any specific treatments that you would not use to treat this problem?

Now you are feeling more confident with questions and questioning, the next step is the physical examination. When carrying out the examination you need to engender an atmosphere of warmth and professionalism helping the woman relax.

PHYSICAL ASSESSMENT

Physical assessment is usually conducted as part of a scheduled screening (e.g., for an annual smear) or for a specific reproductive health problem. The nurse must feel comfortable with the examination of persons of the opposite gender; if the nurse or the person is not comfortable, a nurse of the same gender should be asked to conduct this part of the assessment.

Assessment is by inspection and palpation (to feel by pressing lightly). The woman should void before the examination. Before the examination, collect all necessary equipment and explain the techniques to decrease anxiety. Put on disposable gloves before beginning the examination, wearing them throughout the examination. Ask the woman to remove her clothing and put on a gown. Ensure that the examining room is private and warm. All women have the right to have a chaperone present during any examination, or the performance of any procedure or treatment. This right must be respected.

Explain the procedures thoroughly and in a matter-of-fact way to decrease anxiety and embarrassment. It may help to use charts to demonstrate aspects of the body that will be examined. Show any equipment to be used to the woman. The assessment may be done with the woman in the sitting or supine position (lying on the back) to examine the breasts and in the lithotomy position to assess the external genitalia and internal organs. Expose only those body parts being examined to preserve modesty. Normal age-related findings for the older woman are summarised in Table 15.1.

The examination usually begins with examination of the breasts. The woman is helped to move to the lithotomy position on the examining table, feet in the stirrups and the buttocks even with the foot of the table. Older or frail women may not be able to tolerate this position; if so the woman is examined in the supine position. The internal examination is conducted only by a nurse with advanced practice in the procedure. Nurses are often asked to assist with the examination and should be able to explain the examination to a woman. Breast assessment and assessment of the labia, cervix and vaginal opening is discussed here. The role of the nurse is to act as advocate, to provide comfort and promote dignity.

The assessment of the female reproductive system is complex and the nurse needs to understand the key issues involved in order to provide safe and effective care. Female reproductive system assessments are described on page 573.

Table 15.1 Age-related changes in the female reproductive system

Age-related change	Significance
Breasts: • Atrophy, with sagging of breast tissue. • Linear strands appear from shrinkage and fibrotic changes.	Ageing does not cause breast cancer; the incidence rises in older women; age-related changes may make finding tumours more difficult, for example there may be atrophy, fibrosis and normal age-related changes in breast shape.
External genitalia: • Labia flatten, vulvar adipose tissue and hair decrease. • Decreased collagen and adipose tissues in the vaginal canal, resulting in loss of rugae, shortening and narrowing of vaginal canal. • Reduced vaginal lubrication, epithelium becomes thinner and avascular (without blood vessels). • More alkaline pH of vagina. • Cervix becomes smaller.	Vagina is more easily irritated, increasing the risk of vaginal infections. Lubricants are necessary for comfortable intercourse.
Internal organs: • Uterus shrinks. • Fallopian tubes shrink and shorten. • Ovaries are smaller and thicker. • With menopause, hormone production of oestrogen decreases. • Loss of oestrogen may cause pelvic floor muscles to weaken. • Loss of oestrogen causes changes throughout the body, including loss of skin tone (wrinkling) and growth of facial hair.	With the completion of menopause, the menstrual cycles end and the woman is infertile. Weakening of the pelvic floor muscles may contribute to involuntary incontinence with increased intra-abdominal pressure (as with coughing and sneezing). Skin is dry and thin.

FEMALE REPRODUCTIVE SYSTEM ASSESSMENT

Technique	Abnormal findings
Breast assessment	
Inspect both breasts simultaneously. The woman is seated in the following positions: arms at sides, arms overhead, hands pressed on hips, leaning forward. Inspect breast size, symmetry, contour, skin colour, texture, venous patterns, and lesions. Lift the breasts, and inspect the lower and lateral aspects.	• Retractions, dimpling and abnormal contours suggest benign lesions, but may also suggest malignancy. • Thickened, dimpled skin with enlarged pores (called peau d'orange, orange peel) and unilateral venous patterns are also associated with malignancy. • Redness may be seen with infection or carcinoma.
Inspect the areolae and nipples.	• Peau d'orange may be noted first in the areola. • Recent unilateral inversion of the nipple or asymmetry in the directions in which the nipples point suggests cancer.
Palpate both breasts, axillae and supraclavicular areas. Various palpation patterns may be used as long as every part of each breast is palpated, including the axillary tail, which is the breast tissue that extends from the upper outer quadrant toward and into the axillae. Ask the woman to assume a supine position with a small pillow under the shoulder and the arm over the head, and repeat the systematic palpation sequence. Describe identified masses by location, size, shape, consistency, tenderness, mobility and delineation of borders.	• Tenderness may be related to pre-menstrual fullness, fibrocystic disease or inflammation. Tenderness may also indicate cancer. • Nodules in the tail of the breast may be enlarged lymph nodes. • Hard, irregular, fixed unilateral masses that are poorly delineated suggest carcinoma. • Bilateral, single or multiple, round, mobile, well-delineated masses are consistent with fibrocystic breast disease or fibroadenoma. • Swelling, tenderness, erythema and heat may be seen with mastitis.
Palpate the nipple then compress it between the thumb and index finger. Note the colour of any discharge.	• Loss of nipple elasticity is seen in cancer. • Bloody or serous discharge is associated with intraductal papilloma. • Milky discharge not due to prior pregnancy and found on both sides suggests galactorrhoea (lactation not associated with pregnancy or nursing), which is sometimes associated with a pituitary tumour. • Unilateral discharge from one or two ducts can be seen in fibrocystic breast disease, intraductal papilloma or carcinoma.
Axillary assessment	
Inspect the skin of the axillae. Palpate all sections of both axillae for palpable nodes.	• Rash may be due to allergy or other causes. • Signs of inflammation and infection may be due to infection of the sweat glands. • Enlarged axillary nodes are most often due to infection of the hand or arm but can be caused by malignancy. • Enlarged supraclavicular nodes are associated with lymphatic metastases from abdominal or thoracic carcinoma.
External genitalia assessment	
Help the woman to the lithotomy position with the knees flexed and separated. Inspect and palpate the labia majora.	• Excoriation (skin abrasions), rashes or lesions suggest inflammatory or infective processes. • Bulging of the labia that increases with straining suggests a hernia. • Varicosities (the presence of varicose veins) may be present on the labia.
Inspect the labia minora. Separate the labia majora for better visualisation.	• Inflammation, irritation, excoriation or caking of discharge in tissue folds suggests vaginal infection or poor hygiene. • Ulcers or vesicles may be symptoms of sexually transmitted infection.

FEMALE REPRODUCTIVE SYSTEM ASSESSMENT (continued)

Technique	Abnormal findings
Palpate the inside of the labia minora between thumb and forefinger.	• Small, firm, round cystic nodules in labia suggest sebaceous cysts. • Wart-like lesions suggest condylomata acuminata (genital warts). • Firm, painless ulcers suggest chancre of primary syphilis. • Shallow, painful ulcers suggest herpes infection. • Ulcerated or red raised lesions in older women suggest vulvar carcinoma.
Inspect the clitoris.	• Enlargement may be a symptom of a masculinising condition.
Inspect the vaginal opening.	• Swelling, discoloration or lacerations may be caused by trauma. • Discharge or lesions may be symptoms of infection. • Fissures or fistulae (the pleural of fistula) may be related to injury, infection, spreading of a malignancy or trauma.

Having outlined assessment techniques, the various disorders that may be revealed during assessment will be discussed below.

The woman with sexual dysfunction

The female body maintains the capacity for sexual activity and orgasm long after menopause (see Box 15.1). In a typical sexual event, two physiological sexual responses occur: vasocongestion and myotonia. Sexual stimulation results in vasocongestion in the vagina, causing engorgement, increased lubrication and genital swelling and enlargement. Arousal, or myotonia, increases muscular tension and voluntary and involuntary muscle contraction.

The sexual response cycle has four phases: excitement, plateau, orgasm and resolution. These phases always occur in the same sequence; however, the duration of each phase may vary. Sexual arousal typically ends in orgasm (climax), but sometimes fails to do so. Nurses may not conduct sexual

Box 15.1

Sexual function in the ageing woman

Myths, taboos and stereotypes held by society may foster the belief that older women are no longer interested in expressing their sexuality. Loss of sexual function is not an inevitable result of ageing, but physical changes related to ageing do affect sexual response. Physical changes and chronic conditions in ageing women may alter sexual function. Some medications used to treat the chronic conditions can alter the sexual response.

PHYSIOLOGICAL CHANGES
Changes in the ageing woman's sexual function begin in the perimenopausal period as oestrogen levels decrease. Oestrogen-sensitive cells are involved in the female sexual response. With menopause comes a decrease in the levels of estradiol, affecting nerve transmission and response in the peripheral vascular system. The timing and degree of vasocongestion during the sexual response are affected. Specific changes in sexual response occur in all phases: the plateau phase, the orgasmic phase and the resolution phase.

NURSING CARE
The aim is to assist ageing women reach optimal sexual functioning, discussing the physiological and psychological changes associated with menopause. Women need to be informed about the effects of chronic illness on sexual functioning and the medications used to treat them. Include the importance of maintaining a healthy lifestyle, a balanced diet, weight-bearing and aerobic exercises, stress management and routine health examinations.

Practical advice includes:

● Recommend water-soluble vaginal lubricants or vaginal gels before intercourse for vaginal dryness and dyspareunia, intercourse on a regular basis and oestrogen replacement.
● For joint pain or other musculoskeletal pain recommend adapting positions for intercourse.

Go back to Case Study 1 and think about the ways in which you might sensitively raise a discussion with a woman about her sex life. Can you think of any ways in which you could help women discuss their emotions with the aim of helping to alleviate any feelings that may lead to anxiety and depression?

IN PRACTICE

Guidelines for intravaginal assessment and use of the vaginal speculum and guidelines for bimanual pelvic examination

The size of the speculum that is used for an internal examination of the female reproductive system depends on the age of the woman and size of the vagina. There are narrower types of speculae available which may be used to examine adolescents or adult woman who are virgins, who have never had a baby or who are post-menopausal with vaginal atrophy. The speculum should be warm. If cultures or smears are to be obtained, neither water nor gel should be used to warm or to lubricate the speculum.

The examination is usually deferred if the woman is menstruating or has a vaginal infection.

The general procedure is as follows:

1. Explain the proposed procedure to the woman, gaining her consent.

2. Place the index and middle finger of one hand into the vagina, just inside the introitus, and press the fingers toward the rectum. Hold the speculum in the other hand.

3. Ask the woman to bear down, and insert the closed blades of the speculum into the vagina at an oblique angle until the ends of the blades reach the fingertips. Withdraw the fingers and rotate the speculum to a transverse position.

4. Insert the speculum until it reaches the end of the vagina. Depress the lever of the speculum, opening the blades. If the cervix is not in full view, try closing the blades, withdrawing the speculum about halfway, and inserting it again at a more downward angle. When the cervix is in full view, fix the depressed lever to an open position.

5. Inspect the cervix. Assess colour, position, size, projection into the vagina, surface and shape and any discharge.

6. Throughout the examination, communicate with the woman, explaining to her what you are doing. Observe the woman's non-verbal communication.

If a smear is to be collected, the following procedure may be used:

1. To collect cells from the vaginal pool, roll a sterile applicator on the vaginal wall below the cervix. Paint the smear on the slide and spray the slide with fixative.

2. To collect endocervical cells, place the groove of the spatula snugly against the cervical os, rotate it 360 degrees. In a single stroke, spread the material from both sides of the spatula on a slide, and immediately spray with fixative.

If cultures are to be done, take a specimen from the vagina and/or cervix with a sterile applicator, and then either spread the specimen on a culture plate or place it in a culture container. Follow institutional policy and procedures.

At the end of the examination, loosen the lever control, slowly withdraw the speculum, closing the blades slowly, rotating the speculum while observing all areas of the vaginal wall. Assess the colour of the mucosa and the colour and appearance of any discharge. If needed, offer the woman physical and psychological support. Document findings.

---

counselling, but they should be able to obtain a sexual history, discuss sexual concerns with women and make appropriate referrals.

Pathophysiology of sexual function in women

Disorders of sexual function include **dyspareunia**, inhibited sexual desire and orgasmic dysfunction which will now be discussed.

Dyspareunia

Physical conditions, such as imperforate hymen, vaginal scarring or vaginismus, may cause dyspareunia (pain during intercourse). *Vaginismus* is a rare condition where the vaginal muscles at the introitus contract so tightly that an erect penis cannot be inserted. Early traumatic events, such as sexual abuse, fear of men or rape, may contribute to vaginismus. Dyspareunia may be psychological in origin. The woman develops an anxiety–fear–guilt cycle. Other sexual activity may be pleasurable.

Inhibited sexual desire

This may be a result of pathophysiological processes or psychological in origin. Inhibited sexual desire is related to childhood teaching or experiences that may be painful to recall. Cultural and religious values also affect the processing of sexual stimuli as does fear.

Orgasmic dysfunction

Inhibited orgasm (**anorgasmia**) is the most prevalent sexual problem among women. Fewer than 20% of cases are physiological. Between 8% and 15% of women have never experienced an orgasm in the waking state. Psychologically induced anorgasmia results from unresolved conflicts about sexual activity. Organic causes include the presence of disease resulting in general debilitation that affects the sexual response cycle, and the use of drugs depressing the central nervous system (CNS).

NURSING CARE FOR SEXUAL DYSFUNCTION

Care focuses on identifying the type of sexual dysfunction with a thorough history, including onset, duration, frequency and context or situation in which the problem occurs. The woman's partner should be included in discussions when appropriate.

Teach about varied normal sexual responses, aiming to increase self-awareness and understanding of communication, relationships and sexual desire. Discuss behaviours that men and women consider sexually stimulating. Referral may be required to a sex therapist and group therapy may be encouraged. Sexual dysfunction can occur at any age, and the next section discusses the perimenopausal woman.

The perimenopausal woman

Menopause is the permanent cessation of menses. The *climacteric*, or *perimenopausal*, period is the time during which reproductive function gradually ceases; this can last for several years. It begins with a decline in the production of oestrogen, includes the permanent cessation of menstruation due to loss of ovarian function and extends for one year after the final menstrual period, at which a woman is said to be *post-menopausal*.

Menopause is not a disease or a disorder; it is a normal physiological process. It impacts on the health and wellbeing of women. Hormonal changes occurring can be accompanied by side-effects. Generally, women stop menstruating between 48 and 55 years of age. Earlier menopause is associated with genetics, smoking, higher altitude and obesity (Castledine and Close 2007). Health risks increase after menopause, including heart disease, osteoporosis, macular degeneration (an eye condition), cognitive changes and breast cancer.

Pathophysiology of the menopause

The menopausal period marks the natural biological end of reproductive ability. *Surgical menopause* occurs when the ovaries are removed, dramatically reducing the production of oestrogen and progestins. *Chemical menopause* occurs during cancer chemotherapy, when cytotoxic drugs arrest ovarian function.

As ovarian function decreases, production of estradiol (E_2), the most biologically active oestrogen, decreases and is ultimately replaced by estrone as the major ovarian oestrogen. Estrone is produced in small amounts and has only about one-tenth the biological activity of estradiol. With decreased ovarian function progesterone is also markedly reduced.

Signs and symptoms of the menopause

As oestrogen decreases, breast tissue, body hair, skin elasticity and subcutaneous fat decrease, and changes occur with the ovaries and uterus, the cervix and vagina. This results in problems with vaginal dryness, dyspareunia, urinary stress incontinence, urinary tract infections (UTIs) and vaginitis. Vasomotor instability (dilation and constriction of the blood vessels) often results in hot flushes, palpitations, dizziness and headaches. Other problems include insomnia, frequent awakening and perspiration (night sweats). There may be irritability, anxiety and depression.

Long-term oestrogen deprivation results in an imbalance in bone remodelling and osteoporosis, leading to fractures and kyphosis (curvature of the spine). The risk for cardiovascular diseases increases in response to an increase in atherosclerosis (from an increase in the LDL–HDL cholesterol ratio). Signs and symptoms of the perimenopausal period vary, and are discussed below. Some women experience severe symptoms, others experience moderate symptoms, and some women experience few or no symptoms.

INTERDISCIPLINARY CARE FOR THE MENOPAUSE

Focus is on relieving symptoms and minimising post-menopausal health risks.

Diagnosis

As oestrogen secretion diminishes, levels of FSH and LH rise and remain elevated. A woman who had not menstruated for one full year or who has an increased FSH blood level is considered menopausal (Porth 2009).

Signs and symptoms

Signs and symptoms associated with the perimenopausal period include:

- Menstrual cycles become erratic. Menstrual flow alters in amount and duration and eventually ceases.
- Vaginal, vulvar and urethral tissues atrophy (waste away).
- Vaginal pH rises, increasing risk of bacterial infections.
- Vaginal lubrication decreases, and vaginal rugae decrease in number. This can cause dyspareunia, injury and fungal infections.
- Vasomotor instability occurs, and this may result in hot flushes and night sweats.
- Psychological symptoms may include moodiness, nervousness, insomnia, headaches, irritability, anxiety, inability to concentrate and depression.

Medication

Hormone replacement therapy (HRT) may be prescribed to alleviate severe signs and symptoms of menopause, for a limited amount of time and only after information about known risks is provided. HRT may include oestrogen alone for women who have had a hysterectomy, or a combination of oestrogen and progestin. The addition of progestin stimulates monthly shedding of the interuterine lining, decreasing the risk of uterine cancer. HRT relieves hot flushes and night sweats and decreases problems of vaginal dryness and uro-genital tissue atrophy. Long-term HRT may increase the risk for breast cancer, ovarian cancer, stroke, heart attacks and venous thrombosis (McPhee *et al.* 2007). However, women who have had a hysterectomy and take oestrogen alone do not have an increased risk of breast cancer.

Selective oestrogen receptor modulators (SERMs) (raloxifene (Evista) and Tamoxifen) may be prescribed. Tamoxifen has a beneficial effect on bone mineral density and serum lipids and decreases the risk of invasive breast cancer in women at high risk. SERMs provide an alternative to HRT for preventing osteoporosis.

Alternative and complementary therapies

Non-traditional or alternative therapies have become more popular. Several complementary therapies are available to reduce associated discomforts, and these may include:

- Acupuncture
- Biofeedback
- Massage
- Herbs
- Vitamin supplements
- Meditation and yoga.

Prior to engaging in such approaches it should be recommended that advice and guidance is sought from a reliable source.

NURSING CARE FOR THE MENOPAUSE

Care focuses on minimising the symptoms associated with hormonal changes, reducing the risks and providing information about lifestyle changes important to health and well being.

Health promotion

Frequency of health checkups depends on the individual person. Checkups include examination for cancers of the thyroid, ovaries, lymph nodes, oral cavity, and skin. Others include screening for cervical, breast and colorectal cancer. Information-giving focuses on alcohol and tobacco use, sun exposure, diet and nutrition, exercise, risk factors, sexual practices and environmental and occupational exposures. It is important to discuss the benefits of rest and exercise with the person being cared for. In addition, suggest the following resources for further information:

- Cancer Research UK;
- Health Protection Agency;
- British Menopause Society;
- Association of Reproductive Health Professionals;
- NHS Evidence Women's Health.

Assessment

Data are collected through the health history and physical examination. Be aware of normal changes with ageing.

+ *Health history:* problems with urinary frequency, urgency or incontinence; menstrual history; sexual history; dyspareunia; use of alcohol, nicotine and drugs; medications, sleep patterns, hot flushes, night sweats and changes in emotional responses.
+ *Physical assessment:* height and weight, posture, vital signs, breast examination, pelvic examination, abdominal assessment.

Nursing diagnoses and interventions

Individual interventions often focus on problems with lack of information (deficient knowledge), sexuality, self-esteem and altered body image which are now discussed in turn.

Risk for deficient knowledge

Menopausal signs and symptoms vary widely, and the well-informed woman is better prepared to deal with whatever symptoms are experienced.

+ Discuss physiological signs and symptoms, such as hot flushes and night sweats. The underlying cause of hot flushes is not known (Porth 2009).
+ Provide information about dietary recommendations, including the recommended daily intake of calcium for women over 50 which is 1200 mg.
+ Emphasise the importance of weight-bearing exercise.
+ Provide information about the benefits of HRT. Not every woman will need or want it.
+ Encourage the woman to obtain yearly mammograms, clinical breast examinations and smear tests, and to perform monthly BSE on the same day of each month.

Risk for ineffective sexuality pattern
+ Encourage expression of feelings and concerns about how the menopause is changing her sex life.
+ Suggest ways to increase vaginal lubrication, such as spending more time in foreplay and/or using water-soluble gels (e.g. KY) for vaginal lubrication.
+ Explain that as women age it may take longer for vaginal lubrication and orgasm to occur.

PRACTICE ALERT

Plant oestrogens, found in food such as brown rice, corn, green beans, lemon and orange peels and tofu, are mildly oestrogenic and may improve vaginal dryness.

Risk for situational low self-esteem

Among the factors that may provoke a self-esteem disturbance are the loss of youth, a sense of emptiness as children leave home and the need to redefine one's self-concept and roles as parenting becomes less important.

+ Encourage expression of fears and concerns related to changes in interpersonal and family functions.

+ Suggest volunteer activities or employment for the woman who has extra time.

+ Discuss the importance of a healthy lifestyle. Identify risk factors and high-risk behaviours.

Risk for disturbed body image

The physical changes experienced can include growth of facial hair, excessive perspiration and flushing of the face and weight gain.

+ Encourage the woman to describe her perceptions of her body.

+ Encourage verbalisation of feelings of concern, anger, anxiety, loss and fear over body changes.

+ Stress that certain physical characteristics of a person cannot be changed; emphasise the importance of learning to recognise and appreciate one's own special strengths.

+ Refer, as appropriate, for dietary management, exercise, stress management and cosmetic assistance (e.g., for aggravating facial hair).

Having discussed the menopause we will now move onto address issues concerning menstrual disorders.

MENSTRUAL DISORDERS

There are a number of myths surrounding menstruation; many have been around since women have been menstruating. The nurse has a role to play in correcting any misconceptions concerning menstruation as some of these fallacies may impact on a woman or girl's health and wellbeing.

Monthly menstruation normally involves some minor discomfort, breast tenderness, a feeling of heaviness and congestion in the pelvic area, uterine cramping and lower backache. Many women experience more serious effects. This section discusses **premenstrual syndrome**, **dysmenorrhoea** and abnormal uterine bleeding.

The woman with premenstrual syndrome (PMS)

PMS is a complex of signs and symptoms (e.g., mood swings, breast tenderness, fatigue and depression) that are limited to 3–14 days before menstruation and relieved by the onset of menses. For a small number of women, PMS is so disabling that it is called by the psychiatric label of *premenstrual dysphoric disorder (PMDD).*

The syndrome is seen less frequently during the teens and 20s, peaking in women in their mid-30s. Major life stressors, an age greater than 30 and depression are risk factors.

Pathophysiology of PMS

The pathophysiology of PMS is poorly understood, but hormonal changes, increased prolactin levels and rising aldosterone levels during the luteal phase of the menstrual cycle contribute to the problem. Increased aldosterone results in sodium retention and oedema. Decreased levels of monoamine

oxidase in the brain are associated with depression, and reduced levels of serotonin can lead to mood swings.

Signs and symptoms of PMS

These occur during the luteal phase of the menstrual cycle (7 to 10 days prior to the onset of the menstrual flow), abating when the menstrual flow begins. The multisystem effects of PMS are shown in Figure 15.5. The exact nature of these signs and symptoms and their intensity are individualised for each woman and may even differ from month to month in the same woman.

INTERDISCIPLINARY CARE FOR PMS

When there is no organic cause, the goals of care are to relieve signs and symptoms and to help develop self-care. There are no definitive diagnostic tests for PMS. The regular recurrence of manifestations preceding the onset of menses for at least three months leads to a diagnosis of PMS. The treatment includes regular exercise, avoiding caffeine and a diet low in simple sugars and high in lean proteins (Porth 2009). Many different medications, vitamins and herbal supplements have been used to treat PMS; the most promising appears to be the use of selective serotonin reuptake inhibitors (SSRIs).

Medication

If the signs and symptoms are severe or incapacitating, ovulation may be suppressed by the use of GnRH agonists, oral contraceptives or danazol. Progesterone and antiprostaglandin agents such as non-steroidal anti-inflammatory drugs (NSAIDs) help relieve cramping. Diuretics may be prescribed to relieve bloating. SSRIs such as fluoxetine (Prozac), sertraline (Lustal) and paroxetine (Seroxat) are used to manage mood and some physical symptoms.

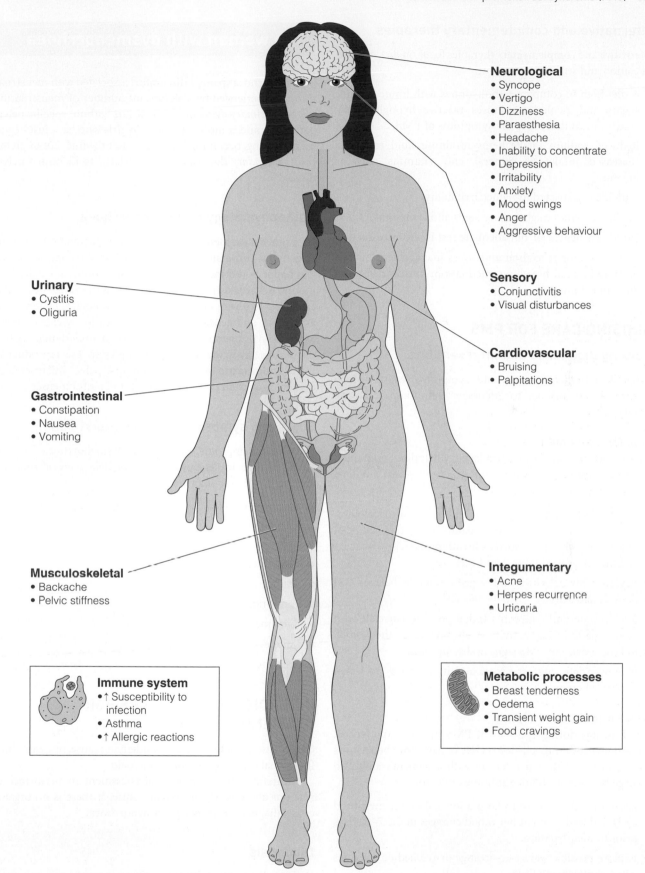

Neurological
- Syncope
- Vertigo
- Dizziness
- Paraesthesia
- Headache
- Inability to concentrate
- Depression
- Irritability
- Anxiety
- Mood swings
- Anger
- Aggressive behaviour

Sensory
- Conjunctivitis
- Visual disturbances

Cardiovascular
- Bruising
- Palpitations

Urinary
- Cystitis
- Oliguria

Gastrointestinal
- Constipation
- Nausea
- Vomiting

Musculoskeletal
- Backache
- Pelvic stiffness

Integumentary
- Acne
- Herpes recurrence
- Urticaria

Immune system
- ↑ Susceptibility to infection
- Asthma
- ↑ Allergic reactions

Metabolic processes
- Breast tenderness
- Oedema
- Transient weight gain
- Food cravings

Figure 15.5 Multisystem effects of premenstrual syndrome.

Alternative and complementary therapies

Alternative and complementary therapies focus on diet, exercise, relaxation and stress management:

- A diet high in complex carbohydrates with limited simple sugars and alcohol minimises reactive hypoglycaemia, which can contribute to the symptoms of PMS.
- Reduced sodium intake helps minimise fluid retention. Increased intake of mineral and vitamins may be helpful.
- Caffeine is restricted to reduce irritability.
- Herbal remedies might relieve signs and symptoms.
- Exercise is beneficial, but adequate rest is also necessary.
- Techniques for relaxation and stress management include deep abdominal breathing, meditation, muscle relaxation and guided imagery.

NURSING CARE FOR PMS

Nursing diagnoses and interventions

Focus is on relieving signs and symptoms. Most women require interventions to manage pain and enhance coping.

Risk for acute pain

There may be pain from headache (including migraine), menstrual cramps, excessive fluid retention, breast swelling, joint and muscle pain, and backache.

- ✚ Teach effective pharmacological and non-pharmacological self-care measures to relieve pain: application of heat, relaxation techniques (such as breathing exercises, imagery techniques or meditation) and exercise.
- ✚ Review daily activities and suggest ways to balance rest periods and activity.
- ✚ Review signs and symptoms and, if possible, correlate with dietary patterns and activity levels. Encourage the woman to keep a diary of PMS signs and symptoms.
- ✚ If appropriate, suggest sexual activity as a way to lessen menstrual cramps.

Risk for ineffective coping

Mood swings during episodes of PMS may be experienced, sometimes exhibiting self-destructive or aggressive behaviours toward others. This can interfere with a woman's ability to manage her responsibilities at home or at work.

- ✚ Encourage the woman to keep a journal of her menstrual cycle and to document her mood changes in the 7–10 days prior to menstruation.
- ✚ Explore possible ways to rearrange or reschedule activities when experiencing PMS.
- ✚ Explore what, if any, self-care measures have helped cope with mood alterations in the past.

The woman with dysmenorrhoea

Dysmenorrhoea (pain or discomfort associated with menstruation) is experienced by a significant number of menstruating women. *Primary dysmenorrhoea* occurs without specific pelvic pathology, and is most often seen in girls who have just begun menstruating, becoming less severe after the mid-20s or giving birth. *Secondary dysmenorrhoea* is related to identified pelvic disease.

Pathophysiology of dysmenorrhoea

In primary dysmenorrhoea, excessive production of prostaglandins stimulates uterine muscle fibres to contract. When this happens uterine circulation is compromised, resulting in uterine ischaemia and pain. Contractions can range from mild cramping to severe muscle spasms. Psychological factors, such as anxiety and tension, may contribute to dysmenorrhoea. Secondary dysmenorrhoea is related to underlying organic conditions involving scarring or injury to the reproductive tract. **Endometriosis**, fibroid tumours, pelvic inflammatory disease or ovarian cancer may result in painful menses.

Signs and symptoms of dysmenorrhoea

Signs and symptoms of primary dysmenorrhoea may be severe enough to disrupt activities of living, sexual function and fertility. These may include:

- abdominal pain beginning with onset of menses and lasting 12–48 hours;
- pain radiating to lower back and thighs;
- headache;
- nausea;
- vomiting;
- diarrhoea;
- fatigue;
- breast tenderness.

INTERDISCIPLINARY CARE FOR DYSMENORRHOEA

Care focuses on identifying the underlying cause, re-establishing functional capacity and managing pain.

A careful history and physical assessment are performed to rule out any underlying organic cause. If there is no organic cause, diagnosis is primary dysmenorrhoea.

Diagnosis

Various diagnostic tests are performed to identify structural abnormalities, hormonal imbalances and pathologic conditions that could cause menstrual pain. Diagnosis is made based on findings from a pelvic examination and diagnostic procedures, including a smear test and cervical and vaginal cultures, ultrasound of the pelvis and vagina and CT scan or MRI to detect structural abnormalities, malignancy or infections. Laboratory tests are used to assess possible causes of dysmenorrhea.

Laparoscopy (also known as keyhole surgery) is used to diagnose structural defects and blockages caused by scarring, endometriosis, tumours and cysts (Figure 15.6). See the box

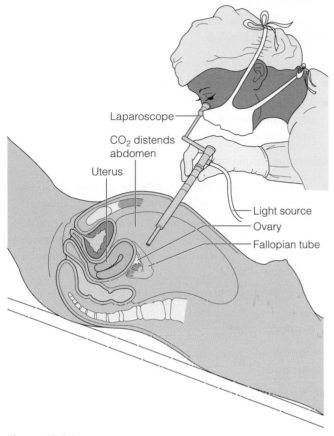

Laparoscope

CO_2 distends abdomen

Uterus

Light source

Ovary

Fallopian tube

Figure 15.6 Laparoscopy.

below for nursing care of the woman having a laparoscopy. A dilation and curettage (D&C) of the uterus may be performed to obtain tissue for evaluation or to relieve dysmenorrhoea and heavy menstrual bleeding.

Medications

Dysmenorrhoea may be treated with analgesics, prostaglandin inhibitors such as NSAIDs, or oral contraceptives. The complementary therapies for the woman with PMS may also be useful for the woman with dysmenorrhoea. Other helpful activities in reducing pain are regular physical exercise, using a heating pad on the abdomen or taking a warm bath.

NURSING CARE FOR DYSMENORRHOEA

Focus is on controlling symptoms and providing education about the normal physiology of the menstrual cycle and self-care measures. Care varies according to the underlying cause and is discussed in this chapter within sections on specific disorders. Nursing interventions previously described for the woman with PMS are also appropriate for the woman with dysmenorrhoea.

The woman with dysfunctional uterine bleeding (DUB)

Dysfunctional uterine bleeding (DUB) refers to vaginal bleeding, usually painless but abnormal in amount, duration or time of occurrence. The types of DUB include primary and secondary **amenorrhoea**, **oligomenorrhoea**, **menorrhagia**, **metrorrhagia** and post-menopausal bleeding.

Many factors may predispose to DUB, including stress, extreme weight changes, use of oral contraceptive agents or intrauterine devices (IUDs) and post-menopausal status.

NURSING CARE PLAN The woman having a laparoscopy

Review Chapter 1 for routine pre- and post-operative care.

Pre-operative care

+ Explain clearly what the procedure is about in order to gain consent.
+ The bladder should be emptied prior to the surgical procedure.
+ Explain that referred shoulder pain or expulsion of gas through the vagina may occur post-operatively. During the procedure, the abdomen is insufflated with carbon dioxide gas to distend the abdomen and facilitate visualisation of the pelvic organs.

+ Explain that pain should be minimal. Instruct the woman to report excessive pain to the nurse or doctor at once.
+ The nurse will be required to help support the woman physically and emotionally during the procedure.

Post-operative care

+ Apply a perineal pad. Teach the woman how to perform perineal hygiene, emphasising the need to change pads at least every four hours. Keep a pad count.
+ Assess for excessive vaginal bleeding.

Dysfunctional uterine bleeding is usually related to hormonal imbalances or pelvic neoplasms, benign or malignant.

Pathophysiology of DUB

The types of DUB include amenorrhoea, oligomenorrhoea, menorrhagia, metrorrhagia and post-menopausal bleeding. Each one is now discussed.

- *Amenorrhoea* is the absence of menstruation. Primary amenorrhoea, absence of menarche by age 16, or by age 14 if secondary sex characteristics fail to develop, may be caused by structural abnormalities, hormonal imbalances, polycystic ovary disease or an imperforate hymen. Anorexia nervosa, bulimia or excessive athletic training can also cause primary amenorrhoea. Secondary amenorrhoea, absence of menses for at least six months in a previously menstruating female, may also be caused by anorexia nervosa, excessive athletic activity or training or a large weight loss. Other causes include hormonal imbalances and ovarian tumours. Normal (physiological) secondary amenorrhoea occurs during pregnancy, breast feeding and menopause.
- *Oligomenorrhoea* (scant menses) is usually related to hormonal imbalances.
- *Menorrhagia* (excessive or prolonged menstruation) may result from thyroid disorders, endometriosis, pelvic inflammatory disease, functional ovarian cysts or uterine fibroids or polyps as well as clotting disorders and anticoagulant medications. A single heavy or long menses is not in itself a cause for concern; however, repetitive long or heavy menses can lead to haemorrhage, excessive blood loss, fatigue and anaemia.
- *Metrorrhagia* (bleeding between menstrual periods) may be caused by hormonal imbalances, pelvic inflammatory disease, cervical or uterine polyps, uterine fibroids or cervical or uterine cancer. Because cancer is a possible cause of metrorrhagia, early evaluation and treatment are essential.
- *Post-menopausal bleeding* may be caused by endometrial polyps, endometrial hyperplasia or uterine cancer. The possibility of cancer makes early evaluation and treatment essential.

Hormonal imbalances, especially progesterone deficiency with relative oestrogen excess, result in endometrial hyperplasia (abnormal multiplication of normal cells). Oestrogen stimulates endometrial proliferation. Without the support provided by progesterone, sloughing occurs, causing vaginal bleeding that may be irregular, prolonged or profuse. Defects in the follicular phase shorten the proliferative phase of the menstrual cycle, resulting in spotting and breakthrough bleeding. Defects during the luteal phase result in excessive amount or duration of flow due to persistence of the corpus luteum, leading to a deficiency of progesterone and vaginal bleeding. *Anovulation*, absence of ovulation, is associated with both oestrogen and progesterone deficiencies. Emotional upsets or stress can cause hormonal imbalances affecting menstruation. Pelvic neoplasms, discussed later, also cause abnormal bleeding.

INTERDISCIPLINARY CARE FOR DUB

Care focuses on identifying and treating the underlying disease. History and physical examination are performed as well as abdominal and pelvic examinations to rule out abdominal masses. The woman may need to keep a menstrual history and basal body temperature chart for several months to determine whether ovulation is occurring.

Diagnosis

A variety of diagnostic tests are used. These are discussed in this chapter and include:

- a cervical smear to rule out or identify cervical carcinoma
- a pelvic ultrasound to identify luteal cysts
- a hysteroscopy to detect abnormalities of the uterine cavity or an endometrial biopsy to obtain endometrial tissue for histological examination.

Laboratory studies may include the following:

- A *full blood count (FBC)* to rule out systemic disease as a contributing factor to DUB and to evaluate its effects.
- *Thyroid function studies*, including measurement of triiodothyronine (T_3), thyroxine (T_4) and thyroid-stimulating hormone (TSH) levels, to rule out hyper- or hypothyroidism as a cause of DUB.
- *Endocrine studies* to evaluate pituitary and adrenal function.
- *Serum progesterone levels* to determine the level of progesterone deficiency.

Medication

For many women, hormonal agents can correct menstrual irregularities. For anovulatory DUB, oral contraceptives may be prescribed for three to six months. Progesterone can help regulate uterine bleeding.

Ovulatory DUB may be treated with progestins during the luteal phase. Oral iron supplements can replace iron lost through menstrual bleeding.

Surgery

The least invasive surgical procedure would be recommended, beginning with a therapeutic dilation and curettage (D&C), then endometrial ablation and, finally, hysterectomy. All of these procedures are outlined below.

Therapeutic D&C

The cervical canal is dilated and the uterine wall is scraped. D&C is used to diagnose and treat DUB and other disorders of the reproductive system. It may be performed to correct excessive or prolonged bleeding. It is contraindicated in any woman who has been taking anticoagulant drugs or whose condition precludes the use of regional or general anaesthesia.

FAST FACTS

Hysterectomy

- Approximately 40 000 hysterectomies are performed each year in the UK in the National Health Service (www.hysterectomy-association.org.uk).
- This surgery is most often performed in women aged between 40 and 44 years.
- The three conditions that most necessitate hysterectomy are uterine **leiomyoma** (fibroids), endometriosis and uterine prolapse.

Endometrial ablation

The endometrial layer (the lining of the uterus) is permanently destroyed using laser surgery or electrosurgical resection. It is performed in women who do not respond to pharmacological management or D&C. This procedure ends menstruation and reproduction.

Hysterectomy

Hysterectomy may be performed when medical management of bleeding disorders is unsuccessful or malignancy is present. In pre-menopausal women, the ovaries are usually left in place; in post-menopausal women, a total hysterectomy, or panhysterectomy, may be performed; this involves removal of the uterus, fallopian tubes and ovaries.

Hysterectomy may involve either an abdominal or a vaginal approach; choice depends on the underlying disorder, the need to explore the abdominal cavity and the preference of the surgeon and woman. Nursing care of the woman undergoing a hysterectomy is described below.

Abdominal hysterectomy is performed when a pre-existing abdominal scar is present, when adhesions are thought to be

NURSING CARE PLAN The woman having a hysterectomy

Review Chapter 1 for routine pre- and post-operative care.

Pre-operative care

- Assess the woman's understanding of the procedure. Provide explanation, clarification and emotional support as needed. Reassure that the anaesthesia will eliminate any pain during surgery and that medication will be administered post-operatively to minimise discomfort.
- Cleanse the abdominal and perineal area and prepare the perineal area in line with evidence-based practice and protocol.
- If prescribed, administer a small cleansing enema (if this is needed) and ask the woman to empty her bladder.
- Administer pre-operative medications.
- Ensure that the informed consent has been gained and that a consent form has been signed.

Post-operative care

- Assess for signs of haemorrhage, for presence of bleeding, low blood pressure, tachycardia, pallor.
- Monitor vital signs as requested and as the woman's condition dictates and, in line with policy and procedure, monitor and measure intake and output.
- If a urinary catheter has been inserted output must be monitored and documented. Once the catheter has been removed, note when urine was passed, measure and record amount.
- Assess for complications, including infection, paralytic ileus, shock or haemorrhage, thrombophlebitis and pulmonary embolus.

- Assess vaginal discharge; assist the woman with perineal care.
- Assess incision and bowel sounds as per policy and procedure.
- Encourage turning, coughing, deep breathing and early mobilisation.
- Encourage fluid intake as tolerated.
- Teach to splint the abdomen and cough deeply.
- Advise the woman to restrict physical activity for four to six weeks post-procedure. Heavy lifting, stair climbing, douching, tampons and sexual intercourse should be avoided. The woman should shower, avoiding taking a bath, until bleeding has ceased.
- Explain she may feel tired for several days after surgery and needs to rest periodically.
- Explain that appetite may be depressed and bowel elimination may be sluggish.
- Teach the woman to recognise signs of complications that should be reported to the doctor or nurse:
  a. temperature greater than 37.7 °C;
  b. vaginal bleeding greater than a typical menstrual period or bright red;
  c. urinary incontinence, urgency, burning or frequency;
  d. severe pain.
- Encourage the woman to express feelings that may signal a negative self-concept. Correct any misconceptions.
- Provide information on risks and benefits of hormone replacement therapy, if indicated.
- Reinforce the need to obtain gynaecological examinations regularly even after hysterectomy.

present or when a large operating field is necessary. The woman with endometriosis is more likely to have an abdominal hysterectomy because endometrial tissue implants that may be present on other abdominal organs need to be removed.

Vaginal hysterectomy, removal of the uterus through the vagina, is desirable when the uterus has descended into the vagina or if the urinary bladder or rectum have prolapsed into the vagina. Vaginal hysterectomy leaves no visible abdominal scar. Laparoscopy-assisted vaginal hysterectomy (LAVH) is most often performed.

NURSING CARE FOR DUB

DUB usually causes the woman anxiety and self-image, sexuality or reproductive capacity may be threatened and she may fear the possibility of cancer.

Nursing diagnoses and interventions

Interventions for the woman with DUB commonly address problems with anxiety and sexual function.

Risk for anxiety

The anxiety associated with abnormal uterine bleeding can be intense. Until the cause of the bleeding is identified and has been addressed, fear of cancer or other life-threatening conditions may exist.

✚ Discuss the results of tests and examinations with the woman.

✚ Provide information about the causes, treatments, risks and long-term effects of treatments, and prognosis.

✚ Evaluate coping strategies and psychosocial support systems. Teach coping strategies if indicated.

Risk for sexual dysfunction

The woman may be unwilling to express herself sexually, particularly if bleeding is frequent or heavy. Fatigue may prevent her from participating in sexual activity.

✚ Offer information about engaging in sexual activity during menstruation. Explain that conception is possible during this time and that orgasm may help relieve symptoms.

✚ Provide an opportunity for the expression of concerns related to alterations in lifestyle and sexual functioning.

✚ Encourage frequent rest periods.

✚ Provide information about alternative methods of sexual expression.

> **PRACTICE ALERT**
>
> If the nurse is not comfortable with frank discussions about sexual activities then it maybe appropriate to refer the woman and her partner to a psychosexual counsellor.

This section of the chapter has demonstrated how dysfunctional uterine disorders can be complex and have the potential to impact negatively on the woman (and her family). The issues discussed are only associated with one aspect of the care of the woman with reproductive disorders. The next section will discuss and describe issues associated with reproductive structural disorders.

STRUCTURAL DISORDERS

These include displacement disorders and fistulae related to the structures of the reproductive system, for example, the vagina or the uterus.

The woman with a uterine displacement

The uterus may be displaced within the pelvic cavity or may descend into the vaginal canal. Displacement within the pelvic cavity is classified according to the direction of the displacement (Figure 15.7):

● *Retroversion* of the uterus is a backward tilting toward the rectum.

● *Retroflexion* involves a flexing or bending of the uterine corpus backwards towards the rectum.

● *Anteversion* is an exaggerated forward tilting of the uterus.

● *Anteflexion* is a flexing or folding of the uterine corpus upon itself.

Prolapse of the uterus into the vaginal canal varies from mild to complete prolapse outside of the body. First-degree, or mild, prolapse involves a descent of less than half the uterine corpus into the vagina. Second-degree, or marked, prolapse involves the descent of the entire uterus into the vaginal canal, so that the cervix is at the introitus to the vagina. Third-degree prolapse, or *procidentia*, is complete prolapse of the uterus outside the body, with inversion of the vaginal canal. Prolapse of the uterus is often accompanied by *cystocele* (herniation of the bladder into the vagina) or *rectocele* (herniation of the rectum into the vagina).

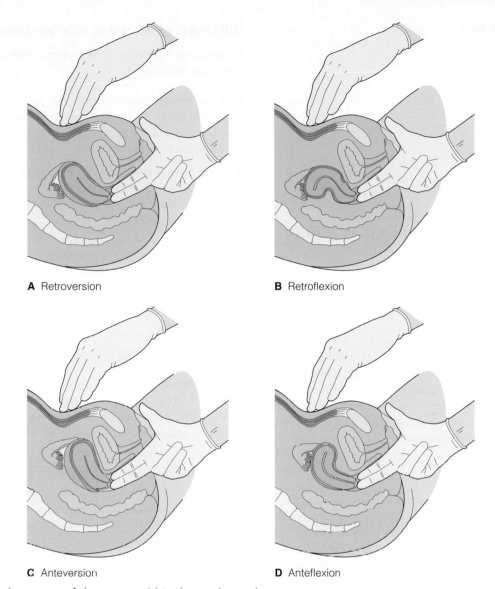

A Retroversion

B Retroflexion

C Anteversion

D Anteflexion

Figure 15.7 Displacements of the uterus within the uterine cavity.

Pathophysiology of uterine displacement

Displacement or prolapse of the uterus, bladder or rectum can be a congenital or an acquired condition. Congenital tilting or flexion of the uterus is rare. More commonly, tilting or flexion disorders in which the uterus remains within the pelvic cavity are related to the scarring and inflammation of pelvic inflammatory disease, endometriosis, pregnancy and tumours.

Downward displacement of the pelvic organs into the vagina results from weakened pelvic musculature, attributed to stretching of the supporting ligaments and muscles during pregnancy and childbirth. Unrepaired lacerations from childbirth, rapid deliveries, multiple pregnancies, congenital weakness or loss of elasticity and muscle tone with ageing may contribute to these disorders.

Signs and symptoms of uterine displacement

The signs and symptoms of displacement disorders are as follows:

Uterine displacement within the pelvic cavity:
- dysmenorrhoea
- dyspareunia
- backache
- infertility

Uterine prolapse:
- backache
- bearing down sensation
- constipation

- urinary incontinence
- haemorrhoids
- dyspareunia

Cytocele/rectocele:

- bearing down sensation
- constipation
- faecal incontinence
- haemorrhoids
- urinary incontinence

INTERDISCIPLINARY CARE FOR UTERINE DISPLACEMENT

Care focuses on identifying the cause of the structural disorder, correcting or minimising the condition, relieving pain, preventing or treating infection and provision of support and education.

A history and physical examination are performed. Diagnosis is made after physical examination. If herniation of the rectum or bladder is suspected, the woman is asked to bear down or cough during the examination so the prolapse can be palpated and any leakage of urine or faeces visualised. A history of infections, multiple pregnancies in rapid succession and rapid labour support diagnosis.

Surgery

There are number of surgical procedures used to repair structural disorders. For those women with a cystocele, anterior colporrhaphy (repair of the cystocele) is the most common procedure. Anterior repair shortens the pelvic muscles, providing tighter support for the bladder. A rectocele is repaired with a posterior colporrhaphy, shortening the pelvic muscles, providing tighter support for the rectum.

A prolapsed uterus may be surgically repositioned and supporting muscles shortened to provide greater support. In post-menopausal women or women with procidentia (also known as or related to a vaginal prolapse), hysterectomy is the preferred treatment.

Pessary

When surgery is contraindicated, a *pessary* may be inserted into the vagina to provide temporary support for the uterus or bladder. At regular intervals, the pessary is removed, cleaned and reinserted.

NURSING CARE FOR UTERINE DISPLACEMENT

Focus is on education about the disorder, proposed treatments and self-care measures to relieve symptoms.

Nursing diagnoses and interventions

Nursing interventions address problems with urinary incontinence and anxiety.

Risk for stress incontinence

Relaxation of the pelvic floor can lead to stress incontinence. This can be troublesome and embarrassing and can increase the incidence of urinary tract infection.

- Teach pelvic floor exercises (sometimes called Kegel exercises); these strengthen perineal muscle tone, minimise urinary leakage and minimise descent of the bladder and rectum into the vagina.
- Suggest the use of perineal pads (ranging from thin panty liners to full-thickness incontinence pads) or special underwear that absorbs urine leakage.
- Explain perineal care and proper use of perineal pads.
- Suggest reducing or eliminating caffeine intake.
- Stress the importance of cleaning the perineal area.
- Offer referral to specialist nurses or physiotherapist.

Risk for anxiety

Anxiety is common among women with a displacement disorder. The nurse can use drawings and models to explain structural disorders and treatment options available if needed.

- Encourage questions from the woman and her partner.
- Explain that the relief from discomfort and fatigue may positively influence sexual expression, and reassure that the capacity for orgasm will not be affected.
- Explore coping mechanisms that have been previously successful.

The woman with a vaginal fistula

A fistula is an abnormal opening or passage between two organs or spaces that are normally separated or an abnormal passage to the outside of the body. Vaginal fistulae may be vesicovaginal or rectovaginal. A *vesicovaginal fistula* is an abnormal opening between the urinary bladder and the vagina, leading to incontinent leakage of urine through the vagina. A *rectovaginal fistula* is an abnormal opening between the rectum and vagina, causing leakage of stool or flatus through the vagina.

Vesicovaginal or rectovaginal fistulae may develop as a complication of childbirth, gynaecological or urological surgery or radiation therapy for gynaecological cancer. Bladder cancer is sometimes involved. The woman with a vaginal fistula often presents with a complaint of involuntary leakage of urine or flatus and symptoms of infection.

INTERDISCIPLINARY CARE FOR VAGINAL FISTULA

Diagnosis is by pelvic examination and can be made by instilling dye into the urinary bladder through a catheter and observing the vagina for leakage. If no leakage is detected, a tampon or vaginal pack is inserted into the vagina, and the woman is asked to mobilise. If an abnormal opening is present, the tampon will absorb the dye. Dye may also be injected intravenously because it is excreted by the kidneys. Urine and vaginal cultures may be performed to rule out infections. Antibiotics are administered if infection is present.

A small vaginal fistula may resolve spontaneously. Otherwise, surgery is performed after inflammation has subsided. Rarely, in the presence of a large, highly inflamed rectovaginal fistula, a temporary colostomy is performed, allowing inflammation and irritation to subside.

NURSING CARE FOR VAGINAL FISTULA

Nursing care is similar to that for the woman with a displacement disorder. Teaching is an important component of nursing care. Stress the importance of careful perineal cleansing to reduce irritation and prevent further tissue breakdown. Suggest perineal irrigation or a bath for cleansing. Perineal pads or special underwear may be used to absorb urine or faecal drainage. For the woman with a rectovaginal fistula, provide information about avoiding gas-forming foods to minimise embarrassment from odour.

This section of the chapter has provided a substantial amount of information concerning the care of women with structural disorders that can have an impact on their health and wellbeing as well as their partner. The next section will provide insight into disorders associated with reproductive tissue.

DISORDERS OF FEMALE REPRODUCTIVE TISSUE

Benign and malignant tissue disorders affect the reproductive system. Benign tumours and cysts include Bartholin's gland cysts, cervical polyps, endometrial cysts and polyps, ovarian cysts and uterine leiomyomas (fibroids). Endometriosis is a condition in which endometrial tissue implants outside the uterus in various locations in the pelvic cavity. Malignant tumours of reproductive tissue include cervical cancer, endometrial cancer, ovarian cancer and vulvar cancer.

The woman with cysts or polyps

A *cyst* is a fluid-filled sac. A *polyp* is a highly vascular solid tumour attached by a pedicle or stem (this is a type of skin flap). Cysts or polyps of the reproductive system can occur in the vulva, cervix, endometrium or ovaries.

Pathophysiology of cysts and polyps

Cysts and polyps can be classified as follows:

- *Bartholin's gland cysts*, the most common vulva cysts, caused by the infection or obstruction of Bartholin's gland.
- *Cervical polyps*, the most common benign cervical lesion in women of reproductive age. They occur in women over age 40 who have borne several children and have a history of using oral contraceptives. The polyp develops at the vaginal end of the cervix, has a stem and is highly vascular.
- *Endometrial cysts and polyps* are caused by endometrial overgrowth and are often filled with old blood. Endometrial cysts are the result of endometrial implants on the ovary and are associated with endometriosis. Endometrial polyps

are intrauterine overgrowths, similar to cervical polyps, and usually have a stalk.

- *Ovarian cysts* are classified as follicular cysts and corpus luteum cysts. Follicular cysts develop as a result of failure of the mature follicle to rupture or failure of an immature follicle to reabsorb fluid after ovulation. Corpus luteum cysts develop as a result of increased hormone secretion by the corpus luteum after ovulation. Most functional cysts regress spontaneously.
- *Polycystic ovarian syndrome* (POS) is an endocrine disorder characterised by an excess of androgens and a long-term lack of ovulation. The cause is unknown. As many as 8 to 10 cysts form in the ovaries from a failure to release ovum. Signs and symptoms include amenorrhoea or irregular menses, hirsutism, obesity, acne, hypertension, sleep apnea and infertility. Women with POS often have insulin resistance and are at increased risk for early-onset type 2 diabetes, as well as heart disease, breast cancer and endometrial cancer.

Signs and symptoms and complications of cysts and polyps

The causes and signs and symptoms of benign cysts and polyps are presented in Table 15.2. Complications include infection, rupture, infertility, haemorrhage and recurrence.

INTERDISCIPLINARY CARE FOR CYSTS AND POLYPS

Focus concentrates on identifying, correcting and preventing the disorder. A history and physical examination are performed. Examination reveals the presence of most cysts and polyps. The menstrual history may reveal menstrual irregularities.

Table 15.2 Benign cysts and polyps

Site	Type	Aetiological origin	Signs and symptoms
Ovary	Functional cysts	Ovulation – include follicular cysts and corpus luteum cysts	May resolve spontaneously; can cause pain, menstrual irregularity or amenorrhoea
	POS	Unknown; possible hypothalamic–pituitary dysfunction	Hirsutism, obesity; amenorrhoea or irregular menses; hyperinsulinaemia; infertility
Vulva	Bartholin cysts	Obstruction or infection of Bartholin's gland	Pain, redness, perineal mass, dyspareunia
Endometrium	Dark brown cysts (chocolate cysts)	Endometrial overgrowth; filled with old blood	
	Endometrial polyps	Unknown	Bleeding between periods
Cervix	Cervical polyps	Unknown	Bleeding after intercourse or between periods

Diagnosis

Diagnostic tests that may be used include a laparoscopy to visualise ovarian cysts, an ultrasound or x-ray to differentiate cysts from solid tumours and a pregnancy test when luteal cysts are suspected. Laboratory analysis will demonstrate elevated LH and testosterone levels, as well as a reverse in FSH/LH in the woman with POS.

Medication

Antibiotics are used for infection or abscess, and oral contraceptives to promote regression of functional ovarian cysts. Clomiphene (Clomid) may be prescribed to stimulate ovulation in the woman with POS who wishes to become pregnant. Dexamethasone suppresses adrenocorticotropic hormone (ACTH) and adrenal androgens, and may be added to increase ovulation.

Surgery

Cervical polyps are visible through a vaginal speculum and are removed with a clamp, using a twisting motion. To remove endometrial cysts or polyps, a transcervical approach is used. The specimen is sent to the laboratory for evaluation, and chemical or electrical cauterisation is applied after cyst removal. For Bartholin's gland cysts and any abscesses, the lesion is incised and drained, and a drainage device is left in place. Follicular cysts may be punctured through laser surgery, or a wedge resection of the ovary may be performed to restore ovulation.

NURSING CARE FOR CYSTS AND POLYPS

Care centres on relieving pain, preventing recurrence and complications. The following should be discussed:

+ The condition, its treatment and measures to relieve pain.
+ The importance of keeping follow-up appointments.

+ Signs and symptoms of infection (for post-surgical care) and the need to notify the doctor should they occur.
+ If cervical polypectomy is performed, advise use of external pads for one week. The woman must be able to state the signs of excessive bleeding and recognise that saturating more than one pad in an hour indicates the need for immediate follow-up.
+ The importance of long-term follow-up care for the woman with POS.

The woman with leiomyoma

Leiomyomas (*fibroid tumours*) are benign tumours originating from smooth muscle of the uterus. They are the most common form of pelvic tumour, occurring in one of every four or five women over 35 years of age (Porth 2009).

Pathophysiology of leiomyomas

The cause is not clearly understood, but there is an association with oestrogen stimulation. Fibroid tumours usually develop in the uterine corpus, and may be intramural, subserous or submucous (Figure 15.8):

● *Intramural fibroid tumours* are embedded in the myometrium, usually presenting as an enlargement of the uterus.
● *Subserous fibroid tumours* lie beneath the serous lining of the uterus, projecting into the peritoneal cavity. They may become pedunculated (on a stem) and displace or compress the ureter or bladder.
● *Submucous fibroid tumours* lie beneath the endometrial lining of the uterus, displacing endometrial tissue and are more likely to cause bleeding, infection and necrosis than the other types.

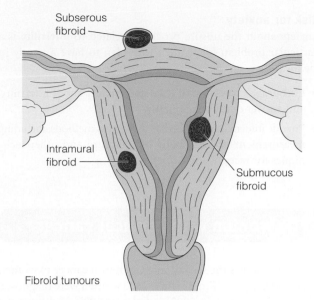

Figure 15.8 Types of uterine fibroid tumors (leiomyomas).

Signs and symptoms of leiomyomas

Small tumours may be asymptomatic (not causing symptoms). The rate of growth varies, and they may increase in size during pregnancy or with use of oral contraceptives or HRT. Large fibroid tumours can crowd other organs, leading to pelvic pressure, pain, dysmenorrhoea, menorrhagia and fatigue. Depending on the location of the tumour, constipation and urinary urgency and frequency may occur.

INTERDISCIPLINARY CARE FOR LEIOMYOMAS

Treatment depends on the size and location of the tumours, severity of the signs and symptoms, age and childbearing status. Tests used may include an ultrasound to differentiate leiomyoma from endometriosis and a laparoscopy to visualise subserosal leiomyomas (leiomyomas located close to the uterus).

In asymptomatic women who wish to bear children, the fibroid tumours are monitored. Follow-up is recommended two to three times annually to monitor growth.

Medication

Leuprolide acetate is used to decrease the size of the tumour if surgery is contraindicated or not desired. Gonadotropin-releasing hormone agonists are also administered.

Surgery

Myomectomy, removal of the tumour without removing the entire uterus, is the surgical procedure of choice for women who wish to retain reproductive capability, and laparoscopic laser technique is used. Hysterectomy is performed if tumours are large, and if bleeding or other problems continue in perimenopausal women. A non-surgical method of treatment is *uterine fibroid embolisation* – a catheter is guided through the femoral artery to the uterus, where tiny particles are injected into the artery supplying the fibroid cutting off the blood supply. This usually requires an overnight hospital stay, returning to normal activities in one week.

NURSING CARE FOR LEIOMYOMAS

If surgery is deferred, teaching should emphasise the importance of regular follow-up assessments to monitor tumour growth. If a hysterectomy is performed, teaching emphasises pre-operative and post-operative care. Dietary modifications to increase iron intake, prevent constipation and promote healing are important.

The woman with endometriosis

Endometriosis is a condition in which multiple, small, usually benign implantations of endometrial tissue develop, most commonly in the pelvic cavity but they may also be found in other areas of the body, such as the lungs. Risk factors include early menarche, regular periods with a cycle of less than 27 days, menses lasting more than seven days, heavier flow, increased menstrual pain and a history of the condition in first-degree female relatives (Porth 2009).

Pathophysiology of endometriosis

The cause is unclear. Metaplasia theory asserts that endometrial tissue develops from embryonic epithelial cells (early-stage epithelial cells) as a result of hormonal or inflammatory changes. The theory of retrograde menstruation suggests that menstrual tissue backs up through the fallopian tubes during menses, implants on various pelvic structures and survives. The transplantation theory asserts that endometrial implants spread via lymphatic or vascular routes.

The abnormally located endometrial tissue responds to cyclic ovarian hormone stimulation, and bleeding at the time of menstruation occurs at the sites of implantation. Scarring, inflammation and adhesions may develop. Endometriosis is a slowly progressive disease, responsive to ovarian hormone stimulation; the implants regress during pregnancy and atrophy at menopause unless the woman is receiving HRT. Progressive scarring may interfere with the ability to conceive, and women are encouraged to have children early if they wish to do so.

Signs and symptoms of endometriosis

Signs and symptoms of endometriosis include:

- heavy, throbbing pain of the lower abdomen and pelvis, radiating down the thighs and around the back;

- feeling of rectal pressure and discomfort when having a bowel movement;
- dyspareunia;
- dysfunctional uterine bleeding;
- infertility.

INTERDISCIPLINARY CARE FOR ENDOMETRIOSIS

Diagnosis may be difficult; a history of dysmenorrhoea, dyspareunia and infertility strongly suggests this diagnosis. Interventions depend on the severity of symptoms, the extent of the disease and age and desire for childbearing. Treatment focuses on pain management and restoring fertility.

Diagnosis

Diagnostic tests rule out other medical conditions and identify the endometrial implants. Tests include a pelvic ultrasound and laparoscopy as well as a FBC with differential ruling out pelvic abscesses and infectious processes.

Medication

Medications include analgesics to control pain and prostaglandin synthesis inhibitors such as NSAIDs. Hormone therapy may include oral contraceptives or progesterone to induce pseudopregnancy or danazol (Danol) to induce amenorrhoea and involution of endometrial tissue (cessation of periods and reduction in the size of the uterus). Prolonged use of danazol may result in masculinising effects. GnRH elevates levels of oestrogen and progesterone and minimises bleeding.

Surgery

This includes laparoscopy with laser ablation (excision or removal) of endometrial implants. Refractory endometriosis may be treated with total hysterectomy.

NURSING CARE FOR ENDOMETRIOSIS

Care includes providing pain relief, providing education about the condition and treatment options and helping the woman cope with treatment outcomes. The severity of the disease and its signs and symptoms are not necessarily related. Advanced disease may exhibit few signs and symptoms; early disease may be quite painful.

Nursing diagnoses and interventions

Interventions for pain, discussed previously, are also appropriate for the woman with endometriosis. A priority diagnosis for disorder is anxiety related to the risk for loss of reproductive function.

Risk for anxiety

Anxiety about the unsure prognosis related to infertility is a particular problem for women who plan to have a family in the future.

✚ Encourage expression of fears and anxiety about infertility, and answer questions honestly.

✚ Provide information on fertility awareness methods, including measurement of basal body temperature and other techniques for recognising ovulation.

The woman with cervical cancer

Cervical cancer is the second most common cancer in women worldwide. In the UK more than 2800 women were diagnosed with cervical cancer in 2007 and almost 1000 died from the disease in 2008. The highest number of cases of cervical cancer occurred in women aged between 30 and 34 years and approximately 70% of cases occurred in women under the age of 60 (Cancer Research UK 2010a).

Effective cervical screening and treatment have reduced the death rate. Hughes (2009) notes that the use of cervical screening programmes in the UK and other countries has reduced the incidence of cervical cancer. Approximately 80% of cervical smears in the UK are performed in the primary care setting; the practice nurse takes most of them. It is essential that those who take smears from women have undergone extensive education and training. If a smear is inappropriately obtained there can be implications for analysis and treatment (Kozier *et al.* 2008).

The terminal illness and death of the reality TV star in the UK Jade Goody and the associated media coverage in 2009 raised the profile of cervical cancer. There was a 12% increase in uptake of cervical smears as result of the media coverage.

Risk factors for cervical cancer

These include infection of the external genitalia and anus with human papillomavirus (HPV), first intercourse before 16 years of age, multiple sex partners or male partners with multiple sex partners, a history of sexually transmitted infections (STIs) and infection with HIV. Other risk factors include smoking and poor nutritional status, family history of cervical cancer and exposure to diethylstilbestrol (DES).

Pathophysiology of cervical cancer

Cancers derive from different tissues in the body; most cervical cancers (90%) are squamous cell carcinomas that begin as neoplasia (the beginning of a tumour) in the cervical epithelium. *Precancerous dysplasia (cervical intraepithelial neoplasia [CIN]), cervical carcinoma in situ* is estimated to occur in one of eight women before the age of 20 and is

Table 15.3 Staging of cervical cancer

Stage 0	Carcinoma *in situ* (pre-invasive carcinoma)
Stage 1	The carcinoma is strictly confined to the cervix (extension to the corpus (the body) should be disregarded) • Stage Ia – invasive carcinoma diagnosed only by microscopy (all macroscopically visible lesions, even with superficial invasion, are stage Ib carcinomas) • Stage Ia1 – stromal invasion of not larger than 3.0 mm in depth and extension of not larger than 7.0 mm (stromal cells are cells associated with connective tissue) • Stage Ia2 – stromal invasion of bigger than 3.0 mm and not larger than 5.0 mm in width, with an extension of not bigger than 7.0 mm • Stage Ib – clinically visible lesion limited to the cervix uteri or pre-clinical cancers greater than stage Ia • Stage Ib1 – clinically visible lesions no larger than 4.0 cm visually • Stage Ib2 – clinically visible lesions larger than 4.0 cm visually
Stage II	Cervical carcinoma invades beyond the uterus but not to the pelvic wall or lower third of the vagina • Stage IIa – no obvious parametrial involvement (the connective tissue of the pelvic floor) • Stage IIb – obvious parametrial involvement
Stage III	The carcinoma has extended to the pelvic wall. On rectal examination there is no cancer-free space between the tumour and the pelvic wall. The tumour involves the lower third of the vagina. All cases with hydronephrosis or non-functioning kidney are included unless they are known to be the result of another cause • Stage IIIa – tumour involves lower third of the vagina with no extension to the pelvic wall • Stage IIIb – extension to the pelvic wall and/or hydronephrosis or non-functioning kidney
Stage IV	The carcinoma has extended beyond the true pelvis, or has involved the mucosa of the bladder or rectum (biopsy proven) • Stage IVa – spread of the growth to adjacent organs • Stage IVb – spread to distant organs

Source: Benedet *et al.* 2000.

often associated with HPV infection. There is also a strong association between precancerous dysplasia and reproductive infections of *Chlamydia trachomatis* (discussed in Chapter 17). Systems of grading of dysplastic changes in the cervix use the *cervical intraepithelial neoplasia (CIN)* system (Table 15.3).

Cancer *in situ* most often develops in a particular area of the cervix – the transformation zone where the columnar epithelium of the cervical lining meets the squamous epithelium of the outer cervix and vagina. Squamous cell cancers spread by direct invasion of accessory structures, including the vaginal wall, pelvic wall, bladder and rectum. Metastasis (spread) is frequently confined to the pelvic area; distant metastasis may occur through the lymphatic system.

Signs and symptoms of cervical cancer

Pre-invasive cancer is limited to the cervix and rarely causes signs and symptoms. Invasive cancer causes vaginal bleeding after intercourse or between menstrual periods, and vaginal discharge increases as the cancer progresses. These changes are subtle, and may be more readily noticed by the postmenopausal woman who will not confuse it with menstrual activity. Signs and symptoms of advanced disease include referred pain in the back or thighs, haematuria, bloody stools, anaemia and weight loss.

INTERDISCIPLINARY CARE FOR CERVICAL CANCER

The goals are to eradicate the cancer and minimise complications and metastasis. Treatment depends on the degree of malignant change, size and location of the lesion and the extent of metastasis.

Consider this . . .

A 12-year-old confides in you that she would like a cervical smear test. After discussing this with her, she informs you that she is sexually active and has read and heard that she can have a test to tell if she has cancer. Her mother has recently been diagnosed with cervical cancer.

Diagnosis

Tests include a cervical smear, colposcopy and cervical biopsy (see above). A loop diathermy technique (LEEP) allows simultaneous diagnosis and treatment of dysplastic lesions found on colposcopy. This can be performed in the out-patients department, using a wire for both cutting and coagulation during excision of the dysplastic region of the cervix. An MRI or CT of the pelvis, abdomen or bones can evaluate the spread of the tumour.

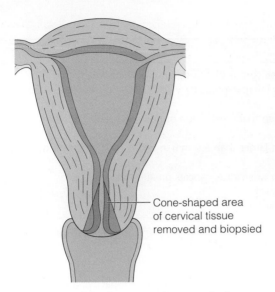

Cone-shaped area
of cervical tissue
removed and biopsied

Figure 15.9 Conisation, the surgical removal of a cone-shaped section of the cervix, is used to treat microinvasive carcinoma of the cervix.

Medication

Chemotherapy is used for tumours not responsive to other therapy, tumours that cannot be removed or as adjunct therapy if metastasis has occurred.

Surgery

When combined with colposcopy, laser surgery is a viable treatment method provided that the cancer is limited to the cervical epithelium. Cryosurgery, which involves the use of a probe to freeze tissue, causing necrosis and sloughing, is also used for non-invasive lesions. Conisation (Figure 15.9) is performed to treat micro-invasive carcinoma when colposcopy cannot define the limits of the invasion. For invasive lesions, hysterectomy or radical hysterectomy is performed.

Pelvic exenteration, removal of all pelvic contents, including the bowel, vagina and bladder, is performed if the cancer recurs without involvement of the lymphatic system. An anterior exenteration is the removal of the uterus, ovaries, fallopian tubes, vagina, bladder, urethra and lymphatic vessels and nodes. An ileal conduit is created for excretion of urine (see Chapter 8). A posterior exenteration is the removal of the uterus, ovaries, fallopian tubes, bowel and rectum. A colostomy is created for excretion of faeces (see Chapter 7).

Radiation therapy

Radiation therapy is used to treat invasive cervical cancer. External radiation beam therapy and intracavity cesium irradiation can be used. Radiation is discussed in Chapter 2.

NURSING CARE FOR CERVICAL CANCER

Nursing care involves helping the woman deal with the physical and psychological effects of a potentially life-threatening illness, providing information needed to make informed deci-

sions and minimising the adverse effects of therapy. Pain relief measures are important, as is the inclusion of bereavement counselling on the part of the woman and family. The woman should be encouraged to perform self-care activities and resume normal everyday activities and sexual functioning to the extent possible.

Health promotion

All women in the UK over 25 years are usually routinely invited to attend for cervical screening (Hughes 2009). Screening should be done every year with regular smear tests or as advised. In 2008 the cervical screening programme in the UK celebrated its 20th year; the programme has screened about 64 million women and detected a significant number of abnormalities. It is estimated that the screening programme saves over 4500 lives each year (National Health Service Cervical Screening Programme (NHSCSP) 2008).

The exact age groups for screening vary between the different countries of the UK. In England, women between 25 and 64 years are screened. In Northern Ireland and Wales, women between 20 and 64 are screened. In Scotland, women between 20 and 60 should be screened every three years (Cancer Research UK 2011a).

Nurses should educate women of all ages about controlling risk factors for cervical cancer and about the importance of screening for this cancer throughout the lifespan. Teach young women about the relationship between early sexual activity, multiple partners and risk for STIs and cervical cancer. Discuss safer sex alternatives and using condoms for protection. Emphasise the importance of continued screening tests for the older woman who may not see a gynaecologist on a regular basis. Encourage women to receive the HPV vaccine. The vaccine is given as three injections over a six-month period and does not protect against HPV in a woman already infected.

Assessment

Collect the following data through a health history and physical examination:

✦ *Health history:* history of STIs, sexual history, partner's sexual history, family history of cervical cancer, vaginal bleeding or discharge, smoking history, maternal treatment with DES.

✦ *Physical assessment:* pelvic examination, abdomen, lymph glands.

Nursing diagnoses and interventions

This section discusses nursing interventions for cervical cancer. Other nursing diagnoses and interventions that may be appropriate for the woman with cervical cancer are considered in the sections discussing other reproductive system cancers.

Risk for fear

Many people believe that cancer equals death; however, this is no longer true in many cases, especially with early diagnosis.

+ The earlier the cancer is diagnosed the better the prognosis (outcome).

+ Allow adequate time for the woman and her partner to express their concerns and to ask questions.

+ Refer for counselling or support groups for additional information.

Risk for impaired tissue integrity

Surgery interrupts the integrity of the skin, providing a potential portal of invasion for bacteria. Radiation therapy causes an inflammatory response in the skin and mucous membranes within the field of radiation, creating further risk of tissue reaction and breakdown.

+ Teach wound and skin care, particularly if pelvic exenteration is performed. Wound care is required based on individual needs. Wound care provision must be evidence-based and in line with local policy and procedure.

+ If appropriate, teach care that may be required with the formation of stoma (an artificial opening on the abdomen for the collection of faeces or urine), and care for the skin surrounding the stoma. (These procedures are discussed in Chapters 7 and 8 respectively.)

+ If the woman wishes to apply non-oil-based lotions to the skin surface, this may minimise itching and help maintain integrity.

+ Advise the woman not to remove the markings used to localise the radiation beam to the target area.

+ Monitor for evidence of fistula formation, and teach the woman to do the same.

COMMUNITY-BASED CARE

Teaching varies according to the stage of the cancer and the treatment selected. Provide information concerning radiation, chemotherapy or surgery, as indicated. Pre-operative teaching focuses on post-operative expectations, including management of faecal or urinary diversion, if indicated (see Chapters 7 and 8 respectively). Help the woman and family recognise signs of infection and understand the importance of follow-up care. Suggest the following resources:

● Cancer Research UK;

● National Cancer Research Institute.

The woman with endometrial cancer

In 2007 in England and Wales, 7536 new cases of endometrial cancer were registered with 1039 deaths. Approximately 90% of cases of endometrial cancer are in women over 50, peaking in the early 70s where declining (Cancer Research UK 2010b).

It is suggested that endometrial cancer is more common in post-menopausal women because of hormonal changes that occur during the menopause. These may make a woman more susceptible to endometrial cancer (NHS Choices 2011).

Risk factors for endometrial cancer

Significant risk factors are prolonged oestrogen stimulation as well as obesity, anovulatory menstrual cycles (having a menstrual cycle without ovulation), decreasing ovarian function, oestrogen-secreting tumours and unopposed oestrogen (e.g., oestrogen therapy without progesterone). Medical conditions that may alter oestrogen metabolism and increase the risk of endometrial cancer are diabetes mellitus, hypertension and POS (Porth 2009). Tamoxifen, a drug blocking oestrogen receptor sites, is used to treat breast cancer, has a weak oestrogenic effect on the endometrium and is also a risk factor.

Endometrial cancer is the most commonly inherited gynaecological cancer.

Pathophysiology of endometrial cancer

Most endometrial malignancies are adenocarcinomas that are slow to grow and spread. These cancers develop in the glandular cells or endometrial lining of the uterus (the same tissue that is shed each month during a normal menstrual period). Endometrial hyperplasia (excessive growth) is a precursor of endometrial cancer. These tumours tend to grow slowly in the early stages.

Tumour growth usually begins in the fundus, invades the vascular myometrium, spreading throughout the female reproductive system. Metastasis occurs by means of the lymphatic system, through the fallopian tubes to the peritoneal cavity, and to the rest of the body via the bloodstream. Target areas for metastasis include the lungs, liver and bone. The International Federation of Gynecology and Obstetrics (FIGO) classification of endometrial cancer is presented in Table 15.4

Signs and symptoms of endometrial cancer

The major sign and symptom is abnormal, painless vaginal bleeding. In menstruating women, this bleeding is manifested as menorrhagia or metrorrhagia. In post-menopausal women, any bleeding is abnormal. Later manifestations include pelvic

Table 15.4 FIGO staging classification for endometrial cancer

Stage	Description
I	Tumour limited to endometrium or myometrium.
II	Endocervical glandular involvement or invasion of cervical stroma.
III	Metastasis or invasion of serosa, adnexae, vagina and pelvic or para-aortic lymph nodes.
IV	Tumour invasion of bladder or bowel mucosa; distant metastases.

cramping, bleeding after intercourse and lower abdominal pressure. In advanced disease, lymph node enlargement, pleural effusion (excessive collection of fluid in the pleural space), abdominal masses and ascites (excessive collection of fluid in the abdominal cavity) may be present.

INTERDISCIPLINARY CARE FOR ENDOMETRIAL CANCER

The goals of care are to eradicate the cancer and minimise complications and metastasis.

Diagnosis

Tests used to diagnose endometrial cancer include a vaginal or transvaginal ultrasound, used to determine endometrial thickening, which may indicate hypertrophy or malignant changes, and an endometrial biopsy or dilation and curettage (D&C) to provide a definitive diagnosis (see earlier in this chapter for further information and nursing care). Other tests include chest x-ray, intravenous urography (an x-ray test used to outline the urinary tract), cystoscopy, barium enema, sigmoidoscopy (examination of the rectum and sigmoid colon using a sigmoidoscope), MRI and bone scans.

Medication

The treatment of choice for primary endometrial carcinoma is surgery; progesterone therapy may be used for recurrent disease. About one-third of women respond favourably, primarily those with well-differentiated tumours (tumours that are well-developed). Chemotherapy is less effective than other forms of therapy, although cisplatin or combination chemotherapy may be used for women with disseminated disease (cancer cells have spread from the original tissues to other tissues).

Surgery

After the diagnosis is confirmed, total abdominal hysterectomy and bilateral salpingo-oophorectomy (surgical removal of both ovaries and both fallopian tubes) is performed for stage I cancer. Radical hysterectomy with node dissection is performed if the disease is stage II or beyond.

Radiation therapy

Treatment with external and internal radiation may be performed as a pre-operative measure or as adjuvant treatment in advanced cases.

NURSING CARE FOR ENDOMETRIAL CANCER

Health promotion

Regular pelvic examinations of perimenopausal and post-menopausal women is advocated. All women at the time of menopause should be informed of the risks and manifestations of endometrial cancer, and should be encouraged to report any unexpected bleeding or spotting to their healthcare provider, i.e. the practice nurse.

Assessment

Collect the following data through a health history and physical examination:

+ *Health history:* abnormal vaginal bleeding, menstrual history, use of oestrogen (without progesterone) to treat menopausal symptoms, breast cancer treated with tamoxifen, child-bearing status, presence of chronic illnesses, family history of hereditary non-polyposis colon cancer.
+ *Physical assessment:* height and weight, pelvic examination, abdomen, lymph glands.

Nursing diagnoses and interventions

Nursing care involves helping the woman deal with the physical and psychological effects of a potentially life-threatening illness, make informed decisions and minimise the adverse effects of therapy. Pain relief is a key component of care, as is bereavement counselling (if appropriate). Encourage the woman to perform self-care and resume normal activities of living.

Risk for acute pain

Total abdominal hysterectomy can involve severe and prolonged pain, from the surgical incision and also from the manipulation of internal organs during surgery.

+ Administer analgesics as prescribed.
+ Encourage mobilisation.
+ Apply heat to the abdomen, and recommend a heating pad at home.

Risk for disturbed body image

For many women, the side-effects of cancer treatment can be almost as difficult and painful as the disease itself. Side-effects of the different therapies vary among individuals; body image and quality of life are always affected. Alopecia (hair loss), nausea, vomiting, fatigue, diarrhoea, stomatitis (inflammation of any structures within the mouth) and surgical scarring disturb body image.

+ Review the side-effects of the treatment regimen proposed, and assist the woman to develop a plan to deal with these effects.
+ Remind the woman and family that side-effects are usually manageable and may be temporary.

Risk for ineffective sexuality pattern

Altered sexuality may result from a feeling of unattractiveness, fatigue or pain and discomfort. The woman's partner may fear that sexual activity will be harmful.

+ Encourage expression of feelings about the effect of cancer on their lives and sexual relationship.
+ Suggest the couple explore alternative sexual positions and coordinate sexual activity with rest periods and times that are relatively free from pain.

COMMUNITY-BASED CARE

Provide information about the specific treatment and prognosis for the cancer. Explain the expected side-effects of radiation implant therapy (see Chapter 2). Pain control measures are also an essential part of the teaching plan (see Chapter 2). The resources listed for the woman with cervical cancer are also appropriate for the woman with endometrial cancer.

The woman with ovarian cancer

This is a common gynaecological cancer. Approximately 6500 women are diagnosed with ovarian cancer annually (Cancer Research UK 2011b). Incidence increases with age, peaking in between the ages of 40 and 80; half of all cases are in the over 65 years age group (Porth 2009). The UK has one of the highest incidences of ovarian cancer in Europe.

Consider this . . .

Why does the UK have one of the highest incidences of ovarian cancer in Europe?

Risk factors for ovarian cancer

Family history is a significant risk factor, with a 50% risk of developing the disease if two or more first- or second-degree relatives have site-specific ovarian cancer. Other inherited risks are breast–ovarian cancer syndrome (first- and second-degree relatives have both breast and ovarian cancer) and family cancer syndrome, in which male or female relatives have a history of colorectal, endometrial, ovarian, pancreatic or other types of cancer (Porth 2009). The breast cancer susceptibility genes *BRAC1* and *BRAC2* are implicated in 5–10% of hereditary ovarian cancers.

Risk factors include having no children or giving birth after age 35, exposure to talc or asbestos, endometriosis and pelvic inflammatory disease. Protective factors include long-term contraceptive use, having a child before the age of 25, tubal ligation, breastfeeding and hysterectomy (Martin 2005).

Table 15.5 FIGO staging classification for ovarian cancer

Stage	Description
I	Growth limited to the ovaries.
II	Growth involving one or both ovaries with pelvic extension.
III	Tumour involving one or both ovaries, with peritoneal implants outside the pelvis or positive retroperitoneal or inguinal nodes.
IV	Growth involving one or both ovaries with distant metastasis.

Pathophysiology of ovarian cancer

There are a number of types of ovarian cancers: epithelial tumours, germ cell tumours and gonadal stromal tumours. Most are epithelial tumours, originating from the surface epithelium of the ovary. It usually spreads by local shedding of cancer cells into the peritoneal cavity and by direct invasion of the bowel and bladder. Cancer cells in peritoneal fluid can implant in the intestines, bladder and mesentery. Further spread occurs through the lymph and blood to the liver, and across the diaphragm involving the lungs. Pelvic and para-aortic lymph nodes may be involved, and tumour cells can block lymphatic drainage from the abdomen, causing ascites. Staging for ovarian cancer is based on surgical and histologic evaluation of biopsy specimens (Table 15.5).

Signs and symptoms of ovarian cancer

In the early stages, ovarian cancer generally causes no warning signs or manifestations. When signs and symptoms do develop, they are vague and mild, such as indigestion, urinary frequency, abdominal bloating and constipation. Abnormal vaginal bleeding occurs if the endometrium is stimulated by a hormone-secreting tumour or if the tumour erodes the vaginal wall. Pelvic pain sometimes occurs. An enlarged abdomen with ascites signals later-stage disease.

Complications of ovarian cancer

Complications of advanced ovarian cancer are outlined in Table 15.6.

INTERDISCIPLINARY CARE FOR OVARIAN CANCER

Care focuses on surgery to determine the stage of tumour and to remove as much of this as possible. As there are no early signs and symptoms, the disease is often well advanced prior to diagnosis. In younger women, an ovarian mass may be monitored for several menstrual cycles; any ovarian mass must immediately be investigated in a post-menopausal woman.

Table 15.6 Complications of advanced ovarian cancer

Complication	Assessments	Treatment
Ascites (accumulation of fluid in the abdominal cavity)	• Abdominal distention • Everted umbilicus • Shiny abdominal skin • Dullness on percussion of dependent areas • Dyspnoea, constipation • Abdominal pain	Paracentesis (removing fluid from the abdomen)
Intestinal obstruction	• Abdominal distention • Abdominal pain • Projectile vomiting • Constipation • Hyperactive bowel sounds	Nasogastric tube insertion, nil by mouth
Deep venous thrombosis	• Leg oedema • Leg pain • Redness, warmth	Anticoagulants
Lymphoedema	• Oedema of leg • Decreased range of motion • Tight, shiny skin on leg	Skin care, range-of-motion exercises, massage or physical therapy, compression bandaging

Diagnosis

Tests used in the diagnosis are transvaginal or abdominal ultrasound and a CT scan of the abdomen and pelvis (discussed earlier).

The blood test most useful is a CA-125 antigen level. CA-125 is a tumour marker that is highly specific to epithelial ovarian cancer. Transvaginal or transabdominal ultrasonography measures ovarian size and detects small masses.

Medication

Surgery is the treatment of choice for ovarian cancer, but chemotherapy may be used to achieve remission. Chemotherapy is not curative. Combination chemotherapy regimens using cyclophosphamide and cisplatin or other agents may be employed. Combination therapy with a platinum compound (cisplatin or carboplatin) is superior to treatment with a single drug, with paclitaxel/carboplatin the preferred regimen (Martin 2005). This may prolong survival. Close monitoring of bone marrow and renal function is vital as chemotherapy has toxic effects.

Surgery

For those with stage I disease who wish to have children, treatment may be limited to removal of one ovary. Usually, total hysterectomy with bilateral salpingo-oophorectomy and removal of the omentum are performed.

Radiation therapy

Radiation therapy using external-beam or intracavitary implants is performed for palliative purposes and is directed at shrinking the tumour.

NURSING CARE FOR OVARIAN CANCER

Nursing care for those with ovarian cancer is similar to the care for women with other gynaecological cancers. The side-effects of treatment of cancer and generally poor prognosis diminish the woman's quality of life involving major psycho-social implications (see Chapter 2).

The woman with cancer of the vulva

There were 1120 cases of vulval cancer registered in 2007, and the cancer occurs most often in women over 50 years (Cancer Research UK 2010c). Prognosis depends on the degree of invasion, general health status of the woman, presence of chronic diseases and ability to withstand treatment.

Pathophysiology of vulvar cancer

The cause is unknown, but there is evidence to associate it with STIs, particularly HPV. Nearly 85% of malignant and pre-malignant cervical and vulvar lesions have been found to contain HPV DNA, HPV structural antigens or both. Herpes simplex type 2 (HSV2) infection has been associated with vulvar cancer. Other risk factors include advanced age, diabetes and a history of leukoplakia (a pre-cancerous lesion on the vulvar mucous membranes characterised by raised white patches).

Most vulvar cancers are epidermoid or squamous cell carcinomas. The primary site is usually the labia majora, but vulvar cancer is also found on the labia minora, clitoris, vestibule and occasionally in multiple locations. Metastasis occurs by direct extension into the vagina, perineal skin, anus and urethra. Cancer also spreads through the lymphatic system.

Signs and symptoms of vulvar cancer

Often vulvar cancer is asymptomatic, lesions are discovered on routine examination or self-examination. Discoloration varies from white macular patches to red painless sores. Lesions may be *exophytic* (proliferating outwardly), *endophytic* (proliferating inwardly), ulcerative or *verrucous* (resembling a wart).

Pruritus is the most common manifestation; often there is a history of prolonged vulvar irritation. Perineal pain and bleeding indicate large tumours and advanced disease. In very advanced disease, dysuria related to urethral involvement may be the presenting symptom.

INTERDISCIPLINARY CARE FOR VULVAR CANCER

Itching, burning or a sore on the vulva merits investigation and biopsy of any lesions. Inguinal lymph nodes may be enlarged. The aim is to eradicate the lesion and reduce the risk of recurrence. Surgical resection is the preferred treatment. If lymph nodes are involved, radiation therapy is used postoperatively. Chemotherapy is reserved for distant metastases.

Diagnosis is based on the results of an excisional biopsy of the lesion. Metastasis can be evaluated by chest x-ray, barium enema, intravenous pyelogram, cystoscopy, CT and MRI scans and proctoscopy. Lymphangiography can also be used.

The specific surgical procedure depends on the stage of the cancer. Early, non-invasive lesions may be treated with laser surgery, cryosurgery or electrocautery. For more advanced disease, vulvectomy may be performed (Figure 15.10). A simple vulvectomy involves the removal of the vulva, labia majora and minora, clitoris and prepuce. A radical vulvectomy is performed if invasion is suspected. This involves removal of all the tissue in a simple vulvectomy, together with the subcutaneous tissue and regional lymph nodes.

NURSING CARE FOR VULVAR CANCER

Nursing care is similar to that for endometrial cancer. The woman fears death as the ultimate outcome as well as the possible pain and suffering that surgery and other treatments may cause. Radical surgery represents a great loss to women of all ages.

Nursing diagnoses and interventions

Disruption of perineal tissue is a priority problem for women with vulvar cancer.

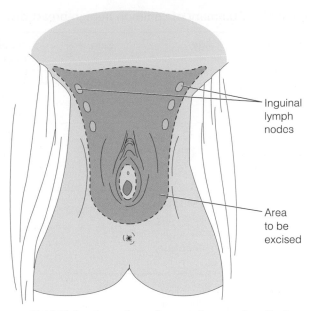

Figure 15.10 Vulvectomy for vulvar carcinoma. A radical vulvectomy involves removal of the vulva, labia majora, labia minora, clitoris, prepuce, subcutaneous tissue, and regional lymph nodes.

Risk for impaired tissue integrity

The woman who has undergone a vulvectomy is at high risk for infection and impaired healing because of proximity of the surgical site to the urinary and anal orifices. Also, the women are often older and may have age-related changes in healing and immune function.

+ Teach the woman and/or her partner or other family member the procedure for irrigation of the vulvectomy. If neither is able to perform this procedure, arrange for the community nurse to carry it out.

+ After irrigation, apply dry heat using a heat lamp positioned about 45 cm from the area; emphasise safety precautions, including use of a low-wattage bulb (40–60 watts).

+ Provide information on maintaining a diet high in protein, iron and vitamin C.

Now that we have covered various disorders associated with the female reproductive tissues, we will go on to look at disorders of the breast.

DISORDERS OF THE BREAST

When a woman discovers a breast lump, her first response is often fear: of breast cancer, of losing her breast and perhaps of losing her life. Many societies view the breast as a significant component of feminine beauty. Problems that threaten the breast often strike at the core of a woman's self-image.

Nurses are central in the care of women experiencing breast disorders by providing education, support and advocacy. The role includes educating women about normal breast tissue, common benign breast disorders, available screening techniques, risk factors and breast self-examination (BSE).

Table 15.7 Summary of common benign breast disorders

Condition	Age	Pain	Nipple discharge	Location	Consistency and mobility	Diagnosis and treatment
Duct ectasia	35–55 years; median age 40	Burning around nipple	Sticky, multicoloured; usually bilateral	No specific location	Retroareolar mass with advanced disease	Open biopsy; local excision of diseased portion of breast
Fibroadenoma	15–39 years; median age 20	No	No	No specific location	Mobile, firm, smooth, well-delineated mass	Mammography, surgical or needle biopsy; excision of the tumour
Fibrocystic changes (FCC)	20–49 years; median age 30 (may subside with menopause)	Yes	May occur	Upper outer quadrant	Bilateral multiple lumps influenced by the menstrual cycle	Needle aspiration; observation; biopsy if there is an unresolved mass or mammographic changes
Intraductal papilloma	35–55 years; median age 40	Yes	Serous or sanguineous; usually unilateral from one duct	No specific location	Usually soft, poorly delineated mass	Smear of nipple discharge; biopsy; wedge resection
Mastitis, acute	Childbearing years	Tenderness, pain	No	No specific location	Generalised redness of overlying skin	Antibiotic therapy; incision and drainage if mastitis progresses to an abscess
Mastitis, chronic	Any age	Tenderness, pain; headache; high fever	No	No specific location	Generalised redness and swelling	Antibiotics, usually penicillin
Fat necrosis	Any age	Tenderness	No	No specific location	Firm, irregular, palpable	Surgical biopsy to rule out cancer

The woman with a benign breast disorder

Benign breast disorders occur frequently in women and may be a source of anxiety. Changes in breast tissue often correspond to hormonal changes of the menstrual cycle. Increased tenderness and lumpiness prior to menses may be noted; therefore, it is best to perform breast self-examination 7–10 days after the beginning of the menstrual period. Changes also occur in response to hormonal, nutritional, physical and environmental stimuli. Benign breast disorders include fibrocystic breast changes, fibroadenomas, intraductal papillomas, duct ectasia, fat necrosis and mastitis (Table 15.7).

Pathophysiology and signs and symptoms of benign breast disorders

Fibrocystic changes (FCC)

Fibrocystic changes (*fibrocystic breast disease*) is the physiological nodularity and breast tenderness that increases and decreases with the menstrual cycle. An estimated 50–80% of all women

experience some of these changes, which include fibrosis, epithelial proliferation and cyst formation. This is common in women 30–50 years of age, and rare in post-menopausal women who are not taking hormone replacement (Porth 2009).

FCC includes many different lesions and breast changes. The more common non-proliferative form does not increase the risk for breast cancer. The proliferative form, accompanied by giant cysts and proliferative epithelial lesions, does.

Non-proliferative changes may be cystic or fibrous. Cystic change refers to the dilation of ducts in the subareolar, lobular or lobe areas. Cysts often go unnoticed unless pain and tenderness is associated with menses. Fibrous changes are infrequent but can occur during the menstrual years.

Women with fibrocystic changes experience bilateral or unilateral pain or tenderness in the upper, outer quadrants of their breasts, and report that their breasts feel particularly thick and lumpy the week prior to menses. Nipple discharge may be present. Pain is due to oedema of the connective tissue of the breast, dilation of the ducts and some inflammatory response. Multiple, mobile cysts may form, usually in both breasts (Figure 15.11). Fluid aspirated ranges in colour from milky white to yellow, brown or green; if it is tinged with blood, there may be malignancy.

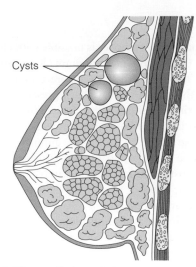

Figure 15.11 Fibrocystic breast changes.

Intraductal disorders

An *intraductal papilloma* is a tiny, wart-like growth on the inside of the peripheral mammary duct causing discharge from the nipple. This may be clear and sticky or bloody. This condition is most common in women in their 30s and 40s. The lesion must be investigated to rule out malignancy.

Mammary duct ectasia (plasma cell mastitis) is a palpable lumpiness found beneath the areola. Duct ectasia involves periductal inflammation, dilation of the ductal system, and accumulation of fluid and dead cells blocking the involved ducts. This usually occurs in perimenopausal women and is difficult to differentiate from cancer.

Signs and symptoms include sticky, thick nipple discharge with burning and itching around the nipple, and inflammation. The discharge may be green, greenish brown or bloody. Nipple retraction is often associated with duct ectasia in post-menopausal women.

INTERDISCIPLINARY CARE FOR BENIGN BREAST DISORDER

Diagnosis of FCC is based on history, physical examination and imaging studies (for example x-rays). A biopsy may be required for diagnosis.

Analysis of nipple discharge, mammography and possibly ductography may be used to diagnose ductal disorders. The duct is excised in an open biopsy procedure. Nursing care is similar to that for any woman with an open biopsy. It is important to reassure the woman that these disorders are not breast cancer.

The treatment is usually symptomatic. Cyst aspiration may relieve pain, and also allows examination of fluid to confirm the cystic nature of the disease. A well-fitting bra that provides good support worn day and night helps relieve discomfort. Aspirin, mild analgesics, local heat or cold and vitamin E may help relieve breast pain.

NURSING CARE FOR BENIGN BREAST DISORDER

When a woman presents with a breast mass, nursing responsibilities include taking a history and facilitating follow-up care. If a palpable mass is present, it is important to ask how long the lesion has been present and if there is any pain associated with the mass, any change in its size and any changes in association with the menstrual cycle.

In many cases, definitive diagnosis of the breast disorder requires surgical biopsy to rule out cancer. The nurse can provide emotional support and education about diagnostic and therapeutic procedures, self-care and comfort measures and resources to help cope with the experience.

The woman with breast cancer

Breast cancer is the unregulated growth of abnormal cells in breast tissue. There are more than 48 000 people diagnosed with breast cancer in the UK annually. The majority of these are women, although approximately 300 are men. Breast cancer is the most common cancer in the UK (after non-melanoma skin cancer). It is the most common cancer in women, and one in nine women will develop breast cancer. Most of the women who get breast cancer are post-menopausal, but almost 8000 diagnosed each year are under 50 years old (Cancer Research UK 2011c).

Risk factors for breast cancer

Some risk factors can be changed and some cannot. Those that cannot are (Cancer Research UK 2011d):

- age and gender;
- genetic risk factors;
- family history of breast cancer;
- personal history of breast cancer;
- previous breast biopsy;
- previous chest irradiation;
- menstrual history.

Lifestyle-related factors and breast cancer risk include using oral contraceptives, not having children or having them after the age of 30, using HRT for more than five years, not breastfeeding, drinking alcohol, obesity, high-fat diets, physical inactivity and (possibly) environmental pollution. Lowering risk factors for breast cancer include breastfeeding, moderate or vigorous physical activity and maintaining a healthy body weight.

Pathophysiology of breast cancer

Possible causes of breast cancer include environmental, hormonal, reproductive and hereditary factors. Two breast cancer susceptibility genes have been identified: *BRCA1* and *BRCA2*. These genes may be responsible for the approximately 10% of women with hereditary breast cancer, with genetic mutations causing up to 80% of breast cancer in women younger than 50 years of age. A woman with identified mutations in *BRCA1* has a lifetime risk of 56–85% for breast cancer and an increased risk for ovarian cancer (Porth 2009).

Breast cancer begins as a single transformed cell and is hormone dependent (depends on the presence of hormone to grow). It is classified as non-invasive (*in situ*) or invasive, depending on the penetration of the tumour into surrounding tissue. Breast cancer may remain a non-invasive disease, or an invasive disease without metastasis, for long periods of time.

Breast cancer may be categorised as carcinoma of the mammary ducts, carcinoma of mammary lobules or sarcoma of the breast. Most breast cancers are adenocarcinomas and appear to arise in the terminal section of the breast ductal tissue. There are many histologic types of breast cancer; only a few examples are described here. The most common type is *infiltrating ductal carcinoma*. Two atypical types of breast cancer are inflammatory carcinoma and Paget's disease. Inflammatory carcinoma of the breast, a systemic disease, is the most malignant form. Oedema with dimpling of the skin, which looks like the peel of an orange (*peau d'orange*) is usually present. *Paget's disease* is a rare type of breast cancer involving infiltration of the nipple epithelium.

Breast cancer can metastasise to other sites. The common sites of metastasis of breast cancer are bone, brain, lung, liver, skin and lymph nodes. Staging is a system of classifying cancer according to the size of the tumour, involvement of lymph nodes, metastasis to distant sites and the presence/absence of distant metastasis. This provides important information for making decisions about treatment options and is used as a basis for prognosis.

Signs and symptoms of breast cancer

These may include a non-tender lump in the breast (upper outer quadrant), abnormal nipple discharge, a rash around the nipple area, nipple retraction, dimpling of the skin or a change in the position of the nipple. There may also be nipple pain, scaliness, ulceration, skin irritation or discharge. Breast cancer is usually painless, but some women report a burning or stinging sensation. There may be no signs and symptoms, and tumours are detected by mammography. Most breast cancers are found by the women themselves or their partner.

INTERDISCIPLINARY CARE FOR BREAST CANCER

Diagnosis begins with detection of asymptomatic lesions discovered through screening or symptomatic lesions discovered by the woman. Any palpable mass requires evaluation. Once the diagnosis is made, a number of treatment options are available. The choice of treatment depends on several factors, such as the stage of the cancer, the age of the woman and the woman's preferences.

Diagnosis

Early detection of breast cancer is possible with clinical breast examination (CBE) and mammogram. Mammography can detect breast tumours two years before they reach palpable size; most of these tumours have been present for 8–10 years. Controversy exists about the ability of screening mammography to improve mortality rates for women under 50. The NHS Breast Screening Programme recommends annual mammograms beginning at age 50 and up to 70 years (Kozier *et al.* 2008).

Other diagnostic tests include a percutaneous needle biopsy to define a cystic mass or fibrocystic changes and specimens for cytologic examination, and a breast biopsy. In aspiration biopsy or fine-needle aspiration biopsy, a needle is used to remove cells or fluid from the breast lesion (Figure 15.12 A). In many facilities, fine-needle aspiration biopsies are performed using a stereotactic biopsy device; mammography and a computer are used to guide the needle.

Medication

Tamoxifen citrate (Nolvadex) is an oral medication interfering with oestrogen activity. It is used to treat advanced breast cancer,

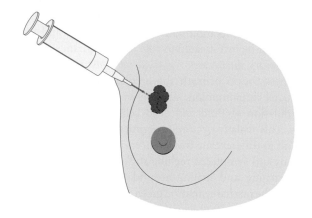

A Aspiration biopsy

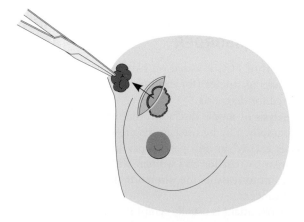

B Excisional biopsy

Figure 15.12 Types of breast biopsy. (A) In an aspiration biopsy, a needle is used to aspirate fluid or tissue from the breast. **(B)** In an excisional biopsy, tissue from the breast lesion is removed surgically.

as an adjuvant for early-stage breast cancer and as a preventive treatment for women at high risk of developing breast cancer.

Immunotherapy, using trastuzumab (Herceptin), is used to stop the growth of some breast tumours. The National Institute for Health and Clinical Excellence (NICE 2006) recommends trastuzumab, given at three-week intervals for one year or until disease recurrence (whichever is the shorter period), as a treatment option for women with early-stage HER2-positive breast cancer following surgery, chemotherapy and radiotherapy (if applicable). Cardiac function should be assessed prior to the commencement of therapy, and trastuzumab treatment should not be offered to women who have a left ventricular ejection fraction (LVEF) of 55% or less, or who have any of the following:

- a history of documented congestive heart failure;
- high-risk uncontrolled arrhythmias;
- angina pectoris requiring medication;
- clinically significant valvular disease;
- evidence of transmural infarction on electrocardiograph (ECG);
- poorly controlled hypertension.

Cardiac functional assessments should be repeated every three months during trastuzumab treatment.

Chemotherapy has become the standard of care for the majority of breast cancer cases with axillary node involvement. In late metastatic disease, chemotherapy becomes the primary treatment to prolong the woman's life. Chemotherapy is discussed in Chapter 2. Adjuvant (additional) systemic therapy following primary treatment for early-stage breast cancer refers to the administration of chemotherapy and other pharmacologic agents. This type of therapy has been widely studied; it reduces the rates of recurrence and death from breast cancer. For example, the drug Avastin, when combined with chemotherapy to treat metastatic breast cancer, has extended cancer-free survival; and Femara (an aromatase inhibitor) has reduced the risk of recurrence after surgery (in some cases more effectively than tamoxifen).

Surgery

Until recently, the treatment of choice for breast cancer was a radical mastectomy. The trend is toward more conservative surgery combined with chemotherapy, hormone therapy or radiation, depending on the stage of the tumour and the age of the woman.

Mastectomy

There are various types of mastectomy. *Radical mastectomy* is the removal of the entire affected breast, the underlying chest muscles and the axillary lymph nodes. *Simple mastectomy* is the removal of the complete breast. *Segmental mastectomy* or *lumpectomy* (Figure 15.13A) is the removal of the tumour and the surrounding margin of breast tissues. *Modified radical mastectomy* is the removal of the breast tissue and lymph nodes under the arm, leaving the chest wall muscles intact (Figure 15.13B). See page 603 for the nursing care of a woman having a mastectomy.

Axillary node dissection is performed during surgery for all invasive breast carcinoma to stage the tumour. This surgery can cause **lymphoedema**, nerve damage and adhesions and, because of the role of the lymph nodes in immune system function, non-surgical methods of detecting lymph node involvement are being used. Sentinel node biopsy prior to a node dissection is conducted by injecting a radioactive substance or dye into the region of the tumour. The dye is carried to the first (sentinel) lymph node to receive lymph from the tumour and would be the node most likely to contain cancer cells if the cancer had metastasised. If the sentinel node is positive, more nodes are removed. If it is negative, further node evaluation is usually not indicated.

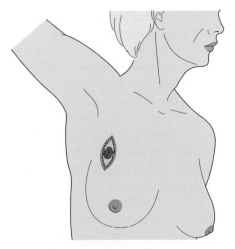

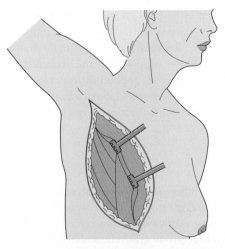

A Lumpectomy   **B** Modified radical mastectomy

Figure 15.13 Types of mastectomy. (A) In a lumpectomy, only the tumour and a small margin of surrounding tissue and removed. **(B)** In a modified radical mastectomy, all breast tissue and the underarm lymph nodes are removed, but the underlying muscles remain.

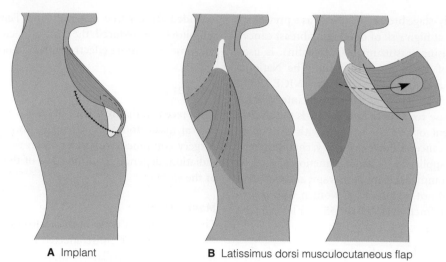

A Implant   **B** Latissimus dorsi musculocutaneous flap

Figure 15.14 Types of breast reconstruction surgeries. **(A)** A breast implant is inserted under the pectoris muscle. **(B)** Autogenous procedures transfer a flap of skin, muscle and fat from the donor site on the woman's body to the mastectomy site. The most frequently used donor muscle sites are the latissimus dorsi and the rectus abdominis (the TRAM flap).

Lumpectomy

Breast conservation surgery (*lumpectomy*) may be defined as excision of the primary tumour and adjacent breast tissue followed by radiation therapy. Many women are candidates for this procedure; however, women who have multicentric breast neoplasms and those who have large tumours in relation to their breast size are unsuitable candidates. Selection of women for this procedure is guided by the need for local control of the lesion, cosmetic results and personal preference.

Breast reconstruction

Post-mastectomy, some women choose to have their breast reconstructed. They report that surgical reconstruction of the breast simplifies their lives and restores a sense of body integrity. Others choose to use a removable breast prosthesis, and some are comfortable without reconstruction or a prosthesis.

Breast reconstruction may be performed during mastectomy or at any time thereafter, depending on preference. A number of procedures may be used for breast reconstruction (Figure 15.14), including placement of a submuscular implant, the use of a tissue expander followed by an implant, the transposition of muscle and blood supply from the abdomen or back, or using the transverse rectus abdominis myocutaneous (TRAM) free tissue flap. Nursing implications for the care of women undergoing breast reconstruction surgery are summarised in the box on page 603.

Radiation therapy

This is typically used following breast cancer surgery to destroy any remaining cancer cells that could cause recurrence or metastasis. If a tumour is unusually large, radiation may be used to shrink the tumour pre-operatively. Radiation therapy is most commonly used in combination with lumpectomy for early stage (I or II) breast cancer. Palliative radiation therapy is used to treat chest wall recurrences and some bone metastases,

helping control pain and prevent fractures. Radiation therapy is administered by means of an external-beam or tissue implants (see Chapter 2).

HEALTH EDUCATION FOR THE WOMAN AND FAMILY

+ Controversy exists about the health effects of silicone. There is no conclusive evidence that silicone implants induce cancer or autoimmune disease, but they are associated with hardening and pain due to contracture of the capsule around the implant. The implant may rupture, releasing silicone gel, or infection may occur. Saline-filled breast implants may be an alternative.

+ Some surgeons believe that delayed reconstruction offers better cosmetic results.

+ Reconstructive surgery can create a natural-looking breast that makes clothes fit better.

+ If a simple mastectomy is done, an implant approximately the same size as the other breast is placed under the pectoral muscle on the operative side, creating a breast mound closely resembling the natural breast.

+ With a simple mastectomy or modified radical mastectomy, a tissue expander may be used to replace the breast. The tissue expander is placed under the pectoral muscle and gradually expands with saline injections every two to three weeks to stretch the overlying skin and create a pocket.

+ With more extensive surgery such as radical mastectomy, a flap of skin, fat or muscle is transferred from a donor site to the operative area. A new nipple may be created by using tissue from the opposite nipple or from the inner thigh.

+ Reconstructive surgery may require multiple surgeries, including all the risks associated with anaesthesia. As the

NURSING CARE PLAN
The woman having a mastectomy and breast reconstruction

Review Chapter 1 for pre- and post-operative care.

Pre-operative care

+ Provide the woman with information in such a manner that she understands what the proposed procedure is, so she is able to give informed consent. A consent form will need to be signed.

Post-operative care

+ Deep-breathing exercises are important. After general anaesthesia, it is difficult for air to reach the lungs, particularly with restrictive surgical dressings that decrease chest expansion.

+ Suction apparatus will be placed in the wound to allow drainage of excess body fluids that accumulate when the lymph nodes are removed. This is usually removed three to five days post-operatively.

+ An IVI will be in place for fluid replacement and antibiotics to reduce the risk of post-operative infection.

+ Control pain by using the patient-controlled analgesia or requesting analgesics before pain becomes severe. Take analgesics before performing recommended exercises to facilitate full movement.

+ Note any signs of bleeding on the dressing or on the bedding.

+ Numbness or feelings of 'pins and needles' in the axillary area are common.

+ Lying on the back or on the side not operated on helps fluid drain from the site.

+ Moving the arm on the operated side helps regain mobility; specific exercises will be prescribed for increasing mobility after the incisions have healed.

+ If fluid builds up after the drains have been removed, it can be aspirated by the surgeon.

+ Use caution about lifting heavy objects with the arm on the operated side.

+ Be careful about injury and infection on the affected side; wear rubber gloves when washing dishes, garden gloves when working outside. Request that caregivers not perform blood pressures or venipunctures on the operative side to reduce the risk of injury and infection.

+ Feelings of anxiety, sadness and fear of looking at the incision are normal; mastectomy means abrupt change in body image.

+ Sexual intimacy can be affected by mastectomy; it often helps to be able to discuss potential sexual problems with the partner, a counsellor or with breast cancer support group.

---

complexity of the procedures increases, so does the risk of complications.

+ To decrease the risk of a fibrous capsule forming around the implant, it is important to perform breast massage as instructed.

Ground-breaking radiation treatment (*intraoperative radiotherapy*) is provided by a single, concentrated dose of radiation. Perioperatively, a probe is inserted into the cavity created by the lumpectomy and radiation equivalent to six weeks of doses is emitted for about 25 minutes. If successful, the treatment could make lumpectomy available to more women and prevent the woman from having six weeks of daily radiation treatments following surgery.

NURSING CARE FOR BREAST CANCER

Breast cancer is not one disease, but many, depending on the affected breast tissue, the tissue's oestrogen dependency, and the age of the person at onset. The psychosocial impact of breast cancer extends beyond the fear and threat of death. The diagnosis may transform the woman's sense of self and lead to reintegration or negotiation of family relationships.

Return to Case Study 3 at the beginning of this chapter. Consider this case in the light of your reading and think of ways in which you might offer support to Rachel.

Health promotion

When a woman reaches 20 years she should be undertaking breast self-examinations. Women should have a clinical breast exam by a healthcare professional (for example a practice nurse) every three years until the age of 40. It is recommended that women do a breast self-exam about a week after the first day of their period, when breasts are no longer swollen and tender due to hormonal fluctuations (Patient UK 2011).

Pre-menopausal women should perform BSE 7–10 days from the first day of their menstrual period, because hormonal changes increase breast tenderness and lumpiness prior to menses. Post-menopausal women should choose one date of the month (for example, the first day of the month) for BSE.

Educational messages about breast cancer screening need to be culturally sensitive to the intended audience. Media campaigns promoting mammography often show young white women, an approach that has proved ineffective among women from black, minority and ethnic groups.

TEST YOURSELF

1. What female structure is analogous to the penis?

   a. ovaries
   b. labia majora
   c. labia minora
   d. clitoris

2. The loss of oestrogen production following menopause may result in elevation of what potentially harmful substance that increases the risk of cardiovascular disease?

   a. uric acid
   b. glucose
   c. cholesterol
   d. testosterone

3. Cessation of menstruation in young women is a normal response to what biological event?

   a. implantation of an embryo
   b. onset of menopause
   c. onset of puberty
   d. beginning spermatogenesis

4. Which of the following diagnostic tests may be used to detect cervical cancer?

   a. colposcopy
   b. mammogram
   c. culture
   d. smear

5. What assessment technique is *primarily* used to determine abnormalities of the breast?

   a. inspection
   b. auscultation
   c. palpation
   d. percussion

6. At what anatomical location would you palpate Bartholin's glands?

   a. above the clitoris
   b. posterior to the labia majora
   c. inferior to the urinary meatus
   d. internal vaginal wall

7. During a health assessment at a local clinic, a woman in her 50s tells you that she is having pain with intercourse. You are uncomfortable discussing this topic with her. What would you say?

   a. 'I know this can be a problem; please discuss it with your doctor.'
   b. 'I don't know anything about that; please ask someone else.'
   c. 'Do you normally enjoy sexual activity?'
   d. 'What do you think is causing your problem?'

8. Long-term oestrogen deprivation results in an increased risk for physical disorders. What are these? (Select all that apply.)

   a. colon cancer
   b. osteoporosis
   c. cardiovascular disease
   d. fractures
   e. cervical cancer

9. You are conducting an educational seminar for post-menopausal women. When discussing calcium intake, you recommend _____ mg per day.

10. An intervention for the woman with a uterine displacement disorder is to teach pelvic floor exercises. These exercises may help reduce:

    a. stress incontinence
    b. menorrhagia
    c. vaginal discharge
    d. retroversion

Further resources

Bladder and Bowel Foundation (B&BF)
www.bladderandbowelfoundation.org
The UK's leading charity providing information and support for people with bladder and bowel disorders, their carers, families and healthcare professionals.

British Association for Counselling and Psychotherapy (BACP)
www.counselling.co.uk
Provides information about aspects of life where therapy can be helpful, and is designed to help assess whether therapy could be of use.

Cancer Research UK
www.cancerresearchuk.org
The world's leading independent organisation dedicated to cancer research, supporting research into all aspects of cancer.

Embarrassing Problems.com
www.embarrassingproblems.com
Independent advice concerning a wide range of embarrassing problems.

Endometriosis UK
www.endometriosis-uk.org
Offers services that enable those with endometriosis to understand their disease and to take control of their condition.

Infertility Network UK
www.infertilitynetworkuk.com
Committed to providing a comprehensive support network to its members and to all those affected by infertility by actively promoting Infertility Network UK services. Provides authoritative information and practical and emotional support, with the aim of raising the profile and understanding of infertility issues in all quarters and strives for timely and consistent provision of infertility care throughout the UK.

PCOS UK
www.pcos-uk.org.uk
This site is the healthcare professional section of Verity (see below), the polycystic ovaries self-help group, and works in

partnership with other organisations to improve the management of this very common and distressing condition.

The Samaritans
www.samaritans.org
Samaritans is a confidential emotional support service for anyone in the UK and Ireland. The service is available 24 hours a day for people who are experiencing feelings of distress or despair, including those which may lead to suicide.

Verity
www.verity-pcos.org.uk
A self-help group for women with polycystic ovary syndrome (PCOS). Established to share the truth about the condition and improve the lives of women living with PCOS.

Bibliography

Abernathy K (2005) Guiding women through menopause—the role of the nurse. *Nurse 2 Nurse*, **4**(11), 36–38, 40.

Albaugh J and Kellog-Spadt S (2003) Sexuality and sexual health: The nurse's role and initial approach to patients. *Urologic Nursing*, **23**(3), 227–228.

Andrist L, Hoyt A, Weinstein D and McGibbon C (2004) The need to bleed: Women's attitudes and beliefs about menstrual suppression. *Journal of the American Academy of Nurse Practitioners*, **16**(1), 31–37.

ARHP (2010) *Talking with Patients About Sexuality and Sexual Health*. Washington DC, Association of Reproductive Health Professionals, available at: http://www.arhp.org/publications-and-resources/clinical-fact-sheets/shf-talking (accessed September 2011).

Ausk K and Reed S (2004) Alternative approaches for treatment of uterine leiomyomas. *Alternative Therapies in Women's Health*, **6**(9), 65–70.

Ballantyne P (2004). Social context and outcomes for the ageing breast cancer patient: Considerations for clinical practitioners. *Journal of Clinical Nursing*, **13**(3a), 11–21.

Benedet J L, Bender H, Jones H, Ngan H Y and Percorelli S (2000) FIGO Staging classifications and clinical practice guidelines in the management of gynecologic cancers. FIGO Committee on Gynecologic Oncology. *International Journal of Gynaecology and Obstetrics*, **7**(2), 209–262.

Bradley P (2005) The delay and worry experience of African American women with breast cancer. *Oncology Nursing Forum*, **32**(2), 243–249.

Buxton-Blake P (2003) Recognizing menopausal symptomatology. *Home Health Care Management & Practice*, **15**(2), 147–151.

Cancer Research UK (2010a) *Cervical Cancer – UK incidence statistics*. London, available at: http://info.cancerresearchuk.org/cancerstats/types/cervix/incidence/?a=5441 (accessed September 2011).

Cancer Research UK (2010b) *Uterus (womb) Cancer – UK incidence statistics*. London, available at: http://info.cancerresearchuk.org/cancerstats/types/uterus/incidence/ (accessed September 2001).

Cancer Research UK (2010c) *Vulval Cancer – UK incidence statistics*. London, available at: http://info.cancerresearchuk.org/cancerstats/types/vulva/incidence/ (accessed September 2011).

Cancer Research UK (2011a) *Cervical Cancer Screening*. London, available at: http://www.cancerhelp.org.uk/help/default.asp?page=2756# (accessed September 2011).

Cancer Research UK (2011b) *Ovarian Cancer – UK incidence statistics*. London, available at: http://info.cancerresearchuk.org/cancerstats/types/ovary/incidence/ (accessed September 2011).

Cancer Research UK (2011c) *Breast Cancer – UK incidence statistics*. London, available at: http://info.cancerresearchuk.org/cancerstats/types/breast/incidence/ (accessed September 2011).

Cancer Research UK (2011d) *Definite Breast Cancer Risks*. London, available at: http://www.cancerhelp.org.uk/help/default.asp?page=3293 (accessed September 2011).

Castledine G and Close A (2007) *Oxford Handbook of General and Adult Nursing*. Oxford, Oxford University Press.

Coward D (2005) Lesson learned in developing a support intervention for African American women with breast cancer. *Oncology Nursing Forum*, **32**(2), 261–266.

Dibble S, Casey K, Nussey B, Israel J and Luce J (2004) Chemotherapy-induced vomiting in women treated for breast cancer. *Oncology Nursing Forum*, **31**(1), Online Exclusive: E1–E8.

Dickerson L, Mazyck P and Hunter M (2003) Premenstrual syndrome. *American Family Physician*, **67**(8), 1743–1752.

Donovan H and Ward S (2005) Representations of fatigue in women receiving chemotherapy for gynecologic cancers. *Oncology Nursing Forum*, **32**(1), 113–116.

Dougherty L and Lister (2009) *The Royal Mardsen Manual of Clinical Nursing Procedures*. (7th edn). Oxford, Wiley-Blackwell.

Eversley R, Estrin D, Dibble S, *et al.* (2005) Post-treatment symptoms among ethnic minority breast cancer survivors. *Oncology Nursing Forum*, **32**(2), 250–256.

Gorem (2004) Gynecologic cancer. *Current Opinions in Oncology*, **16**(5), 477–495.

Higgins C (2007) *Understanding Laboratory Investigations for Nurses and Health Professionals* (2nd end). Oxford, Blackwell.

Hughes C (2009) Cervical cancer: prevention, diagnosis, treatment and nursing care. *Nursing Standard*, **23**(7), 48–56.

Jennings-Sanders A and Anderson E (2003) Older women with breast cancer: Perceptions of the effectiveness of nurse case managers. *Nursing Outlook*, **51**(3), 108–114.

Kee J (2004) *Handbook of Laboratory and Diagnostic Tests with Nursing Implications* (5th edn). Upper Saddle River, NJ, Prentice Hall.

Kozier B, Erb G, Berman A, *et al.* (2008) *Fundamentals of Nursing. Concepts, Process and Practice*. Harlow, Pearson.

Lemaire G (2004) More than just menstrual cramps: Symptoms and uncertainty among women with endometriosis. *Journal of Obstetric, Gynecologic and Neonatal Nursing*, **33**(1), 71–79.

Lyons M and Shelton M (2004) Psychosocial impact of cancer in low-income rural/urban women: Phase II. *Online Journal of Rural Nursing and Health Care*, **4**(2).

Martin V (2005) Straight talk about ovarian cancer. *Nursing*, **35**(4), 36–41.

McCaffrey R and Youngkin E (2004) Sleep disturbances and remedies for perimenopausal and postmenopausal women. *Clinical Excellence for Nurse Practitioners*, **8**(4), 194–202.

McCook J, Reame N and Thatcher S (2005) Health-related quality of life issues in women with polycystic ovary syndrome. *Journal of Obstetric, Gynecologic, and Neonatal Nursing*, **34**(1), 12–20.

McPhee S, Papadakis M and Tierney L M (eds) (2007) *Current Medical Diagnosis & Treatment* (46th edn). Stamford, CT, Appleton & Lange.

Moorhead S, Johnson M and Maas M (2003) *Nursing Outcomes Classification (NOC)* (3rd edn). St Louis, MO, Mosby.

Muscari E (2004) Lymphedema: Responding to our patients' needs. *Oncology Nursing Forum*, **31**(5), 905–912.

NHSCSP (2008) *National Health Service Cervical Screening Programme. Annual Review 2008*. Sheffield, National Health Service Cervical Screening Programme.

NHS Choices (2011) *Uterine (Uterus) Cancer*. Available at: http://www.nhs.uk/conditions/cancer-of-the-uterus/Pages/Introduction.aspx, last accessed August 2011.

NICE (2006) *NICE Issues Final Guidance on Trastuzumab (Herceptin) for Early Breast Cancer*, Press release. London, National Institute for Health and Clinical Excellence.

Oakley E, Buchtel D, Atanosian R and Millar A (2004). Relationship of urinary incontinence to hysterectomy and episiotomy. *Journal of the Section on Women's Health*, **28**(3), 23–30.

O'Connell E (2005) Mood, energy, cognition, and physical complaints: A mind/body approach to symptom management during the climacteric. *Journal of Obstetric, Gynecologic, and Neonatal Nursing*, **34**(2), 274–279.

Patient UK (2011) *Breast Lumps and Breast Examination*. Available at: http://www.patient.co.uk/doctor/Breast-Lumps-and-Breast-Examination.htm, last accessed August 2011.

Porth C M (2009) *Pathophysiology: Concepts of altered health states* (9th edn.). Philadelphia, PA, Lippincott.

Stenchever M (2003) Diagnosing endometrial pathology in women with postmenopausal bleeding. *ACOG Clinical Review*, **8**(2), 10–11.

Wilson B, Shannon M and Stang C (2005) *Prentice Hall Nurse's Drug Guide 2005*. Upper Saddle River, NJ, Prentice Hall.

WHO (2006), *Comprehensive Cervical Cancer Control: A guide to essential practice*. Geneva, World Health Organization.

Yarbo C, Frogge M and Goodman M (2005) *Cancer Nursing: Principles and practice* (6th edn). Sudbury, MA, Jones & Bartlett.

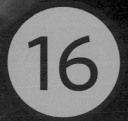

Caring for men with reproductive problems

Learning outcomes

- Describe the anatomy, physiology and functions of the male reproductive system.
- Identify specific topics for consideration during a health history.
- Describe normal variations in assessment findings.
- Identify manifestations of impairment in the male reproductive system, structure or function.
- Explain pathophysiological changes and nursing care.
- Discuss nursing implications and health education required.
- Describe various surgical procedures associated with the male reproductive system

Clinical competencies

- Conduct and document a health history.
- Conduct and document a physical assessment.
- Monitor the results of diagnostic tests and report abnormal findings.
- Assess functional health status of men and monitor, document and report abnormal signs and symptoms.
- Use evidence-based research to provide appropriate care.
- Implement individualised nursing interventions.

CASE STUDIES

Below are two case studies you may wish to consider before, during or after reading the chapter. There are no right or wrong answers, but you should consider the physical, psychological and social implications.

Case Study 1 – Zamir

Mr Zamir Khan, 17 years old, is very nervous, and withdrawn and comes to the general practice where you are working saying he has a pain 'down below'. He tells you he thinks one side of his 'middle part' seems bigger than the other and is aching. He is clearly anxious and acutely embarrassed and asks if there are any male nurses in the practice he could speak with.

Case Study 2 – William

Mr William Turner, a 71-year-old, lives with his wife in a small flat. As his wife had a stroke two years ago, he does all the cooking and housework. He has had good health most of his life, having only 'a small touch' of osteoarthritis in his knees and hands. He noticed a gradual onset of urinary urgency and frequency over the past two years, but has never had incontinence. During a routine checkup, the practice nurse performs a digital rectal examination and palpates a hard nodule on the surface of the prostate. His prostate specific antigen levels are elevated, he is referred to a urologist, who diagnoses prostate cancer. Mr Turner chooses to have surgery, and a radical retropubic prostatectomy and lymph node dissection are performed. Lymph nodes are negative for metastasis. He makes an uneventful recovery. The nurse caring for Mr Turner is concerned about his ability to care for his indwelling catheter because of his arthritis and his wife's physical disabilities. A referral to the district nursing services is made to ensure he can manage at home.

INTRODUCTION

The nurse is in a unique and privileged position to help men who may be experiencing problems. Often people are embarrassed about issues that are related to their reproductive health, for example, when being asked intimate questions and being intimately examined. Explaining things in a language the person understands and taking time to listen can help relieve embarrassment. Return to Case Study 1 at the beginning of the chapter and think of ways in which you might help Zamir feel more relaxed. What words might you choose to use in order to reduce anxiety and enhance the therapeutic relationship? Helping Zamir means you need to understand and empathise with his condition and how he is feeling. There may be moments of embarrassment for both you and for Zamir.

Being explicit about the male reproductive tract can help to save lives. An example of this occurred when a popular daytime television programme in 1999 called the Richard and Judy show, a programme known for approaching controversial issues in innovative ways, addressed the issue of testicular self-examination. The programme aired, live, a man who allowed his testicles to be examined with the aim of publicising the dangers of testicular cancer. This programme pioneered the move towards encouraging frank and open discussion about men's health,

The male reproductive tract

The male reproductive organs, along with the neuroendocrine system, produce hormones that are essential in biological development and sexual behaviour. These organs also encompass and are important to the function of the urinary system. The assessment of the male reproductive and urinary systems can be difficult for both the nurse and the man and calls for sensitivity and understanding on the part of the nurse when discussing intimate issues. Skill is needed when performing physical examinations of a part of the body that is often regarded as private.

Men can experience disorders of the penis, scrotum and testes, prostate gland and breast. These disorders may be inflammatory, structural, benign or malignant. Young men are at increased risk for testicular cancer; as men age conditions of the prostate gland become common. Many of the disorders pose significant risk to the man's fertility, sexual and urinary function; some are life-threatening. This chapter discusses disorders of the male reproductive system, including disorders of sexual expression, for example, **erectile dysfunction**, and the male breast. Treatments and disorders of the male reproductive system have the potential to affect erection and ejaculation.

ANATOMY, PHYSIOLOGY AND FUNCTIONS OF THE MALE REPRODUCTIVE SYSTEM

The male reproductive system consists of the testes, the scrotum, ducts, glands and penis (see Figure 16.1). The breasts are classified as a part of the male reproductive system. The location and functions of the male reproductive organs are summarised in Table 16.1.

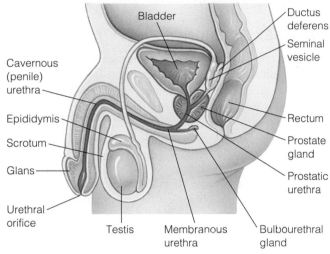

Figure 16.1 The male reproductive system.

THE BREASTS

The male breast comprises primarily an areola (circular pigmented area) and a small nipple, lying over a thin disc of undeveloped breast tissue that may not be overtly different from surrounding tissue. Approximately one in three men have a firm area of breast tissue 2 cm or larger; normal size of this area has not been established (Bickley *et al.* 2009).

THE PENIS

The penis encloses the urethra and is homologous to the clitoris. The penis is composed of a shaft and a tip – the glans – which is covered in uncircumcised men by the foreskin (or prepuce). The shaft contains three columns of erectile tissue: the lateral columns are called the corpora cavernosa and the central mass is called the corpus spongiosum.

Erection occurs when the penile masses become filled with blood in response to a reflex, triggering the parasympathetic nervous system to stimulate arteriolar vasodilation. The erection reflex may be initiated by touch, pressure, sights, sounds, smells or thoughts of a sexual encounter. After ejaculation, the arterioles vasoconstrict and the penis becomes flaccid.

Table 16.1 Location and function of the male reproductive organs

Organ	Location	Function
Penis	Attached to front and sides of the pubic arch, directly continuous with the scrotum.	• Excretes **semen** and urine. Deposits sperm in the female reproductive tract. An organ of pleasure.
Scrotum	Hangs from the body at root of penis.	• Contains testes, epididymis and portions of the vas (ductus) deferens.
Testes	In the scrotal sac.	• Produce sperm and testosterone.
Epididymis	Behind and to the sides to upper aspect of each testicle.	• Stores sperm. • Promotes sperm maturation. • Transports sperm to vas deferens.
Vas deferens (ductus deferens)	Between the epididymis and the seminal vesicle forming the ejaculatory duct.	• Stores sperm. • Transports sperm.
Urethra	Begins at bladder, passes through prostate and penis.	• Serves as passageway for urine or semen.
Prostate gland	Encircles the urethra at the neck of the bladder.	• Contributes to ejaculatory volume. • Enhances sperm motility and fertility.
Seminal vesicles	Lie on posterior bladder wall.	• Contribute to ejaculatory volume. • Contain nutrients to sustain sperm and prostaglandins to facilitate sperm motility.
Bulbourethral (Cowper's) glands	Inferior to the prostate.	• Secrete mucus into urethra. • Neutralise traces of acidic urine in the urethra.

THE SCROTUM

The scrotum is a sac made of two layers. The outer layer is continuous with the skin of the perineum and thighs. The inner layer is made of muscle and fascia (a type of tissue that provides support). The scrotum hangs at the base of the penis, anterior to the anus, regulating the temperature of the testes. The optimum temperature for sperm production is about two to three degrees below body temperature. When the testicular temperature is too low, the scrotum contracts to bring the testes up against the body; when it is too high, the scrotum relaxes allowing the testes to lie further away from the body.

THE TESTES

The testes develop in the abdominal cavity of the foetus, descending through the inguinal canal into the scrotum (akin to the ovaries). They are about 4 cm long and 2.5 cm in diameter, suspended in the scrotum by the spermatic cord and surrounded by two coverings: an outer tunica vaginalis and an inner tunica albuginea. Each is divided into 250–300 lobules (a collection of small lobes), with each lobule containing one to four seminiferous tubules (types of small tubes). They produce sperm and testosterone.

The seminiferous tubules are responsible for sperm production. Leydig's cells (or interstitial cells) lie in the connective tissue surrounding the seminiferous tubules producing testosterone.

THE DUCTS AND SEMEN

The seminiferous tubules (tubes within the testes) lead into the ducts becoming the rete testis; here, thousands of ducts join the epididymis, a long tube that lies over the outer surface of each testicle. The epididymis stores and matures sperm. The epididymis contracts to propel the sperm through the vas deferens where the sperm are stored until ejaculation.

The seminal vesicles produce about 60% of the volume of seminal fluid, but seminal fluid is also made of secretions from the accessory sex organs, the epididymis, the prostate gland and Cowper's glands. Seminal fluid increases sperm alkalinity (an alkaline pH is essential to mobilise the sperm and ensure fertilisation of the ova). Sperm mixed with this fluid is semen. Each seminal vesicle joins the vas deferens to form an ejaculatory duct, which enters the prostatic urethra. During ejaculation, seminal fluid mixes with sperm at the ejaculatory duct and enters the urethra for expulsion.

The total amount of semen ejaculated is 2–4 mL. The total ejaculate of a healthy male contains from 100–400 million sperm.

THE PROSTATE GLAND

The prostate gland is about the size of a walnut encircling the urethra below the urinary bladder (see Figure 16.1). It is made of 20–30 tubuloalveolar glands surrounded by smooth muscle. Prostate gland secretions make up about one-third the volume of semen, entering the urethra through ducts during ejaculation.

SPERMATOGENESIS

Spermatogenesis is related to the formation and development of spermatazoa. This begins with puberty, continuing throughout life, with several hundred million sperm produced daily.

The inner layer of the seminiferous tubules consists of sustentacular cells (or Sertoli's cells), containing spermatocytes (the male germ cell) and sperm in different stages of development. Sertoli's cells secrete a nourishing fluid for the developing sperm, and enzymes help to convert spermatocytes to sperm. Spermatogenesis takes approximately 64–72 days.

MALE SEX HORMONES

These are called **androgens**. Most androgens are produced in the testes, although the adrenal cortex (situated in the adrenal gland) also produces a small amount. Testosterone, the primary androgen, is essential for the development and maintenance of sexual organs and secondary sex characteristics, and for spermatogenesis. It also promotes metabolism, growth of muscles and bone and **libido** (sexual desire).

Now that we have covered the male reproductive system from an anatomical and physiological perspective, the next section outlines methods of assessing the person.

Assessing the male reproductive system

When working in a variety of clinical situations you will be required to assess the needs of the male in order to make a diagnosis, plan care and evaluate interventions. Assessment is associated with the findings from diagnostic tests, a health interview to collect subjective data and a physical assessment to collect objective data.

DIAGNOSTIC TESTS

Understanding these tests will help you to help the person you are caring for in a safer and effective manner. The results of diagnostic tests are used to:

● support a diagnosis;
● provide information to identify or modify treatments;
● help monitor responses to treatment and nursing care interventions.

Diagnostic tests include:

● *Prostate specific antigen (PSA).* A blood test used to diagnose prostate cancer and to monitor treatment of prostate cancer. PSA normal value: less than 4 ng/mL.
● *Prostate ultrasound.* Conducted to identify **testicular torsion** (a teste twists in the scrotum) or masses (for example, cancer), and to evaluate prostate enlargement. A full bladder may be required for the study.

- *Prostate biopsy* (transrectal or transurethral biopsy). Conducted to diagnose prostate cancer. The man should avoid strenuous activity four hours post-procedure. Explain that there may be some discomfort in the area for one to two days, there may be some blood in the urine or from the rectum, semen may appear dark. Following a transurethral biopsy, a urinary catheter may remain for a few hours, and antibiotics will be prescribed. Excess bleeding, pain or signs of infection should be reported to the doctor.
- *Semen analysis*. Performed to assess volume, motility and sperm count, and per cent of abnormal sperm. Normal values of sperm produced, volume: 2–4 mL, sperm count: more than 20 million/mL. A fresh specimen is required within two hours of ejaculation.

The nurse is responsible for explaining the procedure and any special preparation needed, assessing for any medication use that might affect test outcomes, for supporting the man during the examination, for documenting the procedures and for monitoring the results of the tests.

IN PRACTICE

Semen analysis

Two semen specimens are required, and are best collected for immediate assessment in laboratories linked within fertility services (Hirsh 2003). Semen should be collected after 48–72 hours of abstinence from sexual intercourse (and masturbation). The specimen must be kept at body temperature and analysed within one hour of collection. Lubricants should be used only if essential and if required, only small amounts. Some lubricants are spermatotoxic and must be avoided. The most advantageous condition would be to use no lubricant; encourage the man to spend some time during foreplay increasing sexual arousal and natural lubricant.

The semen specimens are produced by masturbation; some men may have difficulty with masturbation or have religious objections. If condoms are used to collect semen avoid using condoms and lubricants that are spermatotoxic.

GENETIC CONSIDERATIONS

During assessment it is important to consider genetic influences on a person's health. Several diseases of the male reproductive system have a genetic component. It is especially important to ask about a family history of testicular or prostate cancer. During physical assessment, assess for any manifestations that might indicate a genetic disorder. If appropriate ask about genetic testing and refer for genetic counselling and evaluation.

Understanding issues concerning genetics and the male reproductive system will help you ask the right questions, developing an awareness of the interplay between genetics and health and illness:

- The exact genetic predisposition for some men to have prostate cancer is unknown, findings have identified a family history as a major risk factor.
- A family history of testicular cancer is a risk factor for testicular cancer.
- Men who have XX chromosomes (instead of XY) often have altered testicular development.

When carrying out the interview:

- Ask about health problems, analyse onset, characteristics and course, severity, precipitating and relieving factors, and any associated symptoms, noting timing and circumstances. You may ask:
  - When did you first notice you were having difficulty urinating?
  - Did you use a different brand of condom before you noticed the rash on your penis?
  - Describe the changes that occurred in your ability to have an erection after taking medicine for high blood pressure.
- Ask about chronic illnesses such as diabetes, chronic renal failure, cardiovascular disease, multiple sclerosis, trauma, thyroid disease. These illnesses and their treatment may cause erectile dysfunction (inability to achieve or maintain an erection).
- The following may cause sexual function problems: antihypertensives, antidepressants, antispasmodics, tranquillisers, sedatives and histamine₂-receptor antagonists.
- Psychosocial stressors such as depression can contribute to erectile dysfunction.
- If the man had mumps as a child, sterility is possible.
- The risk for testicular cancer is greatest in those who have a history of undescended teste, inguinal hernia, testicular swelling with mumps, a family history of testicular cancer.
- Explore lifestyle and social history; the use of alcohol, cigarettes or street drugs may affect sexual function.
- Frequent sexual intercourse, especially if unprotected, increases risk for sexually transmitted infections.
- Ask about sexual preference. Sexual intercourse with same-sex partners increases risk for HIV infection.
- Other questions about sexuality may include number of sexual partners; history of premature ejaculation, erectile dysfunction or other sexual problems; history of sexual trauma; use of condoms or other contraceptives; current level of sexual satisfaction.

HEALTH ASSESSMENT INTERVIEW

This may be conducted during a health screening, and it may focus on a chief complaint (i.e. discharge from the penis) or be part of a total health assessment. Men may be embarrassed to discuss concerns involving their reproductive organs; questions should be asked in a non-threatening, matter-of-fact manner. Consider the psychological, social and cultural factors that affect sexuality and sexual activity. Use words that the man can understand; do not be embarrassed or offended by the words used. Start the interview using less threatening questions, more general questions and then progress to specific questions, giving the man permission to describe behaviours and manifestations. Rather than asking if he has difficulty achieving or maintaining an erection, ask him to describe any changes he has noticed in his erections. Consider a number of other factors, for example, genetics and disorders associated with these and the impact they may have.

To help you structure the assessment process a number of interview questions categorised by functional health patterns are listed in the Functional Health Pattern Interview. You should observe other healthcare professionals you work with noting how they conduct a health interview with men.

FUNCTIONAL HEALTH PATTERN INTERVIEW The male reproductive system

Functional health pattern	Interview questions and leading statements
Health perception–health management	• Have you ever had problems with your reproductive organs (penis, testicles, prostate gland)? Explain. How was the problem treated? • Have you ever had surgery on your reproductive organs? What type, when and what was the outcome? • Have you ever noticed any pain or swelling in your breasts? Explain. • Do you practise testicular self-examination? How often? • Do you smoke? How much and for how long?
Nutritional–metabolic	• Describe your usual daily intake of food and fluids.
Elimination	• Do you now or have you ever had a discharge from your penis? Describe the colour, odour, consistency, amount and frequency. • Have you ever had any bleeding from your penis? Explain. • Have you noticed changes in your urination, like burning, frequency, urgency, difficulty starting the stream, size of the stream, dribbling or getting up frequently at night? Explain.
Activity–exercise	• Describe your usual activity in a 24-hour period. • Do you participate in sports or heavy lifting? If so, do you wear a protective cup or athletic support?
Sleep–rest	• Describe the quality of your rest and sleep.
Cognitive–perceptual	• Describe any pain you have had in the groin area, testicles, penis or scrotum. Where is it? Do you experience it in other parts of your body? How long does it last? What makes it worse or relieves it? • Has there been a change in the condition or colour of the skin on your scrotum or penis? Explain.
Self-perception–self-concept	• Has this problem affected how you feel about yourself? • Are your needs for intimacy and affection being met?
Role–relationships	• Has this condition affected your relationships with others? • Has this condition interfered with your ability to work? Explain. • Has anyone in your family had problems with prostate cancer? Explain.
Sexuality–reproductive	• Are you currently in a sexual relationship? Has this condition interfered with your usual sexual activity? • How long have you been with your current partner? • Have you had any other partners during this time? • What is your sexual preference? • Has this problem affected your relationship with your spouse or sexual partner? • Are you satisfied with your current level of sexual functioning? • Have you ever had any problem with achieving or maintaining an erection or ejaculation? • Do you use any medications to facilitate your sexual ability? Describe. • Do you use condoms?

FUNCTIONAL HEALTH PATTERN INTERVIEW The male reproductive system (continued)

Functional health pattern	Interview questions and leading statements
Coping–stress–tolerance	• Has this condition created stress for you? If so, does your health problem seem to be more difficult when you are stressed? • Have you experienced any kind of stress that makes the condition worse? Explain. • Describe what you do when you feel stressed.
Value–belief	• Describe how specific relationships or activities help you cope with this problem. • Describe specific cultural beliefs or practices that affect how you care for and feel about this problem. • Are there any specific treatments that you would not use to treat this problem?

The health pattern interview questions are presented in list format. Use this only as a guide and tailor the questions you ask.

Now you are feeling more confident with questions and questioning the next step is the physical examination. When carrying out the examination you need to engender an atmosphere of warmth and professionalism helping the man relax.

PHYSICAL ASSESSMENT

Physical assessment may be performed as part of a total assessment or separately for men with known or suspected problems. If part of a total physical assessment, this is usually the final system to be assessed. Problems of the male reproductive system may involve the urinary system, so assessment of both systems is important. If either the nurse or the man is not comfortable, a nurse of the same gender should be asked to conduct the assessment. Normal age-related findings for the older man are summarised in Table 16.2 and assessments of the male reproductive system are given on page 618.

Equipment needed to undertake a physical assessment includes:

● disposable gloves;

● water-soluble lubricant;

● a good light source;

● sterile cotton swabs (for specimen acquisition);

● culture media (a special product to fix specimens).

Assessment is made by inspection and palpation (to touch or feel). A chaperone may be present during the assessment, and the nurse must adhere to local policy and procedure. Explain the procedures for the examination in a matter-of-fact way to decrease anxiety and embarrassment. If the man is unfamiliar with his internal genitalia, charts may be used to demonstrate the parts that will be examined. Ask the man to empty his bladder (to promote comfort); he should remove his clothing and put on a gown or drape. The assessment may be done with the man sitting or standing. Expose only those body parts being examined, preserving modesty. Ensure that

Table 16.2 Age-related changes in the male reproductive system

Age-related change	Significance
Prostate gland: • A number of older men have some degree of **benign prostatic hyperplasia** (this is a prostate condition).	Although ageing does not cause prostate cancer, incidence increases with age.
Penis, testes and scrotum: • Epithelial tissue and mucosa (a type of mucous membrane) of seminal vesicles are thinner with reduced capacity to hold fluid. • Hardening of penile arteries and veins may occur.	Although men may father children throughout life, the sperm count is reduced in some men. Changes in the vascular system of the penis may mean the ageing man takes longer to achieve an erection and ejaculation, or may be impotent.

the examining room is warm and private. Put on gloves before beginning and wear them throughout the examination. In Case Study 1 do you think there may be any value in using charts to help Zamir? What would you need to do to ensure his anxiety levels are reduced? How might you manage the situation if a male chaperone is not present?

The assessment of the male reproductive system is complex and the nurse needs to understand the key issues involved in order to provide safe and effective care.

> **Consider this . . .**
>
> If during the physical examination of the person's genitalia he becomes erect, he is very embarrassed – how will you manage this situation? Go back to Case Study 1 and how this situation could impact on your professional relationship with Zamir.

MALE REPRODUCTIVE SYSTEM ASSESSMENT

Technique/Normal findings	Abnormal findings
Breast and lymph node assessment	
Inspect and palpate breasts, including areola and nipple. *Breast tissue should not be swollen, tender or enlarged.*	• A smooth, firm, mobile, tender disc of breast tissue behind the areola indicates **gynaecomastia**, abnormal enlargement of the breast(s) in men. Gynaecomastia requires additional investigation to determine cause. • A hard, irregular nodule in the nipple area suggests carcinoma (a cancer).
Palpate the lymph nodes under the arms and around the neck. *The nurse should not be able to feel any signs of enlarged lymph nodes.*	• Enlarged axillary nodes are common with infections of the hand or arm but may be caused by cancer. • Enlarged supraclavicular nodes may indicate spreading of cancer (if cancer is present).
External genitalia assessment	
Inspect and palpate the inguinal and femoral area for bulges (located in the groin). Ask the man to bear down or cough as you palpate. *There should be no bulging with coughing or bearing down.*	• A bulge that increases with coughing or straining suggests a hernia.
Inspect the penis. If the man is uncircumcised, retract the foreskin or ask him to do so. *When non-erect, the penis is soft, flaccid and non-tender. The foreskin should be without lesions, of colour equal with the penis, and retract easily. The glans is normally free of lesions.*	• **Phimosis** (tightness of prepuce that prevents retraction of foreskin) may be congenital or due to recurrent balanoposthitis (generalised infection of glans penis and prepuce). • Narrow or inflamed foreskin can cause paraphimosis, retraction of the foreskin that causes painful swelling of the glans. • Balanitis (inflammation of the glans) is associated with infection. • Ulcers, vesicles (a small skin-covered bubble of liquid) or warts suggest a sexually transmitted infection. • Nodules or sores in uncircumcised men may be cancer.
Inspect the external urinary meatus. This will include the glans, penis and the urethral opening. Press the glans between the thumb and forefinger. Replace the foreskin if appropriate. *This is normally in the centre of the glans, without redness or discharge.*	• Erythema (redness) or discharge indicates inflammatory disease. Further assessment is required.
Inspect the skin on the shaft of the penis. *This should be free of redness or lesions.*	• Excoriation (an abrasion or break in the skin) or inflammation suggests lice or scabies.
Palpate the shaft of the penis. *This should not be tender.*	• Induration with tenderness along the ventral surface (towards the front) suggests urethral stricture (narrowing of the urethra) with inflammation.

MALE REPRODUCTIVE SYSTEM ASSESSMENT (continued)

Technique/Normal findings	Abnormal findings
Inspect the scrotum. Further assess any swelling in the scrotum using transillumination: darken the room and place a lighted torch against the skin of the scrotum. *The normal scrotum and epididymis appear as dark masses with regular borders.*	• A unilateral or bilateral poorly developed scrotum suggests cryptorchidism (failure of one or both testes to descend into the scrotum). • Swelling of the scrotum may indicate indirect inguinal hernia, **hydrocele** (accumulation of fluid in the scrotum) or scrotal oedema (swelling). Swellings containing serous fluid will transilluminate. Swellings containing blood or tissue will not transilluminate, that is when a beam of light from a torch is passed through the scrotum the swelling prevents the light shining completely through.
Palpate each testicle and epididymis. *They should not be tender or swollen.*	• Tender, painful scrotal swelling occurs in acute **epididymitis** (inflammation of epididymis), acute **orchitis** (inflammation of the teste), torsion of the spermatic cord and strangulated hernia. • A painless nodule in the testicle is associated with testicular cancer.

Prostate assessment

The prostate gland is assessed by digital rectal examination (DRE).

With a gloved index finger, palpate the posterior rectal wall for the rounded, two-lobed structure of the posterior prostate. *This is normally non-tender, with two lateral lobes that are divided, smooth and about 2.5 cm long.*	• Enlargement (1 cm protrusion into the rectum) with obliteration of the middle aspect of the prostate gland suggest benign prostatic hypertrophy. • Enlargement, asymmetry and tenderness suggest **prostatitis** (inflammation of the prostate gland). • A hard irregular nodule is suspicious of cancer.

Having outlined assessment techniques, the various disorders that may be revealed during assessment will be discussed below.

The man with erectile dysfunction (ED)

Erectile dysfunction (ED) is the inability of the male to attain and maintain an erection sufficient to permit satisfactory sexual intercourse. Impotence which is often used synonymously with erectile dysfunction, may involve a total inability to achieve erection, an inconsistent ability to achieve erection or the ability to sustain only brief erections. Erectile dysfunction has many possible causes (Table 16.3), and may or may not be associated with a loss of libido (sexual desire).

ED can impact on an individual's health and wellbeing. The incidence of ED is difficult to estimate, and many affected men may not report the disorder. This equates to about 26 new cases annually per 1000 men (European Association of Urology 2005). The incidence increases with age. Most problems with erection are the result of a disease, injury or chemical substance (such as prescribed medications, alcohol, nicotine, cocaine or marijuana) that decreases blood flow (European Association of Urology 2005). Because this is a problem primarily of ageing men, the discussion of pathophysiology focuses on this age group. Table 16.3 provides an overview of the pathological and iatrogenic causes.

Pathophysiology of erectile function

Age-related changes involve cellular and tissue changes in the penis, decreased sensory activity, hypogonadism (associated with a deficiency of the hormone testosterone) and the effects of chronic illness. In the penis, a change from elastic collagen to a more rigid collagen causes decreased distensibility (a less rigid erection). This then interferes with the veno-occlusive mechanism, preventing blood from 'leaking' out of the penis into the general vasculature prematurely. Problems with this mechanism result in incomplete erections. Vibrotactile (stimulation of the skin) sensation over the skin of the penis declines with age; this may explain why some older men require longer stimulation to achieve an erection. Hypogonadism results in decreased testosterone levels. There may be a relationship between lower androgen levels (this can result in hair loss and lowered libido) and erectile function.

Many illnesses affect erectile function. Damage to arteries, smooth muscles and fibrous tissues are the most common. Diabetes, kidney disease, chronic alcoholism, atherosclerosis (hardening and narrowing of the arteries) and vascular disease are responsible for organic ED. Innervation and blood flow to the penis may be damaged during surgery. Given the effects of ageing on the blood flow within the penis, the increased incidence

Table 16.3 Causes of erectile dysfunction

Major pathological causes		Major iatrogenic causes	
Neurological	*Arterial*	*Medications*	*Procedures and infections*
Spinal cord injury	Atherosclerosis	*Antihypertensives*	*Surgery*
Stroke	Hypertension	Hydrochlorothiazide	Coronary artery bypass
Parkinson's disease	Aortic aneurysm	Spironolactone	Pelvic lymphadenectomy
Multiple sclerosis	Sickle cell anaemia	Methyldopa	Radical prostatectomy
		Clonidine	Radical cystectomy
Endocrinological	*Mechanical*	Prazosin	Abdominal perineal resection
Diabetes mellitus	Decreased penile distensibility	Propranolol	Sympathectomy
Hypogonadism	Congenital disorders	Reserpine	Aortic aneurysm repair
Hypothyroidism	Morbid obesity		Transplant surgeries
	Hydrocele	*Psychotropic agents*	
Inflammatory	Hip or pelvic fractures	Phenothiazines	*Other*
Prostatitis		Butyrophenones	Severe nosocomial infection
Cystitis	*Psychological*	Tricyclic antidepressants	Radiation therapy to pelvis
	Depression	MAO inhibitors	
Activity intolerance	Stress	Diazepam	
Pulmonary problems	Fatigue	Chlorodiazepoxide	
Anaemias	Fear of failure		
Myocardial infarction		*Endocrinologic agents*	
Congestive heart failure	*Compulsive food disorders*	LHRH agonists	
Hepatic diseases	Compulsive overeating	Oestrogen compounds	
Renal failure	Anorexia nervosa	Progesterone	
	Bulimia		
Substance dependency		*Other*	
Alcohol		Antiparkinsonian agents	
Marijuana		Anticholinergic agents	
Narcotics		Immunosuppressive agents	
Sedatives		Antihistamines	
Tobacco			

of chronic illness and the multiple medications and treatments required to manage those illnesses, it is not surprising that many older men have problems with ED. Effective care means that nurse may need to work with a variety of healthcare professionals in a variety of settings.

INTERDISCIPLINARY CARE FOR ED

The aim is to ensure that the man (and their partner) receives care that is appropriate and effective; understanding what this care incorporates will help the nurse help the person being cared for. The care of men with ED is growing in importance; because the population as a whole is ageing, so incidence is increasing proportionately. Moreover, there is more willingness of men and their partners to discuss sexual concerns. Although sexuality may still be seen by some as a very sensitive and private area, the growing knowledge and help available is causing men to seek answers. The loss of erectile function is not an inevitable part of ageing.

Integrated care pathways and ED

An integrated care pathway (ICP) (also known as care protocol, care pathway, multidisciplinary pathway of care) may be devised for the care of the man with ED, specifying essential steps in the care of the person, illustrating the person's expected

progress. The multidisciplinary team includes the practice nurse, GP, physiotherapist and psychosexual counsellor. The use of uniprofessional care plans (care provided by one professional group only) is unacceptable. Integrated care pathways are able to form all or part of the patient's clinical record, they allow the evaluation of outcomes, and they can be used as a quality improvement tool with respect to clinical governance.

Diagnosis

Diagnostic tests that may be ordered include:

- blood studies;
- penile monitoring;
- penile blood flow.

Blood chemistry, testosterone, prolactin, thyroxine and PSA levels are measured, identifying metabolic and endocrine problems that may cause the dysfunction. Nocturnal penile tumescence (swelling) and rigidity (NPTR) monitoring helps differentiate between psychogenic and organic causes. Tests can be performed in a sleep laboratory, although home testing is an alternative. The number and quality of erections occurring during REM sleep can be determined. Cavernosometry and cavernosography are investigations used to measure pressure and to outline radiographically if there are any problems within the chambers of the penis. The aim is to evaluate arterial inflow and venous outflow of blood in the penis.

Medication

ED can be treated with medications taken orally, injected directly into the penis or inserted into the urethra at the tip of the penis:

- *Oral medications.* These include sildenafil citrate (Viagra), vardenafil hydrochloride (Levitra) or tadalafil (Cialis). Viagra and Levitra, taken an hour before sexual activity, enhance the effects of nitric oxide, facilitating relaxation of the smooth muscle in the penis during sexual stimulation, increasing blood flow. Both drugs should be taken no more than once a day, and should not be taken by men who are prescribed nitrate-based drugs (for health problems) or alpha-blockers (used to treat hypertension and prostate enlargement). Cialis is a selective phosphodiesterase type 5 inhibitor allowing smooth muscle relaxation to facilitate inflow of blood into the penis, lasting for 36 hours. Erection only occurs with sexual stimulation. Cialis should not be taken if the man is also taking nitrates, alpha-blockers, erythromycin or rifampicin (antibiotics), ketoconazole or itraconazole (antifungals), or protease inhibitors (for HIV).

- *Injectable medications.* Hormone replacement therapy with testosterone injections (200 mg IM every three weeks) or topical patches may be used for documented androgen (a hormone) deficiency and for those who do not have prostate cancer. Injectable medications, including papaverine and prostaglandin E injections, may be used. Injected directly into the penis, papaverine relaxes the arterioles and smooth muscles of the cavernosum (these are columns of erectile tissue in the penis), inducing tumescence (swelling). Erection usually lasts from 30 minutes to four hours. Prostaglandin E functions much as papaverine does, but has fewer side-effects. Mode of delivery can be problematic. There is a high attrition rate, and people report

dissatisfaction with lack of spontaneity, loss of interest in sex, physical limitations and, occasionally, pain. Alprostadil (Caverject), another injectable medication, can be used to treat ED.

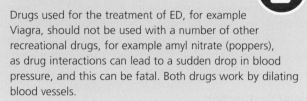

PRACTICE ALERT

Drugs used for the treatment of ED, for example Viagra, should not be used with a number of other recreational drugs, for example amyl nitrate (poppers), as drug interactions can lead to a sudden drop in blood pressure, and this can be fatal. Both drugs work by dilating blood vessels.

Mechanical devices

A frequently prescribed mechanical device for ED is the vacuum constriction device (VCD). This draws blood into the penis with a vacuum, trapping it there with a constricting band at the base of the penis. After the device is removed, a single small band, often called an O-ring, is left at the base of the penis to maintain the erection. If erection can be attained but not maintained, an O-ring alone can be used.

Surgery

Surgical treatment for ED involves either revascularisation procedures (these are procedures that require reconstruction of arteries and/or veins) or implantation of prosthetic devices. Venous or arterial procedures are generally not successful. The result is often temporary, because the underlying cause of the vascular insufficiency is usually not corrected. Implantation of penile prostheses is now common (Figure 16.2). Men are generally satisfied with their prostheses, and they rank the inflatable type highest. Nursing care can be complex and must respond to the individual needs of the man. This will now be outlined.

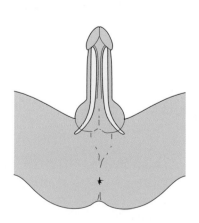
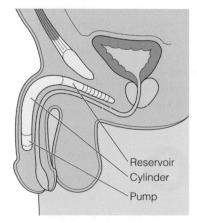
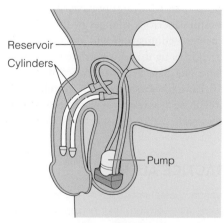

A Semi-rigid   **B** Self-contained   **C** Inflatable

Figure 16.2 Types of penile implants.

NURSING CARE FOR ED

ED can be encountered in any healthcare setting. Through routine examinations or careful assessment of people, their conditions and treatments that may incidentally cause ED can be identified.

Nursing diagnoses and interventions

Assessing a person's health history may reveal ED. Once a problem is known, information and emotional support are given and referral made. There are many possible nursing diagnoses, and this section focuses on nursing care related to sexual dysfunction and self-esteem.

Sexual dysfunction

Those who lose erectile function may not be aware of the cause. The cause may be blamed on unrelated factors, such as age, medications, illness or sexual partner. Not knowing the cause leads to anxiety. The nurse should be aware of the following:

✚ Assess for risk factors for ED. Be especially alert to men who have recently begun medications or had recent surgeries that could cause ED.

✚ Assess for sexual dysfunction. Men have shown increasing willingness to discuss sexual concerns. Be aware of the physiological effects of disease and side-effects of treatment.

✚ Perform a detailed assessment of sexual practices.

✚ Discuss previous methods of coping with ED.

✚ Provide information about treatment options.

Risk for situational low self-esteem

The man with ED often believes himself to be 'less than a man'. A penile prosthesis may result in disturbances in body and you should aim to:

✚ Collect data during the health history, in a non-judgemental manner.

✚ If the man has had a penile implant, teach him and his partner how to use this. Suggest wearing snug-fitting underwear with the penis placed in an upright position on the abdomen and loose trousers.

Having considered the issue of erectile dysfunction, we will now move on to consider disorders of the penis.

DISORDERS OF THE PENIS

The man with phimosis or priapism

Although uncommon, these disorders can cause problems with urination and sexual activity. In some cases, they are considered a medical emergency, because decreased blood flow to the penis may result in tissue ischaemia (reduced blood supply) and necrosis (death of tissue).

Pathophysiology of phimosis and priapism

Phimosis is constriction of the foreskin so that it cannot be retracted over the glans penis. Phimosis may be congenital, or related to chronic infections under the foreskin, leading to adhesions. This condition prevents adequate hygiene, leading to harmful cancerous changes of the penis and can interfere with urinary elimination and intercourse. In paraphimosis, the foreskin is tight and constricted, and is not able to cover the glans. The glans becomes engorged and oedematous and is painful. Paraphimosis may result from long-term retraction of the foreskin, such as occurs in placement of an indwelling urinary catheter (Porth 2009). This can result in ischaemia of the glans.

Priapism is an involuntary, sustained, painful erection not associated with sexual arousal. The prolonged erection may result in erectile dysfunction (Porth 2009). The disorder is either primary or secondary. Primary priapism results from conditions such as tumours, infection or trauma. Secondary priapism is caused by blood disorders (e.g., leukaemia and sickle cell anaemia), neurological disorders (e.g., spinal cord injury or stroke), renal failure and some medications.

FAST FACTS

Illnesses and drugs that may cause priapism

Illnesses/conditions:
● Sickle cell disease
● Leukaemia
● Metastatic cancer
● Spinal cord trauma

Drugs:
● Papaverine
● Psychotropic drugs
● Alcohol
● Marijuana

PRACTICE ALERT

Preventing paraphimosis after catheterisation or assisting a person with their personal hygiene means the nurse must ensure that the man's foreskin is dry and returned to its normal postion.

INTERDISCIPLINARY CARE FOR PHIMOSIS AND PRIAPISM

Severe phimosis or paraphimosis may require surgical circumcision. If infection is present, the appropriate antibiotic is administered. An interdisciplinary approach is advocated across both the primary and secondary care sectors.

Treatment of priapism may include oral terbuataline (acting as a decongestant). Blood may be aspirated from the corpus through the dorsal glans, followed by catheterisation and pressure dressings – dressings used to compress the penis. If necessary, more aggressive surgery to create vascular shunts (implements used to divert the flow of blood) to maintain blood flow is performed. When priapism is prolonged, it increases the risk of subsequent ED.

NURSING CARE FOR PHIMOSIS AND PRIAPISM

Nursing care for priapism focuses on assessing the penis, monitoring urinary output and providing pain control. Assessment of the penis includes inspection for degree of erection and changes in colour due to ischaemia, and palpation of the penis for firmness and degree of rigidity. Monitor urine output, assessing for oliguria (reduced urinary output) or signs of acute urinary retention. Pain is treated with analgesics.

The man usually has moderate to severe anxiety related to pain, the treatment and the threat to his sexual function. The treatment may sound bizarre and painful, especially since the area is already extremely sensitive. The man may be acutely embarrassed by the erection and needs reassurance

that the nurse understands that the erection is not within his control.

The man with cancer of the penis

Cancer of the penis is a rare cancer in the UK with 488 men diagnosed in 2008 (Cancer Research UK 2011c) and is predominantly diagnosed in men over 50 years of age. It is more common in men who live in Asia, South America and Africa. The cause is unknown. Penile cancer is rare in Jewish and Muslim men, populations in which routine circumcision is practised, although the correlation between circumcision and this cancer is unclear. Phimosis and poor genital hygiene are risk factors, as are human papillomavirus HPV (can cause warts and some cancers) and HIV infections. Ultraviolet light exposure (such as that used to treat psoriasis) also may play a role (Porth 2009).

PRACTICE ALERT

Cancer of the penis is rare. Before any decision about treatment is to be made, an opportunity should be given for the man to discuss any issues with all members of the multidisciplinary team. Referal to other specialists, for example a lymphoedema specialist nurse, may be needed.

Having looked at disorders of the penis, we will now consider disorders of the testicles and scrotum.

DISORDERS OF THE TESTIS AND SCROTUM

The man with a benign scrotal mass

Most scrotal masses are benign and can be managed in a manner that is satisfactory to the man. The most common are hydroceles, **spermatoceles** and **varicoceles** (Figure 16.3).

Pathophysiology of benign scrotal masses

A hydrocele is a collection of fluid within the tunica vaginalis. The swelling ranges from slightly larger than the testicle to larger than a grapefruit. The cause in men over the age of 40 years is an imbalance between production and reabsorption of fluid within the layers of the scrotum. Hydroceles also may occur secondary to trauma, infection or a tumour. A hydrocele may be differentiated from a solid mass by transillumination

or ultrasound of the scrotum. If the hydrocele causes embarrassment or pain, fluid is aspirated and an agent is injected into the scrotal sac to sclerose the tunica vaginalis.

A spermatocele is a mobile, usually painless mass formed when efferent ducts in the epididymis dilate and form a cyst. It is thought to result from leakage of sperm due to trauma or infection. Treatment is usually not necessary.

A varicocele is an abnormal dilation of a vein within the spermatic cord. It is commonly caused by incompetent or congenitally missing valves allowing blood to pool in the spermatic cord veins. A soft mass is formed that may be painful. Most occur after puberty on the left side. The condition can decrease blood flow through the testicles, interfere with spermatogenesis and cause infertility. Varicoceles can be felt by palpation. Sonography (an imaging tool) is used for diagnosis. If infertility is a concern, the spermatic vein may be ligated (tied) or occluded (to close) with a sclerosing agent or balloon catheter.

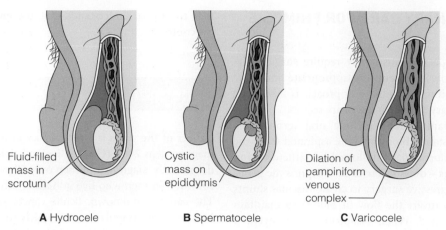

Fluid-filled mass in scrotum

Cystic mass on epididymis

Dilation of pampiniform venous complex

A Hydrocele   **B** Spermatocele   **C** Varicocele

Figure 16.3 Common disorders of the scrotum.

NURSING CARE FOR SCROTAL MASS

This focuses on reducing anxiety and teaching comfort measures. Men are aware of the possible pain associated with scrotal manipulation. Information and reassurance is needed about pain management if surgical treatment is necessary. External bleeding is minimal after surgery; some men develop scrotal haematomas, manifested by scrotal oedema and a purple discoloration.

Give information and allow time to ask questions relieving anxiety and fear. Time should be set aside for this and in private. This is also an important aspect of care when providing support with other reproductive conditions.

The man with epididymitis

Epididymitis is an infection or inflammation of the epididymis. This is often seen in sexually active men who are less than 35 years.

Sexually transmitted urethritis (inflammation of the urethra) caused by *C. trachomatis* or *N. gonorrhoeae* is the usual precipitating factor in younger men. Men who practise unprotected anal intercourse may acquire sexually transmitted epididymitis from *E. coli*, *H. influenzae*, *Cryptococcus* or tuberculosis. In those over 35 years, epididymitis is associated with a urinary tract infection or prostatitis. Chemical epididymitis is associated with an inflammatory response to the reflux of urine into the ejaculatory ducts from urethral strictures, congenital structural anomalies or increased abdominal pressure from excessive heavy lifting.

Infectious epididymis spreads by ascending the vas deferens from an already infected urethra or bladder. Early manifestations include pain and local oedema, progressing to erythema and oedema of the scrotum, especially on the side of the involved epididymis. Complications of the disorder include abscess formation, infarction of the testicles and infertility.

INTERDISCIPLINARY CARE FOR EPIDIDYMITIS

Diagnosis is made with a specimen culture from a urethral swab or epididymal aspiration. Severe epididymitis may be treated with oral or intravenous antibiotics. The man's sexual partner should be treated with antibiotics if the organism is sexually transmitted.

NURSING CARE FOR EPIDIDYMITIS

This involves symptomatic relief and teaching. Ice packs and a scrotal support applied to the scrotum relieve pain. Complete resolution may take weeks to months, and treatment should continue until the infection is gone. Information should be provided about the possibility of infertility.

The man with orchitis

Orchitis is an acute inflammation or infection of the testes, occurring as a complication of a systemic illness or as an extension of epididymitis. Infection may reach the testes through the vas deferens and the lymphatic and vascular channels. Trauma, including vasectomy and other scrotal surgeries, may cause inflammation of the testes.

The most common infectious cause of orchitis in post-pubertal men is mumps; others include scarlet fever or pneumonia. There is sudden onset, usually within three to four days after the swelling of the parotid glands, including high fever, increased white blood cells (WBCs) and unilateral or bilateral scrotal redness, swelling and pain.

PRACTICE ALERT

Help the man to achieve comfort by suggesting he wear supporting underwear, for example briefs as opposed to boxer shorts.

INTERDISCIPLINARY CARE FOR ORCHITIS

Treatment is supportive and symptomatic, including antibiotic therapy if urine cultures are positive. Bedrest, scrotal support and elevation, hot or cold compresses and analgesics for pain are prescribed. If a hydrocele (a collection of fluid in the scrotum) occurs, it is aspirated.

NURSING CARE FOR ORCHITIS

Nursing care is similar to that of the man with epididymitis.

The man with testicular cancer

Testicular cancer accounts for only 1% of all cancers in men; it is the most common cancer in men between the ages of 15 and 40. Approximately 2000 cases are registered each year (ONS 2008). Highest rates of testicular cancer are reported for white Caucasian populations in industrialised countries, in western and northern Europe; it is generally rare in non-Caucasian populations – the New Zealand Maoris being the exception (Ferlay *et al.* 2004). Survival from testicular cancer has improved as a result of treatment with combination chemotherapy.

The cause is unknown, but both congenital and acquired factors have been associated with tumor development. About 5% develop where there is a history of undescended testicle (*cryptorchidism*). Testicular cancer is more common on the right side, paralleling the incidence of cryptorchidism (McPhee and Papadakis 2011).

Risk factors for testicular cancer

Risk factors for testicular cancer include:

- specific age groups;
- cryptorchidism;
- genetic predisposition, especially in identical twins and brothers;
- cancer of the other testicle.

Other risk factors can include occupational risks, presence of multiple atypical naevi (for example, a benign growth like a mole) HIV infection, cancer *in situ (in place)*, extremes of body size, and maternal hormone use (for example, use of oestogen) (Tamimi and Adami 2002).

Pathophysiology of testicular cancer

Approximately 95% of testicular malignancies are germ cell tumours (Porth 2009). Germ cell tumours are classified, depending on their origin and ability to differentiate, as seminomas and non-seminomas. Seminomas are most common, and are believed to arise from the seminiferous epithelium of the testes. Non-seminomas contain more than one cell type; including embryonal carcinoma, teratoma, choriocarcinoma and yolk cell carcinoma. The most common type in men aged 20–30 is embryonal carcinomas. Testicular cancer can arise from specialised cells of the testes. These tumours are named for the cells from which they originate: Leydig cell, Sertoli cell, granulosa cell and theca cell tumours.

Signs and symptoms of testicular cancer

The first sign may be a slight enlargement of one testicle with discomfort. There may also be abdominal aching and a feeling of heaviness in the scrotum. Local spread of the cancer to the epididymis or spermatic cord is inhibited by the outer covering of the testicles, the tunica albuginea. Spread by lymphatic and vascular channels to other organs causes distant disease before large masses develop in the scrotum. Lymphatic dissemination leads to disease in retroperitoneal lymph nodes (lymph nodes located towards the back of the abdomen behind the intestines), whereas vascular dissemination leads to cancerous spread in the lungs, bone or liver. Bilateral (on both sides) presentation is unusual. Manifestations of metastasis include lower extremity oedema, back pain, cough, haemoptysis or dizziness. Human chorionic gonadotropin (hCG) producing tumours may cause breast enlargement. Manifestations of testicular cancer are as follows:

- *Common*:
  - painless swelling on one testicle.
- *Occasional*:
  - dull ache in pelvis or scrotum;
  - painless nodule on one testicle.
- *Uncommon*:
  - acute pain in scrotum.
- *Rare*:
  - infertility
  - gynaecomastia.
- *Metastatic symptoms*:
  - neck mass
  - respiratory symptoms
  - gastrointestinal disturbance
  - lumbar back pain.

INTERDISCIPLINARY CARE FOR TESTICULAR CANCER

Care focuses on diagnosis, elimination of the cancer and prevention or treatment of metastasis. Once suspected, a number of screening tests to help identify the disease and its stage are needed. Stage I is confined to the testicle, stage II is limited to the testicle and regional lymph nodes and stage III involves metastasis or visceral involvement. Often, the man does not undergo biopsy before treatment, but receives a definitive diagnosis after orchidectomy (surgical removal of the testes). Most men treated for testicular cancer will live a normal lifespan.

Diagnosis

Diagnosis is made by laboratory tests. Serum studies (analysis of blood to determine cancer markers) are done to identify tumour markers. Germ cell tumours produce biochemical markers such as hCG and alpha-fetoprotein (AFP). Elevated levels provide strong evidence of testicular cancer. These markers are also measured after surgery to help determine the presence of residual disease. Persistent elevation may indicate the need for further therapy. Serum lactic acid dehydrogenase (LDH) levels are elevated in testicular cancer, and may be significantly elevated when metastatic disease is present.

Treatment

There are number of treatments for testicular cancer including surgery, radiation therapy and medicines. The choice of treatment will depend on each person's individual needs and desires.

Medication

Progress in chemotherapy to treat testicular cancer is one of the chief reasons why most men survive the disease. Men with an advanced disease receive platinum-based combination chemotherapy. Two frequently used combinations are (1) cisplatin, bleomycin and etoposide (BEP), and (2) etoposide plus cisplatin (EP). Side-effects can include nausea, vomiting, hair loss, bone marrow suppression, nephrotoxicity (kidney damage), ototoxicity (damage to hearing) and peripheral neuropathy (damage to the nervous system).

Surgery

Radical orchiectomy is the treatment used in all forms and stages of testicular cancer. A modified retroperitoneal lymph node dissection that preserves the nerves necessary for ejaculation is often performed simultaneously.

Radiation therapy

This is used for stage I seminoma to treat cancer in the retroperitoneal lymph nodes. Side-effects can include diarrhoea, nausea, a decline in bone marrow function, thrombocytopenia or leukopenia. These problems are usually mild and respond to symptomatic treatment or time. Damage to the other testicle is minimised by careful shielding. Pre-treatment and post-treatment analysis of sperm number and function is necessary.

NURSING CARE FOR TESTICULAR CANCER

Health promotion

Most men who develop testicular cancer do not have overt risk factors. Therefore, beginning at the age of 15, all men should perform monthly testicular self-examination, as described in the box below.

Nursing diagnoses and interventions

The nurse must consider the reactions to the diagnosis, change in body image accompanying treatment and sexual and reproductive issues. Chances of a cure are excellent, the long-term effect on quality of life may be extensive, body image may be negatively perceived. There may be a need for changes in life goals, for example, some men may wish to father children. This is still possible, but it may be that alternative approaches are needed.

IN PRACTICE

Testicular self-examination

- Examine testicles when taking a warm shower or bath, or just after. Use a mirror to compare size.
- The scrotum, testicles and hands should be soapy allowing easy manipulation of tissue.
- Gently roll each testicle between the thumb and fingers of each hand (Figure 16.4). If one testicle is substantially larger than the other, or if you feel any hard lumps, contact the GP immediately.
- Just above and behind the testicle is the epididymis. It feels soft and tender, although parts of it may be rather firm. This is normal. The spermatic cord, a small, round, movable tube, extends up from the epididymis. It feels firm and smooth. Any hard lump felt directly on the testicle, even if it is painless, is a concern.
- Choose a day out of each month to examine yourself, such as the first or last day of the month. Star this day on your calendar to help you remember.

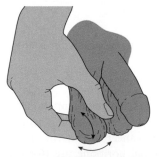

Figure 16.4 Rolling of the testicle.

Risk for deficient knowledge

The nurse initiates and reinforces teaching about what to expect after radical orchiectomy. Assess knowledge about surgery and explain post-operative routines such as early mobilisation (see Chapter 1). The nurse should:

- Explain pain control methods. In addition to analgesics to control post-operative incisional pain, ice bags may be applied to the scrotum. *A scrotal support provides relief, especially when the man mobilises.*

- Teach the signs and symptoms associated with complications. If the incision gapes open, or if there is bleeding beyond slight oozing after 24 hours, the person must inform the nurse, ward or clinic. *Haematoma can occur in the scrotum caused by bleeding from the spermatic cord stump. Rapid scrotal oedema is a sign of this problem.*

Risk for ineffective sexuality patterns

The effect of testicular cancer and its treatment is varied. If the man has retroperitoneal lymph node dissection, severing of the sympathetic plexus may result in **retrograde ejaculation** or failure to ejaculate. Infertility may be caused by ejaculation disorders, surgery, chemotherapy or radiation therapy.

- Assess the man's pre-diagnosis sexual function; establish an atmosphere of openness and permission to discuss sexual concerns. *Men report intense concern about sexual and reproductive issues after diagnosis, which can be relieved by information giving.*

- Discuss the possibility of preserving sperm in a bank prior to treatment.

- Explain that testicular implants can be inserted to preserve appearance.

COMMUNITY-BASED CARE

Families of men with testicular cancer need to be included in teaching. If the man is of reproductive age, his partner may be anxious and will require information. For the teenager, parents need information about the effect on sexual function and are often very involved in post-operative care. The man needs the support of the people he loves, and knowledgeable loved ones can give effective support.

Provide teaching and reinforcement of the need for follow-up, especially if the retroperitoneal lymph nodes were not surgically explored. For men with a risk for recurrence, surveillance with periodic physical examinations, chest x-ray, tumour markers and CT scans of the retroperitoneal nodes could continue for five years and possibly 10 years after orchiectomy.

The nurse must understand treatment modalities and the care required if he/she is to offer support and understanding.

This section of the chapter has provided you with some insight into the key issues concerned with the testicles and scrotum. The next section of the chapter will address some of the issues associated with the prostate gland.

DISORDERS OF THE PROSTATE GLAND

The man with prostatitis

Prostatitis is used to refer to different types of inflammatory disorders of the prostate gland. *Prostatodynia* is a condition in which the man experiences the symptoms of prostatitis but shows no evidence of inflammation or infection.

Pathophysiology of prostatitis

There are a number of types of prostatitis:

- acute bacterial prostatitis;
- chronic bacterial prostatitis;
- chronic prostatitis/pelvic pain syndrome;
- asymptomatic inflammatory prostatitis.

Men with asymptomatic inflammatory prostatitis have no subjective symptoms, but are diagnosed when a biopsy or prostatic fluid examination is conducted.

Acute bacterial prostatitis

This is most often caused by an ascending infection from the urethra or reflux of infected urine into the ducts of the prostate gland. *E. coli* is most often responsible; other causative organisms include *Pseudomonas*, *Klebsiella* and *Chlamydia*.

Manifestations of acute bacterial prostatitis include fever, malaise (a feeling of tiredness), muscle and joint pain, urinary frequency and urgency, dysuria (difficulty passing urine) and urethral discharge accompanied with dull, aching pain in the perineum, rectum or lower back. The prostate is enlarged and painful.

Chronic bacterial prostatitis

There is a history of recurrent urinary tract infections. The causative organisms are most often *E. coli*, *Proteus* or *Klebsiella*. Calculi may form in the prostate and contribute to chronicity.

The manifestations include prostatitis, urinary frequency and urgency, dysuria, low back pain and perineal discomfort. Epididymitis may be associated with the prostatitis.

Chronic prostatitis/chronic pelvic pain syndrome

This is the most common and the least understood of the syndromes (British Prostatitis Support Association 2009). Both types (inflammatory and non-inflammatory) are based on the presence of white blood cells in prostatic fluid.

Signs and symptoms of prostatitis and prostatodynia

Signs and symptoms of prostatitis and prostatodynia include:

● *Acute bacterial prostatitis*:
  – abrupt onset, obstruction, irritation or pain upon voiding, frequency and urgency;
  – positive culture specimens demonstrating infectious organism;
  – non-urinary symptoms – chills, fever, low back and pelvic floor pain.

● *Chronic bacterial prostatitis*:
  – urinary symptoms, similar to those of the acute form, except less sudden, less dramatic or even absent;
  – positive cultures of causative organism not always obtainable as treatment may need to be commenced prior to the test result being available.

● *Chronic prostatitis*:
  – perineal, suprapubic (below the symphysis pubis bone), low back or genital pain;
  – irritation upon voiding;
  – post-ejaculatory pain.

● *Prostatodynia*:
  – pelvic, low back or perineal pain;
  – irritation or obstruction upon voiding;
  – no evidence of inflammation in the prostate;
  – no urinary tract infection;
  – normal prostatic secretions.

● *Inflammatory prostatitis* is believed to be an autoimmune disorder, the cause of which is unknown. There may be low back pain, urinary manifestations, pain in the penis, testicles, scrotum, lower back and rectum, decreased libido and painful ejaculations.

● *Non-inflammatory prostatitis* has manifestations similar to inflammatory prostatitis, but no evidence of urinary or prostatic infection or inflammation can be found. The cause is unknown, but is believed to be the result of a problem outside the prostate gland, such as obstruction of the bladder neck.

INTERDISCIPLINARY CARE FOR PROSTATITIS

Diagnosis

It is difficult to diagnose prostatitis. Urine and prostatic secretion examination and cultures are obtained to determine the presence and type of blood cells and bacteria. X-ray studies and ultrasound to visualise pelvic structures may be useful.

Medication

Bacterial prostatitis is treated with antibiotics. The chronic form requires long-term antibiotics, often up to four months. Non-bacterial prostatitis does not usually respond to drug therapy, although relief from symptoms is possible. Non-steroidal anti-inflammatory drugs are useful for pain, and anticholinergics may reduce voiding symptoms. Prostatodynia is treated symptomatically to relieve muscle tension, usually with alpha-adrenergic blocking agents or muscle relaxants.

NURSING CARE FOR PROSTATITIS

The focus should be on symptom management. Men with acute and chronic bacterial prostatitis should increase fluid intake to around 3 L daily and void often. This helps decrease irritation when voiding. Regular bowel movements help ease the pain associated with defaecation. Local heat, such as taking a bath, may be helpful to relieve pain and irritation. The course of antibiotics must be completed. The condition is not contagious and does not cause cancer (Porth 2009). Referral sources include the British Prostatitis Support Association, Prostate Research Campaign UK and the British Urological Association.

The man with benign prostatic hyperplasia (BPH)

BPH is an age-related, non-malignant enlargement of the prostate gland. It is a common disorder of the ageing male. The prostate, very small at birth, grows at puberty, and reaches adult size around age 20. Benign hyperplasia (increased number of cells) begins at 40–45 years, and continues slowly through the rest of life. Approximately more than one-half of all men over 60 have BPH (Porth 2009). The problem that brings men to a healthcare provider is the associated urinary dysfunction.

Risk factors for BPH

The exact cause of BPH is unknown, but some of the risk factors include:

● age (the older man);
● family history (if a sibling or relative has had BPH);
● race (highest in African Americans, lowest in Asians);
● diet high in meat and fats.

Pathophysiology of BPH

Two necessary preconditions for BPH are age and the presence of testes; those castrated before puberty do not develop BPH.

The androgen (a hormone) mediating prostatic growth, dihydrotestosterone (DHT), is formed in the prostate from testosterone. Although androgen levels decrease in ageing men, the ageing prostate appears to become more sensitive to available DHT. Oestrogen, produced in small amounts in men, appears to sensitise the prostate gland to the effects of DHT. Increasing oestrogen levels associated with ageing or a relative increase in oestrogen related to testosterone levels may contribute to prostatic hyperplasia.

BPH begins as small nodules in the periurethral glands, the inner layers of the prostate. The prostate enlarges through formation and growth of nodules (hyperplasia) and enlargement of glandular cells (hypertrophy). Changes occur over a long period of time. The pathophysiological effects result from a combination of factors, including intravesical (within the urinary bladder) pressure during voiding, detrusor muscle strength (this contracts when passing urine), neurological functioning (for example, spinal injury) and general physical health.

Signs and symptoms of BPH

Growing prostatic tissue compresses the urethra (Figure 16.5) causing partial or complete obstrution of urinary outflow. The detrusor muscles hypertrophy (extend and grow) compensating for increased resistance to urinary flow; however, eventually decreased bladder compliance and bladder instability result. Manifestations of BPH include:

- diminished force of urinary stream;
- hesitancy in initiating voiding;
- post-void dribbling;
- sensation of incomplete emptying;
- urinary retention;
- nocturia;
- frequency;
- urgency;
- urge incontinence;
- dysuria.

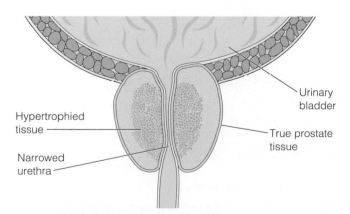

Figure 16.5 Benign prostatic hyperplasia.

Complications of BPH

Unless the enlarging mass is reduced, multiple complications occur. As urine is retained in the bladder, increasing bladder distention occurs causing diverticula (outpouchings) on the bladder wall. Distention may also obstruct the ureters. Infection, more common in retained urine and in diverticula, ascends from the bladder to the kidneys. Hydroureter, hydronephrosis and renal insufficiency are possible complications.

INTERDISCIPLINARY CARE FOR BPH

Focus is on diagnosing the disorder, correcting or minimising the urinary obstruction and preventing or treating complications. Treatment is determined by the severity of the manifestations and the presence of complications. Mild cases are monitored over time, and may remain stable or improve.

Diagnosis

This involves both physical examination and laboratory tests to diagnose the disease and to differentiate it from prostate cancer. A DRE is done to examine the external surface of the prostate; in BPH it is asymmetrical and enlarged. Examination of creatinine levels of the blood is conducted to assess for kidney damage.

The urine is examined for WBCs, RBCs (red blood cells) and bacteria. Urinary function is assessed by measuring residual urine (amount of urine remaining in the bladder after voiding) with ultrasound or post-voiding catheterisation (more than 100 mL is considered high), and through uroflowmetry, measuring urine flow rate; normal is greater than 14 mL/sec. A finding of less than 10 mL/sec indicates obstruction.

Prostate-specific antigen (PSA) levels can rule out prostate cancer. Further information is provided on page 634 under diagnosis of prostate cancer.

The man's own subjective experiences with BPH are included in the diagnosis and treatment. For example, the International Prostate Symptom Score (developed by a group of urologists) uses a scale of 0 (not at all) to 5 (almost always) to collect data about areas such as feeling as though the bladder did not empty with urinating, as well as asking how many times during the night the man gets up to urinate and how the man feels about having the disorder.

Medications

There are several issues that need to be given consideration. The first consideration is usually addressed by treatment for mild prostate enlargement with finasteride (Proscar) or dutasteride (Avodart), anti-androgen agents that inhibit the conversion of testosterone to DHT, causing the enlarged prostate to shrink. These drugs may cause erectile dysfunction, decrease libido and decrease volume of ejaculate.

Excessive smooth muscle contraction may be blocked with the alpha-adrenergic antagonists such as terazosin (Hytrin), doxazosin (Cardura), tamsulosin (Flomax) and alfuzosin (Xatral). These medications relieve obstruction and increase urine flow. They may cause orthostatic hypotension (a low blood pressure in the lying down position). Teaching includes advice about making position changes slowly, avoiding dizziness and accidental falls, how to take and record blood pressure, and to check before taking medications for coughs, colds or allergies (these medications may contain an adrenergic agent that can cause the release of adrenaline or adrenaline-like substances).

In some men it makes sense to initiate combination therapy using finasteride and an alpha blocker such as doxazosin as opposed to using single therapy with the aim of relieving manifestations and to prevent the progression of BPH (Baldwin *et al.* 2001).

Surgery

Men who have urinary retention, recurrent urinary tract infection, haematuria (blood in the urine), bladder stones or renal insufficiency secondary to BPH are candidates for surgical intervention to remove the cause. Surgical treatment may be performed by minimally invasive surgery or through transurethral surgery, open surgery or laser surgery. These treatments are discussed below.

Minimally invasive surgery

Because medications are not effective for all men, procedures have been developed to relieve the manifestations of BPH that are less invasive than traditional surgery.

Microwaves are used to heat and destroy excess prostate tissue in a procedure called *transurethral microwave thermotherapy*. A cooling system protects the urinary tract. It takes about an hour and can be performed on an out-patient basis. Microwave procedures do not cure BPH, but they do reduce urinary manifestations. The procedure does not cause erectile dysfunction or incontinence.

The *transurethral needle ablation (TUNA)* system uses low-level radio frequency through twin needles burning away a region of the enlarged prostate. Shields protect the urethra. TUNA improves the flow of urine through the urethra. It does not cause erectile dysfunction or incontinence.

Transurethral surgery

A *transurethral resection of the prostate (TURP)* is the surgical procedure used most often. Obstructing prostate tissue is removed using the wire loop of a resectoscope and electrocautery, inserted through the urethra (Figure 16.6). No external incision is necessary. During the procedure the resectoscope removes obstructing tissue one piece at a time. The tissue is flushed into the bladder and then flushed out at the end of the operation. There are potential risks, however, including postoperative haemorrhage or clot retention, inability to void and

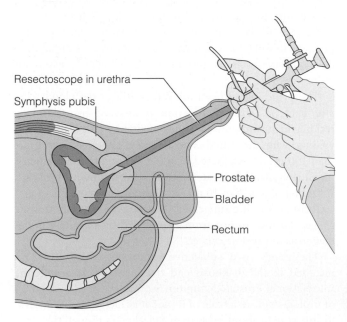

A Transurethral resection of the prostate

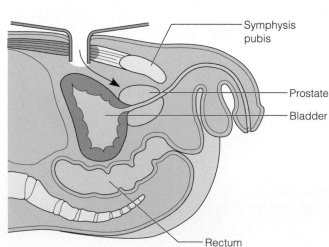

B Retropubic prostatectomy

Figure 16.6 (A) In a transurethral resection of the prostate, a resectoscope inserted through the urethra is used to remove excess prostate tissue. **(B)** In a retropubic prostatectomy, prostate tissue is removed through an abdominal incision.

urinary tract infection. Other complications are incontinence, erectile dysfunction and retrograde ejaculation.

In *transurethral incision of the prostate (TUIP)*, small incisions are made in the smooth muscle where the prostate is attached to the bladder. The gland is split reducing pressure on the urethra. No tissue is removed, and this procedure is most appropriate for men with smaller prostate glands. TUIP can be done on an out-patient basis, and has the advantage of less risk of post-operative retrograde ejacula-tion than is associated with TURP or other prostatectomy procedures.

Open surgery

When the prostate gland is very large, an open prostatectomy may be used. These procedures are discussed in the section on prostate cancer. Nursing care for the man having prostate surgery is outlined in the box below. The aim is to provide safe pre-, peri- and post-operative care.

NURSING CARE PLAN The man undergoing a prostatectomy

Review Chapter 1 for routine pre- and post-operative care.

Pre-operative care

+ Assess knowledge about the surgery.

+ Inform the man that he will have a urinary catheter when returning from surgery and that there may be a drain(s) in his incision. He also will be wearing anti-embolitic stockings.

+ Ensure that a signed consent form is in the notes and all other pre-operative tasks outlined in Chapter 1 are done.

+ Bowel preparation (for example, prescribed enema or suppositories) may be required in line with evidence-based local policy and procedures.

+ Communicate willingness to address any concerns or anxiety.

Post-operative care

+ Maintain the usual post-operative assessments (see Chapter 1). Follow aseptic technique in urinary drainage and irrigation care. Monitor vital signs for the first 24 hours and regularly thereafter.

+ Maintain accurate intake and output records, including amounts of irrigating solution used. Frequently assess patency of any catheters and drains. Monitor colour and character of urine.

+ Assess and manage pain.

+ Maintain anti-embolitic stockings. Assist with leg exercises and ambulation as ordered.

+ Encourage liberal fluid intake of 2–3 L a day

Transurethral resection of the prostate (TURP)

+ First 24–48 hours, monitor for haemorrhage, evidenced by frankly bloody urinary output, large blood clots, decreased urinary output, increasing bladder spasms, tachycardia (increased pulse) and hypotension (low blood pressure). Notify the doctor if any of these manifestations occur.

+ Instruct the man with a three-way indwelling catheter to try to keep the leg straight.

+ Explain that the presence of a urinary catheter will cause the sensation of needing to void; it is important not to strain to try to void around the catheter or when having a bowel movement. Explain that bladder spasms (lower abdominal pressure or pain) and a desire to urinate may occur. This is expected and medications can alleviate this discomfort.

+ If there is continuous bladder irrigation, assess the catheter and the drainage tubing regularly. Maintain the rate of flow of irrigating fluid to keep the output light pink or colourless. Assess the urinary output one to two hourly for colour, consistency, amount, blood clots; assess for bladder spasms.

+ Assess for fluid volume excess and hyponatraemia, called TURP syndrome, manifested by hyponatraemia, hypertension, bradycardia, nausea and confusion. If these occur, notify the doctor.

+ If no continuous bladder irrigation, follow local evidence-based policy and procedure and instructions when irrigating the catheter (usually when the urine is frankly bloody or has larger blood clots, or bladder spasms increase). Using asepsis, the catheter is gently irrigated with 50 mL of irrigating solution at a time, until the obstruction is relieved or the urine is clear. Ensure equal input and output of irrigating fluid.

+ Following catheter removal, assess the amount, colour and consistency of urine. Explain that there may be a feeling of burning on urination and dribbling after urination and that the urine may contain small blood clots after catheter removal.

The man with a retropubic prostatectomy

+ Assess the abdominal incision for the presence of urine. No urine should be found on the dressing.

+ Assess the abdominal incision for increased or purulent drainage, and the man for an increased temperature and pain.

The man with a suprapubic prostatectomy

+ Assess urinary output from the suprapubic and the urethral catheters (suprapubic prostatectomy often has two separate closed drainage systems: one from the suprapubic incision and one from a urethral catheter).

+ Assess the abdominal dressing for urinary drainage, and change saturated dressings frequently.

+ Following removal of the urethral catheter (usually two to four days after surgery) and based on the doctor's instructions,

NURSING CARE PLAN The man undergoing a prostatectomy (continued)

clamp the suprapubic catheter and encourage the man to void. Assess residual urine by unclamping the suprapubic catheter and measuring urinary output after voiding.

The man with a perineal prostatectomy

+ Assess perineal incision for drainage and manifestations of infection.

+ Do not take rectal temperatures or administer enemas.

+ Use a T-bandage or padded scrotal support to hold the dressing in place. Following removal of the dressing and perineal sutures, taking a bath may help.

+ Teach how to perform perineal irrigations with sterile normal saline as ordered and after each bowel movement.

Laser surgery

A cystoscope is used to pass the yttrium aluminium garnet (YAG) laser fibre through the urethra into the prostate vaporising obstructing prostate tissue with several short bursts of energy. An advantage is decreased blood loss and a more rapid recovery time. This method may not be as effective for larger prostates.

New treatments

Newer treatments for BPH include minimally invasive procedures such as balloon urethroplasty and placement of intraurethral stents to maintain patency of the urethra. Balloon urethroplasty is a simple procedure where a balloon-tipped catheter is inserted into the narrowed portion of the urethra and inflated; the balloon widens the urethra, relieving obstruction. These procedures can be done as out-patient surgery.

Alternative and complementary therapies

Phytotherapy is the use of plants or plant extracts for medical treatment. Several plant extracts have been used for years in Europe to treat BPH and are being used more often in the UK. This includes saw palmetto berry, the bark of *Pygeum africanum*, the roots of *Echinacea purpurea* and *Hypoxis rooperi*, and the leaves of the trembling poplar. The mechanisms of the actions of these extracts are unknown.

NURSING CARE FOR BPH

Most men are unsure of the function of the prostate gland and its location, but its relationship to sexual and urinary function is at least generally known. Lack of knowledge and the growing number of treatment options is confusing to many men. There are similarities between the nursing care of men with BPH and men with prostate cancer (see below).

Nursing diagnoses and interventions

This section provides information on nursing interventions related to deficient knowledge, urinary retention, risk for infection and risk for imbalanced fluid volume.

Risk for deficient knowledge

+ Explain the anatomy and physiology of the prostate gland, and normal changes that occur with ageing.

+ Discuss treatment options, including information about effects on erectile function, ejaculation and fertility.

+ Discuss effects of prostate surgery, including urinary retention and urinary incontinence.

+ Explain to the man having a TURP that a catheter will be placed into the bladder and irrigation fluid will be infusing into and out of the catheter for the first 36–72 hours following surgery.

+ Explain that, following removal of the catheter, there may be urinary frequency and urgency and dribbling of urine after voiding. Stress the importance of increasing oral fluid intake and regular pelvic floor exercises.

Risk for urinary retention

+ Teach signs and symptoms of acute urinary retention: dysuria, overflow incontinence, bladder pain and distention, no urine output.

+ Teach that the risk of developing urinary retention increases when the man with BPH takes over-the-counter (OTC) decongestant medications, or prescription medications such as antidepressants, anticholinergics calcium channel blockers, antipsychotics and medications to treat Parkinson's disease.

+ Suggest avoiding intake of large volumes of liquid at any one time.

+ Teach how to use the double-voiding technique: urinate, then sit on the toilet for three to five minutes, then urinate again.

PRACTICE ALERT

In addition to avoiding a large amount of fluids at one time, it is also important to limit liquids that stimulate the passing of urine, such as coffee and alcoholic beverages. Some men, because of the difficulties they may experience with passing urine, may limit their fluid intake. The nurse must be aware of this as it can lead to dehydration and further complications.

Table 16.4 Significance and character of urine after prostatectomy and the related nursing care

Urine colour	Nursing implications
Light red to red	Normal day of surgery and first post-operative day.
Very dark red	May indicate increased venous bleeding or inadequate dilution. Catheter at risk for occlusion. Increase flow rate of irrigant. If urine does not clear, notify doctor.
Bright red	May indicate arterial bleeding. Increase flow rate of irrigant, monitor vital signs, notify the doctor.
Contains blood clots	Occasional blood clot normal. If clots are frequent, catheter may become obstructed. Increase flow rate of irrigant.
Clear to light pink	Normal throughout hospitalisation.

Risk for infection

+ Monitor WBCs and vital signs (body temperature and pulse rate).
+ Maintain sterile procedures when changing irrigation fluids and when emptying the catheter draining bag, adhere to local policy.

Risk for imbalanced fluid volume

Prostatectomy brings increased risk of imbalanced fluid volume (that is, the person may have positive fluid intake with a negative fluid output) as a result of excessive bleeding from the operative site as well as absorption of irrigating fluid. Report manifestations indicating hypovolaemic shock (this is low circulating fluid volume), excess bleeding and/or TURP syndrome immediately.

+ Monitor pulse and blood pressure.
+ Monitor colour of drainage in urinary drainage bag (see Table 16.4).
+ Monitor for manifestations of TURP syndrome: nausea and vomiting, confusion, hypertension, bradycardia and visual disturbances.

Return to Case Study 2 at the beginning of the chapter:

1. Outline a teaching plan for Mr Turner for the risk for altered skin integrity related to urinary incontinence.
2. If you were the district nurse making a home visit and found that Mr Turner had no urinary drainage for 16 hours, what assessments would you make? How would you handle this problem?

The last section addressed a number of issues associated with prostate conditions and in the next section we will move on to the issue of prostate cancer.

COMMUNITY-BASED CARE

Depending on treatment, the procedure may be performed on an out-patient basis. The man having a TURP, although hospitalised for the surgery, may be discharged within two days after surgery if there are no complications. Home care involves care of an indwelling urinary catheter. Teaching how to care for a catheter and drainage bag should include:

● Change from the daytime leg drainage bag to a larger night drainage bag. Larger bag suspended from the bed frame at night permits gravity drainage of urine, preventing reflux of urine back into the bladder.
● Avoid strapping the leg bag on too tightly. This can decrease venous return and increase risk for thrombophlebitis and embolic complications (complications associated with blood clots) such as pulmonary emboli (blood clots in the lungs).
● Place a soft cloth between the leg bag and thigh, decreasing friction and absorbing dampness under the bag, reducing the risk of skin irritation.
● Empty the leg bag every three to four hours during waking hours to prevent overfilling.

Promptly report any unexpected changes in urine colour, consistency, odour, haematuria, evidence of frank bleeding, or large blood clots, as well as a lack of or significant decrease in urine output to the GP.

The man with prostate cancer

Prostate cancer can happen to any man. There are a number of risk factors and these are addressed in this next section. A number of high profile men have succumbed to prostate cancer, for example, Colin Powell (USA politician and retired Secretary of State), Robert De Nero (actor), Nelson Mandela (former President of South Africa), Roger Moore (actor) and Frank Zappa (singer).

This is primarily a disease of older men, increasing in incidence with age, with the majority of cases diagnosed in men older than 65 years. The most common cancer in men in the UK is prostate cancer accounting for nearly a quarter (24%) of all new male cancer diagnoses.

There has been a huge rise in prostate cancer incidence over the last 20 years, but this has not been replicated in mortality rates. The increase in incidence is mainly due to the incidental detection of prostate cancer following TURP and with the increasing use of PSA testing.

In 2008, there were 37 051 new cases of prostate cancer diagnosed in the UK, that is around 90 men every day or one man every 15 minutes (Cancer Research UK 2011a). Prostate cancer is a major health problem for older men, but the death rate is decreasing due to advances in diagnosis and treatment.

When diagnosed early, prostate cancer is curable. Survival rates for prostate cancer have been improving; improvements in survival may be due to more effective treatment, both for early, aggressive prostate cancers and for advanced cases (Kvåle *et al.* 2007).

The five-year relative survival rate for men diagnosed in England in 2001–06 was 77% (Cancer Research UK 2010a), compared with only 31% for men diagnosed in 1971–75 (Coleman *et al.* 2004).

The one- and 10-year prostate cancer survival rates have risen dramatically. Similar increases have taken place in Scotland with the five-year relative survival rates increasing from 47% for those diagnosed in 1980–84 to 80% for men diagnosed in 2000–04 (Information Services Division 2007). The increase in prostate cancer survival rates is particularly pronounced in the 1990s when PSA testing became more prevalent (Quinn and Babb 2002).

Many men are found to have prostate cancer on post-mortem; usually the cancer has produced no manifestations or complications.

Risk factors for prostate cancer

In addition to age, race is a significant risk factor for prostate cancer. Other risk factors being investigated are as follows:

- genetic and hereditary factors, with increased risk in men who have a family history of the disease;
- having a vasectomy, believed to increase the levels of circulating free testosterone;
- dietary factors, including a diet high in animal fat and excessive supplemental vitamin A.

Pathophysiology of prostate cancer

The prostate gland consists primarily of glandular epithelial cells. The exact aetiology of prostate cancer is unknown, although androgens are believed to have a role in its development. Most primary prostate cancers are adenocarcinomas (a specific type of cancer originating in glandular tissue), and develop in the peripheral zones (zones on the outside of the prostate gland). This location increases the risk of local spread to the prostatic capsule. Despite its proximity to the rectum, metastases (spreading) to the bowel are uncommon because a tough sheet of tissue acts as an effective physical barrier.

As the tumour enlarges, it may compress the urethra, obstructing urinary flow. The tumour may metastasise involving the seminal vesicles or bladder. Spread by lymph and venous channels is common.

Signs and symptoms of prostate cancer

Early-stage prostate cancer is often asymptomatic (there may be no symptoms). Pain from metastasis to bones is often noted. Urinary manifestations depend on the size and location of the tumour and stage of the malignancy. They are often much like manifestations of BPH: urgency, frequency, hesitancy, dysuria and nocturia. There may be haematuria or blood in the ejaculate (Porth 2009).

Complications of prostate cancer

Death may occur as a result of debility caused by multiple sites of skeletal metastasis, especially to the vertebrae. Compression fractures of the spine are common, resulting in loss of mobility and bowel and bladder function. Tumours may eventually involve bone marrow, resulting in severe anaemias and impaired immune function.

INTERDISCIPLINARY CARE FOR PROSTATE CANCER

Focus is on diagnosis, elimination or containment of the cancer, and prevention or treatment of complications. There are currently no clinical strategies to prevent the development of prostate cancer. Early detection remains the major emphasis for control of this disease.

Diagnosis

Although an increasing number of men are now diagnosed with no symptoms associated with prostate cancer, many men have either locally advanced cancer (cancer confined close to the prostate) or distant spreading of cancer at the time of diagnosis. The definitive diagnosis can be made only by biopsy; however, other tests may suggest the presence of prostate cancer.

A DRE will find the prostate gland nodular and fixed in prostate cancer. PSA levels are used to diagnose and stage (a way of describing the size and how far the cancer has grown) prostate cancer, and to monitor response to treatment. An increase over time is more significant than one reading (serial measurements determine this). The PSA test is used with a DRE to help detect prostate cancer in men age 50 or older, and is also used to monitor effects of treatment.

There is no one PSA reading considered 'normal' and the use of the PSA test alone can yield insignificant results. PSA values vary from one individual to another and the normal level increases with age. The following values are a rough guide (Cancer Research UK 2010b)

- 3 ng/mL or less is normal for men under 60 years old;
- 4 ng/mL or less is normal for men aged 60–69 years;
- 5 ng/mL or less is normal if the man is aged over 70 years.

A reading higher than these values, but one that is less than 10 ng/mL, is typically due to a benign enlarged prostate. A value that exceeds 10 ng/mL may also just be benign prostate disease, but the higher the level of PSA, the more probable it is to be cancer. A cancer may be diagnosed in a man with a 'normal' PSA reading. The higher the reading, the more probable it is to be cancer. There are some men who have PSA levels in the hundreds (or even thousands) when diagnosed. The higher the level of PSA when the diagnosis is made then the more likely the cancer is to spread quickly.

Transrectal ultrasound (TRUS) may be used when the DRE is abnormal or if the PSA is elevated. In this test, a small probe is inserted in the rectum. The probe gives off sound waves providing a picture of the prostate on a video screen. Guided by this picture, a narrow needle is inserted through the rectal wall into the prostate gland, and the needle removes a sample of tissue for examination. Other tests that may be ordered include urinalysis or cystoscopy (examination of the bladder using a special telescope-like instrument). Bone scan, MRI or CT scans may be performed to determine the presence of tumour metastasis.

IN PRACTICE

Transrectal ultrasound (TRUS)

TRUS can take place in a variety of settings in the primary and secondary care sectors, and a needle biopsy of the prostate gland may also be needed. The role of the nurse is to ensure that the person is safe, to offer support and assist the person carrying out the test. Providing a clear explanation of the test using a language the person understands is vital. Explain that the test should not be painful, but it may be uncomfortable. The nurse assists prior to, during and after the procedure. There may be a requirement to have the bowel empty prior to the examination, and laxatives may have been prescribed. The procedure should take approximately 10 minutes and the man will be awake during this time. Results are usually made available within a week. The nurse assists the man to lie on his side with his knees drawn up to his chest. Physical and emotional support is needed and dignity and privacy must be ensured. After the procedure, assist the man in cleaning his anal area and help him to dress. Allow time for questions. Ensure the man has the contact details of who he can get in touch with should he have any queries concerning his symptoms or the outcome of the investigation.

Grading and staging help to determine prognosis and guide treatment decisions. Grade (cancer cell differentiation) is determined by the pathologist. Prostate cancer is staged with a variety of tests.

Most prostate cancers are adenocarcinomas. Seventy per cent arise in the peripheral zone of the gland, 5–15% occur in the central zone and the remainder in the transition zone (specific area located within the prostate gland). Benign prostate hyperplasia predominantly develops within the transition zone (Kirby and Brawer 2004). Tumours are usually staged using the tumour, node and metastasis (TNM) system. This assesses the size of a primary tumour, if there are lymph nodes

Table 16.5 The Gleason system – prostate cancer grading

Grade 1	Tumours consist of small, uniform glands with minimal nuclear changes.
Grade 2	Tumours have medium-sized acini (a cluster of cells), still separated by stromal tissue but more closely arranged.
Grade 3	Tumours show marked variation in glandular size and organisation and generally infiltration of stromal (a specific type of cells) and neighbouring tissues.
Grade 4	Tumours demonstrate marked cytological atypia (an increase in cell production) with extensive infiltration (meaning that the cancer has infiltrated deeply).
Grade 5	Tumours are characterised by sheets of undifferentiated cancer cells.

Source: adapted from Gleason 1966.

with cancer cells in them and whether the cancer has spread to other parts of the body. Numbers are used to describe the cancer.

The Gleason system is also used to grade prostate cancers and is based on a histological picture (an analysis of cell types under a microscope) assessing the extent to which the tumour cells are arranged into recognisably glandular structures (Gleason 1966) (see Table 16.5).

Schroder *et al.* (1992) describe the tumour, node and metastasis (TNM) classification system, which demonstrates pattern of disease and spread (see Table 16.6).

Those tumours confined within the prostatic capsule are referred to as 'early' disease (T1 and T2). T3/T4 tumours are known as 'locally advanced' disease – the tumour has spread

PRACTICE ALERT

There are number of myths surrounding the prostate gland and prostate cancer. The nurse is in an ideal position to correct any misconceptions, for example:

1. *'I haven't got any symptoms, therefore I can't have prostate cancer'*. Untrue early prostate cancer doesn't cause any symptoms.

2. *'I might pass on prostate cancer to my partner'*. Untrue you cannot pass prostate cancer on to your partner, male or female.

3. *'Prostate cancer is only found in old men'*. It is true that prostate cancer is more common in older men. Prostate cancer is being diagnosed in men in their 40s and 50s.

4. *'Treatment for prostate cancer always cause erectile dysfunction'*. False. This is a possibility, however, there are a variety of procedures used that aim to avoid impotence. There are a number of therapies and aids that can help with erectile dysfunction.

Table 16.6 TNM classification of prostate cancer

Primary tumour		
Tx		Primary tumour cannot be assessed
T0		No evidence of primary tumour
T1		Clinically the tumour is inapparent, neither palpable nor able to be seen by imaging
	T1a	Tumour incidental: histological finding in 5% or less of tissue resected
	T1b	Tumour incidental: histological finding in more than 5% of tissue resected
	T1c	Tumour is identified by needle biopsy (e.g. because of elevated PSA)
T2		Tumour confined within the prostate[1]
	T2a	Tumour involves one lobe
	T2b	Tumour involves both lobes
T3		Tumour extending through the prostate capsule[2]
	T3a	Extracapsular extension (unilateral or bilateral)
	T3b	Tumour invades seminal vesicle(s)
T4		Tumour is fixed or is invading adjacent structures other than seminal vesicles: bladder neck, external sphincter, rectum, levator muscles and/or pelvic wall
Regional lymph nodes involvement		
Nx		Regional lymph nodes cannot be assessed
N0		No regional lymph node metastasis
N1		Regional lymph node metastasis
Distant tumour spread (metastasis)[3]		
Mx		Unable to assess distant metastasis
M0		No distant metastasis
M1		Distant metastasis
	M1a	Non-regional lymph node(s)
	M1b	Bone(s)
	M1c	Other site(s)

1. Tumour found in one or both lobes by needle biopsy, but not palpable or visible by imaging is classified as T1c.
2. Invasion into the prostatic apex or into (but not beyond) the prostatic capsule is not classified as T3, but as T2.
3. When more than one site of metastasis is present, the most advanced category should be used.

Sources: adapted from Cancer Research UK 2010a, Parkinson and Feneley 2004.

beyond the prostate gland and into the surrounding tissue but not to other parts of the body. Metatastic disease (M1) occurs as a result of the tumour despite an increased trend toward early detection.

This section has provided insight into how tumours can be assessed with regard to growth and infiltration. Research has been carried out and continues to carried out in order to help

men with regard to prevention and treatment of prostate disease. This next section considers research activity.

Prostate cancer, research for prevention

Taneja *et al.* (2006) report findings from a study looking at whether the drug toremifene used to treat men with abnormal prostate growth might help prevent the growths from becoming malignant. The drug, which blocks some of the effects of oestrogen, had previously been used to treat advanced breast cancer in women. Men who have prostate intraepithelial neoplasia (PIN) have about a 30% chance of developing prostate cancer in one year and about a 65% chance within two years. Other studies reported that men who took statins (to treat high cholesterol) were less likely to have prostate cancer.

Treatments

There is currently no consensus regarding the best treatment for men with early prostate cancer. Current knowledge does not provide a definitive answer to the options that are available that will result in the most favourable outcome. Table 16.7 outlines some of the treatment options (with intent and drawbacks) for men with localised prostate cancer.

Watchful waiting is not advised for those who are aged less than 60 years; in those aged 60 and 70 years best practice is unclear. The management of early prostate cancer is controversial; it cannot be overemphasised that the man must be fully informed of the options available to him.

Selection of men offered the watchful waiting approach is based on the premise that many of the men are elderly with a

Table 16.7 Some treatment options available for localised prostate cancer

Watchful waiting	Radical prostatectomy (retropubic, perineal or laproscopic)	External radical radiotherapy (external beam, conformal) bracytherapy
Intent and benefit: surveillance; non-invasive.	*Intent and benefit;* aim to cure.	*Intent and benefit:* aim to cure.
Drawbacks: metatastic cancer can develop; uncertainty.	*Drawbacks:* impotence up to 80%*; incontinence up to 20%*; mortality – range between 0.2 and 1.2%; 40% have residual tumour post-surgery.	*Drawbacks:* impotence up to 60%*; incontinence up to 5%*; long-term complications such as diarrhoea/bowel problems in up to 10%*.

* These percentages will vary according to case selection, surgical expertise and the length of follow-up.

Source: adapted from Cancer Research UK 2009, Kirby and Brawer 2004.

relatively short life expectancy, and that their prostate cancer is likely to progress very slowly, may not cause symptoms and will not be their cause of death (Cancer Research UK 2009). The nurse acts as the man's advocate (for example, to liaise on his behalf) and to ensure that he is given enough information to appreciate the rationale for the approach that has been selected for him. The nurse also supports the man in engaging with the process that is undertaken concerning proposed treatment options.

The purpose of treatment concerning 'early disease' (sometimes known as localised disease) (Kirby and Brawer 2004) is to aim to cure. There are two curative choices available, and each option is based on individual evaluation of the person:

- radical prostatectomy;
- radical radiotherapy.

In all approaches, the use of hormone therapy is also considered. Survival rates are high when using all three approaches. Ten-year survival rates are outlined in Table 16.8.

Active surveillance (Cancer Research UK 2009) is another option. A fourth option available entails careful monitoring of localised prostate cancer in attempts to determine its biological aggressiveness with the choice of suggesting curative treatment if the disease extensively progresses.

The nurse should offer reasons why (if appropriate) watchful waiting is the mode of treatment being suggested to the man (NICE 2008). Review includes assessment of PSA levels at frequent intervals. If there is a sequential rise in PSA levels, or the man becomes worried or anxious, he may be offered rebiopsy and the option of commencing therapy. The man needs as much information as possible to make an informed choice. The likelihood and probability of side-effects of treatment must be discussed.

The treatment is complex and depends on the grade and stage of the cancer as well as the age, general health and preference of the man. In some cases, for example, when the man with a slow-growing tumour has a limited life expectancy, watchful waiting is the treatment of choice. Treatments for prostate cancer include surgery, radiation therapy and hormone manipulation.

Surgery

Surgery for prostate cancer includes several types of prostatectomies. For very early disease in older men, cure may be achieved with a simple prostatectomy (a TURP), discussed in the section on benign prostate hyperplasia.

Table 16.8 Ten-year survival rates for three approaches to the management of early prostate cancer

Approach	Estimated ten-year survival
Radical prostatectomy	80–90%
Radical radiotherapy	65–90%
Watchful waiting	70–90%

Sources: adapted from Donovan *et al.* 1999, Cancer Research UK, 2009.

Table 16.9 Potential complications related to radical prostatectomy and radiation therapy

Radical prostatectomy	Radiation therapy
Erectile dysfunction	Erectile dysfunction*
Urethral stricture	Urethral stricture
Fistula/rectal injury	Rectal/anal stricture*
Urinary incontinence	Cystitis
Surgical/anaesthetic risk	Diarrhoea
	Proctitis
	Rectal ulcer
	Bowel obstruction*
	Urinary incontinence

* Delayed complications; may appear months or years after completion of therapy.

- *Radical prostatectomy* involves removal of the prostate, prostate capsule, seminal vesicles and a portion of the bladder neck. Many people experience varying degrees of urinary incontinence and ED (see Table 16.9). A newer treatment is laparoscopic radical prostatectomy (LRP). Small incisions are made in the abdomen and a laparoscope is inserted and used to remove the prostate.
- *Retropubic prostatectomy* may be performed, allowing adequate control of bleeding, visualisation of the prostate bed and bladder neck and access to pelvic lymph nodes.
- *Perineal prostatectomy* is preferred for older men or those who are poor surgical risks. This requires less time and involves less bleeding.
- *Suprapubic prostatectomy* is used when problems with the bladder are expected. Control of bleeding is more difficult because the surgical approach is through the bladder.

For men with stage III, locally advanced (beyond the prostatic capsule) cancer, surgery is controversial because of the likelihood of hidden lymph node metastasis and relapse. TURP is not performed as curative therapy, but it may be used to relieve urinary obstruction for men with advanced disease.

Surgical intervention is available for men with urinary sphincter insufficiency, which is the major cause of incontinence after prostatectomy. An artificial urinary sphincter is surgically implanted (Figure 16.7). The man must be able to manipulate the pump placed in the scrotum and have adequate cognitive function to know when a problem with the appliance occurs.

This section has considered a number of treatment options. For some men, however, their condition may mean (or they may choose) that surgical intervention alone is insufficient. Other treatment modalities are now discussed.

Radiation therapy

This may be used as a primary treatment for prostate cancer. Long-term problems of erectile dysfunction and urinary incontinence may be avoided, and survival rates are often comparable. Radiation may be delivered by external beam or

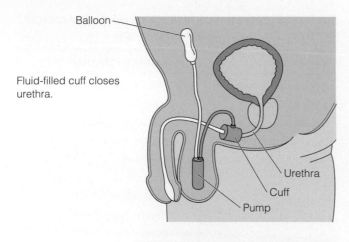

Balloon

Fluid-filled cuff closes urethra.

Urethra

Cuff

Pump

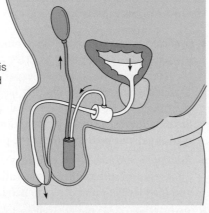

To void, bladder pump is squeezed, drawing fluid from cuff to balloon. Urine drains through open urethra.

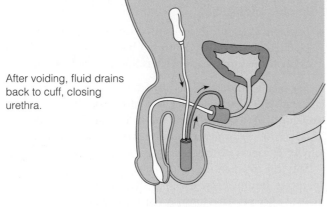

After voiding, fluid drains back to cuff, closing urethra.

Figure 16.7 Method of operation and artificial urinary sphincter.

interstitial implants of radioactive seeds of iodine, gold, palladium or iridium (*brachytherapy*). Interstitial radiation has a lower risk of erectile dysfunction and rectal damage than external-beam radiation. See Chapter 2 for nursing care of the person receiving radiation therapy.

Radiation therapy has a palliative role for men with metastatic prostate cancer, reducing the size of bone metastasis, controlling pain and restoring function, such as continence or the ability to mobilise for those with spinal cord compression. As the cancer increases so does the pain. Cancer pain has many dimensions, including the physical, spiritual, psychological and social; nurses must take these into account when assessing planning, implementing and evaluating pain control measures (SIGN 2008).

Hormonal manipulation

Androgen deprivation therapy is used to treat advanced prostate cancer. Many cells in the growing tumour are androgen-dependent and either cease to grow or die if deprived of androgens. Other cancer cells thrive without androgen and are unaffected by therapy to reduce circulating androgens. Therefore, the effects of hormone manipulations vary from complete but temporary regression of the tumour to no response at all. Strategies to induce androgen deprivation vary from orchiectomy to oral administration of hormonal agents. Table 16.10 compares surgical and hormone therapies. New drugs are being developed that block the effects of male hormones, and research is being conducted to demonstrate what mix of hormones is best.

NURSING CARE FOR PROSTATE CANCER

Nursing interventions vary and may range from teaching to using knowledge and skill in physical care following a radical prostatectomy. A Nursing Care Plan for a man undergoing a prostatectomy can be found on page 631.

Health promotion

Nurses can increase public awareness about early detection of prostate cancer. Every encounter with men and their families is an opportunity to provide information about early detection and identify needs. Studies have shown a positive correlation between increased awareness of and participation in prostate cancer screening procedures. Cancer Research UK has a number of free leaflets and a very extensive web resource available about cancer including the early detection, which can be useful in educating the public (http://www.cancerhelp.org.uk/default.asp).

Men should know that they can lower their risk of prostate cancer by eating less red meat and fat. They should include fruits and vegetables such as tomatoes, pink grapefruit and watermelon which are high in lycopenes helping prevent damage to DNA and which may help lower prostate cancer risk. Other substances that may help are vitamin E and selenium.

Men should be given information about the limitations and benefits of testing for early detection and of treatment so that they can make an informed decision. In the UK, men over 45 years of age can ask their GP or practice nurse for a PSA test, but it is not offered as standard. Currently, approximately 6% of men ask for this test. Digital rectal examination and TRUS are offered to men based on clinical assessment and need. In general practice, for example, some men may approach the nurse requesting assessment of their PSA. The nurse should be prepared to provide advice to those men, helping them to fully understand the potential and limitations of PSA. The approach that may be taken when responding to a man's request for PSA testing is outlined in the In Practice box.

Table 16.10 Surgical and hormone* therapy in the management of advanced prostate cancer

Treatment	Advantages	Disadvantages
Orchidectomy	• Inexpensive. • Immediate effect, i.e. men report diminished pain from metastasis in the recovery room.	• Body image problems due to loss of testicles.
Oestrogen compounds (diethylstilbestrol)	• Inexpensive. • Effects reversible.	• Increased risk of cardiovascular problems. • More likely to cause gynaecomastia, hypertrophy of breast tissue.
Luteinising hormone-releasing hormone agonist (LHRH)	• Effects reversible. • No cardiovascular risk. • Monthly administration.	• Expensive. • Subcutaneous injection route. • Slow onset: up to four weeks.
Steroidal antiandrogens (megestrol [Megace])	• Effects reversible. • No cardiovascular risk. • Inexpensive.	• May not drop testosterone levels sufficiently. • Weight gain.
Non-steroidal antiandrogens (flutamide; often used in conjunction with LHRH)	• Does not alter circulating androgens. • Blocks some side-effects of LHRH. • May be effective if other methods fail.	• Expensive.

* All hormonal manipulations have the potential disadvantage of loss of libido, erectile dysfunction, hot flushes and gynaecomastia.

IN PRACTICE

PSA testing

● The PSA test is not 100% accurate.

● There are no side-effects to having the blood test.

● One in three men who have elevated PSA levels will have prostate cancer.

● Anxiety and worry may be experienced if tests performed later are all negative.

● Usually, even if cancer has been detected nothing can be done until it begins to impact on health and wellbeing Treatment can be recommended but is not without risk.

● There is disagreement relating to the most appropriate way of treating prostate cancer.

● Screening for prostate cancer does not seem to be associated with lower prostate specific mortality.

● In the end, you must decide for yourself what it is you want. Take some time to think over the issues.

Source: adapted from Longmore et al. 2005.

Assessment

Collect the following data through the health history and physical examination. Note that a DRE is an advanced nursing assessment.

✚ *Health history*: risk factors, urinary elimination patterns and manifestations, haematuria and pain.

✚ *Physical assessment*: DRE to assess prostate size, symmetry, firmness and nodules.

Consider this . . .

When assessing the person in relation to prostate cancer he confides in you that he thinks he may have caused this by engaging in anal sex. How do you respond to this?

Nursing diagnoses and interventions

Nursing care must be holistic, sensitive and individualised. The nursing diagnoses discussed for the man with BPH may also be appropriate. This section focuses on problems with urinary incontinence, sexual function and pain.

Risk for urinary incontinence (reflex, stress, total)

This is a disturbing complication following treatment for prostate cancer. Radical prostatectomy and external-beam radiation therapy can cause incontinence, ranging from stress incontinence to no control at all. Older men may experience *urge incontinence*, the involuntary passage of urine soon after a strong sense of urgency to void. The man's reaction to incontinence may be severe even if the incontinence is not great. Many men have significant anxiety at the prospect of incontinence as they feel shame and often guilt about the loss of control.

✚ Assess the degree of incontinence and its effects on lifestyle.

✚ Teach pelvic floor exercises to help restore continence.

✦ Teach methods to control dampness and odour from stress incontinence:
  - do not attempt to prevent accidental voiding by restricting fluids;
  - manage occasional episodes (one to three small-volume accidents per day) with absorbent pads worn inside the underwear and changed as needed – most pads are made with a polymer gel that controls odour.

✦ Refer to a physiotherapist or a continence nurse for additional measures to promote continence.

✦ Explore options such as an external collection device for the man with total incontinence.

✦ Encourage verbalising feelings about the impact of incontinence on quality of life.

Risk for sexual dysfunction

Surgical treatment for prostate cancer may cause ED and changes in ejaculatory function. Hormone therapy for advanced prostate cancer lowers libido and may also cause ED. Diagnosis of cancer and body image changes may lower self-esteem, which can diminish sexual desire and willingness to interact sexually with a partner. Many older men are active sexually and capable of sustaining an erection. They may fear the effect of treatment on their sexual health. A nurse who listens and does not make any prejudgements can encourage open conversation about concerns. They may allow this concern to guide their decision about the treatment, or they may refuse all therapy because of this fear. Reactions vary.

✦ Assess pre-treatment sexual function.

✦ Teach the man about the actual or potential effects of therapy on sexual function.

✦ Provide an opportunity to discuss implications of and concerns about the diagnosis and treatment of sexual function.

✦ Discuss medical and surgical treatments for ED (see page 621).

✦ Refer for sexual counselling as appropriate.

> ### *Consider this . . .*
>
> Men feel that when they go to healthcare settings, these places are often very 'feminine'. Sometimes they feel 'out of place' and are conscious of being male in a predominantly female environment – all the nurses may be female, the receptionist is female and the doctor is also female. Posters on the wall are usually aimed at women and children (breast cancer checks, smear tests, immunisations), the magazines in the waiting room are always female-orientated. They feel that this can put them off coming in and seeking help and advice.
>
> The above issues can deter men from accessing much needed healthcare. What could you do to ensure that access to healthcare facilities are opened up as widely as possible to all men of all ages, sexuality and ethnic background?

Risk for acute/chronic pain

There are many causes of pain associated with advanced prostate cancer. It is not unusual for a man to have three or four distinct pains simultaneously, all from different sources. The most common cause of pain is metastasis to the spinal column. Other sources include fractures, lymphoedema of the lower extremities and muscle spasms. Because most men with prostate cancer are over 65, many also have pain associated with pre-existing conditions, such as osteoarthritis, unrelated to the cancer.

✦ Assess the intensity, location and quality of the pain.

✦ Provide optimal pain relief with prescribed analgesics.

Teach the man and his family non-invasive methods of pain control.

COMMUNITY-BASED CARE

Depending on the type of treatment, the following should be addressed in preparing the man with prostate cancer and his family for home care:

● For a surgical procedure: manifestations of infection and excessive bleeding, catheter care, wound care, pain management.

● For radiation therapy:
  - danger of radiation damage to others (sleep in a room alone for a week, avoid close contact with pregnant women and children);
  - condom use during sexual contact (ejaculate may be discoloured, distressing sexual partner).

● The importance of keeping out-patient appointments and having PSA and rectal examinations as planned.

● If appropriate, community services, such as support groups, district nurses and hospice.

Helpful resources include:

● Cancer Research UK;

● Institute of Cancer Research;

● National Institute for Health and Clinical Excellence.

This section has addressed a number of reproductive health issues and provided insight and understanding. The next section considers issues that the man may experience associated with the breast. Often conditions such as breast cancer are connected with women. Men can and do experience conditions associated with the breast.

MALE BREAST DISORDERS

The man with gynaecomastia

Gynaecomastia, the abnormal enlargement of the male breast, is thought to result from a high ratio of oestradiol to testosterone. It is common during puberty, affecting one breast in as many as 50% of adolescent males, resolving within one to two years. Any condition that increases oestrogen activity or decreases testosterone production can contribute to gynaecomastia. These include obesity, testicular tumours, liver disease and adrenal carcinoma; conditions that decrease testosterone production include chronic illness such as tuberculosis or Hodgkin's disease, injury and orchitis. Drugs such as digitalis, opiates and chemotherapeutic agents are also associated with gynaecomastia. Gynaecomastia after adolescence is usually bilateral. If unilateral, biopsy may be necessary to rule out breast cancer.

No treatment is necessary for the transient gynaecomastia of puberty. If the condition becomes chronic, creating psychological discomfort, surgery may be necessary, removing subcutaneous breast tissue. When related to an underlying disorder, treatment of that disorder is required. In severe cases, tamoxifen is given to decrease oestrogen activity.

Nursing care for the man with gynaecomastia includes education about the cause and treatment of the condition, and emotional support for the psychosocial implications of this feminising condition.

The man with breast cancer

Male breast cancer is rare, accounting for about 1% of all breast cancer cases, but it is as serious to the men who have it as it is to the women. About 300 men in the UK are diagnosed with breast cancer each year, compared to 45 700 cases in women (Cancer Research UK 2011b), accounting for approximately 70 deaths (Cancer Research UK 2011c). The aetiology of male breast cancer is unclear; hormonal, genetic and perhaps environmental factors appear to be important.

Male and female breast cancer are clinically and histologically similar, although lobular cancer is rare in males. Most tumours are oestrogen-receptor positive. Many men believe that breast cancer is only a woman's disease and they delay seeking medical attention for symptoms and may present with advanced disease.

INTERDISCIPLINARY CARE FOR MALE BREAST CANCER

Treatment is much like the treatment of female breast cancer, beginning with modified radical mastectomy, node dissection and staging to determine the therapeutic options. Radiation, chemotherapy and hormonal therapy are the conventional adjuncts to surgery. Surgical removal of the testes is the most successful palliative measure in men with advanced breast cancer, resulting in tumour regression and prolonging life.

PRACTICE ALERT

Some men, just like women, when given a diagnosis of breast cancer may be confused, unbelieving, scared and anxious, and nursing care should take this into account when working with the male with breast cancer. Breast cancer in the male does not mean the man is any less 'manly'. Consideration must be given to any information provided; for example, it must depict issues from a male perspective.

NURSING CARE FOR MALE BREAST CANCER

Nursing care is essentially the same as for the woman with breast cancer (see Chapter 15). The nurse has an opportunity to help the man and his family cope with the psychosocial effects of having breast cancer. He may feel embarrassment or shame about his condition and fear about the life-threatening nature of the disease. Working in a way that demonstrates empathic understanding can alleviate fears and apprehensions. By listening with understanding and empathy, the nurse can help the man and his family resolve feelings and move toward healing.

 CASE STUDY SUMMARIES

We will now consider the outcome for both people in the case studies at the beginning of the chapter.

Case Study 1. A male doctor was found in the practice to examine Zamir. This reduced his anxiety and helped him to relax so that a detailed physical examination could be performed. A testicular lump was evident upon examination on the epididymis; further examination of the local lymph nodes revealed no evidence of lymphadenopathy. An ultrasound examination was booked as matter of urgency and Zamir informed his parents who accompanied him to the x-ray department. Further investigations demonstrated that the lump was caused by a cyst. Surgical excision was performed and Zamir made a good recovery.

Case Study 2. Mr William Turner was visited by the district nurse when he returned home and an assessment of his needs was made. The nurse noted that Mr Turner was finding it difficult to care for his catheter and mobilise and that his elderly wife also struggled to help him. Despite intensive interventions, Mr Turner developed a urinary tract infection, became confused and he was unwilling to mobilise. Arrangements were made to readmit Mr Turner for intravenous antibiotics and further nursing care. After two days on the ward Mr Turner suffered a pulmonary embolism and died despite attempts to resuscitate him. His wife was visiting when the incident occurred; she now lives in sheltered accommodation.

CHAPTER HIGHLIGHTS

- Disorders of male sexual function include erectile dysfunction (ED) and ejaculatory dysfunction. Different illnesses, medications and surgical procedures may affect male sexual function. Treatments include medications, mechanical devices and surgical procedures. It is important for nurses to initiate a discussion of sexual concerns during assessments, recognising that male reproductive treatments and surgeries may result in sexual dysfunction.

- Phimosis and priapism, disorders of the penis, can cause problems with urination and sexual activity and may be considered medical emergencies. The risk of cancer of the penis, although rare, is increased by phimosis, poor genital hygiene and viral HPV and HIV infections.

- Benign scrotal masses include hydrocele, spermatocele and varicocele. Epididymitis may be associated with a urinary tract infection, prostatitis, urethral strictures or a sexually transmitted infection.

- The testes may be infected (orchitis), twisted (testicular torsion) or develop cancer. Testicular cancer is the most common cancer in men between the ages of 15 and 40. Case Study 1 is about a young man with testicular concerns. Monthly testicular self-examination is critical to early detection and treatment of cancer.

- The prostate gland may be inflamed or infected (prostatitis), enlarged (benign prostatic hyperplasia [BPH]) or develop cancer. BPH is a common disorder of the ageing male, causing problems with urination as the enlarging prostate gland constricts the urethra. Treatments include medications and surgery, depending on the size of the prostate and the age and health status of the man.

- Cancer of the prostate is the most common type of cancer and the second leading cause of death in men. When diagnosed early, prostate cancer is curable. Diagnosis is often based on an increasing level of PSA and an abnormal DRE. Reconsider Case Study 2 in light of what you have read in this chapter.

- The male breast may become enlarged (gynaecomastia) or develop cancer.

TEST YOURSELF

1. Sperm and testosterone are produced by the:
   a. epididymis
   b. seminal vesicles
   c. testes
   d. Cowper's glands

2. You are assessing a 65-year-old man. He says, 'I don't understand how having prostate problems can cause me to urinate all the time.' What would you say to begin your explanation?
   a. 'The prostate gland presses on the bladder.'
   b. 'The prostate gland surrounds your urethra.'
   c. 'Your kidneys respond to prostate enlargement.'
   d. 'The prostate glands sit on top of the kidneys.'

3. What blood test may be used to diagnose prostate cancer?
   a. PSA
   b. VDRL
   c. CBC
   d. WBC

4. Suspected abnormalities of the scrotum may be further assessed through:
   a. transillumination
   b. auscultation
   c. palpation
   d. percussion

5. When conducting a health assessment, which of the following statements would most likely elicit information about sexual concerns?

    a. 'Following your prostate surgery, when did you first notice you had problems with sexual intercourse?'

    b. 'Why do you think you should be sexually active at your age?'

    c. 'Do you miss having sex?'

    d. 'Tell me about your experience with sexual function since you developed prostate enlargement.'

6. You are conducting a health teaching session for young men. What topic would be appropriate to reduce the risk of cancer of the penis?

    a. wearing a condom during sexual intercourse

    b. retracting the foreskin of the penis when showering

    c. avoiding tight pants and very hot showers

    d. maintaining a regular testicular self-examination schedule

7. What disease of the male reproductive system is a risk if a man also has a sexually transmitted infection (gonorrhoea)?

    a. epididymitis

    b. hydrocele

    c. erectile dysfunction

    d. gynaecomastia

8. Which of the following statements is true of testicular cancer?

    a. the incidence increases with age

    b. it occurs most between ages 15 and 40

    c. it rarely occurs in brothers

    d. severe pain is the initial manifestation

9. You are teaching a man with chronic prostatitis how to care for himself at home. What measures can be used to decrease discomfort?

    a. take cold showers

    b. wear a scrotal support and take anti-inflammatory drugs

    c. increase oral fluid intake to 3 L/day and void often

    d. increase fibre intake and avoid sexual activity

10. What diagnostic tests are used to differentiate BPH from prostate cancer? (Choose all that apply.)

    a. pelvic ultrasound

    b. digital rectal examination

    c. blood chemistry

    d. PSA level

    e. sperm count

Further resources

Bladder and Bowel Foundation
http://www.bladderandbowelfoundation.org
Charity providing information and support for people with bladder and bowel disorders, their carers, families and healthcare professionals.

British Association for Counselling and Psychotherapy (BACP)
http://www.counselling.co.uk
BACP ensures that it meets its remit of public protection whilst also developing and informing its members. BACP participates in the development of counselling and psychotherapy at an international level.

Cancer Research UK
http://www.cancerresearchuk.org
Cancer Research UK is the world's leading independent organisation dedicated to cancer research, supporting research into all aspects of cancer.

Embarrassing Problems.com
http://www.embarrassingproblems.com
Independent advice concerning a wide range of embarrassing problems.

Everyman
http://www.everyman-campaign.org
A charity providing information to members of the public and healthcare workers. Everyman is dedicated to winning the fight against male cancer.

Infertility Network UK
http://www.infertilitynetworkuk.com
Provides authoritative information and practical and emotional support, with the aim of raising the profile and understanding of infertility issues in all quarters and striving for timely and consistent provision of infertility care throughout the UK.

London Lesbian and Gay Switchboard (LLGS)
http://www.llgs.org.uk
LLGS provides an information, support and referral service for lesbians, gay men, bisexual people and anyone who needs to consider issues around their sexuality.

Orchid Cancer Appeal
www.orchid-cancer.org.uk
The only UK registered cancer charity to focus entirely on the male-specific cancers.

Prostate Cancer Charity
http://www.prostate-cancer.org.uk
The UK's leading voluntary organisation working with people affected by prostate cancer.

The Men's Health Forum
http://www.menshealthforum.org.uk
An independent body working with a wide range of individuals and organisations for the development of health services that aim

to meet men's needs and to encourage men to change their risk-taking behaviours.

The Samaritans
http://www.samaritans.org
Samaritans is confidential emotional support service for anyone in the UK and Ireland. The service is available 24 hours a day for people who are experiencing feelings of distress or despair, including those which may lead to suicide.

Bibliography

Albaugh J and Kellog-Spadt S (2003a) Intimacy issues. Man's search for ultimate sex. Viagra abuse. *Urologic Nursing*, 23(1), 75–76.

Albaugh J and Kellog-Spadt S (2003b) Sexuality and sexual health: The nurse's role and initial approach to patients. *Urologic Nursing*, 23(3), 227–228.

Baldwin K C, Ginsberg P C, Roehrborn C G and Harkaway R C (2001) Discontinuation of alpha-blockade after initial treatment with finasteride and doxazosin in men with lower urinary tract symptoms and clinical evidence of benign prostatic hyperplasia. *Urology*, 58, 203–209.

Bickley L, Szilagyi P and Bates B (2009) *Bates' Guide to Physical Examination and History Taking*. Philadelphia, PA, Lippincott.

BPSA (2009) *Chronic Prostatitis*. British Prostatitis Support Organisation, available at: http://www.bps-assoc.org.uk/info.cfm (accessed September 2011).

Brown C (2004a) Testicular cancer: An overview. *Urologic Nursing*, 24(2), 83–88, 93–94.

Brown O A (2004b) Understanding postoperative hyponatremia. *Urologic Nursing*, 24(3), 197–201.

Calabrese D (2004) Prostate cancer in older men. *Urologic Nursing*, 24(4), 258–264, 268–269.

Cancer Research UK (2009) *Prostate Cancer Symptoms and Treatment*. London: available at: http://info.cancerresearchuk.org/cancerstats/types/prostate/symptomstreatment/ (accessed September 2011).

Cancer Research UK (2010a) *Prostate Cancer – Survival Statistics*. London, available at: http://info.cancerresearchuk.org/cancerstats/types/prostate/survival/#Prostate3 (accessed September 2011).

Cancer Research UK (2010b) *Prostate Cancer Tests*. London, available at: http://cancerhelp.cancerresearchuk.org/type/prostate-cancer/diagnosis/prostate-cancer-tests (accessed September 2011).

Cancer Research UK (2011a) *Prostate Cancer UK Incidence Statistics* London, available at: http://info.cancerresearchuk.org/cancerstats/types/prostate/incidence/#source1 (accessed September 2011).

Cancer Research UK (2011b) *Breast Cancer UK Incidence Statistics*. London, available at: http://info.cancerresearchuk.org/cancerstats/types/breast/incidence/#source1 (accessed September 2011).

Cancer Research UK (2011c) *Latest UK Cancer Incidence (2008) and Mortality (2008) Summary*. London, available at: http://info.cancerresearchuk.org/prod_consump/groups/cr_common/@nre/@sta/documents/generalcontent/cr_072109.pdf (accessed September 2011).

Clinical Resource Efficiency Support Team (2003) *The Management of Hyponatraemia in Adults*. Belfast, CREST.

Coleman M P, Rachet B, Woods L M, *et al.* (2004) Trends and socioeconomic inequalities in cancer survival in England and Wales up to 2001. *British Journal of Cancer*, 90(7), 1367–1373.

Davison B J, Moore K, MacMillan H, Bisaillon A and Wiens K (2004) Patient evaluation of a discharge program following a radical prostatectomy. *Urology Nursing*, 24(6), 483–489.

Dochterman J and Bulechek G (2004) *Nursing Interventions Classification (NIC)* (4th edn). St Louis, MO, Mosby.

Donovan J L, Frankel S J, Faulkner A, *et al.* (1999) Dilemmas in treating early prostate cancer: the evidence and a questionnaire survey of consultant urologists in the UK. *British Medical Journal*, 318, 299–300.

Dorey G, Speakman M, Feneley R, *et al.* (2004) Pelvic floor exercises for treating post-micturition dribble in men with erectile dysfunction: A randomized trial. *Urologic Nursing*, 24(6), 490–497, 512.

European Association of Urology (2005) *Guidelines on Erectile Dysfunction*, Arnhem, EAV, available at: http://www.uroweb.org/fileadmin/user_upload/Guidelines/2005ErectileDysfunction.pdf (accessed August 2011).

Ferlay J, Bray F, Pisani P, Parkin D M and GLOBOCAN 2002 (2004) *Cancer Incidence. Mortality and Prevalence Worldwide*, IARC CancerBase No. 5, version 2.0. Lyon, IARC Press.

Gleason D (1966) Classification of prostatic carcinoma. *Cancer Chemotherapy Reports*, 50, 125–128.

Hirsh A (2003) the ABC of subfertility: male subfertility. *British Medical Journal*, 237, 669.

ISD/NHS National Services Scotland (2007) *Trends in Cancer Survival in Scotland, 1980–2004*. Edinburgh, Information Services Division.

Kee J (2004) *Handbook of Laboratory and Diagnostic Tests with Nursing Implications* (5th edn). Upper Saddle River, NJ, Prentice Hall.

Kirby R S and Brawer M K (2004) *Prostate Cancer* (4th edn). Abingdon: Health Press.

Kvåle R, Auvinen A, Adami H O, *et al.* (2007) Interpreting trends in prostate cancer incidence and mortality in the five Nordic countries. *Journal of the National Cancer Institute*, 24, 1881–1887.

Leonard B (2004) Women's conditions occurring in men: Breast cancer, osteoporosis, male menopause, and eating disorders. *Nursing Clinics of North America*, 39(2), 379–393.

Longmore M, Wilkinson I B and Rajagopalan S (2005) *Oxford Handbook of Clinical Medicine* (6th edn). Oxford, Oxford University Press.

McPhee S J and Papadakis M A (eds) (2011) *Current Medical Diagnosis & Treatment* (50th edn). New York, Lange McGraw-Hill.

Moorhead S, Johnson M and Maas M (2003) *Nursing Outcomes Classification (NOC)* (3rd edn). St Louis, MO, Mosby.

Moyad M (2003) Complementary and preventive medicine. Lifestyle changes to prevent BPH: Heart healthy = prostate healthy. *Urologic Nursing*, 23(6), 439–441.

Mueller N and Mueller E (2004) KTP photoselective laser vaporization of the prostate: Indications, procedure, and nursing implications. *Urologic Nursing*, 24(5), 373–379.

Nash M (2003) Best practice for patient self-cleaning of urinary drainage bags. *Urologic Nursing*, 23(5), 334, 339.

Nazarko L (2007) Bladder pain from indwelling urinary cathertization: case study. *British Journal of Nursing*, 16(9), 511–514.

NICE (2006) *Laparoscopic Retroperitoneal Lymph Node Dissection for Testicular Cancer*. London, National Institute for Health and Clinical Excellence.

NICE (2008) *Prostate Cancer. Diagnosis and Treatment*. London, National Institute for Health and Clinical Excellence.

Oliffe J (2004) Transrectal ultrasound prostate biopsy (TRUS-Bx): Patient perspectives. *Urologic Nursing*, **24**(5), 395–400.

ONS (2008) *Cancer Statistics Registrations: Registrations of cancer diagnosed in 2005, England*, Series MB1 no 35. London, Office for National Statistics.

Parkinson R J and Feneley M R (2004) The PSA debate, in Kirby R S, Carson C C, Kirby M G and Farah R N (eds), *Men's Health* (2nd edn). Oxford, Taylor Francis, 299–313.

Parrott E (2003) TUNA of the prostate in an office setting: Nursing implications. *Urologic Nursing*, **23**(1), 33–40.

Peate I (2007) Men's Health. The Practice Nurse's Handbook. Chichester, Wiley.

Porth C M (2009) *Pathophysiology: Concepts of altered health states* (9th edn). Philadelphia, PA, Lippincott.

Quinn M and Babb P (2002) Patterns and trends in prostate cancer incidence, survival, prevalence and mortality individual countries, *British Journal of Urology International*, **97**(7), 1367–1373.

Schroder F, Hermanek P, Denis L, *et al.* (1992) The TNM classification of prostate cancer, *Prostate*, **4** (supplement), 129–138.

SIGN (2008) *Control of Pain in Adults with Cancer. A National Clinical Guideline*. Edinburgh, Scottish Intercollegiate Guidelines Network.

Tamimi R and Adami H O (2002) Testicular cancer, in Adami H O, Hunter D and Trichopoulos D (eds), *Textbook of Cancer Epidemiology*. Oxford, Oxford University Press.

Taneja S S, Smith M R, Dalton J T, *et al.* (2006) Toremifene – a promising therapy for the prevention of prostate cancer and complications of androgen deprivation therapy. *Expert Opinion on Investigational Drugs*, **15**(3), 293–305.

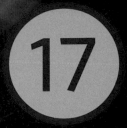

Caring for people with sexually transmitted infections

Learning outcomes

- Explain the incidence, prevalence, characteristics and prevention/control of **sexually transmitted infections** (STIs).
- Compare and contrast the pathophysiology, signs and symptoms, interdisciplinary care and nursing care of a number of STIs.
- Explain the risk factors for and complications of STIs.
- Discuss the effects and nursing implications of medications and treatments.

Clinical competencies

- Assess functional health status of persons with STIs and monitor, document and report abnormal signs and symptoms.
- Determine priority nursing diagnoses and select and implement individualised nursing interventions for persons with STIs.
- Administer topical, oral and injectable medications knowledgeably and safely.
- Integrate interdisciplinary care into the care of persons with STIs.
- Provide teaching appropriate for prevention, control and self-care of STIs.
- Revise plan of care as needed to provide effective interventions to promote, maintain or restore functional health status to persons with STIs.

CASE STUDIES

Below are three case studies that you may wish to consider before, during or after you have read the chapter. There are no right or wrong answers to these case studies, but you should think about the physical, psychological and social implications.

Case Study 1 – Janek

Janek Jaskalainen, a 16-year-old schoolboy, is being treated for **gonorrhoea** and **chlamydia** for the second time in six months. While counselling the young man, the school nurse learns that he has only one sexual partner, but she thinks that his boyfriend might not consider their relationship monogamous. Janek's boyfriend refuses to wear a condom because he says he wants to really enjoy having sex with him and a condom would interfere with that. Janek does not want to confront his boyfriend because he is afraid of losing him. Janek says to the nurse, 'What's the big deal anyway? Gonorrhoea and chlamydia are curable.'

Case Study 2 – Janet

Ms Janet Cirit, a 33-year-old legal secretary, lives in a suburban community. She is unmarried but seeing a man named Jim Adkins, who lives in an adjacent suburb. Ms Cirit visits her gynaecologist because her periods have become irregular and she is experiencing pelvic pain and an abnormal amount of vaginal discharge. Recently she has developed a sore throat. The pelvic pain has begun to disrupt her sleeping pattern, and she is concerned that she might have cancer because her mother recently died of ovarian cancer.

Case Study 3 – Eddie

Mr Eddie Kratz, aged 22 years, works as a porter at a large hotel. For the past year, he has shared a small apartment with Maria Jones, who is five months pregnant with his child. Although he intends to marry Ms Jones before the baby is born, he has continued a previous relationship with a woman named Justine Simpson. His sexual activities with Ms Simpson have increased in frequency as Ms Jones's pregnancy has advanced. Recently, Mr Kratz has noticed a swelling in his groin and a sore on his penis.

INTRODUCTION

Everyone has the right to enjoy good sexual health. Sexual health is an important aspect of health and wellbeing, and it is important that people have the information, confidence and the means to make choices that are right for them. It helps people to develop positive relationships and allows them to protect themselves and their partners from infections and pregnancies that are unintended.

Infections transmitted by vaginal, oral and anal intimate contact and intercourse are referred to as sexually transmitted infections (STIs). Infections transmitted by sexual intercourse are also inappropriately labelled as *sexually transmitted diseases (STDs)* or *venereal diseases*. STIs also include systemic diseases (such as tuberculosis, hepatitis and HIV) that can be transmitted from an infected person to a partner.

Venus the goddess of love

Venereal refers to the sexual contact and the word comes from *Venus* the Roman goddess of love. Venereal disease is not singular, referring to the plural venereal diseases. We are aware that sexually transmitted infections have been around

for hundreds of years. **Syphilis** was one of the earliest identified STIs, an infection which once devastated European society. By the mid-20th century, humans were aware of a number of STIs, many of which became curable with the arrival of penicillin. Towards the end of the 20th century, however, more serious and life-threatening STIs such as HIV emerged, and drug-resistant forms of older STIs began to appear.

In the past, sexually transmitted infections were referred to as sexually transmitted diseases (STDs) or venereal disease (VD), but there has been a move from referring to STIs as STDs or VD. Other euphemisms are also used, for example the clap, pox or social disease. The term STI has a broader meaning. For example, a person may be infected with the possibility of infecting others but may not show the outwards signs of having a disease. The term disease can also carry with it negative connotations. An infection, it could be suggested, can be cured whereas a disease may not. It must be recognised that some STIs can also be contracted through the use of intravenous injections after a needle has been used by an infected person. Sometimes you will find that the terms STI and STD are used interchangeably.

There has also been a concerted effort to move away from the use of the words special clinics or genitourinary medicine (GUM) clinics to refer to care centres where people receive care in relation to various sexually acquired infections. This has been done in an attempt to reduce the stigma that may have been associated with these infections. Some clinics have now been renamed sexual and reproductive health clinics.

Sexual health is one of the six priority areas for Primary Care Trusts (PCTs) to commission comprehensive wellbeing and prevention services to meet the needs of their local population (Department of Health (DoH) 2008a). People are now able to access clinics more quickly than they have in the past, and the range of services they receive has greatly improved in range and quality. The nurse is central in attempting to make sure these improvements are sustained and embedded to ensure that progress being made is faster and, as a result, the rates of STIs and unintended pregnancies will be reduced (DoH 2009).

Developing your understanding of the various STIs will help you help the people you care for in a more confident and competent manner. It may also help you help others to prevent infections that can have a negative impact on health and wellbeing. An overview of a number of STIs will now be provided, incidence and prevalence will be addressed followed by the characteristics of the various STIs, the section concludes with prevention and control.

> ### Consider this . . .
>
> The Nursing and Midwifery Council's *The code*: Standards of conduct, performance and ethics for nurses and midwives (NMC 2008) (the code) states that:
>
> - You must treat people as individuals and respect their dignity.
> - You must not discriminate in any way against those in your care.
> - You must treat people kindly and considerately.
> - You must act as an advocate for those in your care, helping them to access relevant health and social care, information and support.
>
> When working with people in a variety of care settings with a variety of needs you may be helping those who have lifestyles that differ considerably from yours. You may in fact find some elements of their lifestyle, the way they choose to behave, abhorrent, and this may challenge your own values and beliefs (including your religious beliefs). How can you ensure that you uphold the tenets of the code by providing professional care that respects a person and does not discriminate in any way, being kind and considerate and acting as that person's advocate?
>
> Source: NMC 2008.

OVERVIEW OF SEXUALLY TRANSMITTED INFECTIONS

Sexually transmitted infections include those caused by bacteria, *chlamydiae*, viruses, fungi, protozoa and parasites. Portals of entry for these agents of transmission include the mouth, genitalia, urinary meatus, anus, rectum and skin. Sexually transmitted infections have many consequences, and nurses have the responsibility to teach persons who are sexually active how to prevent STIs, regardless of their gender, age or sexual orientation. Nurses have a critical role in the prevention of STIs by teaching people about these infections, their prevention, treatment and potential complications.

INCIDENCE AND PREVALENCE OF STIs

Sexually transmitted infections have reached epidemic proportions in the UK and are on the increase worldwide (DoH 2009). They are the most frequent infections encountered by professionals in the field of reproductive health.

Women and infants are disproportionately affected by STIs. Many STIs are more easily transmitted from a man to a woman than from a woman to a man. Women often experience few early signs and symptoms of the infection, delaying diagnosis and treatment. Furthermore, women are at greater risk for complications of STIs such as **pelvic inflammatory disease** (PID) and genital cancers.

Several factors help explain the escalating incidence of STIs. The so-called sexual revolution of the 1960s and 1970s, fuelled by 'the pill' and the freedom from unplanned pregnancy, led to a more permissive attitude about sexuality and increases in sexual activity and the number of sexual partners. In addition, since oral contraceptives or 'the pill' were

>
>
> ### FAST FACTS
>
> #### A national strategy for sexual health and HIV
>
> The aims of the first national strategy for sexual health and HIV in 2001 were to:
>
> - reduce transmission of HIV and STIs;
> - reduce prevalence of undiagnosed HIV and STIs;
> - reduce unintended pregnancy rates;
> - improve health and social care for people living with HIV;
> - reduce the stigma associated with HIV and STIs.
>
> Source: DoH 2001.

introduced to British women in 1961, they have replaced the condom as a birth control method for many couples. However, oral contraceptives do not protect against STIs, a fact of increasing importance.

STIs affect men and women of all ages, backgrounds and socioeconomic levels. Those aged 16–24 years (young people) are the age group most at risk of being diagnosed with an STI. This age group accounted for 65% of all chlamydia, 50% of genital warts and 50% of gonorrhoea infections diagnosed in GUM clinics across the UK in 2007 (Health Protection Agency (HPA) 2008). Illicit drug use, unprotected sexual activity and sexual activity with multiple partners are also associated with increased incidence of STIs (Blair 2004). Further factors in the increasing incidence are that young people are becoming sexually active at an earlier age and marrying later, and divorce is more common. These factors may result in them having more sexual partners in their lifetime.

The emergence of HIV has created a kind of 'epidemiological synergy' (that is, the interrelationships between HIV and other STIs) among all STIs. Other STIs, such as syphilis, herpes simplex virus (HSV) and chancroid, facilitate the transmission of HIV, and the immune suppression caused by HIV assists in the infectious process of other STIs. In fact, individuals who are infected with STIs are at greater risk of acquiring HIV if they are exposed to the virus. This is the result of several factors: genital ulcers create a portal of entry for HIV, non-ulcerative STIs increase the concentration of cells in genital secretions that can be targets for HIV and infection with both an STI and HIV results in an increased likelihood of having HIV in genital secretions and semen.

CHARACTERISTICS OF STIs

Although STIs are caused by various organisms, they have several characteristics in common:

● Most can be prevented by the use of condoms.

● They can be transmitted during both heterosexual and homosexual activities, including non-penetrating intimate exposure.

● For treatment to be effective, sexual partners of the infected person must also be treated to prevent spread.

● Two or more STIs frequently coexist in the same person.

The complications of STIs in women include PID (a condition involving inflammation of the upper genital tract), ectopic pregnancy (where the fertilised egg remains in the fallopian tube), infertility, chronic pelvic pain, neonatal (relating to the first four months after birth) illness and death and genital cancer. Some bacterial STIs can be cured through appropriate early treatment with antibiotics. Others, such as **genital herpes**, are chronic conditions that can be managed but not cured because they are caused by viruses. The most serious STI is HIV which at this time is incurable. Treatment guidelines for STIs are updated regularly and are available from a variety of organisations including the British Association for Sexual Health and

HIV (BASHH) and Medical Foundation for AIDS and Sexual Health (Medfash). As there is currently no cure for some STIs, the focus must be on prevention and control of transmission. The next section highlights some of the areas where the nurse has a role to play.

PREVENTION AND CONTROL OF STIs

The prevention and control of STIs is based on the principles of education, detection, effective diagnosis and treatment of infected persons; and evaluation, treatment and counselling of sex partners of people who are infected. The ability of the healthcare provider to obtain an accurate sexual history is essential to prevention and control efforts. The way the nurse approaches issues surrounding sexual health can do much to encourage the person to think about safer sex practices and other ways in which transmission can be reduced.

The most effective way to prevent sexual transmission of HIV and other STIs is to avoid sexual intercourse with an infected partner (it must be remembered that there are other ways of transmitting infection, e.g. through the use of contaminated needles). If a person chooses to have intercourse or engage in other forms of sexual activity with an infected partner or one whose infection status is unknown, a new condom should be used for each act of intercourse. This is also important when using injecting materials (for example, new drug-injecting paraphernalia should be used, and these include needles, syringes and spoons).

Prevention teaching for the person who is an injecting-drug user includes:

● Enrol or continue in a drug treatment programme.

● Do not use injection equipment that has been used by another person. If equipment is shared, first clean the syringe and needle with bleach and water (to reduce the rate of HIV transmission).

● If needles can legally be obtained in the community, obtain and use clean needles (needle exchange systems enable used needles and syringes to be replaced by sterile needles and syringes).

Eliminating further transmission and re-infection of STIs is critical to control. For treatable STIs, this means that referral of sex partners for diagnosis, treatment and counselling is essential. Suggested resources for people with STIs are listed in the Fast Facts below.

As you develop your nursing skills and your communications skills are enhanced and honed you will be able to make a positive contribution to the sexual health of people and their partners.

> **Consider this . . .**
> Should nurses be allowed to refuse to care for people with STIs?

COMMUNITY-BASED CARE

Outreach services to sex workers – innovation and creativity: mobile units & mobile clinics

There are some sex workers whose lifestyles are often hectic and solitary, with no permanent place of residence, loneliness and lack of a specific working place. Healthcare professionals therefore need to find new ways to contact the target group and provide them with medical and social services with respect to their health and wellbeing. Mobile units are one way of doing this; these are vans with essential medical equipment where the nurse and other healthcare workers are able to carry out straightforward medical examinations and STI screening and treatment. The vans are kitted out with basic laboratory apparatus allowing the conducting of STI testing as well as HIV and hepatitis testing. The vans also supply services that offer social support; for instance, they can provide educative materials, or at least have discussions with sex workers, attempting to assist and to resolve their problems.

The mobile units can be driven to the areas where street-based sex workers are actually working. The vans have the advantage that they are as mobile as the sex workers; the van moves as the working beat may move. One of the drawbacks with this mobile unit is that it may draw unwanted attention to the sex workers, from the police or local residents, who may be unhappy that sex is being sold in their locality. The van should avoid having obvious external markings on it.

There are alternatives to the van or vehicle and one is to have a mobile or 'satellite' clinic. This is where the nurse and other health professionals can take with them what equipment they need to a non-clinical location, for example a drop-in centre near the working beat, brothel or working flat, providing a basic screening service, with some offer of examinations, testing or treatment. This approach can be seen as more discreet than a mobile unit, whilst still offering the clinical service. It's an innovative way to take the clinic or some of its clinical services out to the target population, with the aim of engaging service users in screening, treatment programmes and interventions.

Source: Gaffney *et al.* 2008.

This next section provides you with an overview of some STIs. The STIs discussed are not a full list. There are more and you are encouraged to delve deeper into the topic area.

The person with genital herpes

Genital herpes has the potential to impact on a person's health and wellbeing. Genital herpes are caused by the herpes simplex viruses HSV-1 and HSV-2. Like most STIs, genital herpes are most commonly found in young, sexually active adults and can be associated with early onset of sexual activity and multiple

FAST FACTS

Resources for person with STIs

- Terrence Higgins Trust (a charity set up to respond to the HIV epidemic with the aim of helping to improve the nation's sexual health).
- Brook (an organisation that provides free and confidential sexual health advice specifically for the under 25s).
- Family Planning Association.
- Herpes Viruses Association.
- National Herpes Hotline.
- British Association for Sexual Health and HIV.

sexual partners. Genital HSV infection is the most common ulcerative STI in the UK and is associated with much physical and psychological morbidity (illness). In 2006, there were 21 698 diagnoses of first attack genital HSV made in GUM clinics in the UK, 13 306 in women and 8392 in men. This is equal to an overall rate of 43 and 29 per 100 000 population in women and men respectively. A substantial number of new diagnoses were also made in general practice (HPA 2008). There is no cure so the treatments are primarily symptomatic; that is, they are aimed at treating the symptoms the person presents with.

Pathophysiology of HSV

Understanding the pathophysiology of HSV can help you help others to prevent transmission. One hundred types of HSV viruses have been identified, with more than 30 affecting the urogenital area (for example the vulva, penis, scrotum). HSV-1 is associated with cold sores, but may be transmitted to the genital area by oral sex (fellatio or cunnilingus) or by self-inoculation through poor hand washing practices, transmitting the virus to other areas. HSV-2 is transmitted by sexual activity or during childbirth (as the child passes through the vaginal canal) from a woman infected with the virus, and is the virus that causes genital herpes. HSV infections begin with an exposure to the virus by contact with infectious lesions (a sore or any area where there is discontinuity of skin) or secretions. The virus then moves into the stratified squamous epithelium (a specific type of tissue), stimulating the replication of the epithelium and infecting the neurones that innervate (supply

IN PRACTICE

Barrier guidelines

Barrier protection	Teaching topics
Male condoms	✓ Use a new condom with each act of sexual intercourse. ✓ Handle carefully to avoid damaging the condom. ✓ Be sure no air is trapped in the end of the condom. ✓ Put the condom on when the penis is erect and before genital contact with partner. ✓ Ensure adequate lubrication exists during intercourse, using only water-based lubricants (e.g., KY jelly). Oil-based lubricants, such as petroleum jelly, massage oil, mineral oil, or body lotions can weaken condoms. ✓ Ensure adequate lubrication during vaginal and anal sex. ✓ Withdraw while the penis is erect and hold the condom firmly against the base of the penis during withdrawal. ✓ Use condoms when sharing sex toys such as dildos.
Female condoms	✓ The female condom is a lubricated polyurethane sheath with a ring on each end that is inserted into the vagina. It is an effective mechanical barrier to viruses.
Vaginal spermicides, sponges, diaphragms	✓ Vaginal spermicides used alone without condoms do not reduce the risk for cervical gonorrhoea, chlamydia or HIV infection. ✓ The diaphragm protects against cervical gonorrhoea, chlamydia and **trichomoniasis**, but not HIV.

with nerves) the area. HSV viruses are neurotropic viruses, meaning that they grow in neurones and can maintain their disease potential even when there are no signs and symptoms. The virus ascends through the peripheral nerves to the dorsal root ganglia (an area of the spinal cord), where it can remain dormant (in a sleeping state – inactive). For unknown reasons, the virus may reactivate and return to the nerve root of the skin, causing lesions. During dormancy, the virus is impervious to treatment. The incubation period (the time taken from initial infection to the development of clinical manifestations) ranges from six weeks to eight months (Porth 2009).

Signs and symptoms of HSV

Within 2–10 days after exposure to the herpes virus, painful red papules (a superficial solid elevation of the skin) appear in the genital area. In men, the lesions generally occur on the glans or shaft of the penis. In women, the lesions commonly occur on the labia, vagina and cervix. Anal intercourse or oral–anal sexual contact may result in lesions in and around the anus.

Soon after the papules appear, they form small painful blisters filled with clear fluid containing virus particles. The blisters break, shedding the highly infectious virus and creating patches of painful ulcers that last six weeks (or longer if they become infected). Touching these blisters and then rubbing or scratching in another place can spread the infection to other areas of the body (this is known as autoinoculation).

The first outbreak of herpes lesions is called *first episode infection*, with an average duration of 12 days. Subsequent

occurrences, usually less severe, are termed *recurrent infections* (average duration of four to five days). The period between episodes is called *latency*, during which time the person remains infectious even though no symptoms are present. During latency, the virus withdraws into the nerve fibres that lead from the infected site to the lower spine, remaining dormant until recurrence, at which time it retraces its path to the genital area.

The signs and symptoms of genital herpes are as follows:

- herpetic lesions (for example, papules and blisters);
- regional lymphadenopathy (for example, enlarged lymph nodes in the groin or neck region);
- headache;
- fever;
- general malaise (a feeling of being generally unwell or run down);
- dysuria (discomfort or pain when passing urine);
- urinary retention;
- vaginal discharge;
- urethral discharge (men).

Prodromal symptoms (these are early non-specific symptoms) of recurrent outbreaks of genital herpes can include burning, itching, tingling or throbbing at the sites where lesions commonly appear. These sensations may be accompanied by pain in the legs, groin or buttocks. Some authorities believe that prodromal symptoms signal increased levels of infectiousness, during which sexual contact should be avoided.

INTERDISCIPLINARY CARE FOR HSV

A diagnosis of genital herpes is based on history and physical examination of the person, including lesions and patterns of recurrence. Because there is no cure for genital herpes, treatment focuses on relieving symptoms and preventing spread of the infection. Person education is essential to prevent further transmission of the disease and to help the person integrate management of a chronic disease into their lifestyle. Any advice offered to the person and, if appropriate, their partners must be given in such a way that the person understands. The nurse should use a variety of media in order to communicate effectively, for example, the use of website addresses and podcasts.

Diagnosis

A definitive diagnosis of HSV requires isolation of the virus in tissue culture. Ideally, tissue specimens should be obtained within 48 hours of the appearance of the blisters.

Medication

Acyclovir helps reduce the length and severity of the first episode and is the treatment of choice for genital herpes. The oral form is considered most effective for first episode as well as recurrences and is given for 7–10 days or until lesions heal. It may also be administered intravenously where the infection is severe. Evidence shows that some strains of HSV are becoming resistant to acyclovir, particularly in those people who are HIV positive. In those cases, foscarnet, another type of antiviral medication is used. Other antivirals used for treatment and prevention are valacyclovir and famciclovir. These will be prescribed according to individual need.

NURSING CARE FOR HSV

Care must be offered in such a way that it reflects individual needs. In planning and implementing nursing care for the person with genital herpes, the nurse needs to consider both short-term and long-term implications. Although the immediate priority is symptom relief and prevention of further transmission, the person needs assistance to deal with the life-changing diagnosis of a chronic disease. The nurse is required to offer physical and emotional care where needed.

Nursing diagnoses and interventions

Nursing diagnoses discussed in this section focus on pain and sexual dysfunction.

Risk for acute pain

Herpetic lesions are very painful and can become infected. Because the virus resides in the nerve ganglia (a mass of nerve tissue), pain may also occur in the legs, thighs, groin or buttocks. Although acyclovir diminishes the pain of herpes

and accelerates the healing process, additional measures can relieve the discomfort further.

+ Teach how to keep herpes blisters clean and dry. Keep the area clean: washing gently once a day is sufficient. Gently bathe the area and avoid scented soap and deodorants. It is best not to use wipes, gel or soap in this area, but if they are used choose an unscented brand. Avoid overwashing as this can increase irritation and delay healing. Dab dry carefully with a tissue after washing or use a hair dryer set at 'cold'. It is important to wear loose cotton clothing that will not trap moisture and to avoid wearing tights and tight jeans. *Keeping the lesions clean and dry reduces the possibility of secondary infection and speeds the healing process.*

+ For dysuria, suggest pouring water over the genitals while urinating. Drinking additional fluids also helps dilute the acidity of the urine; however, fluids that increase acidity, such as cranberry juice, should be avoided. *These measures dilute the acid content of urine and thereby reduce the burning sensation.*

+ Suggest the use of baths (with tepid water) for 15–30 minutes several times a day. *The warm water is soothing and decreases pain from ulcers and an irritated urethral meatus. It also facilitates wound healing.*

Risk for sexual dysfunction

Persons who learn that they are infected with an incurable STI may believe they can no longer have a normal sex life. Fortunately, many people have learned to live with and manage genital herpes without infecting their partners or their children.

COMMUNITY-BASED CARE

Health teaching for persons with genital herpes involves helping them manage this chronic disease with the least possible disruption in lifestyle and relationships. Understanding the disease process and factors that affect it helps the person regain a sense of control and see the potential for future sexual intimacy without transmission of infection. The following topics should be addressed:

● How to recognise prodromal symptoms of recurrence and factors that seem to trigger recurrences (such as emotional stress, acidic food, sun exposure).

● The need for abstinence from sexual contact from the time prodromal symptoms appear until 10 days after all lesions have healed.

● If lesions become infected, use of topical acyclovir (painful lesions can be protected with sterile petroleum jelly or vaseline).

● Use of condoms due to viral shedding at any time and careful hygiene practices (such as not sharing towels or other personal items) even during latency periods.

✚ Provide a supportive, non-judgemental environment for the person to discuss feelings and ask questions about what this diagnosis means to future sexual relationships. *Feelings of guilt, shame and anger are natural responses to such a diagnosis and can lead to a total avoidance of sexual intimacy.*

✚ Offer information about support groups and other resources for people with herpes. *Information about how others cope with this disease can offset feelings of shame and hopelessness.*

This section has provided insight into the keys issues associated with HSV. The next section will address the care people may need if they have **genital warts**.

The person with genital warts

Genital warts (*condylomata acuminata*), caused by the human papillomavirus (HPV), are the most common genital infections in the UK, and are considered epidemic. Genital warts are chronic and, in many people, largely asymptomatic. Currently, they are incurable.

Women are at greater risk for HPV genital infections because they have a larger mucosal surface area exposed in the genital area. Most HPV infections are asymptomatic or un-recognised. In 2006, there were 83 745 diagnoses of first episode genital warts in GUM clinics in the UK, representing 22% of all new STI diagnoses made in this setting. The majority of genital HPV infections are acquired through heterosexual sex. In 2006, however, 3% of new genital warts diagnoses were in men who have sex with men, and this group has shown the greatest percentage increase in new diagnoses (64%) over the past 10 years (HPA 2008).

FAST FACTS

Genital HPV infection

● At least 50% of sexually active men and women acquire genital HPV infection at some point in their lives.

● By age 50, at least 80% of women will have acquired genital HPV infection.

● Most people with a genital HPV infection do not know they are infected; most women are diagnosed by abnormal smear tests.

● Genital HPV is widespread throughout the UK.

Source: HPA 2008.

Although the majority of infected people are asymptomatic, others experience frequent recurrences. Other than recurrences, men are not likely to experience serious physical complications of genital warts. Women, however, face concerns about the increased risk of cervical cancer, with HPV DNA having been identified in almost all cervical cancers worldwide and in approximately 50–80% of vaginal, vulvar and anogenital cancers (Porth 2009).

Consider this . . .

A person you are caring for who has recurrent genital HPV discloses to you that she is getting married soon and she has told her fiancé that she is a virgin. She asks you if she should tell him about the infection or hope for the best. How might you respond?

Pathophysiology of HPV

Genital warts are caused by HPV and are transmitted by vaginal, anal or oral–genital contact. The incubation period (this is the period of time since exposure to the agent and appearance of signs and symptoms) is six weeks to eight months (Porth 2009).

Signs and symptoms of HPV

Although some people with HPV may not have signs and symptoms, others exhibit characteristic lesions: single or mul-tiple painless, soft, moist, pink or flesh-coloured swellings in the vulvovaginal area, perineum, penis, urethra, anus, groin or thigh. In women, the growths may be in the vagina or on the cervix and be apparent only during a pelvic examination.

The four types of genital warts are as follows:

● *Condyloma acuminata:* cauliflower-shaped lesions that appear on moist skin surfaces such as the vagina or anus.

● *Keratotic warts:* thick, hard lesions that develop on kerat-inised skin (a type of horny material on the skin) such as the labia major, penis or scrotum.

● *Papular warts:* smooth lesions that also develop on kerat-inised skin.

● *Flat warts:* slightly raised lesions, often invisible to the naked eye, that also develop on keratinised skin.

INTERDISCIPLINARY CARE FOR HPV

Treatment is directed at removal of the warts, relief of symptoms and health education to reduce the risk of recurrence and future transmission. BASHH (2007) suggest that people should be provided with a detailed explanation of their condition with particular emphasis on the long-term implications for their health and the health of their partners. This should be re-inforced by providing clear and accurate written information as well as allowing the person time to ask questions.

Diagnosis

Genital and anal warts are diagnosed primarily by clinical appearance. Another test, an HPV DNA test, is used to make a definitive diagnosis. Making a definitive diagnosis means having laboratory confirmation; this can be carried out by screening. For the woman this involves a cervical smear.

DIAGNOSTIC TEST HPV

HPV test (HPV DNA test, Genital human papilloma test)

Routinely used as a screening tool for human papillomavirus (HPV) in women after the age of 30. Conducted in conjunction with a pelvic examination and smear. A finding of 'low-grade changes' on the cervical smear with HPV indicates the likely presence of HPV and the need for further testing. A positive test for HPV indicates the presence of a high risk for cancer type of HPV, but does not specify which type is present.

Related nursing care

Explain to the woman that the test should be done during a time when she is not menstruating, and that she should not have intercourse, douche (the introduction of a stream of water into the body for hygiene or medical purposes – a type of irrigation) or use vaginal medications for 36 hours prior to the examination. Ask the woman to void prior to the examination.

Medication

Treatment choice will depend on the morphology (structure, configuration), number and distribution of warts and the individual's preference. Treatment decisions should be made after examining the most suitable options with the person, taking into account their preference and convenience.

Topical agents (medicines applied directly to the skin) used to treat genital warts include podophyllotoxin and imiquimod (both can be applied by the person) or podophyllin and trichloroacetic acid (provider-administered treatments). Podophyllin is contraindicated (not advised) during pregnancy and can have side-effects in any person, ranging from nausea, diarrhoea and lethargy to paralysis and coma.

A vaccine has been developed and is now available to prevent genital warts, pre-cancerous genital lesions and cervical cancer due to HPV. It is administered by three intramuscular injections given over a six-month period. As HPV is so closely associated with cervical cancer, the government has recommended that the vaccine be targeted for females aged 12–13. The vaccine has now been introduced to the national immunisation programme (DoH 2008b). The vaccine does not protect against an existing HPV infection.

Other treatment options

Genital warts may also be removed by cryotherapy (the therapeutic use of cold, freezing), electrocautery (the therapeutic use of heat, burning), laser vaporisation (the use of laser beams) or surgical excision. Carbon dioxide laser surgery is becoming increasingly common for removal of extensive warts.

NURSING CARE FOR HPV

Health promotion activities for adults of all ages should include information about the causes, treatments and prevention of HPV infections.

Nursing diagnoses and interventions

Nursing interventions are primarily directed toward problems with deficient knowledge, fear and anxiety. The nurse must act as an advocate, providing the person with physical and emotional support.

Risk for deficient knowledge

HPV is spread by contact with infectious lesions or secretions, with up to 70% of genital warts spread by people who do not know they have the infection. Although there is no known cure, it is essential to prevent secondary infections. The provision of information can help prevent transmission, but this must be provided in such way that the person understands and retains the information. The nurse may provide the person with written materials, for example using diagrams and terminology the person is familiar with.

+ Discuss the need for prompt treatment and the necessity for sexual abstinence until lesions have healed, or using a condom while lesions are present. *This reduces the risk of reinfection and further transmission of the disease. Some studies have found that using condoms promotes the regression of HPV lesions in both men and women (Winer et al. 2006).*

+ For the woman, discuss the increased risk of cervical cancer and the importance of an annual cervical smear. *Understanding the risk, the person will be more motivated to seek annual screening.*

+ Stress the importance of thorough handwashing. *Handwashing is essential to prevent the spread of HPV.*

Risk for fear

Surgery engenders some degree of fear in most people: fear of the procedure itself and of pain and possible complications. Surgery or cryotherapy in the genital area involves all of these fears plus fear of possible impaired sexual function. The skilled nurse has the ability to reduce fear and alleviate anxiety.

+ Allow the person to express specific fears and feelings about the procedure. Explain the procedure, approximate recovery time, possible complications and ways to avoid them, and ways to cope with complications that do occur. *Knowing what to expect reduces the person's fear and helps the person feel a greater sense of control.*

+ Explain that the procedure is performed with a local anaesthesia. *Being awake during surgery gives the person a greater sense of participation in the treatment process.*

PRACTICE ALERTS

Medication administration: the person with genital warts

Podophyllin and trichloroacetic acid

Cryotherapy using liquid nitrogen or a cryoprobe (a surgical instrument used to apply extreme cold to tissues) is more commonly used to treat genital warts. However, podophyllin preparations are sometimes used. Podophyllin is applied topically to the warts by the nurse or doctor once a week for three to five weeks or as the person's condition dictates.

Podophyllin is contraindicated during pregnancy; the alternative is cryotherapy. Podophyllin is also contraindicated in cervical, urethral, oral or anorectal warts. It is important to avoid contact of podophyllin resin with the eyes.

Adverse effects of podophyllin include local irritation, severe ulceration of surrounding tissue, nausea, diarrhoea, lethargy, paralysis and coma.

Nursing responsibilities

- Explain fully to the person what actions are to be taken and why.
- Only nurses who are deemed competent to apply topical treatments should do so.
- Establish baseline data, including psychological status, vital signs and weight.

- Document and report any existing lesions (genital, anal or oral).
- Cover the tissue surrounding the warts with petrolatum or a paste of baking soda and water to protect the tissue from the caustic treatment solution.

Health education for the person and family:

- Wash off the treated area thoroughly within one to four hours after the first application; gradually increase this period to six to eight hours after the second and subsequent applications.
- Return for regular treatment until warts are gone.
- Refer partners for examination and any necessary treatment.
- Report any adverse effects (nausea, diarrhoea, local irritation, lethargy, numbness).
- Avoid sexual activity until you and your partners have been free of disease for one month.
- Use condoms to prevent future infections, but be aware that some of the treatment used can disintegrate the condom.
- Return for an annual cervical smear.

Risk for anxiety

The woman with an HPV infection faces an increased risk of infection of her newborn during delivery. The neonatal infection can range from asymptomatic to widely disseminated fatal disease. Transmission occurs during passage through the vaginal canal. The risk is highest during the first episode of infection.

+ Discuss with women of childbearing age that caesarean delivery can prevent transmission of infection to the neonate. In women without signs and symptoms of recurrence, vaginal delivery is possible. *Understanding that infection of the neonate can be prevented helps relieve anxiety.*

COMMUNITY-BASED CARE

Health teaching for HPV emphasises the need for the person and infected partners to return for regular treatment until lesions have resolved, and to use condoms to prevent reinfection. Because of the increased risk of cervical cancer, annual cervical smears are essential for women.

HPV is a common STI affecting both men and women of all ages. The next section will consider vaginal infections, providing you with insight and understanding of a number of infections that can negatively impact on a person's health and wellbeing as well as the health and wellbeing of their partner and children.

The woman with a vaginal infection

The vagina may be infected by yeasts, protozoa or bacteria. These infections can be sexually transmitted, but the male partner does not usually have signs and symptoms of the infection. Risk factors include the use of hormonal contraceptives or broad-spectrum antibiotics (these are antibiotics that are suitable for a wide range of disease-causing bacteria), obesity, diabetes mellitus, pregnancy, unprotected sexual activity and multiple sexual partners. Signs and symptoms of vaginal infections are outlined in Table 17.1.

Preventive measures include educating women about personal hygiene practices and safer sex. Women need to avoid frequent douching and wearing nylon underwear and/or tight pants/underpants. Unprotected sexual activity, particularly with multiple partners, increases the risk of vaginal infections.

Table 17.1 Vaginal infections

Infection	Type of discharge	Typical signs and symptoms	Nursing care
Candidiasis (Moniliasis, yeast infections)	Thick white patches adhering to cervix and vaginal wall, resembling cottage cheese; little odour.	Itching of vulva and vaginal area, redness, painful intercourse.	Teach perineal hygiene and proper use of vaginal applicators. Instruct the woman to complete the entire treatment.
Simple vaginalis (bacterial vaginosis, *Gardnerella* vaginosis)	Thin, white, 'milk-like', or grey with fishy odour, especially when mixed with potassium hydroxide.	None to mild itching or burning in vulvar area; clue cells on microscopic examination.	Teach proper perineal hygiene. Instruct the woman to complete treatment. Teach woman relationship of infection to PID.
Trichomoniasis	Frothy, yellow or white, foul odour.	Burning and itching of vulva.	Teach perineal hygiene.
Atrophic vaginitis (senile vaginitis)	Thin, opaque discharge, occasionally blood tinged, odourless; pale, smooth, thin, dry vaginal walls.	Painful intercourse, itching, vaginal dryness.	Counsel woman on symptoms of menopause and sexual techniques to minimise trauma.

Pathophysiology and signs and symptoms of vaginal infection

Alterations in pH, changes in the normal flora (these are healthy micro-organisms) and low oestrogens levels are conducive to the development of vaginal infections. When conditions are favourable, micro-organisms invade the vulva and vagina.

Bacterial vaginosis

Bacterial vaginosis (non-specific vaginitis) is the most common cause of vaginal infection in women of reproductive age. *Gardnerella vaginalis* is one of the causative organisms, but others are also implicated. The relationship of sexual activity to this infection is not clear. The primary manifestation is a vaginal discharge that is thin and greyish-white, and has a foul, fishy odour. Complications include PID, premature labour, premature rupture of the membranes and postpartum endometritis in pregnancy (this is an infection of endometrium during pregnancy) (Porth 2009). The infection is treated with oral or intravaginal (pessary) antibacterial agents.

Candidiasis

Candidiasis (moniliasis or yeast infection) is caused by the organism *Candida albicans*, which has several strains of different virulence. Candida organisms are part of the normal vaginal environment in up to 50% of women (Porth 2009), causing problems only when they multiply rapidly. When antibiotics, diabetes mellitus, faecal contamination or other factors alter the normal vaginal flora, the organism proliferates, resulting in a yeast infection. The signs and symptoms include an odourless, thick, cheesy vaginal discharge. This is often accompanied by itching and irritation of the vulva and vagina, dysuria and **dyspareunia** (pain during or after sexual intercourse). Uncircumcised men may develop a yeast infection over the glans penis, manifested by itching and dysuria. The infection in women is treated with oral or intravaginal

antifungal agents, in men treatment may be oral or topical (applied to the skin).

Trichomoniasis

Trichomoniasis is caused by *Trichomonas vaginalis*, a protozoan parasite. It is the most common curable STI in young, sexually active women. Symptoms usually appear within 5–28 days of exposure. It most commonly infects the vagina in women and the urethra in men. Most men are asymptomatic, but when symptomatic may complain of dysuria and urethral discomfort. Women have a frothy, green–yellow vaginal discharge with a strong fishy odour, often accompanied by itching and irritation of the genitalia. A woman with HIV who becomes infected has an increased risk of transmitting HIV to her sex partner. Trichomoniasis is usually treated with a single oral dose of metronidazole.

INTERDISCIPLINARY CARE FOR VAGINAL INFECTION

Interdisciplinary care focuses on identifying and eliminating the infection and preventing recurrence.

Diagnosis

Diagnostic tests vary with the suspected organism. Cervical cultures are examined to diagnose the causative organism. Trichomonas is identified by microscopically examining a specimen of vaginal discharge in saline. A culture can be performed to identify vaginal organisms, such as trichomonas (see below).

Medication

The pharmacological treatment varies with the organism, as previously described, and with respect to individual preference.

DIAGNOSTIC TEST

Trichomonas, bacteria, candidae (yeast)

A culture is performed to identify vaginal organisms or blood cells. A specimen of vaginal discharge is obtained with a swab, placed in solution and examined under the microscope immediately after it is collected (referred to as a wet-mount).

Related nursing care

Request not to douche before the examination.

The sexual partner of a woman with a trichomonas infection must also be treated to prevent reinfection. Some antifungal agents are available without prescription, which can lead to self-medication with the incorrect agent or allow repeated infections to go unreported.

NURSING CARE FOR VAGINAL INFECTION

Nursing care focuses on teaching the woman and, if necessary, her sexual partner to adhere with the treatment regimen, use safer sex practices and prevent future transmission of the infection. Careful history taking may also reveal high-risk sexual practices (sexual intercourse without a condom) that require intervention, particularly if the woman has had repeated infections. The initial presenting symptom for many HIV-positive women is vaginal candidiasis, which may not respond to over-the-counter treatments. Treatment with some antibiotics destroys normal vaginal flora, resulting in superinfection with yeast.

Nursing diagnoses and interventions

Although each nursing care plan must be individualised, nursing diagnoses that often apply to women with vaginal infections are deficient knowledge and acute pain.

Risk for deficient knowledge

Many women are unaware of the causes of vaginal infections and the self-care measures to prevent and treat these infections. If possible, both the woman and her sexual partner should be taught the information.

✚ Explain the transmission of the infection. Many infections are transmitted most easily during menstruation; some can also be transmitted by towels or other inanimate objects, or by certain types of sexual activity. *A frank and sensitive discussion of disease transmission and prevention with the woman and her partner can reduce the risk of reinfection.*

✚ The need to complete the course of treatment. *Many infections are asymptomatic in one partner. Incomplete treatment allows for recurrence of the infection and reinfection of the partner.*

Risk for acute pain

The symptoms of vaginitis can include dysuria, painful excoriation (loss of skin continuity, for example, as occurs when the skin is shed excessively) or ulceration of tissue and painful intercourse. Often these symptoms can be relieved by relatively simple self-care measures. See the Fast Facts box below for additional comfort measures.

✚ Suggest the use of cool compresses (for example, a flannel soaked in cold water). *Cool compresses relieve itching.*

✚ Recommend baths to alleviate discomfort. *Baths cleanse the perineal area and the warmth is soothing to inflamed, irritated skin and membranes.*

✚ Wear cotton underwear. *Cotton absorbs moisture and allows better air circulation than other types of material.*

✚ If infected with trichomonas (this is a type of STI) avoid sexual contact until treatment is completed. *Treatment of the infected woman and her partner as well as sexual abstinence are necessary to facilitate healing and to prevent reinfection.*

FAST FACTS

Self-care comfort measures

● Do not wear tights; wear loose-fitting pants/underpants, trousers or skirts.

● Double-rinse underwear; do not use fabric softener on underwear.

● Do not use bubble bath, perfumed soaps or feminine hygiene products.

● Use 100% cotton menstrual pads and tampons.

● Use white, unscented toilet paper.

● Use a water-soluble lubricant for intercourse.

● Apply ice or a frozen blue gel pack wrapped in a towel to the vulva after intercourse to relieve burning.

● Rinse vulva with cool water after passing urine and intercourse.

In this section you have been provided with information that should be able to help you help the people you care for in an effective and safe way. Providing people with information concerning vaginal infections can help them to enjoy a healthier sexual life as well as helping to reduce the risks of transmission. The next section will outline issues associated with chlamydia.

The person with chlamydia

Chlamydia are a group of STIs, caused by *Chlamydia trachomatis*, a bacterium that behaves like a virus, reproducing only within the host cell (as viruses do). It is spread by any sexual contact and to the newborn child by passage through the vaginal canal of an infected mother. The infections caused by chlamydia include acute urethral syndrome, nongonococcal urethritis, mucopurulent cervicitis and PID.

In 2006 there were 112 473 chlamydia diagnoses identified from laboratory reports in England and Wales and 17 962 in Scotland. In England and Wales most cases were diagnosed in the GUM clinic setting, but notably, for women, 29% of reports came from general practice. This was similar for Scotland (HPA 2008).

Because chlamydia is asymptomatic in most women until the uterus and fallopian tubes have been invaded, treatment may be delayed, resulting in devastating long-term complications. Nearly a third of men with urethral chlamydia are also asymptomatic. Chlamydia is a leading cause of preventable blindness in the newborn.

The National Chlamydia Screening Programme

The National Chlamydia Screening Programme (NCSP) in England was set up in 2003 with the aim of controlling chlamydia through the early detection and treatment of asymptomatic infection, thus avoiding the development of sequelae (this is a condition following as a consequence of a disease) and reducing disease transmission.

The NCSP was rolled out in three phases. Phase one was launched in 2003 with 10 programme areas. In 2004, 26 new programme areas came on board and in 2007/08 the national rollout of the NCSP was completed. Currently 86 programme areas are in operation in England covering all 152 PCTs, with a total of 11 377 screening venue sites registered (NCSP and HPA 2008).

Risk factors for chlamydia

Risk factors for chlamydial infection are as follows:

- personal or partner history of STI;
- pregnancy;
- adolescent sexual activity;
- oral contraceptive use;
- unprotected sexual activity;
- multiple sexual partners.

Pathophysiology of chlamydia

Chlamydia trachomatis is an intracellular bacterial pathogen that resembles both a virus and bacteria. The organism enters the body in such a form as it is capable of entering uninfected cells. The infection begins when the organism enters a cell and changes into a reticulate body. The reticulate body divides within the cell, bursting the cell and infecting adjoining cells.

Signs and symptoms of chlamydia

The incubation period is from one to three weeks; however, chlamydia may be present for months or years without producing noticeable symptoms in women. Chlamydia typically invades the same target organs as gonorrhoea (cervix and male urethra) and results in similar signs and symptoms (dysuria, urinary frequency and discharge). Patients may be asymptomatic; however, they are still potentially infectious.

Potential complications of chlamydia

If a chlamydial infection in women is not treated, it ascends into the upper reproductive tract, causing such complications as PID, which includes endometritis (infection of the endometrium) and inflammation of the fallopian tubes (salpingitis). Chronic pelvic pain may result. These infections are a major cause of infertility and ectopic pregnancy, a potentially life-threatening disorder in women. Complications of chlamydial infections in men include epididymitis (inflammation of the epididymis), inflammation of the prostate gland (prostatitis), infertility and Reiter's syndrome (syndrome comprising a triad of conditions: urethritis, conjunctivitis and arthritis).

INTERDISCIPLINARY CARE FOR CHLAMYDIA

C. trachomatis is treated with medications to eradicate the infection. Its prevalence, particularly in younger populations, makes widespread screening necessary if the disease is to be controlled. Because chlamydia is often asymptomatic, treatment is often begun on a presumptive basis – based on the history the person gives.

Diagnosis

The diagnostic tests that may be ordered include staining (for analysis under the microscope) of discharge from the female endocervix and urethra or from the male urethra to look for poly-morphonuclear leucocytes (considered evidence of infection).

Tests for antibodies to chlamydia, such as the direct fluorescent antibody (DFA) test and an enzyme-linked immunosorbent assay (ELISA), as well as polymerase chain reaction (PCR) or ligase chain reaction (LCR) tests, are highly sensitive and specific tests performed on cervical and urethral swab specimens. However, nucleic acid amplification tests (NAATs), also performed on cervical and urethral swab specimens, have become the diagnostic method of choice (Porth 2009). NAATs provide the most sensitive and specific tests for *C. trachomatis*. These first-catch urine and vulvo-vaginal swabs are the least invasive of tests and the easiest means of self-sampling. After the self-test has been taken, it usually takes approximately 10 days to receive the result.

Medication

The antibiotic recommended by BASHH for chlamydial infections in men and non-pregnant women is azithromycin, used orally in a single dose, or doxycycline, used orally for seven days. Erythromycin or ofloxacin can be given to those who are unable to use azithromycin or doxycycline. Both sexual partners must be treated at the same time or prior to resuming sexual intercourse.

NURSING CARE FOR CHLAMYDIA

Nursing care of the person with chlamydia focuses on eradication of the infection, prevention of future infections and management of any chronic complications. Nursing diagnoses for the person with chlamydia are the same as for persons with any STI. Interventions are similar to those discussed later in the chapter for gonorrhoea and previously for genital herpes.

COMMUNITY-BASED CARE

Health teaching for the person with chlamydia centres on the need to comply with the treatment regimen, referring partners for examination and necessary treatment and the use of condoms to avoid reinfection. If the infection has progressed to PID (discussed later), the person needs additional information on self-care and health promotion. Regular screening for chlamydia for persons who are young, sexually active and do not use condoms correctly with every act of sexual intercourse is advocated.

There are a number of different places within the community setting where an individual can go to have a chlamydia test:

- Sexual health clinics which provide contraceptive and genitourinary services.

- GUM clinics which provide genitourinary services and STI testing and advice. These clinics offer a free and confidential service. Specialist facilities for testing and systems for contacting, testing and treating sexual partners are available. Clinics are completely confidential and will not inform the GP unless the person specifically asks them to.

- GP surgery.

- The NCSP. This service offers free tests to men and women under 25 who have been sexually active. The screening takes place in a variety of community settings, including GP surgeries, military bases, contraceptive clinics, sexual health and GUM clinics, pharmacies, gynaecology departments, universities and youth centres. The screening programme is usually advertised locally.

- Pharmacists. A chlamydia test kit can be purchased to do the test at home; however, some tests may be more reliable than others. Seek advice from the pharmacist.

Having discussed chlamydia, a common STI that can have an impact on the male and female reproductive systems, the next STI to be discussed is gonorrhoea. This can also have a negative impact on the reproductive system.

The person with gonorrhoea

Gonorrhoea, also known as 'GC' or 'the clap', is caused by *Neisseria gonorrhoeae*, a gram-negative diplococcus. Gonorrhoea is a common communicable disease. The HPA (2008) report that gonorrhoea is the second most common bacterial STI in the UK which, if left untreated, can lead to complications, for example chronic pelvic pain, PID, ectopic pregnancy and infertility in women. In 2006, it was reported that there were 19 007 diagnoses of uncomplicated gonorrhoea in GUM clinics in the UK, 13 627 in men and 5380 in women. This translates to an overall rate of 46 and 18 per 100 000 population in men and women, respectively.

Pathophysiology of gonorrhoea

Understanding the pathophysiological issues associated with gonorrhoea can help you provide safe and effective nursing care. The causative organism of gonorrhoea is a pyogenic (pus-forming) bacteria that causes inflammation characterised by purulent exudates (a pus-like discharge). Humans are the only host for the organism. Gonorrhoea is transmitted by direct hetero- and homosexual sexual activity (including sexual intercourse – vaginal and anal – cunnilingus and fellatio) and during delivery as the baby passes through the vaginal canal. The portal of entry can be the genitourinary tract, eyes, oropharynx, anorectum or skin. The incubation period is two to seven days after exposure. The organism initially targets the female cervix and the male urethra. Without treatment, the disease ultimately disseminates (spreads widely) to other organs. In men, gonorrhoea can cause acute, painful inflammation of the prostate gland, epididymis and periurethral glands and can lead to infertility. In women, it can cause PID, endometritis, salpingitis and pelvic peritonitis.

Signs and symptoms of gonorrhoea

Signs and symptoms of gonorrhoea in men include dysuria and serous (this is term that is used for a number of bodily fluids, usually pale yellow and transparent), milky or purulent discharge from the penis. Some men also experience regional lymphadenopathy (swelling of local lymph nodes, i.e. those in the groin). About 20% of men and 80% of women remain asymptomatic until the disease is advanced. Women with symptoms experience dysuria, urinary frequency, abnormal menses (increased menstrual flow or dysmenorrhoea), increased vaginal discharge and dyspareunia (painful sexual intercourse).

Anorectal gonorrhoea is seen most often in homosexual men, but not exclusively. The signs and symptoms include itching (pruritus), mucopurulent (discharge that is composed of mucus and pus) rectal discharge, rectal bleeding and pain and constipation. Gonococcal pharyngitis (throat infection caused by gonorrhoea) occurs primarily in homosexual or bisexual men or heterosexual women after oral sexual contact (fellatio) with an infected partner. The signs and symptoms include fever, sore throat and enlarged lymph nodes.

Complications of gonorrhoeal infection

The complications of untreated gonorrhoea in both men and women may be permanent and serious. They include:

- PID in women, leading to internal abscesses, chronic pain, ectopic pregnancy and infertility.
- Blindness, infection of joints, and potentially lethal infections of the blood in the newborn, contracted during vaginal delivery.
- Epididymitis and prostatitis in men, resulting in infertility and dysuria.
- Spread of the infection to the blood and joints.
- Increased susceptibility to and transmission of HIV.

INTERDISCIPLINARY CARE FOR GONORRHOEA

The goals of treatment for the person with gonorrhoea include eradication of the organism and any coexisting disease, and prevention of reinfection or transmission. It is essential to emphasise the importance of taking all medications as prescribed and abstaining from sexual contact (and this will include masturbation) until the infection is cured in both patient and partners. Condom use to prevent future infections is essential, particularly for pregnant women whose partners may be infected.

Diagnosis

Diagnosis of gonorrhoea is based on cultures from the infected mucous membranes (cervix, urethra, rectum or throat), examination of urine from an infected person and a Gram stain to visualise the bacteria under the microscope. Testing for other STIs (especially chlamydia and syphilis) at the same time is recommended. Pregnant women are routinely screened during their first pre-natal visit.

IN PRACTICE

Taking a throat swab (a specimen) for microbiological analysis

Specimens are required for a number of reasons, for example to detect and confirm the presence of gonorrhoea in the throat. The nurse must understand the reason why the specimen is needed and ensure that local policy and procedure are adhered to. This is important so that the laboratory can identify pathogens correctly and the right treatment can be commenced if the specimen is positive.

A request for microbiological analysis of a specimen must have the following information attached to it:

- Name of person
- Department/ward
- Hospital identifier (hospital number)
- Date and time the specimen was collected
- Diagnosis (or provisional diagnosis)
- Relevant signs and symptoms and history
- Any antibiotics being taken by the person
- Details (names) of nursing/medical staff requesting the specimen

The information above should be provided on the appropriate request forms and filled in using a black ink (not felt-tipped) pen. Some forms are carbon duplicated so the nurse must ensure that he/she writes firmly on the form ensuring that the information is copied on to all pages. The form must be dated and signed.

EQUIPMENT REQUIRED
Ensure you have all of the equipment ready and to hand prior to performing the procedure.

- Gloves and apron
- Tongue blade
- A light source (pen torch or anglepoise lamp)
- Sterile cotton-tipped swab
- Sterile culture tube with or without transport medium as required (swabs for culture should be taken with transport medium)
- Tissues
- Forms

PERFORMING THE PROCEDURE

- Check this is the correct person for this procedure.
- Explain to the person the need for the swab and how it will be collected. Explain that the collection of the swab from the throat may make the person gag, but the procedure will be over quickly.
- Ensure dignity by closing the door or curtain and covering the person with a blanket.
- Offer tissues.
- Again, explain the procedure and reiterate that the person may gag, but the procedure will take less than a minute to perform.
- Sit the person upright, if possible on the edge of the bed/sofa/chair, and ask the person to face you.
- Wash hands (or use bactericidal gel), don apron and gloves.
- With the person facing you, ask him/her to open the mouth. With the tongue depressor gently depress the tongue and shine the light into the mouth; note any areas of inflammation.

- Communicate (verbally and non-verbally) with the person throughout, asking him/her to breathe deeply.
- Quickly but gently, using the sterile cotton-tipped swab, wipe the tonsillar area from side to side including any inflamed areas or purulent sites. Avoid touching the tongue or cheeks.
- Withdraw swab immediately and place in culture tube, ensuring that the specimen is secured and bagged appropriately.
- Stop and restart the procedure if the person becomes distressed, allowing time for recovery.
- Inform the person that the procedure is over and offer physical and emotional support.
- Remove gloves and apron and safely dispose of them, then wash hands.

- Explain to the person when the result will be ready and how they will be informed of the outcome.

AFTER THE PROCEDURE
- Send the specimen to the laboratory as per policy and procedure. If the specimen needs to wait for collection then it should to be stored in the appropriate place (usually a specimen fridge) until collection.
- Document the procedure in the person's notes and detail the type of and date of specimen sent, the microbiological test requested and any instructions given to the person, i.e. when the result is due and how this will be communicated. Note the condition of the throat and any adverse observations. Date and sign the entry.

Medication

Because of the many penicillin-resistant strains of *N. gonorrhoeae*, an alternative antibiotic, such as ciprofloxacin or ofloxacin, is used to treat gonorrhoea. Ciprofloxacin is often prescribed because it is inexpensive, can be administered orally and a single dose is all that is required. However, because of increased prevalence of fluoroquinolone-resistant *N. gonorrhoeae* in Asia, the Pacific Islands and California, antimicrobial therapy should take account of local patterns of antimicrobial sensitivity to *N. gonorrhoeae*. All sexual partners within 60 days before diagnosis of the infection also need to be treated.

NURSING CARE FOR GONORRHOEA

Care must be provided on an individual basis, taking into account the person's unique needs. In planning and implementing care for the person with gonorrhoea, the nurse considers the possible coexistence of other STIs such as syphilis and HIV, the impact of the disease and its treatment on the person's lifestyle and the likelihood of non-compliance.

Nursing diagnoses and interventions

Nursing diagnoses discussed in this section focus on concordance and impaired social interaction.

Gonorrhoea and concordance

Concordance is a term that refers to an agreement that the person being cared for and the nurse have come to about their therapeutic goals. This includes the medication they have been given and safer sex activities they have been given advice about. Although one-time treatment with the recommended antibiotic is highly effective in curing gonorrhoea, non-compliance with the doxycycline regimen may leave any coexisting chlamydial infection unresolved. Non-compliance with recommendations for abstinence, follow-up meetings or condom use fosters a high rate of reinfection. Failure to refer partners for examination and treatment also leads to reinfection.

✦ Reinforce the need to take all medications as directed and keep follow-up appointments to be sure no reinfection has occurred. Discuss the prevalence of gonorrhoea and the potential complications if it is not cured. *The person who understands the complications of incomplete or failed treatment is more likely to adhere to the medication regimen.*

✦ Discuss the importance of sexual abstinence until the infection is cured, referral of partners and condom use to prevent reinfection. *Understanding that cure is possible and reinfection is avoidable helps the person cope with the disease and its treatment and is likely to increase compliance.*

✦ Explain that condoms must be used during treatment, even if other methods of birth control are used. *Oral contraceptives increase the alkalinity of the vaginal pH, facilitating the growth of the gonococcal bacteria, and intrauterine devices alter the endometrial barrier, favoring persistent gonococcal infections (Blair 2004).*

Risk for impaired social interaction

Diagnosis of any STI can make patients feel 'dirty', ashamed and guilty about their sexual behaviours, and unworthy to be with others.

✦ Provide privacy, confidentiality and a safe, non-judgemental environment for expression of concerns. Help the person understand that gonorrhoea is a consequence of sexual behaviour, not a punishment, and that it can be avoided in the future. *Being treated with respect and privacy helps the person realise that the disease does not change an individual's worth as a person. This knowledge enhances the person's ability to relate to others.*

This section of the chapter has outlined issues associated with chlamydia and gonorrhoea, which are STIs affecting men

Case Study 2 – Janet
NURSING CARE PLAN Gonorrhoea

The care plan below is for Ms Janet Cirit. Return to Case Study 2 at the beginning of the chapter to familiarise yourself with her history.

Assessment

When Ms Cirit arrives for her appointment with the gynaecologist, Marsha Davidson, the nurse practitioner, interviews her. Ms Davidson completes a thorough nursing, medical and sexual history, including questions about her menstrual periods, pain associated with urination or sexual intercourse, urinary frequency, most recent cervical smear, birth control method, history of STI and drug use and types of sexual activity. Ms Cirit reports her symptoms and her concern about ovarian cancer. She also indicates that she is taking oral contraceptives and therefore sees no need for her boyfriend (Mr Adkins) to use a condom because she believes their relationship is monogamous.

Physical examination reveals both pharyngeal and cervical inflammation, and lower abdominal tenderness. Her temperature is 37.0 °C. There is no evidence of pregnancy.

The gynaecologist orders a cervical smear and cultures of the cervix, urethra and pharynx to evaluate for gonorrhoea and chlamydial infection. Blood is taken for a full blood count (FBC) [this will include white blood cells (WBC)]. Test results are positive for gonorrhoea and negative for chlamydia. The WBC is slightly elevated, indicating possible salpingitis. Because Mr Adkins has been Ms Cirit's only sexual partner, it is clear that he is the source of infection and needs to be treated as well.

Diagnoses

+ *Acute pain* related to the infectious process.
+ *Anxiety* related to fear about possible cancer.
+ *Situational low self-esteem* related to shame and guilt because of having an STI.
+ *Ineffective sexuality patterns* related to the impaired relationship and fear of reinfection.

Expected outcomes

+ Experience relief of pain, indicating that the infection has been eradicated.
+ Verbalise that she has nothing to be ashamed of and that she has been wise to seek treatment as soon as symptoms occurred.
+ Verbalise that she will insist her partner use condoms during future sexual activity.

Planning and implementation

+ Administer antimicrobials as prescribed.
+ Emphasise the need for regular cervical smears and pelvic examinations because of the family history of ovarian cancer.
+ Discuss feelings and concerns about the diagnosis of gonorrhoea. Stress that such a diagnosis does not reflect on one's self-worth as a person.
+ Teach how to talk with a future sexual partner about condom use.

COMMUNITY-BASED CARE

Health teaching for the person with gonorrhoea focuses on helping patients understand the importance of:

● taking any and all prescribed medication;
● referring sexual partners for evaluation and treatment;
● abstaining from all sexual contact until the person and partners are cured;
● using a condom to avoid transmitting or contracting infections in the future.

Patients also need to understand the need for a follow-up visit four to seven days after treatment is completed.

and women. Having read this section, you should be more confident and competent with the care you offer people with chlamydia or gonnorhoea. The next section will consider the care required for those people who have syphilis.

The person with syphilis

Syphilis is a complex systemic STI caused by the spirochete (a thin, spiral-shaped moving organism) *Treponema pallidum*, and it can infect almost any body tissue or organ. It is transmitted from open lesions during any sexual contact (genital, oral–genital or anal–genital) The organism is highly susceptible to heat and drying, but can survive for days in fluids; thus, it may also be transmitted by infected blood or other body fluid such as saliva. The incubation period ranges from 10–90 days, averaging 21 days. If not treated appropriately, syphilis can lead to blindness, paralysis, psychiatric illness, cardiovascular damage and death. Syphilis often occurs with one or more other STIs, such as HIV or chlamydial infection.

There has been a considerable rise in numbers of diagnoses of infectious syphilis in the UK, from 301 in 1997 to 3702 in 2006. The majority of cases in men were among those men who have sex with men. Almost 25% of those with infectious syphilis in 2006 were also co-infected with HIV. In 2006, men were six times more likely to be diagnosed with infectious syphilis than women. At first, the majority of syphilis cases were mostly accounted for by outbreaks in London and the North West of England; however, more recently, growing numbers have been seen throughout the UK (HPA 2008).

The Tuskegee syphilis experiment

From 1932–1972 in the USA, the Public Health Service at that time conducted an experiment on 399 black men in the late stages of syphilis. Many of these men came from one of the poorest counties in Alabama and were never told about their diagnosis (syphilis) and the disease they were suffering from; neither were they informed of its seriousness. The men were merely informed that they were being treated for 'bad blood'. The research project meant there was never any intention of curing the men of syphilis at all, despite the fact that effective treatment was available.

One of the aims was to determine what would happen if treatment was not given and syphilis was left to run its full course. Data for the experiment were to be collected from post-mortems carried out on the men who were deliberately left to degenerate under the devastation of tertiary syphilis. Another aim of the study was to determine if syphilis affected black men differently from white men.

This study was an infamous clinical study that has become a byword for racist and unethical medical experimentation. Those men that did survive finally received financial compensation

and in 1997 US President Bill Clinton announced 'on behalf of the American people, what the United States government did was shameful'.

Pathophysiology of syphilis

Any break in the skin or mucous membrane is vulnerable to invasion by the spirochete. Once it has entered the system, the spirochete is spread through the blood and lymphatic system. Congenital syphilis is transferred to the foetus through the placental circulation.

Signs and symptoms of syphilis

Syphilis is generally characterised by three clinical stages: primary, secondary and tertiary. Each stage has characteristic signs and symptoms (see Box 17.1). The person with syphilis may also experience a latency period when no signs of the disease are evident.

- Primary syphilis is the first stage of the condition and ulcers can appear about two to three weeks after having sex with an infected person.
- Secondary syphilis usually occurs two to eight weeks after the initial ulcer has healed.
- Tertiary syphilis can occur years after having been infected.

Box 17.1

Signs and symptoms of syphilis

REPRODUCTIVE

Primary (the first stage of the condition)
- Genital **chancre** (may be internal in female)

Secondary (usually occurs after 2–8 weeks)
- Condyloma lata (a type of wart-like growth)

THE SKIN

Secondary
- Rash on palms of hands and soles of feet

Tertiary
- Granulomatous lesions involving mucous membranes and skin

GASTROINTESTINAL SYSTEM

Secondary
- Anorexia
- Oral mucous patches inside the mouth

NEUROLOGICAL SYSTEM

Secondary
- Asymptomatic
- Meningitis

- Headache
- Cranial neuropathies [these are a number of conditions that may occur, for example facial paralysis, diplopia (double vision)]

Tertiary
- Asymptomatic
- Tabes dorsalis
- Neurosyphilis
- Seizures, hemiplegia (paralysis of half of the body)
- Personality changes, hyperactive reflexes, Argyll Robertson pupil (an abnormality associated with the shape of the pupil), decreased memory, slurred speech, optic atrophy

MUSCULOSKELETAL SYSTEM

Secondary
- Arthralgia (joint pain)
- Myalgia (muscle pain)
- Bone and joint arthritis
- Periostitis (pain over a bone)

Tertiary
- Gummas (a rubbery type of lesion)

CARDIOVASCULAR SYSTEM

Tertiary
- Aortic insufficiency
- Aortic aneurysm
- Stenosis (narrowing) of openings to coronary arteries

RENAL SYSTEM

Secondary
- Glomerulonephritis (a kidney infection)
- Nephrotic syndrome (a condition affecting the kidney's ability to filter)

OTHER

Primary
- Regional lymphadenopathy (a specific swelling of lymph nodes)

Secondary
- Generalised lymphadenopathy (a generalised swelling of lymph nodes)
- Fever
- Hepatitis
- Malaise
- Alopecia

Primary syphilis

The primary stage of syphilis is characterised by the appearance of a chancre (this is a small painless ulcer-like lesion) and by regional enlargement of lymph nodes; little or no pain accompanies these warning signs. The chancre appears at the site of inoculation (such as the genitals, anus, mouth, breast, fingers) three to four weeks after the infectious contact. In women, a genital chancre may go unnoticed, disappearing within four to six weeks. In both primary and secondary stages, syphilis remains highly infectious, even if no symptoms are evident.

Secondary syphilis

Signs and symptoms of secondary syphilis may appear any time from two weeks to six months after the initial chancre disappears. These symptoms can include a skin rash, especially on the palms of the hands or soles of the feet; mucous patches in the oral cavity; sore throat; generalised lymphadenopathy; condyloma lata (flat, broad-based papules, unlike the pedunculated structure of genital warts) on the labia, anus or corner of the mouth; flu-like symptoms; and alopecia. These signs and symptoms generally disappear within two to six weeks, and an asymptomatic latency period begins.

Latent and tertiary syphilis

The latent stage of syphilis begins two or more years after the initial infection and can last up to 50 years. During this stage, no symptoms of syphilis are apparent, and the disease is not transmissible by sexual contact. It can be transmitted by infected blood, however; thus, all prospective blood donors must be screened for syphilis. In two-thirds of all cases, the latent stage persists without further complications. Unless treated, the remaining one-third of infected people progress to late-stage or tertiary syphilis. In the presence of HIV infection, disease progression seems to be more rapid.

Two types of late-stage syphilis occur. Benign late syphilis, of rapid onset, is characterised by localised development of infiltrating tumours (*gummas*) in skin, bones and liver, generally responding promptly to treatment. Of more insidious onset is a diffuse inflammatory response that involves the central nervous system and the cardiovascular system. Though the disease can still be treated at this stage, much of the cardiovascular and central nervous system damage is irreversible.

INTERDISCIPLINARY CARE FOR SYPHILIS

Nursing care interventions endeavour to provide comfort, educate and prevent transmission. The goals of treatment are to inactivate the spirochete and educate the person about how to prevent reinfection or further transmission. Treatment includes antibiotic therapy and identification and referral of partners for testing and treatment if necessary, follow-up testing and education about condom use to prevent reinfection of self and transmission of disease to partners. In addition, patients should be screened for chlamydial infection and advised to have an HIV test.

Diagnosis

Diagnosis of syphilis is complex because it mimics many other diseases. A careful and detailed history and physical examination are obtained, as well as laboratory evaluations of lesions and blood.

The VDRL (venereal disease research laboratory) and RPR (rapid plasma reagin) blood tests measure antibody production. People with syphilis become positive about four to six weeks after infection. However, these tests are not specific for syphilis, and other diseases may also cause positive results. Additional tests are required for definitive diagnosis. These additional tests are decided upon on a case-by-case basis with the person being cared for acting as a partner in his or her care.

The FTA–ABS (fluorescent treponemal antibody absorption) test is specific for *T. pallidum* and can be used to confirm VDRL and RPR findings. It may be used for persons whose clinical picture indicates syphilis but who have negative VDRL results. In immunofluorescent staining, a specimen is obtained from early lesions or aspiration (removal of exudates for examination) of lymph nodes and is specially treated and examined microscopically for the presence of *T. pallidum*. Darkfield microscopy involves examining a specimen from the chancre for the presence of *T. pallidum* using a darkfield microscope.

Medication

The treatment of choice for all stages of syphilis in adults is penicillin G, given intramuscularly (IM) in a single dose. Patients allergic to penicillin are given oral doxycycline or tetracycline for 28 days.

> ### PRACTICE ALERT
>
> Treatment of syphilis may result in a severe reaction called the *Jarisch–Herxheimer reaction*, involving fever, musculoskeletal pain, tachycardia (an increased heart rate usually above 100 beats per minute) and sometimes hypotension. This is not a reaction to the penicillin itself, but to the sudden and massive destruction of spirochetes by the penicillin and the resulting release of toxins into the bloodstream. The Jarisch–Herxheimer reaction generally begins within 24 hours of treatment and subsides in another 24 hours. Treatment should not be discontinued unless symptoms become life-threatening.

NURSING CARE FOR SYPHILIS

In planning and implementing nursing care for the person with syphilis, the nurse needs to consider the person's age, lifestyle, access to healthcare and educational level. Although each person has individualised needs, nursing diagnoses for the person with syphilis would be the same as for any person with an STI. A nursing care plan for a person with syphilis is on p. 666.

Nursing diagnoses and interventions

Nursing diagnoses discussed in this section focus on risk for injury, anxiety and self-esteem.

Risk for injury

If syphilis is not diagnosed and treated promptly and effectively, it can have devastating effects on all body systems, particularly the neurological and cardiovascular systems, eventually leading to death.

✚ Teach the importance of taking any prescribed medication. *Taking the prescribed antibiotic is important to ensure eradication of the infecting organism.*

✚ Encourage referral of any sexual partners for evaluation and any necessary treatment. *Without treatment of both partners, reinfection can occur or the disease may be transmitted to other people through sexual activity.*

✚ Teach abstinence from sexual contact until the person and their partners are cured and to use condoms to prevent future infections. *Abstinence until the organism is eradicated prevents reinfection. Condoms provide barrier protection, reducing the risk of infection during sexual activity.*

✚ Emphasise the importance of returning for follow-up testing at three- and six-month intervals for early syphilis, and six- and 12-month intervals for late latent syphilis. *Follow-up testing is performed to ensure eradication of the disease.*

✚ Provide information about signs and symptoms of reinfection. *Successful treatment of the disease does not prevent possible subsequent infections.*

Risk for anxiety

The diagnosis of syphilis understandably causes the person anxiety, not only about personal wellbeing but about the wellbeing of partners and, in the expectant woman, her foetus.

✚ Emphasise that syphilis can be effectively treated, preventing the serious complications of late-stage disease. *This information provides a sense of control and helps decrease anxiety.*

✚ Teach the pregnant woman that taking medications as directed and returning each month for follow-up testing will help ensure the wellbeing of her baby. *Knowing that treatment can reduce the risk to her baby relieves anxiety and possibly increases compliance.*

Risk for low self-esteem

Living with any chronic disease can be damaging to a person's self-esteem. However, the person with syphilis needs additional support to cope with the stigma of this kind of infection. Unfortunately, the populations most affected by STIs can often lack family and other social support networks.

✚ Create an environment where the person feels respected and safe to discuss questions and concerns about the disease and its effect on the person's life. *Being treated with respect helps enhance self-esteem.*

✚ Provide privacy and confidentiality. *Patients are often embarrassed to discuss the intimate details of their sex lives.*

COMMUNITY-BASED CARE

The nurse has an important role to play in caring for the person with syphilis from a variety of perspectives. Education is an essential part of nursing care for the person with any STI, and syphilis is no exception. The nurse emphasises that syphilis is a chronic disease that can be spread to others even though no symptoms are evident. The nurse should be prepared to address the following topics:

● Taking all prescribed medication.

● Referring sexual partners for evaluation and treatment.

● Abstaining from all sexual contact (this includes masturbation).

● Using a condom to avoid transmitting or contracting infections in the future.

● The need for follow-up testing (at three and six months for patients with primary or secondary syphilis, and at six and 12 months for those with late-stage disease). If patients are HIV positive, follow-up visits are recommended 1, 2, 3, 6, 9 and 12 months after treatment.

Case Study 3 – Eddie
NURSING CARE PLAN Syphilis

The care plan below is for Mr Eddie Kratz. Return to Case Study 3 at the beginning of the chapter to familiarise yourself with his history.

Assessment

When Mr Kratz comes to the clinic, he is interviewed by the Nurse Practitioner, Paul Morovitz. He takes a thorough nursing, medical and sexual history, including questions about drug use, allergies, difficulty with urination, urinary frequency, itching or discharge from the penis, recent sexual activities, precautions taken against infection, history of STIs and sexual function. He determines that Mr Kratz has been having unprotected sex with both Ms Jones and Ms Simpson. Mr Kratz believes that Ms Jones is not having sex with anyone except him, but he is not sure.

Physical assessment reveals a classic syphilitic chancre on the shaft of the penis and regional lymphadenopathy. A specimen of exudates from the chancre is sent for darkfield examination. The nurse discusses with Mr Kratz the likelihood that he has syphilis and the need to tell both Ms Jones and Ms Simpson so that they can be tested and, if necessary, treated. The nurse also suggests that Mr Kratz be tested for HIV since he has been having unprotected sex with two women, at least one of whom may be sexually active with other partners. He agrees, and blood is taken for an ELISA test. Darkfield analysis of the chancre exudate confirms the diagnosis of syphilis; the ELISA results are negative for HIV.

Diagnoses

+ *Risk for injury* to the person, his partners and the infant, related to the disease process.
+ *Ineffective health maintenance* related to a lack of knowledge about the disease process, its transmission and the need for treatment.
+ *Interrupted family processes* related to the effects of the diagnosis of syphilis on the couple's relationship.
+ *Anxiety* related to the effects of the infection on the unborn child.

Expected outcomes

+ Prompt treatment will cure the syphilis.
+ Verbalise understanding for the need to abstain from sexual contact during treatment, complete all medications, return for follow-up visits and use condoms to prevent reinfection.
+ Verbalise ability to cope with the effect of diagnosis and treatment on the relationship.
+ Verbalise decreased anxiety following education and treatment.

Planning and implementation

+ Administer IM injection of penicillin G as prescribed.
+ Discuss the importance of abstaining from sexual activity until he and his partners are cured, and of using condoms to prevent reinfection.
+ Explain the need to return for follow-up testing in three months and again at six months. Provide a copy of the STI prevention checklist, and document that reminders need to be sent at three- and six-month intervals.
+ Notify sexual partners that they need to come to the clinic for testing.
+ Refer to a health adviser for counselling about the effect of the disease on their relationship if appropriate.
+ Teach the couple about the importance of treatment to the health of their infant.

Evaluation

At the three-month follow-up visit, the chancre on Mr Kratz's penis has healed, and he reports that he is using a condom any time he has sex. Ms Jones has also tested positive for syphilis and negative for HIV, so she, too, is given penicillin G, and verbal and written follow-up instructions, including follow-up until the infant is born. The couple is meeting every other week with the health adviser and say that their relationship is improving. Ms Simpson has received similar test results and is given a prescription for doxycycline because she is allergic to penicillin.

+ Let patients know that the nurse and other healthcare providers care about them and the successful treatment of their disease. *Feeling valued enhances self-esteem.*

Whilst syphilis affects both sexes, PID in the next section only affects women, but it can have a detrimental impact on the health and wellbeing of both sexes. This section discusses the issues you will need to understand in order to offer safe and effective care.

The woman with pelvic inflammatory disease (PID)

It must be remembered that not all cases of PID are sexually transmitted. Many myths and misconceptions abound with regards to PID, for example IUDs cause PID. PID is a term used to describe infection of the pelvic organs, including the fallopian tubes (*salpingitis*), ovaries (*oophoritis*), cervix (*cervicitis*), endometrium (*endometritis*), pelvic peritoneum and the pelvic vascular system. PID can be caused by one or more infectious agents, including *Neisseria gonorrhoeae*, *Chlamydia trachomatis*, *Escherichia coli* and *Mycoplasma hominis*. These are responsible for as much as 80% of PID; dual infection with both agents is common.

A range of complications are associated with genital chlamydial infection, including PID, chronic pelvic pain, ectopic pregnancy, infertility, epididymitis, prostatitis, proctitis and Reiter's syndrome. In the UK PID may be caused by infection with *C. trachomatis* or *Neisseria gonorrhoeae*. Approximately 40% of cases are thought to be caused by *C. trachomatis*. The majority of diagnosis and treatment of PID usually occurs in general practice. The incidence of PID was estimated at 1.7% in reproductive-age women attending general practice in England and Wales in 1992, with rates highest in women aged 16–19 (2230/100 000 person years) and 20–24 (2510/100 000 person years) (HPA 2008). The disease may also cause pelvic abscesses and chronic abdominal pain.

Sexually active women age 16–24 years are most at risk. Risk factors include a history of STI (especially gonorrhoea and chlamydia), bacterial vaginosis, multiple sexual partners, douching and previous PID. Barrier contraceptive devices such as condoms reduce the risk of PID.

The prognosis depends on the number of episodes, promptness of treatment and modification of risk-taking behaviours. Prevention includes educating women, especially young women, regarding the causes and transmission of infection and methods of self-protection, such as avoiding unprotected sexual activity.

Pathophysiology of PID

PID is usually polymicrobial (caused by more than one microbe) in origin, with gonorrhoea and chlamydia being common (but not exclusively) causative organisms. Pathogenic micro-organisms enter the vagina and travel to the uterus during intercourse or other sexual activity. They can also gain direct access to the uterus during childbirth, termination of pregnancy or surgery of the reproductive tract. The organisms ascend from the endocervical canal to the fallopian tubes and ovaries.

Signs and symptoms of PID

Signs and symptoms of PID include fever, purulent vaginal discharge, severe lower abdominal pain and painful cervical movement. However, the signs and symptoms may be so mild that the infection is not recognised or noticed by the woman.

Complications of PID

Complications may include pelvic abscess, infertility, ectopic pregnancy, chronic pelvic pain, pelvic adhesions (bands of fibrotic scar tissue in the pelvis), dyspareunia and chronic pelvic pain. Abscess formation is common.

INTERDISCIPLINARY CARE FOR PID

The nurse should aim to promote comfort and offer the woman physical and emotional support. Goals of treatment are to eliminate the infection and prevent complications and recurrence. The physical examination may reveal abdominal, adnexal (these are the accessory or adjoining organs of the female reproductive tract) and cervical pain.

Diagnosis

Tests used in the diagnosis of PID may include a FBC with differential, which will show markedly elevated WBCs and an increased erythrocyte sedimentation rate (a blood test used to detect inflammation). If a laparoscopy (a light source inserted into the abdomen to visualise the contents) or laparotomy (a surgical incision into the abdomen) is carried out, it may reveal inflammation, oedema or hyperaemia (excessive redness) of the fallopian tubes, or tubal discharge and, possibly, generalised pelvic involvement, abscesses and scarring.

Medication

Combination antibiotic therapy with at least two broad-spectrum antibiotics administered IV or orally is the typical treatment for PID. If PID is not acute, out-patient antibiotic therapy is prescribed. In acute cases, however, the woman may be hospitalised. Analgesics are given and the effects monitored, and antibiotics and fluids are administered intravenously. Commonly prescribed antibiotics include cefoxitin, or clindamycin, plus gentamicin (Garamycin) or doxycycline.

Surgery

The surgeon may insert a drain into an abscess, if present, and remove any adhesions. If the woman does not respond to conservative therapy, surgical removal of the uterus, fallopian tubes and ovaries may be necessary.

NURSING CARE FOR PID

The goals of nursing care are to treat the infection and to prevent complications, such as scarring and infertility. The woman who is hospitalised maintains bedrest and the person is placed in a semi-upright sitting position (45–60 degrees) and may have knees either bent or straight to promote drainage and to localise the infectious process in the pelvic cavity.

Nursing diagnoses and interventions

Nursing diagnoses that apply to the woman with PID include a risk for injury and deficient knowledge.

Risk for injury

PID can have severe, even life-threatening, complications. Scarring of fallopian tubes can lead to ectopic pregnancy or

9. The infective organism responsible for gonorrhoea *initially* targets what body parts?

    a. male urethra and female cervix
    b. female vulva and vagina
    c. male prostate
    d. male and female external genitalia

10. Which of the following would you teach a person about syphilis?

    a. syphilis is caused by a virus
    b. syphilis is a local genital infection
    c. syphilis is a systemic infection
    d. syphilis has no effect on the developing foetus

Further resources

British Association for Counselling and Psychotherapy (BACP)
www.counselling.co.uk
BACP is the largest and broadest body within the sector. BACP ensures that it meets its remit of public protection whilst also developing and informing its members. Their work with large and small organisations within the sector ranges from advising schools on how to set up a counselling service, assisting the NHS on service provision, working with voluntary agencies and supporting independent practitioners. BACP participates in the development of counselling and psychotherapy at an international level.

Cancer Research UK
www.cancerresearchuk.org
Cancer Research UK is the world's leading independent organisation dedicated to cancer research. This charity supports research into all aspects of cancer through the work of more than 4500 scientists, doctors and nurses.

Embarrassing Problems.com
www.embarassingproblems.com
Independent advice concerning a wide range of embarrassing problems.

Family Planning Association (FPA)
www.fpa.org.uk
The FPA is the UK's leading sexual health charity. Their purpose is to enable people in the UK to make informed choices about sex and to enjoy sexual health.

Health Protection Agency (HPA)
www.hpa.org.uk
The HPA is an independent UK organisation set up by the government in 2003 to protect the public from threats to their health from infectious diseases and environmental hazards. The HPA does this by providing advice and information to the general public, to health professionals such as doctors and nurses and to national and local government.

Infertility Network UK
www.infertilitynetworkuk.com
Committed to providing a comprehensive support network to its members and to all those affected by infertility by actively promoting Infertility Network UK services. Provides authoritative information and practical and emotional support, with the aim of raising the profile and understanding of infertility issues in all quarters, and strives for timely and consistent provision of infertility care throughout the UK.

London Lesbian and Gay Switchboard (LLGS)
www.llgs.org.uk
LLGS provides an information, support and referral service for lesbians, gay men, bisexual people and anyone who needs to consider issues around their sexuality.

The Samaritans
www.samaritans.org
Samaritans is a confidential emotional support service for anyone in the UK and Ireland. The service is available 24 hours a day for people who are experiencing feelings of distress or despair, including those which may lead to suicide.

The Terrence Higgins Trust
www.tht.org.uk
The Terrence Higgins Trust is the leading and largest HIV and sexual health charity in the UK.

Bibliography

Ali M, Cleland J and Shah I (2004) Condom use within marriage. A neglected HIV intervention. *Bulletin of the World Health Organization*, **82**(3), 180–186.

Anderson M, Klink K and Cohrssen A (2004) The rational clinical examination: Evaluation of vaginal complaints. *Journal of the American Medical Association*, **291**(11), 1368–1379.

Blair M (2004) Sexually transmitted diseases: An update. *Urology Nursing*, **24**(6), 467–473.

BASHH (2007) *United Kingdom National Guideline on the Management of Ano-genital Warts*. London, British Association of Sexual Health and HIV, available at: http://www.bashh.org/documents/86/86.pdf, last accessed August 2011.

DoH (2001) *Better Prevention, Better Services, Better Sexual Health. The National Strategy for Sexual Health and HIV*. London, Department of Health.

DoH (2008a) *A High Quality Workforce: NHS Next Stage Review*. London, Department of Health.

DoH (2008b) *Statutory Directions for the Routine Human Papillomavirus Vaccination Programme*.

London, Department of Health, available at: http://www.dh.gov.uk/prod_consum_dh/groups/dh_digitalassets/documents/digitalasset/dh_087340.pdf (accessed September 2011).

DoH (2009) *Moving Forward: Progress and Priorities – Working Together for High-quality Sexual Health*. London, Department of Health.

Farley T, Cohen D, Kahn R, *et al.* (2003) The acceptability and behavioral effects of antibiotic prophylaxis for syphilis prevention. *Sexually Transmitted Diseases*, **30**(11), 844–849.

Gaffney J, Velcevsky P, Phoenix J and Schiffer K (2008) *Practical Guidelines for Delivering Health Services to Sex Workers*. Amsterdam, Foundation Regenboog AMOC.

HPA (2008) *Sexually Transmitted Infections and Young People in the United Kingdom: 2008 Report*. London, Health Protection Agency.

Jungmann E (2004) Clinical evidence concise. Genital herpes. *American Family Physician*, **70**(5), 813–815, 912–914,.

Klebanoff M, Schwebke J, Zhang J, *et al.* (2004) Vulvovaginal symptoms in women with bacterial vaginosis. *Obstetrics and Gynecology*, **104**(2), 267–272.

McCormack O and Nguyen L (2005) What is the role of herpes virus serology in sexually transmitted disease screening? *Journal of Family Practice*, **55**(5), available at: http://www.jfponline.com/Pages.asp?AID=4108&UID, last accessed August 2011.

NCSP and HPA (2008) *NCSP: Five Years. Annual Report of the National Chlamydia Screening Programme in England 2007/08*. London, National Chlamydia Screening Programme and Health Protection Agency.

Ness R, Hillier S, Kip K, *et al.* (2004) Bacterial vaginosis and risk of pelvic inflammatory disease. *Obstetrics and Gynecology*, **104**(4), 761–769.

NMC (2008) *The Code*. London, Nursing and Midwifery Council.

Nursing Times (2005) Drop-in service cuts wait for STI clinic. *Nursing Times*, **101**(10), 9.

Porth C M (2009) *Pathophysiology: Concepts of altered health states* (9th edn). Philadelphia, PA, Lippincott.

Robertson P and Wiliams O E (2005) Young, male, and infected: the forgotten victims of chlamydia in primary care. *Sexually Transmitted Infections*, **81**, 31–33.

Sterk C, Klein H and Elifson K (2004) Predictors of condom-related attitudes among at-risk women. *Journal of Women's Health*, **13**(6), 676–688.

Tierney L M, McPhee S J and Papadakis M A (eds) (2004) *Current Medical Diagnosis & Treatment* (43rd edn). Stamford, CT, Appleton & Lange.

Wilson B, Shannon M and Stang C (2005) *Nurse's Drug Guide 2005*. Upper Saddle River, NJ, Prentice Hall.

Winer R L, Hughes J P, Feng Q, *et al.* (2006) Condom use and the risk of genital human papillomavirus infection in young women. *New England Journal of Medicine*, **354**, 2645–2654.

Answers to Test Yourself Questions

Chapter 1
1. b
2. a
3. c
4. d
5. b
6. d
7. a
8. c
9. d
10. a

Chapter 2
1. c
2. c
3. d
4. b
5. b
6. a
7. b
8. b
9. c
10. d

Chapter 3
1. a
2. d
3. a, c, d
4. b
5. a
6. c
7. c
8. b
9. b
10. d

Chapter 4
1. a
2. a, c, d
3. d
4. a, b, c
5. a, c
6. b
7. d
8. a, c, d
9. b
10. b

Chapter 5
1. a
2. c
3. b
4. c
5. False
6. Any from the list on page 153
7. a
8. Clean, clean contaminated, contaminated, dirty infected
9. d
10. Pressure, shear and friction

Chapter 6
1. b
2. c
3. a
4. c
5. b
6. b
7. d
8. c
9. b
10. d

Chapter 7
1. a
2. c
3. b
4. b
5. d
6. d
7. c
8. d
9. c
10. d

Chapter 8
1. d
2. d
3. c
4. c
5. b
6. a
7. c
8. a
9. d
10. b

Chapter 9
1. a
2. b
3. b
4. c
5. d
6. b
7. b
8. c
9. b
10. a

Chapter 10
1. c
2. b
3. a
4. d
5. c
6. d
7. b
8. a
9. a
10. c

Chapter 11
1. d
2. a
3. a, c
4. b
5. d
6. b
7. b
8. c
9. b
10. a

Chapter 12
1. c
2. d
3. a
4. c
5. d
6. c
7. a
8. c
9. c
10. b

Chapter 13
1. d
2. c
3. c
4. a
5. b
6. d
7. b
8. a
9. a
10. c

Chapter 14
1. a
2. b
3. b
4. a
5. c
6. c
7. b
8. c
9. b
10. d

Chapter 15
1. d
2. c
3. a
4. d
5. c
6. d
7. d
8. b, c, d
9. 1000
10. a

Chapter 16
1. c
2. a
3. a
4. a
5. d
6. d
7. a
8. b
9. c
10. a, b, c, d

Chapter 17
1. b
2. a
3. a, b, d, e
4. d
5. a
6. d
7. b
8. c
9. a
10. c

Glossary

accommodation the process by which the eyes focus

acquired immunity immunity acquired by coming into contact with infectious micro-organisms

acute coronary syndrome (ACS) an umbrella term for a group of conditions that result in coronary artery disease

acute illness describes an illness with a sudden/rapid onset which is severe in nature

acute respiratory distress syndrome (ARDS) severe difficulty in getting adequate oxygenation despite significant effort to breathe

acute wound a wound that is new or relatively new in injury and occurs suddenly

afterload the force required by the ventricles when they contract to force the blood out

allergy an overreaction of the immune system to normally harmless environmental substances. These substances are then known as allergens

amenorrhoea the absence of menstrual period

amines organic compounds that contain nitrogen

amputation the surgical removal of a limb

anaphylaxis an extreme form of hypersensitivity

androgens hormones such as testosterone responsible for the development and maintenance of masculine characteristics

anions negatively charged ions

anorgasmia an inability to reach orgasm during sexual intercourse

anosmia the inability to smell; may be seen with lesions of the frontal lobe

anterior front

antibody a protein that is produced to fight infectious micro-organisms (also known as an immunoglobulin)

anticipatory grieving grieving before the loss has occurred

antigen a substance that causes an antibody response by the body (e.g. antibody generation)

anuria absence of urine

aphasia defective or absent language function

arthritis a group of degenerative diseases affecting joints

asthma a condition where there is widespread narrowing of the bronchial airways brought on by a number of stimuli

ataxia a lack of coordination and a clumsiness of movements

atelectasis the failure of part of the lung to expand

atherosclerosis a progressive disease characterised by atheroma (plaque) formation, which affects the intimal and medial layers of large and mid-sized arteries

aura a symptom experienced before a migraine or seizure e.g. flashing lights

autoimmunity an abnormal immune response to the body's own cells, which act as self-antigens

autosome a non-sex chromosome

azotaemia an elevation of blood urea nitrogen

bacterial vaginosis a common cause of vaginal discharge

benign prostatic hyperplasia (BPH) an overgrowth of cells in the prostate gland

bile a bitter yellowish, blue and green fluid secreted by hepatocytes from the liver

biotherapy the modification of the biological processes in malignant cells, by enhancing the person's own immune responses

breakthrough pain pain that exceeds baseline treated or untreated pain

bronchiectasis the widening of the bronchi or their branches

bronchitis inflammation of the bronchi

Brudzinski's sign flexion of the neck that causes the hip and knee to flex

bursitis the inflammation of small sacs of synovial fluid that cushion and protect bony areas that are at high risk for friction, such as the knee and the shoulder

calculi stones

calyces small funnel-shaped cavities formed from the renal pelvis

candidiasis a yeast infection

cardiac output the amount of blood pumped by the ventricles into the pulmonary and systemic circulation in one minute

cardiac reserve the heart's ability to work harder and faster when challenged as in exercise

cardiovascular disease (CVD) a generic term for disorders of the heart and blood vessels, including coronary heart disease

cataract a clouding of the lens within the eye

cations positively charged ions

cellulitis the localised infection of the dermis and subcutaneous tissue

cerumen ear wax

chancre a small type of painless ulcer

cheilosis an inflammatory lesion at the corner of the mouth

chelation the process of breaking down excess iron

chemoreceptors receptors that respond to changes in the chemical environment

chemotherapy medication used to treat cancers

chlamydia the most common sexually transmitted infection

chronic bronchitis a long-term condition with excessive mucous production

chronic heart failure a progressive disease that results when the heart cannot function because of damage sustained through cardiovascular diseases

chronic illness long-term on going illnesses often increasing in severity over time

chronic obstructive pulmonary disease (COPD) a disease of adults predominantly over 45 years of age with a history of smoking or inhaling airborne pollutants

chronic pain pain which lasts more than 6 months and frequently lacks the objective manifestations of acute pain, primarily because the autonomic nervous system adapts to this chronic stress

chronic wound a wound that digresses from the normal order of repair in terms of length of time

Chvostek's sign a test for neuromuscular irritability. Chvostek's sign is done by tapping the facial nerve 2 cm anterior to the earlobe. A positive response is ipsilateral (same side) twitching of the facial muscles

chyme a semi-fluid substance of the stomach

compartment syndrome a syndrome that occurs when excess pressure in a limited space of the muscle compartment constricts the structures within it, reducing circulation to muscles and nerves leading to necrosis

compartments spaces

complement a system of proteins that work with (complement) antibodies to fight bacteria

concordance describes the action of people who readily follow prescribed treatments and medication

conjunctivitis inflammation or infection of the conjunctiva

contralateral located on the opposite side of the body (brain)

contusion bleeding into soft tissue that results from a blunt force, such as a kick or striking a body part against a hard object

convergence the inward movement of both eyes

corneal reflex the blink reflex

coronary heart disease (CHD) a disorder of the blood vessels serving the heart in which damage has been caused to them by the formation of atherosclerotic plaques (also known as coronary artery disease)

cor pulmonale the enlargement of the right ventricle of the heart resulting from lung disease

critical thinking the action of focused self-directed thinking

Cushing's syndrome a metabolic disorder resulting from excessive production of cortisol

cyanosis a bluish tinge to the skin and mucous membranes resulting from inadequate levels of oxygen in arterial blood

cystic fibrosis (CF) an hereditary disorder affecting cells of the endocrine system

cytokines chemical messengers released by cells to instruct other cells to undertake various functions.

cytotoxic any cell or other substance that kills or damages cells (e.g. bacteria or viruses)

dehiscence when the opposite edges of a surgical wound open spontaneously

dehydration excessive fluid loss from the body

dermis the second, deeper layer of skin

detoxification the removal of toxic substances from the body

diabetes insipidus a condition where the kidneys cannot conserve water as a result of lack of ADH

diabetic retinopathy a common diabetic eye disease

differentiation a process by which cells go through stages of development to maturity

diplopia double vision due to lack of parallelism

disease disorder with specifically defined signs and symptoms

diuresis excess urine production

duct tube

dysarthria difficulty speaking

dysfunctional uterine bleeding the most common cause of abnormal vaginal bleeding

dysmenorrhoea severe pain during menstruation

dyspareunia painful sexual intercourse

dysphagia difficulty swallowing (common with impaired blood flow to the brain)

dyspnoea laboured or difficult breathing

dysuria painful urination

ecchymosis bleeding under the skin

electrocardiogram (ECG) a graphic record of the heart's activity depicting the electrical impulses produced during a cardiac cycle and portraying them as a wave on graph paper through a heated stylus

electrolytes substances that dissociate in water to form ions

emphysema disease of the lungs where alveoli are enlarged and damaged

end-diastolic volume the volume of blood in the ventricles before they contract

endocrine gland a ductless gland that secretes hormones into the bloodstream

endometriosis the condition in which cells similar to those lining the uterus are found elsewhere in the body

end-systolic volume the volume of blood left in the ventricles after they have contracted (the ventricle is never completely empty)

epidermis the surface or outermost part of the skin

epididymitis infection and inflammation of the epididymis

erectile dysfunction (ED) an inability to get and maintain an erection that is satisfactory for sexual activity

erythema reddening of the skin

erythropoietin a hormone produced by the kidneys that regulates red blood cell production

excretion the elimination of waste products of metabolism

exocrine refers to a group of cells that secrete hormones through a duct into a blood vessel

extracellular space outside the cell

exudate fluid rich in protein and cellular elements that oozes out of blood vessels due to inflammation and is deposited in nearby tissues

fasciculations spontaneous firing of an axon resulting in a visible twitch of all the muscle fibres it contacts

fat embolism syndrome a syndrome characterised by neurological dysfunction, pulmonary insufficiency and a petechial rash on the chest, axillae and upper arms

fibrocystic changes changes that occur in the breast and can be felt as lumps

fibromyalgia a disease associated with rheumatoid arthritis in which people have low levels of serotonin and high levels of Substance P, leading to symptoms of pain and fatigue

filtration a passive transport system

flail chest instability of a segment of the ribcage due to fracture of ribs. Ribs may puncture lungs

fracture a break in the bone

genital herpes a genital infection cause by the herpes simplex virus

genital warts a sexually transmitted infection caused by the human papillomavirus

gingivitis inflammation of the gums

glands the skin contains sebaceous (oil) glands, sudoriferous (sweat) glands and ceruminous (earwax) glands. Each of these glands has a different function

glaucoma a condition in which the optic nerve becomes damaged leading to progressive and irreversible loss of vision

glomerulus a network of capillaries found in the Bowman's capsule

goitre a hypertrophic thyroid gland

gonorrhoea a sexually transmitted infection caused by bacteria

gout an arthritis that arises from inflammation that is caused following a buildup of serum uric acid which precipitates as sodium monourate crystals in the joints causing erosion of cartilage and bone

grading an evaluation of the amount of differentiation (level of functional maturity) of the tissue

grief the emotional response to loss and its accompanying changes

growth factors naturally occurring substances capable of stimulating cellular growth, proliferation and cellular differentiation. Usually it is a protein or a steroid hormone. Growth factors are important for regulating a variety of cellular processes

gynaecomastia an enlargement of male breast tissue

haematoma abnormal localised collection of blood in which the blood is usually clotted or partially clotted and situated within an organ or a soft tissue space, such as within a muscle

haematopoiesis the formation of red blood cells in the bone marrow

haematuria blood in the urine

haemoptysis blood-stained sputum

haemothorax blood in the pleural cavity

health state of individual wellbeing

health behaviour individual response to health activities

health–illness continuum theoretical line between health and illness

hemianopia the loss of vision in one half of the visual field

hemiparesis weakness on one side of the body

hemiplegia paralysis of one-half of the body vertically

hilum a small indented part of the kidney

holistic healthcare all-encompassing care

hormones chemical messengers

human immunodeficiency virus (HIV) a virus that can cause a severe and often fatal immunodeficiency if untreated.

humoral pertaining to elements in the blood or other body fluids

hydrocele a collection of fluid in the scrotum

hyperaemia increased blood flow to the skin

hyperglycaemia higher than normal amount of blood glucose

hyperkalaemia high potassium level in the blood

hyperlipidaemia high levels of fat

hypermetabolism an abnormal increase in metabolic rate

hyperopia long sightedness

hypersecretion excessive production

hypersensitivity oversensitivity of the immune system to certain normally harmless environmental substances

hypertension high blood pressure

hyperthyroidism condition characterised by overactivity of the thyroid gland

hypertonic a solution that has a high concentration of solutes

hypoglycaemia lower than normal amount of blood glucose

hyponatraemia low sodium level in the blood

hypophysis refers to the posterior pituitary gland

hyposecretion low production

hypothyroidism condition characterised by underactivity of the thyroid gland

hypotonic a solution that has a low concentration of solutes

hypoxaemia reduced oxygen concentration in arterial blood

illness state of individual deterioration of health

immune system the system responsible for providing protection against infectious micro-organisms, tumours, foreign bodies and a whole host of potential problems

immunisation the process of protecting against certain infectious diseases without having to have been infected

inflammation the body's immediate reaction to tissue injury or damage.

innate immunity the immunity we are born with (also known as non-specific immunity, giving all-round protection)

integrated care pathways multi disciplinary plan for delivering health and social care to individuals with established health breakdown

intracellular space inside the cell

ipsilateral located on the same side of the body (brain)

ischaemia the inadequate supply of blood to an organ or part of the body as from an obstructed blood flow

isotonic solution that has the same osmolality as the body fluids

keloid scars elevated, irregularly shaped, progressively enlarging scars

Kernig's sign the inability to extend the knee while the hip is flexed at a 90-degree angle

kidneys organs situated in the posterior wall of the abdominal cavity

leiomyoma a benign change (often in the uterus) associated with the soft tissue

libido sexual desire

loss an actual or potential situation in which a valued object, person, body part or emotion that was formerly present is lost or changed and can no longer be seen, felt, heard, known or experienced

lymphocytes a class of white blood cells (leucocytes) that are part of the acquired immune system

lymphoedema a collection of lymph fluid that does not drain away from the tissues

lymphoid system a blood cell system that is made up of the lymphocytes

mediator cells cells of the immune system that do not kill invading micro-organisms, but rather help other cells to do so.

memory cells T- and B-cell lymphocytes that can remember previous infection by a particular micro-organism, therefore quickly involving the immune system in destroying them if subsequently infected by the same micro-organism

Ménière's disease a rare disorder that can affect the inner ear

menopause the cessation of female reproductive ability and the ending of menstruation

menorrhagia heavy menstrual blood loss

menstrual cycle a cycle of female reproductive changes

metabolism a set of chemical reactions that happen in living organisms to sustain life

metrorrhagia irregular menstrual bleeding, e.g. bleeding between periods

micturition the act of voiding urine

myopia ability to see near objects clearly but faraway objects appear blurred

myringotomy a tiny surgical incision in the eardrum

nausea an unpleasant sensation that produces a feeling of discomfort in the region of the stomach with a feeling of a need to vomit

nephron functional unit of the kidney

neurohypophysis refers to the anterior pituitary gland

neutrophils white blood cells of the innate immune system involved in the process of phagocytosis

nociceptive painful

nociceptors nerve endings that are stimulated either by persistent mechanical, chemical or thermal stimuli to the cell, or by the local release of biochemicals secondary to cell injury

nocturia excessive urination at night

nonunion failure of the bones to heal

nuchal rigidity stiff neck

nursing ethics code of principles governing nursing behaviour

nursing process an individualised problem-solving approach to the nursing care of individuals

nutrition relates to nutrients

nystagmus an involuntary movement of an eye that may be horizontal, vertical or rotary

oedema abnormal accumulation of fluid in the interstitial space

oestrogen a general term for a female sex-related hormone

oligomenorrhoea infrequent menstruation

oliguria diminished urine output

oncology the study of cancer (the term come from a Greek word oncoma which means 'bulk')

opsonins substances that help the immune system to function, playing an important role in phagocytosis

orchitis infection and inflammation of the testes

orthopnoea shortness of breath (dyspnoea) which occurs when lying flat, causing the person to have to sleep propped up in bed or sitting in a chair. It is the opposite of platypnoea

osmosis the movement of water through a selective permeable membrane from an area of high volume to an area of low volume

osmotic pressure pressure created by water as it moves across through a selective permeable membrane

ossification the deposition of calcium to harden the bones

osteoarthritis (OA) the most commonly occurring of all forms of arthritis; characterised by loss of articular cartilage in articulating joints and hypertrophy of the bones at the articular margins

osteomyelitis an infection of the bone which can be acute, sub-acute or chronic

osteoporosis a metabolic disorder where bone cells are lost leading to fragile bones which can fracture easily

otitis externa inflammation or infection of the external ear canal

otitis media inflammation or infection in the middle ear

ovarian cycle the normal sex cycle that includes the development of an ovarian follicle, rupture of the follicle and discharge of the ovum

Paget's disease an age-related, progressive metabolic skeletal disorder that results from excessive metabolic activity in bone, with excessive bone reabsorption followed by excessive bone formation

pain the subjective response to both physical and psychological stressors. All people experience pain at some point during their lives. Although pain is usually experienced as uncomfortable and unwelcome, it serves a protective role. For this reason, pain is increasingly referred to as the fifth vital sign

palliative wound a wound that cannot be classified as acute or chronic and whose outcome of wound healing is considered both challenging and unattainable

pancreatitis inflammation of the pancreas

papilloedema swelling of the nerve head in the optic discs seen in raised intracranial pressure

paraesthesia an abnormal sensation, typically tingling or pricking (pins and needles)

parasympathetic part of the autonomic nervous system

parenchyma soft tissue of the kidney involving the cortex and the medulla

parenteral the administration of a drug intravenously or intramuscularly

passive immunity immunity given either via the umbilical cord pre-birth or as an infusion in the case of an immune deficiency

pelvic inflammatory disease a condition involving inflammation of the upper genital tract

peristalsis wave-like symmetrical contraction and relaxation of muscles of the intestine

phagocytosis destruction and consumption of invading micro-organisms and other non-self matter by elements of the immune system

phimosis a tight foreskin

photophobia an abnormal intolerance to light, usually associated with eye pain

plasma the fluid component of blood

pleuritis inflammation of the pleura

pneumonia an acute lung infection

pneumothorax air in the pleural cavity

polymerisation the grouping and sticking together in twisted bundles of haemoglobin molecules due to haemoglobin deoxygenating in sickle cell disease, eventually distorting the shape of the red blood cell

posterior behind

preload the capacity the ventricles have to stretch when filling up with blood during diastole

premenstrual syndrome the name given to a set of physical, emotional and psychological symptoms that appear in the days preceding a woman's period

presbyopia the diminished ability of the eye to focus on near objects with age

priapism a condition in which the penis does not return to its flaccid state

primary immunodeficiencies deficiencies of the immune system for which there is no external cause, i.e. they are genetic in origin

prodromal premonitory symptoms that occur hours to days before the episode

progesterone a hormone predominantly produced in the ovaries

proptosis projecting forward of the eyeball

prostatitis infection and inflammation of the prostate gland

proteinuria protein in the urine

ptosis drooping of the upper eyelid

pulmonary embolism a clot in the blood vessels of the lungs

pupillary light reflex a reflex that controls the diameter of the pupil

pyrexia fever

pyuria presence of white blood cells in the urine

quality assurance review and assessment against an established set of benchmarks

radiotherapy a treatment using high energy x-rays to destroy cancer cells

receptors proteins on cells that can send and receive messages from other cells via cytokines, as well as allowing other cells (and micro-organisms) to attach to cells

refraction the bending of light rays as they pass from one medium to another medium of different optical density

renal artery blood vessel that takes blood to the kidney

renal cortex the outermost part of the kidney

renal medulla the middle layer of the kidney

renal pelvis the funnel-shaped section of the kidney

renal pyramids cone-shaped structures of the medulla

renal vein blood vessel that returns filtered blood into circulation

renin a renal hormone that alters systemic blood pressure

retrograde ejaculation when semen passes into the urinary bladder as opposed to along the urethra

rheumatoid arthritis (RA) a common inflammatory disorder

scleroderma an umbrella term that incorporates a group of rare conditions that may be either localised, affecting the skin only, or generalised (systemic sclerosis), with both skin and visceral organ involvement

secondary immunodeficiencies deficiencies of the immune system caused by an external source

semen a whitish/grey liquid emitted from the penis on ejaculation

sexually transmitted infections infections transmitted through intimate sexual activity

specific gravity density

spermatocele a cyst that becomes distended in the scrotal sac

sphincter a ring-like muscle fibre that can constrict

sprain a stretch and/or tear of one or more ligaments surrounding a joint

stem cell an undifferentiated cell whose daughter cells may differentiate into other cell types (such as blood cells)

strain a stretching injury to muscle or muscle and tendons by mechanical overloading

stridor vibrating sound during respiration

stroke volume the difference between the end-diastolic volume and the end-systolic volume; the exact amount pumped from the ventricle to the aorta in one beat

subcutaneous tissue a layer of subcutaneous tissue called the superficial fascia lies under the dermis

sympathetic part of the autonomic nervous system

syncope a sudden and temporary loss of consciousness

synovitis inflammation of the synovium

synthesised produced

syphilis a sexually transmitted infection caused by bacteria

systemic lupus erythematosus (SLE) a chronic inflammatory connective tissue disease affecting mainly women of childbearing age. It frequently affects the musculoskeletal system but also affects kidneys, lungs, heart, skin and central nervous system

testicular torsion twisting of the spermatic cord, which cuts off the blood supply to the testicle and surrounding structures within the scrotum

thoracentesis aspiration of fluid from the pleural space

thyroidectomy surgical removal of the thyroid gland

tinnitus the perception of sound within the ear without the corresponding external sound

tremor involuntary, rhythmic oscillatory movements about a fixed point due to alternating or synchronous contractions of agonist and antagonist muscles

trichomoniasis a common type of infection that can occur in men and women

Trousseau's sign Trousseau's sign is carried out by placing a blood pressure cuff on the arm, inflating the cuff slightly above the systolic pressure, leaving the cuff inflated for two to three minutes and deflating. A carpal spasm is a positive response

tuberculosis (TB) an infectious disease caused by *Mycobacterium tuberculosis*

tumour markers protein molecules detectable in serum or other body fluids which can be used as a biochemical indicator of the presence of a malignancy. Small amounts of tumour marker proteins are found in normal body tissues or benign tumours and are not specific for malignancy

tympanoplasty reconstructive surgery for the eardrum

ureters membranous tube that drains urine from the kidneys to the bladder

urethra muscular tube that drains urine from the bladder

urgency feeling of the need to void urine immediately

varicocele a type of varicose vein of the small veins close to the testes

venous stasis slow blood flow of the veins

vertigo the sensation that you or the environment around you is moving or spinning

voluntary can be controlled

vomiting a disagreeable experience that occurs when the stomach contents are reflexively expelled through the mouth or nose

Index

Glossary entries are shown in **bold**